Companion to Primary Mental Health

Edited by
Gabriel Ivbijaro
MBE MBBS FRCGP FWACPsych MMedSci MA
Chair of the Wonca Working Party on Mental Health and Medical Director,
Waltham Forest Community and Family Health Services,
The Wood Street Medical Centre, London, UK

President of   *nd Professor of*
Family Medici   *blic Health, USA*

Senior Vice   *Professor and*
Executive Vice   *avioral Sciences,*
Baylor Colleg   *tric Association*

Direc   *nission*

President, Wo   *Vice Chair and*
Director of Clir   *ioral Sciences,*
Mill   *USA*

Wonca and Radcliffe Publishing
London • New York

Radcliffe Publishing Ltd
33–41 Dallington Street
London
EC1V 0BB
United Kingdom

www.radcliffepublishing.com

The World Organisation of Family Doctors
7500A Beach Road
#12-303 The Plaza
Singapore 199591

www.GlobalFamilyDoctor.com

British Library Cataloguing in Publication Data

A catalogue record for this book is available from the British Library.

ISBN-13: 978 184619 976 9

New research and clinical experience can result in changes in treatment and drug therapy. Readers of this book should therefore check the most recent product information on any drug they may prescribe to ensure they are complying with the manufacturer's recommendations concerning dosage, the method and duration of administration, and contraindications. Neither the publisher nor the author accept liability for any injury or damage arising from this publication.

The paper used for the text pages of this book is FSC® certified. FSC® (The Forest Stewardship Council®) is an international network to promote responsible management of the world's forests.

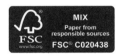

Typeset by Phoenix Photosetting, Chatham, Kent, UK
Printed and bound by Hobbs the Printers, Totton, Hants, UK

Contents

Contributors

Niloufer Sultan Ali MBBS DCH MCPS FCPS
Associate Professor, Department of Family Medicine, The Aga Khan University, Karachi, Pakistan

Abdullah Dukhail Al-Khathami MBBS ABFM FFCM MSC MedEd (Cardiff)
Director of the Saudi Postgraduate Family Medicine Programme; Supervisor of the Primary and Community Mental Health Programme, The Eastern Province MOH, Saudi Arabia

Mohammed T Abou-Saleh MPhil PhD FRCPsych
Chief Executive Officer Qatar Addiction Treatment and Rehabilitation Centre (QATRC) Project, Aspetar, Aspire Zone Doha, Qatar; Professor of Psychiatry and Consultant in Addiciton Psychiatry, Division of Mental Health, St George's, University of London, UK

David C Agerter MD
Consultant in Family Medicine, Austin Medical Center, Mayo Clinic Health System, Austin, Minnesota; Associate Professor of Family Medicine, College of Medicine, Mayo Clinic; Director, Central Region of the Mayo Clinic Health System, Rochester, Minnesota, USA

Olatunji F Aina MBBS FWACP
Associate Professor and Consultant Psychiatrist, College of Medicine of the University of Lagos, Nigeria

James B Anderson PhD
Post-doctoral Fellow in Clinical Health Psychology in Primary Care, University of Massachusetts Medical School, Department of Family Medicine and Community Health, USA

Nuzhat Anjum BA(Hons) MA
Head of Public Health Commissioning, NHS Redbridge, Ilford, UK

Macaran A Baird MD MS
Professor and Head, Department of Family Medicine and Community Health, University of Minnesota Medical School, Minneapolis, Minnesota, USA

Elizabeth Alexandra Barley BSc PhD CPsychol RGN
Senior Lecturer, Florence Nightingale School of Nursing, King's College London, UK

Bryanne Barnett AM MD MBChB FRANZCP
Professor (conjoint), School of Psychiatry, University of New South Wales, Sydney, Australia

Jill Benson MB BS DCH FACPsychMed MPH
Director, Health in Human Diversity Unit, Discipline of General Practice, University of Adelaide; Senior Medical Officer, Migrant Health Service, Adelaide; Medical Director, Kakarrara Wilurrara Health Alliance, Australia; WHO consultant, PIMHNet, Vanuatu

Somashekhar Bijjal MBBS DPM (MD)
Junior Resident in Psychiatry, National Institute of Mental Health and Neurosciences, Bangalore, India

Pedro Camacho MD PhD
Professor of Psychopathology, Centro de Estudios Superiores Monte Fénix, Mexico City, Mexico

Prabha Chandra MD FRCPsych
Professor of Psychiatry, National Institute of Mental Health and Neurosciences, Bangalore, India

Vincent Chin-Hung Chen MD PhD
Assistant Professor, Department of Psychiatry, Chung Shan Medical University; Visiting Staff, Department of Psychiatry, Chung Shan Medical University Hospital, Taiwan

Jen-Yu Chou MD PhD
Assistant Professor, Department of Medical Humanities, Taipei Medical University, Taiwan; Faculty Member, Seattle Psychoanalytic Society and Institute, USA

David D Clarke MD
Clinical Assistant Professor Emeritus, Oregon Health and Science University, Portland, OR, USA

José Miguel Caldas de Almeida MD PhD
Professor of Psychiatry and Head, Department of Mental Health, Faculty of Medical Sciences, Nova University of Lisbon, Portugal

Raúl Martín del Campo MD
Chief, Estado de México Mental Health Coordination, Mexico

Joseph Deltito MD
Clinical Professor of Psychiatry, New York Medical College, Valhalla, New York, USA; Senior Consultant, Gianfranco De Lisio Institute for Behavioral Research, Pisa, Italy

Carlos Augusto de Mendonça Lima MD DSci
Head of the Department of Psychiatry and Mental Health, Centro Hospitalar do Alto Ave, Portugal; Professor of the Portuguese Catholic University, Lisbon, Portugal

D Edward Deneke MD
Fellow in Psychosomatic Medicine, University of Michigan Health System, Ann Arbor, USA

Geetha Desai MD DNB
Associate Professor of Psychiatry, National Institute of Mental Health and Neurosciences, Bangalore, India

Tom Dodd RMN Cert MH Cert Management
Senior Manager, Nene Commissioning, Northampton; Formerly London Regional Manager for IAPT, UK

Tony Dowell MBChB FRCGP FRNZCGP
Professor of Primary Health Care and General Practice, Department of Primary Health Care and General Practice, Wellington School of Medicine and Health Sciences, University of Otago, Wellington South, New Zealand

Christopher Dowrick BA MSc MD FRCGP
Professor of Primary Medical Care, University of Liverpool, UK

Todd M Edwards PhD
Associate Professor and Director, Marital and Family Therapy Program, School of Leadership and Education Sciences, University of San Diego, California, USA

Kay Eilbert DrPH MPH FFPH
Acting Director of Public Health, NHS ONEL Waltham Forest, London, UK

Yaccub Enum BSc MSc Dip(HE) Nurse
Head of Public Health Partnerships, NHS Outer North East London, UK

Jane Fisher BSc(Hons) PhD MAPS
Professor of Women's Mental Health; Director, Jean Hailes Research Unit, School of Public Health and Preventive Medicine, Monash University, Victoria, Australia

Sandra Fortes MSc PhD
Associate Professor of Mental Health and Medical Psychiatry, School of Medical Sciences, University of Rio de Janeiro State, Brazil

Patt Francioisi PhD
Psychologist, Past President of the World Federation for Mental Health, Chair of World Mental Health Day, USA

Luis Galvez MD PhD
Family Physician, El Palo Heath Centre, Family Medicine Teaching Unit of Malaga, Spain

Preston J Garrison BA
Secretary-General and Chief Executive Officer (Retired), World Federation for Mental Health, USA

Priyabrata Ghosh MB ChB MRCPsych
Senior Registrar, South London and Maudsley NHS FT Rotation Scheme, UK

Karinn Glover MD MPH
Instructor, Department of Psychiatry, Albert Einstein College of Medicine; Attending Psychiatrist Montefiore Medical Center, Bronx, New York, USA

David Goldberg KB DM FRCP FRCPsych
Professor Emeritus, Institute of Psychiatry, King's College, London, UK

Janna S Gordon-Elliott MD
Assistant Professor of Psychiatry, Department of Psychiatry, Weill Cornell Medical College; Assistant Attending Psychiatrist, New York Presbyterian Hospital, New York, USA

Jane Gunn MBBS(Melb) DRANZCOG FRACGP PhD(Melb)
Head of Department, Chair of Primary Care Research, General Practice and Primary Health Care Academic Centre, The University of Melbourne, Australia

Sheila Gunn MB Bch BAO MRCGP DCCh DMH
General Practitioner, Saintfield Health Centre, Saintfield, Co Down, Northern Ireland, UK

Michelle Haling RN MC C&FHN Mast IMH CMHN
Mental Health Practitioner, St John of God Health Care, Sydney, Australia

Susan E Hamilton MS
Research Specialist, Women's Mental Health and Infants Program, Department of Psychiatry, University of Michigan, Ann Arbor, USA

Latha Hapugoda MBBS DFM MSc MD (Sri Lanka) Grad Dip Health Promotion (Australia) FFPH (UK)
Consultant in Public Health Medicine; Associate Director of Public Health, Waltham Forest Public Health, NHS Outer North East London, London, UK

Iona Heath FRCGP FRCP
President, Royal College of General Practitioners, London, UK

Carol Henshaw MD FRCPsych FHEA
Consultant in Perinatal Mental Health, Liverpool Women's Hospital; Honorary Visiting Fellow, Staffordshire University, UK

Richard Holt MB Bchir MA PhD FRCP FHEA
Professor in Diabetes and Endocrinology, University of Southampton, Faculty of Medicine; Honorary Consultant in Diabetes and Endocrinology, University Hospital Southampton Foundation Trust, Southampton General Hospital, Southampton, UK

Shou-Hung Huang MD
Visiting Staff, Taipei Medical University Hospital, Taiwan

Yen-Hsun Huang MD
Visiting Staff, Department of Psychiatry, Taipei City Hospital, Taiwan

Steve Iliffe FRCGP FRCP
Professor of Primary Care for Older People, Department of Primary Care and Population Health, University College London, UK

Gabriel Ivbijaro MBE MBBS FRCGP FWACPsych MMedSci MA
Chair, Wonca Working Party on Mental Health; Editor in Chief, *Mental Health in Family Medicine*; Medical Director, Waltham Forest Community and Family Health Services, The Wood Street Medical Centre, London, UK

Rachel Jenkins MA MB BChir MD FRC Psych
Director, WHO Collaborating Centre for Research and Training; Professor of Epidemiology and International Mental Health Policy, Institute of Psychiatry, King's College London

Gene A Kallenberg MD
Chief, Division of Family Medicine, University of California, San Diego School of Medicine, USA

Gustav Kamenski MD
General Practitioner, Department of General Practice, Medical University, Vienna; Karl Landsteiner Institute for Systematics in General Medicine, Austria

Allan S Kaplan MD FRCP(C)
Chief of Clinical Research, Center for Addiction and Mental Health; Vice Chairman for Research and Professor of Psychiatry; Director of the Institute of Medical Science, Faculty of Medicine, University of Toronto, Canada

Sherry Katz-Bearnot MD
Assistant Clinical Professor of Psychiatry, Department of Consultation-Liaison Psychiatry and Behavioral Medicine, Columbia University College of Psychiatrists and Surgeons, New York, USA

Felix Kauye BMedSc(Hons) MBBS FCPsych(SA) PhD
Clinical Lecturer in Psychiatry, Department of Mental Health, College of Medicine, Malawi

Moira Kessler MD
House Officer, Northwestern University, Chicago, USA

Akwatu Khenti MA PhD candidate
Director of International Health Programs, Center for Addiction and Mental Health; Assistant Professor, Dalla Lana School of Public Health, University of Toronto, Canada

Tawfik AM Khoja MBBS DPHC FRCGP FFPH FRCP(UK)
Professor, Family Physician Consultant; Director General, Executive Board of the Health Ministers Council for Cooperation Council States, Riyadh, Kingdom of Saudi Arabia

Michael Klinkman MD MS
Professor, Department of Family Medicine, University of Michigan Medical School, USA; Chair, Wonca International Classification Committee

Lucja Kolkiewicz MBBS MRCPsych
Consultant Psychiatrist and Associate Medical Director for Recovery and Well-being, East London NHS Foundation Trust, London, UK

Albert Lee MBBS(Lond) MD(CUHK) MPH FRACGP(Aus) FRCP(Irel) FFPH(UK) FHKAM(FamMed) DCH(Irel)
Professor (Clinical), School of Public Health and Primary Care, The Chinese University of Hong Kong

Meng-Chih Lee MD PhD
Professor, Institute of Medicine and Department of Family and Community Medicine, Chung Shan Medical University; Superintendent and Visiting Staff of the Department of Family Medicine, Taichung General Hospital, National Department of Health, Taiwan

Pei-Chin Lee OTR EdD
Assistant Professor, School of Occupational Therapy, Chung Shan Medical University, Taiwan

Christos Lionis MD PhD HonFRCGP
Professor of General Practice and Primary Health Care; Head of Clinic of Social and Family Medicine, Faculty of Medicine, University of Crete, Greece

Deborah Maguire
Director of Administration, World Federation for Mental Health, Occoquan, VA, USA

Brendan McLoughlin MA RMN CertBehPsych PGCE
Mental Health Project Manager, London Mental Health Models of Care Project, London Health Programmes, UK

Juan M Mendive MD
Family Physician, La Mina Primary Health Care Centre, Catalan Institute of Health, Teaching Unit of Family Medicine, Barcelona, Spain; Member of GRAPISAM (Research Group of Mental Health in Primary Care in Barcelona), Spain; Member of Wonca Working Party on Mental Health

Alberto Minoletti MD
Psychiatrist, University of Chile and Royal College of Physicians and Surgeons of Canada; Professor of Mental Health Policies and Services, School of Public Health, Medical Faculty, University of Chile, Santiago, Chile

Shameem Mir BPharm(Hons)
Chief Pharmacist, East London NHS Foundation Trust, London, UK

Caroline Morris BPharm MSc PhD MRPharmS MPS
Professional Practice Fellow, Department of Primary Health Care and General Practice, Wellington School of Medicine and Health Sciences, University of Otago, Wellington South, New Zealand

Maria Muzik MD MS
Assistant Professor and Director, Parent-Infant-Program, Women's Mental Health and Infants Program, Department of Psychiatry; Assistant Research Scientist, Center for Human Growth and Development, University of Michigan, Ann Arbor, USA

Irwin Nazareth MBBS LRCP DRCOG MRCGP FRCGP PhD
Professor of Primary Care and Population Science; Vice Dean of Primary Care, University College London, UK

Sammy Ohene MB ChB FWACP FGCP
Head of Department of Psychiatry, University of Ghana Medical School; Consultant Psychiatrist, Korle-Bu Teaching Hospital, Accra, Ghana; Chief Examiner in Psychiatry, West African College of Physicians

Francis Ibe Ojini MBBS MSc FMCP
Associate Professor, Neurology Unit, Department of Medicine, College of Medicine
University of Lagos, Lagos, Nigeria

Eleni Palazidou MD PhD MRCP FRCPsych
Honorary Consultant Psychiatrist, East London Foundation Trust, London, UK

Henk Parmentier MD DFFP
GP, Purley; Medical Director Patient Care 24, Croydon, UK; UK Representative Wonca Working Party on Mental Health

Vesna Pirec MD PhD
Assistant Professor and Program Director, Women's Mental Health, Department of Psychiatry, University of Illinois at Chicago, USA

Jill Rasmussen MBChB FRCGP FFPM DObst RCOG Dip Ther
General Practitioner, Moat House Clinic Surrey; GPSI Mental Health and Learning Disability Surrey PCT and EsyDoc Clinical Commissioning Group, UK

Norman H Rasmussen EdD ABPP
Consultant and Assistant Professor of Psychology, Departments of Psychiatry and Psychology and Family Medicine, Mayo Clinic and Mayo College of Medicine, Rochester, Minnesota, USA

Stefania Rescalli MD MB SB MMC MSC
Specialist in Abdominal Surgery; former non-dependent GP; Clinical Sonographer, Casa di Cura "La Madonnina" (Nursing Home), Milan, Italy

Michelle Riba MD MS
Professor and Associate Chair of Integrated Medical and Psychiatric Services, Department of Psychiatry, University of Michigan, Ann Arbor, MI; Associate Director, Michigan Institute for Clinical and Health Research (MICHR); Director, PsychOncology Program, University of Michigan Comprehensive Cancer Center; Associate Director, University of Michigan Comprehensive Depression Center; Past President, American Psychiatric Association; Secretary for Publications, World Psychiatric Association, USA

Carol Roberts MRPharmS Dip Prescribing Science
Pharmacy and Prescribing Lead, East of England SHA, Cambridge, UK

Tamsen Jean Rochat PhD
Senior Clinical Psychologist, Africa Centre for Health and Population Studies, University of KwaZulu-Natal, Mtubatuba, Republic of South Africa

Helen Rodenburg MB ChB FRNZCGP (Dist) Dip Obst FRACGP
General Practitioner, Island Bay Medical Centre, Wellington; Clinical Director, Primary Mental Health, Compass Health, Wellington; Medical Educator RNZCGP; Visiting Lecturer, Department of Primary Care and General Practice, University of Otago, Wellington School of Medicine, New Zealand

Graciela Rojas MD
Professor of Psychiatry, Psychiatric Clinic, Medical Faculty, University of Chile, Santiago, Chile

Christine N Runyan PhD ABPP
Associate Clinical Professor; Director of Fellowship in Clinical Health Psychology in Primary Care, University of Massachusetts Medical School, Department of Family Medicine and Community Health, USA

Brian Rush PhD
Professor, Department of Psychiatry, University of Toronto; Senior Scientist and Group Head, Health Systems and Health Equity Research Group, Centre for Addiction and Mental Health, Toronto, Canada

Jaime C Sapag MD MPH PhD candidate
Special Adviser and Project Coordinator, Office of International Health, Centre for Addiction and Mental Health, Ontario; Lecturer, Department of Psychiatry, University of Toronto, Canada

Joseph Scherger MD MPH
Vice President, Primary Care and Academic Affairs, Eisenhower Medical Center, Rancho Mirage, CA, USA

Julie M Schirmer MSW LCSW
Director, Behavioral Medicine; Assistant Director, Boston University Family Medicine Global Health Collaborative, Boston, MA, USA

Peter Selby MBBS CCFP FCFP DipABAM MHSc
Clinical Director, Addictions Program, Centre for Addiction and Mental Health; Associate Professor, Departments of Family and Community Medicine and Psychiatry and the Dalla Lana School of Public Health, University of Toronto, Toronto, Canada

Pratima Singh MBBS, MRCPsych, PGCert(Health Management and Leadership)
Specialist Registrar in Psychiatry, London Strategic Fellow in Clinical Leadership, South London and Maudsley NHS Foundation Trust, UK

John Spicer MBBS MA FRCGP FHEA
Head of School of General Practice, London Deanery, UK

Wolfgang Spiegel MD
General Practitioner, Certified Physician for Psychosomatic Medicine, Senior Researcher and Lecturer, Department of General Practice, Center for Public Health, Medical University of Vienna, Austria

Anthony Stern MD
Assistant Clinical Professor, Departments of Psychiatry and Family Medicine, Albert Einstein College of Medicine, New York, USA

Geraldine Strathdee OBE MB BCh BAO MRCPsych
Consultant Psychiatrist and Associate Medical Director and SHA Lead for Mental Health, NHS London, UK

Jung-Chia Su PsyD
Licensed Clinical Psychologist, Taiwan Institute of Psychotherapy, Taiwan

Igor Švab MD PhD FRCP(hon)
Head of Department of Family Medicine, Medical Faculty, University of Ljubljana, Slovenia

Allan Tasman MD
John and Ruby Schwab Chair, Professor and Chairman, Department of Psychiatry and Behavioral Sciences, University of Louisville School of Medicine; Editor Asia Pacific Psychiatry; Past President, American Psychiatric Association, Kentucky, USA

Graham Thornicroft MB BS MA MSc PhD FAcadMedSci
Professor of Community Psychiatry, Health Service and Population Research Department, King's College London, Institute of Psychiatry, London, UK

J Thornton BSc (Hons)
Clinical Lead Speech and Language Therapist (voice, head and neck oncology), Royal Hallamshire Hospital, Sheffield, UK

Bill Travers MB BS FRCPsych MRCGP
Consultant Psychiatrist, North East London NHS Foundation Trust, UK

Himanshu Tyagi MB BS MRCPsych
Locum Consultant Psychiatrist (CBT) in Body Dysmorphic Disorder Service National OCD/BDD Unit, South West London and St George's Mental Health Trust, London, UK

André Tylee MBBS MD FRCGP MRCPsych
Professor of Primary Care Mental Health and Academic Director, Mood Anxiety and Personality Clinical Academic Group, Institute of Psychiatry and South London and Maudsley Foundation Trust, King's Health Partners, King's College London, UK

Elizabeth Wainwright BSC(Hons)
Occupational Therapist, Porterbrook Clinic, Michael Carlisle Centre, Sheffield, UK

Kevan R Wylie MD FRCP FRCPsych FRCOG
Consultant in Sexual Medicine, Porterbrook Clinic and Urology, Royal Hallamshire Hospital, Sheffield and Honorary Professor, Sheffield Hallam University, UK

Zeynep Yilmaz
PhD candidate, Institute of Medical Science, University of Toronto, Clinical Research Program, Centre for Addiction and Mental Health, Toronto, Canada

Filippo Zizzo MD MB SB, MCP MS
Specialist in Psychiatry; Specialist in Criminology; Hypnotherapist; Sexologist; Member of the Italian Society of Criminology; non-dependent GP, Milan, Member of the Italian Society of General Medicine (SNAMID); Lecturer of psychiatric subjects in General Medicine Course, 'Bicocca' University in Milan, Italy; Founding Partner of SIICP (Italian Interdisciplinary Society for Primary Care); Member of the National Scientific Board of *Italian Journal of Primary Care*; Direct Wonca Member, Italy

Abbreviations and acronyms

AA	Alcoholics Anonymous
AACAP	American Academy of Child and Adolescent Psychiatry
AAP	American Academy of Pediatrics
AAS	American Association of Suicidology
ac	ante cibum (before food)
ACE	Adverse Childhood Experiences (study)
ACE	angiotensin-converting enzyme
ACS	anxiety clinical specialist
ACTH	adrenocorticotropic hormone (corticotropin)
ADHD	attention-deficit hyperactivity disorder
ADHD-RS-IV	ADHD Rating Scale IV
ADI	Adolescent Drinking Index
ADIS	Adolescent Drug Involvement Scale
AeSOP	Aetiology and Ethnicity of Schizophrenia and Other Psychoses
AFSP	American Foundation for Suicide Prevention
AHP	allied health-care professional
AIDS	acquired immunodeficiency syndrome
AIMS	Assessment Instrument for Mental Health Systems (WHO study)
AIMS	Abnormal Involuntary Movement Scale
AJCEE	American Joint Committee on Standards for Educational Evaluation
ALT	alanine aminotransferase
AN	anorexia nervosa
APA	American Psychiatric Association
APQ	Alcohol Problems Questionnaire
ART	antiretroviral therapy
ASAM	American Society of Addiction Medicine
ASD	autism spectrum disorder
ASEBA	Achenbach System of Empirically Based Assessment
ASQ-3	Ages and Stages Questionnaires Third Edition
ASQ-SE	Ages and Stages Questionnaires – Social and Emotional
AST	aspartate transaminase
ATC	Anatomical Therapeutic Chemical (classification)
AUD	Australian dollars
AUDIT	Alcohol Use Disorders Identification Test
BA	behavioural activation
BAS	Barnes Akathisia Scale
BASC-2	Behavior Assessment System for Children second edition
BBFC	British Board of Film Classification
bd	bis die (twice daily)
BDI	Beck Depression Inventory
BDNF	brain-derived neurotrophic factor
BED	binge eating disorder
BH	behavioural health
BHU	basic health unit
BITSEA	Brief Infant Toddler Social and Emotional Assessment
BMD	bone mineral density

BME	black and minority ethnic
BMI	body mass index
BN	bulimia nervosa
BNF	*British National Formulary*
BPRS	Brief Psychiatric Rating Scale
BSDS	Bipolar Spectrum Diagnostic Scale
BUN	blood urea nitrogen
CAGE-AID	CAGE questionnaire Adapted to Include Drugs
CALM	Coordinated Anxiety Learning and Management (study)
CAM	complementary and alternative medicine
CAM	Confusion Assessment Method
CAMHS	child and adolescent mental health services
CATCH-IT	Competent Adulthood Transition with Cognitive-behavioral, Humanistic and Interpersonal Training (project)
CATIE	Clinical Antipsychotic Trials in Intervention Effectiveness
CBCL	Child Behavior Checklist
CBT	cognitive-behavioural therapy
CCBT	computerized cognitive-behavioural therapy
CCMHI	Canadian Collaborative Mental Health Initiative
CCNC	Community Care of North Carolina
CD	conduct disorder
CDC	Centers for Disease Control and Prevention
CES-D	Center for Epidemiological Studies – Depression Scale
CGT	complicated grief treatment
CHAT	Checklist for Autism in Toddlers
CHD	coronary heart disease
CHW	community health-care worker
CI	confidence interval
CIDI	Composite International Diagnostic Interview
CIHI	Canadian Institute for Health Information
CIS-R	Revised Clinical Interview Schedule
6CIT	Six-Item Cognitive Impairment Test
CIWA-A(r)	Clinical Institute Withdrawal Assessment of Alcohol Scale (revised)
CKD	chronic kidney disease
CMACE	Centre for Maternal and Child Enquiries
CMD	common mental disorder
CMH	community mental health
CMHT	community mental health team
CNS	central nervous system
COMT	catechol-O-methyltransferase
COPC	community-oriented primary care
COPD	chronic obstructive pulmonary disease
CPHI	Canadian Population Health Initiative
CPN	community psychiatric nurse
CQI	continuous quality improvement
CRH	corticotropin-releasing hormone
CSC	collaborative stepped care
CSDH	(WHO) Commission on Social Determinants of Health
CT	computerized tomography
CVD	cardiovascular disease

DALY	disability-adjusted life-year
DANIDA	Danish International Development Agency
DAP	Drug and Alcohol Problem Quick Screen
DASH	Dietary Approaches to Stop Hypertension
DC: 0–3R	Diagnostic Classification of Mental Health and Developmental Disorders of Infancy and Early Childhood
DELTA	Depression in Elderly with Long-Term Afflictions (study)
DEXA	dual X-ray absorptiometry
df	degrees of freedom
DH	Department of Health (UK)
DISC-IV	Diagnostic Interview Schedule for Children-IV
DQOL	Diabetes Quality of Life
DSM	*Diagnostic and Statistical Manual of Mental Disorders*
DSM-IV-PC	4th edition of the DSM for Primary Care
DSM-IV-TR	4th edition of the DSM, text revision
DTs	delirium tremens
DUSI-R	Drug Use Screening Inventory – Revised
EARL-20B	Early Assessment Risk List for Boys
EARL-21G	Early Assessment Risk List for Girls
EAT	Eating Attitudes Test
EBT	evidence-based treatment
ECG	electrocardiogram
ECT	electroconvulsive therapy
EDNOS	eating disorder not otherwise specified
EE	expressed emotion
EEG	electroencephalography/electroencephalogram
EMDR	eye movement desensitization and reprocessing
EPA	Enduring Power of Attorney
EPDS	Edinburgh Postnatal Depression Scale
ESR	enhanced specialist referral
EST	empirically supported treatment
EU	European Union
EURODEM	European Community Concerted Action on the Epidemiology and Prevention of Dementia
FAS	fetal alcohol syndrome
FASD	fetal alcohol spectrum disorder
FDA	Food and Drug Administration
FEV1	forced expiratory volume in 1 s
GAD	generalized anxiety disorder
GAD-7	7-item Generalized Anxiety Disorder scale
GAPS	Guidelines for Adolescent Preventive Services
GASS	Glasgow Antipsychotic Side-effect Scale
GDP	gross domestic product
GP	general practitioner
GTT	gamma-glutamyltransferase
GHQ	General Health Questionnaire
GISAH	Global Information System on Alcohol and Health
GMHAT/PC	Global Mental Health Assessment Tool – Primary Care Version
GnRH	gonadotrophin-releasing hormone
GP	general practitioner
GPCOG	General Practitioner Assessment of Cognition

GRADE	Grading of Recommendations Assessment, Development and Evaluation
HAD	HIV-associated dementia
HADS	The Hospital Anxiety and Depression Scale
HAM-A	Hamilton Anxiety Rating Scale
HbA$_{1c}$	haemoglobin A$_{1c}$ (glycated haemoglobin)
HBIGDA	Harry Benjamin International Gender Dysphoria Association
HBSC	Health Behaviours in School Children (WHO network)
HBV	hepatitis B virus
HCL	Hypermania Checklist
HCV	hepatitis C virus
HDI	Human Development Index
HDL	high-density lipoprotein
HIV	human immunodeficiency virus
HKD	hyperkinetic disorder
HPA	hypothalamopituitary-adrenal (axis)
5HT	5-hydroxytryptamine (serotonin)
5HTT	serotonin transporter gene
5-HTTPLR	serotonin-transporter-linked polymorphic region
HV	health visitor
IAPT	Improving Access to Psychological Therapies
IC	integrated care
ICD	*International Classification of Diseases*
ICD-9-CM	ICD-9 Clinical Modification
ICD-10-PHC	10th edition of the ICD-10 for Primary Health Care
ICD-10-TR	Text revision of the ICD-10
ICF	International Classification of Functioning, Disability and Health
ICG	Index of Complicated Grief
ICIDH-2	International Classification of Functioning and Disability
ICPC	International Classification of Primary Care
ID/MR	intellectual disabilities/mental retardation
IDS	Inventory of Depressive Symptoms
IHTSDO	International Health Terminology Standards Development Organisation
IL-6	interleukin-6
INR	international normalized ratio
IPC	Integrated Perinatal Care (programme in Australia)
IPT	interpersonal therapy
IQ	intelligence quotient
IQR	interquartile range
LDQ	Leeds Dependence Questionnaire
LHW	lady health worker
LPA	Lasting Power of Attorney
LSD	lysergic acid diethylamide
LUNSERS	Liverpool University Neuroleptic Side-Effect Rating Scale
MAOI	monoamine oxidase inhibitor
MASC	Multidimensional Anxiety Scale for Children
MAST	Michigan Alcoholism Screening Test
MAT	Memory Alteration Test
MBCT	mindfulness-based cognitive therapy
M-CHAT	Modified Checklist for Autism in Toddlers
MCI	mild cognitive impairment

MCPAP	Massachusetts Child Psychiatry Access project
MDD	major depressive disorder
MDG	millennium development goal
MDMA	3,4-methylenedioxymethamphetamine (ecstasy)
MH	mental health
MHG	mutual help group
mhGAP	mental health Gap Action Programme (WHO)
MI	motivational interviewing
MIG	*mhGAP intervention guide*
MIS	Memory Impairment Screen
MMSE	Mini Mental State Examination
MoCAM	models of Care for Alcohol Misusers
MRI	magnetic resonance imaging
MSDD	multisystem developmental disorder
MUS	medically unexplained symptoms
NA	Narcotics Anonymous
NESDA	Netherlands Study of Depression and Anxiety
NFP	Nurse–Family Partnership
NGO	nongovernmental organization
NHDS	National Hospital Discharge Survey (USA)
NHS	National Health Service (UK)
NIASA	National Initiative for Autism Screening and Assessment
NICE	National Institute for Health and Clinical Excellence
NMDA	*N*-methyl-D-aspartic acid
NMP	non-medical prescribing
NRT	nicotine replacement therapy
NSAID	non-steroidal anti-inflammatory drug
NWW	New Ways of Working for Primary Care
OCD	obsessive–compulsive disorder
od	omne die (once daily)
ODD	oppositional defiant disorder
ODIN	Outcome of Depression International Network
ODIN	Overcoming Depression on the Internet (software package)
OECD	Organization for Economic Co-operation and Development
om	omni mane (every morning)
on	omni nocte (every night)
OR	odds ratio
OSHA	Occupational Safety and Health Administration
OTC	over-the-counter (medication)
PAH	polycyclic aromatic hydrocarbon
PAHO	Pan American Health Organization
PAID	Problem Areas in Diabetes
pc	post cibum (after food)
PC	primary care
PCARE	Primary Care Access, Referral and Evaluation (study)
PCMH	patient-centred medical home
PCMH	primary care mental health
PCO	primary care organization
PCOS	polycystic ovary syndrome
PCP	primary care physician

PCT	primary care trust
PD	panic disorder
PDD	pervasive developmental disorder
PDDST-II	Pervasive Developmental Disorders Screening Test, second edition
PEDS	Parents' Evaluation of Developmental Status
PEP	psycho-educational package
PESQ	Personal Experience Screening Questionnaire
PG	Prolonged Grief (index)
PGD	patient group direction
PGD	prolonged grief disorder
PHC	primary health care
PHCC	primary health care centre
PHQ	Patient Health Questionnaire
PHQ-A	Patient Health Questionnaire – Adolescent version
PMDD	premenstrual dysphoric disorder
PMHC	primary care mental health care clinic
PMS	premenstrual syndrome
PMTCT	prevention of mother-to-child transmisison (of HIV)
POSIT	Problem Oriented Screening Instrument for Teenagers
PPGHC	Psychological Problems in General Health Care (WHO study)
PPP	Positive Parenting Programme
PRIME-MD	Primary Care Evaluation of Mental Disorders
PRISM-E	Primary Care Research in Substance Abuse and Mental Health for the Elderly (study)
prn	pro re nata (when required)
PSC	The Pediatric Symptom Checklist
PST	problem-solving therapy
PST-PC	problem-solving treatment in primary care
PTSD	post-traumatic stress disorder
PUFA	polyunsaturated fatty acid
PWP	psychological well-being practitioner
QALY	quality-adjusted life-year
qds	quater die sumendus (to be taken four times daily)
qhs	quaque hora somni (every night at bedtime)
QOF	Quality and Outcomes Framework
RA	rheumatoid arthritis
RAPI	Rutgers Alcohol Problem Index
RBPC	Revised Behavior Problem Checklist
RCT	randomized controlled trial
RET	rational emotive therapy
RR	risk ratio
RRMHS	Rural and Remote Mental Health Service (Australia)
SA	substance abuse
SACS	Substances and Choices Scale
SAD	seasonal affective disorder
SAD	social anxiety disorder
SADQ	Severity of Alcohol Dependence Questionnaire
SAVRY	Structured Assessment of Violence and Risk in Youth
SCARED-R	Screen for Child Anxiety Related Emotional Disorders – Revised
SCID-CT	*Structured Clinical Interview for DSM-IV – Clinical Trials Version*
SCL	Symptom Checklist

SDOH	social determinants of health
SDQ	Strengths and Difficulties Questionnaire
SES	socioeconomic status
SESCAM	Side-Effects Scale/Checklist for Antipsychotic Medication
SF-12 MCS	Short Form 12-item Mental Component Summary
SF-36	Short Form 36-item health survey
SFP	Strengthening Families Programme
SFPS	solution-focused problem-solving
SHA	strategic regional health authority
SIADH	syndrome of inappropriate antidiuretic hormone secretion
SIGN	Scottish Intercollegiate Guidelines Network
SIT	self-instructional training
SMD	severe mental disorder
SMI	severe mental illness
SMR	standardized mortality rate
SMPCL	Substance Misuse Primary Care Liaison Service (Wandsworth, London)
SNAP-IV	Swanson, Nolan and Pelham IV questionnaire
SNOMED	Systematized Nomenclature of Medicine
SNOMED-CT	SNOMED – Clinical Terms
SNRI	serotonin and noradrenaline reuptake inhibitor
SPC	summary of product characteristics
SPMI	serious and persistent mental illness
SRP	Self-Report of Personality
SSRI	selective serotonin reuptake inhibitor
stat	immediately, at once
T_3	tri-iodothyronine
T_4	thyroxine
T-ASI	Teen Addiction Severity Index
TB	tuberculosis
TCA	tricyclic antidepressant
TCBT	therapist-led cognitive-behavioural therapy
TD	tardive dyskinesia
tds	ter die sumendus (to be taken three times daily)
TEACCH	treatment and education of autistic and related communication-handicapped children
TFCBT	trauma-focused cognitive-behavioural therapy
THP	Thinking Healthy Program (Pakistan)
TIA	transent ischaemic attack
tid	ter in die (three times daily)
TNF-A	tumour necrosis factor
TRIPS	Training for Interactive Psychiatric Screening
TRF	Teacher Report Form
TSF	12-step facilitation
TSH	thyroid-stimulating hormone
UGT	uridine 5'-diphosphate glucuronosyltransferase
UK	United Kingdom of Great Britain and Northern Ireland
UKNSC	United Kingdom National Screening Committee
UNICEF	United Nations Children's Fund
USA	United States of America
USPSTS	United States Preventive Services Task Force
VA	US Department of Veterans Affairs

VARS	Vanderbilt ADHD Rating Scale
VNTR	variable number of tandem repeats
WFMH	World Federation for Mental Health
WHO	World Health Organization
WMHDay	World Mental Health Day
Wonca	World Organization of Family Doctors
WPA	World Psychiatry Association
YGTSS	Yale Global Tic Severity Scale
YLD	years lost due to disability
Y-PSC	Youth-Reported Pediatric Symptom Checklist

Four-word foreword: it's about the relationship

It is not possible to practise in family medicine without knowledge of mental health issues and their ramifications. The *Companion to Primary Care Mental Health* seeks to equip primary doctors and their teams with an overview of the field.

My nurse approached me late one afternoon and said, "I need to speak with you about David". I knew David and his family quite well. For two decades, I had looked after him and his wife Betty, who died 3 months earlier of ovarian cancer. I was also the family doctor to David's son and his two teenage children, David's only grandchildren.

David was a 71-year-old man who had retired from the postal service 4 years earlier. He had chronic atrial fibrillation and diabetes mellitus, type 2, for which he was on warfarin and metformin, respectively. He was diligent about coming in to our practice each month to have his international normalized ratio (INR) checked, to assure therapeutic, and not excessive, anticoagulation. Once every 3 months, he also had a glycated haemoglobin (HbA_{1c}) test, to assess his glucose control. His HbA_{1c} hovered persistently around 9%, considerably above goal and undoubtedly worsened by his body mass index (BMI) of 32 kg/m². Both the INR and HbA_{1c} blood tests were obtained by finger stick, with the results available within 5 minutes using point-of-care testing technology.

Our team divided our duties and alternated visits with David. My nurse saw David two successive months, during which she monitored the INR and adjusted the warfarin dose on the spot, before David left our clinic. When I saw him on the third month to assess his anticoagulation and diabetes, I was also able to recommend changes in his diabetes and anticoagulation regimen at the time of our visit, because of the point-of-care results.

I asked my nurse about her concern regarding David. She said she thought that he was depressed and that she had scheduled David to see me the next morning. I had seen David one month earlier for a diabetes check, at which time he seemed to be coping reasonably well with Betty's death. At that time, he had a reassuringly low score of 6 on the PHQ-9 (Patient Health Questionnaire), a screening instrument for depression that we use regularly for those with diabetes and other chronic conditions. My nurse went on to describe that David was not joking with the nurses as he liked to do; he seemed tired and to have low energy

When I saw David the next morning, he was a very different man than the one I had seen a month earlier. Usually carefully groomed, he was unshaven and wearing rumpled clothes. He mentioned several times that he was not sleeping very well and that at night he would see "Betty's angels coming to get me". I went through a mental checklist of questions. Was he safe? He seemed to be. He denied thoughts of suicide. His weight had remained stable so he was eating. There was no evidence that he was out wandering about at all hours. What was his most important concern? He wanted relief from his new and significant insomnia. What were my concerns? I was worried about his depression due to his bereavement and the relative social isolation since Betty's death.

Without a personal history of mental health problems, new-onset schizophrenia or bipolar disorder seemed unlikely, especially at his age. He had not shown any previous signs of dementia. Delirium was possible, but tests of his glucose, chemistries, blood count and drug and alcohol screen made that unlikely as well.

As our interview progressed, it became clear that he was lucid and his thought processes were well organized, but he was depressed. I concluded that he was suffering from depression, with psychotic features related to his lack of sleep. Since his delusions and hallucinations were quite limited, he did not pose an immediate risk to himself or others and was therefore not a candidate for involuntary hospitalization. When I raised the issue of psychiatric consultation, he was very adamant that he "was not crazy" and refused to see a psychiatrist. Further complicating a consultation was the reality that he would have to travel 40 km to get to the nearest psychiatrist.

We focused on sleep restoration and I prescribed an antidepressant and arranged to have David's teenage grandson spend the night with him for several weeks. Night lights were placed strategically in his bedroom and bathroom. Over the next week, my nurse or I spoke briefly each day with him by telephone. The following week, we were able to persuade him to go to the local senior centre for lunch. Eventually, he joined a walking club through the centre and, after a month of significant improvement in sleep and mood, he agreed to continue to take the antidepressant. As of this writing, David continues to do well, lives independently, and has become a regular at the centre.

I share this brief story about David not because it is unusual, but because it is so common in primary care. It features many of the challenges of primary care: several chronic comorbid conditions, physical and mental health issues, polypharmacy, social barriers, and limited resources, even in the relatively resource-rich environment in which I am privileged to practice. It also included many of the key assets and aims of primary care: early detection, multimodal intervention, practical problem-solving, and an acute awareness of the patient and his context.

Family doctors, better than most, understand the importance of context when sorting out symptoms and offering treatments. We are mindful of the impact of an important life event, such as the death of a spouse; the backdrop of education, occupation, and social class; and individual attributes such as resilience or vulnerability. We must take account of all these factors, and more, as we translate symptoms into diagnosis and convert concepts into treatment actions.

Yet, the proper philosophical framework and good intentions are not enough. We need to be ever watchful, easy to access, and comprehensive in our perspective. Most important, we need to establish and maintain a trusted therapeutic relationship. The relationship that my nurse and I had with David and his family allowed us to keep him in his home and enable him to recover from what could have been a tragic outcome. We were able to use that relationship to leverage change, on David's part (joining the senior centre), on his family's part (staying temporarily with him in his home), and on our part (connecting with him more frequently during his acute illness).

While the relationship can be everything, it is not the only thing. We must know, and do, more. We need best science and practices to apply the best treatment, so that we can be comprehensive in our approach to care. We need ready access to resources that are relevant to our setting and expand our knowledge base. This book is that resource on mental health issues in primary care. It can serve as the resource companion to our relationship-based and person-centred care. We should nurture our patient relationships. We should use this book.

Professor Richard Roberts
President of the World Organization of Family Doctors (Wonca) and
Professor of Family Medicine, University of Wisconsin School of Medicine and Public Health, USA

Foreword

The *Companion to Primary Care Mental Health* is a much-needed, invaluable resource for physicians and other health-care professionals, worldwide, who provide primary care and family medicine. Its value is not limited, however, to primary care settings, since it serves as a roadmap to guide psychiatrists and other behavioural health clinicians toward effective person-centred care. The international scope of the book, furthermore, informs us of the vast differences in medical care throughout the world, from over-specialized medicine in high-income countries to the underresourced status of medicine in many low- and middle-income countries.

A century or more ago, medical care in developing nations such as the United States of America (USA), even when available, was provided by the family doctor. My grandfather was a family physician in a small town in Oklahoma, where his initial licence to practise medicine was issued by the Creek Indian Nation before Oklahoma achieved statehood. Patients arrived at his door for him to deliver a baby, set a broken bone, heal an infection, or prevent a suicide – to name but a few of the needs he was challenged to meet. In many parts of the world today, where medical care is sparse, these conditions persist. In other areas, medicine has become so super-specialized that a "generalist" such as a primary care physician or family medicine physician is hard to find. In many ways, of course, these changes reflect great progress. The USA is one of many countries where the face of medicine has become defined by specialty care, driven by remarkable advances in medical research. As a result, astounding new technologies and discoveries have profoundly increased our ability to understand, treat and prevent illnesses of all kinds. And although we would not want to have it any other way, there have been some unintended consequences of this progress.

In my current role as President of the American Psychiatric Association (APA), I was asked to identify a "theme" for my presidential year, and to outline my top priorities. I chose "Integrated care" as my theme, reflecting my conviction that we need to partner with primary care and family medicine to provide the best treatment for patients with psychiatric (brain) disorders, which are often in themselves complex medical conditions, and which commonly co-occur with illnesses such as heart disease, diabetes, hypertension and many others. I believe it is important to emphasize that (1) psychiatry is part of the house of medicine; (2) patients have a right to receive evidence-based quality care; (3) fragmented care is not quality care; and (4) research and education are our best blueprint for a strong future.

Numerous studies are summarized in this book, which demonstrate the high worldwide prevalence of psychiatric disorders such as depression, alcohol or substance use, and many others. The landmark report entitled *The global burden of disease*, published by the World Health Organization (WHO), the World Bank and the Harvard School of Public Health, called attention to the fact that these conditions are leading causes of disability – not just among psychiatric disorders, but among all medical conditions.[1] Another global study by WHO surveyed almost a quarter of a million individuals from 60 countries and reported that consistently, across all countries, those with depression comorbid with one or more other chronic conditions (such as asthma, arthritis or diabetes) had the worst health scores of all of the disease states studied.[2] Recently in the USA, the National Quality Forum identified the 20 high-impact medical conditions that accounted for 95% of Medicare costs. These 20 conditions were prioritized based on dimensions such as cost, prevalence, improvability and disparities; the condition that was ranked as the number one priority was major depression, above ischaemic heart disease, diabetes, stroke, Alzheimer disease, rheumatoid arthritis, lung cancer and many others.[3]

There is an enormous amount of information in this volume that conveys the same message as the reports described above – i.e. that patients with psychiatric disorders can be seriously disabled and that patients with these conditions frequently have significant physical illness as well. Recognizing these facts helps us understand the need for integrated care. All of us, as patients, do not just neatly sort ourselves into single-disease categories and then seek out a specialist in that category; rather, we become ill in ways that can be complex and confusing, and that often call for a broad range of medical skills. It is estimated that more than 20% of primary care patients have diagnosable psychiatric disorders (and this is an extremely conservative estimate), and about 50% of primary care visits are for stress symptoms such as headache, insomnia or fatigue.[4] The isolated lone physician in a remote location in a low-income country needs access to specialty psychiatric knowledge, tools and advice, just as the busy primary care physician in a high-income country needs to have psychiatrists or other behavioural health specialists working, ideally, at his or her side. The APA produced a report on integrated care in 2009, which advised that, at least in the USA, integrated care must be more than simple co-location of two distinct services. It requires interdisciplinary communication, collaboration and coordination of service delivery, where psychiatrists at the very least should serve as team supervisors or consultants.

New models of integrated care are emerging, such as medical homes, and these are described in great detail in this *Companion to Primary Care Mental Health*. In the introductory chapter, for example, three models of collaborative care are described. We are advised that "fragmented care should be a 'never' event", and we are warned that "any approach to integration will have to be clinically sound, operationally functional, and financially viable. If an approach fails in any of these ways, it fails". In subsequent chapters, approaches to treatment of major categories of psychiatric disorders in primary care settings are described in rich detail.

In some countries, such as the USA, the costs of health care are staggering, and there is an urgent need to rein in those costs. Yet health-care reform has proved to be highly contentious and complex. Today's economic challenges mandate, however, that efforts to scale back the costs of medical care are redoubled, not only in the USA but also in many other countries throughout the world. This volume does not pretend to provide those solutions. However, if we in the medical profession can agree about how to provide the best health care possible, across all countries whether rich or poor in resources, patients will receive more efficient, comprehensive and effective care. Workforce productivity and quality of life will increase, and disability will decrease, and in those countries where health-care costs are exorbitantly high, these costs should go down. The *Companion to Primary Care Mental Health* provides welcome wisdom that will help us work towards and achieve many of these goals.

References

1   Murray C, Lopez A, eds. *The global burden of disease*. Boston MA, Harvard School of Public Health, on behalf of the World Health Organization and the World Bank, 1996.

2   Moussavi S et al. Depression, chronic diseases, and decrements in health: results from the World Health Surveys. *The Lancet*, 2007, 370(9590):851–858.

3   *Webinar. Prioritization of high impact conditions and measure gaps*. Washington, National Quality Forum, 2010 (http://www.qualityforum.org/Calendar/2010/03/Webinar__Prioritization_of_High_Impact_Conditions_and_Measure_Gaps.aspx, accessed 4 January 2012).

4   Sorel E et al. *American Psychiatric Association Position Statement. Psychiatry and primary care integration across the lifespan*. Arlington VA, American Psychiatric Association, 2009 (http://www.psych.org/Departments/EDU/Library/APAOfficialDocumentsandRelated/PositionStatements/201004.aspx, accessed 4 January 2012).

John M Oldham
Senior Vice President and Chief of Staff,
The Menninger Clinic and Professor and
Executive Vice Chair Menninger Department of
Psychiatry and Behavioral Sciences,
Baylor College of Medicine and Past President,
American Psychiatric Association

Foreword

Mental health is an essential building block of health and is directly related to personal, family and community well-being. However, the burden of mental illness is often underestimated, in spite of its significant impact on mortality, morbidity and disability throughout all life-stages.

Therefore, the resources to confront and treat mental illness are frequently insufficient and inappropriately distributed. In many countries, the care model is still focused around the psychiatric hospital. This creates a treatment gap – a high proportion of people who require care do not receive it. Other barriers to care include stigma and discrimination towards the mentally ill.

Mental and neurological disorders represent 21% of the total disease burden in Latin America and the Caribbean, and the Pan American Health Organization (PAHO) works with Member States to strengthen national capabilities and implement national mental health policies and plans. Special attention has been devoted to the reorganization of mental health services. In particular, mental health should be integrated into the general health-care system, and the majority of mental disorders should be addressed in primary care settings.

In 2008, the World Health Organization (WHO) launched the Global Program of Action in Mental Health. The goal of this programme is to reduce the burden of mental and neurological disorders, as well as substance abuse disorders, throughout the world. The programme focuses on low- and middle-income countries that have a high prevalence rate of disorders and lack resources. PAHO supports and actively participates in this initiative.

The 49th Directing Council of the Pan American Health Organization/World Health Organization (PAHO/ WHO) adopted a resolution on the Strategy and Plan of Action on Mental Health in 2009. This significant milestone clearly puts mental health on the agenda of the governments of the Americas and becomes a guide for work over the next 10 years. The resolution expresses the political and technical will to prioritize and continue to promote the processes of change required in this field. It also calls attention to the need to accelerate the implementation of reforms in most countries.

A community mental health model is grounded on the basic principles adopted in the regional strategy to organize service delivery. Decentralization, social participation and the inclusion of a mental health component in primary health care are among its cornerstones.

Despite the enormous challenges that lie ahead, including the delivery of technical cooperation, there are reasons to be optimistic. When we look back, the achievements are many, there are innovative experiences in Latin America and the Caribbean, and many lessons have been learnt. We have proven that we can overcome myths, stigma, discrimination and contentment with the status quo, and the political will of governments and the awareness and involvement of society is growing.

I wish to express my appreciation to the World Organization of Family Doctors (Wonca) and all those who have contributed to the preparation of this book, which aims to become a companion for all family doctors and general practitioners in their everyday practice. I do hope that it will become a practical tool for planning and implementing interventions in the mental health field at primary care level.

Mirta Roses Periago
Director, Pan American Health Organization

Foreword

According to the World Health Organization's 2008 study on the global burden of disease, mental disorders represent 23% of the total population who suffer from a disease in the European Union (disability adjusted).

A 2010 Eurobarometer survey revealed that 15% of respondents had sought help for a psychological or emotional problem in the past year, and 11% of those surveyed had talked to their general practitioner (GP) about it.

As the first contact point for patients, family doctors and GPs need to feel that they are adequately prepared to deal with these visits, which constitute a significant percentage of their consultations. In turn, the people who turn to these frontline health professionals for help with their emotional problems must feel confident that they will be provided with state-of-the art advice and medical care.

Therefore, I very much welcome this initiative by Wonca, the World Organization of Family Doctors, to produce this *Companion to Primary Care Mental Health*. The book offers a comprehensive summary of the current knowledge of mental disorders and their cure, building on contributions from many distinguished contributors.

I am confident that this book will quickly become a valuable resource for family doctors and GPs, supporting them in their training and in their everyday experiences with the broad variety of mental health conditions among patients.

The *Companion to Primary Care Mental Health* is also welcome as a contribution to the implementation of the European Pact for Mental Health and Well-being. Through the Pact, the European Commission works together with Member States and nongovernmental partners to raise awareness about mental health challenges, and to identify and disseminate good practices in tackling them.

I thank Wonca for being an active partner in the implementation of the European Pact for Mental Health and Well-being, and wish the *Companion to Primary Care Mental Health* the wide dissemination and the impact it deserves.

Paola Testori Coggi
Director-General Health and Consumers, European Commission

Foreword

The *Companion to Primary Care Mental Health* admirably conceptualizes the most important topics, clinical issues and programmatic components related to the interface between primary care and mental health. The interrelationship between mental health and primary care is, without question, the most critical and important one, insofar as it affects access to care worldwide, as well as comprehensive care within the context of service quality; this is particularly true in those areas of the world where subspecialty care is almost non-existent. From this point of view, this book offers new perspectives to both the field of mental health and also the field of primary care.

The four sections of the book were well chosen and address the most critical and essential topics for today's experiences in relation to the role of primary care vis-à-vis mental illness and mental health conditions. Key issues, such as the conceptualization of this book; the determinants of health and mental health; the essential role of advocacy and stigma; the influences of religion; and the role of ethics are well addressed in this text. The essential role of access to care from a public health point of view, and the interface of mental health and primary care in an ambulatory setting are also presented most effectively. The key principles of primary care intervention within the context of mental health are also fully covered. From a clinical viewpoint, the most relevant treatment initiatives within the context of primary care are also well discussed and reviewed in this textbook.

Finally, the professional contributors to this volume create an impressive list of individuals who are highly respected in the fields of mental health and primary care. Undoubtedly, this book is a major contribution on behalf of the patients who suffer from mental health conditions and require access to appropriate treatment in a primary care environment.

My congratulations to the Editor and his excellent group of collaborators, who have worked together to make this book an outstanding tool for diagnosis and treatment of those who suffer from mental illness within the realm of primary care – especially those patients with limited access to health care and mental health care.

With much respect and admiration.

Pedro Ruiz
President, World Psychiatric Association; Professor and Executive Vice Chair and Director of Clinical Programs, Department of Psychiatry and Behavioral Sciences, Miller School of Medicine, University of Miami, Florida, USA

Acknowledgements

The *Companion to Primary Care Mental Health* is based on the clinical experience of, and literature reviews carried out by, a group of general practitioners, psychiatrists, policy-makers, mental health professionals and mental health advocates. I would like to thank everyone who supported this project.

This book was the result of a collaboration. Each chapter was assigned to a team and the team leader coordinated the information provided by other members of the team. Each chapter was then subjected to a two-stage peer review process, initially by the Editor, and two other contributors, to ensure that the content was relevant to primary care and would provide readers with mental health knowledge relevant to primary care. Feedback was provided to each of the team leaders, who then re-drafted their chapter. Each re-drafted chapter was then submitted to a group review process, initially using a small group of three or four people, followed by whole-group discussion, taking into account the following criteria:

- is the chapter written for a primary care audience?
- does it cover the life-span of the disorder and age range relevant to the chapter?
- does it take a biopsychosocial or holistic approach?
- will it support general practitioners and their teams in their daily practice?
- are the key messages:
  - included in the submission?
  - consistent with the chapter content?
  - fit for purpose?
- does the chapter support and reflect the complexity and systems within primary care?
- are there copyright issues?
- is the chapter internally consistent?
- are there any factual errors?
- are there any chapters that need to be merged to present a more coherent picture?

The members of this group review team included:

Professor José Miguel Caldas de Almeida, Professor of Psychiatry and Head, Department of Mental Health, Faculty of Medical Sciences, Nova University of Lisbon, Portugal; *Professor Carlos Augusto de Mendonça Lima*, Chair, International Psychogeriatric Association, Head of Department of Psychiatry and Mental Health, Centro Hospitalier de Alto Ave, Guimaraes, Portugal; *Professor Sir David Goldberg*, Professor Emeritus, Institute of Psychiatry, London, UK; *Sarah Haspel*, Assistant Operations Director, North East London Foundation Trust, London; *Dr Gabriel Ivbijaro*, Editor; Medical Director, Waltham Forest Community and Family Health Services, The Wood Street Medical Centre, London, UK; *Professor Rachel Jenkins*, Director, WHO Collaborating Centre for Research and Training; Professor of Epidemiology and International Health Policy; Head of Section, Mental Health Policy, King's College, London, UK; *Dr Lucja Kolkiewicz*, Consultant Psychiatrist and Associate Medical Director for Recovery and Well-being, East London NHS Foundation Trust, London, UK; *Professor Christos Lionis*, Professor of General Practice and Primary Health Care; Head of Clinic of Social and Family Medicine, University of Crete, Greece; *Dr Juan Mendive*, Family Physician, La Mina Primary Health Care Centre, Catalan Institute of Health, Teaching Unit of Family Medicine, Barcelona, Spain; *Dr Eleni Palazidou*, Honorary Consultant Psychiatrist, East London Foundation Trust, London, UK; *Dr Henk Parmentier*, General Practitioner and Medical Director, Patient Care 24, Croydon, UK; *Professor*

Michelle Riba, Past President American Psychiatric Association; Associate Chair of Integrated Medicine and Psychiatric Services, University of Michigan; Associate Director Michigan Institute for Clinical and Health Research; Director, PsychOncology Program, University of Michigan Comprehensive Cancer Center; Associate Director, University of Michigan Comprehensive Depression Center, USA; *Dr Wolfgang Spiegel*, General Practitioner; Certified Physician for Psychosomatic Medicine; Senior Researcher and Lecturer, Department of General Practice, Center for Public Health, Medical University of Vienna, Austria; *Dr Geraldine Strathdee*, Consultant Psychiatrist and Associate Medical Director of Mental Health for London; SHA Lead for Mental Health, NHS London, UK.

The feedback from this group review process was provided to each of the team leaders, who amended their chapters accordingly.

I would like to thank all the reviewers for their time and support. I would also like to express gratitude to all the contributors, including the project manager and copy-editor Penny Howes; the team at Radcliffe Publishing, especially Gillian Nineham and Andrea Hargreaves; and all those who have worked to produce this volume. I would like to thank all the members of the Wonca Working Party on Mental Health for all their support. I am also grateful to Jürgen Scheftlein from the European Commision (DG Health and Consumers) and Professors Michael Kidd and Nabil Kurashi and Drs Alan Cohen and Dragana Nalic for all their help and support and extend special thanks to Drs Henk Parmentier and Lucja Kolkiewicz and to my children Efe and Ese.

Gabriel Ivbijaro
Editor

Photo credits

Page 1: A primary care centre in Walthamstow, London, UK. Courtesy of Dr Gabriel Ivbijaro

Page 95: Professor David Goldberg. Courtesy of Professor David Goldberg

Page 153: Mount Meru Regional Hospital, Arusha, United Republic of Tanzania. Courtesy of Louisa Hiu Yu Ho

Page 281: Collage of social networks associated with mental health well-being – Navigator Team, Waltham Forest, London, UK. Courtesy of Dr Todd Edwards

Page 283: wider determinants of health. Courtesy of Waltham Forest Navigator Team, London, UK

Page 337: 'I am here' (2009–2012). Made in response to the experience of living in a run-down inner city housing estate. Andrea Luka Zimmerman, Fugitive Images. Courtesy of Andrea Zimmerman

Page 363: Hawaii, USA. Courtesy of Dr Lucja Kolkiewicz

Page 385: Masai Huts, United Republic of Tanzania. Courtesy of Dr Penny Howes

Page 419: Serengeti Landscape, United Republic of Tanzania. Courtesy of Peter Howes

Page 455: Tranquility-Canal, Agde, Southern France

Page 517: Temporary clinic site in rural village of Garagusain, Himachal Pradesh, India. Courtesy of Dr Harriet Edge

Page 569: Mount Meru Regional Hospital, Arusha, United Republic of Tanzania. Photo courtesy of Louisa Hiu Yu Ho

Page 609: Investiture of an African Chief, The Arure of Iyede, Delta State Nigeria. Courtesy of Dr Gabriel Ivbijaro

Cover photos

Mount Meru Regional Hospital, Arusha, United Republic of Tanzania. Courtesy of Louisa Hiu Yu Ho

Temporary clinic site in rural village of Garagusain, Himachal Pradesh, India. Courtesy of Dr Harriet Edge

Hawaii, USA. Courtesy of Dr Lucja Kolkiewicz

A primary care centre in Walthamstow, London, UK. Courtesy of Dr Gabriel Ivbijaro

Section A

Primary care mental health: the context

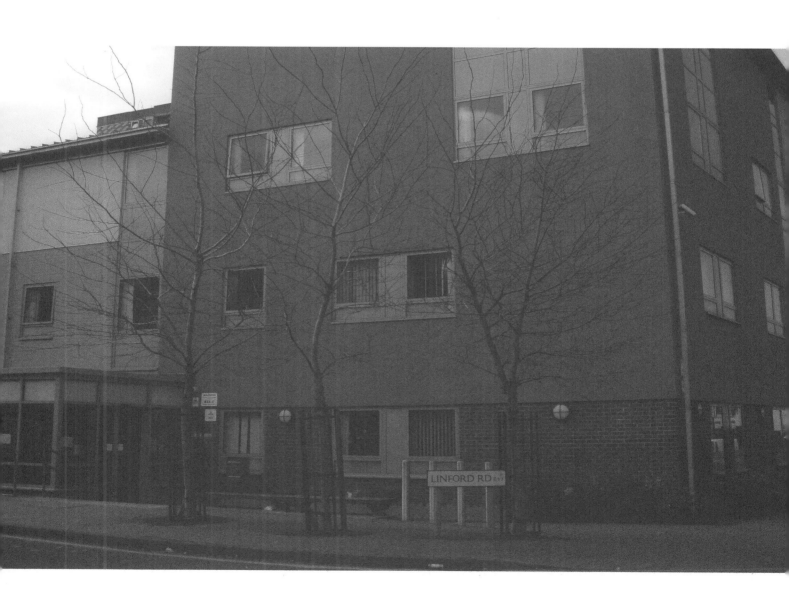

1 Aims, concept and structure of the book

Dr Gabriel Ivbijaro – editor

The *Companion to Primary Care Mental Health* aims to provide the best available evidence for the management of patients with mental health conditions in the primary care setting. It draws on the expertise of a range of experts from primary and secondary care, who have translated information from the literature and their own clinical experience so that it can be applied to everyday family practice globally.

The World Health Report 2008. Primary health care (now more than ever),[1] and the 2008 joint World Health Organization (WHO) and World Organization of Family Doctors (Wonca) publication, *Integrating mental health into primary care. A global perspective,*[2] highlighted the need to strengthen primary care capability in order to improve access to care and the outcome of those patients who are managed in primary care. The WHO/Wonca book also highlighted that patients with mental health problems, and their carers, prefer to be managed within the primary care setting because this supports integration and reduces the stigma associated with mental health problems. This volume presented some good examples of mental health integration in primary care, but this is not universal. There remains a need to support primary care staff to improve their skills and knowledge, so that they can rise to the challenge of providing the best possible care to their patients. The *Companion to Primary Care Mental Health* aims to do this.

There exists a range of evidence-based treatment and management options in mental health, but patients often do not receive these interventions. This has been termed the "science-to-service gap".[3] A literature review of unmet need for mental health care for schizophrenia showed that, even in high-income countries, patients still do not receive the best evidence-based practice despite the availability of knowledge.[4] In low- and middle-income countries, the application of evidence-based knowledge is worse. Patients with mental illness continue to die prematurely, on average 15 to 20 years earlier than their contemporaries who are not mentally ill – a fact that we cannot continue to ignore.[2]

One way of narrowing the "science-to-service gap" is to equip primary care to deliver and demand evidence-based practice for all patients, so they can enjoy good mental health. The *Companion to Primary Care Mental Health* is based on the conviction of the authors, contributors and reviewers that this can happen, and it covers a range of conditions that present to primary care – those that are common and those that are not so common.

Structure

The book is structured to enable individuals to understand the complex network of factors that contribute to mental health (see Figure 1.1). Each chapter opens with a box of short key messages that highlight the most important points it aims to convey.

Sections A and B provide family doctors and their teams with the foundation of knowledge necessary to support the development of fully integrated systems to promote good mental health. This includes the need to harness the wider determinants of health and mental health and to tackle stigma through advocacy, spirituality and ethical practice. The role of public health and the management of the many interfaces associated with providing good mental health are also covered in these sections, which provide practitioners with the tools required to evaluate their services.

Section C describes the tools for assessment, including classification and risk assessment, and the general principles required to enable a biopsychosocial approach to care.

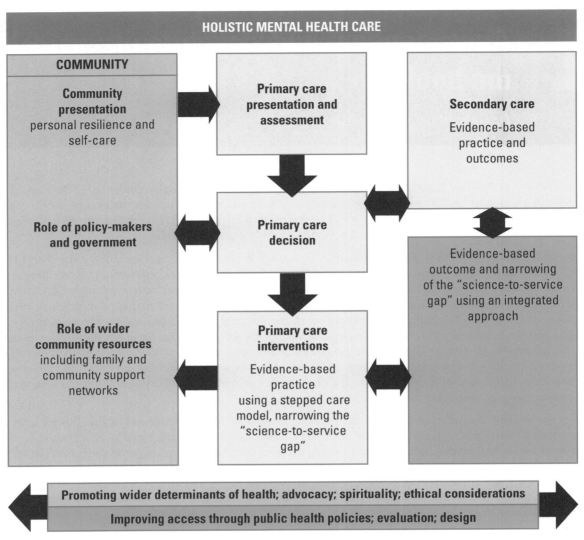

Figure 1.1 The interrelationships between elements of holistic mental health care

Section D considers the individual mental health conditions that family doctors and their teams are likely to encounter during the course of their practice. As comorbidity and the management of complexity are very common in primary care mental health, these are also considered in the final chapters of the book.

References

1 *The World Health Report 2008. Primary health care (now more than ever).* Geneva, World Health Organization, 2008.

2 World Health Organization and Wonca. *Integrating mental health into primary care. A global perspective.* Geneva, World Health Organization, 2008.

3 Drake RE, Essock SM. 2009. The science-to-service gap in real-world schizophrenia treatment: the 95% problem. Schizophrenia Bulletin, 2009, 35:677–678.

4 Mojtbai R et al. Unmet need for mental health care in schizophrenia: an overview of the literature and new data from a first-admission study. *Schizophrenia Bulletin*, 2009, 35:679–695.

2 The wider determinants of health and mental health in primary care

David Goldberg, Kay Eilbert, Akwatu Khenti and Graham Thornicroft

Key messages

- Over the last 30 years, the concept of health has changed from a lack of disease mainly influenced by cure by the medical sector to one where physical and mental health result from interactions of biology and the conditions in which people live and work. The determinants of health and public mental health frameworks define the factors that shape health, calling for more effective partnerships across organizations and levels of society to address those factors.

- A consensus exists that it is the combination of risk and protective factors rather than factors taken individually that determines the impact on mental health. Because the foundation for good mental health later in life is laid in early childhood, interventions that target the early years should be a priority.

- In many high-income countries, a stepped care approach has been adopted, in which patients whose depression is of moderate or severe intensity benefit from a range of both psychological and drug treatments, while those with mild depression benefit from a range of low-cost interventions. A range of cost-effective interventions are described. Nurses and others can also be effective in treating episodes of common mental disorders.

- In low- and middle-income countries, the majority of the population receive no mental health care; insufficient funds are devoted to the necessary staff and the drugs necessary to support treatment for both severe and common mental disorders. It is essential that basic mental health services are provided in primary care.

- In low- and middle-income countries, specially trained health-care workers can administer a range of effective treatments, including problem-solving, psycho-education and some forms of psychotherapy, and more severe cases respond well to antidepressants. Approaches such as cognitive-behavioural therapy and problem-solving can be simplified and adapted for delivery in primary care and through paraprofessionals.

- The World Health Organization has recently formulated the mental health Gap Action Programme (mhGAP) and published an intervention guide intended for use by primary care and community practitioners in these countries. Closer collaboration between the specialist mental health services and primary care services is necessary if scarce resources are to have optimal use, and several patterns are described.

- It is necessary to recognize the social determinants of health, and work towards a change in health-care and social systems, as well as in the education of doctors. This would mean that clinicians consider not only presenting symptoms but also the influences on health – the environment in which people live and the importance of work, for example – in assisting patients to return to good health.

Introduction

This review is in five parts, starting with the wider determinants of physical and mental health. In the second part we deal with mental health in primary care in low- and middle-income countries, where it becomes clear that, at present, training is inadequate both at undergraduate level and in later training, particularly in lower-income countries. Yet if basic mental health services are to reach the wider population, they must do so in primary care. In the third part, we consider practices in primary care mental health services that have been shown to be cost effective, before describing the WHO programme aimed at improving mental health in low-

and middle-income countries (the "mental health Gap Action Programme" (mhGAP)). In the fourth part, we describe the various forms of collaboration between specialist mental health services and primary care, aimed at improving outcomes for people with mental disorders. Finally, we consider measures that can be taken to prevent mental disorders across the life-course.

The determinants of physical and mental health

Summary

- Over the last 30 years, the concept of health has changed from that of a lack of disease, mainly influenced by cure by members of the medical sector to one where physical and mental health result from interactions of biology and the conditions in which people live and work. The social determinants of health (SDOH) model posits that genetic endowment interacts with social and physical environments to determine individual biological and behavioural responses that are influenced by access to and quality of health-care services. These are the conditions in which people are born, grow, live, work and age, and which are shaped by the distribution of money, power and resources at the global, national and local levels.[1] The SDOH framework defines the factors that shape health, calling for more effective partnerships across organizations and levels of society to address those factors. These influences include lack of income, inappropriate housing, unsafe workplaces, and lack of access to health systems, for example. Public mental health uses these approaches in the field of mental health.

- Research has increasingly highlighted the interaction between a genetic predisposition and an environmental trigger and the environmental influences acting directly on gene expression.

- Given the foundation for good mental health later in life, attention needs to focus on key developmental stages and transition points, with additional priority accorded to the importance of a healthy start in the early years.

- Many mental health problems have common risk factors; interventions that successfully address these risk factors may have beneficial effects for a number of disorders.

- A better understanding of the environments in which patients live and that contribute to poor health outcomes is an important aspect of primary care. Primary care practitioners have the most frequent access to patients and, as such, have opportunities for early detection and treatment of signs of mental distress that result from an individual's environment. In addition, general practitioners (GPs) and their primary health-care teams play a central role in promoting physical and mental well-being for all age groups.

Over the last 30 years, the concept of health has changed from that of a lack of disease, mainly influenced by cure by the medical sector to one where physical and mental health result from interactions of biology and physical and social environments. While early public health interventions focused on improving the physical environment through clean water and sanitation, for example, this focus was lost during the last half of the 20th century, with the advent of increasing numbers of medical advances to cure illness once it had developed. The publication of the Canadian *Lalonde Report* in 1976 reintroduced the role of environmental influences on health.[2] The World Health Organization (WHO) *Ottawa Charter for Health Promotion* in 1986 called for working at multiple levels to improve health, combining individual, community and societal interventions.[3] More recently, Sir Michael Marmot's reports, *Closing the gap in a generation*,[1] and *Fair society, healthy lives: a strategic review of health inequalities in England*,[4] set the problems of health inequalities in the widest possible context, recognizing that disadvantage starts before birth and accumulates across the life-course.

The social determinants of health (SDOH) model posits that genetic endowment interacts with social and physical environments to determine individual biological and behavioural responses that are influenced by access to and quality of health-care services. These are the conditions in which people are born, grow, live, work and age, and that are shaped by the distribution of money, power and resources at the global, national and local levels.[1] The SDOH framework (Figure 2.1) defines the factors that shape health, calling for

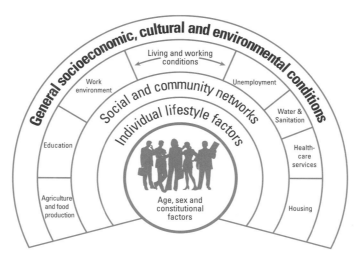

Figuae 2.1 Social determinants of health. Reproduced, with permission, from Dahlgren G, Whitehead M. *Policies and strategies to promote social equity in health.* Stockholm, Institute for Futures Studies, 1991[7]

more effective partnerships across organizations and levels of society to address those factors. The greatest advances in health have been made through a combination of structural change and the actions of individuals.[5] Recommendations from the WHO Commission on Social Determinants of Health centred on improving the conditions of daily life and reducing the inequitable distribution of power and resources that drive daily living conditions. The Commission concluded:

> The conditions in which people live and work can help create or destroy their health – lack of income, inappropriate housing, unsafe workplaces, and lack of access to health systems are some of the social determinants of health leading to inequalities within and between countries.[6]

As early as 1948, recognizing that mental health and physical health are intimately linked, WHO, defined health as:

> a state of complete physical, mental and social well-being and not merely the absence of disease or infirmity.[8]

An emerging concept of public mental health builds on the WHO definition of mental health:

> The successful performance of mental function, resulting in productive activities, fulfilling relationships with other people, and the ability to adapt to change and to cope with adversity; from early childhood until later life, mental health is the springboard of thinking and communication skills, learning, emotional growth, resilience, and self esteem.[9]

Prevention offers opportunities not only to improve the quality of life but also to reduce health-care costs. There is a growing recognition that there is a need to move away from the disproportionate emphasis on treatment, releasing resources for prevention and early detection and management, while maintaining high-quality treatment services for those who cannot be managed in the community. In most parts of the world, at least until recently, the treatment of mental illness was alienated from the rest of medicine and health care, and "incurable" patients were often isolated in asylums. Mental health is now viewed as the foundation for well-being and effective functioning for individuals and for communities. Yet the emphasis remains on acute treatment, placing mental health and mental illness outside the public health tradition that health and illness are multifactorial in origin and therefore often amenable to prevention or management in the community.[5]

Public mental health is a recent development in the field of mental health, combining public health approaches, the social determinants of health and mental health promotion. Public mental health has been defined as "the science, art and politics of creating a mentally healthy society". What is considered healthy can change with the social context in any given historical period.[10] Public mental health is an emerging field that covers prevention, protection and enhancement of mental health and well-being. Prevention of mental disorder focuses on reducing risk factors and enhancing protective factors that are related to the determinants of mental health, and thus becomes the responsibility of all sectors of society.[11] As with public health, public mental health is concerned with beliefs, attitudes and behaviours of individuals, and with socioeconomic and environmental determinants. It, too, concerns itself with a defined population and takes an ecological perspective of the complex interaction between the human as a biological organism with psychological, social and environmental factors. A life-course perspective informs public mental health, which integrates mental health closely with physical health.[12]

It has become clear that the way forward for promotion of mental health and prevention of mental disorder involves integrated models across multiple sectors. Two models have been highlighted in systematic reviews of the literature:[13]

- *the MacDonald and O'Hara model for mental health promotion* (1998) builds on the Albee model that focused on individual factors; this model adds in aspects of mental health promotion. Social conditions are considered, along with individual and environmental factors
- Desjardins[13] adopted the MacDonald and O'Hara model[14] for mental health promotion, combining the previous elements of the MacDonald and O'Hara model. The adapted model suggests that good mental health results from the interaction of individual and environmental factors, as well as recognizing that mental health in later life is influenced by developments at critical or transitional phases earlier in life.

Evidence – across the life-course

The Marmot *Review of health inequalities in England* combined the social determinants of health model with a life-course framework, stating that risk and protective factors start accumulating before birth and continue into old age.[4] Key stages in the life-course include prenatal/early childhood, adolescence, adulthood and older adult life. Priority should be placed on early childhood development, with efforts continuing throughout life to break the links between early disadvantage and poor outcomes.[15]

Given the foundation for good mental health later in life, attention should be focused on key developmental stages and transition points, with additional priority accorded to the importance of a healthy start in the early years. Key developmental stages include reproductive decisions; the prenatal/postnatal period and infancy; the transition to school; adolescence; the transition to independence and adult life, including family and work; and retirement.[16]

Traditional explanations for the link between health risk factors and mental illness involve learned behaviour and a physiological response (heightened neuroendocrine and immunological response) to chronic stress brought about by feelings of low status and decreases in trust and social capital, for example.[17] Psychiatric theories posit that brain mechanisms that evolved to assess environmental threats underlie psychiatric disorders, because similar brain structures are affected in psychiatric symptomatology and in threat assessment and self-defence.[18] Research on maternal attachment in animals has shown its importance in the developing infant and later in life. While genes clearly play a mediating role, influences in the environment can contribute to the way genes express themselves in the adult. For example, the effects of maternal stress and care translate into physiological outcomes in the offspring. These interactions help explain the pathways between genes, the environment, behaviour and genotype that can influence mental health outcomes.[19]

Research has increasingly highlighted the interaction between a genetic predisposition and an environmental trigger and the environmental influences acting directly on gene expression. These gene–environment interactions can confer risk and protective effects that are additional to separate genetic or environmental risks.[20] Figure 2.2 displays these interactions.[20]

Risk/protection factors

A number of influences on mental health have been proposed that act as either risk or protective factors (characteristics at the biological, psychological, family, community, or cultural level that precede and are associated with a higher (risk) or lower (protective) likelihood of problem outcomes). Many mental health problems have common risk factors; interventions that successfully address these risk factors may have beneficial effects for a number of disorders. Poverty and child abuse are common links to depression, anxiety

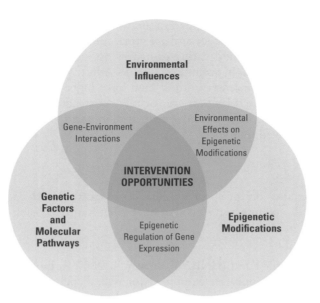

Figure 2.2   The interaction of environmental influences, genetic factors and epigenetic modifications. Reproduced, with permission from the National Academies Press, from O'Connell M, Boat T, Warner K, eds. *Preventing mental, emotional and behavioral disorders among young people: progress and possibilities*. Washington DC, National Academies Press, 2009[20]

and substance abuse. Interventions that successfully address poverty and child abuse can be expected to have an impact on all three of these disorders. A consensus exists that it is the combination of risk and protective factors rather than factors taken individually that determines the impact on mental health. An effective approach to prevention of mental disorder therefore addresses risk factors and nurtures protective factors across the life-span.[13]

This chapter focuses on the socioeconomic determinants of mental health that are malleable and responsive to public policies and interventions. These are presented in Box 2.1. Determinants such as age, sex and genetic factors, which cannot be changed, are excluded from the discussion.

Box 2.1   Risks/protective factors (influences are additive from previous stages)[1,16,20,21]

Prenatal life
- Prenatal exposure to maternal diet, smoking, alcohol; maternal depression

Early childhood to age 12 years
- Stress, preterm birth, low birth weight, socioeconomic status/poverty, teenage mothers, family conflict or family disorganization; abuse, housing, parenting style, nurturing environment, parental mental illness, lifestyle choices (e.g. nutrition, exercise)

Adolescence
- Failure at school, increased vulnerability to drugs and alcohol, increased risk taking; peer pressure/rejection

Adulthood
- Unemployment, work stress, education, transport, housing, crime, violence, discrimination, community networks and support, civic participation, religion

Old age
- Chronic disease, sense of feeling valued for contribution to family/community, isolation and alienation

---

Differences in mental health outcomes are apparent between males and females. In childhood, conduct disorders are the most common mental disorder and are more common among boys. Girls, on the other hand, have a higher prevalence of depression and eating disorders during adolescence. Girls also attempt suicide more often but boys are more successful in attempted suicide. Adult women have a higher prevalence of most affective disorders and non-affective psychosis. Adult men have higher rates of substance use disorders and antisocial personality disorder. Gender roles that are socially constructed (responsibilities, power and status) interact with biological differences to influence how men, and, in particular, men affected by mental disorders seek health and how they are viewed by society.[16]

Life-stages

The discussion that follows focuses on the specific influences associated with each life-stage. The final part of this chapter sets out evidence-based interventions that have been found to be effective.

Pregnancy and early childhood

A recent United Nations Children's Fund (UNICEF) survey in 2007 examined six dimensions of child well-being in rich countries. Among 21 countries examined for overall performance on child well-being, Spain, Switzerland, the Netherlands and Scandinavian countries ranked top, while the United States of America (USA) and the United Kingdom of Great Britain and Northern Ireland (UK) were ranked at the bottom.[16]

The early years are the most important life-stage because mental health challenges have roots in early childhood, starting in the womb. The prenatal and first years of life are important in establishing the foundations of an individual's mental health across the life-course. The extent to which these are positive or negative will help determine whether an individual is more vulnerable to, or resilient in, the face of life's events.[16] Maternal care has been shown to influence gene expression through hippocampal development in females, but not in males. This environmental influence has been shown to work through expression of the gene responsible for the metabolism of serotonin (an important inhibitory neurotransmitter), which is associated with the sensitivity of the adult to external stress.[19] The mental health impact of adversity later in life is mediated by social factors and psychological robustness developed during the early years.

Mental and physical health are inseparable, as are brain and physical development. During the prenatal period, environmental factors can affect the developing brain and impair behaviour and cognition development in early childhood. Goldberg, in 2009 reported several important research findings:[19] research by Caspi et al. in 2003 showed that adults with the short version of the gene *5HTT* promoter polymorphism were more susceptible to stressful life events and increased depressive symptoms, diagnosable depression, and suicidal thoughts; and in 2004, Kaufman et al. confirmed these results in children, extending the findings to show that maltreated children with no social supports, who also had the short allele had the highest depression ratings.[19]

Other factors influencing the prenatal period include low levels of the B vitamin folic acid, exposure to infections such as influenza, and exposure to toxins such as lead and mercury, insecticides, tobacco smoke and alcohol.[20] There is strong evidence for the negative impact during pregnancy of maternal smoking, alcohol consumption and drug use, which increase the risk of premature deliveries, low-birth-weight infants and later behavioural, emotional and learning problems.[15] In additional research reported by Goldberg,[19] Kahn and co-workers in 2003 showed that prenatal maternal smoking was linked through the dopamine transporter genotype with hyperactivity in childhood, and in 2005 Caspi et al. showed that cannabis use was linked with schizophrenia through the catechol-O-methyltransferase (*COMT*) gene.[19] In addition, it is known that parents who use alcohol or drugs after the birth of a child have less emotional availability and less-consistent parenting practices.[13]

Being born prematurely and with a low birth weight are known risk factors for adverse mental health outcomes and psychiatric disorders.[21] Early emotional and behavioural problems predict later school failure, unplanned pregnancy and crime.

Poverty is a risk factor for childhood mental disorders. Child poverty rates in the UK (19.4%) and the USA (22.4%) are among the highest in the Organization for Economic Co-operation and Development (OECD) countries. Other OECD countries such as Belgium, Norway and Sweden have child poverty rates below 5%. A graded relationship has been shown between household income and emotional and behavioural problems in children, as evidenced in Figure 2.3, based on the 1997 Health Survey for England study on young people.[22]

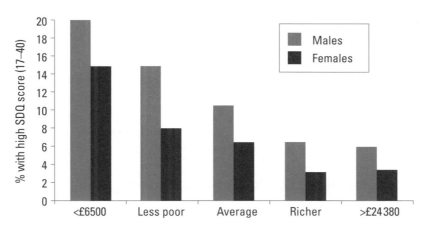

Figure 2.3 Proportion aged 4–15 years with high Strengths and Difficulties Questionnaire (SDQ) total deviance score (17–40) by equivalent household income quintile and sex[22]

Poverty affects childhood development through multiple pathways; i.e. the quality of the home environment (access to resources to stimulate children); the level of stress experienced by parents and subsequent behaviour (insufficient parental resources to cope with life events); and through poor neighbourhoods and schools (limited resources and exposure to additional risk factors).[20]

Teenage pregnancy is associated with poor outcomes for both the infant and the teenager. Rates of live births to teenage women are high in North America and Canada (55 per 1000 women aged 15–19 years and 25 per 1000 in the USA and Canada, respectively). European countries report much lower rates, for example France (7 per 1000 women aged 15–19 years) and the Netherlands (5 per 1000 women aged 15–19 years). Pregnant teenagers often drop out of school, losing opportunities to learn skills necessary for employment and survival as adults. Teenage pregnancy is associated with deprivation levels and premature and low-birth-weight babies.[16]

The principal driving force of childhood development is relationships – secure attachments that allow the child to explore his/her environments. One of the strongest risk factors for mental disorders involves mistreatment of children by primary caregivers, which is also associated with poverty and parental mental illness.[20]

A literature review of evidence of the association between postpartum depression and a poor mother–infant relationship pointed to poor infant-development outcomes.[23] Reviews have identified a range of factors that predict postpartum depression – prenatal depression, low self-esteem, child-care stress and prenatal anxiety.[16] Mothers with depression are more likely to act with hostility, withdraw or use inconsistent parenting practices. The children of mothers who have suffered from postpartum depression have a higher risk of developing behavioural problems and mental disorders.[13]

A study of 14 700 mothers of 9-month-old infants in deprived neighbourhoods in England confirmed that poor maternal mental health placed infants at risk for developmental and behavioural problems. Neighbourhood characteristics were found to be associated with maternal mental health but were less salient than family and maternal characteristics. Place affects mental health through anxieties with regard to safety and antisocial children.[24]

Nutritional deficiencies in early life are linked to poor mental health. While an association between breastfeeding and healthy mental development has not been established, breastfeeding during the early months provides opportunities for the infant to bond and form positive attachments – important protective factors for the developing infant.[17] Researchers recognize that adequate nutrition in early childhood helps prevent mental health problems later in life.[13] Studies of the effectiveness of the Supplemental Nutrition Program for Women, Infants and Children in the USA suggest positive impacts such as: increased absorption of nutrients by women and children; improved birth outcomes (reduction in low birth weight), reduced health-care costs, and increased use of health-care services.[20] Studies have identified important nutrients for child development. The relationship between iron deficiency and subsequent behaviour was noted in a 10-year follow-up study, with parents and teachers noting problems with anxiety, depression, socialization and attention. US Hispanic children and overweight children are particularly vulnerable.[20]

Developing fetuses and young infants are particularly susceptible to harm from hunger and malnutrition. While these are not common in developed countries, the 2001 Canadian Community Health Survey found that 8.16% of British Columbia residents reported sometimes or often not having enough to eat. Studies conducted across 10 USA jurisdictions found that children from families reporting food insufficiency and hunger were more likely to show behavioural, emotional and academic problems. These data do not point to causality but do indicate the need to address issues of hunger and malnutrition.[16]

Early childhood development influences basic learning, school success, employment participation, social activities and health. Risk/protective factors for this period include parental education, parental mental illness, family conflict, poor housing (overcrowding, fuel poverty, homelessness), primary caregivers and single-parent households.[15]

Childhood adversity may lead to maladaptive patterns of attachment (difficulty in forming trusting social relationships), which may result in aggressive or violent behaviour and social isolation later in life. Both childhood adversity and depression are associated with behavioural risk factors for medical illness, such as obesity, smoking, excessive alcohol consumption and sedentary lifestyles. A vicious cycle of poor physical and mental health can develop, where depression leads to unhealthy risk behaviours that result in chronic disease, leading potentially to an inability to exercise, poorer quality of life, and further maladaptive health behaviours, such as increased alcohol consumption. Each of these factors, separately or in combination, can increase the risk of depression.[13]

A systematic review of the genetic and environmental determinants of psychiatric comorbidity, focusing on four of the most prevalent types of psychopathology (anxiety disorders, depression, conduct disorder and substance abuse) confirmed an association between childhood adversity and mental problems. Genetic factors play a particularly strong role in comorbidity between major depression and generalized anxiety disorder or post-traumatic stress disorder. Affective disorders are influenced more by the environment, including childhood adversity/life events, family and peer social connections, and socioeconomic and academic difficulties.[25] A Finnish study using a national representative sample of 18–39-year-old adults confirmed a strong relationship between self-reported health and psychological distress and childhood adversity, as defined by parents with mental health problems, chronic/long-term illness, financial problems and family conflict. Men reported poorer physical health, while women reported higher psychological distress and somatic morbidity.[26]

An important life-course transition, for both the child and family, involves starting primary school. Children between the ages of 5 and 12 years experience rapid development of physical, cognitive, emotional and social skills. Not only do they gain skills to read, write, count and solve problems, but they also develop social skills and resilience to develop good interpersonal relationships, manage conflicts and their emotions and respond appropriately to their social environment. Results from this skill-building period will influence later mental health.

The broader social context of schools and communities affects childhood development. Children may be exposed to victimization, bullying, academic failure and association with deviant peers during their school years. Neighbourhoods and communities can provide settings for learning (libraries) and social and recreational activities (green space). Community norms and values influence children's development through a shared sense of engagement and social controls to prevent antisocial behaviour and violence.[13]

A particular at-risk group involves looked-after children, who may be stigmatized as if at fault when they are looked after because of dysfunctional families.[27]

Adolescence

Adolescence covers the ages from 12 to the mid-twenties. During this period the child transitions to secondary school and enters puberty. The WHO Health Behaviours in School Children (HBSC) network undertakes research to track changes over time and across countries. A cross-national study has provided comparative data covering the period 1998–2006 on the experience of mental well-being as described by self-reported health, life satisfaction and subjective health complaints. While most children reported good mental health, a sizeable minority reported either fair or poor health and experienced a number of recurring health complaints. In 2002, the geographical differences were substantial, with high scores in Finland and the Netherlands and low scores by comparison in Latvia, Lithuania and Ukraine. Case-studies from Belgium (Flanders), Finland and Slovenia confirmed that these general patterns remained consistent in 2006.[28]

Adolescence is characterized by a growing need for independence, increased influence of peers, and challenges related to the development of one's identity and sexual orientation and those associated with school success. This is the period when most mental disorders start manifesting themselves. It is a period of higher risk taking and vulnerability to drugs and alcohol, which can lead to dependence, a mental disorder itself, and lead to other mental disorders. Conduct disorders comprise the largest mental disorder for children. In young children, risk factors include family conflict, failure at school, bullying and early use of substances. A cohort study in New Zealand found that for late onset in adolescence, conduct problems are attributed more to frustrations due to a "maturity gap" (physical maturity before independence) and to social mimicry of deviant peers.[13]

Further studies using HBSC data show:

- *the relationship between bullying and psychosocial adjustment* – despite large country variation (9% of young people reported being involved in bullying in Sweden, compared to 54% in Lithuania), there was a consistent relationship between bullying and psychosocial adjustment. Bullies and victims demonstrated significant problems with health, emotional adjustment and school adjustment

- *acceptance by peers as a key factor in young people's health* – those who are not accepted by peers are far more likely to have emotional problems. Interactions with friends tend to improve social skills and strengthen the ability to cope with stressful events

- *the links between supportive and inclusive neighbourhoods and young people's mental well-being* – results from the England 2001/2002 HBSC survey found that factors associated with neighbourhood social capital were highly predictive of mental well-being, even after controlling for age, sex and family affluence. For example, young people who had no involvement in the local community were twice as likely to report poorer health; those who rarely felt safe in the neighbourhood were almost four times as likely to report being unhappy and twice as likely to feel low at least once a week.[28]

Adulthood

The transition to adulthood involves both significant life changes and changes in the nature of risk and protective factors. For many, childbearing and parenting must be juggled with the demands of employment. Factors that can protect against stress and mental problems include the ability to cope with stress, the ability to deal with adversity, problem-solving skills, literacy, social support from family and friends, and social and conflict-management skills. On the other hand, convincing evidence is available for the link between depression and low socioeconomic status, stressful events, exposure to violence and crime, chronic physical ill health, low education levels, conflict, disasters, poor working environments and female sex and sex inequality. There is reasonable evidence linking mental health with discrimination, income inequality, food insecurity, hunger, unemployment, toxins, urbanization, poor housing, overcrowding, low social capital, poor built environment, and minority ethnicity. For education, there is a strong dose–response relationship: higher education reduces vulnerability to mental health issues and vice versa. Alcohol consumption has a direct influence on mood.[16]

Family breakdown can lead to social isolation, feelings of loss, learned negative behaviours, marginalization and economic difficulties. Migration and urbanization bring changing cultural norms that can lead to loss of identity. Evidence suggests that deprived individuals have reduced access to early mental health treatments. This may also be associated with belief systems that delay a person seeking help where mental health is stigmatized.[29]

A large evidence base confirms the relationship between deprivation, inequality and poor health outcomes across all levels of the social hierarchy. Inequality is associated with increased social position/status competition and insecurity. This in turn affects health through perceptions and emotions that lead to stress, hostility and lack of control over ones' life, which translate into physiological assaults on neuroendocrine and immune systems, exacerbated by the unhealthy lifestyle behaviours that may be adopted.[17]

Deprivation/income and education are the most important influences on health. Together they represent the resources required to meet basic needs, such as housing, healthy food and the ability of parents to provide a safe environment for their children. People living in poverty are not only exposed to conditions that are adverse to their health but they are also more likely to be negatively affected by those conditions. The disadvantaged are over-represented among people with mental disorders.[27]

Using a cross-sectional nationally representative household survey in England, Scotland and Wales, researchers examined the association between mental disorders, poverty and debt. The association between income and mental disorders was confirmed but was largely mediated by debt, after adjusting for income and other socioeconomic variables. Those with larger debts were more likely to have a mental disorder.[30]

The way in which people think is influenced by values and culture (how things are done) and how they are distributed (economic and fiscal policy). Inequalities in health are related to social and economic policies that lead generally to better health for those with higher incomes and better education. Health equity is defined as "the absence of unfair and avoidable or remediable differences in health among population groups defined socially, economically, demographically and geographically".[1] In the west, for example, priority for fiscal and economic growth may undermine family and community relationships.[31] Once societies reach the level of affluence found in developed countries, further improvements in absolute standards make little difference in improving health. Differences in health at that stage begin to reflect differences in income distribution or income inequality. What is important is how rich or poor individuals feel in relation to others in their society.[32]

Employment and work confer access to income and social contacts, as well as a sense of purpose, and social inclusion, all of which impact on mental health.[33] Higher levels of parental employment are associated with lower rates of child poverty and family stressors, and with overall child well-being. On the other hand, the stress of work has the potential to lead to mental illness or to exacerbate an existing mental health problem. Psychosocial factors that can create stress and mental health problems in the workplace include control (autonomy, participation, skill use and development), workload (quantity, complexity, time constraints), roles (conflicts, ambiguity), relationships with others (social support, harassment, recognition), career prospects (promotion, precariousness, demotion), organizational climate and culture (communications, hierarchical structure, equity), and the interaction between work and one's private life.[13]

Issues of work–life balance can be a source of family stress, hampering the emotional availability of parents to their children and increasing the risk of family conflict and of the child developing mental health problems. There is currently no systematic evaluation of the impact of measures to reconcile work and family life on the health of children and families.[13]

A meta-analysis of psychosocial work stressors and mental disorder provided robust evidence that high-demand and low-decision work and high-effort and low-reward work can act as risk factors for mental health.[34] A systematic review and meta-analysis examined the association between job satisfaction and health. The correlation with various mental health issues (range from $r = 0.478$ to 0.420) was stronger than that for physical health ($r = 0.287$). The authors concluded that job satisfaction is an important factor influencing the health of workers, and should be addressed.[35]

The Whitehall II cohort study of the British civil service examined the effect of adverse changes in dimensions of work (effort–reward balance, high job demands, and work social support and control over work). Both an imbalance in effort–reward and high job demands were predictive of psychiatric disorder, while social support at work was found to have a protective effect on mental health. The authors of this study concluded that these associations may be causal.[36]

The rapidly changing nature of work can influence the mental health of workers. Globalization, new technologies, decreased work security resulting from a shift from a manufacturing to a service/knowledge economy, long hours, intensification of work and decreased work–life balance all create stress. At the same time, workers' mental health is influenced by increased employee expectations for more control over work and working arrangements, bullying in the workplace and increased competitiveness versus needs of the workforce to cope with change. These influences are translated into stress, a major cause of absenteeism.[27] The ability to adapt to these increasing stressors is determined by perceptions of work demands and the ability to cope with them.[37]

Individuals in the UK work the longest hours in the European Union. Long hours are common, with one in eight people working over 60 hours per week and one in 10 experiencing a mental health problem in any one year. Half of the days lost at work are due to work-related stress.[12] A meta-analysis examined the link between long hours of work and psychological health problems, pointing to small but significant correlations between overall health – both physiological and psychological symptoms – and long hours.[38]

In a longitudinal cohort study using a random sample of people aged 25–65 years, the global economic crisis has been shown to be associated with increased prevalence of mental disorders, especially in men in relationships.[39]

An important determinant of mental health is education. Education is linked to the ability to earn higher incomes, and acts as a protective factor for cognition across the life-course. For example, success or failure at school is strongly related to a propensity to commit crime or engage in antisocial behaviour.[40] Infants born to less-educated mothers are more likely to have a low birth weight, which is associated with developmental delays, at least in part because these mothers have fewer resources for antenatal care. Completion of at least 10 to 12 years of formal education appears to be a significant protective factor, pointing to the importance of efforts to reach and retain those who are at risk for school leaving in formal educational programmes.[29]

Low literacy and low levels of education severely limit the ability of individuals to access economic opportunities. While there have been impressive gains in improving literacy levels in most countries through better educational programmes targeting children, there is much less effort directed to today's adult illiterates. It is expected that programmes aimed at improving literacy, targeting adults in particular, may have tangible benefits in reducing psychological strain and promoting mental health.[21]

Mental health status is associated with lifestyle behaviours at all stages of life. A body of evidence indicates that the social factors associated with mental ill health are also associated with alcohol and drug use, crime and dropout from school.[5] While individuals make lifestyle choices, their ability to make healthy choices may be limited by their own mental health. Chronic systemic inflammation is a predisposing factor for depressive mood and cognitive impairment, and may make it difficult to assimilate and act on health messages, because of loss of interest in a healthier lifestyle.[33] Poor/risky lifestyle behaviours may not only result from lack of knowledge or beliefs but also reflect the social environment that increases/decreases one's freedom to choose healthy behaviours. For example, unlike the UK and the USA, the diet in Mediterranean countries is not associated with privilege but with a traditional culture where females prepare meals. While this healthy diet confers health benefits, the expectation of the traditional culture for women to stay at home may have negative influences on their mental health.[41]

Areas under study related to nutrition and mental health include the potential effect of large amounts of sugar on the occurrence of attention-deficit hyperactivity disorder (ADHD) and the relationship between vitamin D and brain development and function, as well as the link between sunlight and seasonal affective disorder.[20] Evidence suggests that for pregnant and lactating women, n-3 polyunsaturated fatty acid (PUFA) supplementation can be beneficial for preterm infants and longer-term cognition. Breastfed infants have higher IQ scores, presumably because of the fatty acids uniquely in breast milk. The epidemiological evidence linking specific nutrients such as n-3 PUFA, B vitamins and antioxidants, however, is inconclusive, given the small and short-term nature of the randomized clinical trials conducted so far to test the effectiveness of dietary supplementation on cognition-related parameters. Increased fatty acids in older age may slow ageing-related decline.[42]

Although the causal relationship between physical activity and cardiovascular health is well established, the relationship between physical activity and mental health is less well known. Work by Stathopoulou et al. in 2006, reported by Desjardin et al.,[13] hypothesized that physical activity protects individuals from mental disorders by acting on metabolism, neurotransmitters and sleep regulation. In addition, physical activity may produce a positive psychosocial effect by promoting the development of a feeling of self-efficacy and self-esteem.[13] A meta-analysis of trials of low methodological quality showed a significant positive effect of exercise on depression but not on anxiety.[13] A review of evidence by Bauman in 2004 of more recent longitudinal studies of better methodological quality showed mixed results.[20]

Alcohol consumption is related to genetics and culture. In countries where higher consumption is tolerated, alcohol-related violence is higher.[43] Alcohol consumption increases a person's vulnerability to mental ill health, and people with pre-existing mental health conditions may use alcohol to self-medicate. There is sufficient evidence of the link between alcohol consumption and depression.[44]

Housing may influence health through overcrowding, fuel poverty and homelessness, and is a marker for poverty. A review of studies on the link between housing and mental health showed that six of the seven studies that included mental health confirmed a positive impact of improvements to warmth and energy efficiency.[45] Poor housing is a key factor associated with children's mental development, although it is not known whether the association is causal. Housing quality may be a proxy measure for the quality of the home-learning environment – e.g. lack of resources, disruptive family circumstances, lower-quality social support networks. Children living in poorer-quality housing have also been shown to have higher levels of stress hormones and behavioural problems.[27]

High-rise housing may have a harmful effect on the psychological well-being of women with small children. Factors that may contribute involve poor-quality, residential crowding and loud and exterior noise. These effects are concentrated among the poor and ethnic minorities.[46]

Neighbourhood can be an important influence on health and well-being, through the level of social organization that connects people.[17] Increasing violence and crime in cities isolates people, increases fear and insecurity, and reduces trust, leading to poor mental health and affecting the poor disproportionately.[47] A survey of neighbourhoods in a large US city found that those places with fewer stressors had higher levels of participation, which leads to better mental health. An interesting finding in this study involved neighbourhoods with high stressors, where the isolation associated with anonymous blocks resulted in lower anxiety.[48]

Spatial planning is important to well-being, since planning can create access or barriers to social networks, which is especially important to the elderly, disabled and unemployed. Perceptions of safety, the ability to interact, traffic levels and access to local facilities facilitate these interactions. Planning often exacerbates inequalities by building large social housing developments in less-desirable locations, for deprived people.[49]

Domestic violence can result in short- and long-term effects on both physical and psychological health. These harmful effects may persist long after the abuse has ended. Low self-esteem, depression, anxiety, drug and alcohol abuse and a history of physical or sexual abuse increase the risk of being both a victim and a perpetrator.[13]

Mental health is produced socially. Culture affects how we experience and cope with mental symptoms, how well we are supported by family and the community, our willingness to seek treatment, and our ability to communicate to mental health providers. The United Nations estimated in 2008 that over 3% of the global population comprised international migrants. This points to the increasing importance of understanding culture and cultural differences.[50]

Some policy-makers contend that culture is under-emphasized in the social determinants of health model, which concentrates on poverty and inequalities. The impact of culture may increase the effect of socioeconomic status on well-being. For example, individualism and materialism might accentuate the costs of being poor by making money more important to social position, decreasing group identity. Western culture promotes a "good life" that serves economic growth through marketing, for example to make us dissatisfied with what we have and who we are, and that may not meet our psychological needs.[31] This model de-emphasizes the family and community relationships that protect mental health across all social classes.[17]

A review of mental health and ethnicity commissioned by the NHS Centre for Reviews and Dissemination concluded that the study of mental health and disorders is a Eurocentric discipline. Ethnicity and culture influence the interpretation of mental health and the way people are perceived and treated. In western countries, the mental health of the white population is seen as the norm, thus leading to discrimination against those who do not conform to this norm. The racism and discrimination faced by those who are seen to deviate from the prevailing norm are associated with mental health morbidity. People from black and minority ethnic (BME) groups who seek treatment not only face communication barriers but are treated based on western norms that seek to bring deviations in line with prevailing norms. Less-educated and more-deprived BME groups make up the largest proportion of people in mental hospitals. For example, while African Caribbean males have lower rates of mental illness than others in the UK, inpatient data show higher levels of schizophrenia among first- and second-generation individuals. This is unexpected, especially in the second generation, and is not repeated elsewhere in other countries (e.g. African Americans). "Deviant" African Caribbean individuals are dealt with through the criminal justice system rather than through primary care, where they have lower rates of mental health referral, although they have the same rate of GP registration. It is not clear if this is a communication or other type of barrier.[51]

A literature review of immigrants to Canada revealed that they tended to be healthier at the time of immigration but that they lost that advantage over time. Discrimination was posited as the driver for increased depression.[52] A study by Qureshi concluded that, perhaps because of limited cultural competency on the part of health-care providers, migrants were under-represented in mental health care, had more diagnostic errors, and experienced more coercive measures and less psychotherapy.[53] A study of undocumented immigrants in Spain found these immigrants to be more vulnerable to accidents and psychosocial distress from poor working and living conditions, social exclusion and discrimination.[54]

In a cross-sectional study of the link between self-assessed mental and physical health and discrimination, Stuber and co-workers found that discrimination was linked to increased stress and depression but that this was ameliorated by strong social networks and support to increase resilience in poor Black neighbourhoods but not in poor Latino neighbourhoods.[55]

A growing literature links religion with better mental health outcomes. Religion is shaped by social context and culture, binding individuals to society.[56] Religion can provide social support, a sense of purpose and coherent belief system, as well as a clear moral code, although religion is clearly not the only source of a moral code. Although the USA is the most religious of developed countries, it experiences poor health outcomes and other social indicators compared to other developed nations. The lack of an association may mean that other factors such as the lack of universal health care and elements of the US culture, such as the emphasis on personal consumption and self-gratification, play a more important role.[57]

A number of systematic reviews of religion, spirituality and mental health suggest an association between religion and increased skills for coping with stress and less depression, suicide, anxiety and substance abuse. Healthy normative religious beliefs appear to be stabilizing.[58] Most research in this area is US based and involves Judeo-Christian religions. In addition to social effects, religion may reduce risky behaviours (alcohol and drug use, smoking, risky sexual practices). On the other hand, religion as part of culture is sometimes associated with hatred and exclusion of those who refuse to conform or are different.[59]

A literature review confirmed that although poor children are at greater risk of mental health problems, ethnic poor children have a lower prevalence of mental health problems, perhaps due to religion as a protective factor, where Black children reported higher rates of religiosity with increased social relationships.[60]

Terms that are associated with good health outcomes for individuals and places include empowerment, social cohesion and resilience. Empowerment is defined as a "process by which people, organisations and communities gain mastery over their affairs".[61] There is limited evidence that empowerment improves individual psychological well-being through increased confidence, control, knowledge and awareness, sense of community and networks.[62] Resilience is the ability to deal with life's adversities and to adapt when things go wrong. Places that have promoted empowerment and are resilient may act as buffers to adversity and lead to better health outcomes. For example, Kerala, Costa Rica, and Sri Lanka have promoted land reform and female education and have better health outcomes than some richer places.[17]

Evidence shows that countries that experience sustainable development and prosper have a high degree of social cohesion. This social cohesion involves a concept of social capital, a resource made up of social relationships and networks that involve high levels of trust and shared norms and values, which in turn have a positive influence on health. Putnam states that social capital is characterized by community and personal networks; civic engagement; a sense of belonging; norms of cooperation; and a sense of obligation to help others and trust in the community.[63]

Evidence of the association between social capital and mental health is mixed. A review of research on the relationship between social capital and common mental disorders found that at the individual level there was evidence for an inverse relationship but that at an ecological level, the studies included were too diverse to draw conclusions.[64] A national cross-sectional survey in Japan studied the relationship between mental health and cognitive social capital (trust) and structural social capital (membership in sports and groups). The authors concluded that social capital is associated with better mental health after adjusting for age, sex, income and education.[65] A study of schoolchildren in England aged 11 to 15 years established a link between social capital and young people's health, although the strength of the association varied across health behaviours and social capital indicators.[66]

Old age

Old age brings important changes; retirement and becoming a grandparent may confer positive benefits, while chronic illness or death of a loved one may increase risks to mental health. Further risks are associated with social isolation and loss of meaningful social roles. Social support from family and friends and opportunities for new productive social roles have been shown to protect mental health in older age.[16]

Approximately one-quarter of people with physical illness develop mental health problems such as depression, as a consequence of the stress of their physical condition. The way that people perceive illness is a predictor of depression, with those who perceive it as more threatening than others being at higher risk. Major depression itself increases the risk of chronic illness; for example, depression doubles the lifetime risk of developing type 2 diabetes and has been proven to be a risk factor for heart disease.[11]

A review of studies between 1970 and 1998 on social relationships and health among older people found that social relationships have potential health-promoting or health-damaging effects. Biologically plausible pathways involve the negative effects of the social environment that result in elevated stress hormones, increased cardiovascular activity and depressed immune function.[67]

Implications for primary care practitioners

- A better understanding of the environments in which patients live and that contribute to poor health outcomes is an important aspect of primary care.

- Effective primary care involves understanding patients' beliefs and expectations, which will allow for an agreement with patients on management of their condition.

- Primary care practitioners have the most frequent access to patients and, as such, have opportunities for early detection and treatment of signs of mental distress that result from people's environment.

- GPs and their primary health-care teams play a central role in promoting physical and mental well-being for all ages.

Mental health in primary care in low- and middle-income countries

Summary

- Growing numbers of people are affected by mental health or neurological problems. These problems are particularly acute in poorer regions of the world where few receive the care and support they need. This treatment gap is compounded by stigma, insufficient public education, inadequate funding, low governmental priority and a lack of trained personnel, to name a few ongoing and pervasive challenges.

- The potential of low-cost drugs and treatments is seldom harnessed fully to address eminently treatable conditions. Individuals with the conditions face the additional burden of having to fund their own treatment and to rely heavily upon their families for ongoing support.

- Considerable evidence attests to primary care as the most feasible means of meeting burgeoning needs. Strategies that have demonstrated efficacy include training and retraining, establishing new guidelines, and implementing a range of monitoring tools.

- Adequate infrastructure development is critical for sustainable change including mechanisms to train, supervise and support health professionals, as well as tools for effective assessment, referrals, treatment and follow-up. Better integration with other tiers of care and increased funding are also essential for long-term efficacy.

Mental health or neurological problems affect 450 million people worldwide and the number is steadily increasing.[1] Those in low-income countries are disproportionately affected by mental health problems due to persistent poverty, rapid social change, armed conflict and natural disasters. Poor mental health also contributes significantly to the cycle of poverty in low-income countries. More than 75% of individuals in low-income countries receive no mental health treatment or care.[68] Poor funding for mental health services, inadequate numbers of mental health professionals, and lack of mental health training for primary health-care providers, compounded with a cultural stigma about mental disorder, are major obstacles to accessing mental health care.[69,70]

Most low-income countries have not implemented mental health education programmes for the general population,[71] leading to widespread stigma about mental illness. Stigma is fuelled by cultural beliefs and views about the aetiology of mental illness,[70] especially supernatural and religious beliefs.[72] A common stereotype of people with mental health problems as 'dangerous' also contributes to stigma and discrimination, as does fear of contagion. The pervasiveness of cultural stigma often prevents people from seeking help when it is available.

Mental health care is often a low health priority in low-income countries. For example, only 50% of African countries have a mental health policy, and a third of the African population is not covered by any mental health policy.[73] Despite the potential of low-cost drugs and psychosocial treatments to treat mental disorders successfully, the majority of those in need do not receive even the most basic mental health care.[1,74] The treatment gap for people with mental disorders is extremely high – near 90% in the least-resourced countries, where fundamental resources are inaccessible or unavailable.[75,76] In 2007, WHO found that more than half of low-income countries provide no community-based care for persons with mental disorders.[7] When formal mental health services are available, rates of use are generally low, due to cultural stigmas,[75] and treatment is usually sought from traditional and spiritual healers.[69,77–79]

Inappropriate financing is a primary barrier to the provision of mental health services in low-income countries: 79% of African countries and 63% of Asian countries allocate less than 1% of their total health budget to mental health.[80] Out-of-pocket payment is the primary method of financing in 38.6% of African countries and 30% of South-East Asian countries,[73] further reducing the use of mental health services.[81] Social insurance is the second most common method of financing mental health in 16% of African countries, while no South-East Asian countries use social insurance to finance mental health care.[73] Private health insurance is not available in most low-income countries: mental health care is largely hospital based, and the transition to community care would require additional funds. Only 52% of low-income countries provide community-based care:[75] care is primarily provided by family members, who face a huge financial burden.[82]

Low-income countries also lack mental health professionals: they average only 0.05 psychiatrists and 0.16 psychiatric nurses per 100 000 people, about 200 times less than high-income countries (WHO, 2005) (Table 2.1).[83] Many countries in sub-Saharan Africa and other low-income countries elsewhere have only one psychiatrist for every million people, compared with 137 per million in the USA.[84] In 2002, Uganda had a population of 24.2 million and only 12 psychiatrists;[69] Chad, Eritrea and Liberia each have only one psychiatrist in the whole country. Furthermore, existing training programmes and facilities for mental health professionals in low-income countries are inadequate.[75,74]

Table 2.1 Mental health manpower (per 100 000 population) by wealth of country[83]

Type of country	Psychiatrists	Nurses	Psychologists	Social workers
Low-income	0.05	0.16	0.04	0.04
Low-middle income	1.05	1.05	0.60	0.28
Higher-middle income	2.70	5.38	1.80	1.50
High-income	10.5	33.0	14.0	15.7

Mental health care through primary care

Incorporating mental health services into primary care is the most feasible way to ensure that people in low-income countries receive the mental health care they require. Successful initiatives have been implemented in several African countries, demonstrating how integrating mental health into general health care results in more accessible, affordable and acceptable services and care. A modest investment of resources into primary care has the potential to reduce the burden of mental disorders considerably.[1,75] Uganda is one successful example. Having identified mental health as a priority, small mental health units are being constructed at regional hospitals; other reforms include curriculum changes and substantial training and retraining of health-care providers, new guidelines, training manuals, monitoring tools, and support supervision teams, increased supply of psychotropic medications, and mass public education. Uganda's integration of mental health into primary care and investment of resources has improved access to affordable, and less stigmatizing, mental health care.[85]

Despite the presence of successful examples, many barriers remain. The primary care system in many low-income countries is incapable of providing mental health care and treatment. Some countries lack even basic primary care infrastructure and services.[1,73,86] Lack of knowledge about mental illness among health-care professionals is a continuing challenge that results in common mental disorders, including depression and anxiety, remaining largely neglected or undiagnosed.[30,87,88] Primary care workers require appropriate training, supervision and continuous support to assess, identify, treat and refer people with mental disorders.[1,74,85,88] Figure 2.4 shows that only 2% of undergraduate training hours in lower-income countries are devoted to mental health issues, and the situation is only slightly better in middle-income countries. To meet the challenge of mental illness, primary health care in low-income countries needs to be strengthened.[75,89]

Figure 2.5 shows that in low-income countries, no doctors, and only 1% of nurses, had attended a two-day refresher course on mental health issues, and it has been estimated that only 60% of low-income countries train primary care workers in mental health.[70] Figure 2.6 shows that most clinics in lower- and lower-middle-income countries are not able to prescribe psychotropic drugs.

For example, Nigeria allocates less than 1% of its total health budget to meet the needs of people with mental disorders. It has no national health insurance and no social welfare programmes, so most patient cost comes directly from consumers as out-of-pocket payments. Gureje and co-workers explored the cost-effectiveness

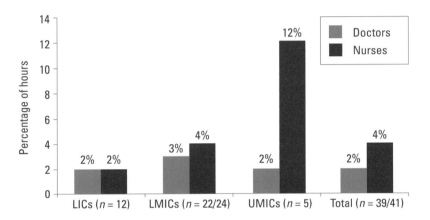

Figure 2.4 Proportion of undergraduate training hours devoted to mental health, by country income group. LIC = lower-income countries; LMIC and UMIC lower- and upper-middle-income countries. Data derived, with permission, from *Mental health systems in selected low- and middle-income countries: a WHO-AIMS cross-national analysis*. Geneva, World Health Organization, 2010[90]

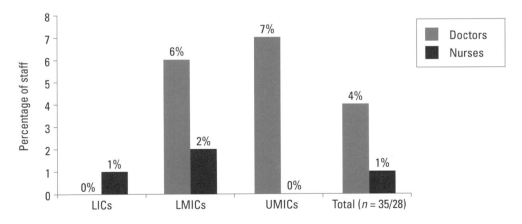

Figure 2.5 Percentage of medical doctors and nurses that received 2 days of refresher training in mental health, by country income group. LIC = lower income countries; LMIC and UMIC lower- and upper-middle-income countries. Data derived, with permission, from *Mental health systems in selected low- and middle-income countries: a WHO-AIMS cross-national analysis*. Geneva, World Health Organization, 2010[90]

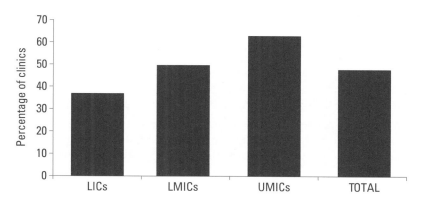

Figure 2.6 Percentage of primary health-care clinics in which psychotropic medicines are available, by country income group. LIC = lower-income countries; LMIC and UMIC lower- and upper-middle-income countries. Data derived, with permission, from *Mental health systems in selected low- and middle-income countries: a WHO-AIMS cross-national analysis.* Geneva, World Health Organization, 2010[90]

of selected interventions for common mental disorders at the primary care level.[86] They found that existing primary health-care services are insufficient to deliver these interventions: effective response for individuals with mental disorders will require better training for health-care providers, better integration of primary care services with those offered at other tiers, and increased funding for health.

Despite these barriers, the delivery of mental health care through primary care services remains the most feasible option. The global imperative is to implement what we know works, all the while striving for further innovation.

Implications for primary care practitioners

- Even 5 minutes of positive interaction with persons with mental health or neurological problems can contribute to recovery and behaviour changes over the long term.
- Continuing medical education is critical for both professional and personal growth. It is a cost-effective means of reducing the stigma that diminishes both the accessibility and quality of services provided to those with mental health and/or neurological conditions.
- There is a wide array of mental health tools freely available online that can be incorporated into primary care practices, with few additional resources.

Which treatments are best for mental disorders in primary care?

Summary

- Many episodes of common mental disorders (CMDs) will resolve by themselves with time, but treatment of the more severe episodes will shorten the duration of symptoms. Although the episode may remit, one year after an episode of CMD about half of patients will be in an episode once more.

- Despite the fact that many episodes of CMD are missed by clinicians in primary care, it is only worthwhile to screen populations known to be at high risk, where the prevalence will be higher than among random patients.

- The cost-effectiveness of treatments partly depends on how much resource is devoted to mental disorders in different countries. In all countries, a stepped care approach, with more expensive treatments being reserved for more severe cases, has been shown to be effective.

- In high-income countries, patients whose depression is of moderate or severe intensity benefit from a range of both psychological and drug treatments, while those with mild depression benefit from a range of low-cost interventions. Several studies have shown that nurses and others can also be effective in treating episodes of CMD. Techniques such as problem-solving can be readily taught, and computerized cognitive-behavioural therapy (CBT) has also been shown to be effective. In those with a chronic physical illness, collaborative care between medical and non-medical staff is effective.

- In low- and middle-income countries, specially trained health-care workers can administer a range of effective treatments including problem-solving, psycho-education and some forms of psychotherapy, and more severe cases respond well to antidepressants. In both Chile and India, lay workers have been shown to make an effective contribution to the treatment of depression.

- The WHO mental health Gap Action Programme (mhGAP) published the *mhGAP intervention guide* in 2010. This is based upon a large-scale overview of recent systematic literature reviews and 93 newly commissioned literature reviews.

- The intervention guide for the mhGAP is intended for use by primary care and community practitioners in low- and middle-income countries and is currently undergoing country adaptation in many countries worldwide prior to implementation.

The natural history of undetected psychological disorder

For most episodes of depression, the natural history is one of remissions and relapses – the major achievement of treatment being to speed up remission by shortening the mean duration of each episode. Thus, the very solid evidence that treatment is effective is generally from studies conducted over a few months.

There have been two well-conducted surveys of confirmed but untreated depression in primary care – WHO's Psychological Problems in General Medical Settings,[91] and the Netherlands Study of Depression and Anxiety (NESDA).[92] In the WHO study, the World Mental Health Composite International Diagnostic Interview (CIDI) was administered to 5500 primary care patients in 14 centres round the world, and patients were re-examined with the CIDI one year later, and by questionnaire at 3 months.[93] Patients with a confirmed *Diagnostic and Statistical Manual of Mental Disorders* (DSM)-III diagnosis of major depression were divided into four groups: those whose depression was detected and treated with antidepressants by the GP, those who were treated with sedatives, and two groups whose illnesses were initially milder: those not treated with any drugs, and those whose illness was not detected by their doctor. Results are presented in Table 2.2.

Both groups treated with drugs had been equally severely depressed at onset, but those treated with antidepressants had fewer symptoms at 3 months; however, at one year the difference was no longer significant. Those who were not treated with drugs or were undetected had milder illnesses at onset, and also had fewer symptoms at one year. The rate at which symptoms were lost was the same in all groups. However, very few of the patients had taken antidepressants for longer than 6 weeks.

The Dutch study also had baseline and one-year follow-up data on 594 patients with anxiety or depression (see Figure 2.7).[94] They confirmed that those whose depressions were undetected had less-severe illnesses

Table 2.2 Initially depressed patients in primary care assessed one year later: WHO's Psychological Problems in General Health Care (PPGHC) study in 11 countries[93]

Treatment by GP	Recovered, %	Subthreshold, %	Another common mental disorder, %	Still depressed, %
Antidepressants	31.0	6.3	10.9	54.6
Sedatives	24.5	16.3	14.3	44.9
No drug (milder disorders)	39.5	10.9	24.4	25.2
Not detected by GP (milder)	41.7	14.0	20.0	28.3

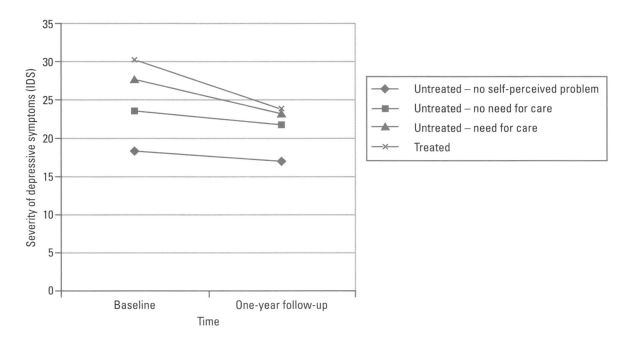

Figure 2.7   The course of depression in patients with a CIDI diagnosis of a depressive disorder at T0, in the treatment/non-treatment groups (*n* = 573) (range: 0–84). IDS = Inventory of Depressive Symptoms. Reproduced from van Beljouw IM et al. The course of untreated anxiety and depression, and determinants of poor one-year outcome: a one-year cohort study. *BMC Psychiatry*, 2010, 10:86[94]

at outset. In depression, treated and untreated patients with a perceived treatment need showed more rapid symptom decline but greater symptom severity at follow-up than untreated patients without a self-perceived mental health problem or treatment need. Despite a wide range of factors measured at onset that predicted a poor outcome, only increased loneliness and the presence of a comorbid anxiety disorder maintained their significance in predicting a poor outcome in depression when baseline symptom severity was controlled for.

A smaller telephone survey in the USA, of 98 patients with major depression who had made a visit to their GP in the past 6 months showed that one-third remained undetected after 1 year, and about a half of these had suicidal ideation.[95] The authors conclude that quality-improvement efforts directed at improving detection without improving management of detected patients may not improve outcomes.

Is screening for depression worthwhile in primary care?

Numerous surveys have shown that many cases of mental disorder are missed by GPs.[100] Some have argued directly from this that screening must be beneficial, but this over-simplifies a complex situation. Patients found to have the various symptoms of common mental disorders typically complain of somatic symptoms, and hope that their doctor will find the cause of these symptoms. Many patients want their doctor to exclude a serious cause for their symptoms and prescribe symptomatic remedies for any pains or discomforts.

Since somatic symptoms are what most doctors typically attend to, their patients are generally well satisfied, despite the fact the GP has missed the mental disorder. Indeed, patients often resist the idea that they have a mental disorder, even when they have many symptoms. Verhaak and co-workers used the CIDI to interview 743 people in the community who had diagnoses of depression or anxiety disorders, also assessing the respondents' views of their need for care.[96] They found that younger patients, and those that rated their health-care provider as having better communicative abilities, were more likely to receive care, and concluded that receiving help for common mental disorders depends not only on the objective need of the patient but also, at least as much, on the patients' own recognition that their problems have a mental health origin.

Many studies have merely provided GPs with feedback of high scores on screening questionnaires, and have not resulted in increased recognition.[97] In 2002, Pignone and colleagues showed that 50% of trials led to increased recognition, but not to increased treatment.[98] However, they also calculated that 110 patients would need to be screened to obtain one extra remission after 6–12 months' treatment. Even this is not enough – it is necessary to show that such increased provision of treatment is affordable, since the screening procedure itself generates costs, as well as producing false-positive results. The usual way to do this is to calculate the cost per quality-adjusted life-year (QALY) gained as a result of the screening procedure. Three studies have done this, but produced conflicting results.

In 2010, Paulden and co-workers used a hypothetical cohort of patients with postnatal depression and found that the cost per QALY gained was $67 130.[99] Understandably, they did not consider that this represented good value for money. However, Morrell et al., in 2009, carried out a cluster trial with training of health visitors to identify postnatal depression and to deliver psychologically informed interventions, followed by an 18-month follow-up, and showed that it was highly cost effective, irrespective of whether they chose to take a cognitive-behavioural approach or a person-centred approach – both with an option of offering antidepressants if they were indicated.[100,101] Finally, Valenstein and co-workers compared the wisdom of offering screening for depression to a hypothetical cohort of 40-year-old primary care patients, using the perspective of the person paying for health care.[102] If screening were to be carried out annually, the cost per QALY would be $192 444; if every 5 years, the cost would fall to $50 988; but single screening would cost only $32 053. The reason is that re-screening previously healthy people produces few additional cases, yet screening an unknown population is bound to produce cases. The authors conclude that single screening is cost effective, and should the quality of treatment improve it would be even more so.

In general, it is easy to see that it will be far more cost effective to screen populations known to have a high prevalence of depression, for example people with a disability produced by a chronic physical illness or old age, and women around childbirth, since the positive predictive value of a high score must necessarily be much better than that found with standard populations. Thus, the National Institute for Health and Clinical Excellence (NICE) argued in 2003 that screening should be carried out in special populations such as post-puerperal women, those with disability produced by chronic physical illness, those with dementia and those with a past history of depression.[103] Whooley argues that screening is worthwhile in patients with chronic cardiac disease.[104]

However, two other things are also necessary, involving both the health-care provider and the patient. The doctor must have the ability to both diagnose and assess the severity of the depression, and must be able to provide effective treatment. It is also helpful if he or she is perceived by the patient as someone with whom it is easy to communicate. The patient must be prepared to admit that they have a need for an intervention, be allowed to choose what treatment they receive, and be willing to invest both time and cooperation in such treatment.

Cost-effective treatments for common mental disorders

Any novel treatment typically costs more money, at least in the short term. Where health costs are free at the point of delivery, or are largely reimbursed by medical insurance companies, it makes sense to offset any advantages gained by the new treatment against the cost of it – as in the case of a screening procedure, as discussed above. Before one can transfer the cost of a QALY from one country to another, one must establish that health costs for items of service are comparable, and that the amount of money devoted to health care is also equivalent. The amount a rich country is prepared to pay for a QALY is by no means the same as a poor one. But in a poor country, individual items of care may cost much less, and this will affect the amount they are prepared to pay for each QALY. Whereas a high-income country like the UK spends 10% of its health budget on mental health, lower-income countries spend only 2% (range 1–3%;[90] see Figure 2.8 between pages 34 and 35). We will therefore separate this account by the rough amount of wealth in three groups of countries – high-, medium- and low-income countries.

High-income countries

Treatments for depression

Episodes of depression and anxiety respond to a wide range of both psychological and pharmacological interventions that shorten the length of episode, and the evidence for this is best summarized in the NICE

Clinical Guidelines – notably the *Update on the treatment of depression in adults, including those with chronic physical illness* (NICE 2009).[105] The type of intervention offered should be determined by the severity of any depression and the patient's preference for mode of treatment. At the mild level of severity of major depression, the disorder responds to a wide range of interventions, including physical exercise, computerized CBT, problem-solving, self-help manuals and sleep hygiene. Patients with moderate depression also respond to problem-solving and computerized CBT, but may also benefit from antidepressants or from a range of more complex psychological interventions including CBT, interpersonal therapy, behavioural activation or couples therapy from a trained therapist – provided that one is available. In terms of treatment costs, drug treatments are cheaper, and when they are effective, they are also quicker. With complex and severe depression, treatment should be within the specialist mental health services, and may involve drugs and electroconvulsive treatment.

While most studies have found broadly comparable outcomes for antidepressants and CBT, some have found that drugs are more cost effective because they cost much less.[106] Indeed, this study in depressed adolescents found an incremental cost over placebo of $24 000 per QALY for treatment with fluoxetine and $123 000 per QALY for fluoxetine plus CBT; CBT alone actually had fewer net benefits than a drug placebo in severe depression.[115] However, two other studies did not support either the higher cost or the worse outcome in severely depressed patients.[107,108] These calculations may assume greater amounts of GP time than are actually encountered in drug treatment of depression, and since the cost of the drug is relatively negligible compared with the substantial amounts of psychologist time required for CBT, it seems likely that, in practice, CBT is a more expensive alternative.

A meta-analysis of 17 studies involving over 1000 subjects showed that behavioural activation was superior to brief psychotherapy, supportive treatment and control treatments, and equally as effective as CBT.[109] A later paper tested the "parsimony hypothesis" that if it is as effective as antidepressants and CBT, yet is a conceptually much simpler procedure, it should be preferred to it.[110]

Where moderate and severe depression are concerned, Simon and co-workers have shown that a combination of antidepressants and CBT is more effective but also more expensive – with a cost of £4056 for each successfully treated patient; but a QALY for a severely ill patient cost £5777, while a moderately ill patient cost £14 540 per QALY.[111] The study concluded that combination therapy was justified in severe depression, but the evidence was insufficient in moderate depression. Training GPs on the best management of anxiety has no such beneficial effects on patient outcome.[112]

In 2009, Wiley-Exley and her colleagues discussed the cost-effectiveness of integrated care (IC) for elderly patients with depression, anxiety or substance abuse.[113] A behavioural health professional was located in primary care, with enhanced specialist referral (ESR), meaning that patients were referred to mental health specialists outside primary care, and the specialist took over the treatment of the patient.[114] The authors found IC was only superior to ESR in the US Department of Veterans Affairs (VA) clinics. They speculated that since the VA system has policies to promote integration, it is more likely to promote integrated service.

Subthreshold depression

Two studies have addressed treatment of subthreshold depression. Smit and co-workers tried a "minimal intervention" consisting of a self-help manual and instructions on mood management supplemented by six telephone calls with a prevention worker.[115] They were able to reduce the risk of developing a diagnosable depressive episode from 18% in controls to only 12%, while over the next year annual per capita cost decreased from a mean of £8614 to one of £6766. Wells and colleagues also claim to have shown an intervention described as "enhanced usual care" is effective in both depressive episodes and subthreshold depression: however, separate data are not shown for these two groups, and the authors admit that there is a lack of evidence for efficacy of treatments for subthreshold depression.[116] The NICE Guideline for the treatment of depression in chronic physical illness concluded that where these patients suffered from persistent subthreshold symptoms of depression, they should be treated with a wide range of non-pharmacological measures, including sleep hygiene, physical exercise, group-based peer support and computerized CBT.[105] Antidepressants should be reserved for those with a past history of moderate or severe depression, depressive symptoms that have not remitted after 2 years and persist after other interventions, and cases where the mild depression is complicating the management of a physical disorder.

Contributions of others to mental health work in primary care

Rost and co-workers have drawn attention to the added value a practice nurse can make to improving the quality of mental health care.[117] They describe "enhanced care", which consists of providing 2 years of high-quality treatment to all depressed patients, starting with a choice between psychotherapy and antidepressants. The practice nurse provides care management, using regular telephone calls and visits and providing primary care physicians with monthly summaries of each patient's symptoms. Patients whose symptoms have not resolved are advised to raise this problem with their primary care doctor at their next visit. Patients with and without such care were followed for 2 years, and the intervention showed excellent results in remission of their depression, as well as both physical and emotional functioning.

Graduate mental health workers have been trained to deliver psychological therapy and psychosocial interventions to patients in primary care. Harkness and Bower reviewed 42 studies to examine the effects they have had on the professional practice of primary health-care providers.[118] Although they found some evidence that the interventions caused a reduction in GP behaviour, they concluded that the changes are modest in magnitude and inconsistent, do not generalize to the wider patient population, and their clinical or economic significance is unclear.

Ekers and co-workers have shown that behavioural activation is effective, even when practised by two mental health nurses without previous psychotherapeutic experience, after a 12-hour training course extending over 3 months.[110] Since cognitive-behavioural therapists are scarce, and their training is protracted in comparison with this, this procedure is of great importance to the whole world, but especially to middle- and low-income countries.

Problem-solving

Problem-solving is also a simple form of psychotherapy that can readily be taught to the intelligent layman. It was shown to be as effective for major depression when given by a practice nurse as by a GP.[119] The combination of problem-solving and an antidepressant is no more effective than problem-solving alone. It had earlier been shown to cost more than treatment by a GP, although this was more than offset by savings in the cost of days off work.[119] This may partly reflect the fact that many different treatments are equally effective in mild (yet diagnosable) depression.

The conclusion of these various studies is that common mental disorders are often chronic or prone to relapses, and that all treatments have their limitations over the longer term. Antidepressant drugs are typically prescribed for longer periods in specialist care than in primary care – but even in the latter, prolonged treatment may be necessary to provide better long-term outcomes. Kendrick and colleagues confirm that problem-solving is more expensive than treatment as usual by the GP, and produces similar outcomes.[120] The important point is that problem-solving is suitable for patients who do not wish to have drug treatment, and involves the health professional discussing the patient's current life problems, rather than merely issuing a prescription.

Making treatment more widely available

Several studies have addressed the problem of making CBT more readily available. Kessler et al. provided treatment from an online psychologist, and showed that a greater proportion of patients had recovered when compared with usual GP care (48% recovered after 8 months with online CBT against only 26% in the controls),[121] and Hollinghurst and colleagues carried out a cost-effectiveness study on these data and showed that online CBT was more expensive than usual care, although the outcomes for the CBT group were better, with a cost per QALY gained of £17173.[122]

Even more widely available than online CBT with a live therapist, are the fully computerized versions (CCBT). Kaltenthaler and co-workers identified 20 studies and found some evidence that CCBT is as effective as therapist-led CBT (TCBT) for the treatment of depression/anxiety and phobia/panic, and is more effective than treatment as usual (TAU) in the treatment of depression/anxiety.[123] The results of the model for the depression software packages in terms of incremental cost per QALY (compared with TAU at £30000 per QALY), were best for *Beating the Blues*, at a cost of £1801, and the chance of it being cost effective was 86.8%, while *Cope* was £7139 and 62.6% and *Overcoming Depression* was £5391 and 54.4%.[124] A further paper reviews randomized controlled trials (RCTs) of three different CCBT packages, *Beating the Blues*, *MoodGym* and *Overcoming*

Depression on the Internet (ODIN),[125] and concludes more cautiously that there is "some evidence" to support the effectiveness of CCBT for the treatment of depression, but there were considerable dropout rates. Nevertheless, NICE recommended *Beating the Blues* and *MoodGym* as an option for delivering CBT in the management of mild and moderate depression.[126,127] Gerhards et al. compared CCBT with treatment as usual and a combination of CCBT and treatment as usual.[128] They found no difference in clinical effectiveness or quality of life, and concluded that CCBT constitutes the most efficient treatment strategy.

Prevention of future episodes of depression

Stant and co-workers devised a psycho-educational package (PEP) in an attempt to prevent future episodes of depression.[129] Depressed patients in Dutch primary care were recruited to the study and assigned to one of four groups: (1) usual care; (2) PEP only; (3) CBT followed by PEP; and (4) a consultation with a psychiatrist followed by PEP. The primary outcome measure was the proportion of depression-free time. The patients were followed up over 36 months, when it was found that groups 3 and 4 had a slightly lower chance of a future episode than groups 1 and 2, but with such a small difference that the authors concluded that PEP was not cost effective, and would not be adopted by the health system.

Treatment of other common mental disorders

Durham and co-workers studied the long-term outcome of 10 studies of treatment of anxiety disorders using CBT.[130] Once more, they found that good outcomes with CBT over the short term are no guarantee of good outcomes over the longer term, and that extending treatment to greater than the standard 10 sessions offered no additional advantage. Konig et al. provided a special training to GPs in the management of anxiety, and were unable to show any differences in outcome of anxiety disorders when compared with untrained GPs.[112]

McCrone and colleagues assessed the cost-effectiveness of CBT, GP therapy and a self-help book and graded exercise therapy for chronic fatigue.[131] They found that while the cost of providing therapy is higher than usual GP care plus a self-help booklet, the outcome is somewhat better. CBT was cost effective only if society is prepared to pay a lot for fatigue-free days.

Low- and middle-income countries

Many effective treatments for depression are inexpensive, and these include antidepressants, problem-solving and behavioural activation. A specially trained lay health-care worker is capable of delivering effective mental health interventions. In 2003, Araya et al. (2003) allocated 240 low-income female patients with severe depression in Santiago, Chile to usual care, or care administered by a 3-month, multicomponent intervention led by a non-medical health-care worker, which included a psycho-educational group intervention, structured and systematic follow-up, and drug treatment.[132] At 6-months' follow-up, 70% of the intervention group compared with 30% of the usual-care group had recovered. A study in rural Uganda by Bolton et al. allocated depressed adolescents either to group interpersonal psychotherapy or creative play.[133] The psychotherapeutic treatment produced a reduction in depressive symptoms in girls only.

A study by Patel and co-workers, in India (see Figures 2.9 and 2.10 between pages 34 and 35),[134] assigned patients with common mental disorders to either collaborative stepped care (CSC) by lay health counsellors or enhanced usual care. The CSC condition meant that all patients with high scores on a screening questionnaire were given psycho-education by the lay counsellors, but patients with higher scores were offered an antidepressant by the primary care physician. Psycho-education taught patients strategies to alleviate symptoms, such as breathing exercises for anxiety symptoms and scheduling activities for symptoms of depression. Moderately or severely ill patients who were offered drug treatment could also have group interpersonal psychotherapy from the lay health-care worker.

Those who failed to respond to the more active treatments, or who were actively suicidal, were referred on to a mental health-care specialist. For the control intervention, physicians and patients in usual-care practices received screening results and were given the treatment manual prepared for primary care physicians. As in the Wiley-Exley study described earlier,[112] the CSC intervention turned out to be effective in the public clinics, but not in private clinics. The authors observe that in the public clinics, larger numbers of patients tend to be seen for shorter periods by a doctor, and the privacy needed to discuss interpersonal difficulties is not always possible.

Severe mental disorders in low-income countries

Two studies have addressed the treatment of severe mental disorders in low-income countries. A study by Ran and colleagues in Chengdu, China, assigned families with a member suffering from schizophrenia to three groups: drug management plus family intervention; drug management only; and a control condition where medication was neither encouraged nor discouraged.[135] This showed that the combined intervention was effective in that relatives' attitudes to the patients and cooperation with medication was improved, and, most importantly, the relapse rate over 9 months in this group (16.3%) was much less than in either the drug-only group (37.8%) or the control group (61.5%). Chatterjee et al. showed that patients with chronic schizophrenia in rural India had a superior response to community-based rehabilitation compared to usual outpatient care.[136]

Evidence-based interventions in middle- and low-income countries: the "mental health gap"

As the evidence above suggest, most people in the world who have mental illnesses receive no effective treatment.[137] At the national level, the proportion of people with diagnosable mental disorders who receive health-care interventions ("coverage") is at best between 27% and 30.5% across Europe[138,139] and the USA[140] respectively, and at worst this has been documented as a treated annual prevalence rate of 2% in Nigeria.[141] Especially since the 2007 *Lancet* series of mental health papers,[151] the significance of this "treatment gap" is increasingly appreciated worldwide. The Department of Mental Health and Substance Abuse at the WHO has recognized the importance of this challenge by launching as its centrepiece the mental health Gap Action Programme (mhGAP) in 2008.[143] The first major product of this programme is the *mhGAP intervention guide* (MIG) published in 2010.[144] This is a landmark mental health publication by the WHO, as it is a document designed for direct use by first- and second-level practitioners (district medical officer, and primary care staff) and, until this time, WHO had more often focused upon providing government-level technical assistance and advice.

The MIG contains case-finding and treatment guidelines for nine categories of mental and neurological disorders that are common in low-income settings and that have a major public health impact:

1 depression
2 psychoses
3 epilepsy/seizures
4 developmental disorders
5 behaviour disorders
6 dementia
7 alcohol use disorders
8 drug use disorders
9 self-harm/suicide.

The MIG is based upon very thorough use of existing literature reviews, and upon 93 newly commissioned systematic reviews addressing important clinical questions where there was uncertainty. The procedures used were those recommended by the WHO for creating transparent, evidence-based guidelines using the *Grading of Recommendations Assessment, Development and Evaluation* (GRADE) methodology.[145] The draft MIG proposals were then modified in light of a detailed feasibility exercise, and subject to scrutiny in relation to their acceptability to service users and carers, and their human rights implications.[146] The MIG was published by the WHO in October 2010.[144] It is therefore reasonable to consider the MIG as being simplified treatment guidelines specifically designed for primary care/district-level non-specialist staff, which are based upon the strongest possible current evidence of effective mental health interventions in low- and middle-income settings.

Yet the fundamental public health questions go beyond the formulation of guidelines and include: (1) can such guidelines be put into practice in routine clinical settings; (2) if so, do they confer patient benefit; and (3) does their use contribute to an increase in the treated prevalence (coverage) rates for specified conditions? In short, it is clear from over two decades of research that the creation of guidelines is necessary but not sufficient for evidence-based practice. As a consequence, there has been a recent rapid development of "implementation science",[147] with some applications in the field of mental health.[148] A recent review has summarized the factors that have been identified as facilitators or barriers to the implementation of mental-illness-related clinical guidelines,[149] and distinguished between: (1) the adoption in principle of guidelines; (2) early implementation; and (3) their sustained use over time. It is therefore now timely to focus effort in low- and middle-income countries less upon national-level policies alone, but more upon the implementation by non-specialist staff of clear and simple treatment guidelines in primary and community care settings.

Implications for primary care practitioners

- A wide range of interventions have been shown to be cost effective in the treatment of common mental disorders.

- The choice of treatment should take the patient's preference into account but may include various kinds of psychological interventions or drug treatments. Both are equally effective in moderate depression, and may suit different patients.

- Many psychological interventions may be administered by staff other than doctors. This is especially important in low- and middle-income countries.

Closer collaboration between primary care and specialist mental health services

Summary

- *Stepped care* is an arrangement in which only the most severe cases of CMD are referred to specialist mental health services, but most cases are treated entirely in primary care, with less-costly interventions for milder disorders. It has been shown to be effective in several countries.

- *Shared care* refers to involving primary care in the management of those with severe mental disorders. It has also been shown to be cost effective in a range of countries, and is an appropriate response to the de-institutionalization of those with chronic severe mental disorders. In some settings, the specialist service can contribute to management electronically.

- *Collaborative care* is a somewhat more involved version of shared care, and may be applied to those requiring specialized psychological interventions and those with chronic physical illnesses. It has now been evaluated in both high- and low-income countries, and has also been shown to be cost effective.

As a wider range of both psychological and pharmacological treatments for mental disorder become available, it has become clear that treatments of both kinds must be targeted on people who will derive most benefit from them. There has been an increasing realization that much useful work can be done not only by behavioural scientists, but by nurses and even lay workers attached to primary care. An additional reason has been that as the chronic mentally ill have been released from mental hospitals, it has become clear that close collaboration is required between primary care and the mental health services.

Different forms of collaboration between the two services

Stepped care

Stepped care refers to offering an inexpensive treatment to mildly ill patients, a more elaborate and more expensive treatment to moderately or severely ill patients, and referral to a mental health professional in a separate service only for those who have not responded to a treatment in primary care, or those who are actively suicidal. At each level, there are usually specific indications for a movement to the next stage. In the context of depression, it may refer to health information, CCBT, or physical exercise for the mildly ill; an active psychological or pharmacological treatment for the moderately or severely ill; and specialist referral only for those few patients who have not responded. It can be seen that stepped care is particularly suited for government- or insurance-funded services, where cost reduction is important – therefore it is routinely used by NICE in the UK, for example.

Shared care

Shared care refers to efforts to involve primary care in the routine management of people with *severe mental disorders* (schizophrenia or bipolar illness) who are maintained on stable medication. The mental health service offers support from a specialized nurse to the GP, and undertakes to readmit the patient should a severe relapse occur. Care from primary care is much less stigmatizing for the patient, and the mental health service is able to continue to accept new referrals from primary care, since it is not faced with an ever-increasing load of psychotic patients.

Collaborative care

Collaborative care is a somewhat more elaborate version of shared care, and typically has three components:

- a dedicated coordinator of the intervention, supported by a multiprofessional team
- joint determination of the plan of care
- long-term coordination and follow-up coordination of both mental and physical health care.

The dedicated coordinator is typically located within the primary care team, rather than being an emissary of the mental health team. Indeed, help is often provided by a behavioural scientist, typically a clinical psychologist in high-income countries, but often a lay health-care worker in low-income countries. Nor need the collaboration refer necessarily to the mental health service at all – in collaborative care of diabetes for example, it may refer to the specialist service for diabetes.

Evaluations of stepped care

In countries with developed mental health services that do not have to be paid for by the patient, it has been known for many years that only a small minority of patients with mental illness known to their GP are referred to specialist services, usually because they have not responded to treatment, or have requested such a referral.[150] The studies of Araya et al.[132] and Patel et al.[134] described earlier are examples of evaluations of stepped care in low-income countries. Reiss-Brennan and co-workers have described a three-tier stepped-care service for depression, with routine care by the GP for mild cases, collaborative care for moderate depression and depression comorbid with chronic physical illness, and specialist care by a mental health professional for severe cases and cases where there is a risk to life.[151] This study gives before-and-after satisfaction ratings by both patients and staff. To be effective, stepped care implies that from time to time patients will be elevated to a higher form of care: Figure 2.11 indicates that this is often not the case in lower-income countries.

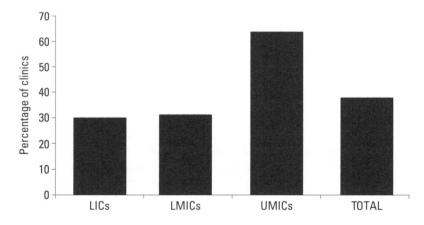

Figure 2.11 Percentage of clinics where primary care physicians make at least one monthly referral to a higher level of care, by country income group. LIC = lower-income countries; LMIC and UMIC lower- and upper-middle-income countries. Data derived, with permission, from *Mental health systems in selected low- and middle-income countries: a WHO-AIMS cross-national analysis.* Geneva, World Health Organization, 2010[90]

Evaluations of shared care

In the past 20 years, there has been a growing appreciation that patients who at one time would have been cared for in a mental hospital are now cared for both in community mental health (CMH) teams and in GPs' clinics, and are receiving suboptimal care for their mental health problems. Early papers were all from the UK, but in the past 15 years the movement has spread to other countries. An early paper by Nazareth et al. showed that the care of former long-stay patients was passing to GPs, in addition to the after care they received from the CMH service.[152] The main reason for contact with the GP was for administration of depot medication. GPs were generally in favour of a shared care record with the mental health service, and most would welcome closer liaison within their practice. Gater et al. described the care of patients with chronic schizophrenia with a community psychiatric nurse (CPN) working within the practice, working closely with both a community psychiatrist and the GP.[153] They compared patients receiving shared care with matched patients who were cared for by the mental health service and primary care without such close collaboration. Two years after it was established, patients with shared care had fewer unmet needs; and were more satisfied with the care they had received. They had more service contacts and had received more interventions.

In 1998, Meadows described a new service in Melbourne, Australia, in which private GPs were persuaded to take over the routine care of former long-stay mental patients, with support from the MH service.[154] In the 2 years since it was set up, the new service had facilitated the transfer of over 90 clients from the area mental health service into shared care with 28 GPs, including GPs from each participating practice. One year after transfer to GP care, 60% of the patients felt their physical health care had improved with the increased GP input. In some 20% of cases, review of GP case notes showed that newly identified physical health problems had been treated.

In 2001, Sharma and colleagues described the impact of a shared-care plan by a multidisciplinary mental health team in close association with five general practices in Liverpool, England 5 years after its inception.[155] The new service was compared with control practices where the two services worked independently of one another. The study evaluated referral rates, waiting times, attendance rates, GP and patient satisfaction, and general measures of patient health and social functioning (the Health of the Nation Outcome Scale). The number of new referrals remained the same over 3 years. The use of inpatient beds dropped by 38% in the same period, compared with an increase in the control practices. No-show rates in the intervention practices dropped from 32% to 18%, compared with a stable rate of 32% in the control practices. GP satisfaction with waiting times, access to CPNs, overall communication, and service delivery were significantly higher in the intervention practices compared with the control practices. After 6 months of intervention, there was an improvement in health and social functioning, with a larger effect in patients with severe mental health problems.

In 1996, a paper by Goldberg and Gournay advocated a new pattern of working for mental health professionals caring for patients with severe mental disorders (SMDs) in close association with GPs.[156] Instead of a given GP having his or her patients with SMD cared for by a range of different CPNs from the CMH team, a dedicated CPN would care for all the SMD patients registered with that practice. Rajagopal and colleagues carried out a postal survey of CMH teams in England and found that the practice of having a single, identified mental health worker for a given practice was becoming widespread, and found that such practices reported greater satisfaction compared to those that did not have this arrangement (91% versus 54%) ($P < 0.05$).[157]

Byng et al. randomized 23 urban general practices to a shared-care arrangement called "Mental Health Link", in which customized shared-care agreements were developed between the primary care team and the local CMH team, or to a control condition.[158] Inevitably perhaps, the degree of implementation varied greatly, with some practices being considerably more active than others. Nevertheless, patients from the shared-care practices had fewer psychiatric relapses than control patients (mean = 0.39 versus 0.71, respectively, $P = 0.02$), and doctors were more satisfied and services improved significantly for intervention practices. There was a modest increase in direct mental health-care costs in the practices with shared care, and no significant differences in patients' perceptions of their unmet need, satisfaction or general health.

A health-economic evaluation of shared care showed that extra costs were lower only for those receiving a low level of care in terms of contacts with their psychiatrist or social worker, and these patients used residential care less than those with higher levels of shared care.[131]

Electronic variations in shared care

Closer collaboration between the two services can also be achieved by enhanced telephone contact, or by telemedicine. Kates et al. describe a closer link between MH and primary health-care services by providing a back-up service by telephone to 18 family physicians in five practices.[159] In the course of a year, 128 calls were made, of which 57% were considered to be routine management in medication issues, while the remainder were considered urgent, but only one required immediate admission. The calls took on average 8 minutes, so that the psychiatrist was only occupied for 20 minutes each week. Berardi et al. describe a broadly similar service in Bologna, Italy, where two psychiatrists and a psychologist were available by telephone for 2 days a week, to 54 GPs.[160] A follow-up study with the GPs 6 months later showed that most were satisfied with the service. A study by Simon and co-workers of the treatment of depression in primary care showed that telephone feedback by a nurse of visits to doctors and prescriptions, when combined with "care management", based upon a population-based clinical information system, monitoring of adherence to treatment, and systematic follow-up care, led to substantial advantages to patients in depression scores, and a lower probability of a diagnosis of major depression, at a modest cost of $80 per patient.[161]

A study by Pyne et al., in rural parts of the deep South of the USA, investigated the effects of introducing a closer liaison with seven small VA clinics by using telemedicine.[162] These widely dispersed sites find that it is difficult or impossible to work more closely with mental health services. In the evaluation, 395 patients were enrolled in an evaluation of the new service and, after baseline measures, allocated to either usual care or an intervention by GPs supervised by telepsychiatrists, nurses or off-site pharmacists. The supervising team made recommendations for management for one year after inception of an episode. Those in the "usual care" arm of the study were offered an interactive video and access to the web site. The new service turned out to offer no advantages in "depression-free days", but the incremental cost was prohibitively expensive – at $85 600 per QALY. This study is important, since much of the world consists of care from dispersed clinics located far away from possible supervision: it must be hoped that a future study will report lower costs.

Evaluations of collaborative care

A comprehensive review of collaborative care up to 2006 can be found in Craven and Bland's monograph,[163] which points out that enhanced patient education about mental disorders and their treatment (usually by a health professional other than the primary care physician) was a component of many of the studies with good outcomes that they reviewed.

The full version of collaborative care involves a care manager in primary care, with supervision available from members of the mental health team. Campo et al. describe three tiers of adolescent patients with major depression in practices in rural Pennsylvania, USA:[164] mild cases managed by the primary care physician (PCP) and practice nurse in primary care – generally appropriate for relatively straightforward, uncomplicated patients or those on a stable treatment; on-site mental health co-management by the PCP in collaboration with the primary care-based social worker from the specialty mental health team – such an approach might be appropriate for patients who failed earlier treatment by the PCP or patients of intermediate complexity or severity; and off-site specialty mental health referral for patients with more complicated and/or severe disorders and psychosocial circumstances likely to render management within the primary care setting unsuccessful. This approach has been well received by PCPs, patients and families. Approximately two-thirds (66%) of newly evaluated patients are triaged to routine services delivered by the PCP with support from the practice nurse; 20% are managed on site by the PCP and the social worker; and the remainder are referred to off-site specialty mental health services.

A study by Hunkeler et al. offered collaborative care to elderly depressed patients in primary care in eight US health-care organizations, and followed the patients up for 2 years.[165] Treatment options included antidepressant drug treatment or problem-solving psychotherapy, and therapy was delivered by a team consisting of the PCP, the practice nurse, a liaison primary care doctor and a psychiatrist. The psychiatrist saw about 10% of the patients in the trial, mainly non-responders to the treatments offered so far. Control patients offered usual care could use all the treatments available (antidepressants, counselling by the doctor, and referral to specialty mental health care). During the initial year, 57% of these patients used antidepressants, 25% reported using psychotherapy or specialty mental health care, and 62% reported using either antidepressants or psychotherapy. Results were dramatic: patients who had had collaborative care fared significantly ($P < 0.05$) better than controls regarding continuation of antidepressant treatment, depressive symptoms, remission of depression, physical functioning, quality of life, self-efficacy, and satisfaction with care at 18 and 24 months. One year after the extra resources were withdrawn, there was a significant difference in SCL (Symptom Checklist) – 20 scores (0.23, $P < 0.0001$) favouring the collaborative care programme.

Simon and co-workers described the collaborative care of depressed patients with diabetes, in a study where patients were randomly assigned to usual care or a multicomponent depression-management programme based in the primary care clinic.[166] Here, the lowest level of stepped care was drug therapy or psychotherapy (problem-solving), depending on patients' expressed preference; step two consisted of addition of the other modality; while for those not responding in 12 weeks, the final step was a direct interview with a psychiatrist. The intervention produced a significant and sustained increase in days free of depression, and reduced outpatient health-services costs by approximately $300 per patient. An investment of approximately $800 in additional depression-treatment costs was offset by a decrease of approximately $1100 in costs of general medical care. Katon et al. argue that the collaborative care of depressed patients with diabetes produces high clinical benefits at no greater cost than usual care.[167] Relative to usual care, patients receiving collaborative care experienced more depression-free days over 24 months. Total outpatient costs were $25 higher during this same period. The incremental cost per depression-free day was 25 cents (–$14 to $15) and the incremental cost per QALY ranged from $198 to $397. An incremental net benefit was $1129 ($692 to 1572).

Collaborative care for depressed patients with a chronic physical illness is so uniformly successful that NICE carried out a meta-analysis of all the high-quality studies found, and showed a significant treatment effect of collaborative care (overall effect $z = 5.91$; $P < 0.00001$).[105]

Implications for primary care practitioners

- Collaborative care refers to a wide range of therapeutic arrangements, but they have in common that care is provided by a non-medical health-care professional who works in association with both the physician in primary care and the mental health service.
- Collaborative care as described above is a good method of management of depression in primary care in high-income countries, but the studies by Araya and colleagues and Patel quoted earlier,[132,134] have shown that impressive results can also be obtained in low-income countries, using lay health-care workers.
- In high-income countries, very good results have been reported for patients with chronic physical disorders whose depression has not responded to the usual treatments, but there is thought to be a relationship between the two disorders.

Prevention of episodes of mental disorder

Summary

- Based on evidence of best practice, there are a number of interventions that have been found effective to prevent mental disorders. These range from national public campaigns to interventions in settings such as schools and one-on-one support.
- Promoting health and well-being demands a wide partnership between individuals, clinicians and community groups, among others.
- Early childhood lays the foundation for good mental health later in life; interventions that target the early years should therefore be a priority.
- Although it is difficult to evaluate complex interventions in the community, where it is impossible to control for all influences, there is a need to adopt the promising findings from quasi-experimental research designs.

Effectiveness of public campaigns

In recent years, national campaigns have been launched to increase public awareness of depression in the USA,[168] the UK,[169] Germany,[170] and Australasia.[171]

These have generally succeeded in raising public awareness of depression – although these changes are not dramatic, so that serial surveys over some years show increases of around 10% in some cases[169] and just over 20% in others.[172] It has generally been found to be more effective if such campaigns are carried out at several levels, and all surveys have concentrated on GPs as well as the population at large. In the UK survey, two-thirds of GPs were aware of the campaign and 40% had definitely or possibly modified their clinical practice.[173] The authors of the latter study argue that it is necessary to do more to improve clinical practice in terms of local and practice-based training activities.

Priest and co-workers found that members of the public generally seemed to be sympathetic to those with depression, but were reluctant to consult their GPs themselves if depressed.[174] Most believed counselling to be effective but believed antidepressants to be addictive. Hegerl and Schafer report that a campaign that was carried out at four levels – teachers, priests and those caring for elderly people, as well as support and self-help activities – in addition to the two levels reported above, has now been extended to 17 European countries.[175] They claim a reduction in suicide rates as a result of their campaign.

Interventions across the life-course

The following discussion sets out evidence-based interventions that have been found to be effective for influences operating at each life stage.

Pregnancy and early childhood

There is strong evidence that improving nutrition in socioeconomically disadvantaged children can lead to healthy cognitive development, improved educational outcomes and reduced risk for mental ill-health, especially for those at risk or who are living in impoverished communities. The most effective intervention models are those that include complementary feeding, growth monitoring and promotion. These models combine nutritional interventions (such as food supplementation) with support to the mother's child-care skills, counselling and psychosocial care (e.g. warmth and attentive listening).[15,21]

Examples of effective interventions to prevent mental disorders in children and to promote positive mental health include:

- effective prenatal interventions to support healthy pregnancy – e.g. fortification of foods with folic acid and programmes that encourage pregnant women to stop smoking and drinking
- during the early years, home visitation, parenting skills training and high-quality preschool sessions, which offer effective interventions to prevent development of child mental disorders.

Examples are listed next.

- The *Nurse-Family Partnership* (NFP) is a home-visiting programme for first-time mothers that has shown positive results in experimental evaluations. While the NFP is delivered through specially trained nurses, a similar programme delivered by paraprofessionals demonstrated positive outcomes in an RCT. These programmes provide evidence of improved pregnancy outcomes and maternal caregiving and reduced physical abuse and harsh parenting.[16,20]
- *Parenting skills training programmes* have been shown in experimental trials and meta-analyses to reduce child maltreatment and to produce positive outcomes such as improved parent–child relationships and increased parenting consistency. Positive parenting can act as a buffer against adversity, including poverty and peer pressure, and may improve child abuse environments.[28] These programmes have been shown to reduce aggressive or antisocial behavior and to improve school outcomes. A meta-analysis by MacLeod and Nelson of programmes to reduce child maltreatment (home visiting, preschool education or child care and multicomponent community projects) concluded that child maltreatment could be prevented.[176] Parents using positive practices are twice as likely to have children with no behavioural problems. Conversely, children whose parents use punitive practices are more likely than others to behave aggressively. A controlling parental style increases the risk of

Health spending around the world, 2007 *
(share of gross domestic product, %)

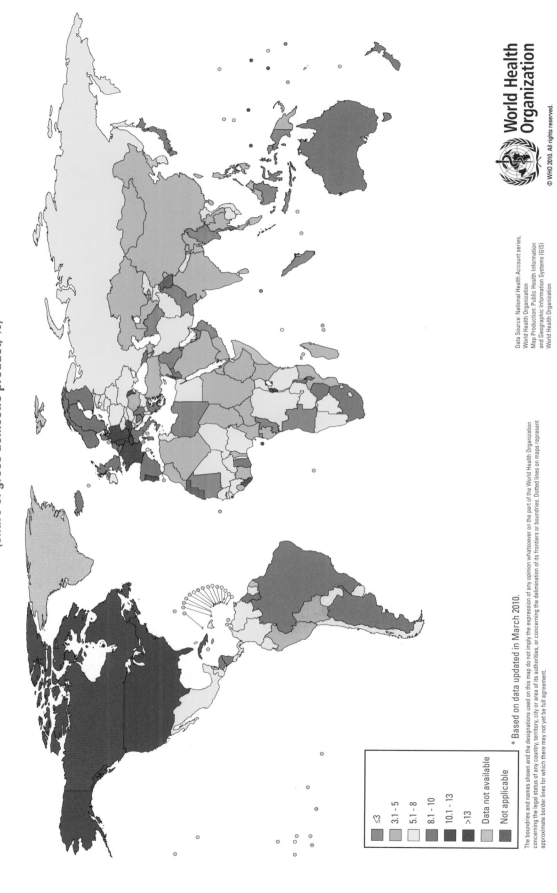

≤3
3.1 - 5
5.1 - 8
8.1 - 10
10.1 - 13
>13
Data not available
Not applicable

* Based on data updated in March 2010.

The boundries and names shown and the designations used on this map do not imply the expression of any opinion whatsoever on the part of the World Health Organization concerning the legal status of any country, territory, city or area of its authorities, or concerning the delimitation of its frontiers or boundries. Dotted lines on maps represent approximate border lines for which there may not yet be full agreement.

Data Source: National Health Account series,
World Health Organization
Map Production: Public Health Information
and Geographic Information Systems (GIS)
World Health Organization

World Health Organization

Figure 2.8 Expenditure on health as a fraction of the gross domestic product (GDP) in each country, WHO data updated to 2010. Reproduced, with permission, from *Mental health systems in selected low- and middle-income countries: a WHO-AIMS cross-national analysis*. Geneva, World Health Organization, 2010[90]

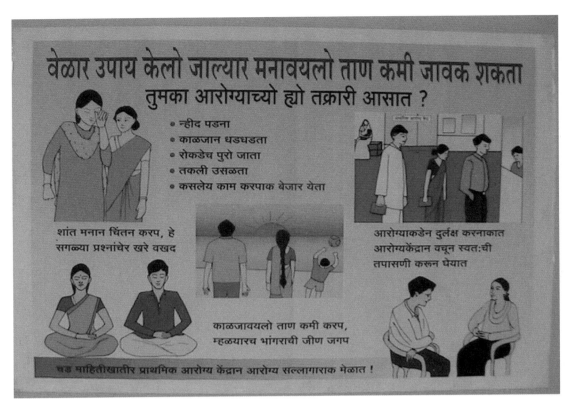

Figure 2.9 Poster in the waiting room in Goa, India, from a service described by Patel et al. (2010);[134] supplied by, and reproduced with permission from, Vikram Patel

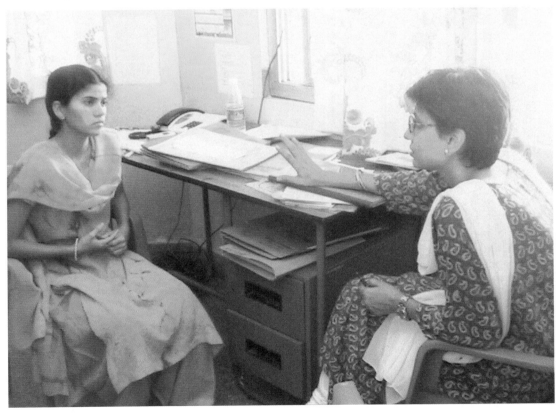

Figure 2.10 Goa, India: a lay counsellor (on the left) receiving monthly supervision on collaborative care from a psychiatrist (on the right); supplied by, and reproduced with permission from, Vikram Patel

depression and anxiety in the child. Children at risk due to deprivation and low educational levels of parents have fewer behavioural problems where positive parenting is used.[13]

- *A Cochrane review* of the relationship between parenting programmes and measures of maternal depression, anxiety and self-esteem confirmed that parenting programmes can be effective in improving a range of aspects of maternal psychosocial functioning. All of the programmes reviewed were successful in producing positive change in maternal psychosocial health.[177]

- *Early education programmes* have been shown to reduce child maltreatment and to lead to higher levels of education completed. An RCT by Love et al. (2005; reported by O'Connell et al.[20]) of 3000 families of the Early Head Start programme in the USA provided evidence that 3-year-old participants scored significantly higher than those not participating in a mental-development measure, and had significantly lower levels of aggressive behaviour. A meta-analysis by Nelson et al. (2003; also reported by O'Connell et al.[20]) of pre-school programmes found significant effects on social–emotional functioning that were sustained through secondary school. Multicomponent interventions to increase social competence through teaching interpersonal problem-solving skills, such as the Perry Preschool Program, demonstrated positive effects on academic performance and social adjustment when followed up to the age of 19 and 23 years, including lower arrest rates and self-reported fighting, and higher rates of secondary school completion.[16]

Multi-pronged interventions with school-based training in social skills and home-based parent training have been used to enhance social competence and academic achievement. A recent review of trials suggested that exercise has positive short-term effects on self-esteem in children and young people, and concluded that the use of exercise may be an important universal approach to improving children's self-esteem, which in turn may help prevent the development of psychological and behavioural problems in children and adolescents. In addition, some interventions trialled training of elementary grade teachers in the use of effective instructional methods, including the use of interactive and mastery teaching methods (see below), to use the results of frequent assessments to adjust instruction or provide more intensive support to increase the academic and cognitive development of all students, including those at risk of poor achievement.[16]

Community epidemiological preventive intervention (an experimental community-based study)

The Mastery Learning and Good Behavior Game (a universal programme that promotes positive behaviour and rule compliance in the classroom through reinforcement) used mastery learning methods in Grade 1 classrooms in 19 sociodemographically diverse public schools in Baltimore, USA. The study found positive effects on reading achievement, mainly among students initially showing depressive symptoms and those with initially low reading scores. This suggests that this universal intervention may have greater benefits for those at risk for depressive disorders. Positive effects from the Good Behavior Game programme were found to reduce aggressive and shy behaviour, with the largest effects found in the most aggressive children.[16]

Adolescence

Interventions

Characteristics of individuals, families, schools and communities combine to influence the risk of an adolescent developing a mental disorder or adopting risky behaviours such as unsafe sex or substance misuse. A solid body of research demonstrates that it is possible to impact young people's lives positively and prevent many mental disorders. The prevention agenda points to establishing appropriate limits and rules, as well as opportunities to develop positive social norms, values and relationships and a sense of identity and of belonging.

Schools are the primary institution for socialization in many countries. They are second in importance to families in exerting influence over adolescents. Schools provide a convenient setting and social context where adolescents can develop academic achievement, rule compliance, and peer relations. School-based programmes focus on individual skill development and on universal interventions to change the school structure.[20] Schools have thus become one of the most important settings for health-promotion and preventive interventions for children and youth. Schools also provide access to parents.[13]

- The *Healthy Schools programme* uses a whole-system approach with families, primary health-care services, and other organizations that work with youth. As well as promoting physical health, a Healthy

School works at the level of the school environment, to change conditions to support prevention of mental disorder for at-risk adolescents, and early interventions for those with symptoms of mental disorders. Studies show that a quality, healthy, stimulating and safe school environment is associated with better physical and emotional health and the adoption of safe behaviours. Participation in school activities fosters social inclusion and is associated with better perceived health, positive socio-emotional development, better self-perception, and a feeling of independence.

Although there has not been an evaluation of the Healthy School approach with all its components, a systematic review by Lister-Sharp et al. (1999), reported by Barlow et al.,[178] identified eight evaluation studies on interventions resembling those of health-promoting schools. The interventions included activities in the school curriculum, school ethos and the school–family–community partnership. The authors concluded that the approach can influence the health and well-being of a young person and the school environment. A systematic review by Wells et al. (2003), also reported by Barlow et al.,[178] of universal approaches to mental health promotion in schools concluded that there is sufficient evidence of the effectiveness of these programmes. Outcomes include academic improvement, increased problem-solving skills and social competence, as well as reductions in depressive symptoms, anxiety, bullying, substance use and aggressive and delinquent behaviour.[21]

- *Classroom behaviour-management programmes* attempt to help children better meet the social demands of the classroom through the overt encouragement of desired behaviours and the discouragement of undesired behaviours. These programmes attempt to provide children with cognitive skills that may help them cope better with difficult social situations.

The Good Behavior Game (described above) has been shown across several RCTs in the USA and the Netherlands to lead to significant reductions in aggressive behaviour up to 5 years after the intervention in those boys with moderate to high aggressive behaviour at baseline.[21]

Evidence from the USA provides support for services for at-risk youth that include smaller classes, intensive counselling, and accelerated instruction aimed at helping students catch up with their peers. Alternative settings such as "schools-within-schools" and alternative schools with their own settings focus on educational achievement, as well as connecting schools, families and community services to work on and monitor malleable risk factors through strong relationships with adult counsellors and formal coaching in specific problem-solving strategies, for example.[21]

- The *Strengthening Families Program* (SFP) and the *Strengthening Families Program: for Parents and Youth* 10–14 (SFP 10–14), a video-based adaptation of the original SFP programme, help families develop the skills, values, goals and interaction patterns needed to avoid substance use and other problem behaviours. RCT evaluations showed positive outcomes on reducing substance use and delinquent behaviour by changing parent–child interaction patterns.[16]

- A large Australian RCT by Bond et al. (2007), reported by O'Briain,[16] evaluated the *Gatehouse Project* in 26 secondary schools in the greater Melbourne area, Australia, involving a combination of classroom, whole-school and school/community strategies. Students with good school connectedness, including relationships with peers, teachers and the learning process, as well as good social connectedness, were less likely to experience subsequent mental health issues and be involved in health-risk behaviours, and were more likely to have good educational outcomes.

- *Parent-focused programs* to improve parenting skills and deal with emotions associated with divorce have improved mother–child relationship quality and reduced mental problems in the children. A 6-year randomized follow-up study by Woilchik et al. (2002), also reported by O'Briain,[16] found that 11% of adolescents in the experimental group had a 1-year prevalence of diagnosed mental disorders, compared with 23.5% in the control group.

- Meta-analyses by Tobler et al. (2000) and Faggiano et al. (2005), reported by Desjardins et al.,[13] show that effective school-based drug-abuse-prevention programmes target interpersonal skills, seeking to change the school environment and involving teachers and parents; they also show that programmes to educate youth on the physical, psychological and social effects of drug abuse show very little impact.[13]

Effective regulatory interventions to reduce substance-use disorders operate at the international, national, regional and local jurisdictional levels and include taxation, restrictions on availability, and total bans on all forms of direct and indirect advertising. It has been estimated that every 10% increase in media campaign expenditure has reduced cigarette sales by 0.5%.[21]

Adulthood

Deprivation

Economic risk factors can be modified by government policies, and some experimental studies have demonstrated that such modifications lead to a reduction in emotional and behavioural problems in children. A recent study for the OECD found that successful anti-poverty strategies included a balance of improved benefits where necessary, and improved structural incentives for increased employment.[16]

Work

- *JOBS programme* – randomized trials in the USA have demonstrated positive effects on rates of re-employment, the quality and pay of jobs obtained and increases in job satisfaction. This type of programme combines basic instruction on job-search skills with enhancing motivation, skills in coping with setbacks and social support among job searchers.[21]

- Employment insurance can mitigate risk factors and protect the mental health of those who lose their jobs, as suggested from epidemiological evidence that links involuntary job loss with increased mental health problems, particularly symptoms of depressive and anxiety disorders. Although empirical evidence is lacking, common sense points to a link between employment insurance programmes and reduction in finance-related stress following job loss.[70]

- A meta-analysis by Van der Klink et al. (2001), reported by Desjardins et al.,[13] on different approaches to prevention of mental disorder in the workplace suggested that cognitive-behavioural approaches significantly improve perceived quality of life in the workplace, self-esteem, the feeling of effectiveness, and work-related skills. A further systematic review on workplace stress among nurses concluded that cognitive interventions providing social support were the most effective.[13]

Education

Some evidence for lifelong learning for adults exists to show the link with improved mental health. While priority has been given to improving education among school-aged children, little attention has been given to illiterate adults. Some evidence exists to show that there are benefits from improving literacy in terms of improving mental health. Literacy benefits go beyond acquiring new skills, to include greater confidence and a reduction of barriers to accessing opportunities, all of which contribute to reducing risks for mental disorders.[21]

Lifestyles

- Older people may be more vulnerable to poor nutrition as they become more isolated. Lunch clubs have been recognized as an effective means of ensuring that older people not only have at least one nutritious meal, but also access the social side of the clubs.[179]

- A systematic review by Kaner et al. (2007), discussed by O'Briain,[16] found that brief interventions and advice in primary care settings can reduce high-risk alcohol use and hazardous drinking patterns. Incorporating brief assessments and interventions into standard primary care protocols can have a significant population-level impact, with relatively little investment of time and resources.

- Regulatory interventions for addictive substances at international, national, regional and local levels, including taxation, restrictions on availability and total bans on all forms of direct and indirect advertising can prevent substance-use disorders. A tax increase that raises tobacco prices by 10% reduces both the prevalence and consumption of tobacco products by about 5% in high-income countries and 8% in low- and middle-income countries. A 10% increase in the price of alcohol can reduce the long-term consumption of alcohol by about 7% in high-income countries and, although there are very limited data, by about 10% in low-income countries.[21]

Housing

A British systematic review suggested improvement in housing was linked with improvement in self-reported physical and mental health and reduced mental health strain, as well as broader positive social impacts on factors such as perceptions of safety, crime and social and community participation. Of the 18 studies included, one involved a large prospective controlled study that found a dose–response relationship between the extent of housing improvement and the degree of improvement in mental health.[45]

A systematic review by Bridge et al. in 2007, discussed by O'Briain,[16] confirmed the association between housing improvements (quality, location and suitability of housing) and positive physical and mental effects. Indoor air quality, poor heating, insulation, ventilation and plumbing were also found to be very important factors linked to poor health outcomes. The authors also found a potential negative impact of housing, where people's sense of control was diminished where they were not consulted.

Neighbourhood, crime and violence

The most common community approach involves strengthening community networks by working on multiple levels to foster a sense of social responsibility. Other approaches involve complementary work on public policy, work on school organization and practices, family support through parent training, and individual social-competence skills.[70]

The Communities that Care programme developed in the USA has been replicated in Australia, the Netherlands and the UK. The programme adopts a whole-community approach, working with residents to undertake a local assessment and prioritize goals in crime prevention and mental health promotion and mental-disorder-prevention programmes, particularly for children and adolescents.[16]

Empowerment, social cohesion and resilience

A literature review of empowerment interventions to improve the health of excluded populations concluded that the participatory processes underlying empowerment must be accompanied by capacity and skills building among individuals and community organizations. The most effective empowerment strategies involve real decision-making by the community members themselves.[62]

Community development is defined as a process of voluntary cooperation, mutual support, and building social connections between residents and local community institutions. Community-development approaches seek to help individuals and communities increase their sense of control over their own health and provide the means to improve it. Supporting community development enhances the social capital of communities.[13]

There is little evidence of the effectiveness of community-development approaches, given the difficulties in evaluating these complex interventions. In the scientific literature, Communities that Care (see above), shows promise. The intervention adopts a community-development approach to increase the participation of local leaders and citizens to find solutions to violence in their communities. Evaluations of the US interventions using a quasi-experimental design showed an increase in the ability of participants to identify risk and protective factors and to implement effective measures to address them.[13,21]

Old age

Exercise interventions have been shown to have positive effects on the mental health of older people. Cross-sectional studies and controlled trials show that exercise, such as aerobic classes and t'ai chi, provides both physical and psychological benefits in older populations. Benefits include greater life satisfaction, positive mood states, lower blood pressure, and reductions in psychological distress and depressive symptoms.[21] A review to assess the potential role of the serotonin system in affecting sensitivity to the health-related effects of the social environment concluded that the serotonin system, as indexed by *5HTTLPR* (serotonin-transporter-linked polymorphic region), is an important link between the social environment and health.[180]

One quasi-experimental outcome study by Stevens and van Tilburg (2000), reported by Hosman et al.,[21] confirmed that befriending programmes for older women can significantly reduce loneliness and increase the making of new friends.

Other promising preventive interventions include the use of patient-education methods that teach about the prognosis and management of chronic conditions. These strategies have been shown to have short-term beneficial effects such as reductions in depression. Early screening and interventions in primary care, and programmes using life-review techniques, have also shown promise.[16]

Implications for primary care practitioners

- Research has shown that brief interventions by primary care practitioners are one of the most effective means of bringing about patient behaviour change for unhealthy behaviours such as smoking and alcohol and for taking up secondary prevention such as screening services.

- Primary care practitioners have the most frequent contact with patients and are able to promote mental health and detect signs of physical and mental health problems early, for treatment or referral, as appropriate.

- Links into their communities through schools or community organizations would enable primary care practitioners to develop a sound understanding of the environmental influences on patients' mental health and of available services such as those discussed above, for referral.

Chapter summary

Overall determinants of mental health

Recent reviews have found suggestive evidence of the links between the social determinants of health and mental health.[181] A review by the US Institute of Medicine of child mental health suggested that the key is to identify risks – biological, psychological and social factors – that may increase a child's risk of mental disorders. These risks reside not only in the individual and family but also in the social environment and include poverty, violence, lack of safe schools, and lack of access to health care.[20] Yet the approach to mental disorder has largely been to wait until a disorder is established.

The key message is that prevention, early diagnosis and treatment now have the potential to yield substantial long-term benefits. In particular, early intervention could ensure that evidence-based treatment to reduce distress and disability is made available at the earliest possible stage.[27] The Royal College of Psychiatrists statement in 2010 on the social determinants of health,[11] recognized the need for a change in doctors' attitudes towards the social determinants of health and broader public health and a change in health-care and social systems, as well as in education of doctors.

The UK Foresight study (2008) on "mental capital and well-being" recommended that primary care should ensure early diagnosis and referral to integrated services for social, psychological and occupational needs.[27] Moving beyond physical and mental health to include the influences on mental health, advice needs, for example, to include improving financial situations and debt, and advice on employment and housing.

Developments in the delivery of mental health services in primary care

Irrespective of income, similar developments are occurring in primary care services across the world. The GP has been joined by other staff – practice nurses, behavioural scientists and closer liaison with mental health services in the developed world, and multipurpose health-care workers and trained lay workers in the developing world. While CBT, couple therapy and behavioural activation have been favoured in high-income countries, problem-solving has usually been used in middle- and low-income countries. However, there is no reason why behavioural activation and motivational interviewing should not be simplified and adapted for primary care, and also taught to paraprofessionals working in this setting. In addition to drug therapy, these techniques are cheap to administer and equally effective as psychological treatments for most mild to moderate depression. However, many "treatment-resistant" patients can be helped by a combination of both treatments. In all countries, it is important that, as mental hospitals are drastically reduced in size, treatments are available for those with severe mental illnesses as well as for people with depression and substance-use problems. For this to happen, there would need to be a massive expansion in mental health training in low-income countries, together with greater empowerment of lay health-care workers.

References

1   Committee on Social Determinants of Health. World Health Organization. *Closing the gap in a generation. Health equity through action on the social determinants of health*. Geneva, World Health

Organization, 2008 (http://www.searo.who.int/LinkFiles/SDH_SDH_FinalReport.pdf, accessed 31 October 2011).

2   Lalonde M. *A new perspective on the health of Canadians*. Ottawa, Health and Welfare, 1974.

3   World Health Organization. *Ottawa Charter for Health Promotion* First International Conference, Ottawa, 21 November 1986 (WHO/HPR/HEP 95.1) Geneva, World Health Organization, 1986 (http://www.who.int/hpr/NPH/docs/ottawa_charter_hp.pdf, accessed 31 October 2011).

4   Marmot M. Fair society, healthy lives. *Strategic review of health inequalities in England post-2010*. London, Department of Health, 2010.

5   Herrman H, Saxena S, Moodie R, eds. *Promoting mental health concepts. Emerging evidence, and practice*. Geneva, World Health Organization, 2004.

6   *Commission on Social Determinants of Health*. Geneva, World Health Organization, 2006 (http://www.who.int/social_determinants/resources/csdh_brochure.pdf, accessed 31 October 2011).

7   Dahlgren G, Whitehead M. *Policies and strategies to promote social equity in health*. Stockholm, Institute for Futures Studies, 1991.

8   *Constitution of the World Health Organization* (1948) (http://www.who.int/governance/eb/who_constitution_en.pdf, accessed 31 October 2011).

9   *World Health Report. Mental health: new understanding, new hope*. Geneva, World Health Organization, 2001 (http://www.who.int/whr/2001/en/whr01_en.pdf, accessed 31 October 2011).

10 Friedli L. *Mental Health Improvement 'concepts and definitions': briefing paper for the National Advisory Group. Mental health, mental wellbeing, mental health improvement: what do they mean? A practical guide to terms and definitions*. Edinburgh, Scottish Executive, 2004 (http://www.taysidemindset.org.uk/documents/Terms%20&%20Definitions.pdf, accessed 31 October 2011).

11 No *health without mental health. Position statement and the supporting evidence*. London, Royal College of Psychiatrists, 2010.

12 *Choosing mental health. A policy agenda for mental health and public health*. London, Mental Health Foundation, 2005.

13 Desjardins N et al. *Science advisory report on effective interventions in mental health promotion and mental disorder prevention*. Quebec, Gouvernement du Quebec, 2010 (http://www.inspq.qc.ca/pdf/publications/1116_EffectiveInterMentalHealthPromoMentalDisorder.pdf, accessed 31 October 2011).

14 MacDonald G, O'Hara K. *Ten elements of mental health, its promotion and demotion: implications for practice*. Birmingham, Society of Health Education and Health Promotion, 1998.

15 Irwin L, Siddiqi A, Hertzman C. *Early childhood development. A powerful equalizer*. Geneva, World Health Organization, 2007.

16 O'Briain W. *Evidence review: prevention of mental disorders*. British Columbia, British Columbia Ministry of Health, 2007.

17 Friedli L. *Mental health, resilience and inequalities*. Geneva, World Health Organization, 2009.

18 Flannelly K et al. Beliefs, mental health, and evolutionary threat assessment systems in the brain. *The Journal of Nervous and Mental Disease*, 2007, 195:996–1003.

19 Goldberg D. The interplay between biological and psychological factors in determining vulnerability to mental disorders. *Psychoanalytic Psychotherapy*, 2009, 23:236–247.

20 O'Connell M, Boat T, Warner K, eds. *Preventing mental, emotional and behavioral disorders among young people: progress and possibilities*. Washington DC, National Academies Press, 2009.

21 Hosman C, Jane-Llopis E, Saxena S. *Prevention of mental disorders: effective interventions and policy options*. Geneva, World Health Organization, 2004.

22 Spencer N. Social, economic, and political determinants of child health. *Pediatrics*, 2003, 112:704–706.

23 Stewart DE et al. Postpartum depression: literature review of risk factors and interventions. Toronto, University Health Network Women's Health Program, 2003

24 Barnes JJ et al. Neighborhood characteristics and mental health: the relevance for mothers of infants in deprived English neighborhoods. *Social Psychiatry and Psychiatric Epidemiology*, 2010, 6 October, epub ahead of print.

25 Cerda M et al. Genetic and environmental influences on psychiatric comorbidity: a systematic review. *Journal of Affective Disorder*, 2010, 126:14–38.

26 Kestila L et al. Determinants of health in adulthood: what is the role of parental education, childhood adversities and own education? *European Journal of Public Health*, 2005, 6:305–314.

27 Jenkins R et al., Foresight Mental Capital and Wellbeing Project. *Mental health: future challenges.* London, Government Office for Science, 2008.

28 Morgan A et al. *Health and social inequalities in English adolescents: exploring the importance of school, family and neighbourhood. Findings from the WHO health behaviour in school-aged children study.* London, National Institute for Health and Clinical Excellence, 2006.

29 Patel V et al. Mental disorders: equity and social determinants. In: Blas E, Kurup AS, eds. *Equity, social determinants and public health programmes*. Geneva, World Health Organization, 2010:115–134.

30 Jenkins R et al. Debt income and mental disorder in the general population. *Psychological Medicine*, 2008, 38:1485–1493.

31 Eckersley R. Is modern western culture a health hazard? *International Journal of Epidemiology*, 2006, 35:252–258.

32 Wilkinson R, Pickett K. *The spirit level. Why more equal societies almost always do better*. London, Allen Lane Penguin Group, 2009.

33 Beaulieu A et al. Le travail comme determinant social de la sante pour les personnes utilitrices des services de santé mentale. *Santé Mentale au Quebec* 2002, 27:177–193.

34 Stansfeld S, Candy B. Psychosocial work environment and mental health – a meta-analytic review. *Scandinavian Journal of Work, Environment & Health*, 2006, 32:443–462.

35 Faragher E, Cass M, Cooper C. The relationship between job satisfaction and health: a meta-analysis. *Occupational and Environmental Medicine*, 2005, 62: 105–112.

36 Stansfeld SA et al. Work characteristics predict psychiatric disorder: prospective results from the Whitehall II Study. *Occupational and Environmental Medicine*, 1999, 56:302–307.

37 Van den Berg et al. The effect of psychosocial factors at work and lifestyle on health work ability among professional workers. *International Archives of Occupational and Environmental Health*, 2008, 81:1029–1036.

38 Sparks K et al. The effects of hours of work. *Psychology*, 1997, 70:391–408.

39 Wang, JL et al. The prevalence of mental disorders in the working population over the period of global economic crisis. *Canadian Journal of Psychiatry*, 2010, 55:598–605.

40 Feinstein L et al. *The social and personal benefits of learning a summary of key research finding*. London, Institute of Education, 2008.

41 Bartley M et al. Resilience as an asset for healthy development. In: Morgan A, Davies M, Ziglio E. *Health assets in a global context theory, methods, action*. New York, Springer, 2010:101–115.

42 Ordovas J, Foresight Mental Capital and Wellbeing Project. *Mental capital and wellbeing state of science review: SR-E18 nutrition and cognitive. Foresight Mental Capital and Wellbeing Project*. London, Government Office for Science, 2008.

43 Belles M, Hughes K, Hughes S. *Alcohol and interpersonal violence*. Policy Briefing. Geneva, World Health Organization, 2005.

44 Cornah D. *Cheers? Understanding the relationship between alcohol and mental health*. London, Mental Health Foundation, 2006.

45 Thompson H et al. The health impacts of housing improvement: a systematic review of intervention studies from 1887 to 2007. *American Journal of Public Health*, 2009, 99(S3):S681–S692.

46 Evans GW. The built environment and mental health. *Journal of Urban Health*, 2003 80:536–555.

47 Kjellstrom T. *Our cities, our health, our future. Acting on social determinants of health, equity in urban settings*. Geneva, World Health Organization, 2008.

48 Dupere V, Perkins DD. Community types and mental health: a multilevel study of local environmental stress and coping. *American Journal of Community Psychology*, 2007, 39:107–119.

49 Barton H. 2009 Land use. Planning and health and well-being. *Land Use Policy*, 2009, 26S:S115–S123.

50 Bhugra D, Jones P. Migration and mental illness. *Advances in Psychiatric Treatment*, 2001, 7:216–222.

51 Cochrane R, Sashidharan SP. Mental health and ethnic minorities: a review of literature and implications for services. Birmingham, University of Birmingham and Northern Birmingham Mental Health Trust, 1995.

52   DeMaio FG. Immigration as pathogenic: a systematic review of the health of immigrants to Canada. *International Journal of Equity in Health*, 2010, 9:27.

53   Qureshi A, Moussaoui VD. Position statement environment network on mental health and migration. *Annals of General Psychiatry*, 2010, 9(Suppl 1):S237.

54   Sousa E et al. Immigration, work and health in Spain: the influence of legal status and employment contract on reported health indicators. *International Journal of Public Health*, 2010, 55:443–451.

55   Stuber J et al. The association between multiple domains of discrimination and self-assessed health: a multilevel analysis of Latinos and Blacks in four low-income New York City neighborhoods. *Health Services Research*, 2003, 38:6.

56   Roff L, Cavanaugh R. Religiousness/spirituality and mental health among older male inmates. *The Gerontologist*, 2008, 48:5.

57   Eckersley R. Culture, spirituality, religion and health: looking at the big picture. *Medical Journal of Australia*, 2007, 186(10 Suppl):S54–S56.

58   Koenig HG. Research on religion, spirituality and mental health: a review. *Canadian Journal of Psychiatry*, 2009, 54:283–291.

59   William D, Sternthal MJ. Spirituality, religion and health: evidence and research directions. *Medical Journal of Australia*, 2007, 186(1 Suppl):S47–S50.

60   Samaan R. The influences of race, ethnicity, and poverty on the mental health of children. *Journal of Health Care for the Poor and Underserved*, 2000, 11:100–110.

61   Woodall J et al. *Evidence summary: empowerment and health and wellbeing.* Leeds, Centre for Health Promotion Research, 2010.

62   Wallerstein N. *What is the evidence on effectiveness of empowerment to improve health?* Geneva, World Health Organization, 2006.

63   Putnam R. *Bowling alone. The collapse and revival of American community.* New York, Simon & Schuster, 2000.

64   De Silva M et al. Social capital and mental illness: a systematic review. *Journal of Epidemiology and Community Health*, 2005, 59:619–627.

65   Hamano T et al. Social capital and mental health in Japan: a multilevel analysis. *PLoS ONE*, 2008, 5: e13214.

66   Morgan A, Haglund BA. 2009. Social capital does matter for adolescent health: evidence from the English HBSC study. *Health Promotion International*, 2009, 24:363–372.

67   Seeman TE. Health promoting effects of friends and family on health outcomes in older adults. *American Journal of Health Promotion*, 2000, 14:362–370.

68   Poznyak V, Saraceno B, Obot IS. *Breaking the vicious cycle of determinants and consequences of alcohol use.* Geneva, World Health Organization, 2007 (http://www.who.int/bulletin/volumes/83/11/editorial21105html/en/, accessed 31 October 2011).

69   Ndyanabangi S et al. Uganda mental health country profile. *International Review of Psychiatry*, 2004, 16(1–2):54–62.

70   Saxena S, Jane-Llopis E, Hosman C. Prevention of mental and behavioural disorders: implications for policy and practice. *World Psychiatry*, 2006, 5:5–14.

71   Saraceno B et al. Barriers to improvement of mental health services in low-income and middle-income countries. *The Lancet*, 2007, 370:1164–1174.

72   Lauber C, Rössler W. Stigma towards people with mental illness in developing countries in Asia. *International Review of Psychiatry*, 2008, 19:157–178.

73   *Atlas. Psychiatric education and training across the world.* Geneva, World Health Organization, 2005. (http://www.who.int/mental_health/evidence/Atlas_training_final.pdf, accessed 31 October 2011).

74   Beaglehole R et al. Improving the prevention and management of chronic disease in low-income and middle-income countries: a priority for primary health care. *The Lancet*, 2008, 372:940–949.

75   Saxena S et al. Resources for mental health: scarcity, inequity and inefficiency. *The Lancet*, 2007, 370:878–889.

76   Patel V et al, Zonal, WPA and Member Society Representatives. Reducing the treatment gap for mental disorders: a WPA survey. *World Psychiatry*, 2010, 9:169–176.

77 Kilonzo GP, Simmons N. Development of mental health services in Tanzania: a reappraisal for the future. *Social Science and Medicine*, 1998, 47:419–428.

78 Adewuya A, Makanjuola R. Preferred treatment for mental illness among Southwestern Nigerians. *Psychiatry Services*, 2009, 60:121–124.

79 Ofori-Atta A, Read UM, Lund C. A situation analysis of mental health services and legislation in Ghana: challenges for transformation. *African Journal of Psychiatry*, 2010, 13:99–108.

80 Raja S et al. Mapping mental health finances in Ghana, Uganda, Sri Lanka, India and Lao PDR. *International Journal of Mental Health Systems*, 2010, 4:11.

81 Lewin S et al. Supporting the delivery of cost-effective interventions in primary health-care systems in low-income and middle-income countries: an overview of systematic reviews. *The Lancet*, 2008, 372:928–939.

82 Karim S et al. Pakistan mental health country profile. *International Review of Psychiatry*, 2004, 16:83–92.

83 *Mental health atlas*. Geneva, World Health Organization, 2005 (http://www.who.int/mental_health/evidence/atlas/global_results.pdf, accessed 23 November 2011).

84 Miller G. Mental health in developing countries. The unseen: mental illness' global toll. *Science*, 2006, 311:458–461.

85 Kigozi F. Integrating mental health into primary health care: Uganda's experience. South Africa Psychiatry review, 2007, 10:17–19.

86 Gureje O et al. Cost-effectiveness of an essential mental health intervention package in Nigeria. *World Psychiatry*, 2007, 6:42–48.

87 Jenkins R et al. Integration of mental health into primary care in Kenya. *World Psychiatry*, 2010, 9:118–120.

88 Saraceno B et al. Barriers to improvement to mental health services in low-income and middle-income countries. *The Lancet*, 2007, 370:1164–1174.

89 Mwape L et al. Integrating mental health into primary healthcare in Zambia: a care provider's perspective. *International Journal of Mental Health Systems*, 2010, 4:21.

90 *Mental health systems in selected low- and middle-income countries: a WHO-AIMS cross-national analysis*. Geneva, World Health Organization, 2010 (http://whqlibdoc.who.int/publications/2009/9789241547741_eng.pdf, accessed 31 October 2011).

91 Ustun TB, Sartorius N. *Mental disorders in general health care*. Chichester, Wiley, 1995.

92 Penninx BW et al. The Netherlands Study of Depression and Anxiety (NESDA): rationale, objectives and methods. *International Journal of Methods in Psychiatric Research*, 2008, 17:121–140.

93 Goldberg DP et al. The effects of detection and treatment on the outcome of major depression in primary care: a naturalistic study in 15 cities. *British Journal of General Practice*, 1998, 48:1840–1844.

94 van Beljouw IM et al. The course of untreated anxiety and depression, and determinants of poor one-year outcome: a one-year cohort study. *BMC Psychiatry*, 2010, 10:86.

95 Rost K et al. Persistently poor outcomes of undetected major depression in primary care. *General Hospital Psychiatry*, 1998, 20:12–20.

96 Verhaak PF et al. Receiving treatment for common mental disorders. *General Hospital Psychiatry*, 2009, 31:46–55.

97 Gilbody SM, House AO, Sheldon TA. Routinely administered questionnaires for depression and anxiety: a systematic review. *BMJ*, 2001, 322:406–409.

98 Pignone MP et al. Screening for depression in adults. A summary of the evidence for the US Preventive Services Task Force. *Annals of Internal Medicine*, 2002, 136:765–776.

99 Paulden M et al. Screening for postnatal depression in primary care: cost effectiveness analysis. *BMJ*, 2010, 340:253.

100 Morrell CJ et al. Clinical effectiveness of health visitor training in psychologically informed approaches for depression in postnatal women: pragmatic cluster randomised trial in primary care. *BMJ*, 2009, 338:a3045.

101 Morrell CJ, Warner R, Slade P. Psychological interventions for postnatal depression: cluster randomised trial and economic evaluation. The PoNDER trial. *Health Technology Assessment*, 2009, 13:i–153).

102 Valenstein M et al. The cost-utility of screening for depression in primary care. *Annals of Internal Medicine*, 2001, 134:345–360.

103 *Management of depression in primary and secondary care*. London, National Institute for Health and Clinical Excellence, 2003.

104 Whooley MA. To screen or not to screen? Depression in patients with cardiovascular disease. *Journal of the American College of Cardiology*, 2009, 54:891–893.

105 The treatment and management of depression in adults with chronic physical health problems (Partial update of CG23). London, National Institute for Health and Clinical Excellence, 2009 (CG91) (http://guidance.nice.org.uk/CG91, accessed 23 November 2011).

106 Domino ME et al. Cost-effectiveness of treatments for adolescent depression: Results from TADS. *American Journal of Psychiatry*, 2008, 165:588–596.

107 Bower P et al. Randomised controlled trial of nondirective counselling, cognitive-behaviour therapy, and usual general practitioner care for patients with depression. II: Cost effectiveness. *BMJ*, 2000, 321:1389–1392.

108 Vos T et al. Cost-effectiveness of cognitive–behavioural therapy and drug interventions for major depression. *Australian and New Zealand Journal of Psychiatry*, 2005, 39:683–692.

109 Ekers D, Richards D, Gilbody S. A meta-analysis of randomized trials of behavioural treatment of depression. *Psychological Medicine*, 2008, 38:611–623.

110 Ekers D, Richards D, McMillan D. Behavioural activation delivered by a non-specialist: phase 2 of a randomized trial. *British Journal of Psychiatry*, 2011, 198:66–72.

111 Simon J et al. Treating moderate and severe depression with antidepressant therapy or combination of antidepressants and psychological therapy: decision analysis supporting a clinical guideline. *British Journal of Psychiatry*, 2006, 189:494–501.

112 Konig H-H et al. Cost-effectiveness of a primary care model for anxiety disorders. *British Journal of Psychiatry*, 2009, 195:308–317.

113 Wiley-Exley E et al. Cost-effectiveness of integrated care for elderly depressed patients in the PRISM-E study. *Journal of Mental Health Policy and Economics*, 2009, 12:205–213, 217, 220.

114 Bartels SJ et al. Improving access to geriatric mental health services: a randomized trial comparing treatment engagement with integrated versus enhanced referral care for depression, anxiety, and at-risk alcohol use. *American Journal of Psychiatry*, 2004, 161:1455–1462.

115 Smit F et al. Cost-effectiveness of preventing depression in primary care patients: Randomised trial. *British Journal of Psychiatry*, 2006, 188:330–336.

116 Wells KB et al. Cost-effectiveness of quality improvement programs for patients with subthreshold depression or depressive disorder. *Psychiatric Services*, 2007, 58:1269–1278.

117 Rost K et al. Managing depression as a chronic disease: a randomised trial of ongoing treatment in primary care. *BMJ*, 2002, 325:934.

118 Harkness EF, Bower PJ. On-site mental health workers delivering psychological therapy and psychosocial interventions to patients in primary care: effects on the professional practice of primary care providers. *Cochrane Database of Systematic Reviews*, 2009, (1):CD000532.

119 Mynors-Wallis LM et al. Randomised controlled trial of problem solving treatment, antidepressant medication, and combined treatment for major depression in primary care. *BMJ*, 2000, 320:26–30.

120 Kendrick T et al. Cost-effectiveness of referral for generic care or problem-solving treatment from community mental health nurses, compared with usual general practitioner care for common mental disorders: Randomised controlled trial. *British Journal of Psychiatry*, 2006, 189:50–59.

121 Kessler D et al. Therapist-delivered internet psychotherapy for depression in primary care: a randomised controlled trial. *The Lancet*, 2009, 374:678.

122 Hollinghurst S et al. Cost-effectiveness of therapist-delivered online cognitive-behavioural therapy for depression. Randomised controlled trial. *British Journal of Psychiatry*, 2010, 197:297–304.

123 Kaltenthaler E et al. Computerised cognitive behaviour therapy for depression and anxiety update: a systematic review and economic evaluation. *Health Technology Assessment*, 2006, 10(33):iii, xi–xiv, 1–168.

124 Proudfoot J et al. Clinical efficacy of computerised cognitive–behavioural therapy for anxiety and depression in primary care: randomised controlled trial. *British Journal of Psychiatry*, 2004, 185:46–54.

125 Kaltenthaler E et al. Computerised cognitive–behavioural therapy for depression: systematic review. *British Journal of Psychiatry*, 2008, 193:181–184.

126 *Guidance on the use of computerised cognitive behavioural therapy for anxiety and depression. Review of Technology Appraisal 51*. TA97. London, National Institute for Health and Clinical Excellence, 2006.

127 Christensen H, Griffiths KM, Jorm AF. Delivering interventions for depression by using the internet: randomised controlled trial. *BMJ*, 2004, 328:265.

128 Gerhards SA et al. Economic evaluation of online computerised cognitive-behavioural therapy without support for depression in primary care: randomised trial. *British Journal of Psychiatry*, 2010, 196:310–318.

129 Stant AD et al. Cost-effectiveness of a psychoeducational relapse prevention program for depression in primary care. *Journal of Mental Health Policy and Economics*, 2009, 12:195–204, 216–217, 220.

130 Durham RC et al. Long-term outcome of cognitive behaviour therapy clinical trials in central Scotland. *Health Technology Assessment*, 2005, 9(42):1–128.

131 McCrone P et al. Economic implications of shared care arrangements – a primary care based study of patients in an inner city sample. *Social Psychiatry and Psychiatric Epidemiology*, 2004, 39:553–559.

132 Araya R et al. Treating depression in primary care in low-income women in Santiago, Chile: a randomised controlled trial. *The Lancet*, 2003; 361:995–1000.

133 Bolton P et al. Group interpersonal psychotherapy for depression in rural Uganda. A randomized controlled trial. *JAMA*, 2003, 289:3117–3124.

134 Patel V et al. Effectiveness of an intervention led by lay health counsellors for depressive and anxiety disorders in primary care in Goa, India (MANAS): a cluster randomised controlled trial. *The Lancet* 2010, 376:2086–2095.

135 Ran M-S, Xiang M-Z, Chan CL-W. Effectiveness of psychoeducational intervention for rural Chinese families experiencing schizophrenia. A randomised controlled trial. *Social Psychiatry and Psychiatric Epidemiology*, 2003, 38:69–75.

136 Chatterjee S et al. Evaluation of a community-based rehabilitation model for chronic schizophrenia in rural India. *British Journal of Psychiatry*, 2003, 182:57–82.

137 Thornicroft G. Most people with mental illness are not treated. *The Lancet*, 2007, 370:807–808.

138 Alonso J et al. Population level of unmet need for mental healthcare in Europe. *British Journal of Psychiatry*, 2007, 190:299–306.

139 Wittchen HU, Jacobi F. Size and burden of mental disorders in Europe – a critical review and appraisal of 27 studies. *European Neuropsychopharmacology*, 2005, 15:357–376.

140 Kessler RC et al. Lifetime prevalence and age-of-onset distributions of DSM-IV disorders in the National Comorbidity Survey Replication. Archives of General Psychiatry, 2005, 62:593–602.

141 Wang PS et al. Use of mental health services for anxiety, mood, and substance disorders in 17 countries in the WHO world mental health surveys. *The Lancet*, 2007, 370:841–850.

142 Saxena S et al. Resources for mental health: scarcity, inequity and inefficiency. *The Lancet*, 2007, 370:878–889.

143 *Mental health Gap Action Programme – scaling up care for mental, neurological, and substance use disorders*. Geneva, World Health Organization, 2008.

144 *mhGAP intervention guide for mental, neurological and substance use disorders in non-specialized health settings: mental health Gap Action Programme (mhGAP)*. Geneva, World Health Organization, 2010.

145 Hill S, Pang T. Leading by example: a culture change at WHO. *The Lancet*, 2007, 369:1842–1844.

146 Barbui C et al. Challenges in developing evidence-based recommendations using the GRADE approach: the case of mental, neurological, and substance use disorders. *PLoS Medicine*, 2010, 7:e1000322.

147 Madon T et al. Public health. Implementation science. *Science*, 2007, 318:1728–1729.

148 Thornicroft G, Lempp H, Tansella M. The place of implementation science in the translational medicine continuum. *Psychological Medicine*, 2011, 15:1–7.

149 Tansella M, Thornicroft G. Implementation science: understanding the translation of evidence into practice. *British Journal of Psychiatry*, 2009, 195:283–285.

150 Goldberg DP, Huxley PJ. *Mental illness in the community. The pathway to psychiatric care*. London, Tavistock, 1980.

151 Reiss-Brennan B et al. Mental health integration: rethinking practitioner roles in the treatment of depression: the specialist, primary care physicians, and the Practice nurse. *Ethnicity and Disease*, 2006, 16(S3):37–43.

152 Nazareth I, King M, Davies S. Care of schizophrenia in general practice: The general practitioner and the patient. *British Journal of General Practice*, 1995, 45:343–347.

153 Gater R et al. The care of patients with chronic schizophrenia: A comparison between two services. *Psychological Medicine*, 1997, 27:1325–1336.

154 Meadows GN. Establishing a collaborative service model for primary mental health care. *Medical Journal of Australia*, 1998, 168:162–165.

155 Sharma VK et al. Developing mental health services in a primary care setting: Liverpool primary care mental health project. *International Journal of Social Psychiatry*, 2001, 47:16–29.

156 Goldberg DP, Gournay K. *The general practitioner, the psychiatrist and the burden of mental health care*. Maudsley Discussion Paper No.1. London, Institute of Psychiatry, 1996.

157 Rajagopal S, Goldberg D, Nikolaou V. The relationship between mental health services and primary care services in the UK: a postal survey. *Primary Care Psychiatry*, 2003, 8:131–134.

158 Byng R et al. Exploratory cluster randomised controlled trial of shared care development for long-term mental illness. *British Journal of General Practice*, 2004, 54:259–266.

159 Kates N et al. Sharing care: the psychiatrist in the family physician's office. *Canadian Journal of Psychiatry*, 1997, 42:960–965.

160 Berardi D, Menchetti M, Dragani A. The Bologna Primary Care Liaison Service: first year evaluation. *Community Mental Health Journal*, 2002, 38(6):439–445.

161 Simon GE et al. Randomised trial of monitoring, feedback, and management of care by telephone to improve treatment of depression in primary care. *BMJ*, 2000, 320:550–554.

162 Pyne JM et al. Cost-effectiveness analysis of a rural telemedicine collaborative care intervention for depression. *Archives of General Psychiatry*, 2010, 67:812–821.

163 Craven M, Bland R. Better practices in collaborative mental health care: an analysis of the evidence base. *Canadian Journal of Psychiatry*, 2006, 51(Suppl 1).

164 Campo JV et al. Managing pediatric mental disorders in primary care: a stepped collaborative care model. *Journal of the American Psychiatric Nurses Association*, 2005, 11:1–7.

165 Hunkeler EM et al. Long term outcomes from the IMPACT randomised trial for depressed elderly patients in primary care. *BMJ*, 2006, 332:259–263.

166 Simon GE et al. Cost-effectiveness of systematic depression treatment among people with diabetes mellitus. *Archives of General Psychiatry*, 2007, 64:65–72.

167 Katon W et al. Cost-effectiveness and net benefit of enhanced treatment of depression for older adults with diabetes and depression. *Diabetes Care*, 2006, 29:265–270.

168 Regier DA et al. The NIMH Depression Awareness, Recognition, and Treatment Program: structure, aims, and scientific basis. *American Journal of Psychiatry*, 1988, 145:1351–1357.

169 Paykel ES et al. Impact of a national campaign on GP education: an evaluation of the Defeat Depression Campaign. *British Journal of Psychiatry*, 1998, 173:519–522.

170 Althaus D et al. [Veränderungen in der häufigkeit von suizidversuchen: ergebnisse nach neun monaten intervention des "Nurnberger Bundnis gegen Depression".] *Psycho*, 2003, 29:28–34.

171 Hickie I. Can we reduce the burden of depression? The Australian experience with beyondblue: the national depression initiative. *Australasian Psychiatry*, 2004, 12:S38–S46.

172 Jorm AF, Christensen H, Griffiths KM. Changes in depression awareness and attitudes in Australia. The impact of beyondblue: the national depression initiative. *The Australian and New Zealand Journal of Psychiatry*, 2006, 40:42–46.

173 Rix S et al. Impact of a national campaign on GP education: an evaluation of the Defeat Depression Campaign. *British Journal of Psychiatry*, 1999, 49:99–102.

174 Priest RG et al. Lay people's attitudes to treatment of depression: results of opinion poll for Defeat Depression Campaign just before its launch. *BMJ*, 1996, 313:858.

175 Hegerl U, Schafer R. From the Nuremberg Alliance against Depression to a European Network (EAAD) – extending community-based awareness-campaigns on national and European level. *Psychiatrische Praxis*, 2007, 34(3 Suppl):S261–S265.

176 MacLeod J, Nelson G. 2000. Programs for the promotion of family wellness and the prevention of child maltreatment: a meta-analytic review. *Child Abuse and Neglect*, 2000, 24:1127–1149.

177 Barlow J, Coren E, Stewart-Brown S. 2009. Parent-training programmes for improving maternal psychosocial health (Review). *Cochrane Database of Systematic Reviews*, 2009, (1):CD002020.

178 Barlow J et al. A systematic review of reviews of interventions to promote mental health and prevent mental health problems in children and young people. *Journal of Public Mental Health*, 2007, 6:25–32.

179 Eating well for older people. *Practical and nutritional guidelines for food in residential and nursing homes and for community meals*, 2nd ed. St Austell, The Caroline Walker Trust, 2004.

180 Way BM, Taylor SE. 2010. Social influences on health: is serotonin a critical mediator? *Psychosomatic Medicine*, 2010, 72:107–112.

181 Bambra C et al. Tackling the wider social determinants of health and health inequalities: evidence from systematic reviews. *Journal of Epidemiology and Community Health*, 2009, 64:284–291.

3 Advocacy and overcoming stigma in primary care mental health

Preston J Garrison, Gabriel Ivbijaro, Yaccub Enum,
Deborah Maguire, Julie M Schirmer and Patt Francioisi

Key messages

- The emergence of mental health advocacy has contributed to changing society's perceptions of people with mental disorder, and hence reducing stigma, but more needs to be done.
- Advocacy for mental health is needed at all levels of the health-care system and government.
- Overcoming stigma in primary care mental health should involve interventions beyond primary care, and involve people with mental health problems in their design and delivery.
- To effectively tackle stigma in primary care, primary care professionals need to improve their effectiveness at helping people with mental health problems.
- The media play a key role in shaping people's attitudes and should be a key ally in tackling mental health stigma.

Introduction

Stigma is a Greek word meaning "marked". Over the years, it has acquired a more sinister meaning. Stigma has been defined as "a mark of disgrace or discredit that sets a person aside from others".[1] It is often based on misunderstanding and can lead to discrimination. *Cambridge Dictionaries Online* defines discrimination as "treating a person or a particular group of people differently, especially in a worse way from the way in which you treat other people, because of their skin, colour, religion, sex, etc" (reproduced with permission from *Cambridge Dictionaries Online* (http://dictionary.cambridge.org/dictionary/british/discrimination_1?q= discrimination).[2]

About 4000 years ago, the ancient Egyptians believed that all diseases had physical causes, and they did not distinguish between physical and mental illness. With time, mental illness became associated with the "mind". This led to victims being blamed for such things as moral weakness or spirit possession. These perceived causes of mental illness led to people with mental illness being stigmatized and ostracized from society.[3]

> They were not recognised as sick people and were accused of having abandoned themselves to shameful and forbidden practices with the devil.[3]

They were often persecuted and the few doctors who tried to help them often risked their reputations. It has been suggested that the origins of stigma could be attributed to the 19th century separation of the mental health treatment system from the medical treatment system and the building of asylums.[4]

Advocacy is speaking up for, or acting on behalf of, yourself or another person. Advocacy in mental health primarily aims to tackle stigma and discrimination against people with mental disorders and enhance their human rights. According to the World Health Organization (WHO):

> Mental health advocacy includes a variety of different actions aimed at changing the major structural and attitudinal barriers to achieving positive mental health outcomes in populations.[5]

Mental health advocacy began with the families of people with mental disorders making their voices heard. This was followed by contributions from people with mental disorders themselves, and then supported by mental health professionals and various organizations.[5]

WHO further notes that:

> Advocacy is an important means of raising awareness on mental health issues and ensuring that mental health is on the national agenda of governments. Advocacy can lead to improvements in policy, legislation and service development.[5]

The emergence of mental health advocacy has contributed to changing society's perceptions of people with mental disorders, and hence reducing the stigma associated with mental disorders. People with mental health problems, particularly in high-income countries, are increasingly participating in decisions about their health and social care. Consequently, even though stigma still exists in high-income countries, it is not as persistent as in some low-income countries where mental health advocacy is less well developed, with poorer outcomes for people with mental disorders.

Primary advocacy concerns that will have to be addressed as mental health services are integrated into primary care are:

- the danger that adequate and effective diagnosis, treatment and recovery of people living with mental illness will not receive a parity level priority within the general and primary health-care system
- the potential that primary health-care workers in all disciplines (particularly in low-income countries) will not receive adequate training and education that is necessary to effectively diagnose and treat people with mental health problems, especially the more serious disorders such as severe depression, bipolar disorder and schizophrenia
- the complexities of providing culturally competent mental health services to ethnic minorities and immigrant groups in increasingly multicultural communities and service settings.

Each of these advocacy concerns is significant in its own right. Together, they offer potential major public-policy and service-delivery barriers to effectively integrating mental health services into the primary health-care systems of countries. All will require well-planned and united advocacy on the part of all sectors of the primary care and mental health communities, if accessible and affordable mental health services are to be available to those who need them.

The engagement of patients and families, who carry much of the responsibility for helping people living with mental illnesses to manage in the community, and of the advocates who work to influence mental health policies, is critical during this time of change, reform and limited resources. This issue presents a major challenge for many primary care practitioners, who may not be familiar, or comfortable, with the activist nature of many mental health service users and their family members. This chapter discusses advocacy and strategies for overcoming stigma in primary care mental health.

Advocacy

This section offers useful background information about the need and relevance of integrating mental health services in primary health-care services. It also describes the reasons why informed and concerted advocacy will be required to create the necessary public policy, education and service-delivery system that will support effective integration and service improvement for people who experience mental health problems and serious mental disorders.

Integrating mental health in primary care: task shifting to scale-up services for people with mental disorders

In 2008, the world commemorated the 30th anniversary of the landmark declaration by representatives from 134 countries in Alma-Ata, committing themselves to achieving "health for all by the year 2000" through strengthening primary care.[6] In 2011, the world is very far from achieving this aspiration, but the declaration was a significant juncture in global health, as it emphasized the importance of health care near people's homes, the need to integrate promotive and preventive health-care interventions alongside medical care, and the understanding that mental health is an integral component of health.

In 2008, WHO and the World Organization of Family Doctors (Wonca) published a report on the global perspective on integrating mental health in primary health care, to mark this anniversary.[7] The year before, *The Lancet* had published a series of articles to focus global attention on the massive treatment gap for people with mental disorders in most parts of the world, particularly in low- and middle-income countries.[8] *Primary health care was identified as the most crucial setting for delivery of health care to close this treatment gap.*

The next part of this section describes how evidenced-based mental health care can be integrated into primary care through the WHO-Wonca report,[7] *The Lancet* series call to action on global mental health care,[8] and the Movement for Global Health goals launched on World Mental Health Day (WMHDay) 2008.[9] This call for action speaks directly to the core message of the Alma-Ata declaration's aspiration for health for all, built on the principles of equity and social justice, community participation, appropriate use of resources and intersectoral action.

The WHO-Wonca report[7] provides an excellent review and summary of the strategies needed to integrate mental health in primary care (see Box 3.1). However, there are two critical challenges that need to be addressed to achieve realistic, sustainable integration.

- The first is the tension between strengthening horizontal initiatives (i.e. strengthening health systems) versus vertical programmes (for example, for specific mental health-care programmes).
- The second is the tension between community-based care with active involvement of non-professional health-care workers and facility-based care provided by specialist health-care workers.

Although we speak with a collective voice for the need to integrate mental health in primary care, does this mean we advocate for a vertical mental health-care programme to have a primary care component or for a comprehensive primary care programme with a strong mental health-care component?

The integration of primary care into mental health programmes is not likely to achieve success, given the extremely weak primary care system in many countries, particularly in terms of human resources and poor financial coverage of most basic health-care interventions. Historically, mental health care has been viewed by primary health-care workers to be alien to their day-to-day work, and a vertical mental health-care programme will continue to perpetuate this perspective.

Box 3.1   Ten strategies for integrating mental health in primary care

1   Policy and plans need to incorporate primary care for mental health.
2   Advocacy is required to shift attitudes and behaviour.
3   Adequate training of primary care workers is required.
4   Primary care tasks must be limited and doable.
5   Specialist mental health professionals and facilities must be available to support primary care.
6   Patients must have access to essential psychotropic medications in primary care.
7   Integration is a process, not an event.
8   A mental health service coordinator is crucial.
9   Collaboration with other government non-health sectors, nongovernmental organizations (NGOs), village and community health workers, and volunteers is required.
10 Financial and human resources are needed.

Reproduced, with permission, from World Health Organization and Wonca. *Integrating mental health into primary care. A global perspective.* Geneva, World Health Organization, 2008.[7]

On the other hand, not having a vertical programme runs the risk that mental health care will simply disappear from the agenda in the face of strong competition for limited resources from other health interventions. The most feasible strategy will be to support a vertical programme for resource allocation (especially financial resources), but to emphasize the utilization of these resources through the existing primary health-care systems, thereby strengthening the system rather than creating a parallel mental health-care system. The WHO-Wonca report provides some excellent examples of case-studies of how such integration has been achieved.

The second challenge relates to concerns of specialist mental health professionals about the devolution of mental health care to non-specialists with a focus on community-oriented care delivery.

In many parts of the world, this concern is largely irrelevant, as there are no specialists or facilities to deliver mental health services in any case. Even where these do exist, they are scarce, inequitably distributed with less access to poor and marginalized groups, often unaffordable, associated with stigma and, in some instances, with profound violations of basic human rights. So, the answer to this challenge is that the front-line delivery of mental health care can be carried out by non-specialists for reasons of acceptability, feasibility and affordability. As countries' economies improve, specialty care can start to be developed, as is occurring in Viet Nam.

But are there models to show how this can be done in a manner that is both effective and safe?

Task shifting, which refers to the strategy of the redistribution of health-care tasks among health workforce teams, has become a popular method to address specialist health human resource shortages.

Specific tasks are moved, where appropriate, from highly qualified health workers to health workers with shorter training and fewer qualifications, in order to make more efficient use of the available human resources for health. The evidence base for task shifting in mental health care in developing countries is growing and is consistent in its findings. Lay people or community health workers can be trained to deliver psychological and psychosocial interventions for people living with depressive and anxiety disorders, schizophrenia and dementia, in a diverse range of low- and middle-income countries.

A critical element of these task-shifting interventions, and a significant departure from earlier efforts to improve primary mental health care, is the extension of the role of mental health specialists well beyond the training phase of primary care and community health workers, to providing continuing supervision, quality assurance and support.

Integrating mental health in primary care has been a slogan for many decades, but there has been only limited success in achieving this aspiration, in some part due to the challenges addressed in this commentary (of course, there are others too, not least of which is the very low political will to address mental health conditions).

We now have a reasonably strong evidence base on how to scale-up services for mental disorders through primary care while, simultaneously, contributing to strengthening the primary care system. The role of non-specialists, in particular community and primary health workers (physicians, all levels of nurses, social workers and other clinical staff), is central to this strategy and specialists must play a larger public health role to make the aspiration of mental health for all a reality.[10,11]

The relevance of delivering mental health services in primary care settings

Mental health disorders are a significant issue for every country, regardless of its level of economic development and resources. Prevalence rates for mental health disorders are increasing globally, as health-care systems in developing countries make the epidemiological shift from predominantly treating communicable diseases and injuries to treating chronic diseases. This shift is associated with an increase in longevity and an increase in the prevalence of mental health disorders. The prevalence rate of depression in low- and moderate-income countries varies from 2–15% among people with no disease, to 9–23% among people with one or more chronic diseases.[12] The prevalence rate for anxiety disorders varies from 2.2–28%, with only about 25% receiving any kind of treatment.[13,14]

Mental health disorders account for 12% of the WHO global burden of disease and constitute a larger burden than acquired immunodeficiency syndrome (AIDS), tuberculosis (TB) and malaria combined.[15] By the year 2020, major depression will be second only to ischaemic heart disease in contributing to the loss of life-years in terms of productivity and social functioning. At any given moment, 10% of the general population and 20% of primary care patients will have a mental health disorder.[15]

Effective treatments for mental health disorders are available. Medication interventions are as cost effective as antiretroviral therapy for human immunodeficiency virus (HIV)/AIDS.[10] Yet, only 52% of low-income countries provide community-based mental health care, including mental health care that is part of primary care services. One in four countries does not provide basic antidepressant medicine in primary care settings. Most people with mental health conditions do not get treatment for their symptoms. Nearly two-thirds of individuals with any mental health condition do not seek help for their symptoms.[15]

Mental health disorders are more prevalent in people with chronic and communicable diseases, and are associated with risk factors such as smoking, poor diet, obesity, hypertension and treatment avoidance. Mental health disorders place individuals at risk for the development of communicable and non-communicable disease and injury. Patients with mental health disorders are twice as likely to have a substance abuse disorder, be it alcohol, drugs or tobacco. All of these factors contribute to the decreased quality of life and reduced lifespan experienced by persons living with untreated mental health conditions. Effective primary care counselling and education methods are available to help patients make the changes they need to improve their health.

Persons with mental health disorders are more likely to seek medical care than mental health care. Mental health treatment in primary care has been shown to be effective. Numerous low- and middle-income countries have successfully integrated mental health and primary health care by providing training and specialty support through psychiatrists or specialty care nurses at the district or community levels of care. Integrating mental health into primary care saves money by providing care to patients within their own community and in less-costly health-care settings, thereby decreasing the extent and severity of disability and increasing productivity in persons with mental health conditions.[7]

Barriers to achieving effective integration

- No national policies or monies legislated for providing mental health care to all communities.
- No national policies or monies legislated for mental health workforce development. This includes the training of specialists (psychiatrists, psychologists, social workers) and training of primary health-care workers (primary care physicians, nurses, midwives, village health workers, and others).
- Treating mental illness and substance abuse as "social evils", with persons with these issues being institutionalized and separated from the rest of the population. This removes them from the possibilities of leading a vital life and contributing to society.
- Allowing only psychiatrists to prescribe psychotropic drugs. This prohibits the provision of medications in primary care settings and sets up competition between primary care providers and psychiatrists.
- Legislators and health-care administrators being more interested in protecting their budgets than in working together to promote the health of their population.
- As services are developed, not investing in communications campaigns to decrease the stigma of mental illness and to improve communities' openness to seeking treatment.
- In specific cases, a reimbursement system that separates or "carves out" mental health care from medical care. This creates two separate billing and coding systems, with different rules, regulations and processes. It promotes competition for funds and excessive administrative costs.
- A health and mental health-care reimbursement system where payments are based solely on episodes of care, as opposed to reimbursing for improvements in the health and productivity of a population. An episodic care-reimbursement structure rewards providers for seeing as many patients as possible, as opposed to reimbursing a team of providers for improving the health of a population.

Strategies for promoting integration of primary care and mental health-care delivery

- *Country- and community-specific epidemiological studies* that illustrate the prevalence and impact of mental health disorders on a particular society. This informs policy-makers and administrators of the extent of the problem.

- *Legislation related to mental health workforce development* that ensures mental health care at the community, or primary health care, level of care.

- *Long-term (5–10-year) consortiums of in-country and out-of-country experts* that can develop relationships and continually share and learn from each other in relation to curriculum development, outcome measurements and programme design. The continuity relationships leads to in-depth understanding and trust, which enhances integration projects.

- *Pilot projects that integrate mental health and primary health care* and link these services to specialty mental health care for education, supervision, consultation and support. Champions in these pilot projects need to measure clinical, quality and cost outcomes, which can then inform policy-makers and legislators.

- *Collaborative team-based education processes* that bring together different members of the health-care team, at all levels of their training, in the classroom and at the point of care. In Viet Nam, certificate courses are provided to faculty groups from family medicine, psychiatry, public health, social work and nursing. Conversations are ongoing to develop a clinic that brings together students from family medicine, social work and nursing to provide primary health care to vulnerable populations in a major urban area in Viet Nam.

- *Brief, doable treatment models and protocols* that delineate the roles and responsibilities of all members of the health-care team.

- *Mental health and counselling training materials* pertinent to the health-care systems and cultures in specific countries. Although universal principles can be found in many publications,[16,17] it is extremely important to have materials written by and for persons as close to one's own community as possible.

- *Public health campaigns* to decrease stigma and educate communities about mental health and substance abuse conditions and treatment options.

Strategies for effectively delivering mental health services and promoting effective self-care into primary care delivery systems

Start where the health-care system and culture is at the time and do NOT create projects that are too advanced for existing systems. For example, most health systems in low- and middle-income countries do not pay for annual preventative examinations. Primary care outpatient visits are similar to "acute care" visits and last anywhere from 3 to 8 minutes. Development needs incremental steps to be widely adopted and funded. It is important to have mental health service-delivery models that are close enough to the present system, to be seen as doable and sustainable by legislators and policy-makers. As the WHO/Wonca report notes,[7] mental health/ primary health-care integration is a process, not an end-point.

Self-care and prevention campaigns can start in childhood and can be a collaborative process with schools, given that "well-child examinations" are often not the norm. Teaching children how to develop habits of living that lead to good health is extremely important and leads to psychological resiliency, or the "ability to recover from or adjust easily to misfortune or change".[18] Evidenced-based "healthy living or wellness" strategies are available, such as the "formula for preventing paediatric obesity"[19] or the "formula for good health".[20]

Empower all members of the health-care team to have a role in identifying, treating and managing mental health issues. Train them in motivational interviewing principles and practices. Develop protocols with them for brief interventions and "stepped care", which matches interventions to the severity of patients' problems.

Self-care strategies of providers and staff are extremely important to integrating mental health into primary health care. The stress of a demanding schedule and constantly seeing patients who are in crisis can result in compassion fatigue and burn-out, which affect one's ability to identify and manage psychological distress in others. Burn-out is a pathological "syndrome of emotional and physical exhaustion and severe pessimism that results from prolonged exposure to stress".[21] Compassion fatigue is a form of burn-out and is "a deep sense of emotional exhaustion accompanied by emotional pain".[21]

A medical work culture that promotes a positive work environment and responds to burn-out in a supportive, non-threatening way is important for the health of care team members. Adequate sleep, rest and nutrition are essential ingredients to mental health and to supporting resilience, which is the ability to bounce back from stress and trauma. The American Psychiatric Association describes ways to nourish individual resiliency.[22] These are listed below:

- make connections with family, friends and groups
- avoid viewing crises as insurmountable problems
- accept that change is part of living
- set realistic goals and move towards them
- take decisive action in adverse situations
- look for self-discovery opportunities
- nurture a positive view of yourself
- keep things in perspective – avoid blowing things out of proportion
- maintain an optimistic outlook
- take care of yourself physically, emotionally and socially
- add ways of strengthening your resilience, such as recreation activities, meditation and the arts.[22]

The LIFE Curriculum[23] is a free, Internet-based curriculum for health-care providers and is one way for systems to support resiliency and the health of workers.

What the future primary care workforce will need to look like in order to achieve successful integration of mental health and primary care services

The vision for successful mental health/primary health-care integration is to have proactive multidisciplinary primary health-care teams with the knowledge and skills to have productive conversations with activated patients; to identify and manage mental health issues; and to promote resiliency and empower patients to live the most vital and meaningful lives possible. Mental health/primary health-care integration holds the most promise for patients receiving the right care, by the right provider, at the right time.[24]

Advocacy strategies for mental health and primary care integration can increase mental health promotion, prevent mental health problems, and reduce the worldwide burden of disease caused by mental health disorders.

Advocacy is needed at all levels of the health-care system and government. This includes government ministries, health-care administrators, teachers and providers at the national, provincial, district and community levels. Advocacy is also needed for funders and NGOs, which tend to promote "siloed" projects for specialized health issues that do not cut across communities. Advocacy content needs to include:

- the extent of the problem in the specific country, with epidemiological studies and stories
- the value of mental health/primary care integration on the health, quality of life (functioning, productivity) and medical costs of populations
- the risks of not addressing mental health issues.

The World Federation for Mental Health's (WFMH) 2009 WMHDay global awareness campaign, *Mental health in primary care: enhancing treatment and promoting mental health*,[9] was the first global public-awareness effort to focus attention on the need to fully integrate mental health care into primary health-care service delivery. The campaign theme stressed the continuing need to "make mental health issues a global priority" and on the all too-often neglected fact that mental health is an integral element of every individual's overall health and well-being. The campaign, supported by national and grassroots awareness and educational activities in over 100 countries during October 2009, drew worldwide attention to the growing body of information and knowledge focusing on the need and value of integrating mental health in primary health care.

In planning and conducting the WMHDay campaign, WFMH collaborated closely with Wonca. This collaboration built upon the landmark release, in September 2008, of *Integrating mental health into primary care: a global perspective*, by WHO and Wonca,[7] which signalled a major step in fostering a global effort to integrate mental health into primary care.

The WMHDay 2009 campaign highlighted the opportunities and the challenges that integrating mental health services into primary health care will present for people living with mental disorders and poor mental health, their families, caregivers, and health-care professionals.

This current movement to improve the way in which mental health services are delivered is not the first such reform effort. Lessons learnt from the past inform us that achieving parity in how mental health services are addressed in countries around the world is not an easy struggle. The effective integration of mental health into primary care at a level of priority appropriate to the documented burden of care of mental illnesses will be a major undertaking in a time of global economic and social difficulty.

The next section describes the stigma associated with mental health disorders, its effect on health-seeking behaviours, and strategies for overcoming stigma.

Stigma

Mental illness has been ill defined and poorly understood for centuries; and those affected have been sidelined and "stigmatized". Despite the major advances made in our understanding of mental health issues and the availability of effective treatments, the general public remains either wary or dismissive of people with mental health problems. The stigma associated with mental health problems can make it difficult for people to seek help and to be hired or continue to work. The attitude of the media, employers and the general population to mental health problems, consciously or unconsciously reinforces a cycle of exclusion and stigma.

An Australian study[25] noted that attitudes on help-seeking for mental health problems were influenced more by perceived stigma than by the levels of impairment caused by illness. New Zealand has one of the largest publicly funded anti-stigma campaigns, which notes that:

> One of the biggest barriers to recovery is discrimination. That's why stopping discrimination and championing respect, rights and equality for people with mental illness is just as important as providing the best treatments and therapies.[26]

Efforts to tackle the stigma and discrimination associated with mental illness have ranged from small-scale local projects to national and international campaigns. However, the stigma of mental illness persists today. In many countries, greater knowledge, understanding and government policy have not ensured the eradication of stigma for mental health problems.

Compared to issues such as race or sexuality, mental health has lagged behind and has not benefited from the successes in tackling stigma. Tackling stigma is the responsibility of society as a whole. Strategies to tackle stigma in primary care mental health clinics should be complemented by public education at all levels and systems of a society.

Stigma and discrimination in mental health

- Almost 9 out of 10 people (87%) with mental health problems have been affected by stigma and discrimination.[27]
- More than two-thirds of people with mental health problems (71%) say they have stopped doing things they wanted to do because of stigma.[27]
- 73% of people with mental health problems say they have stopped doing things they wanted to do because of fear of stigma and discrimination.[27]
- 53% of carers of people with mental health problems also say they feel unable to do things they want to do because of stigma and discrimination.[27]
- A 1993 UK survey found that 92% of the general public agreed that there was a need to be more tolerant of people with mental health problems. Ten years later, this had dropped to 83%![28]
- Another UK survey found that a quarter of the population still think that people with mental health problems should not have the same rights to employment as others.[29]
- An international survey across a number of countries found that 47% of people with schizophrenia had experienced stigma.[30]

The relevance of stigma to the delivery of mental health services in primary care

Most people with mental health problems in both high- and low-income countries are cared for in primary care rather than in specialty care. Nevertheless, mental health service users report stigma within primary health care and specialist mental health services. In the UK, 44% of people with mental health problems reported discrimination from general practitioners (GPs).[28]

Ethnic minority communities in multicultural inner-city settings tend to distrust mental health services. This distrust, alongside stigma and fear, often leads to members of ethnic minority communities accessing mental health services further down the line when their symptoms are more severe.[31] Addressing mental illness stigma from primary care would encourage people to access care earlier.

Primary care professionals' possible fears or misunderstanding of mental illness might inadvertently reinforce stigma experienced by patients with mental health problems. This could be overcome by the professionals familiarizing themselves and learning more about mental illness and how to engage with people with mental health problems.

One way of tackling stigma associated with mental disorders is to promote contact between people with and without mental health problems.[32] In the UK, the annual "Get Moving" events promote physical activity undertaken jointly by people with and without mental illness. This contact breaks down some of the barriers, and helps to reduce the stigma associated with mental health problems.

Primary care is an important player in tackling stigma associated with mental health problems, as it is often the first point of contact with health services. Primary care also provides a good opportunity for contact between people with and without mental health problems, accessing health care for a variety of health issues.

Description of a "gold standard" approach

Following successful pilots in a number of areas in England, the Tackling Stigma Framework[33] identifies a number of advocacy domains that can be applied to a range of settings. This framework is based on research on mental health service users' perceptions of mental health and stigma. Providing information alone is not effective in tackling stigma.[34] A multifaceted approach is required. The domains should therefore be implemented together to achieve maximum impact. Even though this framework was developed for child and adolescent mental health services (CAMHS), it can be applied to primary care. Its eight domains are listed below, followed by a more detailed description of each domain.

- Mainstreaming
- Language and definition
- Information
- Education
- Communication
- Effective systems and accessible services
- Media as allies
- Citizenship and participation

Mainstreaming

Mainstreaming is seen as the foundation of the Tackling Stigma Framework. To effectively tackle stigma in primary care mental health clinics, treatment programmes need to be mainstreamed into primary care services rather than being stand-alone.

> Mainstreaming approaches to tackle stigma involve embedding the framework and associated actions as a philosophy that underpins all structures and related actions and ensuring that they are continually considered in planning and development.[33]

For example, instead of having special "mental health clinics" within primary care, people with mental health problems should be seen by health professionals in generic clinics. Integrated primary care is less threatening for patients with mental health problems than going to a separate site for treatment.

At a service level, mainstreaming involves a multifaceted process that ensures that patients and carers/family are part of the process of tackling stigma. This would include a change of policies and strategies where relevant, and commitment from primary care professionals.

Language and definition

All services providing mental health care, including primary care clinics, should work with an agreed definition of mental health and related terminology. The 2001 *World Health Report* identifies the challenges of giving a comprehensive definition of mental health.[15] There are now a number of good definitions of positive mental health. It is therefore important that countries adopt a definition that takes account of the breadth of mental health issues and cultural aspects of mental health.

According to the Tackling Stigma Toolkit,[33] confusion about the terminology used to describe mental health and mental health problems contributes to the reluctance in accessing services. Developing age-appropriate and culturally appropriate explanations of mental health and mental health problems will facilitate more open discussions about mental health. This will help towards a shared understanding of mental health issues and will improve help-seeking behaviour.

In order to achieve this, it is important to involve all stakeholders (administrators, commissioners, health professionals, those affected by mental health problems, and their caregivers) in agreeing upon shared definitions of mental health and mental illness, which should be publicized and used consistently.

Information

The general public is often unclear about the level of mental health care provided in primary care and what to expect. This can contribute to the fear and stigma experienced by people with mental health problems and their families. To overcome this, commissioners and providers of primary health care should develop age-appropriate and culturally appropriate information about primary care mental health provision. This would include information about general mental health awareness, location of services, access or referral routes, and interventions offered.

There is some evidence that attitudes towards community-based mental health clinics could be improved by providing information about mental disorders and their treatment, as well as contact with persons who suffer from those disorders.[35] Provision of information should be done in a strategic and coordinated rather than piecemeal manner, to ensure consistency.

Information to tackle stigma should be provided in a variety of formats, depending on the setting and available resources. These could include leaflets, web sites, drama, multimedia (DVD), and face-to-face outreach work. In the UK and USA, many primary care practices have an information screen in waiting areas that streams information to patients. These screens could be used to convey relevant messages about stigma associated with mental health problems.

Local areas should explore the best format for their local population, considering literacy levels and cultural appropriateness. This is particularly important in multicultural inner-city settings.

There should be a combination of generic mental health information for the general public, as well as specific information targeting people with mental health problems and their families. It is important to involve all stakeholders in the development and design of information.

Education

There is a need to develop robust, local education programmes in order to promote early recognition of mental health problems and to increase primary care professionals' knowledge and capacity to detect them early. Education should be tailored to the needs of the community – public, professional or postgraduate primary care students – and should include "information about stigma, its impact and the stigmatisation process".[33]

Providers should consider how people with mental health problems would be involved in the design, delivery and evaluation of the educational programmes. For example, a mental health seminar on recovery in persons with schizophrenia, co-taught by a mental health service user and a professional, led to more favourable perceptions of treatment for mental illness.[36]

Education not only tackles negative attitudes towards mental illness but also tackles stigma towards treatment. There is some evidence that increasing people's knowledge about mental illness through courses like "mental health first aid" improves adherence to treatment.[37]

All educational programmes should include evaluation to assess the impact on mental health awareness, and attitudes towards people with mental health problems, including health professionals and the public.

Communication

People with mental health problems are sometimes unclear about the role of primary care within the mental health system. They can feel left out about their treatment plans and decisions directly affecting them, which can reinforce fears about mental health treatment. The Care Programme Approach in secondary care mental health services in England ensures that patients are involved in planning their care. Insurers in the USA will not pay for behavioural health counselling at a primary care site unless a treatment plan is in place and has been signed by the patient, the behavioural health provider and the physician. However, there is no such system for the majority of patients with mental health problems who are only cared for by a primary care provider. Primary care providers can involve patients in their care by keeping them and their families (where appropriate) well informed about all aspects of their care, and collaborating with patients on decisions regarding treatment and referrals to specialist services.

Effective systems and accessible services

It is important to ensure that primary care mental health services are accessible, and timely, without long waiting times. All primary care professionals should have at least basic mental health awareness training, including an awareness of local services, in order to be able to refer patients appropriately.

There need to be clear care pathways, with referral criteria covering the whole mental health system. The more people understand about the mental health system, the less fear and stigma will be attached to mental health problems and services.

Effective non-stigmatizing services could include providing primary care mental health services in other community settings such as community centres, or integrating support services, such as welfare advice, into primary care. This would help "normalize" primary care mental health clinics and hence reduce the stigma associated with them. It would also provide ready access to other support services that patients need in addition to health care, and free up the time that health professionals spend negotiating access to other services.

A project in Bradford, UK placed advisers focusing on debt, housing, employment and immigration rights within GP practices and found that the scheme saved time for GPs and nursing staff, reduced stress levels and improved quality of life for clients.[28]

The Improving Access to Psychological Therapies (IAPT) programme in England has enabled some primary care mental health services to be provided in collaboration with other agencies such as employment and welfare benefits. This would help improve access to both health care and the relevant support services.

Media as allies

The media can be very powerful in influencing public attitudes. Many people who have no contact with anyone with mental health problems tend to get mental health information from the media. The media portrayal of people with mental health problems often focuses on the negative aspects and stereotypes. Primary care commissioners, administrators and providers need to work with the media to portray more positive information about people with mental health problems and mental health services.

It is important to involve the press in anti-stigma campaigns, so that positive stories can be reported about mental health issues and the damaging effects that stigma can have on people with mental health problems. The local press can provide factual information about mental health problems and services, to increase public awareness. There should be universal as well as targeted coverage, depending on local circumstances. All relevant media should be utilized depending on local circumstances – print, radio, television and the Internet. For example, the media can be used to target radio or television stations that are popular with particular target groups, such as young people, men or specific ethnic groups.

Citizenship and participation

This requires service providers and professionals to identify opportunities to involve service users as partners in decision-making regarding service provision. It should be a core aspect of primary care mental health service provision, with funding set aside for participation. The active involvement of service users influences the way services are provided, helping to improve access and reduce stigma.

What the primary care workforce needs to look like to achieve the best outcomes

The New Ways of Working (NWW) for Primary Care subgroup in the UK considered evidence from a number of sources and produced a briefing document that recommends key practice and operational changes to improve the effectiveness of the primary care mental health workforce, as shown in Table 3.1.[38]

In addition, the primary care workforce needs to develop new ways of working to be effective at helping people with mental health problems. The NWW group recommends the following new roles for primary care professionals and administrators:

- *GPs* – developing specific skills such as the basics of cognitive-behavioural therapy (CBT)
- *practice nurses* – screening for anxiety and depression in high-risk groups
- *practice administrators/receptionists* – facilitating access to appointments with professionals and responding empathetically to those experiencing distress. Practice receptionists are often the first primary care staff that patients come into contact with. It is important that they have a basic mental health awareness training, to help them communicate appropriately with people with mental health problems.

Other professionals attached to general practice teams include:

- *health visitors* – using screening tools to recognize and manage a parent's mental distress in the postnatal period
- *district nurses* – screening for and identifying mental health problems such as depression and dementia
- *midwives* – incorporating psychosocial interventions in working with prenatal women.

Table 3.1 Key changes that would make a real difference to the primary care mental health workforce	
Five practice changes	**Five operational changes**
1 Increase confidence in mental health issues for primary care team members	1 Develop career pathways for primary care mental health workers
2 Develop more flexible use of mental health specialists	2 Support the development of networks to promote self-management and recovery for those with enduring mental or physical health problems
3 Increase the use of low-intensity interventions	3 Encourage partnership working between voluntary and statutory services along care pathways, including health and social care
4 Adopt a single patient record for specialists and generalists working together in primary care	4 Enable the commissioning of flexible mental health services based on local need
5 Develop referral pathways from primary care for people with long-term mental health problems	5 Develop a mental health and personal well-being component of education within the core curriculum of professionals who may go on to work in primary care

Source: New Ways of Working. *New ways of working for primary care in mental health* (http://www.newwaysofworking.org.uk/content/view/56/467/).[38]

Developing these roles will improve the effectiveness of the primary care workforce in managing mental disorders, help to improve access to mental health care within primary care, and reduce the stigma associated with mental disorders.

The necessary key stakeholders to deliver the "gold-standard" approach

As already mentioned, tackling stigma is the responsibility of everyone – administrators, service providers, health professionals, NGOs, media, patients and the general public.

Through effective monitoring, evaluation and feedback from patients, primary care commissioners and administrators need to ensure that the services are inclusive and do not reinforce stigma. Commissioners and administrators should also work with service providers, the media and NGOs to raise mental health awareness within the general public. Primary care professionals should ensure that patients with mental health problems are not disadvantaged in accessing services, care or treatment because of their mental illness.

NGOs usually work with local communities and are best placed to develop community outreach anti-stigma programmes. These should include culturally appropriate workshops designed to increase awareness of mental health problems and challenge stigma.

The implications of stigma for mental health promotion

Tackling stigma should be at the heart of mental health promotion, as stigma can be a barrier to successful mental health promotion. Mental health promotion should aim at increasing people's knowledge and understanding of mental health issues. It should be culturally appropriate and challenge myths and misconceptions surrounding mental illness and mental health services. WHO notes that:

> Public education and awareness campaigns on mental health should be launched in all countries. The main goal is to reduce barriers to treatment and care by increasing awareness of the frequency of mental disorders, their treatability, the recovery process and the human rights of people with mental disorders.[15]

Overcoming stigma about mental illness through mental health promotion should include children, by involving people with experience of mental health problems in delivering school-based mental health awareness sessions. These sessions should be interactive and encourage children to explore any ideas that they have about mental illness and mental health services.

People from different backgrounds will have different beliefs and understanding of mental well-being. Administrators and providers of mental health promotion interventions should understand these beliefs and how they influence people's attitudes towards mental ill health and help-seeking behaviour. Mental health promotion should then be tailored around the relevant beliefs and understandings.

For example, through a health equity audit, mental health commissioners and service providers in Tower Hamlets, an inner-city borough in London, UK, identified poorer access to primary care mental health services among the minority ethnic groups (predominantly Muslims) compared to the indigenous white population. Further qualitative work with Muslim groups identified stigma as an important barrier to accessing services.

To help understand the mental health needs of the Muslim population and improve access to primary care, the primary care trust commissioned mental health awareness training for local faith leaders (who are sometimes the first source of help for people experiencing mental health problems) and involved them in developing mental health promotion resources for the community. This was complemented by workshops for faith leaders and mental health professionals to share ideas. Understanding attitude to mental ill health and challenging stigma were important parts of the training and workshops. The faith leaders involved in these sessions gave positive feedback about the sessions.

Strategies for overcoming stigma should also include training for people with mental health problems, to enable them to challenge stigma, and to deliver mental health awareness sessions.

Steps for successfully tackling stigma in primary care

Interventions to tackle stigma must be implemented strategically. Tackling stigma is not a one-time event. It must involve a number of activities or interventions implemented over a sustained period, and requires the availability and sustainability of resources. The following list is a nice summary of a practical step-by-step strategy for tackling stigma.[33]

1 Make all primary care partners aware of stigma and its effects.
2 Investigate levels of stigma and its impact at local level.
3 Gain support at a strategic level.
4 Develop an action plan.
5 Enhance areas of strength first.
6 Incrementally implement the remaining elements of the framework.

The first step in tackling stigma is to ensure that all relevant stakeholders understand stigma and its effects on people with mental health problems and their families. It is then important to work with stakeholders, including people with mental health problems, family members and caregivers, to establish how stigma affects their lives and health-seeking behaviours. To gain support at a strategic level, there is a need to embed tackling stigma in all relevant strategies and policies. Based on the needs, an action plan should be developed that enhances areas of strength first, then incrementally addresses the remaining needs of the community.

WHO provides case examples of advocacy work in low-, medium- and high-income countries leading to stigma reduction associated with better outcomes for people with mental health problems. For example, a local NGO in Mexico focused on the rehabilitation of persons with mental disorders, and utilized several methods for advocacy.[5] It "denounced human rights violations, promoted consumer participation in mental health facilities, implemented pilot projects and provided community services. It is also an example of advocacy that has influenced policy-makers, leading to changes in mental health policy, the direct collaboration of members of a nongovernmental organization with government". This made it possible to improve the quality of life of patients.

A call to action for citizens, society, and health-care practitioners

WHO's 2008 publication *Primary health care – now more than ever* supports the need for resourcing and development of primary care globally.[39] We can no longer afford to neglect primary care or service-user needs and perspectives. The WHO/Wonca 2008 publication, *Integrating mental health into primary care: a global perspective,*[7] enables us to focus sharply on the problems and suffering that people with mental health problems are subject to when mental health is not part of primary care. It celebrates the success and voices of service users when mental health integration is achieved.

All stakeholders must work together to deliver the goals and aspirations of all service users and their families. We call on countries, governments, individuals, human rights groups and other NGOs, academies and colleges of family medicine, and nursing and other health-care professionals to come together and be the champions of mental health. Together we can publicly recognize that mental health is essential for achieving person-centred holistic primary care in the following ways:

- by demanding that mental health is an essential part of primary care and family medicine, and that mental health should be included in all primary health-care services
- by providing mental health care in the least restrictive setting and recognizing that family and community provide the majority of support to patients with mental health disorders and are where mental health interventions and treatment should take place
- by acknowledging that psychological, social and environmental interventions and resources are essential components of mental health for all, and that access should be promoted for all
- by ensuring that mental health training is facilitated and made available to all who work within primary health care

- by guaranteeing the availability of essential pharmacological therapy for those mental health patients who truly require it
- by demanding an end to mental health stigma and discrimination, and monitoring and protecting the human rights of all people at all times
- by facilitating the provision and support of specialist services for those whose needs cannot be met in primary care alone
- by guaranteeing continuity of care for those with mental health difficulties, through primary care.

The WMHDay 2009 campaign provided grassroots organizations around the world with an opportunity to reaffirm the advantages that primary care mental health integration can provide. Through the campaign, thousands of citizens, advocates, service users, families, health-care professionals and public policy-makers were informed about these pressing needs and issues. The landmark reports referred to in this chapter, including the WHO *Primary health care – now more than ever,* WMHDay report[39] and the WHO/Wonca *Integrating mental health into primary care: a global perspective,*[7] provide background and guidance for effective education and advocacy for change in the way that mental and physical health-care funding and service delivery can be improved in countries across the globe. The blueprint for change has been well developed and the time for change has come! This call to action recognizes that mental health for all cannot be achieved solely by an individual, nor can it be achieved through the existing 'separate but unequal' systems of physical and mental health care that exist in most countries today. By communicating and working together, by adopting the principles of respect, dignity and humanity across all sectors and groups, strength can be found and progress achieved.

Primary care provides the first formal contact with health services in most health systems. Those who work in primary care should see themselves as ambassadors and advocates for service users and act accordingly. Those who commission primary care services must include mental health as a key component of the services they commission and must recognize and fund the important components of self-care and advocacy.

Remember that mental ill health can affect anybody. It could be you or your loved ones. We all deserve the best possible care.

What should I do now?

This chapter provides all of those who are engaged in, or who are concerned with, efforts to improve integration of mental health services into primary health clinics the chance to be heard.

- *Service users, their families, carers and advocates*: discuss this *call to action* with all those who provide health care in your area, including health professionals, politicians, charities and other NGOs. Ask them how they intend to use this call to action to encourage policy-makers and health-care planners to focus on these issues. Demand to participate in how your health care is being designed and delivered, as it is your right and entitlement.
- *Primary health-care practitioners and teams*: benchmark yourselves against the principles included in this *call to action*. Develop practical action plans to address identified gaps.
- *Professional colleges*: include your members and benchmark yourselves against the principles included in this *call to action*. Develop practical action plans to address identified gaps.
- *Those who commission health services*: urgently review your service specifications and ensure that contracts embrace the principles of this *call to action*.
- *Governments, politicians and opinion leaders*: demand that those who commission and procure primary health-care services demonstrate to you that they are engaging with the principles of this *call to action*.

Conclusion and future opportunities

On the whole, life expectancy worldwide is improving. Yet, with this increase in longevity has come an increase in the number of people with mental health problems. The gains in mental health care have not kept pace and are patchy. Many people who suffer from mental health problems continue to suffer stigma and discrimination. They have poor access to both physical health care and mental health care and their life expectancy is worse.

Stigma is a very important barrier to accessing mental health services in both high- and low-income countries. In addition to advocacy, a number of strategies have been presented. Even though this chapter is about primary care mental health, the approach taken goes beyond primary care. This is to ensure that mental health awareness and advocacy are embedded within the general population.

Strategies and interventions to tackle stigma should aim to challenge people's fears and misconceptions about mental illness and mental health services. Increasing the effectiveness of the primary care workforce in dealing with mental health issues will increase patients' confidence and help reduce stigma.

There can be no health without mental health, and nobody is immune to mental illness. All of us need to work together to address the gap between reality and aspiration, the gap between the "haves and the have nots" and the stigma and discrimination that continues to dog us, both as professionals and service users with an interest in mental health.

Further reading

- Beaglehole R et al. Improving the prevention and management of chronic disease in low-income and middle-income countries: a priority for primary health care. *The Lancet*, 2008, 372:940–949.
- Lancet Global Mental Health Group. Scaling up services for mental disorders – a call for action. *The Lancet*, 2007, 370:1241–1252.
- Walley J et al. Primary health care: making Alma-Ata a reality. *The Lancet*, 2008, 372:1001–1007.

References

1   Byrne P. Psychiatric stigma. *British Journal of Psychiatry*, 2001, 178:281–284.

2   *Cambridge Dictionaries Online* (http://dictionary.cambridge.org/dictionary/british/discrimination_1?q= discrimination, accessed 23 November 2011).

3   Bipolar World. *History of mental illness and early treatment in a nutshell* (http://www.bipolarworld.net/ Bipolar%20Disorder/History/history.html, accessed 2 November 2011).

4   *Mental Health: a report of the surgeon general* (http://www.surgeongeneral.gov/library/mentalhealth/ chapter1/sec1.html, accessed 2 November 2011).

5   *Advocacy for mental health*. Geneva, World Health Organization, 2003 (http://www.who.int/mental_ health/resources/en/Advocacy.pdf, accessed 2 November 2011).

6   *Declaration of Alma-Ata*. International Conference on Primary Health Care, Alma-Ata USSR, 6–12 September 1978 (http://www.who.int/hpr/NPH/docs/declaration_almaata.pdf, accessed 2 November 2011).

7   World Health Organization and Wonca. *Integrating mental health into primary care. A global perspective*. Geneva, World Health Organization, 2008.

8   Movement for Global Mental Health. Lancet series on global mental health (http://www. globalmentalhealth.org/articles.php?id=16&menu_id=0, accessed 2 November 2011).

9   *World Mental Health Day October 10, 2009. Mental health in primary care: enhancing treatment and promoting mental health*. Woodbridge, VA, World Federation for Mental Health, 2009 (http://www. wfmh.org/WMHD%2009%20Languages/ENGLISH%20WMHD09.pdf, accessed 2 November 2011).

10 Patel V et al. Treatment and prevention of mental disorders in low-income and middle-income countries. *The Lancet*, 2007, 370:991–1005.

11 Wiley-Exley F. Evaluations of community mental health care in low- and middle-income countries: a 10 year review of the literature. *Social Science and Medicine*, 2007, 64:1231–1241.

12 Moussavi S et al. Depression, chronic disease, and decrements in health: results from the World Health Survey. *The Lancet*, 2007, 370:851–858.

13 Price D et al. The treatment of anxiety disorders in a primary care setting. *Psychiatric Quarterly*, 2007, 7:31–45.

14 World Health Organization. *Mental disorders in primary care*. Geneva, World Health Organization, 2008 (http://whqlibdoc.who.int/hq/1998/WHO_MSA_MNHIEAC_98.1.pdf, accessed 2 November 2011).

15 *The World Health Report 2001. Mental health: new understanding, new hope*. Geneva, World Health Organization, 2001 (http://www.who.int/whr/2001/en/whr01_en.pdf accessed 2 November 2011).

16 Schirmer JM, Montegut AJ. *Behavioural medicine in primary care: a global perspective*. Oxford, Radcliffe Publishers, 2009.

17 Patel V. *Where there is no psychiatrist: a mental health care manual*. London, Gaskell, 2003.

18 *Merriam-Webster dictionary* (www.merriam-webster.com/dictionary/resilience, accessed 2 November 2011).

19 *5-2-1-0 The pediatric obesity clinical decision support chart*. Elk Grove Village, IL, American Academy of Pediatrics, 2007.

20 Kopes-Kerr C. Preventive health: time for change. *American Family Physician*, 2010, 82:610–614.

21 Pfifferling JH, Gilley K. Overcoming compassion fatigue. *Family Practice Management*, 2000, 7:39–45.

22 American Psychological Association. *The road to resilience*. http://www.apa.org/helpcenter/road-resilience.aspx, accessed 2 November 2011).

23 Adonlsek KM, Cefalo RC. *LIFE curriculum: learning to address impairment and fatigue to enhance patient safety* (http://www.lifecurriculum.info/default.aspx, accessed 2 November 2011). 2011).

24 Strosahl, K. *The primary behavioural care services practice manual (version 2.0). Produced for the Behavioral Health Optimization Project. US Air Force Medical Operations Agency Population Health Support Division (AFMOA/SGZZ). Office for Prevention and Health Services Assessment (OPHSA)*. Texas, Brooks AFB, 2002 (http://www.integratedprimarycare.com/Air%20Force%20Manual/primary%20care%20practice%20manual.pdf, accessed 2 November 2011).

25 Wrigley et al. Role of stigma and attitudes towards help-seeking from a general practitioner for mental health problems in a rural town. *Australian and New Zealand Journal of Psychiatry*, 2005, 39:514–521.

26 Like Minds. Like Mine (http://www.likeminds.org.nz/page/5-Home, accessed 2 November 2011).

27 *Stigma shout: service user and carer experiences of stigma and discrimination*. London, Time to Change, 2008.

28 Social Exclusion Unit. *Mental health and social exclusion*. London: HMSO, 2004.

29 Lauber C et al. Do mental health professionals stigmatize their patients? *Acta Psychiatrica Scandinavica Supplementum*, 2006, 429: 51–59.

30 Thornicroft et al. Global patterns of experienced and anticipated discrimination against people with schizophrenia: a cross-sectional survey. *The Lancet*, 2009, 373:408–415.

31 *Breaking the cycles of fear*. London, The Sainsbury's Centre for Mental Health, 2002.

32 Corrigan PW et al. Challenging two mental illness stigmas: personal responsibility and dangerousness. *Schizophrenia Bulletin*, 2002, 28:293–310.

33 *Tackling stigma: a practical toolkit*. York, National CAMHS Support Service, 2010 (http://www.chimat.org.uk/resource/item.aspx?RID=96731, accessed 2 November 2011).

34 Luty J et al. Effectiveness of Changing Minds campaign factsheets in reducing stigmatising attitudes towards mental illness. *Psychiatric Bulletin*, 2007, 31:381–384.

35 Wolff G et al. Public education for community care. A new approach. *British Journal of Psychiatry*, 1996, 168:441–447.

36 Coodin S, Chisholm F. Teaching in a new key: effects of a co taught seminar on medical students' attitudes toward schizophrenia. *Psychiatric Rehabilitation Journal*, 2001, 24:299–302.

37 Kitchener BA, Jorm AF. Mental health first aid training in a workplace setting: a randomized controlled trial. *BMC Psychiatry*, 2004, 15:23.

38 New Ways of Working. *New ways of working for primary care in mental health* (http://www.newwaysofworking.org.uk/content/view/56/467/, accessed 2 November 2011).

39 *The World Health Report 2008. Primary health care (now more than ever)*. Geneva, World Health Organization, 2008 (http://www.who.int/whr/2008/en/index.html, accessed 2 November 2011).

4 Spirituality in primary care mental health

Anthony Stern and Allan Tasman

> **Key messages**
>
> - Many patients relate better to spiritual concepts than to medical, scientific or psychological concepts.
> - In this light, spiritual language can help build a bridge of trust between doctors and patients.
> - Supporting patients in their spiritual life by being open to what they say about it can be an important element in holistic care and healing.
> - The art of listening well to patients involves its own implicit spiritual dimension.
> - The art of encouragement reinforces the spiritual value of hope in patients' lives, and sayings and stories from sacred traditions can serve as tools that bolster this hope.

And why, after all, may not the world be so complex as to consist of many interpenetrating spheres of reality, which we can approach in alternation by using different conceptions and different attitudes ... On this view religion and science, each verified in its own way from hour to hour and from life to life, would be co-eternal. (William James, *The varieties of religious experience*, 1902, pp.120–121)[1]

Our faith has our humanity as its foundation and our humanity has our faith as its foundation. (Martin Buber, *A believing humanism*, 1969, p. 117)[2]

Introduction

By their very nature, spiritual realities and views elude satisfactory definition, but one succinct attempt refers to spirituality as "the search for existential meaning".[3] A longer attempt calls it "that vast realm of human potential dealing with ultimate purposes, with higher entities, with God, with love, with compassion, with purpose";[3] a third effort names it as "an overarching construct that involves personal beliefs or values that provide a sense of meaning and unity with self, people, nature and universe".[4] Transcending the self and connecting with the other (or Other) beyond oneself are usually seen as central features of spirituality.

Why consider this topic as an important matter for primary care clinicians? There is abundant evidence that the best clinical outcomes occur in the context of a trusting and collaborative doctor–patient relationship. Developing such a relationship depends not only on understanding the illness, but also on understanding *who* is the person with the illness. For many people in every country, the individual defines himself in part by spiritual beliefs.

A spiritual orientation in primary mental health care is holistic and all-encompassing, stretching between the poles of science and religion. It includes psychology but goes beyond its usual borders. Individual clinicians need to find their own comfort level in any conversations with patients about the sacred dimension of life; this position, which will vary from doctor to doctor, arises from an honest assessment of one's own outlook and inclinations.

Spirituality and religion

Spirituality and religion differ, though they overlap. "Spiritual beliefs" arise from the inevitable human search for meaning, and "spirituality" refers to any inclination that seeks an ultimate good or a basic set of beliefs that give meaning to our existence. Thus, spirituality is a universal drive. Religions are more culture-bound and community-oriented modalities, where many individuals participate in common intergenerational beliefs and rituals. Many of us value religion as a way to express the spiritual search and to share it in a communal way. Others have concluded that formal religion is not personally of value, yet still embrace spirituality in some way in their own lives.[3]

The mutual search for healing and wisdom

The basic premise of our discussion is that medical science and the spiritual traditions have always been animated in every culture in the world by *a search for meaning, healing and truth*. Historically this quest has not been explicitly shared, but in the last few decades, these two worlds have discovered each other in an unexpected yet natural set of encounters.[5–22] It could be said that the spiritual impulses stirring in all human beings have run parallel with the aspirations of the scientific community, and that this implicit mutual search has recently grown into a more open and conscious dialogue.[23–44]

At the beginnings of the modern mental health field in the west, Freud tried to steer us as far from the compelling pull of spiritual ideas and experiences as possible, thus establishing a mainstream early 20th century position of antipathy toward religion.[45–49] Other prominent thinkers, however, have been interested in rational and non-rational states of mind as more or less equally valid points of view. William James' 1902 classic, *The varieties of religious experience*,[1] concludes:

> The whole drift of my education goes to persuade me that the world of our present consciousness is only one out of many worlds of consciousness that exist, and that those other worlds must contain experiences which have a meaning for our life also; and that although in the main their experiences and those of this world keep discrete, yet the two become continuous at certain points, and higher energies filter in.[1,50]

Other major figures like Robert Assagioli, Wilfred Bion, Victor Frankl, Eric Fromm, Carl Jung and Abraham Maslow have since echoed this appreciation of a higher power in their own distinct idioms.[51–62] Eastern philosophers and their influences on medicine have embodied these principles for centuries.

The last few decades have now seen the mainstream of psychiatry and psychology in what are considered the western societies shift to a new stance that honours religious thought, where the spiritual dimension has attracted increasing attention among doctors and others in the helping professions (although such concerns have for centuries been considered integral parts of Asian approaches to healing). This can be understood as a return of clinical medicine to its roots in the healing traditions and premodern models of mind and body,[63–77] integrating for us today, at least potentially, the best of science and religion.[78–95] Another way of thinking about this shift is greater consideration being given in western medicine to eastern philosophies.[96,97]

The simple fact that many patients speak the language of religion and spirituality and are invested in finding higher ground in their own lives has been one enormous reason that doctors have reawakened to the legitimacy of spirituality as a component of holistic care. As medicine has moved slowly from a more patriarchal model to a more collaborative alliance between doctor and patient, we have come to appreciate the necessity to meet patients more where they are, not where we wish them to be. Where patients are, quite frequently, involves a fairly strong sense of walking a spiritual path, of being on a spiritual journey.

One distinct example of this patient reality is the worldview of indigenous peoples. They usually rely on traditional healers, even when modern medical care is available, and they often hold beliefs about sacred powers within the natural world, the holy significance of ancestors, and the non-linearity of time that affect their mental and spiritual well-being.[4,64,65,98,99] Both a knowledge and an appreciation of such matters provides a bridge between the world of modern medicine and the world where the patient lives and thinks and suffers.[100]

It should be added that the recent convergence of mental health and spiritual interests can be seen as one instance of our global and ecumenical age. We live at a time when religious denominations in particular, and world cultures in general, have increasingly been opening doors to each other. It makes sense that this process of communication would also flourish across the many traditions that share a common concern for the inner development of human beings.

Where science and religion diverge

Along with the recognition that science and religion are both expressions of the hunger for healing and truth, let us also be aware of the differences between them. First, science remains largely concerned with "what" questions, and the spiritual traditions focus on "why" questions. Science deals with facts, whereas the spiritual life deals with values. This separation grows murkier when we turn to the "facts" of human psychology that are so intertwined with the subjective quest for meaning, yet it still holds as partially valid.[101–104]

Second, scientists and disciples of evidence-based medicine tend to enthrone the power of human reason even today, more than many adherents of a spiritual path. Philosophers and religious writers in particular are fond of reminding us that the human intellect is a great servant but a poor master. In the view of many of them, the mind can fancy itself in control but be in way over its head, as it were; at times, they believe, our rational faculty can be like the sorcerer's apprentice, scrambling to keep up with the magic and mystery all around him, but succeeding quite miserably at keeping it all straight. More scientific types, of course, tend to see all such talk as fuzzy and misleading nonsense.

A third point where the scientific world and the spiritual traditions tend to part company has to do with their attitude toward suffering, loss and death.[105–108] Scientists and other secular humanists often have little use for devoting much attention to the experience of suffering, whereas most spiritual teachings see some value in it, especially in the event where human beings manage to turn and face it. Religious faith of various denominations tends to view loss as a potential doorway into a fuller life, if and when approached in the right spirit.

In this light, health-care clinicians still err mostly in our noble, yet at times misbegotten, attempts to eliminate, or at least reduce, all suffering at all costs. (In end-of-life care, these costs in economic terms are increasingly viewed as unsustainable.) Some individuals with a single-minded religious approach can perhaps, at times, honour these unavoidable facts of life too fervently. Indeed, when clergy and other spiritual leaders err, it usually lies in a unitary focus on suffering and death that does not make room for human joy, creativity and fulfilment, or in a backlash against such rigidity.

In other words, doctors are rightly committed to beating back the claims of death and suffering, whereas more religiously inclined thinkers tend to be aware of the potential inner growth inherent in pain, and in the facing of unsettling facts about self, other, and reality. The mental health field in general, and its early embodiment in the west in Freud's and Jung's schools of thought (and all the branches of therapy that followed), may well be the closest we have come to a mainstream health-care arena where suffering that is dealt with in the right way and under the right circumstances tends to be valued.

To sum up, the two grand cultural forces of science and religion have both grown out of the depths of what it means to be human, and have taken on remarkable lives of their own as our collective life has evolved. Although there have always been attempts to reach a glimmer of a fruitful complementarity, even through their friction, in recent years they have begun to converge in a mutual search for healing and truth. Hence, there is, at present, an unusually strong momentum of ongoing conversation between them. At the same time, distinctions as described above need to be kept in mind. These differences can enhance rather than detract from the dialogue itself.

Implicit and explicit spirituality

As we turn from the abstractions of our introduction to how these trends apply in daily clinical practice, it will be helpful to draw a distinction between *implicit* and *explicit* spirituality. To the extent that what we do as doctors is motivated by the desire to serve and heal other human beings, an implicit spirituality could be said to underlie all our work. Implicit spiritual values are present whenever there is goodness, service, or the reaching for meaning in life. Implicit spirituality is always a good thing. (The particular connection with a sense of meaning is especially relevant in any clinical effort to treat conditions of depression and anxiety, since these both involve a diminished ability to tap into a sense that life has meaning, and these both improve to one degree or another when a sense of meaning or goodness is restored.)

Explicit spirituality is a somewhat other matter, and a trickier one in the clinical situation. Once a conversation with a patient or family member about religion and spirituality becomes explicit, care needs to be taken as to the context and attunement with the patient. At such a moment, an awareness of one's own role and boundaries properly comes into play. Explicit spirituality can be useful and helpful, but to be a positive contribution to an individual's health care, it requires both clinical wisdom and inner wisdom. Mistakes can easily be made when the clinician becomes mired in either over-avoidance or over-involvement in this arena.

One frequently encountered example involves the question of praying with a patient. Under most circumstances, it is safe to say that it crosses a line that is best not crossed to suggest this idea oneself, as a health professional. If, however, a patient asks to pray with you, and if you can assent to this request comfortably, this is an option to be considered.

Rapport building

As described in our introduction, for most of the 20th century, patients who held religious convictions often felt judged by their doctors, particularly in the areas of mental health and psychology, and they generally kept silent about their spiritual life. We are now in a different era, where the ideal of a non-judgemental view of a patient's thoughts and feelings extends naturally to their religiosity as well. When patients sense we support their spiritual journey as an important part of themselves, they feel we are "on their side", and they can communicate more freely about their inner life, including whatever tradition or self-creation provides a sense of meaning for them.

The simplest clarifying questions, like "Do you have spiritual or philosophic beliefs that are meaningful to you, or that help you get through this struggle?", can let patients know that you are open to this side of their lives, and that you care about what brings meaning to their existence. If and when you can take the next step of offering encouragement about the search for meaning that patients are engaged in, then they usually feel all the more confirmed. This applies to the questions as well as the answers that patients live with and live within: their doubts, their convictions and all the shadings of thought and feeling in between these two poles.

Even when there is no overt mention of spirituality, the therapeutic alliance between doctor and patient brings an implicit spiritual dimension into play. The arts of *listening* and *encouragement* provide the main ingredients of the rapport-building process that undergirds this alliance. Indeed, as any doctor already knows, for this reason, they are the foundation of effective clinical care. They also form the basis of a spiritual orientation as well as psychotherapeutic approaches in general.

Caring curiosity leads to listening

Excellent tools are readily available that can guide an interview in a spiritual direction, and the reader is encouraged to study and review them.[109–113] Koenig and Pritchett recommend the mnemonic FICA as a brief screen to be kept in mind: F for faith (do you have a religious faith or belief in something?), I for influence (how do your beliefs influence your life?), C for community (do you belong to a faith-based community?), and A for address (are there spiritual needs to be addressed in the clinical setting?).[114]

But whether explicit spirituality is addressed or not, our taking interest in a patient as a person, even briefly, can work its own quiet magic. At the risk of stating the obvious, we all know what it is like when we ask ourselves, who is this patient sitting here? Who is this person? What is he or she going through? The medical educator Lawrence Dyche identifies caring and curiosity (along with respect) as the core attitudes that can lead to skilful communication with patients.[115] We have all had experiences with this clinical fact: that when *caring curiosity* takes over as the central motive force in our history-taking, the patient is put at ease, and all then tends to flow smoothly in the session. This flow can be remarkable at times. It results from a joining together of heart (hence the *caring*) and head (hence the *curiosity*).

Over the centuries, such a joining has always been one of the goals of spiritual work: to bring heart and head together in harmony.

The art of careful listening

Especially when we are involved with counselling our patients, or with anything approaching psychotherapy, *the art of careful listening* makes up much of what we do. Even when taking a medical history or trying to obtain further clarification of a physical symptom, this is the case.

Historically, the different sacred traditions over the centuries, and the more recent psychotherapeutic schools, have had much to say about the fine art of listening, of opening to another human being in dialogue.[116–118]

To become aligned and in tune with a patient is similar to the process of learning to appreciate a piece of music. When we listen with a careful and carefree spirit to a musical selection, we begin to catch its rhythm. Then, and only then, might we be ready to dance with the music, or to join the music in song.

For the same reason, listening carefully to a patient needs to come first and to be kept as the first priority. As and when this is established, speaking can come from a place of greater empathy and attunement.[9,119]

Listening, as we are using this word, means more than listening with the two ears. The mystical writers of various traditions speak of listening with the ears of the heart. For instance, the Sufi poet Rumi refers us to "the ear at the center of the chest".[120] Theodor Reik, one of Freud's direct disciples, calls this fine tuning "listening with the third ear".[121]

Listening includes listening to oneself, to one's own responses, to one's own thoughts and feelings.

One of the rarer things about listening is the ability to continue to listen well even as we speak. We tend to get lost in the active "doing" of speaking and thereby lose the receptive sensitivity of the listening stance. To aspire to keep both listening and speaking alive at the same time is a highly worthwhile aspect of our own inner work in the clinical setting. We can help our patients in deeper ways as we develop this art.

When listening, we become more and more attuned, and this simple act can begin to take on an implicit sacred dimension, as suggested by the I–Thou relation described by Martin Buber: "I–Thou" arises when two people truly "connect".[122–125]

Careful listening implies being more fully in the present and more fully present to the other.[126–128] In this light, the following words from Buber are worth pondering: "Being true to the being in which and before which I am placed is the one thing that is needful".[129]

Eugene Gendlin has developed a method called *focusing*, which is one systematic way for clinicians and patients alike to learn this art of being present, of listening with the ears of the heart. As a colleague of Carl Rogers at the University of Chicago, Gendlin conducted research on what works in psychotherapy. He discovered that the most critical variable was how well a given patient could tune into a *felt body sense* of his or her situation. Based on this finding, he worked out a series of steps for people to learn this inner skill.[130–133] This can be learnt in a stepwise manner and can be applied in our own practices as one method of stepwise care.

Let's conclude this overview of careful listening with two further quotations to mull over. The first is from the Harvard psychoanalyst Elvin Semrad: "If you can't sit with the patient until he can feel it in his own body, you're in the wrong business".[134] The second is another passage from Buber: "To be aware of a person . . . means to perceive the dynamic center which stamps his every utterance. . . . Such an awareness . . . is only possible when I step into an elemental relation with the other, that is, when he becomes present to me".[135]

The art of encouragement

We have already pointed out that listening and encouragement comprise much of what we do as doctors. In fact, these are major tools for any healer, whether a trained health professional or otherwise. In the religious world, this would include pastors, pastoral counsellors, and spiritual teachers of all sorts, including saints and sages.

Any form of encouragement based on concern for the other is implicitly spiritual, especially one that is grounded in careful listening and empathy. Effective encouragement could well be said to bolster the other's sense of faith, in the most generic use of that word.[136]

"Encouragement" is actually a vast topic that may include far more than may first appear to the reader. One word of caution brings us back to careful listening and being fully present to the patient: as most psychotherapists learn in their training, supportive words can easily take on a tinge of impatience, as if the clinician is saying, "Now pull yourself together, look on the bright side, things could be a lot worse". If we are not fully accepting of a patient's fear or pain, the tone and content of our encouraging efforts will transmit this lack of compassion. (How often, for instance, are many of us tempted to interrupt a patient's bout of tears, rather than being present and letting them happen?) Often the most helpful thing one can say is little or nothing; when we listen more and speak less, the patient can be left with a greater sense of being understood, accepted and supported. There is no hard and fast rule here, by any means; but experimenting with "less is more" can lead to deeper levels of non-judgemental listening.

As we offer support related to spirituality, it pays to be attentive to healthy and unhealthy factors in the inner life of the patient. Pargament,[35] as well as Josephson and Peteet,[137] distinguish protective coping mechanisms from problem areas in religion and spirituality. Rizzuto describes one common difficulty: when patients see God as punitive, this often reflects an upbringing by punishment-prone parents or other caregivers.[138]

While there are many instances where religion works well or poorly in people's lives, most of the time we can discern some mixture of elements; it is rarely a case of either/or. Along these lines, we frequently encounter the situation where a patient has a religious worldview that brings with it some dismissal of medical or psychological thinking. For example, a patient may be inhibited to discuss symptoms of depression or suicidality openly, or even to be clearly aware of them. Clinicians need to recognize that psychiatric problems can be masked by outright and subtle taboos, as well as subcultural factors in general.

At times, if the doctor has comfort speaking of the divine, it may make sense to make a sort of bridging manoeuvre. Specifically, here is a sample of potential comments in this vein: "Strange as it may seem, perhaps God has brought this medicine to you, to help you on your healing journey"; "I know it may seem unlikely, but is it possible that the higher power has intended this meeting? Whatever the reasons, maybe one of them is for you to get help"; "You have heard the saying, the Lord works in mysterious ways? Maybe the fact that we're talking now is one of those mysterious ways"; "The Lord works in all kinds of ways. Perhaps that includes a little talk therapy". Needless to say, each health professional needs to come up with a particular version of what feels most right to say in such circumstances; these possibilities can give some sense of the ballpark to place oneself in.

This point leads to an overarching consideration that cannot be stressed too strongly: while writings like this chapter can offer general and specific recommendations, every clinician needs to find his or her own way. In any case, what we say to encourage patients is inevitably founded upon our own worldview, as well as our own clinical understanding.[112,137,139,140] It does make sense to think through our beliefs and our wishes regarding the engagement with patients about spirituality. Peteet offers a useful framework for such self-reflection.[112] Even when we improvise in the clinical setting, honesty with ourselves about our own comfort zone is an indispensable guide.

How do we listen to another, especially someone in distress? How do we re-invigorate someone's flagging sense of hope through an empathic, encouraging stance? These two related arts can draw upon recent scientific findings, but they also rely on the inner work practised in various traditions over the centuries. We would do well to study them.

The art of encouragement: a few recommendations for interventions involving explicit spirituality

At times, it may be appropriate to offer encouragement in explicitly spiritual terms, if and when the patient has conveyed something about a religious or philosophical understanding of his struggle. The following is a small "grab-bag" of suggestions, with, once again, the caveat that some ideas, methods, schools and techniques may fit your own style as well as the clinical situation, while many will not.

- If you know 12-step language from the alcoholics anonymous (AA) programme, or offshoots of AA, consider using it when appropriate with someone who relates to this language.

- If there is a specific school of therapy or spiritual practice you know about, you can discuss an idea from that source that relates to the patient's situation.
- If you are drawn to the literature of the spiritual traditions, consider sharing stories, sayings and poems from this world in your clinical work, when appropriate.

In addition to the illustrations offered in the previous section ("The art of encouragement"), the following are four examples of sayings that AS (the first chapter author) has used at times.

The first is usually well known and appreciated by patients who have been in 12-step programmes like AA or Narcotics Anonymous (NA):

> God grant me the serenity to accept the things I cannot change, The courage to change the things I can, and the wisdom to know the difference. (*The serenity prayer*, written by theologian Reinhold Neibuhr, 1987)[141]

> If I am not for myself, who will be for me?
> If I am only for myself, what am I?
> If not now, when? (a well-known saying of Rabbi Hillel)[142]

For spiritually-oriented patients who are struggling with overwhelming guilt or shame, I often refer them to the counsel of Mother Teresa of Calcutta:

> Let's allow that [our mistakes, our guilt] to help us grow closer to God. Let's tell him humbly, "I know I shouldn't have done this, but even this failure I offer to you".[143]

The last saying is paraphrased from the spiritually oriented psychiatrist Thomas Hora:

> Some people see the glass as half-empty, others as half-full. But maybe it's just best to be grateful for the water, no matter how much it fills up the glass.[144]

Here is one example of a spiritual story used by AS. I have found it especially helpful on occasion when speaking with angry teenagers, sometimes with their family members present. (Teenage boys like stories about warriors!)

> A samurai warrior travels to the Zen master and bows to him. "Tell me, master, is there a heaven and a hell?" The master looks at his visitor and replies, "Once upon a time, the samurai were a noble tradition. But I can see from your rude manners, it has gone terribly downhill". The samurai cannot believe his ears. Where a moment before he was bowing, now his sword is already held high, glittering in the sun, and the Zen master is about to pay with his life for his insult. But the split second before being beheaded, he declares, "Right here and right now you have opened the gate of hell". The samurai takes this in, and his face relaxes slowly from its mask of rage, and slowly relaxing now from the shame underneath the rage … dumbfounded, he returns the sword to its sheath. Then the master says, "Right here and right now, you have opened the gate of heaven".[145,146]

- For terminally ill patients and their family members, you can provide a CD resource of inspiring statements ("spoken wisdom") that are set to music entitled *Graceful passages*. This CD features Thich Nhat Hanh, Elizabeth Kubler-Ross, and other familiar teachers. It can be applied to any difficult transition, not only death. Go to www.wisdomoftheworld.com. (The creators of *Graceful passages* offer related resources, including one CD entitled *Healing your life after the death of a loved one* and another called *Care for the journey, a self-renewal tool for health-care professionals*.)
- Relaxation techniques with a non-sectarian spiritual component to them can be taught to patients. (Good resources for guided meditation CDs include Dean Sluyter (www.deansluyter.com) and Tara Brach (www.tarabrach.com). If you Google Tara Brach beliefnet, you will find a downloadable meditation by this teacher, called *A moment of calm*.)
- If you are already inclined to prayer, you may wish to consider setting aside time when you are alone to pray for your patients. If you are drawn to meditation, you may wish to take time to meditate over them.

Two case examples

More often than not, patients come to us with a spiritual worldview. As we have stressed above, if we take an open stance to these beliefs, they can enter meaningfully into our sessions. The two cases that follow not only provide a sense of how this can happen, but they also help to drive home the central importance of careful listening and encouragement that we have emphasized in the chapter thus far. They also put this emphasis into fuller perspective.

These two cases present two quite different clinical situations. They may not apply entirely to most primary care situations, but they reinforce some of the key points we have made. In both cases, we have avoided many details about specific *Diagnostic and Statistical Manual of Mental Disorders* (DSM) diagnostic categories or psychotherapeutic terminology, as these are beyond the purview of this chapter overview. (Both patients were seen by AS.)

Case-study 1

Ms W is a 52-year-old survivor of a traumatic marriage. Her husband had abused her physically and mentally, and she had left him 10 years ago. She has relied heavily on her Christian faith to survive emotionally, both during the active abuse and afterwards. She shows very little interest in any way of looking at her problems except as tests of her faith, yet she had developed a good therapeutic alliance with her primary care doctor in the clinic over a number of months (Dr C), because of the doctor's caring help in relation to the patient's medical problems. Dr C had also listened supportively to her stories of abuse, deepening the patient's trust.

Nonetheless, Ms W described such consistent symptoms of anxiety, agoraphobia, insomnia and paranoia, that an attempt was made to refer her to the social worker therapist and myself. This initially failed, but when she came to see Dr C next, I joined the session. (For some hours each week, I am co-located at the clinic.) Nearly immediately, the patient announced that she only trusted in God, not in people, after all she had been through. When I motioned to her doctor and asked, "What about her? Do you trust her?", Ms W was happy to say that Dr C was the single exception. I appealed to the idea of teamwork, on two levels: "Well, Dr C and I are a team, and she has asked me to see you . . . Also, I'd like to think that we are both on God's team, to try to help you in your work to get over the pain and fear you still feel; do you think that is possible?" Ms W liked this idea, but she wanted to make it clear that she is not sick. I responded, "No one is saying you are sick; it's just that we are here to offer some help in your own healing, your own spiritual journey, in relation to all the pain you have been through". These comments provided some tenuous common ground between the patient and the mental health-care world. Where before Ms W was unwilling to see a therapist or a psychiatrist (me), after listening to this appeal, she agreed to go and see us. Her ambivalence and distrust remain, but explicit spiritual language has been a bridge where we can meet halfway. It has given us a beginning, however fragile, for a working alliance.

Here, both listening and encouragement in a spiritual key have served positive roles. An appeal to explicit religious language has been quite crucial for laying a beginning groundwork of rapport.

Case-study 2

Mr T is a 38-year-old former divinity student who had been seeing me for help with his depression for almost 2 years. He was working as a high school English teacher. He dated intermittently but "hadn't found the right woman". He had originally come to me for treatment with antidepressant medication, but after a year was off the antidepressant and no longer nearly as depressed as he had been. Yet he had a basic fear of being happy, a suspicion about what the world would hand him next.

The first clear turning point was when I began to realize that I was nodding along automatically with whatever he was telling me. This clued me into the fact that I was having trouble listening fully. In fact, despite my ideal of wholehearted listening, I felt he was droning on. I realized that I was not indeed wholeheartedly present. (*A crucial piece of listening is listening to yourself, to where **you** are.*)

What he often droned on about was his spiritual life, the openings and synchronicities he experienced on a regular basis. Once I saw my own inattention, my basic intervention was to interrupt him somewhat more frequently, to question and clarify what he was really saying, and once in a while to confront him quite seriously about his behaviours and his feelings.

This went on for several months, with my seeing him every 2 or 3 weeks. Two specific conversations brought our work deeper. One involved his saying he "had taken care of himself" by not returning someone's phone call. I let this slide initially but then caught myself and brought it up again with him 10 minutes later, in the spirit of "let's look carefully at this together". I confronted him gently about what such self-care really meant. Did he need to ignore the other's call in order to feel good? Was there any middle ground he had overlooked? How was he feeling then; how is he feeling now? The patient was defensive initially, but he responded well to a non-judgemental sense of exploration.

The second conversation some months later involved his forthcoming 40th birthday. His mother had died a few months before, and he had pushed aside his grief to a significant degree.

Some friends and family members were planning a bit of a birthday bash for him. He remarked that this was all so trivial, this fuss about himself, and he wished they would put half as much energy into their prayer lives. I asked him if he was feeling down about anything. He shot back, "Yeah, I get down when you give me grief . . . why do you assume I'm down? You cause me to be down". This led to my reminding him of the comments he had made about his birthday party, and his tendency to blame me for feelings he was already expressing. He began to speak of how much he missed his mother, how much he was sorry she wouldn't be there. We turned to considering how much self-celebration and self-transcendence are the same: "When we get over ourselves, we can begin to celebrate everything, including ourselves".

Here we can begin to see more of the complexity in the role of listening as well as the role of religious thinking. When is it good to stop listening, to interrupt and to confront? This case provides one illustration of answers to these questions. The main take-home point is that careful listening does not mean that one always sits back passively and does not remain active in the session. It is all too easy to become *overly* supportive and therefore neither truly supportive nor wholehearted in one's approach.

Further considerations

We began this chapter with the statement that spirituality is holistic and all-encompassing, but then we immediately narrowed the discussion to a focus on the clinical encounter. Let us return to where we started and add that spiritual considerations, like aesthetic ones, touch on everything involved with the primary care clinic, from the architecture and lay-out of space, to the scheduling of patients and doctors and other health professionals; from what kind of music is played in the waiting room, to how community ties are built beyond the clinic walls. From the vast array of concerns, we make the following final recommendations as a brief sample list to stir further thinking.

- Outreach to local clergy to discuss common concerns can be helpful. This can be facilitated by designating one or two clinicians or administrators in this role.

- Community-building efforts can include joint programmes with local houses of worship, whether they be yoga classes, spiritual movies nights, spiritual stories nights, informational seminars, AA groups or other activities.

- The co-location of pastoral counsellors as members of a mental health team in the clinic is highly recommended where feasible. Martial arts instructors can also introduce simple meditative concepts and practices to young people, and martial arts classes located at the clinic, or at least affiliated with it, are another recommended venue.

- An ongoing spiritual discussion group is a possibility worth exploring. One excellent example would be one modelled after the work of Nancy Kehoe, who is both a clinical psychologist and a Catholic nun.[109,147]

- Other groups can involve staff alone or staff and patients together. One suggestion would be a weekly or monthly dream group based on Montague Ullman's pioneering work.[148] Another suggestion would be an intuition-based group involving John Cogswell's method of "Walking in one's shoe's".[149] Along similar lines, "focusing" can also be applied in a group setting.[150]

- Creativity in general, and art and music in particular, can be powerful avenues connected with spirituality. See Barclay Goldstein[151] and Wooden[152] for two of the many potential entry points into this arena.

- If clinic administration is committed to supporting a spiritual component in primary care, even a modest financial outlay for weekend workshops and other trainings would be worthwhile. In any case, clinicians need to know that some investment of time is required in order to develop, refine and keep alive this different vocabulary and skill set, just as it is for any sphere of learning.

Further reading

Three journal issues devoted to spirituality

- Rudnick S, ed. Buddhism and psychoanalysis. *American Journal of Psychoanalysis*, 1999, 59 (1).
- Sperry L, ed. Spirituality and clinical practice. *Psychiatric Annals*, 2000, 30(8).
- Spero MH, Cohen M, Ingram DH, eds. God and psychotherapy. *Journal of the American Academy of Psychoanalysis and Dynamic Psychiatry*, 2009, 37(1).

Other spiritually-oriented publications by the co-authors

- Josephson AM, Nicholi AM, Tasman A. Religion and psychoanalysis: past and present. In: Verhagen P et al., eds. *Religion and psychiatry: beyond boundaries*. New York, World Psychiatric Association/Wiley, 2010:283–304.
- Josephson AM, Peteet JR, Tasman A. Religion and the training of psychotherapists. In: Verhagen P et al., eds. *Religion and psychiatry: beyond boundaries*. New York, World Psychiatric Association/Wiley, 2010:571–586.
- Stern T. The light of faithful awareness. In Cooper P, ed. *Into the mountain stream: psychotherapy and buddhist experience*. New York, Jason, 2007:59–75.
- Stern, T. Psychosis and religious conversion. *Academy Forum*, 2002, 46(1): 10–11.
- Stern A, Stein J. Leboyer's gentle childbirth. *Birth Psychology Bulletin*, 1981, 2:20–28.
- Stern A. The sunflower: confession, silence and forgiveness. Academy Forum, 2009, 53(2):12–14.
- Stern A. An answered prayer. In Dale Salwak D, ed. *The power of prayer*. Novato California, New World Library, 1998.

References 128, 136 and 143 in the reference list that follows are also relevant.

References

1   James W. *The varieties of religious experience*. New York, The Modern Library/Random House, 1902.
2   Buber M. *A believing humanism: gleanings by Martin Buber*, translated by Friedman M. New York, Simon and Schuster, 1969.
3   Zinnbauer B, Pargament K. Religiousness and spirituality. In: R.F. Paloutzian RF, Park CL, eds. *Handbook of the psychology of religion and spirituality*. Guilford, New York, 2005:21–42.
4   Tse S et al. Exploration of Australian and New Zealand indigenous people's spirituality and mental health. *Australian Occupational Therapy Journal*, 2005, 52:181–187.
5   Jones JW. *Contemporary psychoanalysis and religion: transference and transcendence*. New Haven, Yale University Press, 1991.
6   Finn M, Gartner J. *Object relations theory and religion*. Westport, CT, Praeger Publishers, 1992.
7   Friedman MS. *A heart of wisdom: religion and human wholeness*. Albany, New York, State University of New York Press, 1992.
8   Halligan FR, Shea JJ, eds. *The fires of desire: erotic energies and the spiritual quest*. New York, Crossroad, 1992.
9   Rubin J. *Psychotherapy and buddhism: toward an integration*. New York, Plenum Press, 1996.
10   Welwood J, ed. *Awakening the heart: east/west approaches to psychotherapy and the healing relationship*. Boulder, Colorado, Shambhala, 1983.

11   May G. *Will and spirit*. San Francisco, Harper and Row, 1983.

12   Meissner WW. *Psychoanalysis and religious experience*. New Haven, Connecticut, Yale University Press, 1984.

13   Peck MS. *The road less travelled*. New York, Simon and Schuster, 1978.

14   Moore T. *Care of the soul*. New York, Harper Collins, 1992.

15   Epstein M. *Thoughts without a thinker*. New York, Basic Books, 1995.

16   Walsh F, ed. *Spiritual resources in family therapy*. New York, Guilford, 1999.

17   Argyle M. *Psychology and religion: an introduction*. London, Routledge, 2000.

18   Weiner MB, Barbre C, Cooper PC, eds. *Psychotherapy and religion: many paths, one journey*. Lanham, Maryland, Jason Aronson, 2004.

19   Morris K. Oedipal flowers: through poetics to "O". *Psychoanalytic Review*, 2008, 95:501–514.

20   Cooper PC. *The Zen impulse and the psychoanalytic encounter*. London, Routledge, 2009.

21   Jennings P. *Mixing minds: the power of relationship in psychoanalysis and Buddhism*. Boston, Wisdom Publications, 2010.

22   Verhagen P et al., eds. *Religion and psychiatry: beyond boundaries*. New York, World Psychiatric Association/Wiley, 2010.

23   Karasu TB. *The art of serenity*. New York, Simon and Schuster, 2002.

24   Shorto R. *Saints and madmen: how pioneering psychiatrists are creating a new science of the soul*. New York, Henry Holt, 1999.

25   Schwartz T. *What really matters: searching for wisdom in America*. New York, Bantam, 1995.

26   Robinson LH, ed. *Psychiatry and religion: overlapping concerns*. Washington DC, American Psychiatric Press, 1986.

27   Lothane Z. *In defense of Schreber: soul murder and psychiatry*. London, Routledge, 1992.

28   Friedman MS, ed. *Martin Buber and the human sciences*. Albany, New York, State University of New York Press, 1996.

29   Kalsched D. *The inner world of trauma: archetypal defenses of the personal spirit*. London: Routledge, 1996.

30   Podvell E. *Recovering sanity*. [Original title, 1990: *The seduction of madness*.] Boulder, Colorado, Shambhala, 2003.

31   Roland A. *Cultural pluralism and psychoanalysis*. New York and London, Routledge, 1996.

32   Miller WR, ed. *Integrating spirituality into treatment: resources for practitioners*. Washington, DC, American Psychological Association Press, 1999.

33   Ulanov A. *Finding space: Winnicott, God, and psychic reality*. Louisville, Westminster John Knox Press, 2001.

34   Koenig HG, ed. *Handbook of religion and mental health*. San Diego, California, Academic Press, 1998.

35   Pargament KI. *Spiritually integrated psychotherapy: understanding and addressing the sacred*. New York, Guilford Press, 2007.

36   Molino A, ed. *The couch and the tree: dialogues in psychoanalysis and Buddhism*. New York, North Point Press, 1998.

37   Mann DW. *A simple theory of the self*. New York, WW Norton, 1994.

38   Wilber K. *The essential Ken Wilber*. Boulder, Colorado, Shambhala, 1998.

39   Shafranske EP, ed. *Religion and the clinical practice of psychology*. Washington, DC, American Psychological Association, 1996.

40   Sperry L, Shafranske P, eds. *Spiritually oriented psychotherapy*. Washington, DC, American Psychological Association, 2005.

41   Safran J, ed. *Psychoanalysis and Buddhism*. Boston, Wisdom Publications, 2003.

42   Paloutzian RF, Park CL. *Handbook of the psychology of religion and spirituality*. New York, Guilford, 2005.

43   Magid B. *Ordinary mind: exploring the common ground of Zen and psychoanalysis*. Boston, Wisdom Publications, 2005.

44   Nelson JM. *Psychology, religion, and spirituality*. New York, Springer, 2009.

45   Nicholi AM. *The question of God: CS Lewis and Sigmund Freud debate God, love, sex, and the meaning of life*. New York, The Free Press, 2002.

46   Fuller AR. *Psychology and religion*, 4th ed. Lantham, Maryland, Rowfield and Littlefield, 2007.

47   Gay P. *Freud, atheism, and the making of psychoanalysis*. New Haven, Connecticut, Yale University Press, 1987.

48   Kung H. *Freud and the problem of God*, translated by Quinn E. New Haven, Yale University Press, 1979.

49   Verhagen P. General introduction: religion and science. In: Verhagen P, ed. *Religion and psychiatry: beyond boundaries*. New York, World Psychiatric Association/Wiley, 2010:1–10.

50   Barnard GW. *Exploring unseen worlds: William James and the philosophy of mysticism*. Albany, New York, State University of New York Press, 1997.

51   Jung CG. *Memories, dreams, reflections*. New York, Vintage, 1965.

52   Jung CG. The difference between eastern and western thinking. In: Campbell J, ed. *The portable Jung*. New York, Viking, 1971:480–504.

53   Frankl V. *The doctor and the soul*. New York, Vintage Books, 1955.

54   Frankl V. *Man's search for meaning*. New York, Washington Square Press, 1959.

55   Maslow AH. *Religions, values, and peak-experiences*. Columbus, Ohio, Ohio University Press, 1964.

56   Fromm E. Psychoanalysis and Zen Buddhism. In: Molino A, ed. *The couch and the tree*. New York, North Point Press, 1998:65–71.

57   Bion WR. *Cogitations*. London, Karnac, 1992.

58   Symington J, Symington N. *The clinical thinking of Wilfred Bion*. London, Routledge, 1996.

59   Grotstein J. *A beam of intense darkness: Wilfred Bion's legacy to psychoanalysis*. London, Karnac, 2007.

60   Nachmani G. Psychoanalysis and spirituality – catastrophic change and becoming "O". *Journal of the American Academy of Psychoanalysis and Dynamic Psychiatry*, 2009, 37(1):137–152.

61   Assagioli R. *Psychosynthesis*. New York, Penguin, 1971.

62   Assagioli R. *Transpersonal development: the dimension beyond psychosynthesis*. London, Thorsons, 2007.

63   Frank JD. *Persuasion and healing*. Baltimore, Maryland, Johns Hopkins University Press, 1961.

64   Ellenberger H. *The discovery of the unconscious*. New York, Basic Books, 1970.

65   Halifax J. *Shamanic voices: a survey of visionary narratives*. New York, EP Dutton, 1979.

66   Grof S. Realms of the human unconscious. New York, Viking Press, 1975.

67   Dean SR, ed. *Psychiatry and mysticism*. Chicago, Nelson-Hall, 1975.

68   Khan PVI. *Introducing spirituality into counseling and therapy*. Lebanon Springs, New York, Omega Press, 1982.

69   Houston J. *The search for the beloved: journeys in mythology and sacred psychology*. New York, Tarcher/Putnam, 1987.

70   Berends PB. *Coming to life: traveling the spiritual path in everyday life*. New York, Harper and Row, 1990.

71   Fleischman PR. *The healing spirit: explorations in religion and psychotherapy*. St Paul, Minnesota, Paragon House, 1990.

72   Eigen M. *The psychoanalytic mystic*. London, Free Association Books, 1998.

73   Richards PS, Bergin AE. *Handbook of psychotherapy and religious diversity*. Washington, DC, American Psychological Association, 2000.

74   Leder D. *Games for the soul*. New York, Hyperion, 1998.

75   Leder D. *Sparks of the divine: finding inspiration in our everyday world*. Notre Dame, Indiana, Sorin Books/Ave Maria Press, 2004.

76   Miller WR, Delaney HD, eds. *Judeo-Christian perspectives on psychology: human nature, motivation, and change*. Washington, DC, American Psychological Association, 2005.

77   Cooper P, ed. *Into the mountain stream: psychotherapy and Buddhist experience*. Northvale, New Jersey, Jason Aronson, 2007.

78   Low A. *The iron cow of Zen*. Wheaton, Illinois, Quest Books, 1985.

79 Forman RKC, ed. *The innate capacity: mysticism, psychology, and philosophy*. Oxford, Oxford University Press, 1998.

80 Jones JW. *Waking from Newton's sleep: dialogues on spirituality in an age of science*. Eugene, Oregon, Wipf and Stock, 2006. (Don't miss the recommendations for further reading at the end.)

81 Josephson AM, Peteet JR, eds. *Handbook of spirituality and worldview in clinical practice*. Washington, DC, American Psychiatric Publishing, 2004.

82 Farber L. Martin Buber and psychotherapy. In: Schilpp PA, Friedman M, eds. *The philosophy of Martin Buber*. LaSalle, Illinois, Open Court, 1967:577–602.

83 Shainberg D. *The transforming self*. New York, Intercontinental Medical Book Corp, 1973.

84 Fowler JW. *Stages of faith*. New York, HarperCollins, 1981.

85 Comfort A. *Reality and empathy: physics, mind, and science in the 21st century*. Albany, New York, State University of New York Press, 1984.

86 Loder J. *The transforming moment*. New York, Harper & Row, 1981.

87 Loder J. *The logic of the spirit: human development in theological perspective*. San Francisco: Jossey-Bass, 1998.

88 Boehnlein JK, ed. *Psychiatry and religion: the convergence of mind and spirit*. Washington, DC, American Psychiatric Press, 2000.

89 McCullough ME, Pargament KI, Thoresen CE, eds. *Forgiveness: theory, research, and practice*. New York, Guilford Press, 2000.

90 Goleman D. *Destructive emotions: a scientific dialogue with the Dalai Lama*. New York, Bantam Dell, 2003.

91 Boorstein S, ed. *Transpersonal psychotherapy*. Albany, New York, State University of New York Press, 1996.

92 Wilber K, Engler J, Brown D, eds. *Transformation of consciousness: conventional and contemplative perspectives on human development*. Boston, Shambhala, 1986.

93 Gilkey L. *Nature, reality and the sacred: the nexus of science and religion*. Minneapolis, Fortress Press, 1993.

94 Morrison NK, Severino SK. *Sacred desire: growing in compassionate living*. West Conshohocken, Pennsylvania, Templeton Foundation Press, 2009.

95 Jeeves M, Brown WS. *Neuroscience, psychology and religion: illusions, delusions, and realities about human nature*. West Conshohocken, Pennsylvania, Templeton Foundation Press, 2009.

96 Watts AW. *Psychotherapy east and west*. New York, Pantheon, 1961.

97 Aurobindo G. *The life divine*. New York, Sri Aurobindo Library, 1949.

98 Njenga F, Nguithi A, Gatere S. Psychiatry and African religion. In: Verhagen P et al., eds. *Religion and psychiatry: beyond boundaries*. New York, World Psychiatric Association/Wiley, 2010:143–158.

99 Appiah KA. *In my father's house: Africa in the philosophy of culture*. Oxford, Oxford University Press, 1992.

100 Verhagen P, Cox J. Multicultural education and training in religion and spirituality. In: Verhagen P et al., eds. *Religion and psychiatry: beyond boundaries*. New York, World Psychiatric Association/Wiley, 2010:587–614.

101 Polanyi M. *Personal knowledge*. Chicago, Illinois, University of Chicago Press, 1958.

102 Maslow AH. *The psychology of science*. Washington, DC, Henry Regnery, 1970.

103 Low A. *The butterfly's dream: in search of the roots of Zen*. Boston, Tuttle, 1993.

104 Low A. *Creating consciousness*. Ashland, Oregon, White Cloud Press, 2002.

105 Young-Eisendrath P, Muramoto S. *The gifts of suffering*. Reading, Massachusetts, Addison-Wesley Publishing Company, 1996.

106 Kramer P. *Against depression*. New York, Viking/Penguin, 2005.

107 Davies J. *The importance of suffering*. London, Routledge, 2011.

108 Davies J. The rationalization of suffering. *Harvard Divinity Bulletin*, 2011, Winter/Spring:48–56.

109 Kehoe N. *Wrestling with our inner angels*. San Francisco, Jossey-Bass/Wiley, 2009.

110 Josephson AM, Peteet JR. Talking with patients about spirituality and worldview: practical interviewing techniques and strategies. *The Psychiatric Clinics of North America*, 2007, 30: pp.181–197.

111 Josephson AM, Wiesner I. Therapeutic implications of worldview. In: Josephson AM, Peteet JR, eds. *Handbook of spirituality and worldview in clinical practice.* Washington, DC, American Psychiatric Publishing, 2004:15–30.

112 Peteet JR. Therapeutic implications of worldview. In: Josephson AM, Peteet JR, eds. *Handbook of spirituality and worldview in clinical practice.* Washington, DC, American Psychiatric Publishing, 2007:47–62.

113 Griffith JL, Griffith ME. *Encountering the sacred in psychotherapy: how to talk with people about their spiritual lives.* New York, Guilford, 2002.

114 Koenig HG, Pritchett J. Religion and psychotherapy. In: Koenig HG, ed. *Handbook of religion and mental health.* San Diego: California, Academic Press, 1998.

115 Dyche L. Interpersonal skill in medicine: the essential partner of verbal communication. *Journal of General Internal Medicine,* 2007, 22:1035–1039.

116 Lindahl K. *The sacred art of listening.* Woodstock, Vermont, Skylight Paths, 2002.

117 Steidl-Rast D. *A listening heart.* New York, Crossroad, 1999.

118 O'Hara N. *Just listen.* New York, Broadway Books, 1997.

119 Karasu TB. *Wisdom in the practice of psychotherapy.* New York, Basic Books, 1992.

120 Barks C, Green M. *The illuminated rumi.* New York, Broadway Books, 1997.

121 Reik T. *Listening with the third ear.* New York, Farrar, Straus, 1952.

122 Buber M. *I and thou.* New York, Charles Scribner's Sons, 1958.

123 Buber M. *Between man and man.* New York, MacMillan, 1965.

124 Friedman MS. *Martin Buber: the life of dialogue,* 4th edn. London, Routledge, 2002.

125 Agassi JB, ed. *Martin Buber on psychology and psychotherapy.* Syracuse, New York, Syracuse University Press, 1999.

126 Tolle E. *The power of now.* Novato, California, New World Library, 1999.

127 Almaas AH. *The unfolding now: realizing your true nature through the practice of presence.* Boulder, Colorado, Shambhala, 2008.

128 Stern A. The narrow ridge: insights from Zen, Judaism, and psychoanalysis. *Academy Forum,* 2006, 50:6–10.

129 Buber M. *Pointing the way.* New York, Harper and Row, 1957.

130 Gendlin ET. *Focusing.* New York, Bantam, 1981.

131 Gendlin ET. *Focusing-oriented psychotherapy: a manual of the experiential method.* New York, Guilford, 1996.

132 Hinterkopf E. *Integrating spirituality into counseling: a manual for using the experiential focusing method.* Alexandria, Virginia, American Counseling Association, 1998.

133 Campbell P, McMahon E. *Biospirituality: focusing as a way to grow.* Chicago, Loyola University Press, 1985.

134 Semrad E. In: Rako S, Maxer H, eds. *Semrad: the heart of a therapist.* S. Rako, H. Mazer (eds.) Northvale, New Jersey, Jason Aronson, 1980:107.

135 Buber M. *The knowledge of man: a philosophy of the interhuman.* Atlantic Highlands, New Jersey, Humanities Press International, 1988.

136 Stern A. Faith and denial. *Journal of the American Academy of Psychoanalysis,* 1996, 24:545–554.

137 Josephson AM, Peteet JR. (2004). Worldview in diagnosis and case formulation. In: Josephson AM, Peteet JR, eds. *Handbook of spirituality and worldview in clinical practice.* Washington, DC, American Psychiatric Publishing, 2004:31–46.

138 Rizzuto AM.*The birth of the living god: a psychoanalytic study.* Chicago, University of Chicago Press, 1979.

139 Nicholi AM. Introduction: definition and significance of a worldview. In: Josephson AM, Peteet JR, eds. *Handbook of spirituality and worldview in clinical practice.* Washington, DC, American Psychiatric Publishing, 2004:3–14.

140 Freud S. The question of a weltanschauung. In: Strachey J, ed. *The standard edition of the complete psychological works of Sigmund Freud,* vol. 22. London, Hogarth Press, 1962.

141 Sifton E. *The serenity prayer: faith and politics in times of peace and war.* New York, WW Norton & Company, 2005.

142 Buxbaum Y. *The life and teachings of Hillel.* Northvale, New Jersey, Jason Aaronson, 1995.

143 Stern A, ed. *Everything starts from prayer: Mother Teresa's meditations on spiritual life for people of all faith,* 2nd ed. Ashland, Oregon, White Cloud Press, 2009.

144 Hora T. *One mind: a psychiatrist's spiritual teachings.* New York, PAGL Foundation, 2001.

145 Reps P, Senzaki N, eds. *Zen flesh, Zen bones.* Boston, Charles E Tuttle, 1957.

146 Martin R, Soares M. *One hand clapping: Zen stories for all ages.* New York, Rizzoli International, 1995.

147 Expanding connections. *Bridging gaps* (www.expandingconnections.com, accessed 2 November 2011).

148 Ullman M. *Appreciating dreams: a group approach.* New York, Cosimo, 2006.

149 Cogswell JF. Walking in your shoes: toward an integrating sense of self with sense of oneness. *Journal of Humanistic Psychology,* 1993, 33:99–111.

150 McGuire K. *Focusing in community: how to start a listening and focusing support group.* Eureka Springs, Arkansas, Creative Edge Focusing, 2007.

151 Barclay Goldstein V. *The magic of mess painting: the creativity mobilization technique.* Sausalito, California, Trans-Hyborean Institute of Science, 1999. (This book has a very good annotated bibliography on pp.211–217.)

152 Wooden VL. *The music lesson: a spiritual search for growth through music.* New York, Berkley/Penguin, 2006.

Ethics in primary care mental health

John Spicer, Iona Heath and Tawfik Khoja

Key messages

- Mental health care is beset with definitional problems, of which retaining control of 'normality' is the greatest.
- Ethical analysis in primary care can be undertaken with traditional models and frameworks, of which virtue theory is the most relevant and appropriate.
- Stigma and discrimination of the mentally disordered patient remain challenges to clinical practice and equity.
- Context and issues of cultural relativism are key problems for primary care.
- Primary care clinicians should never lose their advocacy role.

Introduction

Mental illness, primary care and society are locked together in a multiplicity of reciprocal relationships. All three are broad concepts with a host of different potential meanings, understood in quite different ways by different people at different times and in changing circumstances. Some of those people are the various professionals who work in the primary care environment and who may share some common concerns about the ethical foundations of such work.

Individuals (psychiatrists, social workers, case managers, nurses, psychologists, peer counsellors, primary care physicians) who serve on the front line of community mental health clinical and social services find that they must deal, on a daily basis, with significant ethical dilemmas that involve personal, social and policy matters – overstepping personal boundaries, risking coercive practices, dealing with violence in the home and in the workplace, breaching confidentiality – while all the time attempting to ensure the rights and welfare of vulnerable individuals.

Traditional ethical perspectives

Ethics is about doing the right thing, or living in the right way. As such, medical ethics are simply a subset of ethical mores associated with the achievement of those two states. Medical ethical thinking, particularly in the western world, is now predominantly secular, though cognisant and respectful of its religious antecedents. So before examining modern ethical analysis, we will take account of and summarize some of those transcendent ethical frameworks from around the world.

Confucian ethics, from China, are part of a worldview that includes a concern and care for all living things, a reverence for others that is formalized into careful rules of conduct and an ethos of self-improvement to an ideal.

Buddhism, again from the Asian continent, is a complex religion of many schools, which defines eight moral *paths* (being the right speech, actions, efforts, etc.); following these paths lead to intuitive wisdom in the individual.

Islamic ethics flow from interpretations of the *Qur'an*, considered by Muslims to be the word of Allah. As such, a *fiqh,* or understanding, of medical practice has been developed over time to link modern practice with verses of the *Qur'an*, and the ways of living they require.

Judeo–Christian ethics are also essentially instructions from God, illustrated by the Ten Commandments, and interpreted over centuries by priests and ministers.

These four religious approaches to ethics, and they are merely four of many more, are the traditional sources of moral rules, or ways of amplifying the two statements at the start of this section.

They are important to bear in mind, not simply because they can determine the way people of the relevant parts of the world might approach medical problems, but also because our modern cities, particularly in the west, are full of many differing populations who would reflect the diversity of the communities from which they come.

Case-study 1

Maria is an Italian woman living in Northern Europe, to where she had emigrated some years ago. She became unexpectedly pregnant in her 44th year, and both she and her husband were delighted at the prospect of a child at this stage of their lives. In a booking appointment at her primary care centre, the midwife recommended antenatal testing for Down syndrome as Maria's age conferred a high risk. The midwife was surprised when Maria refused, indicating that she would never countenance a termination of pregnancy should she have conceived a Down syndrome fetus. The consultation became somewhat testy, and finished inconclusively. In discussion with her colleagues later that day, the midwife revealed she just could not understand how anyone might continue a pregnancy that might be affected by serious congenital disease.

Questions to consider

- Why might Maria refuse antenatal screening or termination of pregnancy?
- How should the midwife rationalize the difference of view?
- Might there be emotional sequelae if patients like Maria are coerced into screening?

Before addressing the particular issues in mental health care, it would be fruitful to review some of the substructure of ethical analysis as it is most commonly done. This analysis is held to be independent of any particular deontological approach, such as summarized in the religious ethics listed above.

Principle-based ethics, developed by Beauchamp and Childress,[1] popularized by Gillon,[2] and summarized below seem to have most purchase in ethical analysis by clinicians. When considering the ethical content of a given clinical situation, professionals are advised to pay attention to four principles.

- *Autonomy*: autonomy, self-government or free will represents a core individual right that encompasses the capacity to deliberate upon reasons, make and change decisions, and act on the basis of those decisions.
- *Beneficence*: beneficence encompasses the notions of virtue and duty that require individuals and institutions to pursue goals that positively shift the balance of good over harm. Beneficence represents a key individual ethic that is the basis of professional altruism and has provided the raison d'être for clinical freedom in medical practice. Services should be provided purposively to do good to the client or patient. Some moral theories, notably utilitarianism, elevate beneficence to the supreme moral obligation, drawing on Bentham's notion of "the greatest good to the greatest number".[3]
- *Non-maleficence*: the principle of non-maleficence is closely related to beneficence, exhorting decision-makers not to impose harm or evil upon those affected by their actions. This is a clear enough ethical rule to follow in terms of deliberate violation of accepted medical practice, and therefore violation

also of patients' rights. It is less apparent when maleficence can be imposed (perhaps unwittingly) on a particular patient by the use of risky or unevaluated interventions (such as in clinical trial settings), or indeed in the pursuit of benefit for the majority (for instance, unpleasant side-effects of psychotropic drugs administered to individuals who pose a risk to others).

■ *Justice*: considerations of justice or fairness revolve around the ideas that each person must be given their due, and equals must be treated as equals. On what basis, and from what starting point this collective notion of justice is assessed, is a source of much theoretical debate: egalitarian approaches emphasize the social basis of justice by arguing for the distribution of equal shares of a commodity such as health care, while libertarian approaches, by contrast, argue for consumer sovereignty and willingness to pay as the measures of the direction of society's preferences with respect to health care. Debates on justice or equity at a policy level have typically concentrated on the distribution or redistribution of (scarce) resources, which, in the context of mental health care, is typically determined by need and expressed in terms of access to or utilization of services.

At this point, a crude summary of the application of these four principles to the world of primary mental health care might run, in reverse order, thus: equity and justice have never, in any jurisdiction, been manifested in the allocation of resources to mental health. Deciding on the balance of doing good and avoiding harm is particularly difficult for the mental health patient in view of the close association with autonomous reasoning. All these issues will be considered in more depth later, but for now it should be noted, if not already obvious, that conceptions of personal autonomy can be radically altered by psychiatric processes and treatments. Moreover, the modern nostrum that a patient's best interests (approximating to the beneficence/non-maleficence balance) can be considered without personal autonomous decision-making remains open to ethical challenge.

The four-principles analysis also lays claim to being both a summary of moral theory up to the 20th century and a culturally neutral framework.

However, the notion that it is the best framework available to us for ethical analysis is debatable. It is certainly the most generally used but other perspectives should be considered too. Moral theory offers us several other approaches, but we will identify those arising from theories of virtue as being probably the most salient.[4]

Virtues are the personal moral qualities and attributes that can be realized or cultivated by clinicians in everyday practice, and it is argued that such qualities are vital to mental, and primary, health care. Consider the following list:

■ *empathy*: the ability to communicate understanding of another person's experience from that person's perspective

■ *sincerity*: a personal commitment to consistency between what is professed and what is done

■ *integrity*: commitment to personal straightforwardness, honesty and coherence in dealings with others

■ *resilience*: the capacity to work with the client's concerns without being personally diminished

■ *respect*: showing appropriate esteem for others and for their understanding of themselves

■ *humility*: the ability to assess accurately and to acknowledge one's own strengths and weaknesses

■ *competence*: the effective deployment of the skills and knowledge needed to do what is required

■ *fairness*: the consistent application of appropriate criteria to inform decisions and actions, without bias or favour

■ *wisdom*: the exercise of sound practical judgement in applying theoretical constructs to unique individuals

■ *courage*: the capacity to act in spite of known fears, risks and uncertainty.

It is a daunting list, expressed in this rather stark form. Perhaps the best most clinicians can claim is the daily application of some, with the daily aspiration to all. Nonetheless, the care of the patient in mental distress or disorder might justifiably be better delivered by a practitioner offering all these virtues of clinical practice. Demonstrably among the moral theories available, virtue analysis considers the attributes of the individual practitioner, rather than the clinical dilemma itself, and so perhaps provides the most solid grounding for the daily reality of clinical practice.

Consider, for example, a patient presenting to a primary care clinician. He is suffering from psychological distress in the aftermath of a family bereavement. It is a common enough presentation, and apart from the clinical skills that might be relevant (recognition of suicidality, knowledge of patterns of bereavement and appropriate use of medicines, to name a few),[5] we should consider the moral perspective of the case. The four principles offer some insights. However the list of attributes above might be more valuable. It is easy to understand empathy, resilience and humility and several others as worthwhile virtues in the rendering of care to this distressed patient. It is perhaps easier to admit that the clinician approaching a bereaved patient cannot render such care without dispositions such as these. There is a separate discussion to be had elsewhere as to whether such dispositions can be learnt, acquired or even assessed.

Case-study 2

Ricardo has a history of violent behaviour. He has a criminal record for actual bodily harm, alcohol-related offences and domestic violence. His partner, Edie, often comes to the primary care clinic and reveals accounts of a chaotic and dangerous life. They have two children who have never been harmed physically by Ricardo. When he presents for care he is often demanding and aggressive, and none of the primary care staff like dealing with him.

Questions to consider

- What is the extent of the duty of care to Ricardo?
- What qualities might be needed in looking after him, or his family?
- Might a long-term relationship with Ricardo be of value?

Illness, disease and health: the mental dimension

Ethical challenges arise in the interstices of our concepts of the subjective symptoms of illness, the theoretical constructs of disease, and the broader notion of health. Mental illness describes an individual's perception of a sense of mental distress, a perception of things not being quite right – of feeling inexplicably sad, exhilarated or persecuted, or at odds with the world and others around. Defined in this way, mental illness is a universal experience, which usually resolves spontaneously as the stresses of daily living are adjusted and, at least temporarily, mitigated. It becomes absolutely clear that mental illness, perhaps even more than its physical counterpart, can be caused both by disease and unhappiness. Coleridge described:

> . . . a compressing and strangling Anguish, made up of Love, and Resentment, and Sorrow – quarreling with all the Future & refusing to be consoled for the Past.[6]

TS Eliot wrote:

> . . . the sorrow before morning,
> In which all past is present, all degradation
> Is unredeemable.[7]

Almost everyone experiences such feelings; relatively few are suffering disease.

Mental disease, in contrast, is a theoretical abstraction that groups together very diverse experiences of suffering into broad categories that seem to have some features in common,[8] and that seem to respond to particular treatments. Mental health is quite different again and has much to do with a sense of self-esteem and self-determination, and of life having a purpose and a worth.

Various authors have offered a theoretical understanding of health – Nordenfelt historically suggests a sense of "balance" exemplifies health.[9] From a Galenic humoral balance to a modern homeostasis runs a clear line of thought. Or, health can be described in functional terms, as a sense of well-being, or of having the ability to achieve personal goals. By inference, both illness and disease can limit or undermine any of these attributes.

Across the whole range of illness and disease, that which presents to formal health-care services represents the tip of the hidden symptom iceberg.[10] Fulford defines illness as an "action failure" or an inability to "just get on and do",[11] and this action failure often makes it more difficult for people with mental rather than physical symptoms to initiate contact with health-care services. Shifting the definition of mental illness back to the patient, as a decision to consult a primary care physician, offers an attractive shorthand, but risks missing many who are profoundly troubled but who nonetheless do not manage to consult. With greater emphasis on primary care's responsibility for the needs of populations as well as individuals, this becomes more important.

The shifting sands of definition – the impossibility of precise diagnosis

The borderline between symptoms caused by unhappiness and disease is very blurred and is often scarcely distinguishable. This blurring is manifested in the research finding that more than half of unselected patients in a primary care waiting room in the United Kingdom of Great Britain and Northern Ireland (UK) have symptoms that fulfil a definition of clinical depression.[12] Such a finding must raise fundamental ethical questions about definitions of normality and disease and whether there is any constructive purpose to be served by a definition of disease that includes such a large proportion of the population. A core task of primary care is to resist the medicalization of all illness, and this seems to apply with even greater force to mental illness where symptoms are a universal response to existential distress. As primary care practitioners, we must constantly ask ourselves: "at what point does it become helpful to the patient to concretize their mental distress as mental disease?".[13]

In 1917, the American Psychiatric Association recognized 59 psychiatric disorders. With the introduction of the *Diagnostic and Statistical Manual of Mental Disorders*, the DSM, in 1952, this rose to 128. The second edition in 1968 had 159, the third in 1980 227, and the revision of the third (DSM-III-R) in 1987 had 253. Now we have DSM-IV, which has 347 categories, and DSM-V is in preparation. What does this mean?

Does it represent the progress of science or, somewhat less honourably, an epidemic of medicalization that threatens to engulf an ever-greater proportion of the population?[14] And is the contemporary degree of definition helpful to the sufferers or does it merely provide intellectual exercise for researchers and specialist clinicians? In the lay press quite recently, a retired United States (US) professor of psychiatry argued that behind the preparation of DSM-V lay the societal risk of overdiagnosis and overtreatment. Binge eating disorder, paraphilic coercive disorder and hypersexuality disorder are all cited as examples of "disorders" vulnerable to "psychiatric mission creep". This would reflect a challenge for primary care in the interpretation of such definitions.[15]

The normative nature of much psychiatric diagnosis is given a further twist by the superimposition of moral judgement. Over the centuries, we have interpreted behaviour and disease differently, and attached moral value to both. In the 19th century, the now evidently infectious disease cholera was seen as a moral hazard that: "exposed relentlessly political social and moral shortcomings".[16] Conversely, at a time when homosexuality was becoming pathologized and available for medical "treatment", Benjamin Britten, in his opera of the Thomas Mann novella *Death in Venice*, explored the comparisons to be made between cholera and the morality of certain sexual behaviour. None of this holds either intellectual or moral weight in the early 21st century.[16] Most societies now accept that there are no moral hazards in same-sex relationships, or in cholera, though the latter is still a marker for the breakdown of basic services within society, such as the provision of clean water and effective sanitation, as was seen most recently in post-earthquake Haiti.

The journey to being a patient

Many primary care clinicians have the extraordinary privilege of knowing patients and families over many years and several generations. They see mental illness and disease being generated slowly and inexorably, and encroaching on the patient's life from a long distance. They watch with a terrible sense of helplessness, which often leads to a disturbing sense of moral detachment, as individuals are progressively damaged by the actions and attitudes of families, strangers, the wider society and themselves.[17] Not all of this is malevolent, but the gradual undermining of coherent meaning and self-esteem within the story of a life is profoundly pernicious. The resources that constitute mental health are systematically eroded and the process is disturbing and distressing to witness.

Farmer and colleagues have adopted the term "structural violence" from Latin American liberation theology:[18]

> The term "structural violence" is one way of describing social arrangements that put individuals and populations in harm's way. The arrangements are structural because they are embedded in the political and economic organization of our social world; they are violent because they cause injury to people (typically, not those responsible for perpetuating such inequalities).

They identify racism, gender inequality, poverty, political violence and war as the main drivers of such structural violence, and all of these pose ethical challenges within primary mental health care.

Mad or bad

The ethical position of clinicians is further challenged by the murky hinterland between madness and badness that pervades the conceptualization of mental illness. The effective practice of medicine depends on the clinician's ability to imaginatively understand the patient's predicament. Only in this way can the central virtue of empathy be enacted and the patient's crucial subjective experience of their symptoms be properly scrutinized. Effective imaginative identification depends on positive regard – an actively fostered willingness to think well of a patient's aspirations and intentions. This is perhaps even more important, and more difficult to sustain, in primary care where relationships with patients may need to be kept going over long periods of time. Positive regard implies the rejection of judgemental or condemnatory attitudes and underpins an attempt to make sense of the patient's attitudes and actions in terms of the realities of their particular life situation. The increasingly blurred boundary between madness and badness, combined with the enduring moral disjunction between the two, challenges all this and perhaps explains the ever-increasing medicalization of all forms of non-conforming or deviant social behaviour. Historically, the criminal and the insane have too often been treated equally badly by society, and often within the same institutions. The development of psychiatry has been a great force for good in improving the life opportunities and experience of those suffering from psychiatric illness. But today, we seem to have arrived at a point where psychiatric discourse has been extended to become the only acceptable means of humanizing society's attitudes to the bad. The result is the terrible conundrum of the "personality disorder".[19,20]

Clinicians, and perhaps particularly doctors, tend always to extend the remit of medicine and use a medical model of reasoning to explain behaviour that is otherwise unacceptable. It is probable that this does a disservice to those whose psychiatric morbidity is beyond doubt, and it certainly sets us an impossible task. Nonetheless, until the criminal justice system in many countries is rendered more humane and rehabilitation more effectively included within punishment, the tendency to try to hold people within the medical system will continue.

The tag "sad" is often added to the two adjectives that head this section, as though disordered thought and behaviour in psychological distress can be categorized in one, or more, of these three ways: sad, mad or bad. However, where such a set of adjectives may be of value is in analysing the voluntariness of some patients' behaviour. The traditional analysis of an autonomous decision is that is should be informed, competent and free. These factors are raised into law in almost all jurisdictions around the world. It is worth thinking about how clinicians might regard, say, the patient misusing substances or alcohol in everyday practice. The tenor of this chapter and most clinical practice generally, is that we should regard such patients as in need, in distress and in some way entitled to relevant "treatment".[21] Often in primary care, we will know such patients and families over many years, and therefore understand the life events surrounding such behaviour. We should, as stated above, attempt to act as virtuous practitioners. But a slightly deeper moral consideration might include reflecting on how the standard descriptors of personal autonomy apply. Is the decision to progressively destroy oneself with alcohol over years a rational, affective or morally culpable form of behaviour? Are the early exposures to alcohol injurious to self-control by virtue of its chemical addictive properties? Are young people sufficiently aware of the potential harms of long-term alcohol use? Is it reasonable to proscribe alcohol as a dangerous drug on consequentialist grounds? How can we in primary care help patients to make positive choices around alcohol use?

These are essentially moral questions that the reader is asked to consider, and there are no easy answers. Certainly we should be aware of best clinical practice in the management of alcohol-related disease – a subject beyond the scope of this chapter – but perhaps more important is a consideration of the regard we should offer the patient involved in substance misuse. That it should be positive is an argument we espouse, but in coming to that position, some thinking on the approaches to these questions is of value.

That primary care clinicians most usually find themselves fortunate, and their patients unfortunate, in their relative positions across the consulting room can be held to be, among other things, a matter of luck.

Moral luck

The notion of moral luck, first discussed by Bernard Williams in 1981,[22] and further explored by Thomas Nagel,[23] is deeply entangled in the distinction between madness and badness, and in the impact of structural violence. Nagel described moral luck as follows:

> Where a significant aspect of what someone does depends on factors beyond his control, yet we continue to treat him in that respect as an object of moral judgment, it can be called moral luck.[23]

We all try to make sense of our lives by finding explanations for the events that befall us. We search out explanations for the behaviour of ourselves and others and, crucially, we hold each other responsible for attitudes and actions. In so doing we make moral judgements about them. A plea of illness is one of the few socially sanctioned grounds for being excused this responsibility for our own attitudes and actions, and thereby the moral judgements of others. Those who become criminal and those who suffer serious psychiatric illness tend to share life stories that have been subject to violence, abuse and loss. Do those who have had the moral luck of life stories free of such deep scars, have the right to condemn? When does an explanation of violence condone it, and when does it not? Such insistent ethical questions arise whenever a clinician, often favoured with considerable moral good luck, meets a patient, burdened by an excess of moral bad luck.

Case-study 3

Jonquil, at 45 years old, lost the mother she had always lived with, and in latter years had cared for. She had no other real relationships, and spent most of her time watching television and walking her dog. For the last year she had been visiting her general practitioner (GP) in consultation, where all she did was weep, consumed with grief for her loss. Though not formally depressed, Jonquil had been offered antidepressants and bereavement counselling without effect. Eventually she and her GP fell into a pattern of monthly planned meetings, which became shared with a community mental health nurse. The consultations moved from accounts of her sorrow and present state, to discussions of her early life with her mother. Though she continued to weep almost uncontrollably, her mood seemed to improve over time.

Questions to consider

- How might the relationship between Jonquil and the primary care team influence her mood?
- How might the two primary care staff work together?
- Might they need supervision in dealing with Jonquil?

The abuse of psychiatry

The lack of a clear demarcation between madness and badness also goes some way to explaining psychiatry's peculiar susceptibility to political abuse. Per Fugelli maintains that:[24]

medicine = biology × individuality × culture × politics squared

and the preponderance of political influence is underlined by our increasing understanding of the power of the socioeconomic determinants of health. Poorer people live shorter and sicker lives. There is a socioeconomic gradient for the prevalence of almost every major disease, and these gradients are often steepest for psychiatric diseases.[25] But at what point does psychiatry become an agent of social control and, beyond that, a tool of political repression? The history of psychiatry demonstrates that it is peculiarly susceptible to being used in the medicalization of political, socioeconomic, racial and homophobic oppression – the medicalization of "otherness".

The discontent of the socioeconomically deprived will always have the capacity to drive social unrest. But if the discontented can be described as depressed or found to be suffering from psychological distress, they can be treated with pharmaceuticals or offered counselling. Social unrest is averted, the discontent is subverted and the injustices of society remain untouched. Nothing then disturbs the comfort and complacency of those on the gaining side of injustice. Many clinicians feel implicated in this process,[26] and implicated more deeply with every prescription for a psychotropic medication written to help someone put up with unacceptable or unjust social conditions.

Those struggling to retain their dignity and to cope at the bottom of a steep socioeconomic gradient are marginalized, and excluded from many of the conventional rewards of life. This exclusion may well be reflected in a rejection of "normal" mainstream attitudes, priorities and behaviours, and, at the extreme of this process, behaviours come to be regarded as either mad or bad by the rest of society. There is a constant need to guard against the tendency towards normalization that exists within psychiatry. And these difficulties are further compounded by issues of cultural diversity and the differing understanding of different behaviours in different cultural contexts. The continuing differential rate of compulsory hospital admission for African Caribbean men in Europe and North America remains a major cause of concern, which should drive an ongoing critique of the role played by psychiatry in underpinning the political and cultural hegemony of the powerful.

> It [dysthymic disorder in DSM-III or neurotic depression in the International Classification of Diseases (ICD-9)] may hold coherence in the more affluent West, but it represents the medicalisation of social problems in much of the rest of the world (and perhaps the West as well), where severe economic, political and health constraints create endemic feelings of hopelessness and helplessness, where demoralisation and despair are responses to real conditions of chronic deprivation and persistent loss, where powerlessness is not a cognitive distortion but an accurate mapping of one's place in an oppressive social system, and where moral, religious and political configurations of such problems have coherence for the local population, but psychiatric categories do not.[27]

These factors play out differently around the world and, described with such clarity in the quotation above, reawaken the importance of morality in the consideration of this issue, or at least the distinction between local and universal moralities. Some primary care professionals will deal with populations that are similar, from the perspective of faith, ethnicity or any other descriptor, and it is tempting to think that such populations might share a set of values (collectively, a morality) that defines how they think about challenging behaviours in persons that could be construed as mentally "ill". Other primary care practitioners will look after very diverse populations, described in the same way, and be exposed to many differing sets of patient values all in the same day. London, possibly the most diverse city in the world, illustrates this observation.

So therefore, the competent generalist must steer a course between reliance on universal moral perspectives and an overly great respect for the locally defined, or relative.

The parent who knowingly denies his child who has diabetes access to insulin on grounds seen to be irrational, religious or criminal is only respected by a too-relativist physician. On most accounts, such a parental behaviour cannot but be interrupted within a medical duty of care. On the other hand, few physicians would interfere with a parent's teaching of a child in religious theory and practice. This difficulty is well described in Anne Fadiman's account of clinicians struggling to find common ground with a Hmong family, living in the United States of America (USA), who interpret their daughter's severe epilepsy and mental disorder as the malign intervention of the spirit world.[28]

Such cultural differences between doctor and patient can clearly be difficult to manage. Some overarching principles may be useful in negotiating this divide. While respect for one another's differing moral positions may be easy to declare, it can be challenging to realize. Without doubt, as patients are the object of care, doctors should have respect for their moral positions – and in the case of the US care staff in Fadiman's account,[28] that is evidently present. It is not necessary to disrespect a patient's religious belief, and the moral guidance that may flow from it, to render appropriate care. Local jurisdictions will define the law relevant to the case. So even if the belief system and culture of a parent suggest insulin treatment for a sick child is proscribed, most legal environments will allow, and indeed require, the physician to overrule such a cultural norm in the best interests of the child.

Stigma

Despite much effort, mental illness still carries a significant stigma.[29] Some of this is historical but another part seems to be to do with the fact that mental illness relieves affected individuals of some or all of their responsibilities to the rest of society. In this context, the inevitable subjectivity of mental illness can become a liability. Physical illness is perceived as having a tangible effect on the body, providing apparently objective proof of the existence of illness beyond the control of the sufferer. In contrast, the subjectivity of mental illness makes it much more elusive and much less open to any form of objective verification. Sufferers are excused their responsibilities but also systematically excluded in a way that is no longer as cruel as it once was but that often remains judgemental and condemnatory. The pervasive, atavistic fear of mental illness and disintegration means that apparently "normal" individuals can be very keen to draw a clear demarcation between themselves and those others who suffer mental illness. This barrier nurtures the stigma that many sufferers feel. The public perception that severe mental illness lies at the root of much seriously violent crime further stigmatizes sufferers, and the whole situation is exacerbated by sensationalist media reporting.[30] Stigma is compounded by discrimination and, regrettably, discrimination against those suffering from mental illness remains endemic within the organization of many health-care services. The notion of diagnostic overshadowing, where clinicians do not see the whole patient beyond the impaired mental state, is a recently developed arena, and one that primary care is uniquely empowered to challenge. As research in this field proceeds, the importance of the physical care of the patient with serious mental illness becomes ever more relevant, particularly when they are admitted to hospital with decompensations.[31]

Sensibility and insight

Despite the very widespread stigmatizing and fear of mental illness, there often seems to be a very narrow dividing line between madness and creativity. Many creative artists of undeniable international and historical stature have had serious mental illnesses, and many more ordinary patients with mental illness seem to have an exceptional sensibility and great insight into human nature and its predicament. However, this insight also leaves them vulnerable to the loss of balance that seems to lie at the root of so much mental illness. Many patients seem to be aware of both the rewards and the risks of their sensibility, and have a very accurate appreciation of how much it is blunted by "tranquillizing" psychiatric medication.

> Whenever their lives were set aflame, through desire or suffering, or even reflection, the Homeric heroes knew that a god was at work. They endured the god, and observed him, but what actually happened as a result was a surprise most of all for themselves . . .

> No psychology since has ever gone beyond this; all we have done is invent, for those powers that act upon us, longer, more numerous, more awkward names, which are less effective, less closely aligned to the gain of our experience, whether that be pleasure or terror. . . . What we consider infirmity they saw as "divine infatuation" (áte). They knew that this invisible incursion often brought ruin: so much that the word áte would gradually come to mean "ruin". But they also knew, and it was Sophocles who said it, that "mortal life can never have anything grandiose about it except through áte".[32]

Part of the stereotypical description of a patient suffering mental illness is that they lack insight into their own condition. Gadamer points out what an odd notion this is.[33] Denial has always been part of the human response to illness, and the more serious the illness the more likely the patient is to deny something of its reality. Why is it that such denial is often regarded as courageous in the face of physical illness but profoundly and morally reprehensible in the mentally ill?

Mind and body

The Cartesian distinction of mind and body has had extraordinary reverberating consequences in the centuries since the French Enlightenment. Many have increased our understanding but some remain deeply troublesome. Biomedical science assumes the validity of such a split, but almost all experience of illness denies it. All bodily illness has consequences for the mind, and all mental illness affects the body.

> As living things we are wholly taken up by anger, completely shaken by fear. We are not angry or fearful in just one part of the soul.[32]

The chronically mentally ill have very poor physical health and a significantly reduced expectation of life. The tendency to separate mental health services illustrates and institutionalizes the enduring fiction of the mind–body split. The physical consequences of poor mental health are more and more widely recognized and yet, too often, the specialist care of physical illnesses and mental illnesses occur at geographically separate sites. This runs the risk of systematically distancing those with the most serious mental illness from the physical care that they need. The increasing numbers of patients who suffer both a serious mental illness and a serious physical illness, such as diabetes, epilepsy or asthma, have a very poor prognosis. Yet, there is very little research on the best and most effective ways of managing such patients, particularly when the situation is further compounded by significant abuse of alcohol or drugs. Care based on guidelines formulated for people suffering a single disease is very unlikely to be effective.

Somatization

Some minds seem more than usually resistant to the apprehension of distress and disorder, and when distress becomes intolerable, it is somehow forced to find an outlet in bodily symptoms. These symptoms can be hugely varied and the patient rapidly becomes trapped in a situation of displaced psychological misery now combined with a fear of serious physical illness. Biomedicine's insistence on the clear differentiation of mind and body exacerbates the situation of these patients, as does society's unstated moral judgement that physical illness is somehow more honourable than its mental equivalent. The whole picture is yet further compounded by our knowledge that chronic psychological stress not only causes physical symptoms but also significantly increases the patient's risk of serious physical disease.[34] The clinician has the challenging task of trying to focus on the underlying distress in the hope of finding some way of working with the patient to mitigate it. Yet, at the same time, the clinician must be always vigilant for the signs of serious physical disease, while not adding to the patient's already huge burden of anxiety and apprehension.

Case-study 4

Rafiq presented repeatedly to his primary care team with a variety of physical symptoms, over a year or so. Among other things, he experienced abdominal pain, giddiness, sleep disturbance, tiredness and headache. His GP and the rest of the team offered a sympathetic response that included multiple appointments, physical examinations, blood tests and elementary investigations. No clear physical pathology emerged. There were no obvious stressors or negative life events. Consultations always took a certain course, where symptoms were described in some detail, culminating in a request for more tests "to see what the problem is". He was eventually referred to a psychiatrist, who embarked on reattribution therapy for these medically unexplained symptoms. Over a year he made some progress.

Questions to consider

- Could the diagnosis have been considered by the primary care team?
- If so, could the therapy have been undertaken in primary care?
- What are the resource implications of cases like this?
- Is there a continuing professional education issue for the team?

The clinician can sometimes encourage the patient to locate and describe both the physical manifestations of mental and emotional distress, and the impact of physical symptoms on their state of mind. In this way, the barrier between mind and body can be gently eroded, enabling the patient to describe their experience more fully.

Listening and hearing

We could summarize the ethical duties of the primary care physician in this field in terms of the values he or she should espouse:

- to respect human rights and dignity
- to protect the safety of patients
- to ensure the integrity of practitioner–client relationships
- to enhance the quality of professional knowledge and its application
- to alleviate personal distress and suffering
- to increase personal effectiveness
- to enhance the quality of relationships between people
- to appreciate the variety of human experience and culture.

In holding to all these values, primary care clinicians strive to approach their patients closely – to understand the detail of the experience of illness and distress; not only to listen to stories but to hear them. The challenge is always to approach closely enough; not to delude ourselves about the nature of what we see and hear, and not to seek the shelter of the familiar structures of psychiatric diagnosis before we have recognized and acknowledged the experience that the patient brings. The inevitable yet essential reductionism of biomedical discourse is an impediment to understanding, and needs always to be balanced by a valuing of experience that does not fit.

> I am also convinced
> That you only hold a fragment of the explanation.
> It is only because of what you do not understand
> That you feel the need to declare what you do.
> There is more to understand: hold fast to that
> As the way to freedom.[7]

The whole enterprise of medicine is predicated on the patient being able to communicate the nature of their distress to the doctor. The patient can trust the doctor's intervention and treatment only if he or she feels that their experience of illness has been understood. A too-rapid process of diagnostic labelling can undermine this understanding.

The meanings of illness, the threat, the fear, the suffering and the endurance can only be interpreted, ordered and contained if both doctors and patients can find and agree on the right words. In this, the task of the consultation parallels that of poetry.

> Poetic form is both the ship and the anchor. It is at once a buoyancy and a holding, allowing for the simultaneous gratification of whatever is centrifugal and centripetal in mind and body. And it is by such means that Yeats's work does what the necessary poetry always does, which is to touch the base of our sympathetic nature while taking in at the same time the unsympathetic reality of the world to which that nature is constantly exposed. The form of the poem, in other words, is crucial to poetry's power to do the thing which always is and always will be to poetry's credit: the power to persuade that vulnerable part of our consciousness of its rightness in spite of the evidence of wrongness all around it, the power to remind us that we are hunters and gatherers of values, that our very solitudes and distresses are creditable, in so far as they, too, are an earnest of our veritable being.[35]

Language has evolved to mirror human experience, and to find meaning in it that can be shared with others to make us feel less alone. Poets and novelists make use of the whole resource of language, and

> . . . that sedimented reason which resides in all use of language[32]

and doctors need a similar aspiration. Any restriction of language to a particular discourse closes off the possibility of understanding. At its best, the consultation allows both the "buoyancy" of a detailed exploration of individual suffering and the "holding" of a careful setting of that suffering within the context of our shared human experience of a frequently hostile world.

Understanding the distorted and tumultuous experience of the psychotic mind poses particular challenges.

> O that awful privacy
> Of the insane mind![7]

> The final difficulty of reading madness . . . is that in the act of doing so, one dissociates oneself from it or associates oneself with it, and in either case becomes disqualified as an interpreter. To read madness sanely is to miss the point; to read madness madly is to have one's point be missed.[36]

Yet, the universality and inclusiveness of language[37] will always have the potential to make the connections necessary to at least begin a dialogue.

> What takes place here between doctor and patient is a form of attentiveness, namely the ability to sense the demands of an individual person at a particular moment and to respond to those demands in an appropriate manner. . . . It is an attempt to set in motion once again the communicative flow of the patient's life experience and to re-establish that contact with others from which the person is so tragically excluded.[32]

Context

This chapter will conclude with a practical set of recommendations as to how mental health care could be better delivered, on a firmer ethical foundation, but first we must consider the context of care and the locus of delivery.

Society, and therefore primary care, tends to be divided between the town or the countryside. Contexts will vary widely around the world, but essentially patients and their physicians are situated in either urban or rural environments. These locations have implications for morbidity in mental health, and the care that primary care physicians are able to offer.

Modern cities concentrate persons in mental distress together and this situation is exacerbated by socioeconomic disadvantage, the breakdown of extended family structures and the predicament of refugees and asylum seekers. This was demonstrated in Amsterdam in 1998,[38] and there is no reason to think anything has changed for the better. Many studies have demonstrated the clear over-representation of mental illness of all types in urban as compared to rural environments. Primary care clinicians in cities will usually have case-loads in which mental health care is over-represented, especially in socially deprived neighbourhoods.

Rural clinicians face different obstacles in delivering an appropriate standard of care to their patients with mental health problems. People who live in more remote frontier regions appear to be especially affected by geographic and climatic barriers; shortages of clinicians, facilities and specialized services; and sociocultural issues in care delivery. Rural clinicians encounter particular ethical challenges, especially in relation to care for stigmatizing illnesses. These challenges pertain to overlapping personal and professional relationships, confidentiality, balancing patient and community needs, resource limitations, and giving care beyond one's usual scope of clinical competence. Finally, professional ethics codes may be ill-attuned to the ethical aspects of rural life, which has a different character from that of resource-enriched, less interdependent urban communities.

Care for rural patients with mental illnesses poses further problems, such as addressing patients' potential for self-harm and violence, dealing with the heightened social stigma associated with mental disorders, protecting vulnerable patients from potential abuse or exploitation, and grappling with care planning for individuals with impaired decision-making capacity. These ethically rigorous issues are universal but are often more acute in rural or isolated health-care settings, primarily because usual practices to ensure ethical conduct are narrowed by the scarcity of health-care resources. Certainly the availability of primary care teams to form and work together is constrained by the distances of the countryside, in a way that is not normally problematic in urban areas.

So both town and country have their individual issues in the delivery of primary care mental health: differing but always demanding.

Joe was released from prison after serving a 6-month sentence for drug offences. He moved to a new area of the city in an attempt to avoid his old haunts and the people in the drug scene he used to associate with. He tried to access primary care in this new area but found it difficult to find a GP who would take him on. Primary care administrative staff did seem to find reasons why a doctor's appointment could not be offered. Eventually, his probation officer prevailed upon the local health authority to require a GP to care for him, and he was able to enter drug-misuse follow-up and get some physical health problems sorted out.

Questions to consider

- Why did Joe find primary care hard to access?
- Is such a difficulty consistent with a general right to health care?
- Is the duty of care different in substance misuse?
- How could this situation have been prevented?

How could things be better?

We need a mental health service that:

- is grounded in the notion of positive regard
- is built on listening and "enabling"[39]
- provides a response to all degrees of seriousness of mental ill health and tries to prevent less serious problems becoming much more serious over time
- provides an accessible service to all subgroups within the population – particularly the most vulnerable – adolescents, the homeless, some members of ethnic minority communities, refugees and asylum seekers, the old, single unemployed men, etc.
- is aware of the genesis of much mental ill health within damaged and damaging families and attempts to provide intensive therapeutic support to such families
- provides an adequate response to the very steep socioeconomic gradient in mental ill health
- is properly integrated with services for those who misuse drugs and alcohol
- is balanced in the supply of services to geographical areas
- is aware that many of those suffering chronic mental illness also suffer physical ill health
- is multidisciplinary, involves all members of the primary health-care team and extends beyond that team to make use of resources within local communities, local authorities and patients themselves
- uses medication frugally, sceptically and in an appropriately evidence-based manner, and reassesses the continuing need for medication at regular intervals
- enables equity of access to the psychological and psychotherapeutic treatment modalities
- is aware of the dangerous potential for abuse within psychiatry
- acknowledges the differing values patients bring to the primary care interaction.

The main barriers to achieving such a service are the lack of time, trust and resources, and the background of an unjust society which distributes opportunity and hope in a profoundly inequitable manner. The ethical imperative is that primary care professionals and mental health professionals work together to maximize the former and to advocate at every opportunity for the alleviation of the latter.

References

1   Beauchamp TL, Childress JF. *Principles of biomedical ethics*, 6th ed. Oxford, Oxford University Press.

2   Gillon R. Medical ethics: four principles plus attention to scope. *British Medical Journal*, 1994, 309:184.

3   Rachels J. Elements of moral philosophy, 2nd ed. New York, McGraw Hill, 1997.

4   Toon P. *Towards a philosophy of general practice: a study of the virtuous practitioner.* Occasional Paper 78. London, Royal College of General Practitioners, 1999.

5   Nagraj S, Barclay S. Bereavement care in primary care: a systematic literature review and narrative synthesis. *British Journal of General Practice*, 2011, 61:53–58.

6   Holmes R. *Coleridge: darker reflections.* London, Harper Collins, 1998.

7   Eliot TS. *The family reunion.* London, Faber & Faber, 1939.

8   Robert JS. Schizophrenia epigenesis? *Theoretical Medicine and Bioethics*, 2000, 21:191–215.

9   Nordenfelt L. *On the nature of health*, 2nd ed. Dordrecht, Kluwer, 1995.

10   Eavy G. Defining illness as action failure: a response to McKnight. *Journal of Applied Philosophy*, 2000, 17:290–297.

11   Fulford KWM. *Moral theory and medical practice.* New York, Cambridge University Press, 1989.

12   Kessler D et al. Cross sectional study of symptom attribution and recognition of depression and anxiety in primary care *BMJ*, 1999, 318:436–440.

13   Heath I. There must be limits to the medicalisation of human distress. *BMJ*, 1999, 318:440.

14   Wessely S. The medicalisation of distress. *RSA Journal*, 1998, 4:79–85.

15   Frances A. It's not too late to save normal. *Los Angeles Times*, 1 March 2011.

16   Hutcheon L, Hutcheon M. Opera: desire, disease and death. Lincoln and London, University of Nebraska Press, 1996.

17   Kirkengen AL. *The lived experience of violation – how abused children become unhealthy adults.* Bucharest, Zeta Books, 2010.

18   Farmer P et al. Structural violence and clinical medicine. *PLoS Medicine*, 2006, 3(10):e449.

19   Mullen P. Dangerous people with severe personality disorder. *BMJ*, 1999, 319:1146–1147.

20   Eastman N. Who should take responsibility for antisocial personality disorder? *BMJ*, 1999, 318:206–207.

21   Metzl JM, Kirkland A. Not fit for purpose. *New Scientist*, 2010, 20 November:28–29.

22   Williams B. *Moral luck.* Cambridge, Cambridge University Press, 1981.

23   Nagel T. *Moral luck in mortal questions.* Cambridge, Cambridge University Press, 1991.

24   Fugelli P. Rød resept. Essays om perfeksjon, prestasjon og helse. Oslo, Tano Aschehoug, 1999:14.

25   Thornicroft G. Social deprivation and rates of treated mental disorder – developing statistical models to predict psychiatric service utilisation. *British Journal of Psychiatry*, 1991, 158:475–484.

26   Berger J, Mohr J. *A fortunate man: the story of a country doctor.* London, Allen Lane, The Penguin Press, 1967.

27   Kleinman A. Anthropology and psychiatry: the role of culture in cross-cultural research on mental illness. *British Journal of Psychiatry*, 1987, 151:447–454.

28   Fadiman A. *The spirit catches you and you fall down.* Chicago, Farrar, Straus and Giroux, 1998.

29   Porter, R. Can the stigma of mental illness be changed? *The Lancet*, 1998, 352:1049–1050.

30   Ferriman A. The stigma of schizophrenia. *BMJ*, 2000, 320:522.

31   Miller BJ. Hospital Admission for schizophrenia and bipolar disorder. *BMJ*, 2011, 343:596–597.

32   Calasso R. *The marriage of Cadmus and Harmony.* London, Vintage, 1994.

33   Gadamer H-G. *The enigma of health. The art of healing in a scientific age.* Stanford, Stanford University Press, 1996.

34   Dinan TG. The physical consequences of depressive illness. *BMJ*, 1999, 318: 826.

35   Heaney S. *Crediting poetry: the Nobel lecture 1995.* Oldcastle, The Gallery Press, 1995.

36 Neely CT. 'Documents in Madness': reading madness and gender in Shakespeare's tragedies and early modern culture. *Shakespeare Quarterly*, 1991, 42:315–338.

37 Roberts G. The rehabilitation of rehabilitation: a narrative approach to psychosis. In: Holmes J, Roberts G, eds. *Healing stories. Narrative in psychiatry and psychotherapy*. Oxford, University Press, 1999.

38 Reijneveld SA, Schene AH. Higher prevalence of mental disorders in socioeconomically deprived urban areas in The Netherlands: community or personal disadvantage? *Journal of Epidemiology and Community Health*, 1998, 52:2–7.

39 Howie JGR et al. Quality at general practice consultations: cross sectional survey. *British Medical Journal*, 1999, 319:738–743.

Section B

Access and primary care mental health

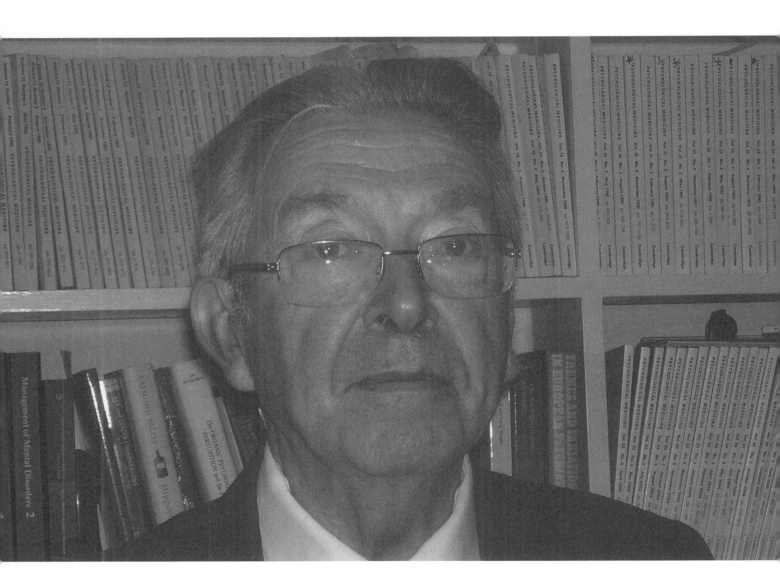

6 Public health aspects of integration of mental health into primary care services

Rachel Jenkins, Moira Kessler, Michelle Riba, Jane Gunn and Felix Kauye

Key messages

■ The availability of specialist resource relative to the ubiquity of mental illness is key in understanding the importance of primary care, and in how specialist care can support primary care.

■ The impact of the mental health burden in low-income countries is exacerbated because of the restricted services, lack of access, poor financing and limited availability of even the most basic treatments, and the high burden borne by the family in out-of-pocket expenses.

■ There is now a considerable knowledge base for effective interventions (health promotion, prevention, treatment, rehabilitation and prevention of mortality) for many mental and neurological conditions in the developed world. However, this knowledge is not implemented in many parts of the world for a variety of reasons, including lack of mental health policy, lack of specialist services, lack of skills in primary care and lack of availability of essential medicines and treatments.

Introduction

The important contribution of mental capital for nations is becoming increasingly apparent, and therefore underscores the need for national strategies to promote mental capital and to address the burden of mental disorders.[1] The need for such national strategies to include the integration of collaborative mental health care into primary health care stems from the burden of mental disorders (prevalence, disability, chronicity and mortality), both in the community and in primary care, and their public health, economic and social cost to society, the restricted availability of specialist care, and the unique positioning of the primary care team. This rationale is persuasive in high-income countries like the United Kingdom of Great Britain and Northern Ireland (UK), the United States of America (USA) and Australia, but is even more so in low- and middle-income countries, especially in Africa.

The definitions of integration, collaboration and collaborative care that we will use in this chapter are as follows:

■ *integration* of mental health into primary care occurs where primary care staff undertake direct assessment, diagnosis and management of mental disorders themselves, albeit ideally with guidelines, support and supervision from specialist staff visiting from the district level

■ *collaboration* occurs when two sectors or two levels of the same sector meet to discuss service issues to improve service coordination in general

■ *collaborative care* occurs when two sectors or two levels of the same sector work together to support specific clients.

Epidemiology of mental disorders

The magnitude of mental disorders may be described in terms of prevalence, disability, chronicity and mortality. In the UK, the one-week prevalence figures are: common mental disorders 15%, psychosis 0.4%, alcohol abuse 5.9% and drug abuse 3.4%;[2] in the USA, the 12-month prevalence is anxiety 18.1%, mood disorders 9.5%, impulse control 8.9%, substance misuse 3.8% and any mental disorders 26.2%.[3] In Australia, 14.4% (2.3 million) of those aged 16–85 years had a 12-month prevalence of anxiety disorder,[4] 6.2% (995 900) had a 12-month prevalence of affective disorder and 5.1% (819 800) had a 12-month prevalence of substance use disorder.[5] However, within those overall figures there is wide regional variation, so, for example, psychosis rates vary from 0.2% to 0.9% in different regions within the UK and vulnerable groups have increased rates of disorder.

Contrary to prevalent misconceptions, mental disorders are at least as common in low-income countries as in established market economies,[6] and are not simply a problem of rich countries or indeed of rich populations in poor countries, as is sometimes erroneously argued. The prevalence of psychosis is around 0.5% to 1%, and the prevalence of common mental disorders (mostly depression and anxiety) is between 10% and 20% in most studies,[6] with a number of studies finding substantially higher rates in relatively poor populations.[7] The prevalence of substance abuse is highly culture specific, but is a growing problem in many countries. Recent studies in the United Republic of Tanzania found rates of 17.2%, 8.7% and 0.8% for alcohol, tobacco and cannabis use respectively. The prevalence of hazardous alcohol use was 5.7%.[8–10] Post-traumatic stress disorder (PTSD) is an additional problem in post conflict situations, but researchers and donors often, unfortunately, focus on this to the exclusion of the overall mental health needs of the population.[11] In general, rates of mental disorder are increased in populations subject to poverty, conflicts, displacement, and high rates of human immunodeficiency virus/acquired immunodeficiency syndrome (HIV/AIDS).

Some authors have suggested that more than 25% of the world's population will develop at least one mental disorder in their lifetime.[12–15] Studies have demonstrated the severity, duration,[16,17] and accompanying disability of depression and anxiety. The costs of depression and anxiety are immense in terms of repeated general practitioner (GP) consultations,[16] sickness absence,[18] labour turnover,[18] reduced productivity, and impact on families and children.

Increased physical morbidity of people with mental illness

Studies have found that more than half of those with mental illness also suffer from physical illness,[20] and that as the number of chronic conditions experienced by an individual increases, the likelihood of an affective disorder increases. It is also emerging that the combination of multiple conditions is worse for mental health than a particular single condition.[21] Specifically, many studies have found a higher prevalence of diabetes, respiratory disease, hepatitis B and C and HIV in this population. With such a high rate of physical comorbidities, one would hope and expect these individuals to receive a high quality and quantity of medical care; however, there is a severe discrepancy in the need for and the receipt of medical care in the mentally ill. For example, although people with schizophrenia have the highest mortality rates from cardiovascular disease, they have low rates of surgical interventions such as stenting or bypass grafting.[22] Additionally, studies have found that the mentally ill with diabetes are likely to receive a lesser standard of diabetes care than that of the general population. A meta-analysis of the quality of medical care for those with comorbid mental and medical illness demonstrated a significant inequality in the receipt of medical care for the severely mentally ill.[22] Specifically, individuals have been found to receive poor routine preventative service,[23] which is especially concerning given that the majority of mortality is secondary to preventable illnesses. Decreased medical care is harmful both to patients' medical health and to their mental health. Studies have found that a combination of medical and psychiatric illness is associated with increased functional and occupational disability, poorer quality of life and accelerated mortality.

Increased mortality of people with mental illness

People with mental illness have a higher mortality rate than the general population.[24] Suicide is one of the leading causes of global mortality, with national rates varying between 70 per 100 000 per year and 10 per

100 000 per year.[25] It used to be thought that suicide was largely a problem in high-income countries and was mostly unknown in low-income countries. This is now known not to be the case, and the few studies carried out in Africa indicate suicide rates akin to those in the west.[26]

The increased mortality of people with mental illness is caused not just by suicide and accidents, but also by physical illness, especially cardiovascular disease, respiratory illness and cancer.[22] A US study looking at individuals receiving public mental health care found that these patients died as much as 25 years earlier than the general population, again mainly from medical causes. In fact, this study found that the gap in mortality between people with severe mental illness and the general population is increasing over time.[23] Individuals with schizophrenia have been found to have proportional mortality ratios of two or more. Cardiovascular disease is reportedly responsible for at least 50% of this excess mortality.[27,28] One identifiable risk factor for cardiovascular disease in this population is antipsychotic drugs, many of which increase the risk of diabetes and other metabolic abnormalities.[22,27] Additionally, many modifiable risk factors such as substance use, smoking, and other unhealthy lifestyles, are more prevalent in the severely mentally ill.[22,28]

The public health and economic significance of mental disorders

Mental disorders matter because of their impact on human capacity, poverty, social capital, economic productivity and the achievement of the millennium development goals (MDGs).[29] Mental disorders attack the intrinsic human abilities to think, feel and communicate, and they erode social and physical functioning in all areas of life. A recent systematic review of large-scale epidemiological studies in the west has found a consistent relationship between rates of mental illness and indicators of social disadvantage, including low income, poor education, unemployment, and low social status.[30,31]

Children with emotional disorders and learning disabilities are often not recognized; they are frequently the ones who repeat classes, drop out or perform poorly. Orphans and other vulnerable children such as ex-combatants, street children and children in child-headed households have increased rates of mental disorder due to the risks they live with daily and the lack of social supports. Mental health also impacts on infant and child mortality, antenatal care, vaccination programmes, prevention and treatment of infectious diseases and rehydration therapy for watery diarrhoea. Treating maternal depression improves compliance with vaccination, nutrition, oral rehydration and hygiene regimes, to reduce infectious diseases in children. Treating maternal depression also reduces maternal mortality through decreased rates of suicide and cancer (less smoking, better nutrition) and improved physical health through better mental well-being. HIV infection rates for the 17–24-year age group are reduced because improved mental health reduces unsafe sex and levels of drug usage and addiction.

As well as actual comorbidity between mental and physical disorders, many people with depression and anxiety present with somatic symptoms that may be misdiagnosed as physical disease. In high-income countries, this misdiagnosis may be of influenza, while in low-income countries it may be of malaria, typhoid or amoebiasis. If not properly diagnosed and treated effectively, there is a high rate of repeat consultations and inappropriate treatments, placing an additional burden on health-care systems. Furthermore, treating a depressed person with physical aches and pains for malaria, when they have no parasites, contributes to drug resistance.

It is important to recognize that in all countries physical illnesses are given a higher priority than mental illnesses, and there is a common view that primary care should not dilute its efforts in tackling physical illness by taking on mental disorders as well. Clearly, psychosis is a severe illness and few people, if any, would argue that individuals with psychosis do not need treatment and rehabilitation. However, it has often been argued by those responsible for developing health systems that the non-psychotic disorders of depression and anxiety may be common but that their consequences are not as severe as those of physical illness, and that therefore they can be safely ignored. Such an argument is misguided, as the impact of mental illnesses on disability and mortality, as well as on economic productivity, is such that attention to them is imperative, and it is important to research sustainable ways of preventing and treating these disorders in different health-system contexts.

There is now a considerable knowledge base for effective interventions for many mental and neurological conditions in the developed world (health promotion, prevention, treatment, rehabilitation and prevention of mortality), as well as a growing number of studies in low-income countries, although studies of cost-effectiveness are particularly sparse.[32] However, this knowledge is not implemented in many parts of the world for a variety of reasons, including, for example, lack of mental health policy, lack of specialist services, lack of skills in primary care and lack of availability of essential medicines and treatments.

Caring for people with mental health problems – the need for integration of mental health in primary care

Primary health care has been defined by the World Health Organization (WHO) as:

> . . . essential health care made accessible to individuals and families in the community by means acceptable to them, through their full participation and at a cost that the community and the country can afford. It forms an integral part of the country's health system of which it is the nucleus, and of the overall social and economic development of the community.[33]

The high prevalence of mental disorders in those who consult primary care has been well documented over the last several decades in high-income countries,[34–38] and more recently in low- and middle-income countries.[6,39]

There is a significant amount of undetected morbidity and much untreated morbidity in primary care. A major WHO collaborating study in 15 primary care sites in developed and low-income countries round the world found that overall primary care physicians identify 23.4% of the attenders as being a "case" with a psychological disorder, while an interview using a research instrument identifies 33%.[39] The primary physicians reported that they provided treatment to 77.8% of the cases whom they identified as having a psychological disorder (around half are given counselling, a quarter sedative medication and only one-sixth receive antidepressants).

There are a number of reasons why people with severe mental illness have difficulty accessing care. These include amotivation or cognitive limitations, poverty, stigma, not knowing where or how to get care, difficulty interpreting physical symptoms, difficulty caring for self, and lack of available resources.[28,40,41]

A national US comorbidity survey found that more than half of the individuals with some form of mental illness – largely depression – receive treatment through primary care.[14,42] This means that primary care staff need training about mental health issues, and this need is highlighted in studies showing that opportunities for prevention of suicide are being missed in primary care. For example, a US study showed that for older adults, which is the population with the highest rate of suicide, 70% visited primary care within one month of committing suicide.[43] Similar opportunities for prevention of suicide are also being missed in UK primary care.[44] In the US, fewer than 3% of older adults report seeing a mental health professional for their treatment, and instead seek care with their primary care physician (PCP).[43] However, a focus-group study of US PCPs found that few used any formal screening tools to detect mental health problems, and they often only screened new patients for mental health; furthermore, when mental health issues were identified, they often did not refer patients to a mental health professional.[14]

PCPs have identified various barriers to adequately treating mental illness in the primary care clinic, including stigma, time pressure, limited reimbursement, lack of well-organized mental health systems and regarding physical complaints of the mentally ill as psychosomatic symptoms.[22,41,45]

On the other hand, many individuals with severe mental illness may only receive their health care through a mental health professional.[28] In these cases, patients also receive suboptimal medical care, as studies have shown the rate of preventive medical services provided at psychiatric visits to be about 11%.[46] Various barriers identified by mental health professionals include lack of knowledge or comfort in medical issues and lack of time and resources to address these issues. In some cases, when patients are seeing both psychiatrics and PCPs, it is unclear which physician is screening the patient for medical problems related to their psychiatric medications.

The advantages of integrating mental health into primary care have been well documented and include:

- *achievement of good clinical and social outcomes for people with a mental disorder who may not be able to gain access to a specialist*: in relatively rich countries this includes the majority of people with a common disorder such as depression and anxiety, while most if not all individuals with a psychotic illness would expect to be able to see a specialist. In low-income countries where there may not be a specialist within hundreds of miles, it will also include most people with psychosis

- *meeting physical health-care needs*: physical and mental illness frequently co-exist, so exclusive preoccupation with a single speciality may be disastrous for the individual patient. People with severe mental illness have relatively high standardized mortality ratios from physical diseases such as cardiac disease, respiratory disease, malignancy and, in low-income countries, infectious diseases
- *meeting social needs*: many psychiatric disorders are connected with family problems and social difficulties, and are only understandable when viewed against this background. Primary care teams, with their continuing contact with their local population, are well placed to have such detailed knowledge. The co-location of social workers with, or working in association with, primary health-care teams may be helpful in delivering integrated health and social care
- *continuity of care*: primary care teams are well placed to provide long-term follow-up and support without frequent changes of personnel
- *the patient's perspective*: many people with mental disorders do not consider themselves to be in need of psychiatric care and there may be less perceived stigma for the patient if they are seen in primary care.

Description of gold standard approaches

Having emphasized the vast scale of the problem, the advantages of the primary care setting and the scope for prevention in primary care, how can the busy primary care team possibly deliver on mental health, in the midst of all the other competing demands?

The WHO identified the crucial aspects for the successful design and implementation of a primary mental health-care programme,[47] which include:

- national policy formulation on mental health and the establishment of a mental health department or unit within each country's national or regional government
- financial provision for:
  - data collection and research
  - a network of facilities, including transport
  - the adequate supply of essential medicines
  - the recruitment, training and employment of human resource
- decentralization of mental health services, integration of mental health services with the general health services, and the development of collaboration with non-medical community agencies
- use of non-specialized mental health workers including primary health workers, nurses, medical assistants and doctors, for certain basic tasks of mental health care
- training of mental health professionals in this new task of training and supporting non-specialized health workers.

This list remains just as relevant today, and the main addition to be added to it is the use of good practice guidelines by primary care teams, to support their diagnosis, management and referrals.[48–50] These crucial elements will be discussed in turn.

Support for primary care from national policy

National mental health policies historically have tended to focus on the care of people with severe mental illness by the specialist services, and particularly on the care of mentally disordered offenders, but have tended to ignore the care of people with less severe disorders in primary care, and have also ignored the role of primary care in relation to the physical health care of people with mental illness. Such an approach is highly flawed, because the lack of attention to common mental disorders by primary care (which if not adequately treated greatly increase the burden to health services) will always compromise the care that can be targeted at people with severe mental illness, as well as generating immense costs for society. It is essential, therefore, that government policy should cover all the main categories of mental disorders, namely psychosis, depression and anxiety, childhood emotional and conduct disorders, PTSD, dementia, substance abuse, learning disabilities and epilepsy (which is a neurological disorder but is usually considered with the mental disorders because of the lack of neurological services).

It is crucial to have a mental health presence inside the ministry of health, in order to ensure that mental health is integrated into the health-sector reform plans, the essential package of health services, and the health management information system. There will need to be close liaison between the directorate of mental health and the directorates of primary care, curative services, preventive services, health management information systems and human resources. There will also need to be close liaison at government level between the directorate of mental health and the other relevant ministries of social welfare, education, criminal justice, etc.[51]

Each country has its own unique health-care-delivery system, and what makes sense in one country may not make sense in another. In the development of policy on integration of mental health into primary care, it is important to examine the existing primary care and secondary care systems, staffing, basic and continuing training for each of the professional groups involved, and the system of information collection. It is outside the scope of this review to provide a comprehensive account of the different organizational models of health-care delivery, financing and coverage; the different degrees of provision of specialist care; the degree to which it has moved from a hospital-based system to a community system; and the role of primary care in each country. Nonetheless, these are important contextual factors for primary care integration and will be referred to below.

Specialist human resource available to support primary care and take referrals

The USA and UK now have, on average, around 1 psychiatrist per 10 000 population, with 1.5 per 10 000 in Australia, having built up these ratios from 1 per 100 000 over the last 40 years or so. On the other hand, one psychiatrist per 1 000 000 population is a common scenario in low-income countries, especially sub-Saharan Africa. Some countries operate at one psychiatrist per five million, or even no psychiatrist at all. This situation is exacerbated by the fact that the distribution of specialists is not equitable relative to the distribution of the population, with most psychiatrists concentrated in the main cities for a variety of reasons, including the availability of private practice, the availability of academic links and posts, and the availability of schools and other facilities for families. For example, in the United Republic of Tanzania, over half the country's psychiatrists live and work in Dar es Salaam, leaving four or five psychiatrists to care for 29 million people.[52] In Egypt, where there is a much higher proportion of psychiatrists, nonetheless they are mostly in Cairo and Alexandria, leaving many governorates with only one or two psychiatrists to look after populations of 3 million.[53] Thus, access to a specialist is frequently geographically impossible in low-income countries, and sometimes even in the remote rural areas of high-income countries.

In low-income countries with restricted availability of specialist doctors, could their role, especially in the districts across the country concerned, be played by specialist nurses? In sub-Saharan Africa, specialist mental health nurses have, for several decades now, been trained to fulfil the role of doctors in that they are trained to assess, diagnose, treat and refer as appropriate. They are also expected to provide clinical leadership and management to district-level services. In countries where there are very few doctors, this leadership role for nurses is pretty much accepted and valued, whereas in more middle-income countries, for example Egypt and Iraq, such a leadership role for nurses has not previously been supported for a variety of reasons (including historical cultural attitudes to women), and this has hindered the development of accessible services for all districts, especially in the more remote areas away from large cities.

Therefore, in order to support community mental health programmes, training of psychiatrists should include supervised experience in the above areas. As recommended by WHO:

> specialized mental health workers should devote only a part of their working hours to the clinical care of the patients; the greater part of their time should be spent in training and supervision of specialized health workers who will provide basic health care in the community. This will entail significant changes in the role and training of the mental health professionals.[54]

Thus, the district mental health professional will need to devote a proportion of his or her working week to visiting, supporting and supervising local primary care teams, for example, establishing that each team is visited once a month.

To ensure the most effective use of specialist resources and to guarantee that those in greatest need are not neglected, attention needs to be paid to appropriate targeting of specialist resources at the more severe and difficult-to-treat disorders.[55] This requires development of agreed criteria for referral to the specialist services, taking into account the diagnosis, severity of symptoms, duration and risk of harm to self or others, as well as evolving safe methods of shared care, including medication, physical health care and health promotion.[56,57]

Primary care human resource

The composition of the primary care team varies from country to country. In the UK, the primary care team consists of the GP, practice manager, practice nurse, possibly a counsellor, and linked community nurses such as health visitors and district nurses. In low-income countries, primary care may contain no doctors and possibly a few medical assistants, and be largely staffed by nurses and health workers with brief periods of training. In Kenya, primary care is staffed by nurses and clinical officers (medical assistants with 3 years' training). These staff are supplemented by volunteer village health workers who have had no formal training but who receive ad hoc sessions of topic-based training from their primary care training centre. In Malawi, primary care is staffed mainly by medical assistants with 2 years' training, and these are supported by health surveillance assistants who undergo a 6-week course, while in the United Republic of Tanzania, primary care is staffed mostly by nurses, sometimes along with assistant medical officers (who have had a 3-year training).[52] In Egypt, primary care is staffed by doctors (who are given specific postgraduate training for primary care) and nurses.[53]

Key questions to ask when considering primary care human resource include: whether primary care doctors and nurses are in the front line of assessment and treatment or whether there is another tier in the frontline; whether the lead professional in the primary care team is a doctor or a medical assistant or a nurse, and what their respective roles are; what the basic training for each tier and professional in the primary care unit consists of and how much, if any, mental health training is included; what continuing professional development is available and how much mental health is included in the regular continuing education.

For example, in Iran, health workers with only 6–9 months' training are in the front line dealing with screening and case-finding, assessment and treatment for a population of around 2000. They refer if necessary to the primary care doctor or nurse, who may look after a population of 10000.[58] In mainland Tanzania, the front-line worker is a first aid worker who carries a first aid box and looks after 50 households. The second tier is the dispensary, which is staffed by nurses and looks after a population of 2000. The third tier is the primary care centre, which is staffed by nurses and sometimes assistant medical officers and looks after 10000 population.[52] In Zanzibar, the first tier is the primary health care unit which usually contains a medical assistant, and several male and female nurses,[59] while in Malawi the health surveillance assistant is the front-line worker and looks after a number of villages. In Kenya, the front-line worker is the village health worker (with no formal training apart from ad hoc days), looking after 100–200 households. The second tier is the dispensary and the third tier is the primary care centre. In practice, there is no formal relationship between the dispensary and the primary care centre, and people merely attend the closest facility.[60] In Pakistan, the first tier consists of health workers, usually married women with grown-up children, who receive a short training; the second tier is the primary care doctor.[61]

The lead professional in primary care in sub-Saharan Africa is usually a clinical officer with 3 years' training – if they are present – but otherwise will be a nurse with 3–4 years of training. This is in contrast to the UK, where the front-line worker is the GP, who is also the lead professional in primary care. Most GPs in the UK now work in groups or partnerships of three to five partners, and employ one or two primary care nurses between them. They also collaborate with a community nursing structure of district nurses and health visitors, who are specialist nurses for older people and young mothers with pre-school children respectively.

In the USA and Australia, the front-line worker has traditionally been a private primary care physician, but even this model is changing. Throughout the USA, nurse practitioners and physician assistants are increasingly taking a lead role in providing front-line primary care. These physician extenders are especially useful in geographically rural areas where it might be difficult to see a physician. In addition, new ways of using telemedicine have helped to link these clinicians with physicians who can help guide and provide additional consultation.

In Australia, the front-line worker is most commonly a GP who works either in private practice or a community health centre, although Australians can obtain direct access to a psychologist or counsellor via their workplace or, if they are able to pay, without going via a GP. Despite this, most people visit their GP as the first level of care. Australia recognizes the enormous challenge that depression care brings, and considerable policy attention and substantial investment in primary care began in 2001 with the "Better Outcomes in Mental Health Care" initiative and the 2006 "Better Access to Mental Health" programme, which allows GPs to conduct a mental health plan and to refer to psychology for up to 12 government-subsidised sessions per eligible individual, per calendar year. There has been enormous uptake of this initiative; in 2008–2009, the Medicare Benefits Schedule subsidized expenditure of 234 million Australian dollars (AUD) for access to psychological services and AUD167 million for GP-completed mental health plans.

In Iran, health workers receive several months' training in a few priority topics, which include reproductive health, infectious diseases, tuberculosis (TB), schizophrenia and the common mental disorders such as depression and anxiety. Addiction has recently been added to this list. These health workers are taught to screen and case-find by routine visits to homes, and to perform basic assessments, diagnoses and treatments in those conditions, using good practice guidelines. They follow agreed criteria for referral to the primary care nurse and doctor, who form the second tier of care, looking after a population of 10 000. In Zanzibar, the College of Health Sciences runs a 4-year basic nursing course, of which the fourth year for women is midwifery and the fourth year for men is psychiatry. (The college has recently decided to add some psychiatry to the midwifery course as well.) A similar situation exists in mainland Tanzania, so that both countries (linked as the United Republic of Tanzania, but with separate ministries of health) now have a substantial population of primary care nurses who have received basic training in psychiatry. In the UK, USA and Australia, the front-line doctors receive a 5- or 6-year medical training and often a further 3 years of training as a general physician.

In most countries, the continuing education programmes focus largely on physical illness, and any mental health continuing education is an optional extra rather than an integrated component received by all front-line health professionals. In Australia, the "Better Outcomes in Mental Health Care" initiative has invested heavily in providing extra voluntary training for GPs in mental health, including training-focused psychological strategies, and almost AUD 900 million of government funding has been dedicated to this since 2001.

Information systems in primary care

Adequate planning is not possible without good systems for information collection in primary care. In Iran, health workers routinely collect basic data every year on the prevalence and outcome of the priority disorders, which include infectious diseases, schizophrenia, epilepsy, depression and anxiety. These data are summarized into an annual table and displayed on the wall of the health centre, so that they are readily available to all staff, who then have the data and their implications for their work at their fingertips and can compare them with preceding years. In some low-income countries, a stroke form is used for collecting consultation data in primary care. However, while containing 34 categories for separate physical disorders, it only contains one all-inclusive category for mental disorder. In Zanzibar, this stroke form has now been revised to include six categories of mental disorder. As part of current health-sector reforms, new health management information systems are being developed in a number of African countries, so that key categories of mental disorders will be included as integral parts of the information system.[62] In Australia, despite the widespread use of electronic medical records in general practice, there is no uniform coding of consultations, and the capacity of the information systems to be used as part of a continuous quality-improvement system is extremely poor for mental health conditions.[63]

Transport for outreach and supervision

A key consideration here is how far the work of the primary care team is proactive or reactive. Does the primary care team mostly concentrate its time on those individual patients who actively consult, or does it take a more population-based approach and seek to find and treat the common disabling conditions in that population?

In many countries, especially in rural areas with little or no public transport, outreach from primary care to the community, and from secondary care to primary care and to the community, is not systematically possible unless transport is available; this may need to be provided or subsidized, and needs to be appropriate to the terrain and linked to maintenance contracts. With the focus on integration of services and a move away from vertical programmes, it is hard to argue for transport specifically dedicated to mental health but, on the other hand, practical experience indicates that shared transport schemes for district health services rarely include the mental health teams. There is a need, then, for considerable advocacy with district health-management teams, to ensure that the district transport matrix includes prioritization of mental health needs for supervision to primary care and outreach.

Supply of essential medicines

If primary care teams are to look after the majority of people with mental disorders effectively, they need an adequate supply of essential medicines. This is not normally a problematic issue for developed countries, but in low-income countries it is common to find that primary care units – each looking after a population of roughly 10 000 people, including, for example, 50 people with chronic schizophrenia, 50 people with epilepsy and several hundred people with severe depression – may have little or no access to medicines for their patients. It is possible using basic epidemiological data to calculate the requirements for essential medicines for a population of say 10 000 people, served by a primary health-care unit. Basic medicines are required for depression (e.g. amitryptyline and imipramine), psychosis (chlorpromazine and haloperidol), for side-effects (benzhexol), and epilepsy (phenobarbitone, phenytoin and tegretol). Valium is usually available in primary care for pre-eclampsia and status epilepticus but is misused for depression and anxiety, because of the lack of availability of antidepressants. It is not remotely affordable for the public health services to supply the new antipsychotics or the new antidepressants on a routine basis (even now it is barely affordable for high-income countries). What is crucial is to ensure an adequate supply of basic medicines and to establish the implementation of good practice guidelines in their usage, including the capacity to explain and manage the side-effects. Primary care teams also need access to occupational rehabilitation services and to psychosocial intervention skills.

Good practice guidelines

Primary care and secondary care are more efficient and effective if there is good communication between them, agreed criteria for referral and discharge, agreed guidelines and mutual support. This is likely to entail regular meetings between primary health-care teams and specialist staff to discuss criteria for referral, discharge letters, shared care procedures, need for medicines, information transfer and any other coordination issues, training, good practice guidelines and consideration of appropriate research. Good practice guidelines are helpful educational tools for ensuring that best practice is routine, yet many of those that currently exist have failed to take account of the complexity of patients presenting to primary care, and none have dealt adequately with the co-occurrence of multiple physical health problems.[64] They may cover assessment, diagnosis, management and criteria for referral. The WHO International Classification of Diseases (ICD)-10 primary care guidelines have been useful, and have been adapted for a variety of high- and low-income countries.[48,48,65] WHO has now issued a new set of treatment guidelines, which will be adapted by respective regions and countries.

Is there any scope for quality monitoring of standards in primary care?

In Iran, health psychologists perform a quality-monitoring role for the health workers, visiting every month to support, supervise and check on the quality of the work.[66] In the United Republic of Tanzania, supervision of mental health in primary care is provided by psychiatric nurses,[52] while in Kenya it is by a combination of district psychiatric nurses and district public health nurses.[60]

Linkages with physical health programmes

The links between physical and mental disorders have already been summarized earlier in the section on public health and the economic significance of mental disorders. Thus, mental health and mental illness issues are so inextricably associated with delivery of physical health targets that it makes sense to address them, both in research and practice, in concert with other physical health priorities such as malaria, HIV and TB. We need a partnership – rather than a competition – between communicable and non-communicable diseases. For example, in advanced HIV, there is chronic loss of general cognitive function, leading to apathy, withdrawal and deterioration of personality. As in other major life-threatening illness, AIDS has a high frequency of adjustment reaction, persistent depression, affective psychosis and suicidal risk. There is a need for more research on mental health promotion in schools to reduce the risk of contracting HIV with unprotected sex or drug use, to support girls to be assertive and confident in ensuring their sexuality and safety, to address particular difficulties in countries where use of condoms is not widely culturally accepted by men, and to encourage abstention from drugs and harm reduction in those who use drugs.

Linkages with non-health sectors

Mental disorders in primary care carry a high incidence of disability and impaired social role performance, which means that primary care should interface well with social care where it exists, both statutory and voluntary; yet in most countries this is a rare occurrence. Primary care has the potential to provide a referral and support service to increase awareness of and access to existing sources of support within the community. This could include facilitating self-help groups, providing access to user and patient support via the Internet, and building links with religious organizations. Strengthening social support reduces the burden on primary care not only by mediating symptoms, but also by reducing the risk of mental health problems developing.

Mental disorders are common in children, and many predispose them to mental disorders in later life. Primary care is uniquely positioned to recognize and address problems in children and to support schools to play their roles, both by liaison and consultation with teachers and by contributing to the curriculum. Mental health promotion should be as integral to education as is physical health education.[67] Schools will need policies on bullying, truancy, supporting teachers, etc. A recent study in Norway showed that being a bully or a victim of bullying at school is a predictor for later problems, including conduct disorders, crime and alcohol abuse (bullies) and depression, anxiety and suicidal behaviour (victims).[68] There is therefore a strong case for including anti-bullying strategies as a key mental health promotion intervention. In some countries, e.g. India and Pakistan, schoolchildren play a vital role in recognizing illness such as epilepsy and schizophrenia in adults and bringing them to medical attention.[69] In other countries, for example Zanzibar, primary care teams include health education workers who link with schools on a local basis.[59]

Mental disorders are common in employed adults in the west,[70,71] and primary care teams often provide the occupational health care for businesses and industries. In Africa, occupational health care is very sparse, but some of the big multinational companies use private doctors to deliver their occupational health care. It is vital that such occupational health care is able to address mental health problems and to work with employers to establish sensible workplace health policies, which address mental health.[70–72] Employers need a greater awareness of the benefits of adopting policies to promote mental health at work. A number of stress-related disorders, as well as anxiety and depression, have been linked to a poor-quality working environment. Lack of control at work also increases the risk of cardiovascular disease.[73] There is growing awareness of the problems of stress and substance abuse in major public-sector professionals such as teachers, the police force, social workers and health professionals, but as yet little or no occupational health provision for them. Mental problems are common in those who have experienced violence or substance use, and the primary care response needs the capacity to deal with these challenging problems.[74]

Occupational rehabilitation

In richer countries occupational rehabilitation of severely ill people back into employment and their other social roles has generally been considered the preserve of the specialist services, and rehabilitation centres have been set up in association with the specialist services. Some excellent examples linked to specialist services are also to be found in low-income countries.[6] However, if occupational rehabilitation is to be available for all severely ill people who need it, it will have to be made available at the primary care level in low-income countries, rather than exclusively at the specialist level. This is because of the great shortage of specialists and because even each primary health-care unit – covering a population of 10 000 people – will have at least

50 people with chronic schizophrenia, 50 people with bipolar disorders and several hundred with severe depression to care for, with little or no access to distant specialist services. Therefore, part of the support that needs to be given to primary care is expertise in stimulating, for example, the development of local community groups and nongovernmental organizations (NGOs) to carry out such rehabilitative tasks in conjunction with the health-care system.

Low-income country examples of integration of mental health into primary care

Given the burden of common mental health problems, the integration of mental health with primary care services has been a significant policy objective in wealthy and low-income areas of the world.[75-77] Different countries are at varying stages of putting in place mechanisms for integrating mental health care into the work of primary care teams. Some of the most well-developed and proactive examples have been pioneered in low-income countries, where the organization has often been closely influenced by WHO and followed a public health model.[78,79]

In those developing countries that have pioneered community approaches to tackling severe mental illness, most have pursued the strategy of integrating such community approaches with primary care. The stimulus for this was the WHO collaborative multicentre international project entitled "Strategies for Extending Mental Health Care 1975–1981", which involved seven developing countries: Brazil, Colombia, Egypt, India, the Philippines, Senegal and the Sudan.[80,81]

Guinea-Bissau

A useful model public mental health programme was evaluated in Guinea-Bissau.[79] Following independence in 1974, Guinea-Bissau transformed its centralized, curative and hospital-based approach into a decentralized and preventive approach, setting up a nationwide primary health-care system. The model programme had three main aspects: firstly, a small-scale psychiatric hospital for referral, training and support of the basic mental health programme; second, participant observation with traditional healers to explore possibilities for collaboration; and third, a public health approach, which was in turn delivered in three stages:

- firstly an epidemiological investigation to discover what percentage of adults and children visiting basic health-care facilities in a rural and an urban area have a mental disorder, what kind of disorder, and whether these problems are recognized by health workers, along with a qualitative and quantitative assessment of the community strengths and impediments to setting up a nationwide intervention programme
- second a training programme for health workers and repetitive supervisory visits to the primary care facilities
- third an evaluation of the programme.

Using the information gathered in the first stage – on prevalence, evidence of community concern, seriousness, susceptibility to treatment, sustainability of the programme, and knowledge and skills of the health workers – it was decided to construct a training programme for health staff working at the level of primary care about psychosis, agitation, neurotic and especially depressive disorders, and epilepsy. The training programme also included the nurses who train and supervise the volunteer village health workers. The intervention also included increasing the supply of essential psychotropic medicines to the health centres. The evaluation in the third stage showed that there was no need for a separate cadre in a basic mental health programme. Primary care nurses were successful in diagnosing and treating severe mental disorder, major depression and epilepsy. However, there was less success with somatizing patients (i.e. those showing symptoms of physical illness as a result of mental health problems). The costs of the basic mental health programme are low, given that the functioning primary health-care system already exists and that buildings and salaries are already funded. The author concluded that the programme only works with supervision. The health workers only started to practise their acquired knowledge after the supervising team had visited them.[79]

Mainland Tanzania

In mainland Tanzania, a pilot programme in two demonstration areas was launched and evaluated.[78] The programme design aimed to take full advantage of Tanzania's existing primary care infrastructure by integrating mental health into the general health services of the country, including the "grassroots" level in the villages and districts. The essential features of the strategy were to integrate mental health care within the general functions of the health workers at village and dispensary level, with the capacity to refer to specialist mental health services at district and regional levels. Five target conditions were designated as programme priorities: acute psychosis, epilepsy, common emotional illness (such as depression, anxiety, somatization), and mental retardation. The strategy was pilot tested in two regions – Morogoro and Moshi. For a period of 3 years, a WHO consultant was posted in each of the two pilot areas, and a third WHO consultant was based at the Mental Health Resource Centre at Muhimbili. It was intended that following the withdrawal of WHO consultants and the reduction of external financial support, the government would extend the programme to other regions of the country. This did not happen in the succeeding years, at least partly because of the government's subsequent financial difficulties. However, in the last several years the programme has been revitalized in half the regions of the country as part of the health-sector reforms.[52]

Zanzibar

In Zanzibar, integration of mental health into primary care was started in the 1980s as part of a Danish International Development Agency (DANIDA)-funded programme, but stopped after a few years due to lack of finance. It was approved by the House of Representatives in 1999 as part of the new mental health policy, and since then there have been systematic continuing education programmes about mental health for primary care teams. Prison nurses and some local traditional healers have also been invited, which has assisted intersectoral collaboration.[59]

Kenya

In Kenya, a programme to train primary care staff about mental health has been rolled out since 2005 – training over 2000 front-line health workers so far – accompanied by provision of good practice guidelines, supervision from the district level (district psychiatric nurses and district public health nurses), provision of essential medicines, and collection of diagnostic data.[82–84]

Malawi

In Malawi, two pilot programmes of training primary health workers in mental health have been carried out, with the aim of rolling out the programmes nationally. In 2008, all primary health workers in one of the 28 districts of Malawi were trained in mental health as part of the evaluation process of a training toolkit for training primary health workers in mental health; and in 2010, a pilot programme of integrating mental health in the activities of health surveillance assistants so that they can carry out early detection, monitoring and psychosocial rehabilitation activities in the community started, and is due to finish in 2011.

Gold standard approaches in high-income countries

Randomized trials that have attempted to improve care by changing one aspect – such as screening, education or feedback from patients – have demonstrated minimal, if any, improvement in patient outcome.[85] These trials have made it more apparent that there needs to be a large structural change in the way care is delivered.[86] Specifically, research has found that integrating mental health services into primary care clinics improves the access to care by patients and improves outcomes, in particular for treatment of depression.[87] Studies have found various common characteristics in successfully integrated models, including a team approach, strong clinical and practice-management leadership, informal knowledge exchange, effective use of midlevel practitioners, a loyal base of consumers, and the ability to serve patients with complicated problems and diverse backgrounds. Models for embedding effective depression care into primary care have been developed and may assist in ensuring sustainability – which has proved difficult to date.[63]

White River Junction model[42]

One form of integrated care is co-located care, where mental health-care providers and primary care providers are in the same practice location. One model that has been very successful and sustainable is the White River Junction model used in the United States Department of Veteran Affairs (VA) system. In fact, this model has been considered the standard of care for the VA system since 2005.

The model first came into being in 2004 as a quality-improvement project; at that point, the waiting time for new psychiatric evaluations was 6 weeks and the no-show rate of patients was over 40%. The goals of the project were to improve efficiency, shorten waiting times, and improve access to care. Focus-group studies involving physicians and patients were carried out prior to initiation of the new model, and found that "ease of access" to care was the most important issue for patients. The focus groups also concluded that most patients' mental health issues could be handled by mental heath experts within the primary care setting, thus reserving specialized clinics and those scarce resources for the more complicated patients. As a result, in 2004, the "primary care mental health care clinic" (PMHC) opened, located entirely within the primary care clinic. Several core principles were identified for this clinic: (1) mental health-care providers should be part of the primary care team; (2) care should be flexible to meet the needs of both patients and providers; (3) care should be immediately accessible without the need for scheduled appointments; and (4) most patients should be able to receive all of their mental health care without the need for referral into a more specialized setting.

Therefore, when the PMHC first opened it was staffed by two mental health clinicians (a therapist and a psychiatrist or advanced nurse practitioner with prescribing privileges) and a clerk. Patients come to the clinic either through self-referrals or referral by their PCP, emergency room staff, or other professionals. Appointments are not necessary prior to arrival, and upon presenting to the clinic patients complete various self-report tools, including the Beck Depression Inventory, The Speilberger State/Trait Anxiety Inventory, The PTSD Checklist-Military, and the Medical Outcome Study 36-Item Short Form Health Survey. The psychotherapist receives a summary of these results and then interviews the patient. Then they review the case with the psychiatrist or psychiatric nurse, who does a medically oriented interview and mental status exam and then formulates a diagnosis. The mental health clinicians and patient then create a treatment plan together, and new medications agreed or medication changes made. If a patient is more complex than can be adequately treated in the PMHC, they make a follow-up appointment in the specialized mental health clinic. Otherwise, patients are then given a "return interval" during which they should come back to the clinic. No specific appointments are necessary. A care manager was later added to the clinic to call patients if there was a lag between appointments and to assess patients over the phone. Other components of this model include national conferences attended by both primary-care and mental-health practitioners, monthly national education teleconferences, and policy development, including procedures and tools for workload tracking.[88]

The results of this project were overwhelmingly encouraging. In the first 3 months of opening, the number of people referred to PMHC who arrived for their initial evaluations more than doubled; additionally, the waiting time to see a mental health professional decreased from a mean of 33 days to 19 minutes; also, the number of patients referred for more specialized mental health care decreased by 74%, and the no-show rate at these specialized clinics decreased from 40% to 12%.[42] In the first year of opening, only 26% of new patients in the PMHC had problems requiring referral to a specialized mental health clinic. In terms of resources required for this clinic, less than 10% of the overall staff of the department provided all the treatment in the PMHC. Perhaps most importantly, 99% of patients seen in the PMHC expressed good to excellent satisfaction with the overall care they received. This clinic in fact won the 2005 American Psychiatric Association gold award for excellence in health services delivery.[87] A very important measure of the success of a model is its sustainability – this model has now been the standard of practice in the VA for over 5 years.

PRISM-E (Primary Care Research in Substance Abuse and Mental Health for the Elderly)[41]

This trial also utilized the co-located integrated care model, showing that this type of model can also work outside of the robust, well-funded VA system. Ten sites were involved, including both primary care and specialty mental health/substance abuse clinics. The trial randomized primary care patients who were aged 65 years or older and were found to have depression, anxiety, or at-risk alcohol consumption. Patients were either assigned to the integrated care group – where mental health and substance abuse providers were co-located with primary care specialists – or to the enhanced referral group, which referred to specialty mental health/substance abuse clinics. In the integrated group, patients had psychiatric assessment, care planning, counselling, case management, psychotherapy and psychopharmacologic treatment, all in the same place.

The mental health/substance abuse treatment was provided by licensed professionals in these areas and there was verbal or written communication between mental health professionals and the patients' PCP. Mental health appointments were arranged within 2–4 weeks following the PCP appointment.

The study found that statistically significantly more patients were likely to engage in mental health services in the integrated care group than in the enhanced referral group. Specifically, depressed patients in the integrated group were 2.86 times more likely to have at least one contact with a mental health specialist than those in the referral group. Additionally, the integrated group had more visits with mental health and substance abuse specialists, averaging three visits per patient, compared to 1.9 visits in the referral group. The study found that for the referral group, engagement in mental health and substance abuse care decreased as the distance between the primary care services and other services increased.

Primary Care Access, Referral and Evaluation (PCARE) model[23]

This is another model involving enhancing primary care and mental health care for individuals attending community health care centres. In the USA, over 3.5 millions adults with mental health problems attend community health care centres. As these centres lack the resources to create a co-located health-care system, this trial embarked on an inexpensive and practical model, involving medical care management. This trial involved 407 individuals with severe mental illness attending an urban community mental health centre. These individuals were randomly assigned to the medical care management intervention or to usual care. The intervention group provided care managers who offered the following types of support: providing communication and advocacy with medical providers; providing health education; and providing logistical help to navigate through the health-care system.

A 12-month follow-up evaluation found that 58.7% of individuals in the intervention group received the recommended preventive services, compared to 21.8% of individuals receiving usual care. This intervention group also received a significantly higher proportion of services for cardiometabolic conditions and was significantly more likely to have a PCP. At this time interval, 11.9% of the intervention group had newly diagnosed medical conditions, most commonly hyperlipidaemia and hypertension, compared with 1.8% of the group receiving usual care.

Collaborative care model – Washington State[89]

This is another type of collaborative care model involving the PCP and a medically supervised nurse that also provided encouraging results. It is but one example of a number of important studies by Kanton and colleagues at Group Health in Seattle, Washington, who have sought to better determine best models for collaborative primary mental health care. The single-blind randomized controlled study involved 214 participants from 14 primary care clinics in Washington State. The patients had poorly controlled diabetes or coronary heart disease, or both, as well as coexisting depression. Patients were randomly assigned to the usual-care group or to an intervention group involving medically supervised nurses. These nurses had experience with diabetes education and also attended a 2-day training course on depression management; behavioural strategies; and glycaemic, blood-pressure and lipid control. In addition to these educational sessions, the nurses had weekly supervisions with a psychiatrist, primary care physician and psychologist, to review both new patients and the progress of old patients. In terms of patient follow-up, patients visited the primary care clinic every 2–3 weeks to monitor progress of both their medical and psychiatric illnesses. During these visits, the patients worked with the nurses and PCPs to create individualized goals for their treatment. The nurses then followed the patients through phone calls to support both self-care and medication compliance. They also provided patients with self-care materials for both depression and their medical issues.

The study found that the intervention group had a greater improvement both medically and psychiatrically. Over 12 months, this group had greater improvements in glycated haemoglobin levels, low-density lipoprotein cholesterol levels, systolic blood pressure, and Symptom Checklist (SCL)-20 depression scores compared to the usual-care group. Additionally, these patients were more likely to have at least one adjustment in their medication regimen, better quality of life, and greater satisfaction with their medical and psychiatric care (all with stastistical significance). As the financial burden of implementing changes in the medical system are always a significant concern, it should be noted that the estimated mean cost per patient for these interventions was only $1224.

This model is extremely beneficial for community health centres that have difficulty with resources and funding. However, one drawback is that this system depends on an accessible place for individuals to receive quality primary medical care in the community. Furthermore, these Seattle trials have been done with highly trained staff rather than within the usual clinic, so generalizing the findings into routine care often proves very difficult.

Barriers to change

The models described above, in high-income countries, demonstrate that integrated care can significantly improve the care of patients both medically and psychiatrically. However, there are still several barriers preventing the implementation of these models in various settings. First of all, many clinics have difficulty with funding and reimbursement of integrated care clinics.[15] Although the VA model has proven sustainable, many other systems do not have the financial means to fund these changes and to maintain them. Even when studies have found improvement in both patient and physician satisfaction with system changes, many models cannot be implemented without continued administrative and financial support once the research period has ended. In primary care settings, reimbursement favours shorter office visits and performance of laboratory tests and procedures, and does not compensate for communicating with colleagues or screening for mental health.[90] Also, the stigma of mental health issues is still very prevalent, and systems that favour sharing information between mental health professionals and PCPs may be thwarted if patients do not want their psychiatric issues shared with their PCPs. Another barrier is the willingness of both primary care providers and mental health professionals to operate differently from how they have been trained and to how they have practised. Various problems cited by mental health-care providers include changing the pace of patient encounters, as they must move more quickly with patients and between patients. Also, the length of treatment tends to be shorter, the use of standardized assessment tools may be more prevalent, and common therapies, such as cognitive-behavioural therapy (CBT) may be too long in this setting. Additionally, these professionals have cited difficulties with loss of autonomy, as they must rely on a care team more than they may be used to.

The barriers to change in low-income countries include low financial and human resource, international migration of health workers,[91] and lack of attention to health and social programmes from international donors.[92]

Necessary stakeholders

The stakeholders for integration of mental health into primary care include national policy-makers, specialist human resource, primary care human resource, and non-health sectors (social welfare, education, criminal justice etc.).

Future directions

Training is a key element for improving patient care, but must be accompanied by systemic change if it is to lead to improved health outcomes. First of all, basic and post-basic training for all health workers needs to emphasise a biopsychosocial approach to assessment, diagnosis and management of disorders, so that general health workers can address mental health issues and mental health workers can address physical health issues, cross-referring as necessary.

Additionally, training programmes for psychiatrists need to provide experience in giving collaborative support to primary care, in working closely with primary care, and in understanding primary care settings. In high-income countries, there may be enough specialist resource for some specialists to work based in primary care. Also, both mental health and primary care practitioners should be required to attend, or at least offered, educational meetings outside of their specialty so as to be more comfortable treating patients with comorbidities and to reduce the stigma of mental illnesses.

Studies have suggested that PCPs be given brief protocols for managing patients with severe mental illness, such as chronic psychoses.[93] Practitioners are often unclear on how to treat patients with psychiatric and medical comorbidities, because research studies often exclude patients with both medical and mental illness. Research is therefore needed in patients with complex comorbidities.

References

1   Beddington J et al. The mental wealth of nations. *Nature*, 2008, 455:1057–1060.

2   Jenkins R et al. The British Mental Health Programme: achievements and latest findings. *Social Psychiatry and Psychiatric Epidemiology*, 2009, 44:899–904.

3   Kessler RC et al. Prevalence, severity and co-morbidity of 12 month DSM-IV disorders in the National Comorbidity Survey Replication. *Archives of General Psychiatry*, 2005, 62:617–627.

4   *National Survey of Mental Health and Wellbeing: summary of results.* Canberra, Australian Bureau of Statistics, 2007.

5   Andrews G, Henderson S. Prevalence, comorbidity, disability and service utilisation. Overview of the Australian National Mental Health Survey. *British Journal of Psychiatry*, 2001, 178:145–153.

6   Jablensky A et al. Neurological, psychiatric and developmental disorders – meeting the challenge in the developing world. In: Press NA, ed. Washington DC, Institute of Medicine, 2001:293–295.

7   Mirza I, Jenkins R. Risk factors, prevalence, and treatment of anxiety and depressive disorders in Pakistan: systematic review. *BMJ*, 2004, 328:794–797.

8   Jenkins R et al. Prevalence of psychotic symptoms and their risk factors in urban Tanzania. *International Journal of Environmental Research and Public Health*, 2010, 7:2514–2525.

9   Jenkins R et al. Common mental disorders and their risk factors in urban Tanzania. *International Journal of Environmental Research and Public Health*, 2010, 7:2543–2558.

10 Jenkins R et al. Prevalence of alcohol consumption and hazardous drinking, tobacco and drug use in urban Tanzania and their associated risk factors. *International Journal of Environmental Research and Public Health*, 2009, 6:1991–2006.

11 Jenkins R et al. Mental health and the development agenda in sub Saharan Africa. *Psychiatric Services*, 2010, 61:229–234.

12 Thornicroft G, Alem A, Dos Santos RA. WPA guidance on steps, obstacles and mistakes to avoid in the implementation of community mental health care. *World Psychiatry*, 2010, 9:67–77.

13 *World Health Report 2001. Mental health: new understanding, new hope.* Geneva, World Health Organization, 2001.

14 Winternheimer L, O'Connell KL, on behalf of the Mental Health Transformation Working Group. *Integration of behavioral health and primary care best practices. International Journal of Environmental Research and Public Health*, 2010, 7:2515–2525.

15 Pomerantz AS, Corson JA, Detzer MJ. The challenge of integrated care for mental health: leaving the 50 minute hour and other sacred things. *Journal of Clinical Psychology in Medical Settings*, 2009, 1:40–46.

16 Lloyd K, Jenkins R, Mann A. Long term outcome of patients with neurotic illness in general practice. *BMJ*, 1996, 313:26–28.

17 Mann AH, Jenkins R, Belsey E. The 12-month outcome of patients with neurotic illness in general practice. *Psychological Medicine*, 1981, 11:535–550.

18 Jenkins R. Minor psychiatric morbidity in civil servants and its contribution to sickness absence. *British Journal of Industrial Medicine*, 1985, 42:147–154.

19 Jenkins R. Minor psychiatric morbidity and labor turnover. *British Journal of Industrial Medicine*, 1985, 42:534–539.

20 Mitchell A et al. Quality of medical care for people with and without comorbid mental illness and substance misuse: systematic review of comparative studies. *British Journal of Psychiatry*, 2009, 194:491–499.

21   Gunn J et al. The association between chronic illness, multimorbidity and depressive symptoms in an Australian primary care cohort. *Social Psychiatry and Psychiatric Epidemiology*, 2010, 25 December epub ahead of print.

22   Lawrence D, Stephen K. Inequalities in health care provision for people with severe mental illness. *Journal of Psychopharmacology*, 2010, 24:s61–68.

23   Druss BG et al. A randomized trial of medical care management for community mental health settings: the Primary Care Access, Referral, and Evaluation (PCARE) study. *American Journal of Psychiatry*, 2010, 167:151–159.

24   Harris EC, Barraclough B. Excess mortality of mental disorder. *British Journal of Psychiatry*, 1998;173:11–53.

25   World Health Organization. *Suicide rates per 100000 by country, year and sex* (http://www.who.int/mental_health/prevention/suicide_rates/en/index.html, accessed 15 November 2011).

26   Moshiro C et al. The importance of injury as a cause of death in sub-Saharan Africa: results of a community based study in Tanzania. *Public Health*, 2001, 115: 96–102.

27   De Hert M et al. Physical health management in psychiatric settings. *European Psychiatry*, 2010, 25:S22–S28.

28   De Hert M, Correll CU. Physical illness in patients with severe mental disorders: I. Prevalence, impact of medications and disparities in health care. *World Psychiatry*, 2011, 10:52–77.

29   Jenkins R et al. *Mental capital and wellbeing: making the most of ourselves in the 21st century. Mental health: future challenges*. London, Government Office for Science, 2008.

30   Fryers T, Melzer, D, Jenkins, R. Social inequalities and the common mental disorders. A systematic review of the evidence. *Social Psychiatry and Psychiatric Epidemiology*, 2003, 38:229–237.

31   Baingana F et al. *Mental health and socio-economic outcomes in Burundi*. Washington, The World Bank, 2004.

32   Shah A, Jenkins R. Mental health economic studies from developing countries reviewed in the context of those from developed countries. *Acta Psychiatrica Scandinavica*, 2000, 101:87–103.

33   *Declaration of Alma-Ata*. International Conference on Primary Health Care, Alma-Ata USSR, 6–12 September 1978 (http://www.who.int/hpr/NPH/docs/declaration_almaata.pdf, accessed 2 November 2011).

34   Shepherd M. *Psychiatric illness in general practice*. Oxford, Oxford University Press 1967.

35   Harding TW et al. Mental disorders in primary health care: a study of their frequency in four developing countries. *Psychological Medicine*, 1980, 10:231–241.

36   Regier DA et al. The "de facto" US mental health service systems. *Archives of General Psychiatry*, 1978, 35:685–693.

37   Goldberg DP, Huxley P. *Mental illness in the community. The pathway to psychiatric care*. London, Tavistock Publications, 1980.

38   Goldberg DP, Huxley P. *Common mental disorders – a biopsychosocial model*. London, Routledge and Kegan Paul, 1992.

39   Ustun TB, Sartorius N, eds. *Mental illness in general health care: an international study*. Chichester, Wiley, 1995.

40   *Achieving the promise: transforming mental health care in America. Final report*. Rockville, MD, New Freedom Commission on Mental Health, 2003.

41   Bradford DW et al. Access to medical care among persons with psychotic and major affective disorders. *Psychiatric Services*, 2008, 59:847–852.

42   Pomerantz AS et al. Improving efficiency and access to mental health care: Combining integrated care and advanced clinical access. *General Hospital Psychiatry*, 2008, 30:546–551.

43   Bartels SJ et al. Improving access to geriatric mental health services: a randomized trial comparing treatment engagement with integrated versus enhanced referral care for depression, anxiety, and at-risk alcohol use. *American Journal of Psychiatry*, 2004, 161:1455–1462.

44   Haste F, Charlton J, Jenkins R. Potential for suicide prevention in primary care? An analysis of factors associated with suicide. *British Journal of General Practice*, 1998, 48:1759–1763.

45   Oxman TE et al. A three-component model for reengineering systems for the treatment of depression in primary care. *Psychomatics*, 2002, 43:441–450.

46   Bradford DW et al. Access to medical care among persons with psychotic and major affective disorders. *Psychiatric Services*, 2008, 59:847–852.

47   *Mental health care in developing countries. Report of a WHO study group*. Geneva, Switzerland: World Health Organization; 1984.

48   World Health Organization Collaborating Centre for Mental Health Research and Training IoP. *WHO guide to mental health in primary care. Adapted for the UK from Diagnostic and Management Guidelines for Mental Disorders in Primary Care (ICD 10 Chapter V) Primary Care Version*. London, Royal Society of Medicine, 2004.

49   *Diagnostic and management guidelines for mental disorders in primary care: ICD-10 Chapter V primary care version*. Seattle, Hogrefe and Huber, 1996.

50   Paton J, Jenkins R, eds. *Mental health primary care in prison. A guide to mental ill health in adults and adolescents in prison and young offender institutions*. London, Royal Society of Medicine Press Ltd, 2002.

51   Jenkins R, McCulloch A. *Developing mental health policy*. Maudsley Monograph 43. London, Psychology Press, Taylor and Francis Group, 2002.

52   Mbatia J, Jenkins R. Mental health policy in Tanzania. *Psychiatric Services*, 2010, 61:1028–1031.

53   Jenkins R et al. Mental health policy and implementation in Egypt. *International Journal of Mental Health Systems*, 2010, 4:17.

54   *Recommendation 10, organization of mental health services in developing countries*. Geneva, World Health Organization, 1975.

55   Kindon D, Jenkins R. *Adult mental health policy. Commissioning mental health services*. London, HMSO, 1996.

56   Strathdee G, Jenkins R. Purchasing mental health care for primary care. In: Thornicroft G, Strathdee, eds. *Commissioning mental health services*. London, HMSO, 1996:71–84.

57   Lloyd K, Jenkins R. The economics of depression in primary care. Department of Health initiatives. *British Journal of Psychiatry Supplement*, 1995, 27:60–62.

58   Mohit A. Mental health in Tehran in the context of Iranian national mental health programme. In: Goldberg D, Thornicroft G, eds. *Mental health in our future cities*. London, Psychology Press, 1998:217–238.

59   Jenkins R et al. Developing and implementing mental health policy in Zanzibar, a low income country off the coast of East Africa. *International Journal of Mental Health Systems*, 2011, 5:6.

60   Kiima D, Jenkins R. Mental health policy in Kenya – an integrated approach to scaling up equitable care for poor populations. *International Journal of Mental Health Systems*, 2010, 4:19.

61   Karim S et al. Pakistan mental health country profile. The International Consortium on Mental Health Policy and Services: objectives, design and project implementation. *International Review of Psychiatry*, 2004, 16:83–92.

62   Ndetei D, Jenkins R. The implementation of mental health information systems in developing countries: challenges and opportunities. *Epidemiologia E Psichiatria Sociale – an International Journal for Epidemiology and Psychiatric Sciences*, 2009, 18:12–16.

63   Gunn J et al. Embedding effective depression care: using theory for primary care organizational and systems change. *Implementation Science*, 2010, 5:62.

64   Hegarty K et al. How could depression guidelines be made more relevant and applicable to primary care? A quantitive and qualitative review of national guidelines. *British Journal of General Practice*, 2009, 59:322–328.

65   WHO Collaborating Centre for Mental Health Research and Training, Institute of Psychiatry. *WHO guide to mental health in primary care in prison*. London, Royal Society of Medicine, 2001.

66   Mohit A. Training packages in developing countries. In: Jenkin R, Ustun TB, eds. *Preventing mental illness – mental health promotion in primary care*. London, Wiley, 1998:253–259.

67   Patton G et al. Pilot whole school intervention to increase students' social inclusion and engagement and reduce substance use. *Health Education*, 2010, 110:252–272.

68   Olweus D. *Bullying at school: what we know and what we can do*. Massachusetts, Blackwell, 1993.

69 Gater R et al. Detection of disabilities by school children in rural Pakistan. *Tropical Doctor*, 1999, 29:151–155.

70 Jenkins R, Corney N. *Prevention of mental ill health at work*. London, HMSO, 1992.

71 Department of Health. *Developing mental health policies in the workplace*. London, HMSO, 1993.

72 Jenkins R. Mental health at work. In: Snashall D, Patel D, eds. *ABC of occupational and environmental medicine*, 2nd ed. London, BMJ Books, 2003:45–52.

73 Marmot MG et al. Health inequalities among British civil servants: the Whitehall II study. *The Lancet*, 1991, 337:1387–1393.

74 Gilchrist G et al. The association between intimate partner violence, alcohol and depression in family practice. *BMC Family Practice*, 2010, 11:72.

75 Lambo T. Socioeconomic change, population explosion and the changing phases of mental health programs in developing countries. *American Journal of Orthopsychiatry*, 1996, 26:77–83.

76 Shepherd M. Mental health as an integrant of primary medical care. *Journal of the Royal College of General Practitioners*, 1980, 30:657–664.

77 Burns BJ et al. Future directions in primary care/mental health care research. *International Journal of Mental Health*, 1979, 8:130–140.

78 Schulsinger F, Jablensky A. The national mental health programme in the United Republic of Tanzania: a report from WHO and DANIDA. *Acta Psychiatrica Scandinavica*, 1991, 83(Suppl 364):132.

79 Jong J. A comprehensive public mental health programme in Guinea-Bissau: a useful model for African, Asian and Latin American countries. *Psychological Medicine*, 1996, 26:97–108.

80 Sartorius N, Harding T. The WHO Collaborative Study on Strategies for extending mental health care/ the genesis of the study. *American Journal of Psychiatry*, 1983, 140:1470–1479.

81 Murthy S, Wig N. A training approach to enhancing mental health manpower in a developing country. *American Journal of Psychiatry*, 1983, 140:1486–1490.

82 Kilma D, Jenkins R. Mental health policy in Kenya – an integrated approach to scaling up equitable care for poor populations. *International Journal of Mental Health Systems*, 2010, 4:19.

83 Jenkins R et al. Integration of mental health in primary care and community health workers in Kenya – context, rationale, coverage and sustainability. *Mental Health in Family Medicine*, 2010, 7:37–47.

84 Jenkins R et al. Integration of mental health into primary care in Kenya. *World Psychiatry*, 2010, 9:118–120.

85 Hendrik SC, Chaney EF. Effectiveness of collaborative care depression treatment in Veterans' Affairs. *Journal of General Internal Medicine*, 2003;18:9–16.

86 Gunn J et al. A systematic review of complex system interventions designed to increase recovery from depression in primary care. *BMC Health Services Research*, 2006, 6:1–11.

87 Watts BV et al. Outcomes of a quality improvement project integrating mental health into primary care. *Quality and Safety in Health Care*, 2007, 16:378–381.

88 Post EP, Van Stone WW. Veteran's health administration primary care – mental health integration initiative. *North Carolina Medical Journal*, 2008, 69:49–52.

89 Katon WJ, Elizabeth HB, Lin MD. Collaborative care for patients with depression and chronic illness. *New England Journal of Medicine*, 2010, 363:2611–2620.

90 Alfano E. *Integration of primary care and behavioral health: report on a roundtable discussion of strategies for private health insurance*. Washington DC, Bazelon Center for Mental Health Law, 2005.

91 Jenkins R et al. International migration of doctors, and its impact on availability of psychiatrists in low and middle income countries. *PLoS One*, 2010, 5:e9049.

92 Jenkins R et al. Mental health and the development agenda in sub Saharan Africa. *Psychiatric Services*, 2010, 61:229–234.

93 Keks NA et al. Collaboration between general practice and community psychiatric services for people with chronic mental illness. *The Medical Journal of Australia*, 1997, 167:266–271.

7 Managing the interface in primary care mental health clinics

Macaran A Baird, Michelle Riba, Albert Lee, Luis Galvez and D Edward Deneke

---

Key messages

- Integration is more feasible if the primary care system is reasonably well organized and uses systematic approaches to screening, diagnosis and management. Health-delivery systems, community agencies and schools can all be involved.

- As the number of local collaborative partners increases, the role clarity of each participant must increase. Each participant must have a clear role and boundaries around the role, but also have clear signals about when to engage other teammates. As the number of collaborative partners increases, the degree of differentiation and integration must also increase.

- Integration is more feasible when conscious attention is given to clinical, operational and financial aspects of integration, so that clinical innovations are supported operationally and so that all of it is supported to some degree by a suitable business model. There are examples of successful collaboration in low- and high-income countries.

- In the United States of America, mental health treatment patterns have become increasingly focused upon psychopharmacology as primary treatment for many disorders, in spite of scant evidence for the widespread benefits of this shift.

- Many kinds of social distress and unhappiness have come to be labelled as clinical depression, even when diagnostic criteria do not suggest that diagnosis.

Introduction

The 2008 World Health Organization/World Organization of Family Doctors (WHO/Wonca) report, *Integrating mental health into primary care: a global perspective*,[1] provides an international summary of activities in specific countries and regions within nations that brings to life the long-desired goal of offering integrated physical and mental health services. This chapter will offer concrete ideas regarding how to manage the interface between mental/behavioural health and medical care, and a case example of an early screening tool for presymptomatic behaviour disorders in children and adolescents. We will review the dilemmas encountered with integrated care, distinguish integrated care from collaborative care and note some examples of integrated care from low-income as well as higher-income countries.

We must start by defining some terms. Recently, others have worked on creating a lexicon or glossary of terms closely related to United States of America (USA) efforts to improve understanding of how to move behavioural health care closer to – or to become integrated with – primary health-care delivery.[2]

The distinction between the terms *integration* and *collaboration* for this area of health care is worthy of exploration. For our purposes in this chapter:

- *integration* is defined by the *Merriam Webster Dictionary*[3] as "the combining and coordinating of separate parts or elements into a unified whole". In the medical field, this usually refers to the general concept and applied effort to create a unified health team with close working day-to-day contact either remotely or directly, and suggests close working relationships with behavioural health-care providers and all types of medical providers. On one end of the spectrum is an individual physician who is also a trained therapist who integrates his or her interactive skills with each patient (but still needs team members to follow through with specific aspects of care). In this unusual case, the care is integrated within the practice of that one individual. More commonly, integration takes the form of therapists/mental health-care providers working in close proximity with primary care providers in a primary care clinic, with shared charts and some shared visits for the same patient and/or family. A very low degree of integration keeps medical and behavioural health entirely separate, except in emergencies or other unusual circumstances

- *collaboration* is defined by the *Collins Dictionary*[3] as "1. the act of working with another or others on a joint project; 2. something created by working jointly with another or others; 3. the act of cooperating as a traitor, especially with an enemy occupying one's own country". Collaboration is a relational concept meaning individuals working together towards a common goal. The lingering negative nuance of this last definition (collaborating with an enemy) may be experienced when medical and mental health clinicians are brought together in the same space, engendering an uncomfortable response in some countries. This has caused some working in this field to avoid the term and prefer "integration" to "collaboration".

There are at least three ways to organize one's thinking about an integrated service model that adds operational detail to implementation of the biopsychosocial model of health care first popularized by George Engel in 1977.[4] We will first review these frameworks and then provide specific ideas for clinicians and health systems to work together to help patients who have long suffered the negative consequences of fragmented care. Fragmented care should be a "never event",[5] similar to other events that should never happen, such as amputating the wrong limb.

The first framework, the "four quadrant model",[6] organizes the level and type of integration by the relative behavioural health and physical health risks and needs of the served population, and suggests operational approaches to integration for each of the resulting "quadrants." The second framework ("levels of systemic collaboration") organizes the approach to integration for a selected population by the level of systemic and cultural collaboration that the collaborating clinicians (medical and mental health) are working within – everything from "a basic collaboration from a distance" to "fully collaborating close collaboration in a fully integrated system".[7] The third framework ("three simultaneous worlds of the health-care organization") is a reminder that any approach to integration will have to be clinically sound, operationally functional and financially viable. If an approach fails in any of these ways, it fails. Only simultaneous success in all three "worlds" will be sustainable.[8] To bring these themes to life, this chapter will present several examples of specific methods of communication, and a case-study of integration.

Frameworks

The four quadrant model

Viewing integration from this perspective encourages provider teams to articulate their primary focus for integration of medical and behavioural health care, based on the needs of the actual population the team is to serve.[6] The four quadrants reflect the relative medical and mental health risks and needs of the clinic population (see Figure 7.1). For example, some primary care clinics provide limited (or no) care of serious and persistent mental illness (SPMI) but are capable of managing onsite care for patients who struggle with their adaptation to a chronic illness, even if most do not have a diagnosable mental disorder (quadrants 1 and 3). For example, in quadrant 1, routine medical outpatient problems might be managed with psychiatric consultation as needed, while quadrant 3 would manage both inpatient and outpatient medical problems of a more complex nature with psychiatric consultation, as needed. Other ambulatory centres provide primarily psychiatric care for those with SPMI but also deliver basic primary medical care onsite (quadrants 2 and 4). Quadrant 2 would be mental health centres, with a primary care physician or nurse practitioner onsite to address routine medical issues, while quadrant 4 could be managing outpatient and inpatient mental health

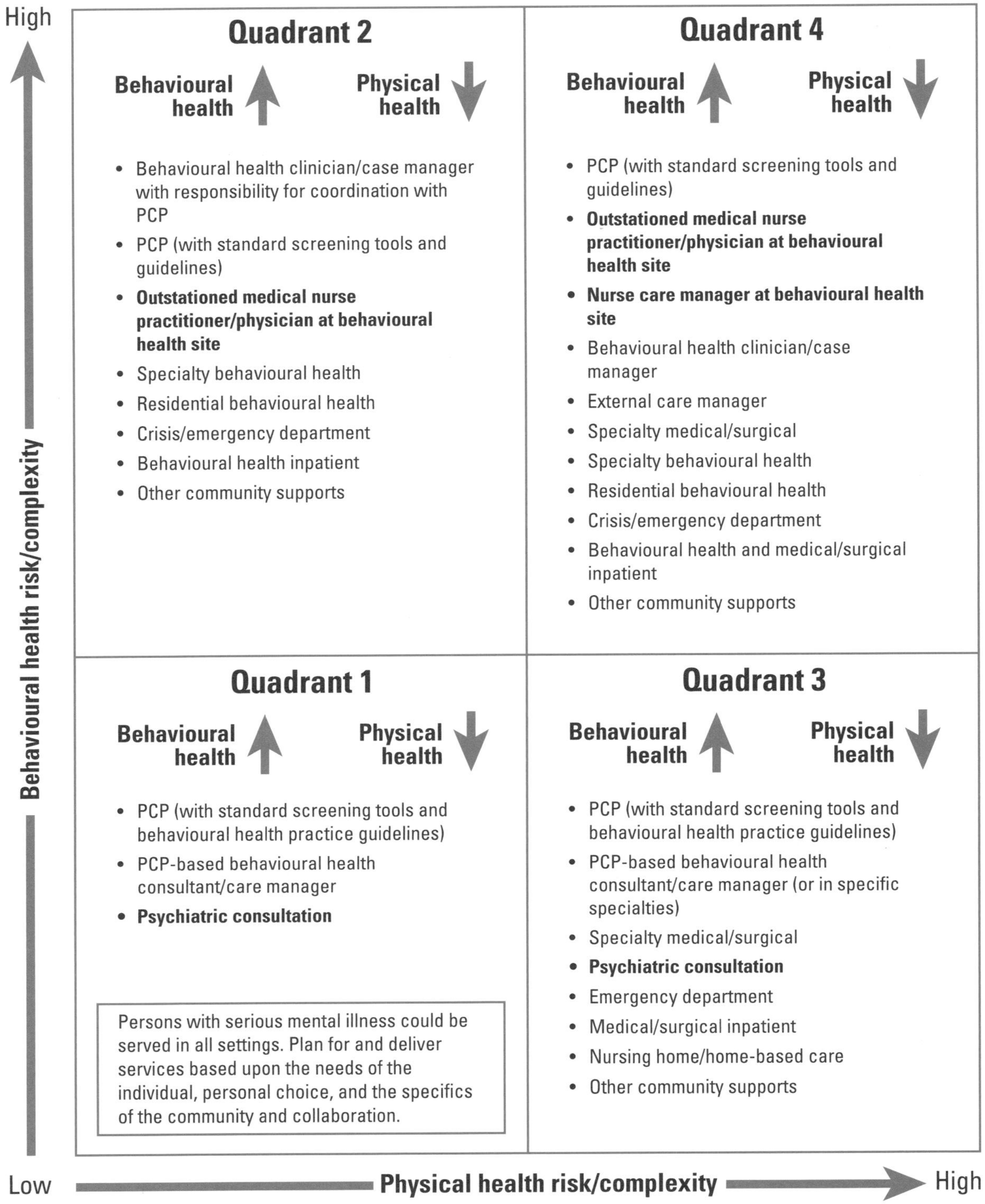

High

Behavioural health risk/complexity

Quadrant 2

Behavioural health ↑   **Physical health** ↓

- Behavioural health clinician/case manager with responsibility for coordination with PCP
- PCP (with standard screening tools and guidelines)
- **Outstationed medical nurse practitioner/physician at behavioural health site**
- Specialty behavioural health
- Residential behavioural health
- Crisis/emergency department
- Behavioural health inpatient
- Other community supports

Quadrant 4

Behavioural health ↑   **Physical health** ↓

- PCP (with standard screening tools and guidelines)
- **Outstationed medical nurse practitioner/physician at behavioural health site**
- **Nurse care manager at behavioural health site**
- Behavioural health clinician/case manager
- External care manager
- Specialty medical/surgical
- Specialty behavioural health
- Residential behavioural health
- Crisis/emergency department
- Behavioural health and medical/surgical inpatient
- Other community supports

Quadrant 1

Behavioural health ↑   **Physical health** ↓

- PCP (with standard screening tools and behavioural health practice guidelines)
- PCP-based behavioural health consultant/care manager
- **Psychiatric consultation**

> Persons with serious mental illness could be served in all settings. Plan for and deliver services based upon the needs of the individual, personal choice, and the specifics of the community and collaboration.

Quadrant 3

Behavioural health ↑   **Physical health** ↓

- PCP (with standard screening tools and behavioural health practice guidelines)
- PCP-based behavioural health consultant/care manager (or in specific specialties)
- Specialty medical/surgical
- **Psychiatric consultation**
- Emergency department
- Medical/surgical inpatient
- Nursing home/home-based care
- Other community supports

Low ═══════ **Physical health risk/complexity** ═══════▶ High

Figure 7.1 The four quadrant clinical integration model. PCP = primary care professional. Adapted, with permission, from Mauer BJ. *Behavioral health/primary care integration: the person-centered healthcare home.* Washington DC, National Council for Community Behavioral Healthcare, 2009[6]

Companion to Primary Care Mental Health

patients, with primary care physicians or nurse practitioners available to manage medical problems. Each clinic has to create its own operational formula for meeting the needs of patients in the four quadrants. The value of the model is to organize thinking about integrating medical and mental health care by understanding the needs of the clinic population.

Most primary care clinics focus on quadrants 1 and 3, which include patients who have medical conditions that are acute and/or chronic, as well as managing their mental health issues, such as moderate depression, anxiety and moderate degrees of compulsivity that are mild to moderately severe (not SPMI). Other specific and common conditions or disorders seen in primary care include:

- common childhood disorders
  - attention deficit hyperactivity disorders
  - moderate degrees of childhood anxiety and depression
  - less-severe autism spectrum disorders
  - child developmental delays
  - behavioural and emotional adaptations to medical illnesses
- common stresses of life
  - work and home strains
  - challenges of raising children
  - coping with a seriously ill family member's rising needs
  - elderly patients with depression and early dementia
- mid-range adult disorders
  - depression
  - anxiety
  - high-risk alcohol and substance abuse
  - somatoform disorders.

This is a very broad spectrum of conditions but many are managed to a variable extent by physicians and nurses in partnership with a range of mental health professionals in primary care settings. Other chapters cover these conditions more specifically. For this chapter, the authors have focused on the practical methods by which a variety of professionals interact collaboratively to the benefit of the patients and families. More severe mental illnesses and conditions are often beyond the scope of primary care integrated mental health. In most industrialized nations, those patients are referred to specialty mental health programmes and clinicians.

Levels of systemic collaboration

A second organizing framework is to view integrated care along a continuum of degrees or levels of collaboration and integration (see Table 7.1).[7] An additional way to meet the needs of the population the team is to serve is through conscious selection of the level of collaboration required for that population. For example, level 1 (minimal collaboration) provides almost entirely separate services for mental health and medical care and little communication between medical and mental health clinicians. The fragmentation generated by this lowest level has been the stimulus for worldwide efforts to move forward with better integration of care. Level 5 (close collaboration in a fully integrated system) describes seamlessly integrated care delivery: one medical record, combined care teams, shared cultural values, and respect for all dimensions of the patient's needs, with neither medical nor mental health themes prioritized unless that is predicated upon the patient's needs. Few clinics function at the highest level of integration in standard primary care models. However, hospice programmes, some geriatric centres, well-organized primary care clinics and some specialty paediatric clinics are examples of being fully integrated in their area of focus.

The authors of this model caution against clinics assuming that the highest levels of collaboration are the most desirable or should automatically become the goal for all clinics.[7] The desired level of collaboration should be chosen based on the needs of the population and the local situation. For example, in some contexts, moving from level 1 (minimal collaboration) to level 2 (basic collaboration at a distance) may represent a large

Table 7.1 Five levels of collaboration

	Model				
	1 **Minimal collaboration**	**2** **Basic collaboration from a distance**	**3** **Basic collaboration on-site**	**4** **Close collaboration in a partly integrated system**	**5** **Close collaboration in a fully integrated system**
Characteristics	• Separate systems • Separate facilities • Communication is rare • Little appreciation of each other's culture: little influence sharing	• Separate systems • Separate facilities • Periodic focused communication, mostly letter, occasionally phone • View each other as outside resources • Little understanding of each others' culture or sharing of influence	• Separate systems • Same facilities • Regular communication, occasionally face to face • Some appreciation of each others' roles and general sense of larger picture, but not in depth • Medical side usually has more influence	• Some share systems • Same facilities • Face-to-face consultation, coordinated treatment plans • Basic appreciation of each others' roles and cultures • Share same biopsychosocial model	• Shared systems and facilities in seamless biopsychosocial web • Patients and providers have same expectation of a team • Everyone committed to biopsychosocial aspects; in-depth appreciation of roles and culture • Collaborative routines are regular and smooth • Conscious influence sharing based on situation and expertise
Handles adequately	Routine, with little biopsychosocial interplay and management challenges	Moderate biopsychosocial interplay, e.g. diabetes and depression with management of each going reasonably well	Moderate biopsychosocial interplay, requiring some face-to-face interaction and coordination of treatment plans	Cases with significant biopsychosocial interplay and management complications	Most difficult and complex biopsychosocial cases with challenging management problems
Handles inadequately	Cases refractory to treatment or with significant biopsychosocial interplay	Significant biopsychosocial interplay, especially when management is not satisfactory to either mental health or medical providers	Significant biopsychosocial interplay, especially those with ongoing and challenging management problems	Complex cases with multiple providers and systems, especially with tension, competing agendas or triangulation	Team resources insufficient or breakdowns occur in the collaboration with larger service systems

Adapted, with permission, from Doherty WJ, McDaniel SH, Baird MA. Five levels of primary care/behavioural healthcare collaboration. *Behavioral Healthcare for Tomorrow*, 1996, 5.25–27.[7]

step forward and substantively reduce fragmentation. Other clinics embedded in other communities or larger organizations may discover that their optimum level of collaboration is at level 3 or 4.

Implicit (but not described in detail here) are variations in the role of behavioural health clinicians in relation to medical clinicians and to patients. For example, in "basic collaboration from a distance" (level 2), the behavioural health clinician may function more as a mental health specialist in familiar ways such as seeing referred patients with mental health disorders. At the other end of the continuum, in highly integrated systems (levels 4 or 5), the behavioural health professional may do some psychotherapy, in addition to helping patients by using brief consultative and skill-building approaches to manage their conditions and helping physicians manage those conditions so that patients can remain in the practice rather than having to be referred out. Some behavioural health clinicians also help with establishing the mental health diagnosis and do some onsite psychotherapy, and others help with managing psychiatric medications. More serious disorders may be outside the scope of primary care clinics and might be referred outside. The mental health clinician may be the person to establish and maintain those referral relationships.

The three-world view

A third organizing perspective was introduced by Peek, when he observed that for successful innovation of any type, especially integrating mental/behavioural health services into primary medical care, one must take a "three world view", that is, balance (and ultimately satisfy) the demands of the clinical, operational, and financial worlds (see Table 7.2).[8,9] The clinical issues are the primary motive and direct much of what the patient needs in order to be more healthy. The operational view clarifies how someone might function, and determines who does the care as well as when. The financial realities must be addressed, or good ideas and noble plans will collapse when human and financial capital as well as operational financial costs are not adjusted to local realities. Understanding the need to balance these interacting factors simultaneously facilitates creating and maintaining more functional and enduring integrated delivery teams and systems. This is especially relevant as we consider integrating care within low-, medium- and high-income regions and countries, as demonstrated in the case summaries and best practices within the 2008 WHO/Wonca report.[1] Taking a three-world view may

Table 7.2 Simultaneous worlds of a health-care organization

	Worlds		
	Clinical	**Operational**	**Financial**
Basic questions	• What care is called for? • Is it high quality?	• What will it take to accomplish care? • Is it well executed?	• How will care best use resources? • Is it a good value?
Object (what you touch every day)	Patients, populations and health	Systems	Numbers
Process	Clinical interactions	Operations	Accounting
Outcome	Achievement (of care and health goals)	Production	Bottom line
Standard	Quality and elegance	Efficiency and facility	Price and value
Relationship	Clinician	Provider	Vendor
	Patient	Customer	Buyer
Relevant principles	Principles of science, healing, and medical ethics	Principles of process and system improvement, business ethics	Principles of business and financial return, business ethics

Reproduced, with permission, from Patterson JE et al. *Mental health professionals in medical settings: a primer.* New York, WW Norton & Company Inc., 2002.[9]

help a clinic decide what level of collaboration is both important and feasible, which of the four quadrants is most important to focus integration efforts on, or, specifically, which methods and tools to select. In the end, any clinic's integrated care efforts must succeed clinically, operationally and financially. Judicious selection of approach can help achieve this goal.

Differences in low-income and highly industrialized and wealthy nations

Differences in operational and financial capabilities in different countries lead to different methods. In highly industrialized and wealthier nations and regions, integrated care teams work closely together, share information (often electronically), connect patients to relevant social and mental health services beyond the primary care clinic, and create the most advanced models of integrated care at this time. Less wealthy countries and regions, as noted in the 2008 WHO/Wonca report on integrated care,[1] use smaller teams and fewer electronic means for communication, and connect to more humble community resources if any are available.

In either high- or low-income environments, a key to improving outcomes for patients and families is that the care system uses a systematic approach to the discovery of mental distress and disorders, uses systematic methods to connect with patients/families before, during and after office visits, and connects routinely to resources outside the individual clinic. The examples that follow reflect ideas as well as concrete examples of this more systematic approach. It is possible to aim to be systematic in either a high- or low-income environment, although the methods and levels of technology will be different.

In either high- or low-income environments and countries, patients with behavioural health disorders often stay within the primary care system. General practitioners (GPs) see and treat the majority of people in the community with mental health problems. Many of these patients are seen in primary care clinics and have relatively mild and self-limiting disorders. In this context, general medical settings represent an important – perhaps the single most important – point of contact between patients with mental disorders and the health-care system. This is especially important because mental disorders frequently co-occur with other medical disorders.

> Numerous studies have assessed strategies to improve care at the interface of general medicine and mental health. Much of this work has been done in the area of depression, because it is one of the most common disorders seen in general medical settings, and because efficacious treatments have existed for several decades. More recently, parallel research has examined strategies to improve care for anxiety and somatoform disorders and for severe and persistent mental illness among patients with comorbid medical disorders.[10]

Collaboration/integrated care

Advantages of collaboration

We have to define roles and responsibilities and look for new ways of learning together.[11] In some European countries, primary and secondary care for patients with mental disorders has traditionally been clearly separated, consisting of communication between GPs and psychiatrists by written correspondence and, less commonly, by telephone. Sometimes they meet in the health centre or during home visits.[12]

Many prior authors have noted the wisdom of integrating mental health/behavioural health services into primary care:

> Collaborative care for a heterogeneous group of persons with common mental disorders seems to be as effective as the usual practice of referral to mental health services for reducing psychopathology, but it is significantly more efficient regarding referral delay, duration of treatment, number of appointments, and related treatment costs.[13]

Collaborative care ensures the optimal use of resources, provides better outcomes for patients and improves the efficiency of the system overall. Gask and Croft have:

> . . . suggested ways of working more harmoniously with primary care. [These] include . . . shared care records such as those already used in pregnancy and diabetes [and] . . . developing local protocols for the management of specific disorders such as depression, anxiety and schizophrenia.[14]

How collaboration works

We observe some underlying principles about the interface of mental health and primary care. For example, integration is more feasible if the primary care system is reasonably well organized and uses systematic approaches for screening, diagnosis and management.[15] As the number of local collaborative partners increases, each participant's role must be clarified. In primary care, physicians, nurses, care coordinators, pharmacists and mental health clinicians might all have some role in the care plan of a complicated patient. To make the teamwork efficient, each participant must have a clear role with boundaries, but also have clear signals about when to engage other teammates. As the number of collaborative partners increases, the degree of differentiation and integration must also increase.[9,16] This is not a linear increase but an almost logarithmic increase when the team expands beyond two or three individuals. Integration is more feasible when conscious attention is given to clinical, operational and financial aspects of integration, so that clinical innovations are supported operationally and so that all of it is supported to some degree by a suitable business model.[8] Integration becomes increasingly important as particular efforts move from being pilots to being mainstreamed implementations.[17]

Collaborative models

There is no single best practice model that can be followed by all countries.[1,18] The practice model has to be adapted to each country's characteristics. In some countries, such as Canada or Australia, people are widely dispersed geographically or they live in areas with a low density of population. In other countries, the populations are fairly homogeneous. However, many nations are becoming more and more culturally diverse, such as in the USA and the United Kingdom of Great Britain and Northern Ireland (UK). On the other hand, there is a big variability in the names given to the same shared activities by mental health and primary care, which make it difficult to compare them; for example, Canadians use the term "shared care".[19,20] Today in the UK, as well as in some areas of Spain, there are three basic models of systematic collaboration.[13] There are two models of collaboration with psychiatrists (not other mental health clinicians):

- *the visiting specialist model*: the psychiatrist goes to the health centre to see patients selected by their GP. Later there is a medical meeting to discuss each patient's diagnosis and treatment with the rest of the team. This model improves patient accessibility to mental health care. There may be shared visits where both professionals visit with the patient and then attend a meeting with the primary care team to discuss these cases. Its main advantage is that the GP acquires knowledge and skills. It also improves the quality of referrals to secondary care, due to the existence of agreed-upon referral criteria. Similar models are used in the USA in federally qualified health centres, in which mental health (and dentistry) are required components of primary medical care

- *the consulting psychiatrist model*: in this approach, the primary care team hires a psychiatrist to work in the health centre, typically to help other providers or care coordinators manage a population of patients with mental health conditions or concerns in the mix. The psychiatrists may see some patients, but mostly support the other providers as onsite specialist consultants rather than filling their schedules with their own patients. Other behavioural health consultants may be onsite, and care for mental health disorders and medical conditions can be coordinated.[21]

In these models there is a face-to-face contact between the psychiatrist who regularly visits the health centre and the members of the primary care team. It is an important step toward providing integrated mental health services in primary care. But in their training experiences, psychiatrists do not often meet face-to-face with their patients' GP. The frequency of the visits will vary depending on the available resources. Many teaching practices in the USA use a similar model. The mental health clinician represents a variety of disciplines: psychology, psychiatry, family therapy and social work. In these models, the GP continues to provide treatment for the patient, achieving continuity in care. Attention by GPs at the primary care level is accessible, affordable and acceptable for the community.

Another advantage of these two models is that some individuals with mental health problems feel less stigmatized if they see a mental health professional in a primary care setting. On the other hand, at the referral level of mental health, the clinician sees patients with more severe mental health problems. In such referral or specialty mental health clinics, more extensive mental health teams can be assembled for patients.

In Spain in the last two decades, there has been an effective integration of mental health in the national health system, but it has not been homogeneous throughout the country. In 75% of the Spanish autonomous communities, there are multidisciplinary teams. The computerized medical record is only implanted in some areas, and it only works between primary care and mental health.[22]

The new vocational training of family medicine programmes in Spain includes three months of a rotation in mental health services. This makes it possible for the trainee to become familiarized with mental health problems and improve shared attention to patients and their families.[23] In the USA, this type of training in family medicine programmes has required one to three months of behavioural health training since 1970.

Medical homes or health-care homes

In May 2008, the USA passed health reform legislation regarding medical homes or health-care homes as

> an approach to providing comprehensive primary care for children, youth and adults. The Patient Centered Medical Home is a health care setting that facilitates partnerships between individual patients, and their personal physicians, and when appropriate the patient's family. . . . [It is a] physician directed medical practice [in which] the personal physician leads a team of individuals at the practice level who collectively take responsibility for the ongoing care of patients.[24]

As industrialized European and Asian nations' health-care systems have become better organized, the progression toward more systematically organized health-care homes[25] in the USA is slowly moving towards integrating behavioural health into primary care settings.[26] The operational definition of a health-care home (medical home) was created by consensus in Minnesota in 2010.[27] More specific operational definitions and consistently understood concepts are being developed for practice and research development in the subfield of behavioural health integration in primary care.[2] As this national experiment unfolds, there are several evolving themes regarding the interface of mental health and primary care. Some are exciting and represent opportunities for improved outcomes and pathways to reduce suffering for patients and families. For example, in health-care homes the patients/families will be systematically invited to help shape care plans for patients with complex problems. Care teams will be connected by design to community resources and have created standardized work processes for screening for mental health disorders. Also, as funding for health-care homes moves toward payment for care coordination and prepayments, there are funds available to support the mental health teams, outreach activities and team meetings for collaborative care planning.

Mental health disorders seen as chronic disorders

As mental health treatment systems continue to evolve, multiple models are being evaluated based on the patient populations served, the nature and chronicity of the mental disorders most prevalent, socioeconomic characteristics, and so on.[28] In the USA, the current and most prominent system of health care has been established around the goals of diagnosing and treating acute illnesses.[29] Further, the current body of evidence suggests that serious and persistent mental illness and some forms of depression are best treated as chronic illnesses. Numerous models, similar in their design and goals, have been shown to improve the overall quality of health care received by the patient.[30–32] The organizational foundation of many of these models can be found in the work of Wagner et al.,[29,33] who looked at models of care designed for the management of chronic illnesses. Wagner and colleagues outline a number of common elements shared among successful programmes. These elements primarily involve reorganization of the health-care practice to better meet the needs of patients with chronic illnesses, and a shift in priority from treatment of acute problems through curative measures to the management of chronic issues through patient education and behavioural-change techniques. Patient care is organized by the primary provider, who then relies on specialists for clinical consultation, supervision and education.

The elements of care established by chronic care models have been adopted by the mental health field, and the concept of collaborative care models in mental health has become quite popular over the past few decades.[34] The models vary based on location, culture and available resources, but common themes exist. The collaborative care team generally consists of the primary care physician; a care manager who serves ancillary roles such as providing patient education and helping to ensure patient follow-up; and a psychiatrist.[35] Use of these models has shown benefits for multiple patient populations. For example, use of collaborative care has been shown to improve medication adherence in patients with depression, and reduced physical symptoms and use of health care in patients with somatoform disorders.[32]

Communication models for integrated care

With multiple team members who are often located at different settings, communication among these team members is integral to the success of the models. Despite living in an age of rapidly advancing technology, including cyberculture, communication among providers remains a potential point of weakness in collaborative care. Collaborative care models demonstrate a variety of mechanisms for communication. For example, some of these mechanisms include face-to-face meetings, tasks forwarded on electronic medical records, phone calls, and emails. Models generally include the primary care physician and the case manager in the same location, but the location of the psychiatrist or other mental health clinician varies. Levels of communication range from the presence of the specialist on site and even physically in the same room as the primary physician, to little to no communication among the collaborative team members; this lack of communication leads rapidly to fragmentation in care.[35]

Co-location of the psychiatrist with the rest of the team has been shown to increase mental health referrals and remains the gold standard in collaborative care.[36] However, this option is usually limited by resources, including the availability of psychiatrists in any given area, reimbursement limitations by insurance companies, and other factors. In rural areas, the distance between a primary care provider and a psychiatrist can be significant. To compensate, systems have incorporated varying levels of technology to bridge this gap, from writing letters between providers to more direct communication via telephone or videoconferencing.

The number of psychiatrists in any given area can vary dramatically, and mental health can suffer in areas with few specialists.[28] Collaborative care models thus make sense in these areas. The majority of mental health care is provided by primary care providers, who are more numerous, while specialists serve in a prominently supervisory role, with possible direct consultation available on more complicated cases. Consultation/liaison psychiatry has a long history in hospital care, in which patients admitted to the hospital with primarily medical diagnoses have comorbid mental health issues for which the on-site psychiatrist is consulted. Bauer et al. postulate that consultation/liaison-trained psychiatrists are well equipped to fill the roles of specialists among underserved populations, given their specific training in areas of education and consultation.[28]

Telepsychiatry has been shown to be an effective method of connecting psychiatrists to patients in a rural area, when compared to face-to-face treatment by a psychiatrist,[37] but can alternative methods of communication prove helpful in extending collaborative care models? Given the general availability of these technologies, it is not surprising that telephone communication has been adapted along with other modes of communication such as videoconferencing and e-mail to help bridge the gap between primary providers and psychiatrists, making these methods of long-distance communication a viable option in collaborative care models. Hilty et al. argue that telephone or e-mail consultation between psychiatrists and primary care providers can decrease the time to treatment and broaden access to mental health care in rural areas.[38] Unfortunately, studies examining the effectiveness of these communication methods are few. However, there is some evidence that utilization of telephone consultations between primary care providers and psychiatrists, with emphasis on providing education to these providers, can lead to a high satisfaction level and improved prescribing habits among primary care providers.[39]

These technologies are naturally well suited for large geographical areas with sparse numbers of psychiatrists. Bauer et al. provide the example of the reorganization of mental health services in Australia and emphasize the importance of communication between the primary provider, serving on the front line of health care, and the psychiatrist, often working from hundreds of miles away.[28] The Rural and Remote Mental Health Service (RRMHS) was developed in South Australia following an identified need for greater mental health coverage in more sparsely populated regions of the country.[40] The psychiatrist in this model serves in several roles, including providing direct consultation services; case-conferencing and supervision on visits to remote areas; and telepsychiatric services to both outpatient and inpatient settings. Given the large area and low density of psychiatrists in South Australia, innovations such as telepsychiatry serve as creative solutions to the problems of communication among team members. These strategies help provide mental health care to a greater percentage of the population, despite a limited number of psychiatrists.

The critical need for greater access to integrated mental health care is apparent worldwide. It seems that consultation/liaison psychiatrists are in a strong position to fill that niche, but the number of psychiatrists will never fill this need without changes in the delivery model. Using the foundations provided by existing collaborative care models, basic access to mental health care has the potential to increase dramatically. As specific geographic locations develop individualized strategies for meeting their particular needs, it is clear that effective communication will remain a key ingredient in the equation. Further, as technologies advance, such as telecommunication, the Internet and social networking, health-care providers will hopefully find a growing number of creative options available to assist in providing quality mental health care in settings of limited resources. In addition, other mental health professionals, such as psychologists, family therapists, advanced practice psychiatric nurses and social workers, are able to be part of the integrated care team. There are examples in more wealthy regions of integrating psychiatry services directly into primary care practices. The following example is consistent with quadrant 3 clinics.

Examples of integrated care in low-income countries

Petersen and colleagues recently reported that efforts to improve mental health in many low-income countries have focused on: shifting some of the diagnostic and treatment tasks to others in the community in order to provide basic mental health services; expanding the numbers of mental health trainees; improving the public's mental health literacy; and moving towards a more socially based model, which includes helping patients with mental health problems stay and function within the community rather than being moved to distant facilities and consultants for expertise.[41] These countries view mental illness as parallel to a developmental disability issue; treatment includes local social support. In these nations, the focus is on serious and persistent mental illnesses such as schizophrenia and manic disorders; these previously had been treated primarily by institutionalization and government-managed facilities. However, these patients can best be cared for in their own communities with local resources including primary care teams. Wright advocated this more community-based approach in England many years ago.[42] However, Petersen and colleagues observed that problems with access to specialty mental health treatment can be exacerbated in low-income countries in Africa, Asia and Central and South America, when primary mental health-care tasks are shifted to medical clinicians and others in the community.[43] This is especially true if there are insufficient specialty resources to which these clinicians can refer. Screening and early treatment of patients locally may increase referrals to specialty mental health-care providers, exacerbating the existing referral bottlenecks. Currently, this shortage of specialty mental health care is very acute in most countries but especially in low-income countries. Existing general health services are not well coordinated with mental health in many instances. The authors suggest more research is needed at a local level to evaluate how to help at more than one level of care to improve overall cost-effectiveness and access.

Over the past decade, substantial political shifts and major changes in the way practices are organized have influenced the scope of primary care services in Eastern Europe. In Slovenia, for example, Albrecht et al. observed that as the political landscape changed to a more democratic model, their primary health-care centres changed significantly.[44] The number of employees in these primary health-care centres decreased by one-third; their relationship to their previous sponsoring municipalities became more complex and less directed from the government body; and private health centres began to compete for patients. In this turbulent climate, the integration of behavioural health into health-care centres was not a prominent theme, but as other specialty medical services were moving into these health centres, they began to provide a more diverse menu of medical services.

Rurik and Kalabay reviewed demographic, socioeconomic and mortality data and interviewed family physicians and patients in the former socialist countries in Eastern Europe.[45] They found similar changes, from publicly funded and government-directed primary health centres to a somewhat chaotic mix of privately funded entrepreneurial practices competing with government primary care practices. Patients were generally satisfied with their care but the physicians felt care was fragmented and poorly coordinated, as the countries shifted from hospital-based care to community-based primary care. Once again, during the tumultuous changes in government and culture, behavioural health integration was not discussed as a priority. However, basic population health statistics and mortality rates improved while expenditures for health increased only slightly.

Collaboration between mental health and primary care clinicians was studied in Bologna, Italy,[46] to gain insight into what aspects of that spontaneous project were working. Without a government stimulus, primary care physicians and psychiatrists in Bologna created a pilot to shift the psychiatrist's role from a distant consultant to an integrated partner in primary care. Some integration was focused geographically inside a primary care centre, while others worked closely by phone with specifically defined hours of access to the primary care clinicians and teams. The primary care physician remains chiefly responsible for the management of the patient, but the psychiatrist can become involved more quickly, with a focus on the patient's most immediate needs rather than a full psychodynamic therapy. Phone and group interactions with primary care physicians in a consultation/liaison model had been implemented in only a few sites at the time the study was published in 1999.[45]

In Kenya, an extensive effort was launched in 2005 to improve the education and skills of primary care physicians, nurses and others in the diagnosis and management of common mental health disorders.[47] This was done in the context of an extreme shortage of psychiatrists in public service (23 psychiatrists and about 500 psychiatric nurses in the whole country). The rates of depression (10%) and psychosis (1%) in the general population suggested a new and more widely dispersed model of care was needed. The goal of this multi-year programme was to make it more realistic and functional for local primary care teams to manage common mental disorders. A customized 40-hour training course emphasizing the national adoption of WHO primary care guidelines was implemented via six regional training sites. Qualitative evaluation of this programme was very positive from more than 1800 who had taken this course, with an emphasis on reduced referrals to the scarce specialty mental health providers while providing improved care locally. The authors describe many obstacles to sustaining this effort,[47] and clinical outcome studies are still needed. Building local treatment capacity was the essential focus of the education, with the goal of improving local knowledge and teamwork among primary care team members, with the knowledge that regional specialty resources would remain very limited.

Other strategies for integrating additional medical services into primary health care in low- and middle-income countries have usually focused on improving prevention, screening, acute care, and long-term management of more direct medical problems such as infectious diseases and improved prenatal care. Improved integration with public health measures to increase rates of immunization, early detection and prevention measures and earlier prenatal care are widely recommended and have positive results in many countries.[48] As those medically focused efforts improve the overall function of local primary care, there may be greater opportunity for realistic efforts to integrate behavioural care into primary care in some low-income countries where such efforts have not received wide attention to date.

Evaluation of integration and effective interventions for several types of mental disorders was the focus of a review by Patel et al., as part of a six-part series on mental health published by *The Lancet* in 2007.[49] That review of interventions in low-income and middle-income countries found that primary care physicians and others in primary care practices can provide cost-effective treatment for depression via use of antidepressant medication or cognitive-behavioural therapy (CBT). Increased informational support and increased sports training combined with CBT was also found to be effective for mild depression. Using protocols to manage gradually increased treatment intensity with steps for increased medication and increasing collaboration with specialty mental health clinicians (stepped care) was as effective for depression as were antiviral drugs for human immunodeficiency virus/acquired immunodeficiency syndrome (HIV/AIDS). In many low- and middle-income countries, schizophrenia has a low incidence but, of course, is a very long-term illness for which late treatment compounds the effects of the disorder. Increased involvement of families and improved public understanding through education has been associated with improved patient adherence to medication treatment. The effectiveness of treatments for other common mental health disorders has not been tested extensively in low- and middle-income countries. For example, treatment often used in higher-income countries, such as increased screening for high-risk alcohol use and brief office interventions by primary care physicians, has not been tested sufficiently in lower-income nations. Public education to reduce the impact of alcohol abuse and addiction has also not been followed up with significant evaluation research in these countries. Similarly, there has been little evaluation of social and medication interventions for children's emotional disorders and developmental disabilities, although some effective treatments are available.

The next section features a case-study of one such intervention in a higher-income country.

Case-study in Hong Kong

Hong Kong has a population of more than seven million, with gross domestic product (GDP) per capita US$45 277, which ranks this metropolitan city/state as number seven in the world next to the USA for per capita income.[50] Hong Kong has around 10 000 doctors in active clinical practice, with a psychiatrist-to-population ratio of 2 per 100 000 or about one-seventh of the Australian ratio.[51] Recent community surveys in different districts in Hong Kong have shown that approximately 15% of the population had emotional problems affecting their work and daily activities. Out of 100 000 persons, 15 000 will have some form of mental health problem but only two psychiatrists will be available to serve them. Psychiatric services would need to expand exponentially to meet those needs. In contrast, in Hong Kong half of all doctors work in primary care settings, so the primary care physician-to-population ratio is 1:1400. Out of 1400 cases, about 200 patients would have mental health problems. This ratio could allow primary care physicians to review their patients' mental health status periodically. The management of mental health disorders would be even more efficient if a variety of mental health professionals, other than psychiatrists, were integrated into the primary care setting.

Primary care delivers primary, secondary and tertiary prevention

Primary health care can deliver the three tiers for prevention of mental illness. Preventing the onset of mental health illnesses will be the most cost-effective way of managing the mental health burden. It is not always an easy task. Ideally, a system of care would try to identify patients with mental illness at an early stage, so they could be managed with less complex treatment. Failing that, it is important to have good rehabilitation services for patients with mental illness, to stabilize their conditions and avoid further deterioration. Figure 7.2 illustrates the three tiers of prevention for mental illnesses (primary, secondary and tertiary prevention). Primary care is the ideal setting to provide services for the full range of care, with effective articulation between different levels of care in a clinic and interfacing with community resources close to the patient when needed.

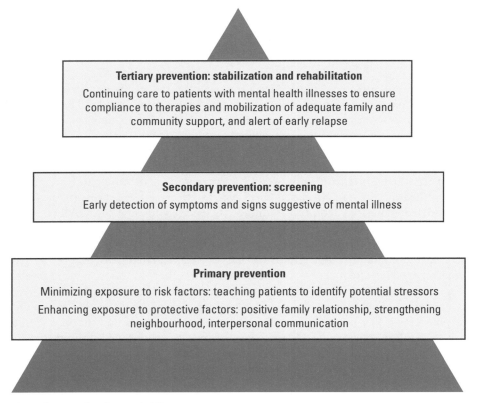

Tertiary prevention: stabilization and rehabilitation
Continuing care to patients with mental health illnesses to ensure compliance to therapies and mobilization of adequate family and community support, and alert of early relapse

Secondary prevention: screening
Early detection of symptoms and signs suggestive of mental illness

Primary prevention
Minimizing exposure to risk factors: teaching patients to identify potential stressors
Enhancing exposure to protective factors: positive family relationship, strengthening neighbourhood, interpersonal communication

Figure 7.2 Three tiers of prevention for mental illness

Continuity with a primary care team helps establish trust. Studies have shown that having a regular source of care for adolescents in rural areas and having health insurance were found to be associated with a twofold increase in receiving preventive care during the previous 2 years.[52] Uptake of paediatric preventive services in community health centres was greater among those identifying the centre as their regular source for both preventive and treatment care.[53] Having a regular source of care was found to be the most important factor associated with receiving preventive care services, even after considering the effect of demographic characteristics, financial status, and the need for ongoing care. Receiving optimal primary care (in terms of availability, continuity, comprehensiveness, and communication) from the regular source of care further increases this likelihood.[54] Research by Lee et al. found that the prevalence rates of good health and hygiene behaviours were higher, and scores in all three main domains on the Child Behavior Checklist[55] – anxious/depressed, somatic complaints and aggressive behaviours – were lower among children with a regular source of primary care doctors; the results were statistically significant after adjusting for socioeconomic status.[56] Good primary care is, therefore, essential for good uptake of preventive services for mental illnesses.

Primary prevention

Primary care can enhance primary prevention by an improved understanding of the normal stresses and strains in families and communities. Building resilience can promote better mental health. Stress is commonly related to distortions in perception, replaying of past events and worry about the future. Primary care providers can educate patients to moderate their perception of demands when they are unrealistic and suggest alternative, less stressful choices. Patients can be advised that relaxation and meditation can reduce the level of emotional and physiological reactivity to daily events and thoughts, enhance the mind's ability to focus and allow the patient to deal more successfully with daily life. Primary care providers can also educate patients to recognize their weaknesses and vulnerabilities, and to seek help and support as needed. Emotional support would be built by establishing effective communication with the families of patients, creating good interpersonal relationship with family members and friends, and involving a supportive neighbourhood. Development of healthy lifestyles such as regular physical activities, healthy diet, family and social connectedness, spiritual support and pleasant living and working environment are all protective factors for mental well-being. Primary care providers are closest to their patients and need to play a more proactive role in health promotion for them. By guiding their patients to an awareness of these protective factors, stressors are minimized.

Secondary prevention

Primary health care can identify diseases at an early stage, as the majority do not seek help until a late stage of illness and also present with non-specific signs and symptoms. Patients with mental health problems usually present with somatic concerns that can easily be mistaken as symptoms of particular systems disorders,[57] for example:

- *cardiovascular*: palpitation, chest pain, fainting, flushing, sweating
- *respiratory*: shortness of breath, hyperventilation
- *gastrointestinal*: choking, lump in throat, dry mouth, nausea/vomiting, diarrhoea
- *neurological*: dizziness, headache, numbness
- *musculoskeletal*: muscle ache, muscle tension, tremor, restlessness.

These symptoms are usually presented to primary care and can be recognized as a signal of mental distress if the primary care physicians adopt the core concept of family medicine, that of providing comprehensive, holistic and continuing care.

Although it is a common assumption that continuity and a trusting relationship facilitate more open discussion of depression and emotional distress, research confirms this belief. Simon et al. found that depressed patients in primary care centres where patients have a relationship with a particular primary care physician were more likely to have a frank presentation of their depression than patients at centres where such a relationship was not characteristic.[58] In this WHO study of 1146 patients with a diagnosis of major depression in 15 primary care centres in 14 countries on five continents, depressed patients in centres without this relationship were more likely to present themselves with somatic symptoms.[58] Good primary care is essential for screening patients with somatic symptoms as possible signals of early onset of mental illnesses.

Tertiary prevention

Improved adherence to treatment plans becomes the focus for tertiary prevention, with the primary goal of slowing the progression of disease. Providers work directly with patients to improve compliance to therapy. Clinics provide easier ways for a patient to stay engaged, with consistent follow-up appointments, phone calls, and e-mails. Even with these efforts, consistent follow-up remains a challenge. Research suggests that one-fifth of patients miss their psychiatric appointments, and those living far away from a hospital are more likely to miss the appointment.[59] If patients with mental health problems were followed in a primary care setting in close proximity to where they live, the default rate of missed appointments could be reduced. Local family and community support would become more important for patients with chronic illnesses and could be engaged in the treatment process more easily if treatment is nearby. Frequent admission to hospitals and excessive demands to review the results of investigations erode the patient's feelings of self-control. Evidence suggests that if the professionals remain in total control, the patient's outcome is worse.[60] Patient-centred care is more likely to yield positive results. It does not imply a lack of input from health professionals but rather that health professionals must encourage and facilitate patients' self-management to improve care outcomes. Patients with strongly positive assessments of their service providers were substantially more confident in self-care.[61] Effective self-care is essential for the long-term management of mental illness, and primary care providers can play a pivotal role in supporting self-care.

Assessment of children and adolescents in Australia

The 2007 Australian National Survey of Children's Health estimated that about 4 out of 10 children would need mental health services for emotional development or behavioural problems but are not receiving this care; more than half of those lacking care are uninsured children.[62] In Australia, the incidence of mental health problems of children and adolescents has been estimated to be about one in seven. Although a large percentage of these adolescents present to their GP at least once a year, their mental health issues are usually somatized and not presented directly as a mental health issue.[63,64] In children, mental illnesses are more likely to be neurodevelopmental than neurodegenerative disorders, with the cognitive and behavioural manifestation as later stages of processes starting early in development.[65] It is constructive to think of some mental disorders as brain circuit disorders caused by developmental processes shaped by complex interactions of genetics and life. There is evidence suggesting greater neural plasticity around puberty, and persistent changes in neural function as a result of external stimuli having a significantly large impact on future health including mental health.[65,66] The physiological processes of puberty interact with the social context to affect an individual's emotional and social development. This has strong implications for the mental health of children and adolescents.[67] High-risk behaviours in youth such as heavy smoking, substance abuse, alcohol drinking, feeling hopeless and early sexual experience were found to be associated with both suicidal thoughts and/or attempts at suicide.[68] The management of emotional problems is complex and requires a multidisciplinary approach. This should be the number one area of concern for improving health outcomes in young people.[69,70] Therefore, we must reorientate ourselves to focus on mental health not simply the absence of mental illnesses. The tripartite interfacing of primary care, school and family becomes very crucial.

Integration of care with parents, families and schools

According to the Guidelines for Adolescent Preventive Services (GAPS) by the American Medical Association,[71] parents or other adult caregivers should receive health guidance at least once during their child's early adolescence, once during middle adolescence and, preferably, once during late adolescence, including information about signs and symptoms of disease and emotional distress. These health, educational and evaluation sessions would allow clinicians and parents/guardians to search for stressors and review youth behaviour at home and school and with peers. This would allow the early identification of mental health problems among children and adolescents and facilitate early intervention.[72,73] Waiting for adolescents to attend a primary care clinic is neither user-friendly nor cost-effective for the optimal identification of early problems. In addition to using this method, Australia has a long history of organizing health activities around settings such as schools, communities and workplaces, which provides the social structures to reach the defined populations and helps deliver health-promotion activities in the context of their families' daily lives.[74,75] An interfacing model can be developed, in which various mental health-promotion activities, including awareness training and early screening, would be visibly demonstrated in the day-to-day setting of children and adolescents, such as at schools and in family settings, facilitated by primary care providers.

One proposal for the psychosocial assessment of students uses observation checklists for parents and teachers, as those areas of concern noted in these models would be unveiled in day-to-day activities. This would enable the primary care providers to have preliminary impressions of those youth at potentially high risk. The primary care team would train a group of health assessors, who do not need to be specialized health-care workers with advanced professional training, in a particular discipline of health. However, they would undergo training in general health studies, with a focus on mental health. Evidence-based guidelines have been published for use by non-specialist health-care workers to provide treatment for eight mental, neurological and substance misuse disorders in a routine health-care setting. Therefore, these less-expensive professionals would also be enhanced in their ability to conduct informative psychosocial interviews.[76] The psychosocial interview for the students can take place in school settings, with prior arrangements with schools in order to be within the context of their daily lives. The multidisciplinary team will consist of health assessors defined as health professionals with training in primary care mental health. Those identified as potential high-risk students will be assessed by more highly trained health professionals. However, the lowest-risk groups would be assessed by health assessors in this model. If the health assessors identify the students at high risk, they will refer them to the health professionals on site for further assessment. These health professionals will assess those students with possible mental illnesses to be seen in primary care clinics for further evaluation. Students with low or no risk will be given appropriate counselling, including practical tips on how to recognize early symptoms and signs of mental health problems and how they would seek help. They will be reviewed periodically.

The involvement of teachers and parents in initial assessment, followed by a school-based evaluation by a primary health-care team with input from trained health assessors, will enable large numbers of students to be screened. Those identified to be at risk would undergo further evaluation. Successful initiatives in mental health promotion of students need to include:

- linking the school, home and community
- addressing the school ecology and environment
- combining a consistency in behavioural-change goals through connecting students, teachers, family and community
- fostering respectful and supportive relationships among students, teachers and parents
- increasing the connections for each student.

The interface of primary care, school and family would facilitate mental health promotion, which would not be done solely by primary health-care providers. This would enhance primary prevention and earlier identification of mental illnesses among children and adolescents. For example, in the USA some clinics are using a standardized screening tool for autism spectrum disorder in toddlers, M-CHAT™ – Modified Checklist for Autism in Toddlers.[77]

Integrated care is not a panacea for improving health

Integrated care implies that health-care teams will work together collaboratively to achieve improved health for patients, without the customary fragmentation between biomedically and psychosocially focused care and clinicians. Finn et al. studied the unintended effects of teamwork in operating rooms and medical records departments, and found that teamwork is difficult to achieve when multiple highly skilled professionals are involved.[78] Teamwork itself does not always yield a satisfactory experience for the team or the patient. For example, lower-paid, lower-status teammates may not be afforded a voice in decision-making. Coordination of technical efforts may cause ambiguity regarding each person's role, and require ever higher levels of coordination and collaboration. As the number of team members increases, there is a need for simultaneously increased levels of collaboration as well as clear differentiation of roles. This paradox requires ever better communication as the team grows in number or distance.

Demonstrating improved clinical outcomes from integrated care is not always the measured result. Positive clinical outcomes were found in Puerto Rico by Vera et al.[79] Patients randomly selected from primary care clinic waiting rooms were screened for having chronic medical conditions as well as depression and then assessed via structured scales and interviews. Equal numbers of usual-care and collaborative-care patients were interviewed. The collaborative-care patients had lower post-treatment depression scores and higher social functioning and were overall four times as likely to show a positive response to treatment.

Sometimes the measurable impact is only marginally positive. A large review sponsored by the Department of Veterans Affairs evaluated the literature for evidence of effectiveness of first-line treatment of depression in primary care settings with brief psychotherapy.[80] It was found that brief psychotherapy had small but significant benefits. It was not possible to verify what number of treatment sessions (6 or fewer versus 6–12 sessions) was most effective for CBT or problem-solving therapy, nor could the authors find a difference based on the professional training of the therapist. They found no standardization of functional treatment outcomes, although the SF-36 (a multipurpose, short-form health survey with 36 questions) was used more than others. Their conclusion was that six to eight sessions of either CBT or problem-solving therapy showed modest positive treatment effects if delivered by a variety of health professionals in a primary care setting. This is not a ringing endorsement of brief psychotherapy delivered in primary care settings, but documenting treatment effects for mental disorders remains a significant challenge for all delivery systems, whether primary care with integrated services or specialty mental health systems.

Conclusion

Some trends in the USA are more challenging and may represent cautions to other nations if they consider redesigning their primary care model to integrate mental health care. The following list represents an informal recognition of problematic trends.

- Interdisciplinary teams must work efficiently with high degrees of integration among teammates with clear roles. Currently, health professional training for nurses, physicians and mental health clinicians is not structured in this highly integrated manner. Students from different fields often do not train or learn together as maturing professionals. Interdisciplinary teamwork is new behaviour and a new social architecture within clinics; it is not automatic behaviour.

- In the USA, mental health treatment patterns have become increasingly focused on psychopharmacology as primary treatment for many disorders, in spite of scant evidence for the widespread benefits of this shift.[81] Primary care physicians in the USA (plus many kinds of psychotherapists) are increasingly adding to the pressure to treat their clients with medications. Since non-psychiatrist mental health clinicians usually cannot prescribe, they suggest patients return to primary care providers to ask for a medication.[82] If highly skilled counselling, psychotherapy, family therapy or other methods of interactive and talk therapy do not yield rapid results (this is common), the fast-paced USA culture feeds the understandable desire by patients/clients for results to be apparent quickly.[81,83]

- Many kinds of social distress and unhappiness have come to be labelled as clinical depression, even when diagnostic criteria do not suggest that diagnosis. Unfortunately, this expanding diagnosis compounds the pressure for medication and is building momentum just as we are learning more and more about the lack of scientific evidence for commonly used medications for depression[84] and bipolar disorder.[85] Similarly, some difficult childhood disturbances are quickly labelled as bipolar disorder[86,87] and treated with potent mood stabilizers and atypical antipsychotic medications. Unfortunately, there is no evidence that such medications are safe or useful in the long run for children. Unfortunate impacts of frequent household moves, parental distress, divorce and serious illness in a family member can be highly influential on the mood of children (and adults) but can be lost in the rush to medication.[81,83]

It is understandable that psychiatrists in the USA are leading this shift towards using psychopharmacologic agents as first-line treatments for conditions common to primary care, in spite of little evidence for such treatment as primary treatment, because patients and their families often see psychotherapy as too slow or inconvenient.[88] Many research psychiatrists or primary care physicians have difficulty obtaining funding for research on non-pharmacologic interventions that need to be evaluated.

There are reasons for caution as we move towards more integrated care. Given these trends to rely on medications to treat so many forms of human distress as a medical diagnosis in industrialized nations such as the USA and Spain, it may be that efforts to integrate mental health care into primary care will not improve the overall health of populations to the degree we desire, if integration is viewed mostly as an expeditious pathway to medications. On the other hand, if integration is designed to truly unite biomedical and psychosocial factors in care plans and how they are carried out by teams (that include patients and families), then integration is much more promising.[85]

We can move forward to improve health by increasing the integration of behavioural health into primary care if we do the following:

- create systems of primary care around the world using systematic modern methods of communicating with patients, families and other professionals
- create systems designed from the ground up to treat health and health care in an integrated fashion (medical and behavioural), and create the kind of teamwork required at the outset rather than waiting until all else fails to improve care
- use systematic and tested methods of screening for distressed children rather than waiting for an overt crisis, to identify youths with mental health needs earlier
- link families with schools, integrated primary care systems and other community resources to help children who suffer from mental disorders, social strains and family distress more effectively.

In summary, we can move forward with integrating mental health services into primary care at the interface of patients/families with collaborative professionals working within a biopsychosocial model. By learning from others around the world, we have the potential to succeed.

References

1   World Health Organization and Wonca. *Integrating mental health into primary care. A global perspective.* Geneva, World Health Organization, 2008.

2   Peek CJ. A collaborative care lexicon for asking practice and research development questions. In: *A national agenda for research in collaborative care: papers from the Collaborative Care Research Network Research Development Conference.* Rockville, Agency for Healthcare Research and Quality, 2011:25–44 (AHRQ Publication No. 11-0067) (http://www.ahrq.gov/research/collaborativecare/, accessed 8 November 2011).

3   Dictionary.com (http://dictionary.reference.com/, accessed 8 November 2011).

4   Engel GL. The need for a new medical model: a challenge for biomedicine. *Science*, 1977, 196:129–136.

5   Baird MA, Meier MA. Depression: what are we really treating? *Society of Teachers of Family Medicine Resource Library* (http://www.fmdrl.org/index.cfm?event=c.beginBrowseD&clearSelections=1&criteria=Baird#3572, accessed 30 November 2011).

6   Mauer BJ. *Behavioral health/primary care integration: the person-centered healthcare home.* Washington DC, National Council for Community Behavioral Healthcare, 2009 (http://www.thenationalcouncil.org/galleries/resources-services%20files/Integration%20and%20Healthcare%20Home.pdf, accessed 8 November 2011).

7   Doherty WJ, McDaniel SH, Baird MA. Five levels of primary care/behavioral healthcare collaboration. *Behavioral Healthcare for Tomorrow*, 1996, 5:25–27.

8   Peek CJ. Planning care in the clinical, operational, and financial worlds. In: Kessler R, Stafford D, eds. *Collaborative medicine in case studies: evidence in practice.* New York, Springer, 2008:25–38.

9   Patterson J et al. *Mental health professionals in medical settings: a primer.* New York, WW Norton & Company, 2002.

10 Unutzer J et al. Tansforming mental health care at the interface with general medicine: Report for the President's Commission. *Psychiatric Services*, 2006, 57:37–47.

11   Lester H, Glasby J, Tylee A. Integrated primary mental health care: threat or opportunity in the new NHS? *British Journal of General Practice*, 2004, 54:285–291.

12   Bower P, Gilbody S. Managing common mental health disorders in primary care: conceptual models and evidence base. *BMJ*, 2005, 330: 839–842.

13   van Orden M et al. Collaborative mental health care versus care as usual in a primary care setting: a randomized controlled trial. *Psychiatric Services*, 2009, 60:74–79.

14   Gask L, Croft J. Methods of working with primary care. *Advances in Psychiatric Treatment*, 2000, 6:442–449.

15   Cummings NA, Cummings JL, Johnson JN. *Behavioral health in primary care: a guide for clinical integration.* Madison CT, Psychosocial Press, 1997.

16   Hunter CL et al. *Integrated behavioral health in primary care: step-by-step guidance for assessment and intervention.* Washington DC, American Psychological Association, 2009.

17   Davis TF. From pilot to mainstream: promoting collaboration between mental health and medicine. *Families, Systems and Health*, 2001, 19:37–45.

18   Blount A, ed. *Integrated primary care: the future of medical and mental health collaboration.* New York, WW Norton & Company, 1998.

19   Kates N, Craven M. Shared mental health. Update from the Collaborative Working Group of the College of Family Physicians of Canada and the Canadian Psychiatric Association. *Canadian Family Physician*, 2002, 48:936–937.

20   Kates N, Mach M. Chronic disease management for depression in primary care: a summary of the current literature and implications for practice. *Canadian Journal of Psychiatry*, 2007, 52:77–85.

21   Katon W et al. Cost-effectiveness and net benefit of enhanced treatment of depression for older adults with diabetes and depression. *Diabetes Care*, 2006, 29:265–270.

22   *Estrategia en salud mental del sistema nacional de salud, 2006.* Madrid, Ministerio de Sanidad Y Consumo, 2007 (http://www.msps.es/organizacion/sns/planCalidadSNS/pdf/excelencia/salud_mental/ESTRATEGIA_SALUD_MENTAL_SNS_PAG_WEB.pdf, accessed 8 November 2011).

23   *Programa de la especialidad de medicina familiar y comnunitaria.* Madrid, Ministerio de Sanidad y Consumo, 2005.

24   American Academy of Family Physicians, American Academy of Pediatrics, American College of Physicians, and American Osteopathic Association. *Joint principles of the patient centered medical home, February 2007.* (http://www.aafp.org/online/etc/medialib/aafp_org/documents/policy/fed/joint principlespcmh0207.Par.0001.File.tmp/022107medicalhome.pdf, accessed 8 November 2011).

25   Stewart EE et al. Implementing the patient-centered medical home: observation and description of the national demonstration project. *Annals of Family Medicine*, 2010, 8(Suppl. 1):S21–32.

26   DeGruy FV, Etz RS. Attending to the whole person in the patient-centered medical home: the case for incorporating mental healthcare, substance abuse care, and health behavior change. *Families, Systems and Health*, 2010, 28:298–307.

27   Peek CJ, Oftedahl G. *A consensus operational definition of patient-centered medical home (PCMH): also known as health care home.* 2010 (Minneapolis, University of Minnesota and Institute for Clinical Systems Improvement (ICSI), 2010 (http://www.icsi.org/health_care_home_operational_definition/health_care_home_operational_definition__.html, accessed 8 November 2011).

28   Bauer AM et al. Tackling the global mental health challenge: a psychosomatic medicine/consultation-liaison psychiatry perspective. *Psychosomatics*, 2010, 51(3):185–193.

29   Wagner EH, Austin BT, Von Korff M. Organizing care for patients with chronic illness. *Milbank Quarterly*, 1996, 74:511–544.

30   Cape J, Whittington C, Bower P. What is the role of consultation-liaison psychiatry in the management of depression in primary care? A systematic review and meta-analysis. *General Hospital Psychiatry*, 2010, 32:246–254.

31   Gilbody S et al. Collaborative care for depression: a cumulative meta-analysis and review of longer-term outcomes. *Archives of Internal Medicine*, 2006, 166:2314–2321.

32   van der Feltz-Cornelis CM et al. Effect of psychiatric consultation models in primary care. A systematic review and meta-analysis of randomized clinical trials. *Journal of Psychosomatic Research*, 2010, 68:521–533.

33 Wagner EH et al. Improving chronic illness care: translating evidence into action. *Health Affairs (Millwood)*, 2001, 20:64–78.

34 Katon WJ et al. Collaborative care for patients with depression and chronic illnesses. *New England Journal of Medicine*, 2010, 363:2611–2620.

35 Katon W et al. Rethinking practitioner roles in chronic illness: the specialist, primary care physician, and the practice nurse. *General Hospital Psychiatry*, 2001, 23:138–144.

36 Annunziato RA et al. Site matters: winning the hearts and minds of patients in a cardiology clinic. *Psychosomatics*, 2008, 49:386–391.

37 O'Reilly R et al. Is telepsychiatry equivalent to face-to-face psychiatry? Results from a randomized controlled equivalence trial. *Psychiatric Services*, 2007, 58:836–843.

38 Hilty DM et al. Use of secure e-mail and telephone: psychiatric consultations to accelerate rural health service delivery. *Telemedicine Journal and E-Health*, 2006, 12:490–495.

39 Hilty DM, Yellowlees PM, Nesbitt TS. Evolution of telepsychiatry to rural sites: changes over time in types of referral and in primary care providers' knowledge, skills and satisfaction. *General Hospital Psychiatry*, 2006, 28:367–373.

40 South Australian Mental Health Service, Division of CHS. *Country mental health services for South Australia: a framework for service delivery*. Adelaide, SA Health Publications, 1993 (http://www.publications.health.sa.gov.au/mhs/9, accessed 21 November 2011).

41 Petersen I, Lund C, Stein DJ. Optimizing mental health services in low-income and middle-income countries. *Current Opinion in Psychiatry*, 2011, 24:318–323.

42 Wright AF. People with long-term mental illness: making shared care work. *British Journal of General Practice*, 1995, 45:338–339.

43 Petersen I et al. Lessons from case studies of integrating mental health into primary health care in South Africa and Uganda. *International Journal of Mental Health Systems*, 2011, 5:8.

44 Albreht T, Delnoij DM, Klazinga N. Changes in primary health care centres over the transition period in Slovenia. *European Journal of Public Health*, 2006, 16:238–243.

45 Rurik I, Kalabay L. Primary healthcare in the developing part of Europe: changes and development in the former Eastern Bloc countries that joined the European Union following 2004. *Medical Science Monitor*, 2009, 15:H78–H84.

46 Berardi D et al. Collaboration between mental health services and primary care: The Bologna Project. *Primary Care Companion, Journal of Clinical Psychiatry*, 1999, 1:180–183.

47 Jenkins R et al. Integration of mental health into primary care and community health working in Kenya: context, rationale, coverage and sustainability. *Mental Health in Family Medicine*, 2010, 7:37–47.

48 Dudley L, Garner P. Strategies for integrating primary health services in low- and middle-income countries at the point of delivery. *Cochrane Database Systematic Review*, 2011, (7):CD003318.

49 Patel V et al. Treatment and prevention of mental disorders in low-income and middle-income countries. *The Lancet*, 2007, 370:991–1005.

50 International Monetary Fund. *World Economic Outlook Database, October 2010* (http://www.imf.org/external/pubs/ft/weo/2010/02/weodata/index.aspx, accessed 8 November 2011).

51 Tsang FK. *Future mental health services in Hong Kong: conceptual and practical*. Paper to Legislative Council, LC Paper No. CB(2)373/07-08(06), November 2007 (http://www.legco.gov.hk/yr07-08/english/panels/hs/papers/hs1122cb2-373-6-e.pdf, accessed 8 November 2011).

52 Ryan S et al. The effects of regular source of care and health need on medical care use among rural adolescents. *Archives of Pediatrics and Adolescent Medicine*, 2001, 155:184–190.

53 O'Malley AS, Forrest CB. Continuity of care and delivery of ambulatory services to children in community health clinics. *Journal of Community Health*, 1996, 21:159–173.

54 Bindman AB et al. Primary care and receipt of preventive services. *Journal of General Internal Medicine*, 1996, 11:269–276.

55 Achenbach TM. *Integrative guide to the 1991 CBCL/4–18, YSR, and TRF profiles*. Burlington, VT, University of Vermont, Department of Psychology, 1991.

56 Lee A et al. Children with a regular FP – do they have better health behaviours and psychosocial health? *Australian Family Physician*, 2007, 36:180–182.

57 Escobar JI et al. Medically unexplained physical symptoms, somatization disorder and abridged somatization: studies with the Diagnostic Interview Schedule. *Psychiatric Developments*, 1989, 7:235–245.

58 Simon GE et al. An international study of the relation between somatic symptoms and depression. *New England Journal of Medicine*, 1999, 341:1329–1335.

59 Charupanit W. Factors related to missed appointment at psychiatric clinic in Songklanagarind Hospital. *Journal of the Medical Association of Thailand*, 2009, 92:1367–1369.

60 Kaplan RM, Chadwick MW, Schimmel LE. Social learning intervention to promote metabolic control in type I diabetes mellitus: pilot experiment results. *Diabetes Care*, 1985, 8:152–155.

61 Greene J, Yedidia MJ. Provider behaviors contributing to patient self-management of chronic illness among underserved populations. *Journal of Health Care for the Poor and Underserved*, 2005, 16:808–824.

62 US Department of Health and Human Services, Health Resources and Services Administration, and Maternal Child Health Bureau. *The National Survey of Children's Health, 2007*. Rockville, Maryland, US Department of Health and Human Services, 2009.

63 Fleming GF. The mental health of adolescents – assessment and management. *Australian Family Physician*, 2010, 36:588–593.

64 Lee A, Tsang KK. Healthy Schools Research Support Group. Youth risk behaviour in a Chinese population: a territory wide youth risk behavioural surveillance in Hong Kong. *Public Health*, 2004, 118:88–95.

65 Insel TR, Wang PS. Rethinking mental illness. *JAMA*, 2010, 303:1970–1971.

66 Stroud LR, Salovey P, Epel ES. Sex differences in stress responses: social rejection versus achievement stress. *Biological Psychiatry*, 2002, 52:318–327.

67 Cameron JL. Interrelationships between hormones, behavior, and affect during adolescence: understanding hormonal, physical, and brain changes occurring in association with pubertal activation of the reproductive axis. Introduction to Part III. *Annals of the New York Academy of Sciences*, 2004, 1021:110–123.

68 Lee A et al. Understanding suicidality and correlates among Chinese secondary school students in Hong Kong. *Health Promotion International*, 2009, 24:156–165.

69 Browne G et al. Effective/efficient mental health programs for school-age children: a synthesis of reviews. *Social Science and Medicine*, 2004, 58:1367–1384.

70 Stewart-Brown S. *What is the evidence on school health promotion in improving school health or preventing disease and specifically what is the effectiveness of the health promoting schools approach?* Copenhagen, World Health Organization, WHO Regional Office for Europe (Health Evidence Network report), 2006 (http://www.euro.who.int/document/e88185.pdf accessed 8 November 2011).

71 American Medical Association, Department of Adolescent Health. *Guidelines for Adolescent Preventive Services (GAPS)*. Chicago, American Medical Association, 2007 (http://www.ama-assn.org/ama/pub/physician-resources/public-health/promoting-healthy-lifestyles/adolescent-health/guidelines-adolescent-preventive-services.page, accessed 8 November 2011).

72 Goldenring JM, Rosen DS. Getting into adolescent heads: an essential update. *Contemporary Pediatrics*, 2004, 21:64–90.

73 Parker A, Hetrick S, Purcell R. Psychosocial assessment of young people - refining and evaluating a youth friendly assessment interview. *Australian Family Physician*, 2010, 39:585–588.

74 Lee A et al. A comprehensive Healthy Schools Programme to promote school health: the Hong Kong experience in joining the efforts of health and education sectors. *Journal of Epidemiology and Community Health*, 2003, 57:174–177.

75 Green LW, Poland B, Rootman I. The settings approach to health promotion. In: Poland B, Green LW, Rootman I, eds. *Settings for health promotion: linking theory and practice*. Thousand Oaks, CA: Sage, 2000:1–43.

76 World Health Organization, 2010. *mhGAP intervention guide for mental, neurological and substance use disorders in non-specialized health settings*. Geneva, World Health Organization, 2010 (http://www.globalmentalhealth.org/downloads/Packages%20of%20Care%20-%20mhGAP%20Implementation%20Guidelines%20%282.79%20MB%29.pdf, accessed 8 November 2011).

77 Robins D, Fein D, Barton M. *M-CHAT*™ (http://www2.gsu.edu/~psydlr/DianaLRobins/Official_M-CHAT_Website.html, accessed 8 November 2011).

78 Finn R, Learmonth M, Reedy P. Some unintended effects of teamwork in healthcare. *Social Science and Medicine*, 2010, 70:1148–1154.

79 Vera M et al. Collaborative care for depressed patients with chronic medical conditions: a randomized trial in Puerto Rico, *Psychiatric Services*, 2010, 61:144–150.

80 Nieuwsma JA. *Brief psychotherapy for depression in primary care: a systematic review of the evidence.* Washington DC, Department of Veterans Affairs, Health Services Research and Development Service, 2011.

81 Horwitz AV, Wakefield JC. *The loss of sadness: how psychiatry transformed normal sorrow into depressive disorder.* New York, Oxford University Press, 2007.

82 Salazar-Fraile J et al. 'Doctor, I just can't go on.' Cultural constructions of depression and the prescription of antidepressants to users who are not clinically depressed. *International Journal of Mental Health*, 2010, 39:29–67.

83 Whitaker R. *Anatomy of an epidemic.* New York, Crown Publishers, 2010.

84 Watters E. The Americanization of mental illness. *New York Times*, 8 January 2010 (http://www.nytimes.com/2010/01/10/magazine/10psyche-t.html?scp=1andsq=Americanizing mental illnessandst=cse, accessed 8 November 2011).

85 Menand L. 2010. Head case: can psychiatry be a science? *New Yorker*, 1 March 2010 (http://www.newyorker.com/arts/critics/atlarge/2010/03/01/100301crat_atlarge_menand, accessed 8 November 2011).

86 Kuehn BM. Studies shed light on risks and trends in pediatric antipsychotic prescribing. *JAMA*, 2009, 303:1901–1903.

87 Harris G. 2008. Use of antipsychotics in children is criticized. *New York Times*, 19 November (http://www.nytimes.com/2008/11/19/health/policy/19fda.html, accessed 8 November 2011).

88 Althoff RR, Waterman GS. Commentary: Psychiatric training for physicians: a call to modernize. *Academic Medicine*, 2011, 86:285–287.

8 Evaluation of primary care mental health

Jaime C Sapag and Brian Rush

Key messages

- Evaluation of primary care mental health services is a critical challenge for continuous quality improvement.
- A comprehensive and holistic evaluation approach should be based on context needs, and consider the use of mixed methods in order to better face system complexities.
- Existing theories, evaluation frameworks and previous evaluations may be relevant to define the best evaluation approach for a particular evaluation need.
- Evaluation strategies for primary care mental health need to recognize the importance of the structure, process and outcomes elements of primary care mental health services, as well as the criteria of effectiveness, efficiency and equity.
- Rather than thinking of evaluation as an isolated event, it is critical to actively work on developing a healthy evaluation culture in primary care mental health services, at all levels.
- An inclusive strategy may enrich the evaluation process. Everybody has a role to play in developing evaluation: policy-makers and decision-makers, clinicians, health promoters, patients and families, and stakeholders.
- Defining and accomplishing a knowledge exchange strategy is critical for having an impact when doing evaluation.

Introduction

This chapter discusses the importance and challenges of evaluating primary care mental health (PCMH) and some of the main concepts and methodological bases that policy-makers, planners, managers and health teams should consider to better address their own local evaluation needs. The hope is that fostering evaluation will support decision-making and resource allocation, aimed at improving the results of PCMH worldwide. A continuous process of improving services and the overall health system requires evaluation capacity to be strengthened, which is essential for obtaining better results and identifying best practices, thus meeting the requirements in the field of service delivery. The sharing of concepts, methods and tools to conduct practice-oriented evaluations in the context of PCMH is urgently needed.

Health services research is a:

> multidisciplinary field of inquiry, both basic and applied, that examines the use, costs, quality, accessibility and delivery, organization, financing, and outcomes of health care services in order to increase knowledge and understanding of structure, processes, and effects of health services for individuals and populations.[1]

In particular, evaluative research and programme evaluation assess how well programmes and services, which have been developed and implemented based on previous descriptive and analytical research, have done in achieving a desired objective,[2] and provide knowledge about the value of programmes that can be used to reduce the social problems to which programmes are relevant.[3] Theoretical rationales and methodological approaches are fundamental to defining the most appropriate design and to applying evaluation research methods in specific situations and contexts for PCMH.

The chapter is organized in seven sections. First, some background regarding mental health integration in primary care is provided, and the need for evaluation is discussed. The following section reviews some important concepts regarding PCMH and evaluation. The next two sections discuss theories and frameworks that are relevant for evaluating PCMH, respectively. The fifth section presents some orientations for defining the appropriate evaluation focus, objectives and guiding questions, followed by a section that analyses some challenges related to evaluation design and methodological approaches. The final section concludes with advice for decision-makers and health teams regarding practical considerations that are important for implementing an evaluation of PCMH.

In this chapter, the term "*mental health*" includes substance use issues. In some cases, to remind the reader of its importance, the terms "addiction" or "substance use disorders" are also explicitly mentioned.

Background

There is a high level of need for mental health care among people who attend primary health care (PHC). The prevalence of mental disorders among consecutive PHC attendees varies between 24% and 69%.[4] Substance use disorders are present in 10–20% of primary care patients, and rates are increasing.[5] Primary care providers already deliver significant levels of mental health care, often to people who would not otherwise reach mental health services. The PHC system has to respond effectively to a high demand from the population. A continuous and systematic improvement process that considers a holistic health approach is required.[6]

As discussed in other chapters, integrating mental health and addictions into primary care is an urgent and important need that involves a health-system transformation.[6] Mental health and physical health problems are interrelated components of overall health, and are best treated in a coordinated care system. Many individuals with serious medical problems also have comorbid psychiatric problems, predominantly depression, anxiety and substance use disorders. Primary care provides a unique opportunity to address mental health and addiction needs. Fostering mental health services in primary care capitalizes on the long-term relationships, frequent routine contact, opportunity for early detection for mental illness, and potential to reduce stigma and barriers to care that characterize this setting.[7]

There is a need to focus on the development of effective, affordable and equitable mental health systems (including substance use) and PCMH. One of the major difficulties related to the achievement of this goal is the lack of evidence for what kinds of PCMH services are more appropriate and effective in varying contexts. It is necessary to incorporate evaluation in order to support decision-makers and their organizations. Evaluation will provide critical information to strengthen PCMH services in terms of access, quality of care and impact on population health status, including mental health. A culture of evaluation may also be critical to foster better use of local resources, as well as to fulfil requirements for transparency and accountability.

However, research and programme evaluation have not played a major role in informing PCMH development in many places. There are some evaluation challenges regarding PCMH.[8] The complexity and variability of approaches, and the deficit of explicit goals when implementing PCMH, in many cases, are barriers to implementing evaluation initiatives. At the same time, limited resources, lack of an evaluation culture in many mental health and primary care settings, as well as a low level of prioritization of mental health and primary care in many countries, make it more urgent to advance in the evaluation area worldwide. Any evaluation endeavour needs to consider all the aforementioned factors, as well as the local context and ongoing changes within it. It should also incorporate existing relevant theoretical models and programme/health services evaluation frameworks.

As the PCMH field grows, health system decision-makers are looking at the key components of successful programmes and how they can be adapted to improve access for particular populations and communities that traditionally underuse mental health services.[9] However, a comprehensive performance evaluation framework for PCMH systems and services has not yet been developed.

In particular, there is a need for organizations that offer PCMH services to strengthen their institutional capacity in the area of programme evaluation. Only by doing so can these organizations engage in a continuous process of quality improvement that will progressively enhance the services they deliver, ensuring that scarce resources are effectively allocated, and that target populations benefit from best practices based on the most recent experiences. In low- and middle-income countries, programme-evaluation constraints are even more pronounced, since these countries must also contend with issues of widespread poverty, inadequate housing, high rates of unemployment, lack of food security, limited access to education, and many other urgent challenges.

There are still many evaluation needs that have not been sufficiently explored in the area of PCMH. For example:[10]

- effective methods of integrating primary care into specialty mental health practice settings (e.g. obesity and depression)
- the use of information technology (e.g. Internet, electronic health records)
- the sustainability of integrated care without external support, such as grant funding
- the effectiveness of the various components of integrated care, including determination of the value added by each component individually and synergistically
- the cost-effectiveness of integrated models at the societal level
- the effectiveness of PCMH for case identification, treatment, and monitoring, focusing on mental health conditions other than depression
- the effectiveness of PCMH in the presence of both general medical comorbidities (e.g. diabetes or chronic pain) and mental health comorbidities (e.g. depression or substance disorders).

Key concepts

To advance the evaluation of PCMH, it is first necessary to review some key concepts and operational definitions. This step is critical, in order to be more precise about the breadth and boundaries of the evaluation initiative, and the process of distinguishing activities, outputs, and expected outcomes of PCMH through the development of a logic model.

Primary care mental health: the "object" of evaluation

There are many definitions of PCMH. For this chapter, PCMH involves a strong primary care component, with providers from different specialties, disciplines or sectors working collaboratively to offer complementary services and mutual support to ensure that individuals/populations receive the most appropriate and effective mental health services with high standards of quality, from health promotion and early detection to diagnosis, treatment and recovery support.

The Canadian Collaborative Mental Health Initiative's (CCMHI's) Collaborative Mental Health Care Framework[11] was developed by the Canadian Collaborative Mental Health,[12] and provides a clear picture of some of the key areas and concepts included in PCMH. This framework has a strong focus on enhancing the relationships and collaboration among the community (including patients, families, and others), health-care providers, and caregivers, in order to foster mental health and well-being by improving prevention, health promotion, treatment and rehabilitation services in primary health-care settings. It puts consumers at the centre and assumes that collaborative mental health care will increase access to mental health services, decrease the burden of illness, and optimize care. It is made up of fundamentals that influence the success of collaborative mental health care, and key elements that are considered critical to providing effective services. The fundamentals are:

- the degree of consistency of legislation, policies and funding structures with the principles of collaborative mental health care
- funds and needs-based research (e.g. identification of best practices) that support it
- community strengths and needs, resources, and readiness to implement it.

The key elements are:

- increasing accessibility to mental health care
- collaborative structures (including the ways in which people have agreed to work together to accomplish certain key functions of collaborative mental health care, such as referral strategies or evaluation instruments)
- richness of collaboration among health-care partners
- consumer (patient or user) centredness (people facing mental health issues and their families should be involved in all aspects of their care).

This conceptual framework can help evaluators to consider the particularities of PCMH in an evaluation approach. However, there are also three other conceptual perspectives, which are very important to take into account when developing any evaluation initiative regarding PCMH:

- *a population health approach* is aimed at improving the health and well-being of the entire population and at reducing health inequities among population groups.[13] In order to reach these objectives, it recognizes the importance and acts upon the broad range of individual and collective conditions that determine health, including social, economic, and environmental factors, personal health practices, individual capacity and coping skills, biology and genetic endowment, early childhood development and health services.[14–16] This broader perspective emphasizes political and community determinants, for example living and employment conditions, income, housing, environment, culture, social inclusion and social capital.[16,17] A population health approach is critical for the development of effective PCMH

- *a system approach*: programmes or interventions occur within a complex system, where structures and relationships are interactive and dynamic. Systems are highly sensitive to initial conditions, so small changes can make a major difference.[18] Facilitating system change is not easy and requires persistent, incremental changes in order to maintain stability, while minimizing disruption. It is also important to consider unintended consequences in formulating a strategy. System thinking theory encompasses ecological models and goes beyond incorporating system dynamics and complexity theory approaches[19]

- *complex problems and the chronic care model*: this is consistent with both the overarching sociocultural context of PCMH and findings regarding the existence of complex challenges, such as competing demands, heavy case-loads, limited resources, and inadequate training in primary care settings.[20] The chronic care model[21] represents a major rethinking of primary care practice.[22] Six key components have been identified to improve effectiveness of chronic care: community resources (including linkages with other services); health-care organization (goals and policies); self-management support; decision support (e.g. clinical guidelines); delivery systems redesign (e.g. case management, primary care teams); and clinical information systems.[23] An evaluation of any PCMH setting should integrate the components of the chronic care paradigm.

When assessing PCMH services, it is also necessary to note that there are different models of collaborative mental health care:[7]

- *community mental health team*: an interface between primary and secondary care, where the aim is to make multidisciplinary mental health treatment more widely available in the community
- *shifted outpatient clinic*: visiting psychiatrists operate clinics within health centres and see both new and follow-up patients
- *attached mental health professional*: many practices have integrated mental health professionals in their primary care teams
- *consultation–liaison*: places greater emphasis on developing close links within a practice between a primary care team and psychiatric staff. Consultation–liaison can be combined with any or all of the three models above, and this is probably the situation in many PCMH settings.

However, it is important to be aware that there is not a rigid or single model of collaborative mental health care,[24] and in many settings there is a mix of models in place in the same context.

Context-specific characteristics of primary care mental health

Some of the barriers or opportunities for effective PCMH are very context specific, for example the population served, local organization and structure of the health system, funding, and specific communication barriers with specialty mental health and addictions agencies. Those unique characteristics are likely to require context-specific solutions.[25] Evaluators should understand the local context in order to address the needs of those who requested the evaluation, as well as the potential sharing of the results locally and beyond. From an equity perspective, it is also relevant to assess if PCMH services are targeting specific subpopulations (e.g. people living in poverty, severe mental illness, the elderly with depression, persons facing substance use issues, high users of medical care).

Evaluation needs will vary according to the specific time and reality of the context, as well as who is interested in the results. For example:

- the director of a health system at the national, provincial or district level might be interested in knowing how cost-effective the mental health programmes are that they have been implementing in PHC (e.g. a depression initiative for women, brief interventions for youth facing alcohol-use disorders, etc.)
- the director and managers of a PHC clinic might have questions about the competencies of the existing human resources working with patients facing mental health issues, the quality of the specific services they are providing, and/or regarding the availability of psychopharmacological medicines for the most prevalent conditions in PHC
- a PHC interprofessional team would like to know how their definition of roles and responsibilities is working in practice, as well as how effective their team functioning is, in order to provide support to patients with mental health needs
- an individual PHC physician might be interested in knowing what is happening with the patients he/she had referred for secondary or tertiary care
- a health-promotion team might be asking about the impact of their community-based efforts to foster positive mental health and prevent mental illness.

These are just some examples and there are many others. An important consideration is to identify the most relevant needs-based questions, in order to improve the practice at the individual, team, organizational and system levels, as well as to consider the feasibility of addressing those questions in practice, according to the context reality.

Quality of care

There is an ongoing and active debate on what *quality of health care* entails. That lack of consensus challenges a comprehensive framework to evaluate the quality of health systems,[26] including PCMH services. Donabedian remarked on the importance of having a clear definition of *quality* and considering specific criteria and standards before assessing quality of care.[27,28] He identified three main dimensions to be assessed regarding quality of care:

- *structure*: focused on the attributes of the setting where health services are provided (e.g. facilities, equipments, etc.)
- *process*: refers to how (methods) health care is delivered or what is done by both patients and practitioners in seeking and providing care, respectively (e.g. use of evidence-based guidelines, referral dynamic, etc.)
- *outcomes*: the effects of health care on individual and population health (e.g. health status, health-care experience, quality of life, mortality, etc.).

A more recent definition of *quality of health care* comes from the Institute of Medicine:[29] "the degree to which health services for individuals and populations increase the likelihood of desired health outcomes and are consistent with current professional knowledge". This definition includes six critical dimensions: safe; effective; patient-centered; timely; efficient; and equitable.

Continuous quality improvement (CQI) is a management philosophy and system that is focused on the continuous improvement of work processes to achieve better outcomes of care. Its goal is to consistently meet or exceed the needs of patients, families, community, and health workers, and it is focused on specific key areas:[28]

- processes of health care and health-care delivery
- people who are served
- continuous monitoring of quality focused on service improvement
- committed leadership necessary to improve quality of services
- education
- long-term commitment.

The main elements of CQI and some of the techniques that it uses are closely related with programme evaluation and monitoring.[31]

The expectation is that evaluation of PCMH will be, directly or indirectly, supporting the process of CQI.

Evaluation and types of evaluation

There are many definitions of what evaluation is. For example, Smith and Glass define it as the process of establishing value judgements based on evidence about a programme or product.[32] For Briones,[33] evaluation is a type of research that analyses the structure, functioning and results of a programme to provide information that derives useful criteria for making decisions regarding its management and development.

Types of evaluation

There are different types of evaluation designs that could be used to assess different aspects or stages of PCMH. The most basic distinction in evaluation types is that between *formative* and *summative* evaluation.[34] *Formative evaluation* is most often conducted during the planning of the early stages of a programme, for the purpose of providing feedback for improvement during the course of the intervention, identifying deficiencies and building on strengths. *Summative evaluation*, in contrast, provides information on the effectiveness of the programme or service (its ability to achieve what it was designed to achieve in the real context) by examining the effects or outcomes of some initiative.

Evaluation involves the systematic collection of feedback about a programme, service or intervention for informing the decision-making. The feedback and specific questions asked can be about different areas, depending on the specific situation (see Figure 8.1):[35]

- *needs*: e.g. what needs exist in the community, related to the problem? This is very important before the programme takes place
- *process*: e.g. what is developing the treatment programme? To what extent is it proceeding as planned? How is the quality of the programme/service implementation or operation?
- *satisfaction*: e.g. what is the patient perspective on treatment and its benefits to them?
- *results*: e.g. how have patients changed and to what extent are these changes attributable to treatment? Have the expected outcomes been achieved?
- *economic*: e.g. what is the cost of each component of treatment? What is the total cost? Is the treatment more efficient than other options?

The evaluation may be focused on different levels depending on need:[35]

- *single case*: focuses on an individual case in clinical practice to generate feedback to solve a particular problem and/or to improve specific interventions for the client
- *activity*: evaluation of a specific treatment or technique (e.g. a certain drug, relapse prevention, etc.). This involves summarizing the participation of a group of patients
- *service or programme*: evaluation of a specific service or programme (e.g. first response plan, outpatient plan, primary care depression programme, etc.) The programme includes more than one activity or modality
- *agency*: the assessment of all those services provided by a single health service

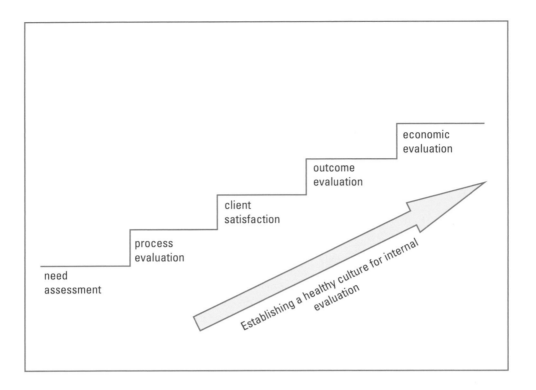

Figure 8.1   Stepped model of treatment service or system evaluation

■   *system*: this level is more complex and has greater sociopolitical significance. It comprises many different activities, programmes and agencies.

Monitoring versus evaluation

These terms are related, but different.[35] *Monitoring* involves a systematic collection and analysis of information of selected aspects of a programme or service as it progresses. It may help to keep the initiatives on track, as well as identify implementation issues and needs for process improvement. On the other hand, *evaluation* considers a kind of comparison of actual impacts of the programme/services against the agreed standards. It will not just use routine sources of information, and may be implemented as a one-time evaluation project with specific objectives and time frame. Both monitoring and evaluation contribute to assessing *effectiveness* (the extent to which a programme or service achieves its specific objectives, in a real context), *efficiency* (the achieved results according with the invested resources) and *impact* (a positive result regarding the health problem or situation because of the intervention/service).

Evaluation theories

Different theoretical approaches have been used to guide evaluation designs and implementation. *Health system evaluation* has evolved in terms of defining how programme efforts and outcomes have been valued; how evaluators justified different kinds of knowledge identified or created by the evaluation process; and how studies have been conducted in order to impact on policies and actions for social change. The evolution of programme and systems evaluation has been closely related to what has been happening in the sociopolitical context where those programmes and systems have been implemented.

There have been different, but not mutually exclusive, stages regarding *programme evaluation*, each of which provides different understandings and methodological approaches. It is possible to identify three stages:[3]

Companion to Primary Care Mental Health

- the first stage can be termed "traditional research methods" (1960–1980) and is represented by evaluators like Scriven and Campbell
- the second is alternative evaluation models (1970–1985), which responded to the limitations of the previous models
- finally, a third stage (1985 until now) develops a comprehensive approach by integrating previous theories and adding new perspectives like system thinking.

First-stage theories, which emerged in the social climate of the 1960s, aimed to identify implementable solutions (programmes) to address social problems. The main theorists who contributed to this stage are Scriven, Campbell and others. Among their assumptions are: (1) interventions would be defined, implemented and evaluated in unambiguous ways; (2) an external world exists, but it can never be fully known; (3) evaluated successful initiatives would be adopted by policy-makers, service/programme managers and deliverers, in order to (4) reduce the social problem. They valued demonstrative programmes as a way to learn and create manipulable solutions, and considered that feedback about programmes would be used by decision-makers to maintain or expand effective programmes or to radically change or stop ineffective programmes. They believed that it is possible to construct more or less valid knowledge about reality, and that biases are a constant threat that should be prevented. Evaluators should maintain distance from stakeholders in order to foster the integrity of the evaluation. Quantitative methods and traditional experimental perspectives have a major role in evaluation.

Theorists such as Weiss, Wholey and Steke led *second-stage theories* in the 1970s, in response to the perception that previous theories had failed in producing useful knowledge to improve programmes. Among their assumptions were:

- the best knowledge should be useful and not just interestingly true
- instrumental use of knowledge (from evaluation) does not occur spontaneously, so evaluators must promote such use, working closely with stakeholders and specific users of each evaluation (not just senior managers and policy-makers) in identifying their needs and supporting them in defining what to do with the evaluation results
- evaluation can provide enlightening information about the nature and causes of social problems, and this information may be helpful to make incremental improvements rather than a total programme change
- methodological pluralism offers new opportunities for evaluation.

Third-stage theories are focused mainly on the synthesis of previous theories and a comprehensive approach. Among the most recognized authors of this wave are Cronbach and Rossi. They indicate that the specific evaluation design and methods should be defined depending on the purposes and different circumstances. That gives space for a variety of evaluation possibilities to address concrete challenges, where previous concepts from first-stage or second-stage evaluation theories might be less appropriate. They value descriptive knowledge about use (second stage) and also the relevance of validity (first stage).

Theorists from the third stage recognize how politics may affect social programmes, and consider that they are subjects of potential incremental changes or improvements (short-term social change), as well as radical changes, when it is necessary and when a longer-term perspective is incorporated. They do not believe in single paradigms to resolve evaluation challenges, and are explicitly open to multiple epistemologies, multiple methods (methodological pluralism), and multiple priorities, in terms of what the important questions are and the kind of knowledge that is relevant. For example, in early stages of programme development, they prioritize discovery and describing the implementation process. When the programme is established, their focus is on monitoring techniques, including the analysis of programme outcomes. When there is a specific hypothesis to be tested, they suggest more sophisticated and experimental methods.

It is important to explicitly identify what theory or theories will be used in designing an evaluation for the specific context of PCMH.

Health services evaluation frameworks

There is a lack of a comprehensive framework to assess PCMH. A complete picture is necessary in order to evaluate PCMH and understand its contribution to health outcomes. It is necessary to evaluate the linkages between the sector's contexts, inputs, activities, outputs and outcomes. In turn, this will require a comprehensive data-collection strategy and the development of information systems that recognize the linkages between primary health care, the other levels of the health system and other sectors. In order to think about alternatives for evaluating, different existing evaluation models and conceptualizations may help.

Aday and colleagues proposed a very useful and comprehensive approach for evaluating health systems.[2] Health policy is crucial in terms of how the health system is organized and how it is working. The *structure*, composed of the delivery system, the population at risk and the environment, is interrelated with the level of access (utilization and satisfaction) as well as health risks, which are considered *process*. Lastly, *outcomes* are the final health and well-being impact at the individual (patients) and population levels (community). The criteria of *effectiveness*, *efficiency* and *equity* provide a broad perspective for assessing the performance of collaborative mental health-care programmes. These three criteria are often complementary.

The *mental health matrix* designed by Thornicroft and Tansella for planning and evaluation of mental health services emphasizes the need for simplicity, and presents a conceptual framework with only two dimensions: the geographical and the temporal.[36] The geographical includes three levels: *country/regional (system)*; *local*; and *patient*. The temporal dimension has three phases: *inputs*; *process*; and *outcomes*. Using these two dimensions, a 3 × 3 matrix is constructed in order to introduce and then measure critical aspects of mental health services. This framework suggests that mental health services should be primarily organized at the local level in order to better focus policies and resources, and that even when outcomes are the most important aspect of service evaluation, they can only be interpreted in the context of their prior phases: inputs and processes.

Performance measurement is something that needs to be considered when evaluating PCMH. There is no agreement in terms of what exactly performance measurement is.[37] Nazdam and Nelos consider the use of both outcomes and process measures to understand organizational performance and to effect positive change to improve care.[38] Performance measurement for health has also focused on the three classical components of health: *structure*, *process* and *outcomes* and at all care levels, from clients to population. It conceptualizes two major issues:[39] aligning with organizational strategic direction; and determining the appropriate scope for the system, considering three dimensions: (1) vertical (level of the health-care organization or system); (2) horizontal (breadth across the continuum of care or business unit); and (3) longitudinal (temporal).

Finally, special attention should also be given to issues related to predisposing, enabling, and need factors associated with health service use,[40] as well as cost-effectiveness.

Defining the evaluation focus, objectives and guiding questions

One key step for a successful evaluation is to clearly define the evaluation focus, as well as the evaluation question(s). Ideally, an evaluation of PCMH should describe key features of the main policies, structural changes, and the new mechanisms and processes introduced as a result of the PCMH programme/service. It should also describe and measure changes in health-system performance and try to establish causal linkages between interventions (the programme or its subcomponents) and outcomes – to assess the extent to which the changes observed can be attributed to the PCMH initiative.

However, in real life it is not easy to establish causal links, given that PCMH services or systems are not isolated experiments in controlled settings. In most cases, it will be more realistic to define the focus of the evaluation on a more specific need for information. Before defining the evaluation questions, it is ideal that the evaluation team meets with key stakeholders and decision-makers in the PCMH setting, in order to have a better understanding of the context and explore the feasibility of responding to different evaluation questions. Of course, funding limitations need to be considered.

A transparent discussion within the specific context has to take place before any decision is made. Next steps are to decide who will be involved in the evaluation and their interest; assess the availability of evaluation resources; and describe the programme for evaluation – with a programme logic model. Analysing the external context and assessing how it affects the likely success of the programme are critical preliminary steps to be addressed before designing the evaluation. Beginning with a participatory development of a logic model of the local PCMH, as well as a clear definition of activities and outcomes is a good starting point. The involvement of the local stakeholders from the outset is critical. They should also participate in defining the evaluation questions. At the same time, it will be essential to explore what kind of information is or is not available, and how feasible it is to collect new information in order to respond to the evaluation questions.

The evaluators will also have to consider the following key questions in order to focus their evaluation:[41]

- what will be evaluated?
- what aspects of PCMH will be considered when judging programme performance?
- what standards (i.e. type or level of performance) must be reached for PCMH to be considered successful?
- what evidence will be used to indicate how PCMH has performed?
- what conclusions regarding PCMH performance are justified by comparing the available evidence to the selected standards?
- how will the lessons learnt from the inquiry be used to improve PCMH?

Then, the evaluators will be ready to start the process of defining the specific questions of a particular evaluation. Some examples of specific evaluation questions are presented in Box 8.1.

Box 8.1 Examples of evaluation questions

- What is the impact of PCMH on the health of the population?
- How cost-effective are PCMH services?
- What is the most effective use of resources, including cost–benefit analyses of PCMH care strategies?
- What components of the PCMH collaborative model work best for which mental health and addiction issues (e.g. care for vulnerable populations, chronic disease management)?
- Which are the barriers and facilitators of collaboration in PCMH?
- What are the optimal roles for family physicians, social workers, and other professionals working together to deliver mental health care?
- How can PCMH strategies be used to improve the care provided for hard-to-serve populations?
- How are PCMH initiatives to be implemented on a large scale?

Evaluation research design and methodological approaches

A critical analysis of evaluation approaches and models is very important to define the best evaluation design, in the hope that evaluators and clients have an evaluation that is able to respond to their evaluation needs and to avoid useless studies. However, there are many options and all of them have their strengths and weaknesses. Stufflebeam and Shinkfield classified and analysed 26 evaluation approaches, concluding that there is no single best evaluation approach for each particular situation.[42] The main implication of this is a need to be open to using one or more of them, as deemed the most appropriate (depending on the particularities of the situation), and to be open to integrating different evaluation approaches.

An ideal evaluation design for PCMH should be one that:

- measures and reports on both the processes and outcomes associated with the PCMH system/services, including all aspects of PCMH (i.e. contexts, inputs, activities, outputs and outcomes) and recognizes the relationships between each of these aspects)
- is population based[13–16]
- is longitudinal
- is comparative
- is based on multilayered perspectives (e.g. linking individual clients to providers, clinics, organizations and systems), including the involvement of key stakeholders.

PCMH programmes or services do not happen in isolation. They are part of a historical process and have a specific context. It is important to see them as dynamic systems with a trajectory of development and change over a period of time. In practice, it is very difficult to separate contextual factors from policy interventions and PCMH, and to clearly establish causal links. There are also issues of collaboration within settings and between settings that need to be considered. Given this, any method used to evaluate complex collaborative care models will have limitations. Nevertheless, a systematic approach to evaluation can yield useful information for drawing plausible conclusions about how to advance and how to use the new information for effective knowledge exchange among researchers, evaluators, stakeholders, decision-makers and clinicians of PCMH.

The evaluation should be composed of concrete interdependent steps that are starting points for tailoring the evaluation (see Figure 8.2).[41,43,44] First of all, it is fundamental to start focusing the evaluation by understanding the evaluation context, engaging key stakeholders to be part of the process of developing the evaluation design from the beginning, clarifying the purpose and the evaluation questions and/or objectives of the evaluation, and describing the programme/services, including (critical assumptions, target groups, components, activities and outcomes), using different approaches (e.g. logic model) to help in building an appropriate evaluation design. Steps 2 to 4 (see Figure 8.2) deal with collecting and analysing data to address the evaluation questions. Finally, step 5 includes interpreting the finding(s), making concrete recommendations and sharing the lessons learnt (dissemination). This five-step approach reinforces the importance of integrating planning and evaluation, and the ongoing, cyclical nature of evaluation.[44]

Quantitative methods probably represent the most dominant evaluation approach. They tend to focus on objectivity, accuracy, and the validity of the obtained information.[45] On the other hand, *qualitative methods* emphasize the importance of observation, the need to retain the phenomenological quality of the context,

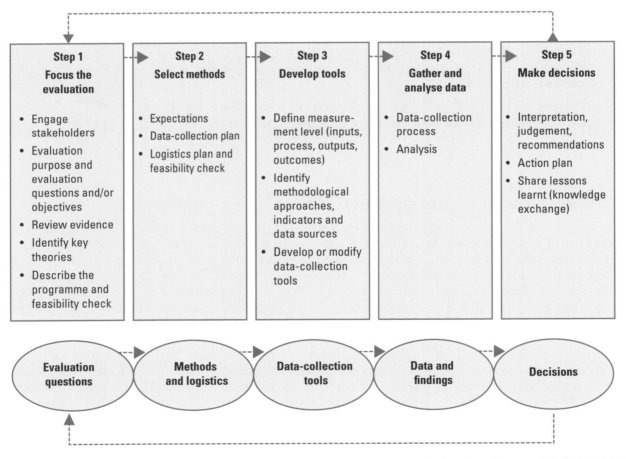

Figure 8.2 Evaluation steps; adapted, with permission from the Canadian Evaluation Society, from Porteous NL, Sheldrick BJ, Stewart PJ. Enhancing managers' evaluation capacity: a case study from Ontario Public Health. *The Canadian Journal of Program Evaluation*, 1999, Special issue:137–154[44]

and the value of subjective human interpretation in the evaluation process.[46] It is beyond the scope of this chapter to describe their pros and cons in detail. Each of the various features may be viewed as a strength or a weakness, depending on the original purpose, context and resources of the evaluation. The analysis of data will depend on the particular methods selected. Mixed methods or multimethod research holds potential for rigorous, methodologically sound studies in PCMH.[47]

A variety of data-collection procedures can be useful in defining and/or implementing an evaluation for PCMH: using clinical records, questionnaires, qualitative interview, focus groups, Delphi group consultation, participant and non-participant observation, document analysis, administrative databases, etc. Some existing instruments may be considered for the data-collection process, when they are appropriate for the evaluation objectives and validated.

Operational and structural context and constraints influence the choice of method. It will be necessary to start by describing PCMH (the object of evaluation) in a particular context and to involve stakeholders from the beginning. It is necessary to be aware of appropriate standards of professional evaluation practice in order to ensure evaluation quality and protect the public from potential harm relating to the evaluation itself.[42,48] There are four fundamental concepts regarding programme-evaluation standards:[48]

- *utility*: seek to ensure that an evaluation will serve the information needs of intended users
- *feasibility*: seek to ensure that an evaluation will be realistic, prudent, diplomatic and frugal
- *propriety*: seek to ensure that an evaluation will be conducted legally, ethically, and with due regard for the welfare of those involved in the evaluation, as well as those affected by its results
- *accuracy*: seek to ensure that an evaluation will reveal and convey technically adequate information about the features that determine the worth or merit of the programme being evaluated.

It is important to ensure that an evaluation will convey technically adequate information about the service's features associated with the benefits of PCMH. These standards should be discussed from the beginning of the process, and are critical for the decision-making regarding each of the evaluation steps.

It is equally important that the measures or indicators of a PCMH evaluation are reliable and valid.[33] Reliability means that the measures must be sensitive to change in a particular characteristic across time and that this can be measured consistently. Validity refers to the measure's ability to accurately assess the characteristic of interest, for example, current drug use. There are many types of reliability and validity, which are related, but will not be discussed in this chapter. Nevertheless, it is noteworthy that in evaluation research the notion of validity applies to the entire evaluation and not just the data.[49] In the case of qualitative studies, the concepts of trustworthiness, quality and rigour may be more appropriate than reliability and validity. The focus of trustworthiness is to support the argument that the research findings are "worth paying attention to".[50]

Conclusion and practical considerations

Evaluation of PCMH services and how they address mental health and addiction issues at the individual and population levels is a critical challenge for *continuous quality improvement*. This chapter proposes that it is essential to adapt a comprehensive and holistic evaluation approach, considering mixed methods, and understanding the particularities of the circumstances, as well as system complexities. In order to propose an evaluation for PCMH, it is fundamental to first analyse the context and know more about its structure, organization and functions, to have a better understanding of its complexities. It is very important also to fully understand the stage of development of each PCMH setting (initial, implementation or established), in order to better define an appropriate design and use the advantages of different types of methodologies and evaluation techniques. Clearly, evaluation strategies for PCMH need to recognize the importance of effectiveness, efficiency and equity.

The need for theories to guide the evaluation process (theory-driven evaluation) has been already emphasized. For example, it is relevant to first identify the main theories underlying primary care and collaborative care models, as well as the specific theory behind the issues on which the evaluation will be focused. This theoretical base will help to define the best way to integrate qualitative and quantitative methods in an appropriate design. There are also existing evaluation frameworks that may be useful.[2,36] At the same time, three specific perspectives have been suggested to connect theories with reality and strengthen the evaluation: population health approach; system approach; and complex problems and the chronic care model.

The following are some of the practical elements that need to be considered when designing and implementing evaluation of PCMH.

- *Budgeting the evaluation*: conducting the evaluation will require investment of valuable resources, including time and money. The amount of resources will be critical in defining the evaluation possibilities and design.

- *Defining the profile of the evaluator(s)*: it is important to define an evaluation team/leader with sufficient experience in the field, according to the evaluation needs, as well as to work with staff to integrate evaluation activities into day-to-day project management and delivery. It is also relevant for the PCMH team not to delegate all evaluation decision-making to the evaluator; they should stay involved and encourage teamwork. An important part of an evaluator's job (internal or external) is to assist in building the skills, knowledge, and abilities of PCMH and stakeholders. Capacity building in the area of PCMH evaluation is a critical need.

- *Participation of the community and stakeholders*: clearly research studies suggest that the usefulness of the final product of an evaluation is improved by the inclusion of relevant stakeholders in the process, as seen in applications of participatory evaluation approaches. However, despite the benefits of involving stakeholders, it is important to define the extent and type of stakeholder involvement in theory evaluation. It would be critical to have a consultation process with the specific PCMH. It is necessary to keep in mind that to be consistent with PCMH as a collaborative care model, an evaluation should include different perspectives: clients, families, community, other partner agencies and providers, among others. A particular emphasis should be given to the participation of clients in the evaluation process, when appropriate.[51]

- *Looking for the best balance of the evaluation design*: the consideration of the evaluation standards developed by the American Joint Committee on Standards for Educational Evaluation (AJCSEE) in 1994,[48] *utility, feasibility, propriety and accuracy*, is highly recommended, in order to ensure that an evaluation will reveal and convey technically adequate information about the features associated with the benefits of the programme being evaluated (PCMH). These standards should be at the discussion table from the beginning of the process, and be critical for the decision-making regarding each of the evaluation steps.

- *Knowledge exchange process*: it is especially important for any evaluation (thinking in terms of real impact) to define and accomplish concrete knowledge exchange outcomes using an appropriate dissemination strategy, considering knowledge synthesis, knowledge exchange (dissemination/adoption) and evaluation stages.

Finally, it is necessary to remark that more than thinking of evaluation as an isolated event, it is critical to actively work on developing *a healthy evaluation culture in PCMH*, at all levels. This culture of evaluation requires the following critical elements: goodwill, buy-in, collaboration, participation, interest among stakeholders, internal champion, use of the findings, management support, resource allocation, and training/capacity building. It is a responsibility of all the actors of PCMH to commit with the development of a healthy evaluation culture in PCMH and to foster its critical elements in order to facilitate a continuous process of quality improvement. That evaluation culture will benefit people in need – patients, families and communities – as well as health workers, who will be able to be protagonists of health-system transformation, where mental health and substance use issues are effectively addressed in primary health care, from mental health promotion and prevention, to early recognition, diagnosis, treatment, rehabilitation and social integration.

References

1   Institute of Medicine. *Health services research: work force and educational issues*. Washington DC, National Academy of Sciences, 1995.

2   Aday A et al. Equity: concepts and methods. In: Aday A et al., eds. *Evaluating the healthcare system: effectiveness, efficiency and equity*. Chicago, AHR, 2003:173–205.

3   Shadish WR Jr, Cook TD, Leviton LC. *Foundations of program evaluation. Theories and practice.* Newbury Park, CA, Sage, 1991.

4   Ustun B, Sartorius N. *Mental illness in general health care.* Chichester, John Wiley, 1995.

5   Malin R. *Substance abuse in office-based practice: an issue of primary care clinics in office practice.* Philadelphia, Saunders – Elsevier – Health Sciences Division, 2011.

6   World Health Organization and Wonca. *Integrating mental health into primary care. A global perspective.* Geneva, World Health Organization, 2008.

7   Gask L, Sibbald B, Creed F. Evaluating models of working at the interface between mental health services and primary care. *British Journal of Psychiatry*, 1997, 170:6–11.

8   Kennedy P, Griffiths H. Mental health 'collaborative' challenges care culture. *Psychiatric Bulletin*, 2003, 27:164–166.

9   Kates N, Gagne M-A, Melville Whyte J. Collaborative mental health care in Canada: Looking back and looking ahead. *Canadian Journal of Community Mental Health*, 2008, 27:1–4.

10   Carey TS et al. *Future research needs for the integration of mental health/substance abuse and primary care.* Future Research Needs Paper No. 3. (prepared by the RTI International University of North Carolina at Chapel Hill Evidence-based Practice Center under Contract No. 290-2007-10056-I) AHRQ Publication No. 10-EHC069-EF. Rockville, MD, Agency for Healthcare Research and Quality, 2010 (http://www.effectivehealthcare.ahrq.gov/ehc/products/234/534/Future03--Abuse-09-23-2010.pdf, accessed 9 November 2011).

11   Canadian Collaborative Mental Health Initiative (http://www.ccmhi.ca/en/who/framework.html, accessed 9 November 2011).

12   Gagné MA. *What is collaborative mental health care? An introduction to the collaborative mental health care framework.* Mississauga, ON, Canadian Collaborative Mental Health Initiative, 2005 (http://www.ccmhi.ca/en/products/documents/02-Framework-EN.pdf, accessed 22 November 2011).

13   Health Canada. Social capital and health: maximizing the benefits. *Health Policy Research Bulletin*, 2006, 12.

14   Health Canada. The population health template: key elements that define a population health approach. Ottawa, Health Canada Population and Public Health Branch, Strategic Policy Directorate, 2001 (http://www.phac-aspc.gc.ca/ph-sp/pdf/discussion-eng.pdf, accessed 9 November 2011).

15   Canadian Population Health Initiative (CPHI). *What is population health?* (http://www.cihi.ca/CIHI-ext-portal/internet/en/document/factors+influencing+health/environmental/cphi_pop_health, accessed 9 November 2011).

16   Commission on Social Determinants of Health. *Closing the gap in a generation: health equity through action on the social determinants of health.* Final report of the Commission on Social Determinants of Health. Geneva, World Health Organization, 2008.

17   Sapag JC et al. Social capital and self-rated health in urban low income neighbourhoods in Chile. *Journal of Epidemiology and Community Health*, 2008, 62:790–792.

18   Gladwell M. *The tipping point: how little things can make a big difference.* Boston, Little, Brown, 2000.

19   Trochim WM et al. Practical challenges of system thinking and modeling in Public Health. *American Journal of Public Health*, 2006, 96:538–546.

20   Munson M et al. Case managers speak out: responding to depression in community long-term care. *Psychiatric Services*, 2007, 58:1124–1127.

21   Wagner EH. Chronic disease management: what will it take to improve care for chronic illness? *Effective Clinical Practice*, 1998,1:2–4.

22   Bodenheimer T, Wagner EH, Grumbach K. Improving primary care for patients with chronic illness. *JAMA*, 2002, 288:1775–1779.

23   Bodenheimer T. Interventions to improve chronic illness care: evaluating their effectiveness. *Disease Management*, 2003, 6:63–71.

24   Kates N et al. The evolution of collaborative mental health care in Canada: a shared vision for the future. *The Canadian Journal of Psychiatry*, 2011, 56:1–10.

25   Cristofalo M et al. Unmet need for mental health and addictions care in urban community health clinics: frontline provider accounts. *Psychiatric Services*, 2009, 60:505–511.

26   Harteloh PPM. The meaning of quality in health care: a conceptual analysis. *Health Care Analysis*, 2003, 11:259–267.

27   Donabedian A. The quality of medical care. *Science*, 1978, 200:856–864.

28   Donabedian A. Quality of care: how it can be assessed? *JAMA*, 1988, 260:1743–1748.

29   *Crossing the quality chasm: a new health system for the 21st century*. Washington DC, Institute of Medicine, 2001.

30   Harrigan M. *Quest for quality in Canadian health care: continuous quality improvement*, 2nd ed. Ottawa, Health Canada, 2000 (http://www.hc-sc.gc.ca/hcs-sss/pubs/qual/2000-qual/index-eng.php, accessed 9 November 2011).

31   *Evaluation of psychoactive substance use disorder treatment: framework workbook*. Geneva, World Health Organization, 2000.

32   Smith M, Glass G. *Research and evaluation in education and the social sciences*. New Jersey, Prentice Hall, 1987.

33   Briones G. *Evaluación de programas sociales. Teoría y metodología de la investigación evaluativa*. [Evaluation of social programs. Theory and evaluation research methods.] Santiago, PIIE, 1985.

34   Scriven M. The methodology of evaluation. In: Tyler RW, Gagné RM, Scriven M, eds. *Perspectives of curriculum evaluation*. 39–83. Chicago, IL, Rand McNally, 1967:39–83.

35   Rush B. The evaluation of treatment services and systems for substance use disorders. *Revista de Psiquaitria de Rio Grande do Sul*, 2003, 25: 393–411.

36   Thornicroft G, Tansella M. *The mental health matrix. A manual to improve services*. Cambridge, Cambridge University Press, 1999.

37   Adair CE et al. Performance measurement in healthcare: Part I – Concepts and trends from a state of the science review. *Health Care Policy*, 2006, 4:85–104.

38   Nazdam D, Nelson M. The benefits of continuous performance measurement. *Nursing Clinics of North America*, 1997, 32:549–559.

39   Adair CE, Simpson E. Performance measurement in healthcare: Part II – State of the science findings by stage of the performance measurement process. *Health Care Policy*, 2006, 2:56–78.

40   Anderson RM. Revisiting the behavioral model and access to medical care: does it matter? *Journal of Health and Social Behaviour*, 1995, 36:1–10.

41   Centers for Disease Control. Framework for program evaluation in public health. *Morbidity and Mortality Weekly Report*, 1999, 48:RR-11.

42   Stufflebeam DL, Shinkfield AJ. *Evaluation theory, models, and applications*. San Francisco, Jossey-Bass, 2007.

43   Finn T. *A guide for monitoring and evaluating population-health-environment programs. USAID-measure evaluation*. Chapel Hill, USAID, 2007 (http://www.cpc.unc.edu/measure/publications/ms-07-25/?searchterm=None, accessed 22 November 2011).

44   Porteous NL, Sheldrick BJ, Stewart PJ. Enhancing managers' evaluation capacity: a case study from Ontario Public Health. *The Canadian Journal of Program Evaluation*, 1999, Special issue:137–154.

45   Punch K. *An introduction to social research: quantitative and qualitative approaches*. London, Sage Publications, 2005.

46   Liamputtong Rice P, Ezzy D. *Qualitative research methods: a health focus*. Oxford, Oxford University Press, 1999.

47   Creswell JW, Fetters MD, Ivankova NV. Designing a mixed methods study in primary care. *Annals of Family Medicine*, 2004, 2:7–12.

48   American Joint Committee on Standards for Educational Evaluation. *The program evaluation standards*, 2nd ed. Newbury Park, CA,Sage Publications, 1994.

49   House B. *Evaluating with validity*. Beverly Hills, CA, Sage, 1980.

50   Lincoln YS, Guba EG. *Naturalistic inquiry*. Beverly Hills, CA, Sage, 1985.

51   Cooper LA. At the center of the decision-making in mental health services and interventions research: patients, clinicians, or relationships? [commentary] *Clinical Psychology: Science and Practice*, 2006, 15:26–29.

Section C

Assessment and the principles of intervention in primary care mental health

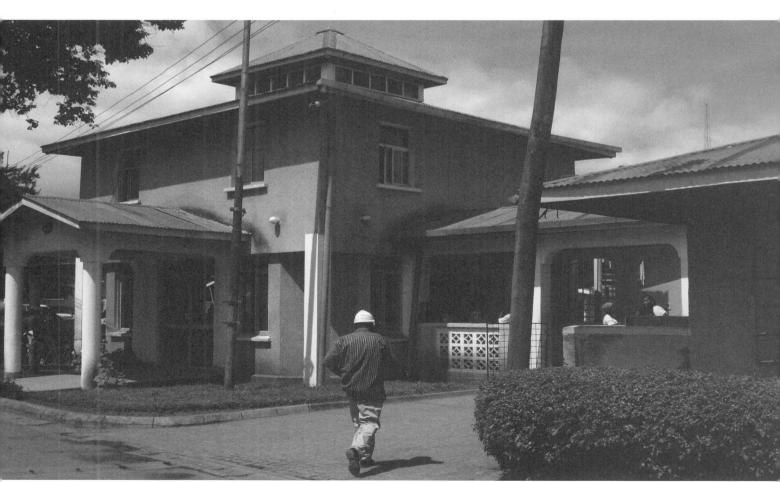

9 History-taking and investigations in primary care mental health

Christos Lionis, Filippo Zizzo, Henk Parmentier, Wolfgang Spiegel, Eleni Palazidou, Gustav Kamenski, Abdullah Al-Khathami and Stefania Rescalli

Key messages

- The mental health history aims to elicit more detail about the patient's illness from a broad perspective, focusing on a biopsychosocial approach. For mental health problems, data gathering simultaneously acts as a diagnostic and a therapeutic tool.

- A list of key symptoms that will assist the doctor's diagnosis of mental health disorders could be used in this stage of the medical history.

- Most of the mental health disorders are familial and it is essential to elicit enough information not only about first-degree relatives but about others too (grandparents, uncles, aunts etc.).

- Personal history is a "collage" of the patient's life, which provides the doctor with an invaluable insight into the person they are assessing and is essential to the final formulation of the patient's condition. An abnormal premorbid functioning may suggest a personality disorder, or a prelude to an illness such as schizophrenia.

- Screening in mental health care is aimed at detecting risk factors, symptoms, or early signs of mental health disorders in a primarily not conspicuous "healthy" population. Screening systems frequently consist of a patient questionnaire intended for screening and a multilevel system of questionnaire modules, which verify or falsify one or more suspected diagnoses.

Introduction

Care of the mentally ill is shifting towards the general practitioner (GP) or family doctor, particularly in high-income countries where there is often a clear separation between primary and secondary or specialist health services. Closure of the asylums, and long-stay hospitals, and the emphasis on community care has resulted in primary care practitioners having a vital role in the management of milder forms of mental disorders but also of severe mental illnesses such as schizophrenia. This is achieved in collaboration with the specialist services in high- and medium-income countries, as well as some lower-income countries, at least in urban areas. The World Health Organization (WHO) and World Organization of Family Doctors (Wonca) encourages a shift of care for the mentally ill worldwide, from specialist to primary care.[1]

In low-income countries, and particularly outside urban areas, all physicians, whether general or specialist, are expected to manage mentally ill patients as well as to cope with mental disorders that are comorbid with physical illnesses. It is essential to acquire the skills necessary for assessment of such patients, and this is recommended during undergraduate training. Medical schools need to review their undergraduate curriculum and place a higher emphasis on the teaching of psychiatry, as well as assessment of mental health when patients consult in primary care.[2]

GPs often say that the patients they see in primary care are different from those seen by the specialist services. This is true, as GPs see all patients who present with conditions from subthreshold, mild or moderate mental health disorder to the more severe mental illness. Of course the majority usually present with physical complaints or hidden problems, and thus are at the mild end of the spectrum and are unlikely ever to be referred to the specialist services.[1] Symptoms and complaints that denote the presence of a mental health disorder present differently in the primary care setting compared to the setting of specialized care. This is an additional reason for GPs to take more responsibility for managing mental illness; therefore they will need to acquire adequate skills to ensure effective treatment of such patients.

This chapter addresses issues of the primary care approach to mental health in general consultation, in relation to clinical medical history-taking and diagnosis.

The consultation

It is essential that the physician in primary care has appropriate consultation skills for history-taking of mentally ill patients, as well as a good diagnostic approach to mental disorders. A comfortable relaxed environment, possibly the presence of a close friend/relative, and a sympathetic, non-judgemental approach will increase the likelihood of a successful encounter. The points that follow should be considered.

Environment

The consultation essentially begins from the moment the patient steps into the physician's premises. The waiting room in the surgery of a primary care physician differs from that of a specialist, as almost all patients have an experience of a GP visit. A busy waiting room and long waiting time can be a problem for the depressed, anxious or paranoid patient. It is a great help if all the primary care staff, including non-clinical members of staff, acquire training regarding how to deal with mentally ill patients. The receptionist is the first contact with the patient and usually continues to observe the patients seated in the waiting area, but this is not the case in all primary care contexts. The receptionist can alert the doctor if a patient becomes agitated, wishes to leave, or behaves strangely (talking to themselves etc.). This may be invaluable information, contributing to the overall assessment. In contexts where such capacity is not available, the GP needs to take into account his/her patient waiting time as well as ensuring they receive regular reassurance that their time concerns and anxiety are receiving the proper attention.

Time allocated

In the primary care setting, the range of diagnostic possibilities with each patient walking through the door is enormous. Yet limited time is available for each consultation. If a patient presents with straightforward symptom(s) like a sore throat, and with no additional problems, it is possible to obtain the information, examine the throat or chest, make a diagnosis, arrange investigation if appropriate, and supply a prescription in 10 minutes. Yet this is not always enough for a patient with a mental illness, particularly on a first visit. Also, patients in primary care usually present with more than one reason for consultation, and even when a mental health problem is suspected by the GP it is not always possible to properly address it in the same consultation. This has been described as the "tyranny of the urgent".[3] Considering this "tyranny of the urgent" helps doctors to understand that one essential skill in primary care is to structure the consultation properly and, if necessary, settle with the patient on an "agenda for the consultation", without missing the important (e.g. a suspicion of presence of an affective disorder) over the urgent (e.g. abdominal pain). In such cases, a preliminary assessment can be followed by a follow-up appointment arranged soon, when enough time will be allocated to carry out a comprehensive assessment.

Getting settled

The interview should be performed in an open area where the visitor can feel comfortable. Patients should be reassured that their consultation will be private and confidential, and that no other health personnel will interrupt their communication. Effective communication is the bridge between the doctor and patient. Therefore, application of communication skills to build rapport, attentive listening and empathy is an essential component of the consultation in mental health care.[4]

Method

History-taking for mentally ill patients generally follows the same format as for any patient in primary care. However, the mental health history aims to elicit more detail about the patient's illness from a broad perspective, focusing on a biopsychosocial approach. Therefore, more attention is paid to the developmental, personal and social history; this can be achieved by focusing on the three elements listed next:[5]

- listening attentively to the patient's complaints – this means not only listening but also encouraging the patient to talk, using open-ended questions and trying to pick up subtle cues to discover the reason for their visit. You may understand the underlying or precipitating factor for the presenting problem, but there may be events that took place in the patient's childhood that are also contributing to mental distress; for example, if a patient starts to cry or is unable to continue talking, it is important to explore all aspects of their life and past events in a sympathetic way

- examination of the patient's appearance, expressions, behaviour, walking and sitting pattern – this could assist in creating discussion even if the problem presented is not related to mental health. At this point, the doctor can provide a direct question related to the observed patient characteristics, to explore any suspected problem

- testing or screening the patient in primary care by using direct or closed questions for common mental health problems such as depression, anxiety disorders, etc. If the patient screens positively for any mental health problem, then the doctor must ask for the major criteria, in order to reach a proper diagnosis.

Taking the history

The medical profession still has the public's confidence and patients readily reveal information to doctors that they may only otherwise confide in a priest/imam/other spiritual leader. The doctor has the responsibility not only to ensure patient confidentiality, but also to assure the patient of this.

History-taking is the key to correct assessment and subsequent management of an illness, whether physical or mental. For mental health problems, data gathering simultaneously acts as a diagnostic and therapeutic tool. Therefore, it is even more important to assess mental health disorders in an appropriate way, since the diagnostic work-up relies almost entirely on verbal interaction and data gathering from the patient. With the exception of organic disorders, there are no blood tests or imaging techniques to facilitate the diagnosis.

Patients with mental health problems who are seeking primary care often present with somatic complaints that are related to their underlying disorder; for example, for mood disorders, the most frequent complaints are fatigue, sleep disorders, dyspepsia, irritable bowel and chronic pain. This can lead to misdiagnoses and symptomatic management rather than dealing with the hidden problem that may also cause these symptoms. GPs must carefully explore the possibility of psychosocial problems or mental health disorder underlying the presented complaints, especially when the patient presents with chronic or atypical symptoms or physical diseases that are difficult to control, such as diabetes or hypertension.

The actual history-taking can be recorded under headings as follows. The interviewer may vary the order depending on how the consultation progresses and what seems more comfortable for the patient. However, after assessing the patient's presenting problem by asking open-ended questions, it is essential to explore the non-visible problem – for example, what ideas, concerns, and worries the patient has and the impact of the presented problem on the patient's life (sleep pattern, relationships, performance, etc.).

It is essential to note that collateral history is almost always necessary in the assessment of mental health disorders. It is also important to find out how the family is coping and what difficulties they are facing in relation to their family member's illness.

The patient's problem

Presenting complaints

Being able to establish rapport with the patient is crucial to the assessment. A sympathetic non-judgemental approach encourages the patient to open up. An example of a general opening question may be "Could you please tell me about what has been worrying or bothering you recently?" or "Could you tell me more about this?". Starting with open-ended questions to identify the general idea of the problem, one can then proceed with more targeted questions to explore further symptomatology and obtain the full picture. It is important to focus on the symptoms' existence, even in cases where they are not presented as the major complaints or not as leading to the consultation. A list of key symptoms that will assist the doctor's diagnosis of mental health disorders could be used in this stage of the medical history.

History of the presenting complaints

Once symptoms are elicited, then further exploration should be made regarding the duration, onset and timing of symptoms (whether they are present all the time or episodic) and how these symptoms affect the person's day-to-day functioning and quality of life. In some cases, this may be for several days', weeks' or months' duration, and in others symptoms may be of more chronic duration.

Explore the patient's ideas about the cause of the problem; concerns and worries the patient has; and the impact of the presented problem on the patient's life (sleep pattern, relationships, performance, etc.). This approach will help both the doctor and patient to identify the non-visible problem.[6] What does the patient expect his/her doctor to do?

Background information

Past mental health history

It is very important to ask about this, as this will lead to a proper diagnosis. This can be explored by knowing whether there were similar episodes in the past or indeed other presentations of mental health disorders. A previous manic episode will shift the diagnosis from that of unipolar to bipolar affective disorder in a patient currently presenting with depression. Patients are usually unable to provide this information to the doctor, and the electronic patient records system is not available in many primary care contexts. In these cases, the doctor could obtain some information if they look for past prescriptions or ask about medicines that the patient has taken in the past.

Past/current history of physical illness

The presence of physical illness in either the present or past may be highly relevant to the present mental health complaints. Neurological disorders (in early life or currently) such as epilepsy, Parkinson disease or others; endocrine disorders such as thyroid disease, Cushing syndrome or others; autoimmune disease, for example systemic lupus erythematosus; chronic conditions such as diabetes, cardiovascular disease, including ischaemic heart disease, chronic obstructive pulmonary disease and chronic pain, are only some examples of physical illnesses that it is important to consider asking about. They may be of aetiological importance, triggers and/or maintaining factors, influencing the choice of drug treatment or response to treatment of the mental health disorder.

Family history

Most mental health disorders are familial and it is essential to elicit enough information not only about first-degree relatives but about others too (grandparents, uncles, aunts etc.). Similar presentation within any family member helps to clarify the nature of the problem. Some behaviour, such as suicide, also tends to be familial, and such information is needed alongside other facts for a reliable suicidal risk assessment. GPs should seek this information with some caution, since patients with a low education level could misunderstand these questions, with an impact on the doctor–patient relationship.

Health beliefs

An experienced primary care physician will always keep in mind that the patient's beliefs concerning possible causes of his/her illness – irrespective of whether they are in line with modern medicine or not – are very important and will influence the course of the illness (those subjective aspects of the disease that matter for the patient). When mental health issues are concerned in all kinds of cross-cultural consultations, this is especially true. For a deeper understanding, please refer to the literature.[7,8]

Personal history

Personal history is a "collage" of the patient's life, which provides the doctor with an invaluable insight into the person they are assessing and is essential to the final formulation of the patient's condition. This background information should start from the perinatal period, include early development (physical/psychological/social) and be followed through childhood, adolescence and adulthood.

Early life stress has a major role in an individual's psychological status in adulthood, and the interplay between genes and early life experiences has been the focus of research activity in recent times, with recognition that this may have more importance in the later development of mental illness, particularly depression, than either factor alone.

It is also important to enquire about the patient's psychosexual development and experience. This leads to exploration of the sensitive question of possible child sexual abuse.

Early life and later ability to sustain relationships, educational achievements, work, etc. are the good indicators of a person's premorbid functioning. Malfunctioning from early life may suggest a neurodevelopmental type of illness, for example schizophrenia. On the other hand, a clear change from normal functioning gives an indication of the time of onset of the mental health disorder, even in the absence of the full picture; for example, a change in social functioning such as social withdrawal, impaired functioning at school/university or at work may be the beginning of a schizophrenic illness, with the psychotic signs emerging later in the course of the disorder.

Premorbid personality

This is very useful information in a variety of ways. An abnormal premorbid functioning may suggest a personality disorder, or a prelude to an illness such as schizophrenia.

The premorbid personality enables the doctor to assess the patient's vulnerability to illness. It also gives a target to work towards, aiming to get the patient well enough so that he/she can return to their premorbid level of functioning, which is what remission should really mean – not just improvement.

In order to get a good picture of the patient's premorbid personality, it is essential, whenever possible, to obtain information from a close relative/friend. The patient's recollection of their premorbid functioning may be skewed by their current mental state. For example, a depressed patient may believe he/she has always been low in mood and have a depressive recollection of their past functioning, while the opposite may apply to a patient in a manic state.

Substance misuse

In most parts of the world, mental illness is complicated by the presence of substance misuse, including alcohol,[9] illicit and non-illicit psychostimulants and other drugs. Such substances may be the cause or trigger of the presenting symptoms, and may be complicating the presenting illness by increasing the patient's morbidity and response to treatment. A detailed history of the duration of use, frequency and amount used, physical and psychological dependence, and craving needs to be explored and the possible physical and cognitive effects of excessive use need to be considered.

It should be remembered that prescribed medications such as codeine, benzodiazepines and others have the potential for misuse and cause dependence, particularly in people with anxiety disorders or chronic pain. It is also appropriate to record the smoking history and alcohol consumption in this part of the medical history. It is important to note that a holistic approach is one of the core competencies of the European definition of general practice/family medicine.[10]

Forensic history

If the doctor explores the previous convictions and behaviour causing police involvement, it is not uncommon to find that people with mental illness are over-represented in the prison population.

Current circumstances (social/other)

The current life status, i.e. living alone or with family, with or without children, working environment, housing, social supports and financial status needs to be assessed, as well as being taken into consideration when deciding a management plan. GPs should take some efforts to develop an understanding of the patient's family cycles and dynamics.

Current medication

Patients with mental illness often have physical illness as well, in particular diabetes, cardiovascular or gastrointestinal problems, amongst others. They are therefore likely to be receiving medication for these and it is essential to check for any adverse interactions. Some medication can directly affect the mood, e.g. a beta-blocker[11] or the oral contraceptive pill.[12] These medications should be stopped and other management options considered. Conversely, certain drugs affecting mood disorders can introduce adverse consequences on the cardiovascular or digestive system, resulting in deterioration of a patient's existing chronic illness.

Collateral history

For many cases of mental illness, more than any other condition, it is important to obtain collateral history; it may not be possible to obtain this from the patient, but it can usually be acquired from the partner, a close friend or family member. For example, a patient in a depressed state may not be able to recall happier times or periods of elation and such information is highly relevant to the diagnosis. This is an additional task that the GP should undertake when monitoring a patient with mental health disorder, and it is particularly important to ensure the patient's family is involved and well informed.

Exploration of the patient's problems

Mental health state assessment

While the history-taking elicits information from the patient, often known as the symptoms of illness, assessment of the mental state is a critical evaluation and examination of this information, which enables the doctor to elicit the presence or absence of signs of illness. The following headings are usually used in mental state assessment.

Mood/affect

Although on face value this appears straightforward, in practice it is generally poorly assessed. Firstly, it is important to separate the description of affect from mood. In a patient with schizophrenia, there may be a reduction in affective expression or flatness of affect, or inappropriate affect. In a depressed patient, the affect may present with low mood or sadness, and there may be irritability or anger.

Thought

Here one needs to examine the content of the patient's thoughts, i.e. what thoughts are preoccupying the patient, while examining the form of thought establishes the presence or absence of abnormalities in the processing of thought. In a patient with mania, for example, there may be flight of ideas with generally happy/grandiose ideas (thought content) that go through the patient's mind in rapid succession so that sometimes it is difficult to follow the flow of thought. Nevertheless, there is always a connection between these thoughts, however tenuous this may be (there may be rhyming, punning, or other connections). In a patient with schizophrenic thought disorder, the thought processing is actually disrupted, and sentences, sometimes even words, do not have a logical connection (word salad).

Other abnormalities of thought that are typical of schizophrenia include thought insertion/withdrawal.

Abnormal beliefs

Abnormal beliefs may be overvalued or delusional ideas, and these can be present in psychotic disorders, which include affective disorders where mood-congruent delusions are sometimes present.

Abnormal experiences

These refer to hallucinations, which can be of any modality. Most commonly in mental illness these are auditory, but visual, tactile, olfactory or gustatory hallucinations may be present. This can be explored by asking a patient "Have you ever had the sensation that you were 'unreal' or that the world had become unreal?" or "Have you ever had the experience of hearing noises or voices when there was no one about to explain it?".

Insight

It is important to assess whether the patient recognizes that he or she is ill, and whether they believe they require treatment. Insight may be intact, partial or completely lost. The less insight the patient has, the more difficult it is to engage in treatment.

It is not always possible to obtain all this information in the first assessment, and the skilled clinician should be able to focus on the key issues relevant to the diagnosis without missing important information that may affect the diagnosis and care plan. The details of the history may be completed at another consultation, which should be undertaken as soon as possible.

Diagnostic consultation

Screening as a diagnostic aid

Screening in mental health care is aimed at detecting risk factors, symptoms, or early signs of mental health disorders in a primarily not conspicuous "healthy" population. However, screening instruments are often used for diagnostic testing. When the patient presents with a history, symptoms or signs denoting the presence of any mental health disorder, the primary care physician is invited to choose a suitable diagnostic instrument to increase the probability of diagnosis at the practice level. There is an important debate on the appropriateness and effectiveness of the screening tools in the primary care setting, and certainly the decision to use a particular tool rests entirely upon the analysis made by the physician, who needs to consider the pretest probability of the supposed mental health disorder.

The utility of any screening measure and diagnostic test for general practice/family medicine, and the question as to whether GPs or any other primary care doctors should screen their patients for mental health disorders, depends not only on the sensitivity and specificity of the instrument and the pretest probability in the respective population, but also on the particular primary care framework conditions. It has, for example, been repeatedly demanded by specialists that patients over a certain age be screened for cognitive impairment, but the United States Preventive Services Task Force (USPSTF), taking into account utility and framework conditions, maintains that the evidence is insufficient to recommend for or against routine screening for dementia in older adults.[13]

Basic ethical and decision-making considerations

Ethical considerations concerning the use of screening measures have been considered by the historical work of Wilson and Junger, published by WHO in 1968.[14] They stressed that early detection and treatment of mental illness in a community should be treated as a high priority in general practices with a high prevalence of those disorders and an annual consultation rate of more than 4% of the total consultation rate for all causes. To achieve this goal, they developed 10 crucial principles which are still valid today. In their principles of detection of early disease, they define the main point, which always accompanies each screening measure – bringing treatment to those with previously undetected disease and avoiding harm to those who are not in need of treatment.

From a bioethical point of view, questions arise concerning the decision to screen or to apply diagnostic testing at an early stage of a disease if early detection and treatment of a clinical or subclinical condition affects its course and prognosis.

In their landmark article on the ethics of screening,[15] Shickle and Chadwick provided some helpful advice on how to avoid the violation of ethical and economic principles by giving special attention to the test's sensitivity and specificity. Tools with high sensitivity but low specificity introduce a high level of anxiety for the patient and his/her family and they are usually followed by unnecessary and costly investigations.

However, current evidence-based analysis and decision-making should consider all ethical, probabilistic and cost-relevant factors, including the preferences of the patient.

Quality standards for screening programmes

The United Kingdom National Screening Committee (UK-NSC) and the USPSTF recommended certain criteria for the rationale of screening.[16] These criteria focus on the kind of targeted population, the resulting diagnostic measures caused by the screening, the chance to detect the targeted condition, the harm caused by screening, the harm caused by the initiated diagnostics and treatment, the intermediate and final benefit, and the status of health with respect to the reduction of morbidity and mortality of the targeted disease. The evidence-based approach that takes into account the balance of benefit/harm is also presented in this publication.[16]

Examples of psychometric tests commonly used in primary care for the detection of mood disorders, anxiety and cognitive impairment

Screening instruments are often constructed in a multilevel fashion. They frequently consist of a patient-questionnaire intended for screening and a multilevel system of questionnaire-modules, which verify or falsify one or more suspected diagnoses. For the *Diagnostic and Statistical Manual of Mental Disorders* (DSM-IV), the *Structured Clinical Interview for DSM-IV – Clinical Trials Version* (SCID-CT) is used as a benchmarking for the evaluation of screening-instruments.[17]

In principle, two strategies have been proposed to increase the recognition rate of common mental health disorders in primary care: (1) the use of screening instruments and (2) extensive psychiatric training for GPs. Spiegel et al. have chosen a "middle-of-the-road" approach when developing their educational interventions to teach GPs by means of a time-saving psychiatric tool named TRIPS (Training for Interactive Psychiatric Screening), a shortened and adapted form of the Primary Care Evaluation of Mental Disorders (PRIME-MD).[18]

TRIPS aims to detect depressive disorders, anxiety disorders and alcohol problems. It covers 12 International Classification of Diseases (ICD-10) disorders and was evaluated as accepted by patients and appropriate for the family practice setting.[18]

Depression is a major cause of morbidity worldwide in general practice/family medicine.[19,20] It is characterized by "loss of interest or pleasure in normally enjoyable activities", also called "anhedonia",[21] by "decreased energy or increased fatiguability", often referred to as "fatigue", and by low mood accompanied by low self-esteem. Actual depressive symptoms can be recognized and quantified through tests such as PRIME-MD,[22] or the Patient Health Questionnaire (PHQ),[23] a self-administered questionnaire of the PRIME-MD; the latter explores mood disorders and panic on the first page, including information about events and psychosocial stressors. The psychometric characteristics of both PRIME-MD and the PHQ have been studied with great care and have proved to be excellent.

As lack of time is always a key issue in primary care and general practice/family medicine, Brodaty and co-workers evaluated suitable instruments for the detection of dementia and cognitive impairment in primary care.[24] The Mini-Cog,[25,26] the Memory Impairment Screen (MIS)[27] and the General Practitioner Assessment of Cognition (GPCOG)[28] are appropriate for the primary care setting and easy to use, with administration times of 5 minutes or less and low misclassification rates in comparison to the Mini-Mental State Examination (MMSE).

Formulation of a diagnosis and care plan

Once all the relevant information is obtained, the clinician should be able to put together a formulation that will include diagnosis, management and prognosis.

Diagnosis

The diagnosis should be made on the basis of the history, symptoms, signs and diagnostic tests elicited from the patient using the ICD-10 criteria. The doctor should not be influenced by speculative aetiological factors. This is a mistake that is often made, particularly in people presenting with depressive symptoms when a depressive disorder is mistaken for existential unhappiness because there are psychosocial reasons that are believed to explain their mood state.

A differential diagnosis needs to be considered unless the case is straightforward, and further information may be sought, investigations undertaken or a specialist opinion obtained.

Aetiological factors (determinants)

Often in mental health disorders, there is no known cause and usually a combination of aetiological factors is present. For example, in a depressed patient there may be genetic vulnerability (family history of depression) as well as recent major stressors. Currently, the term "determinants" has replaced that of "aetiological factors" and it serves better the probabilistic association of the different factors with the nosological outcome rather than the certainty of a causal relationship that the old term implied. There may be additional factors such as chronic physical illness, thyroid abnormalities or others. In a patient presenting with psychosis, there may be family history, substance misuse and life stressors. It is useful to work through a checklist, as this will not only guide further investigation to yield a comprehensive picture of the patient's physical and mental state, but will also help with drawing up an effective care plan.

All possible aetiological factors/determinants that trigger, or reasons contributing to, the illness status need to be addressed to optimize the patient's outcome. Treating a patient with any mental illness with medication, without addressing any physical problems, substance misuse or psychosocial issues, is not likely to achieve any sustained remission. In certain cases, medicines that the patient takes for a long time introduce symptoms that can imitate mental disorders.

Investigations

If not recently done, routine blood tests should be considered, particularly if medication is to be offered, and to exclude physical health problems. Other investigations such as X-rays, a brain scan or electroencephalogram, etc. may be considered, depending on the patient's presentation. The use of screening tools in assessing depression, anxiety and cognitive impairment has already been discussed and we repeat here that they can be used in the primary care setting, with caution and a careful interpretation in association with the patient's symptoms and signs.

Care plan

When deciding upon a care plan, one should consider not only medication but also psychological treatments such as family/marital therapy, cognitive-behavioural therapy, or others. The patient's ideas must be considered, as well as their concerns and expectations. The impact of any psychosocial problems should be included in the management plan as a priority. Dealing with or counselling these problems will help relieve the stresses and hence contribute to effective care. Therefore, the likelihood of a more favourable outcome will be enhanced.[29]

The care plan should include a risk assessment (risk to self or others), and if there is a risk, or if in doubt, a specialist opinion should be sought.

Arrangements need to be made for regular follow-up as required in each individual case until remission is achieved and the treatment discontinued. Unfortunately, not uncommonly, this follow-up is discontinued when the patient feels better and before they have returned to normal, either because the patient fails to attend or the doctor does not consider follow-up or treatment to be necessary any more. Partial remission inevitably leads to relapse or a chronic illness state, with the possibility of achieving remission in the future increasingly reduced.

Prognosis

An attempt should be made to assess the prognosis of the current episode as well as the long-term outcome of the condition, bearing in mind that most psychiatric conditions are chronic relapsing disorders. This will assist in planning follow-up in terms of frequency, duration and whether the specialist services need to be involved.

References

1   World Health Organization and Wonca. *Integrating mental health into primary care. A global perspective.* Geneva, World Health Organization, 2008.

2   Al-Khathami AD et al. Mental health training in primary care. Impact on physicians knowledge. *Neurosciences*, 2003, 8:184–187.

3   Bodenheimer T, Wagner EH, Grumbach K. Improving primary care for patients with chronic illness. *JAMA*, 2002, 288:1775–1779.

4   Silverman J, Kurtz S, Draper J. *Skills for communicating with patients*, 2nd ed. Oxford, Radcliffe Medical Press, 2005.

5   Ivbijaro G et al. Wonca's culturally sensitive depression guideline: cultural metaphors in depression. *European Journal of General Practice*, 2005, 11:46–47.

6   Ong L et al. Doctor–patient communication: a review of the literature. *Social Science and Medicine*, 1995, 40:903–918.

7   Carrillo JE, Green AR, Betancourt JR. Cross-cultural primary care: a patient-based approach. *Annals of Internal Medicine*, 1999, 130:829–834.

8   Pumariega AJ, Rothe E, Pumariega JB. Mental health of immigrants and refugees. *Community Mental Health Journal*, 2005, 41:581–597.

9   McIntosh C, Ritson B. Treating depression complicated by substance misuse. *Advances in Psychiatric Treatment*, 2001, 7:357–364.

10 *The European definition of general practice/family medicine.* Barcelona, Wonca Europe, 2005 (http://www.woncaeurope.org/Web%20documents/European%20Definition%20of%20family%20medicine/Definition%202nd%20ed%202005.pdf, accessed 16 November 2011).

11 Van Melle JP et al. Beta-blockers and depression after myocardial infarction: a multicenter prospective study. *Journal of the American College of Cardiology*, 2006, 48:2209–2214.

12 Kulkarni J, Liew J, Garland KA. Depression associated with combined oral contraceptives – a pilot study. *Australian Family Physician*, 2005, 34(11):990.

13 *Recommendations on screening for dementia.* Rockville MD, US Preventive Services Task Force (USPSTF), 2003 (http://www.uspreventiveservicestaskforce.org/uspstf/uspsdeme.htm, accessed 9 November 2011).

14 Wilson JMG, Junger G. *Principles and practice of screening for disease.* Geneva, World Health Organization, 1968.

15 Shickle D, Chadwick R. The ethics of screening: is 'screeningitis' an incurable disease? *Journal of Medical Ethics*, 1994, 20:12–18.

16 Community Preventive Services Task Force. *Guide to clinical preventive services 2010–2011* (http://www.thecommunityguide.org/about/guide.html, accessed 9 November 2011).

17 First MB et al. *Structured Clinical Interview for DSM-IV-TR Axis I Disorders, Clinical Trials Version (SCID-CT).* New York, Biometrics Research, New York State Psychiatric Institute, 2007 (http://www.scid4.org, accessed 9 November 2011).

18 Spiegel W et al. Learning by doing: a novel approach to improving general practitioners´ diagnostic skills for common mental disorders. *Wiener Klinische Wochenschrift*, 2007, 119:117–123.

19 Mitchell AJ, Vaze A, Rao S. Clinical diagnosis of depression in primary care: a meta-analysis. *The Lancet*, 2009, 374:609–619.

20 Mulrow CD et al. Case-finding instruments for depression in primary care settings. *Annals of Internal Medicine*, 1995, 122:913–921.

21 Sibitz I et al. ICD-10 or DSM-IV? Anhedonia, fatigue and depressed mood as screening symptoms for diagnosing a current depressive episode in physically ill patients in general hospital. *Journal of Affective Disorders*, 2010, 126:245–251.

22 Spitzer RL et al. Utility of a new procedure for diagnosing mental disorders in primary care: The PRIME-MD 1000 Study. *JAMA*, 1994, 272:1749.

23 Spitzer RL et al. Validation and utility of a self-report version of PRIME-MD. *JAMA*, 1999, 282:1737.

24 Brodaty et al. What is the best dementia screening instrument for general practitioners to use? *American Journal of Geriatric Psychiatry*, 2006, 14:391–400.

25 Borson S et al. The Mini-Cog: a cognitive "vital signs" measure for dementia screening in multi-lingual elderly. *International Journal of Geriatric Psychiatry*, 2000, 15:1021–1027.

26 Kamenski G et al. Detection of dementia in primary care: comparison of the original and a modified Mini-Cog with the Mini-Mental State Examination. *Mental Health in Family Medicine*, 2009, 6:209–217.

27 Buschke H et al. Screening for dementia with the Memory Impairment Screen. *Neurology*, 1999, 52:231.

28 Brodaty H et al. The GPCOG: a new screening test for dementia designed for general practice. *Journal of the American Geriatrics Society*, 2002, 50:530–534.

29 Stewart MA. Effective physician-patient communication and health outcomes: a review. *Canadian Medical Association Journal*, 1995, 152:1423–1433.

10 Mental health classification in primary care

Michael Klinkman, Christopher Dowrick and Sandra Fortes

Key messages

- We need a system of classification to help us make sense of the variety of mental health problems found in primary care.

- Mental health classification systems in primary care cannot simply be drawn from those used in psychiatry. The ways in which problems are presented and understood by patients, and the options available for management, are often very different from those found in specialist settings.

- In addition to accurately defining the diseases that may or may not be present, we need tools for classification that address problems and illnesses experienced by those seeking care, the clinical and social context in which those problems occur, and patients' personal preferences, goals and priorities for care.

- A valid primary care mental health classification must capture the dynamic interaction between these factors as it unfolds over time.

Introduction

Since 1980 we have seen the introduction of several classifications of mental health disorders intended for use in primary health care. This list began with the *Diagnostic and Statistical Manual of Mental Disorders* (DSM)-III and has continued through DSM-IV and DSM-IV-PC (Primary Care), the 10th edition of the International Classification of Diseases for Primary Health Care (ICD-10-PHC), and the International Classification of Primary Care (ICPC-2). Development of the "next generation" of primary care mental health classifications is now under way, with work on ICD-11-PC, DSM-V and ICPC-3. Despite considerable efforts at harmonization, there are significant differences in how each of these tools covers the clinical domain of mental health problems.[1]

These differences reveal our lack of understanding about the process of emotional suffering and its relationship to the development of mental disorders, and reflect a fundamental difference between primary care and specialty mental health professionals in the perceived importance of social and cultural factors in understanding and formally diagnosing mental disorders. We seem to be able to agree on a set of criteria to diagnose hypertension, or diabetes, and these biomedical classification standards have been relatively stable over time. But we cannot agree on a stable set of criteria for "depressive disorder": the DSM, ICD, and ICPC definitions will each capture a different group of patients suffering from depressive symptoms,[1,2] and we cannot even agree whether anxiety and depression represents one disorder or two![3,4] What is the problem here? Why have our definitions changed so much in recent years, and why do such differences persist between our major classification tools?

Why do we need mental health classification at all?

The short answer is that *classification is necessary to order a clinical domain*. The ordering principle(s) used to create a classification depend on the boundaries of that domain, as well as the planned uses of the classification. For us, the clinical domain is *primary health care*, so the classification needs to include the full range of mental health problems experienced by persons who seek care in this setting. There are several potential uses for an international classification that covers the domain of mental health problems.

- We need an international classification for *mental disorders*, so that professionals from different parts of the world can communicate between themselves and know exactly what disease they are discussing, or what type of pathology a patient is suffering from. This uniformity is especially important when treatment, including the development of new therapeutic strategies, is involved. For disorders for which treatment guidelines are created, the definition of the disorder needs to be precise and reproducible.
- A classification of mental disorders is also necessary in order to conduct research. If we want to conduct international research into the prevalence of specific disorders or conditions, we must start with a common view about how those conditions are defined.
- A classification of mental disorders is important to the efficient organization of health systems. Payment for consultations and other type of interventions needs to be based on the type of problems addressed, so that treatment (and its payment) can be effectively managed for a defined population.
- We also need an international classification of *mental health problems* that do not qualify as mental disorders (or diseases), so that professionals can communicate clearly between themselves and know exactly what types of problems are being managed, for both clinical and research purposes. This is of particular importance to the domain of primary health care, as problems such as "feeling anxious" or "feeling depressed" are not the same as a "subthreshold" or "minor" mood disorder, and may have different clinical pathways over time.[5,6]

Problems with classification

The last point above points out one of the major difficulties in primary care classification: the issues or problems that lead patients to seek medical consultation involve much more than diseases. Examples include routine check-ups and physical examinations, feeling distressed or overwhelmed with personal problems, experiencing somatic symptoms for which there is no clear medical diagnosis, and a long list of interventions for disease prevention and health promotion. It is very important that systems designed to be used in primary care to classify existing diseases also provide a way to classify issues or problems that bring people in to consult with health professionals in the absence of a specific disease. Both ICD-10 and ICPC include non-disease codes: ICD-10 has a list of social problem and preventive care codes, and ICPC offers a comprehensive list of symptoms, preventive care, and social problem codes.

Even where there is full domain coverage (diseases, problems, other issues), classification systems share several general problems.

Defining disease

The first problem is simply defining a "disease". In simplest terms, a disease is what somebody has when they get sick. That may well be true in many cases, but it leaves a lot of room for error at the margins.

Category or continuum

The conventional approach to defining diseases assumes that you either have or do not have a condition. This works reasonably well for infectious diseases such as tuberculosis, or for acute medical problems such as myocardial infarctions. It does not work very well for most mental health problems, as these are based on common sensations and perceptions that most of us experience from time to time.

It is apparent that the various symptoms that make up the diagnostic categories of mental disorders are distributed widely and variously across the population. We all feel anxious, or low in mood from time to time, and many of us have occasional thoughts about suicide, or wonder if other people are behaving suspiciously towards us. It is also demonstrable that our experience of these symptoms can change quickly, sometimes within a matter of hours or days. Any cut-off in the level or duration of symptoms which is taken to represent a "true" diagnosis is therefore bound to be arbitrary.

So, at what point do a particular group of symptoms emerge as a clinical, pathological or psychiatric disorder? As Rose and Barker succinctly express it: "the real question [. . .] is not 'Has he got it?' but 'How much of it has he got?'".[7] Classification must here involve an arbitrary element, in finding an agreed-upon point along a continuum to label as a disorder. For example, in the classification system adopted in DSM-IV, at least two from a set of nine symptoms have to be present for at least 2 weeks to qualify for a diagnosis of minor depression, and at least five from the same set for 2 weeks to qualify as major depression. But the rationale used to make these arbitrary decisions on symptom counts and duration is not clear. Why not three symptoms for minor depression, or six for major depression? Why 2 weeks' duration? Why not 10 days, or 3 weeks?

Rose and Barker describe four possible solutions to this problem. Firstly, a decision to award clinical status to a condition or set of symptoms may be made on statistical grounds, for instance if they are more than two standard deviations from the age-specific mean of a particular population. Second, clinical status may be granted when a set of symptoms or complications becomes more frequent. Third, a "prognostic" or functional approach awards clinical status when a particular level or amount of something is more likely to cause problems than having a different level or amount of that something. Fourth, an "operational" or utility-based approach awards clinical status to levels of symptoms above which action will improve either symptoms or prognosis. The developers of DSM, ICD and ICPC have used a combination of these methods to define mental health disorders. However, only ICPC has used statistical evidence from the primary care setting in setting its definitions.

Alternative versus biomedical models

Another way to approach definitions for diseases or disorders is to consider different theoretical models for understanding health and disease processes. The biomedical model has dominated scientific research and mainstream medical care for many years, while the alternative medicine model (acupuncture, homeopathy, others) appeals to many who see the shortcomings of biomedicine.

The biomedical model considers that pathophysiological changes are the basis on which to consider and characterize the presence of a pathological process. These changes can be seen directly, or inferred on the basis of a medical history, biomedical imaging or laboratory testing. From this point of view, diseases represent something going wrong within our body that we need to find and fix.[8] The alternative medical model holds that getting sick is just a problem of one's own imbalance; symptoms and diseases simply demonstrate that the internal equilibrium was lost. The problem is not just that there is a part of the body that needs repair, but rather that the whole person is not well and should be given assistance in recovering their health (equilibrium).[9]

All three mental health classifications (DSM, ICD, ICPC) are based upon the biomedical model, listing specific disorders associated with specific changes in pathophysiology. Some effort has been made to map biomedical mental health disorders to traditional or alternative medicine disorders, but this work is in its early stages.

The problem of validity

Disease categories should only be regarded as valid if they can be shown to be discrete entities with natural boundaries that separate them from other disorders.[10] These boundaries may be based on observable differences in symptom clusters, or on specific neurobiological pathways or genetic patterns.

Despite historical and research assumptions to the contrary, there is little evidence to support the contention that currently recognized mental disorders are separated by natural boundaries. Variation in symptoms is continuous between the different mental disorders, and between mental disorders and normality.[11]

Taking depression as a prominent example, a careful examination of its apparent diagnostic boundaries reveals a high degree of uncertainty, disagreement and confusion.[12] This is most apparent in attempts to distinguish between depression and anxiety disorders. There is a view gaining ground within psychiatric circles that anxiety and depression should be regarded as two symptomatic presentations of a common broader underlying vulnerability, or of a common affective disorder, within which the expression of anxiety or depressive symptoms may vary over time.[13] This is supported by the high prevalence of depressive symptoms in patients with anxiety and vice versa,[14] and the strong correlation between anxiety and depression when measured by research rating scales.

There is also considerable overlap of symptoms between common mental and physical disorders. For example, in chronic obstructive pulmonary disease (COPD), somatic symptoms such as fatigue, anorexia and weight loss may be simultaneously attributable to both the medical condition of COPD and the psychiatric diagnosis of depression. This raises substantial risks of diagnostic confusion, particularly in primary care where mental and physical problems frequently coexist.

Even more uncertain are the boundaries between anxiety, depression and somatization in primary care. There is now a considerable amount of empirical evidence suggesting that persistent medically unexplained symptoms frequently coexist with mood or anxiety disorders. This coexistence may be cross-sectional in that all these symptoms appear together at the same time,[15] or it may be longitudinal in that one set of symptoms is followed closely in time by another.[16]

Nor has the quest for neurobiological markers of specific mental disorders had great success. Although some studies have indicated a link between the serotonin transporter (*5HTT*) gene and depression in the context of adverse life events, these findings have to be interpreted with caution. Positive linkage of effects tends to be over-reported in small samples, and the combined analyses of multiple datasets, including a larger number of candidate genes and polymorphisms, will be necessary for an adequate assessment of the presence and impact of depression susceptibility genes (see Chapter 2).[17]

There is already evidence that genetic variations are related to generic rather than specific vulnerability. Associations have been found, for example, between short variations of the *5HTT* gene and predisposition to alcohol disorders,[18] and perhaps schizophrenia.[19] These findings indicate an overlap in genetic susceptibility across the traditional classification systems for mental disorders.

The problem of utility

Mental health disorders may be "valid" but not useful in clinical practice. Conversely, even "invalid" diagnoses may possess high utility by virtue of the information they convey about aetiology, outcome or treatment response.[2]

However, the argument that a diagnosis is useful on the grounds that it offers a rationale for providing or withholding treatment is increasingly open to question. As one example, growing evidence for a substantial placebo effect in treating major depressive disorder suggests that the rationale for active treatment with antidepressant medication is not as strong as previously believed.

In a review of 75 double-blind placebo-controlled trials of antidepressant medication for adults in ambulatory care, Walsh and colleagues found the placebo response to be "variable, substantial and growing".[20] Kirsch and colleagues have analysed antidepressant medication data submitted to the US Food and Drug Administration. Using the Hamilton Depression Rating Scale as their benchmark, they found that the mean overall difference between responses to antidepressant drugs and placebo in this database was two points: although this difference was statistically significant, it is well below accepted levels of clinical importance.[21] They subsequently found that drug–placebo differences increase in relation to initial severity, with conventional criteria for clinical importance reached only for patients at the upper end of the "very severely depressed" category.[22]

The evidence for efficacy of psychological interventions such as cognitive-behavioural therapy is open to equal or even stronger challenge, on the grounds that their precise modes of action have not been adequately tested. Contextual factors, such as the impact of hope generated by an apparently scientific approach to treatment, the effects of therapist personality, or the benefits of time spent with a sympathetic professional, may be equally as important as, if not more important than, the specific formal components of a given therapeutic approach.[23]

Disease versus illness

Another major problem in classifying mental disorders lies at the intersection of patient and caregiver. Kleinman,[24] Helman,[25] and other medical anthropologists have shown that there are often substantial differences between what professionals, especially doctors, consider as disease and what patients mean by the same word. They have denominated these two distinct ways of understanding and representing the process of being sick as "disease" and "illness":

- *disease*: the biomedical conception on which professionals' understanding is based – scientifically based, measurable, involving an individual pathology that can be classified
- *illness*: the patients' perception of their suffering, which is subjective, culturally based and collective.

There is often a large gap between how patients understand and express their suffering and what professionals "count" as symptoms associated with a disease. Patients may in practice be operating from a radically different image of what constitutes a medical problem. They may not consider their problems as being related to their mental health, or, even if they do, may not believe that they are worthy of medical attention.[26] In South Wales, for example, patients do not see problems relating to mood and social function as proper reasons to seek medical care: while it is reasonable to take signs and symptoms of a physical disorder to a doctor, they do not consider that this is the case for emotional distress.[27] From the professionals' perspective, trying to bridge the gap between patient symptoms experienced during an illness and a specific disease that they can treat can lead to significant errors, and "overtreatment" or "undertreatment".[28]

The central role of the patient in the therapeutic process has been determined quite recently, being the basis of new theoretical models underlying health interventions.[29] The movement from a disease-centred to a patient-centred approach is a recent advance for organized medicine, and corresponds to the increasing prevalence of chronic health conditions with a course and prognosis that is dependent on long-term management rather than curative treatment. For example, human immunodeficiency virus (HIV) infection has changed from a lethal disease in the 1980s to a chronic disorder in the 21st century. Successful management of chronic health conditions requires that the patient and provider reach mutual decisions about treatments that will continue over a long period of time, and those decisions must take into account personal factors such as illness beliefs, personal goals and preferences, behavioural activation and patient adherence. Unfortunately, our classification systems do not reach far enough into the "patient side" to capture these factors,

The discrepancy between illness and disease is also affected by cultural patterns and the social context in which illness occurs.

Cultural patterns

Cultural patterns may affect the expression or presentation of recognized mental health disorders, leading to confusion about their proper place in a classification. For example, neurasthenia and chronic fatigue syndrome appear at first glance to be distinct disorders, but a closer look reveals that they may represent the same pathological process, expressed in different ways in different cultures. The entire group of culturally bound syndromes present in DSM-IV can be questioned for the same reason. The term "nerves" has been shown to be just a different way of naming and communicating a type of emotional distress that involves anxious and depressive reactions.[30] Medically unexplained symptoms, can be considered a cultural way of presenting emotional distress, but can also be a core symptom of a somatoform disorder. The boundary between symptoms and distress on the one hand, and psychiatric disorder on the other, is one of the most debatable items in ICD-10 and DSM-IV.

More generally, cultural differences in perceptions of what a mental disorder might be can cause tremendous conflict between doctors and patients. For recent migrants or asylum seekers, distress may be deeply embedded within, and inseparable from, lives fraught with frightening premigration experiences, traumatic escape and profound dislocation and alienation in their new "home". If a health professional tries to apply a rigid biomedical disease-based approach to depression in this situation involving a profoundly communal and structural account of emotional distress, problems are likely to occur.[31]

Context

It is now well accepted that mental health problems arise out of a context that includes predisposing factors, social problems, life events and other circumstances. It is fair to say that context is involved in the causality, evolution and prognosis of mental health disorders. In primary health care, this context also includes the frequent presence of physical health problems and social difficulties. Patients very often see social problems as a major component of their reason for consulting their doctors, and find it impossible to disentangle them from how they are feeling. In everyday clinical practice, simply making a formal diagnosis of a mental health disorder is not sufficient to guide treatment decisions. We must know more. We need to know how severe the symptoms of the disease may be, how long it has lasted, and what levels of disability are associated with it.[32] We also need to know whether other social or medical problems are affecting the person we are trying to help.

Unfortunately, neither culture nor context has been routinely incorporated into any of our mental health classification tools. These aspects will be discussed in more detail later in this chapter.

Classification problems specific to primary care

As mentioned above, mental health disorders are often defined by an arbitrary cut-off point along a continuum of symptoms. For most disorders, the range of relevant symptoms and their cut-off points have been defined based on patients seen by mental health specialists in the United States of America (USA) and similar western settings. While there is some evidence that core symptoms of depressive disorder may be equivalent in western and non-western settings,[33] the "gold standard" for diagnosis generally does not accommodate the range of symptoms and severity experienced by persons in non-western settings, and it may not accurately reflect the range or severity of symptoms experienced by persons seen in western primary care settings.

Persons who present to primary care clinicians may be closer to "normal" than those presenting to specialists, and finding the correct cut-off point to differentiate normality from pathology can be quite difficult. For example, the set of nine cardinal symptoms for depressive disorder includes fatigue and sleep difficulties. These symptoms are predictive of depression in patients seen by mental health specialists, but they have a significantly lower predictive value in primary care – because the prevalence of severe depression is proportionately lower, and because fatigue and sleep concerns are prominent symptoms of patients with other health problems. So, even when DSM-IV or ICD-10 diagnostic criteria are correctly applied in primary care, some patients who "qualify" for the label of major depression will have a less severe disorder, or no disorder at all.

It is still more difficult to determine "gold standards" for problems with behaviour and emotions, where norms may differ across different cultures. How can the limit between normal sadness and the development of a depressive episode be defined for a mother who has lost a child? What is the normal level of anxiety expected for somebody who has lost a job and has no money to feed his family? Once again we go back to context, but when primary care is considered, these are urgent, everyday questions. The twin risks of medicalizing normality, or of normalizing illness processes, are always present.

Making sense of mental health suffering in primary care therefore demands special classification systems. It involves careful thought about the ways in which patients may experience and present their emotional distress, and how their physical and "medical" symptoms may be mixed up with psychological symptoms. It also involves paying attention not only to the presence and severity of a core list of symptoms, but also to their chronicity, associated impairment, and the personal, social, and cultural context in which those symptoms occur. Most importantly, it involves paying careful attention to the meanings that patients themselves may attach to their symptoms.

Towards a new classification for primary care

With these issues in mind, we can see the need to redesign classification and terminology tools to more accurately capture the content areas needed to understand mental health conditions as seen in the primary care setting. These tools must address *problems and illnesses* experienced by those seeking care, the *clinical and social context* in which those problems occur, and patients' *personal preferences, goals and priorities* for care, in addition to accurately defining the *diseases* that may or may not be present. We will discuss each of these areas in turn.

Diseases

We have described the limitations of disease-based classifications developed for specialty mental health care such as DSM-IV and Chapter V of ICD-10. While they provide a high level of diagnostic specificity, the criteria sets used for diagnosis are often of suspect validity in the primary care setting. Two "primary care" diagnostic classifications, ICD-10-PC and ICPC-2, are increasingly used in primary care settings, but each has its limitations. ICD-10-PC was derived from the "parent" ICD-10 and shares some of its validity issues, and ICPC-2 contains a limited number of relatively non-specific diagnostic terms. The conceptual overlap between ICD-10, DSM-IV and ICPC-2 is complex and incomplete, and mapping between these classifications has proven difficult.[1] None of the classifications in current use addresses diagnostic thresholds for disease "caseness" or boundaries between disease categories in a satisfactory way for primary care, although ICPC provides a symptom-level alternative (for example, P03 – "feeling depressed") to assigning a "minor" or "subthreshold" case the label of "depressive disorder".[34]

Work is currently under way to develop the next generation of primary care disease classifications, ICD-11-PC and ICPC-3. These parallel efforts are being coordinated so that core diagnostic content is more closely aligned, to improve clinical validity and utility, and to improve their mapping to the more granular specialty-based classifications. These revised classifications should provide improved coverage of this core content area.

Problems and "illnesses"

Patients in primary care present with problems (or illnesses) until such time as their problems are given a disease label. In many cases, a formal diagnosis of disease is never made – a common situation in primary health care, but one that cannot be accommodated in disease-based classifications! We know that illness behaviour is not always associated with disease; therefore, it is absolutely essential that a primary care mental health classification be able to reliably capture and track problems that have only a "symptom" label, or problems that are not related to the presence of a specific disease.

This capability is a core feature of ICPC-2, which includes a set of rubrics describing common emotional symptoms (such as "feeling anxious", "acute stress") that can be used to capture the patient's reason for encounter or as the "diagnosis" at the end of the encounter. ICD-10 contains some symptom-level "diagnosis" codes scattered across chapters, but these codes provide incomplete coverage and are infrequently used. The multi-axial nature of the full DSM-IV diagnostic classification encompasses a variety of biopsychosocial parameters, but the psychosocial content is only a modifier for a formal "disease" diagnosis.

Clinical and social context

Our current classification tools have limited capacity to capture clinical and social problems, events or circumstances that can influence or cause mental health problems. Chapter XXI of ICD-10 contains some social problem codes, but these are incomplete and rarely used. Chapter Z of ICPC-2 includes a number of common social and personal problems that may be a reason for either encounter or a diagnosis, but use of these rubrics has also been limited. We have not developed classification or terminology tools to capture personal demographics, cultural beliefs, or other social determinants of mental health or care-seeking behaviour.

Much work is needed to fill in the gaps in this content area. While ICPC-2 offers the best current coverage of symptoms and problems, further work to develop content such as a "cultural beliefs" classification or terminology is needed.

Personal preferences, goals, and priorities

In the setting of multimorbidity and increasing prevalence of chronic health problems, the delivery of person-centred health care requires that clinicians understand and respect the goals, priorities and preferences of their patients. For patients with mental health problems, it would be important to know whether patients prefer, or reject, pharmacological treatment for depression – or whether they rank management of their mental health symptoms or problems as a higher, or lower, priority than their other health problems. If known, these preferences would clearly affect treatment and enhance clinician–patient relationships.

We have not developed a system to reliably capture and use patient preferences and goals in primary care; this area remains a high priority for future research.

Putting it all together: classification and terminology tools in a primary care data model

We know that primary care patients frequently present for care with a mixture of psychological, physical and social problems. When we view primary care through a "disease" lens, we first look at the primary "disease", then see other problems that we artificially label as "comorbid" and of secondary importance. But mental health and general medical comorbidities, along with social problems, are the rule rather than the exception in persons coming to see primary care clinicians, and they are certainly not of secondary importance in the process of care. Our understanding of primary care might be enhanced by replacing the term "comorbidity" with "multimorbidity" and focusing effort on the integration of diagnosis and treatment across biomedical, mental health and social domains,[35–37] in a three-dimensional biopsychosocial space. In this space, the severity or level of problems in each domain at a single point in time could, in theory, be plotted as a point on an axis (see Figure 10.1), as a rough estimate of the overall burden of illness. Over time, the position of the point on each axis will change.

As the biopsychosocial model would predict,[38] these three domains are highly correlated. Mental health problems are known to occur more frequently in those with common chronic physical illness, such as diabetes, arthritis and heart disease;[39–43] general medical conditions affect how persons experience and cope with their mental health problems,[44–46] and the presence of social problems or the occurrence of significant life events has a major impact on the severity of mental health problems or outcomes of care for chronic physical illness.[47,48] Over time, changes in the severity of general health problems may create additional social problems or intensify existing mental health problems, and increasing severity of mental health problems may amplify physical symptoms. Understanding and managing these interactions is a core part of the everyday work of a primary care physician.

A valid primary care mental health classification must capture this dynamic interaction as it unfolds over time. Viewed through this integrated lens, and coupled with knowledge of patients' preferences and goals, we will be better able to understand the effectiveness of mental health care provided in the primary care setting. A group of primary care leaders in the USA has produced a first draft of a data model to support the "patient-centred medical home".[49] The model, shown in Table 10.1 includes each of the content areas discussed above, within its seven core components.

- *Patient background*: demographic, social, and geographic information, not currently captured in a standard format.
- *Active problems*: health problems currently known to and being addressed by the health-care team. In a model that adheres to the episode structure, each active problem has a "history" tracing its path from initial reason for encounter (first point of contact with the health system) to current status. This

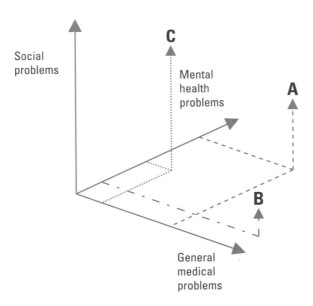

Figure 10.1 The three-dimensional matrix of primary care diagnosis

Point A characterizes a person with a moderate level of general medical problems, a high level of mental health problems, and a fairly low level of social problems.

Point B characterizes a person with a "classic" biomedical illness: a high level of general medical problems, a low level of mental health problems, and a minimal level of social problems.

Point C characterizes a person with a low level of general medical problems, a moderate level of mental health problems, and a very high level of social problems.

feature enables the calculation of specific disease probabilities for presenting symptoms as well as the proportion of symptoms that resolve without formal diagnosis.

- *Clinical modifiers*: previously experienced clinical events or risk factors that are important to the care process but are not active clinical problems. Examples include significant medical events (hysterectomy, cerebrovascular accident) and known risk factors (genetic, biochemical or historical).

- *Patient goals, preferences and requests*: patients' expressed goals, priorities and preferences for care, limits to care (advance directives), and the reasons why patients choose to seek care.

- *Process data*: capturing the decisions made in the course of care; laboratory or ancillary services, referral decisions, procedures performed, pharmacy orders, exception or error reporting and follow-up plans.

- *Time (and the episode structure)*: organizing data longitudinally, for example, following the structure of the episode of care, enables clinical data to be placed in the context of time. Without this structure, clinical data lose much of their meaning and validity.

- *Information-exchange protocols (data interoperability)*: enables structured import and export of data between electronic health records to assist in coordination of care across settings.

Here is one patient example (from the practice of MK) to illustrate the importance of capturing and integrating information from all three domains.

Case-study

MM is a 54-year-old woman, a long-term patient with chronic medical problems including autoimmune pancreatitis, chronic abdominal pain, rheumatoid arthritis (RA), and osteoporosis related to long-term corticosteroid use to control RA. She has a long-term history of anxiety (with panic attacks) and depressive symptoms that wax and wane, sometimes meeting formal diagnostic criteria for a major depressive episode.

Her social history is complex and important to her current care. She grew up in a small town in the southern USA in a family with prevalent substance abuse, depression and suicide. She was married at the age of 18 years but her husband died suddenly a few years later; she remarried several years later, to a man who also struggled with substance abuse. She has a very strong work ethic and continued to work at physical labour tasks long after her RA became crippling, and now feels guilty that she cannot work at a paying job. She has at times been prescribed antidepressant medications, but is strongly opposed to their use because of her religious beliefs and prior experience of family members.

She recently presented to the emergency department with increased abdominal pain, and had a short inpatient hospital admission where her pain was managed with increased doses of narcotic analgesics. The hospital team did not identify the death of her second husband a few months earlier, and her increasing difficulties in sorting out his business affairs, as a primary contributor to distress and increased pain. Her pancreatitis was in fact in remission at the time of her admission. Over a series of encounters, we were able to identify and begin to manage her distress and anxiety as a first step in reducing her narcotic use, with the understanding that her primary short-term goal was simply to maintain function so that she could solve pressing business issues. Although she met formal criteria for major depressive episode when seen in follow-up, we considered this a "false-positive" diagnosis related to recent life events and distress, and she responded well to supportive goal-focused care.

When viewed through a medical lens and from the data available in our electronic health record, "appropriate" care was provided to MM during her hospital admission and "inappropriate" care was provided after, as we did not formally diagnose and aggressively treat a major depressive episode. Viewed through a biopsychosocial lens, *and from the perspective of the patient*, her hospital stay was unnecessary and created harm through additional use of narcotic analgesics, while her follow-up care met her expressed needs. In the absence of available data on clinical modifiers (concerns about business) and patient goals (maintain function, solve business problems and avoid medication), we cannot see – or assess – the proper treatment path for MM.

What tools do we have? What tools do we need to develop?

As seen in Table 10.1, much of the content in the primary care data model can be captured using currently available classification and terminology tools. For some content, several options are available (for example, diagnostic content in the Systematized Nomenclature of Medicine (SNOMED), ICD and ICPC). But in other areas, development is necessary. We do not yet know how to classify or record important *clinical modifiers* such as risk factors (genetic, biochemical or historical), and we have not made good use of existing classifications of social or personal determinants of health. We have not enabled patients to express and record their own goals or preferences for care. We have not captured process data related to mental health care, as much of it occurs outside the primary care practice, and data-exchange standards are not available.

Work is under way to close these gaps. The World Organization of Family Doctors (Wonca), World Health Organization (WHO) and International Health Terminology Standards Development Organisation (IHTSDO) are collaborating on the next generation of classification and terminology standards, and improving and harmonizing the classification of social problems is a high priority. The Wonca International Classification

Table 10.1 Content available for the primary care data model

Components	Available content
Person (background)	ICPC (limited); ICF (limited)
Demographics	
Social structure	
Functional status	
Problem(s)	ICPC; ICD, SNOMED- CT; ICF (limited)
Current/active	
Severity	
Clinical modifiers	ICPC (minimal); ICD (minimal)
Prevention	
Risk factors	
Significant events	
Goals and requests	ICPC (limited); ICNP (limited)
Patient goals	
Patient preferences	
Requests for care	
Process data	ICPC (process codes); national procedure codes; ICNP; ATC; ICHI (in development)
Decisions	
Interventions	
Plans	
Time	ICPC
Episode structure	
Data import/export	
Exchange protocols	

ATC = Anatomical Therapeutic Chemical classification; ICD = International Classification of Diseases; ICF = International Classification of Functioning, Disability and Health; ICHI = International Classification of Health Interventions; ICPC = International Classification of Primary Care; SNOMED-CT = Systematized Nomenclature of Medicine – Clinical Terms.

Committee has begun work on a classification of risk factors and clinical modifiers to supplement ICPC. Discussion on how to best capture patients' goals and preferences has emerged in the past couple of years. Once these tools are available, we will be able to capture mental health in its real-world context in primary care practice.

In the end, the core task of general medical practice is to meet the needs of people living in communities. We must find a way to bring the patient's own voice into our work.

References

1   Lamberts H et al. The classification of mental disorders in primary care: a guide through a difficult terrain. *Internaional Journal of Psychiatry in Medicine*, 1998, 28:159–176.

2   Lamberts H, Hofmans-Okkes IM. The classification of psychological and social problems in general practice: 1. ICPC in relation to ICD-10. *Huisarts En Wetenschap*, 1993, 36(Suppl.):5–20.

3   Brown TA, Chorpita BF, Barlow DH. Structural relationships among dimensions of the DSM-IV anxiety and mood disorders and dimensions of negative affect, positive affect, and autonomic arousal. *Journal of Abnormal Psychology*, 1998, 107:179–192.

4   Preskorn SH, Fast GA. Beyond signs and symptoms: the case against a mixed anxiety and depression category. *Journal of Clinical Psychiatry*, 1993, 54(Suppl.):24–32.

5   van Weel-Baumgarten E et al. Ten year follow-up of depression after diagnosis in general practice. *British Journal of General Practice*, 1998, 48:1643–1646.

6   van Weel-Baumgarten EM et al. Long-term follow-up of depression among patients in the community and in family practice settings. A systematic review. *Journal of Family Practice*, 2000, 49:1113–1120.

7   Rose G, Barker DJ. Epidemiology for the uninitiated. What is a case? Dichotomy or continuum. *BMJ*, 1978, 2:873–874.

8   Camargo KR. *Racionalidades médicas: a medicina ocidental contemporânea*. Rio de Janeiro, Universidade Estadual do Rio de Janeiro/Instituto de Medicina Social, 1993 (Série Estudos em Saúde Coletiva, n.65).

9   Camargo KR Jr. *Biomedicina, saber & ciência: uma abordagem critica*. São Paulo, Editora Hucitec, 2003.

10   Kendell R, Jablensky A. Distinguishing between the validity and utility of psychiatric diagnoses. *American Journal of Psychiatry*, 2003, 160:4–12.

11   Cole J, McGuffin P, Farmer AE. The classification of depression: are we still confused? *British Journal of Psychiatry*, 2008, 192:83–85.

12   Dowrick C. *Beyond depression*, 2nd ed. Oxford, Oxford University Press, 2009.

13   Shorter E, Tyrer P. Separation of anxiety and depressive disorders: blind alley in psychopharmacology and classification of disease. *BMJ* 2003, 327:158–160.

14   Baldwin DS et al. Can we distinguish anxiety from depression? *Psychopharmacology Bulletin*, 2002, 36s2:158–165.

15   Escobar J et al. Somatisation disorder in primary care. *British Journal of Psychiatry*, 1998, 173:262–266.

16   de Waal MW et al. Somatoform disorders in general practice: prevalence, functional impairment and comorbidity with anxiety and depressive disorders. *British Journal of Psychiatry*, 2004, 184:470–476.

17   Levinson DF. The genetics of depression: a review. *Biological Psychiatry*, 2006, 60:84–92.

18   Pinto E et al. The short allele of the serotonin transporter promoter polymorphism influences relapse in alcohol dependence. *Alcohol and Alcoholism*, 2008, 43:398–400.

19   Sáiz PA et al. Association study of serotonin 2A receptor (5-HT2A) and serotonin transporter (5-HTT) gene polymorphisms with schizophrenia. *Progress in Neuro-psychopharmacology and Biological Psychiatry*, 2007, 31:741–745.

20   Walsh BT et al. Placebo response in studies of major depression. *JAMA*, 2002, 287:1840–1847.

21   Kirsch I et al. The emperor's new drugs: an analysis of antidepressant medication data submitted to the US Food and Drug Administration. *Prevention and Treatment*, 2002, 5:Article 23.

22   Kirsch I et al. Initial severity and antidepressant benefits: a meta-analysis of data submitted to the Food and Drug Administration. *PLoS Medicine*, 2008, 5:e45.

23   Parker G. What is the place of psychological treatments in mood disorders? *International Journal of Neuropsychopharmacology*, 2007, 10:137–145.

24 Kleinman A. *Social origins of distress and disease*. New Haven, Yale University Press, 1986.

25 Helman CG. *Culture, health and illness*, 4th ed. London, Arnold, 2001.

26 Kovandžić M et al. Access to primary mental health care for hard-to-reach groups: from 'silent suffering' to 'making it work'. *Social Science and Medicine*, 2011, 72:763–767.

27 Prior L et al. Stigma revisited, disclosure of emotional problems in primary care consultations in Wales. *Social Science and Medicine* 2003, 56:2191–2200.

28 Klinkman MS. Competing demands in psychosocial care. A model for the identification and treatment of depressive disorders in primary care. *General Hospital Psychiatry*, 1997, 19:98–111.

29 Tinetti M, Fried T. The end of the disease era. *American Journal of Medicine*, 2004, 116:179–185.

30 Fonseca MLG et al. Distress and common mental disorders: a bibliographic review. *Revista de Atencao Primaria a Saúde*, 2008, 11:285–294.

31 Kokanovic R et al. Negotiations of distress between East Timorese and Vietnamese refugees and their family doctors in Melbourne. *Sociology of Health and Illness*, 2010, 32:511–527.

32 Gask L et al. Capturing complexity: the case for a new classification system for mental disorders in primary care. *European Psychiatry*, 2008, 23:469–476.

33 Simon GE et al. Understanding cross-national differences in depression prevalence. *Psychologocal Medicine*, 2002, 32:585–594.

34 Wonca International Classification Committee. *ICPC-2-R: The International Classification of Primary Care*, revised 2nd ed. Oxford, Oxford Medical Publications, 2005.

35 van den Akker M et al. Multimorbidity in general practice: prevalence, incidence, and determinants of co-occurring chronic and recurrent diseases. *Journal of Clinical Epidemiology*, 1998, 51:367–375.

36 Fortin M et al. Prevalence of multimorbidity among adults seen in family practice. *Annals of Family Medicine*, 2005, 3:223–228.

37 Batstra L, Bos EH, Neeleman J. Quantifying psychiatric comorbidity – lessons from chronic disease epidemiology. *Social Psychiatry and Psychiatric Epidemiology*, 2002, 37:105–111.

38 Engel G. From biomedical to biopsychosocial. Being scientific in the human domain. *Psychosomatics*, 1997, 38:521–528.

39 Ormel J et al. Mental disorders among persons with heart disease - results from World Mental Health surveys. *General Hospital Psychiatry*, 2007, 29:325–334.

40 Harter M et al. Increased 12-month prevalence rates of mental disorders in patients with chronic somatic diseases. *Psychotherapy and Psychosomatics*, 2007, 76:354–360.

41 He Y et al. Mental disorders among persons with arthritis: results from the World Mental Health Surveys. *Psychological Medicine*, 2008, 39:1639–1650.

42 Scott KM et al. Depression–anxiety relationships with chronic physical conditions: results from the World Mental Health Surveys. *Journal of Affective Disorders*, 2007, 103:113–120.

43 Scott KM et al. Mental disorders among adults with asthma: results from the World Mental Health Survey. *General Hospital Psychiatry*, 2007, 29:123–133.

44 Demyttenaere K et al. Comorbid painful physical symptoms and anxiety: Prevalence, work loss and help-seeking. *Journal of Affective Disorders*, 2008, 1909:264–272.

45 de Graaf R et al. Risk factors for 12-month comorbidity of mood, anxiety, and substance use disorders: findings from the Netherlands Mental Health Survey and Incidence Study. *American Journal of Psychiatry*, 2002, 159:620–629.

46 Gallo WT et al. Involuntary job loss as a risk factor for subsequent myocardial infarction and stroke: Findings from The Health and Retirement Survey. *American Journal of Industrial Medicine*, 2004, 45:408–416.

47 Rasul F et al. Psychological distress, physical illness, and risk of coronary heart disease. *Journal of Epidemiology and Community Health*, 2005, 59:140–145.

48 Rosengren A et al. Association of psychosocial risk factors with risk of acute myocardial infarction in 11 119 cases and 13 648 controls from 52 countries (the INTERHEART study): case-control study. *The Lancet*, 2004, 364:953–962.

49 Phillips RLM et al. *Harmonizing primary care clinical classification and data standards*. Washington DC, American Academy of Family Physicians, 2007.

11 Risk assessment and the management of suicidality in primary care mental health

Geraldine Strathdee, Priyabrata Ghosh, Sheila Gunn, Gabriel Ivbijaro and Lucja Kolkiewicz

Key messages

- Suicide is an act that is a tragedy and brings great sadness to families, carers and treating clinicians.
- Suicide-prevention strategies internationally have mainly focused on high-risk populations in specialist secondary mental health-care services and rates have reduced.
- However, four-fifths of those who commit suicide have consulted their general practitioner in the month before the suicide, and national and international strategies to support primary care are necessary.
- There are well-established methods to reduce suicide with the system of primary care at the level of the individual practitioner, the primary care team, and the practice organization.

Introduction

Suicide is defined as a death with an underlying cause of intentional self-harm or injury or poisoning of undetermined intent. Determination of the prevalence of suicide is complex. International rates of suicide vary and are dependent upon a number of factors, which include the reporting methods, the presence and comprehensiveness of official statistics and the cultural attitudes to death by suicide. Primary care teams play a central role in the assessment and management of suicidality because primary care is often the first port of call for people in distress.

This chapter is written in four sections. In the first section, the prevalence of suicide across the world is explored, and characteristics of the determinants of higher rates of suicide are identified. In the second section, the national policies and health-care system methods that effectively deliver suicide prevention and reduction are delineated. The third section describes the critical role of primary care in developing service-delivery systems, team training and integrated care pathways that reduce suicide. The chapter does not present a comprehensive account of how the clinical antecedents to suicide, especially depression, are best managed, as these are well documented in other chapters of this book (see especially Chapter 17). The final section considers the management of suicidality in areas where primary care is less well developed, such as low-income countries where the role of general practitioners is less well developed. This section places a special emphasis on the role of community health workers, spiritual leaders and other opinion leaders in local communities.

The prevalence of suicide across international cultures

Suicide is a serious international public health problem and is among the top 10 causes of death worldwide.[1] Over the past 50 years, the World Health Organization (WHO) has estimated that global suicide rates have shown a steady increase, and are projected to increase to 1.53 million by the year 2020 – up to 20 million people a year will attempt suicide.[2] An estimated 877 000 lives were lost worldwide through suicide in 2002, representing 1.5% of the global burden of disease, or more than 20 million disability-adjusted life-years, that is years of healthy life lost through premature death or disability.[2]

Beliefs and attitudes towards suicide differ greatly between different cultures and religions. The three major Abrahamic religions (Christianity, Islam and Judaism) consider suicide to be a sinful act. In other cultures, such as in Japan, suicide is considered an honourable act and an appropriate response to a behaviour that may be considered shameful. In ancient Hindu culture, wives would commit suicide by self-immolation, in an act known as Sati, after the deaths of their husbands. Suicide has also been used as an act of war, as long ago as in ancient Greece, where the Spartans had units of fighters who would kill themselves in battle. Japanese pilots killed themselves in the second World War in Kamikaze attacks, and in more recent times of conflict, organizations such as the Tamil Tigers have also used suicide.

Globally, suicide rates are highest in the old Soviet Bloc countries. Lithuania currently has the highest rate in the world. These high rates are thought to be due to high levels of substance misuse, climatic factors and recent political instability. Work has also been done on a possible common "Fino-Ugarian" allele, which may demonstrate a predisposition to suicidal behaviour in these populations.[4] Interestingly, island countries tend to have high rates of suicide, demonstrated by the values shown for Japan and Sri Lanka in Table 11.1.[3] Latin America and Islamic nations tend to have the lowest rates of suicide in the world, due to the strong influence of religion in these parts of the world.[3]

In the United States of America (USA), over 34 000 people commit suicide every year.[5] In the United Kingdom of Great Britain and Northern Ireland (UK) in 2009, there were 4304 male suicides and 1371 female suicides.[6] Statistics also show that across the period 2000–2009, suicide rates were highest among males aged 15–44 years. In fact suicide accounts for approximately 1% of deaths in the UK population over the age 15 years.[6] The leading cause of death in postnatal woman in the UK has been found to be suicide.[7]

Ethnicity has been found to play a major part in suicide. Caucasians are 2.5 times more likely to kill themselves than African Americans, although Native Americans have the highest rates of suicide.[8] In Australia, the indigenous Aboriginal population has historically had higher rates of suicide. In Sweden, first-generation immigrants have higher rates of suicide when compared to the local population, and this risk is even higher for their Swedish-born children.[9] British studies have found higher rates of self-harm in young Asian women[10] and black women.[11] Ethnic minorities are at particular risk when living in an area of low ethnic density.[12]

Table 11.1	Top ten suicide rates per 100 000[3]				
Rank	Country	Year	Males	Females	Total
1	Lithuania	2005	68.1	12.9	38.6
2	Belarus	2003	63.3	10.3	35.1
3	Russia	2004	61.6	10.7	34.3
4	Kazakhstan	2003	51.0	8.9	29.2
5	Slovenia	2003	45.0	12.0	28.1
6	Hungary	2003	44.9	12.0	27.7
7	Latvia	2004	42.9	8.5	24.3
8	Japan	2004	35.6	12.8	24.0
9	Ukraine	2004	43.0	7.3	23.8
10	Sri Lanka	1996	N/A	N/A	21.6

N/A, not available.

The link between war and conflict and suicide rates

Durkheim proposed that societal and cultural factors can influence suicide levels.[13] Periods of war often cause a decline in suicide rates, as there is a greater sense of collective unity, while economic recessions cause the opposite, due to the effects of disintegration of society.

Table 11.2 outlines some of the major risk factors for suicide and describes the sociodemographic characteristics, environmental factors, cultural and life-cycle precipitants.

Table 11.2	People at higher risk of suicide
Variables	**High-risk groups**
Age	All over 65 years; 25–35 years (men); 35–55 years (women)
Sex	Male (3:1)
Marital status	Single, separated, divorced, widowed
Ethnicity	Ethnic minority groups have similar representation in the population in general as they have in suicide statistics. Young Asian women may be at particular risk in the UK, as are some immigrant workers
Social factors	Living alone, unemployment, lack of social support; drop in socioeconomic status; ease of access due to occupation or other reason; living in an area of social unrest
Life events	Recent life events, especially relationship problems and bereavement, and development of physical health problems in individuals aged over 65 years
Physical health	Chronic or terminal conditions, especially with pain or functional impairment. These include malignant neoplasms; human immunodeficiency virus/acquired immunodeficiency syndrome (HIV/AIDS); peptic ulcer disease; haemodialysis; systemic lupus erythematosus; pain syndromes; functional impairment; diseases of the nervous system
Mental health	All mental illness, especially affective disorders and schizophrenia: current acute episode, comorbidity.
Duration of illness	<1 year or >5 years (risk particularly high in new diagnosis in individuals aged under 25 years)
Substance misuse	Alcohol and drug misuse, especially when combined with mental health problems
Past history	Previous self-harm: especially if medically serious (1 in 11 died within 5 years after a serious attempt, >60% by suicide); history of violence; history of sexual abuse
Medication	Distressing side-effects, especially in some ethnic minority populations
Family history	Actual or attempted suicide, especially by a parent; family history of mental illness
Inpatients	The discharge planning period is the most common time; absconders (especially young, unemployed, homeless men) and those under intermittent observation
Service factors	Within 3 months of discharge (especially self-discharge); those who do not access health care

The demographic spectrum of suicide rates

Sex differences in suicide rates have been identified in many studies. Men generally have higher rates of suicide globally. In the UK, while women have higher rates of self-harm events, men have higher rates of completed suicide, at a ratio of 3:1. However, in Asian countries such as India, the gap is greatly narrowed, and in China it is reversed.[14] Those who are unemployed, single, divorced, separated or living alone have higher rates of suicide.

There are *seasonal variations* in suicide rates. Suicide is most likely to occur in the spring and summer in both the northern and southern hemispheres. Life events such as financial hardship and interpersonal relationships also pose an increased risk. Young males are thought to be most at risk after a relationship break-up and are generally a high-risk group.

Age plays a more consistent role in suicide rates. Elderly men have the highest rate of suicide in the USA[15] and the UK.[16] In the USA in 2007, completed suicides in people aged 65 years and over comprised nearly 16% of all suicides, while this age group represented 12.6% of the total USA population. This age group gives few warnings of intent, attempts are more planned and two-thirds have high scores for suicide intent. They are also less likely to survive a suicide attempt, due to the use of more violent and immediate methods. They are more likely to be single, divorced, widowed, socially isolated, experience physical pain or illness or have functional impairments. Seventy-seven per cent are thought to have psychiatric disorders, of whom 63% have depression.

Primary care is the locus of care of long-term conditions and people with long-term physical health conditions are also at considerable risk of suicide. This is especially the case for individuals with neurological conditions such as multiple sclerosis and epilepsy. Conditions with high levels of chronic pain, such as pancreatitis, also result in high suicide rates. Those suffering from HIV/AIDS also have increased rates, but the widespread use of antiretroviral drugs in high-income countries has led to a reduction in suicide rates in this group.

In a British study, a psychological autopsy of 100 suicides in five English counties, on deceased suicide victims aged 60+ years,[16] found that 82% suffered from physical health problems, which was a contributing factor in 62% of suicides; 55% had interpersonal problems, considered to be a contributing factor in 31% of cases; and 47% had "bereavement-related problems". Bereavement was a contributing factor in 25% of cases overall and 15% had financial problems.

Suicide methods

The most common method of suicide in women is poisoning, while in men it is by more violent means. Most western countries follow a similar trend. In the USA, the most common method of suicide is overwhelmingly the use of firearms, while in other western countries hanging is more common. In the USA in those aged over 65 years,[17] over 70% of suicides were committed by firearms, with around 10% commiting suicide by hanging or poisoning. Methods of suicide have been found to vary according to ethnicity. In Malaysia those of Chinese origin are likely to commit suicide by jumping and those of Indian origin by poisoning.[18]

Particular occupations such as working in agriculture or health care indicate that those with the knowledge and access to methods of taking their own life are most at risk. Veterinary surgeons have a four-times higher rate of suicide than the general population,[19] while doctors, pharmacists and farmers have double the rate.[20] Research has shown that it is only female doctors who carry this increased risk.[21]

Determinants of high risk of suicide

Among the high-risk precursors of suicide, mental illness is a major factor. Around 30% of those committing suicide are thought to be depressed, 18% have substance misuse problems and 13% have personality disorders.[22] Around 5% of those suffering from schizophrenia commit suicide, with the risk being highest in young men in the first 5 years of their illness.[23] Evolving levels of insight in the initial years of illness are also thought to result in the development of depressive symptoms and suicide.[24] In particular, those who have previously enjoyed academic success prior to their illness are at higher risk. There is also a link between *deliberate self-harm and suicide*. Around 1% of those presenting with self-harm will have committed suicide within 1 year, and these individuals contribute to 10% of all suicides in total.[25]

Substance misuse, help-seeking and poverty

An example of the complex interaction of high-risk factors is the recent review of suicide and homicide in the Northern Ireland report by the *National Confidential Inquiry into Suicide and Homicide by People with*

Mental Illness.[26] It was found that from 2000–2008 in Northern Ireland, young people who died as a result of suicide were more likely than other age groups to be living in the poorest areas. Young mental health patients who died as a result of suicide tended to have high rates of drug misuse (65%), alcohol misuse (70%) and previous self-harm (73%).[26] They also had the lowest rate of contact with mental health services (15%) compared to young people in other areas of the UK.

Similarly, in a 2002 Estonian psychological autopsy study using primary care information on 427 cases from 1999 (all ages), compared to a living control group,[27] alcohol abuse was found in 10% of suicide cases and alcohol dependence in 51%. In men, alcohol abuse and dependence was a significant predictor of completed suicides. An important education point is that doctors only recognized the symptoms of alcoholism in 25% of cases.

Media impact

The phenomenon of the impact of media on suicide is relatively recent, and given the growing place of media in the lives of people, understanding this new social influence, especially in the younger generations, is important. This is a relatively new and complex research field, where it is often difficult to identify methods that align presentation with outcome, and include the issues of cohort and demographic effect. The study methods, emulating the research of media impact on smoking behaviours, range from reviews of single media format (e.g. television and film) to celebrity copy-cat events. In a major review,[28] Stack found that between 1967 and 2009, around 120 scientific studies were published on the possible link between media depictions of suicide and in vivo suicides. Most studies measured the suicide rate before and after a widely publicized news story (or film) on suicide. For example, Simkin et al.[29] reported that 32% of those who presented at accident and emergency departments with a suicide attempt were aware of a recent suicide on British television and 14% reported it had influenced their attempt. Hawton et al. determined that 20% of suicide attempters reported that a recent suicide on British television had influenced their attempt.[30] In Hungary, Fekete and Schmidtke found that 41% of suicide attempters reported a suicidal role model from the media, compared to 10% of controls.[31]

The power of celebrity

Studies measuring the presence of either an entertainment or a political celebrity were 14.3 times more likely to report a copy-cat effect than other kinds of stories. Published research findings are 4.39 times more likely to report copy-cat effects for youth suicides, than research findings based on other suicide rates.[32] Cheng et al. found that 39% of 438 depressed patients exposed to a media report of a celebrity suicide reported that the media story had an influence on their subsequent suicidal behaviour.[33] In Canada, Tousignant et al. found that 13% of suicides after the highly publicized suicide of a Quebec journalist were influenced by the reporter's suicide.[34]

Stack's conclusion, from his systematic meta-analysis of 293 findings in 42 studies,[28] was that less than half of the findings supported a copy-cat effect. His conclusion was that in large-scale investigations, some of the time, research finds that, after controlling for confounding factors (e.g. season, unemployment), publicized suicide stories are associated with increases in population suicide rates. His view was that there is no automatic relationship between suicide in the news/media and copy-cat suicides, and that there is a need to search for the contexts that maximize or minimize the probability of finding a copy-cat effect. He concluded that newspaper stories that could be reread several times, as opposed to the usual 'ten second' story of TV exposure had a greater impact.

National and international suicide-prevention policies and strategies

In this section, the focus is on the national and international policies and public health strategies that have been involved in suicide reduction, and examples are provided. Figure 11.1 illustrates the range of strategies employed across the world to reduce suicide rates. The strategies fall into three broad categories: firstly, programmes that require government and national-level leadership; secondly, effective service-delivery models in organizations that provide mental health care; and thirdly, individual patient clinical care pathways that increase the identification, assessment and treatment of individuals with high-risk factors for suicide. The individual clinical-level prevention policies in primary care are described in the next section ("The role of primary care in suicide prevention and reduction").

Suicide-prevention strategies

See Figure 11.1.

Policies relating to reduction in access to suicide methods

In the UK, the most common method of suicide was paracetamol poisoning, and thus, in 1997, the government placed restrictions on the sale of paracetamol to 32 tablets from a pharmacist and 16 tablets from retail outlets, with the additional introduction of blister packs. In the following 2 years, suicidal deaths from paracetamol and salicylate overdose fell by almost a quarter, with a 30% reduction in admissions to liver transplantation units. However, there was an increase in ibuprofen overdose in this period but this had no effect on the suicide rate as ibuprofen is a safer drug in overdose.[11]

Restrictions on the prescription and sale of barbiturates in Australia proved to be very successful.[36] Similarly, co-proxamol was withdrawn after a study in 2003,[37] which found that the most popular drug used for suicidal overdoses by both young males and females was co-proxamol (37.1%). Importantly, the same study also found that in 37.6% of young person suicides, alcohol had been consumed shortly before death.[37]

Tougher legislation on access to firearms has seen a fall in suicide rates. In the USA, the Brady Act has been implemented in 32 states; this has introduced background checks and a mandatory waiting period for an individual wishing to buy a firearm. The suicide rate in those aged over 55 years has fallen in the states where the Act has been implemented.[38] In 1996 in Victoria, Australia, there were a number of high-profile shootings. This led to more stringent legislation, with the introduction of a firearms amnesty and a buyback

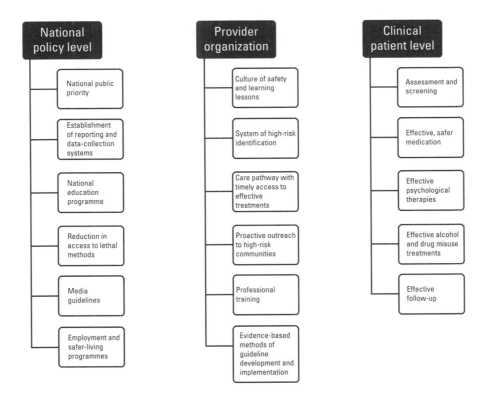

Figure 11.1 National policy, service-provider organizations and clinical suicide strategies

scheme, which led to a significant downturn in firearm-related suicides.[39] Similar findings have been reported in Austria, following introduction of stricter firearms laws.[40]

In Sri Lanka, the suicide rate rose eight-fold from 1950 to 1995, with the preferred method of suicide being ingestion of pesticides. In 1995, the Sri Lankan Government placed strict import controls on WHO Class I pesticides. In the following 10 years, there were almost 20 000 fewer suicides compared with the preceding 10 years. Other factors such as trends in employment or the ongoing civil war did not appear to influence this result.[41]

Switzerland is one of a number of countries that has reduced suicide by detoxifying domestic gas.[42] In the UK, there has been a fall in suicide by car exhaust asphyxiation in all age and sex groups.[43] This change was most marked after the introduction of catalytic converters in 1993. Stringent environmental legislation in Australia that curtailed carbon monoxide emission from motor vehicles has also seen a fall in the suicide rate.[44]

In the Soviet Union in the late 1980s, restrictions were placed on alcohol use during perestroika, which resulted in a 40% reduction in the male suicide rates in all 15 Soviet republics.[45] Interestingly in Iceland, after the legalization of strong beer, there was a reduction in the sale of spirits, which saw a consequent fall in the suicide rate.[46]

Policies relating to awareness and education

Somewhat counterintuitively and disappointingly, evidence suggests that public-awareness campaigns aimed at raising awareness and reducing the stigma around mental illness, and improving recognition of suicide risk have not demonstrated specific reductions in suicide.[47]

Strategies to identify and reduce risk in "hot spots"

The prevention of access to methods of suicides in high-risk situations, or "hot spots", has been a recurrent focus in successful national and local policies. High-level bridges or plunge points are made safer by the construction and erection of barriers at jumping sites. In Bristol, UK, the Clifton Suspension Bridge was a local suicide hotspot, but placing barriers on the bridge cut the suicide rate on the bridge by 50%.[48] A similar strategy was effective in San Francisco in relation to the Golden Gate Bridge.[49]

Inpatient and discharge "hot spots"

There is a higher risk of suicide in those admitted to specialist mental health inpatient facilities, as these are the most seriously ill patients, with severe and enduring illnesses such as schizophrenia, bipolar disorder and depression, as well as concomitant substance misuse. British national suicide-prevention policies[50] have embedded improvements in the care pathway. These involve introducing rigorous assessment and identification of risk on admission and clear and easily comprehensible policies and protocols on observation, aimed at preventing and responding to absconding, including scrapping the use of intermittent observations, during admission. A key learning point is that, for these to be successful, there needs to be a focus on training staff in the use of observation as a therapeutic tool, where the focus is engagement and building a trusting and helpful relationship with the patient, coupled with risk reduction. In addition, making the ward environment safer through ligature-free, collapsible rails and collapsible equipment in bedrooms and bathrooms has been very successful in reducing suicide rates in this setting.

The first six weeks post discharge "hot spot"

The British *National Confidential Inquiry into Suicide and Homicide by People with Mental Illness* found that the first 6 weeks post discharge from a mental health unit carried the greatest risk of suicide, relapse and readmission.[51] Consequently, the government set an operating framework target of 100% patient follow-up through face-to-face contact within 7 days of hospital discharge.

In the Northern Ireland report of the National Confidential Inquiry into Suicide and Homicide by People with Mental Illness,[26] 125 patient suicides (24% of all cases) and nine patient homicides (43%) occurred within 3 months of discharge from hospital. In 129 patient suicides (27%) and 10 patient homicides (53%), the patient missed their final appointment with services. The report therefore recommends the introduction of an assertive outreach function in community mental health services, with staff training, reduced case-loads, and new team structures. Another key recommendation is that there needs to be specific training of staff in recognizing risk, as, at the final contact, immediate risk of suicide had been estimated as low in the majority of the patient suicides (90%) and patient homicides (81%).[26] The report recommends a review of risk-management processes within mental health services and an organizational culture that has an appropriate balance between identifying blame and recognizing the complexities of clinical risk management.

Media guidelines

As described in the first section of this chapter, we live in a world of ever-increasing access to media in many forms. Since the mid-1990s various organizations have produced guidelines to improve the reporting of suicide. WHO and the International Association for Suicide Prevention issued *Preventing suicide: a resource for media professionals* in 2008, with 11 helpful recommendations.[52] These guidelines have been disseminated by many organizations, including WHO, the Centers for Disease Control and Prevention (CDC), the American Foundation for Suicide Prevention (AFSP) and the American Association of Suicidology (AAS).

The 11 key recommendations in the guidelines are:

1. take the opportunity to educate the public about suicide
2. avoid language that sensationalizes or normalizes suicide, or presents it as a solution to problems
3. avoid prominent placement and undue repetition of stories about suicide
4. avoid explicit description of the method used in a completed or attempted suicide
5. avoid providing detailed information about the site of a completed or attempted suicide
6. word headlines carefully
7. exercise caution in using photographs or film footage
8. take particular care in reporting celebrity suicides
9. show due consideration for people bereaved by suicide
10. provide information on where to seek help
11. recognize that media professionals themselves may be affected by stories about suicide.

The two key questions are: to what extent are the guidelines effective in preventing or reducing the impact of copy-cat suicides, and to what extent has there been compliance with the guidelines. Evaluation of the use and impact of these guidelines suggests that the media can be selective about which ones they follow. For example, in Switzerland, sensationalist presentations almost glamorizing suicide reduced the incidence of suicide, although the number of reports on suicide actually increased. An Australian study likewise found that in 410 press reports, front page headlines and sensationalist reporting reduced the incidence of suicide,[53] but found that only 6.5% of reports provided information on where to seek help, e.g. suicide hotline number as recommended in the WHO guideline.[52]

Whole-systems national policies

In order to make a real impact on suicide prevention and reduction, a whole-systems policy programme is of most value. Senior government focus and commitment to a programme of prevention is likely to lead to the greatest success, as a range of methods can be employed and resourced. The example chosen to illustrate an integrated whole-systems approach is that of the UK.

UK as an example

In the UK, in 1999, senior policy leadership set ambitious targets for suicide reduction. These were set out in *Saving lives: our healthier nation*[54] and reinforced within the *National Service Framework for Mental Health*.[55] The aim was to reduce the death rate from suicide and undetermined injury by at least one-fifth by the year 2010. To achieve a focus on delivering this goal, a *National Suicide Prevention Strategy in England* was published in 2002.[56]

The strategy recognized that a combination of approaches was necessary, and a programme with a focus on six areas was developed. These six areas were to:

- reduce risk in key high-risk groups
- promote mental well-being in the wider population
- reduce the availability and lethality of suicide methods
- improve reporting of suicidal behaviour in the media
- promote research on suicide and suicide prevention
- improve monitoring of progress towards the targets of *Saving lives: our healthier nation*.[54]

The successful outcomes of this multifaceted approach have shown that in the UK, since 2000, the number of suicides in people aged 15 years and over has gradually decreased.[54] However, some patterns have remained consistent, in that there are more suicides among males than females. Between 2000 and 2009, the highest suicide rates in the UK were among men aged 15–44 years. The rate for this age group in 2009 was 18.0 per 100 000. The lowest male suicide rates between 2000 and 2009 varied between those aged 45–74 years and 75 years and over, and by 2009 the rate for 75 years and over was 13.6 per 100 000, while for men aged 45–74 years, the rate was 17.4 per 100 000. There has been less variation in suicide rates across the female age groups. Since 2005, rates have been highest among women aged 45–74 years, although they decreased from 6.7 per 100 000 in 2005 to 5.8 per 100 000 in 2009. Suicide rates were lowest among women aged 15–44 years until 2008, although they were not significantly different from those for women aged 75 years and over. In 2009, the rates for these groups were 4.9 and 4.7 per 100 000 respectively.

Establishment of suicide data-collection methods and learning reports

One of the greatest challenges to suicide reporting that enables lessons to be learnt is having agreed definitions of suicide recording and reporting systems. A commitment in the UK policy was to improve the collection of data relating to suicide, and the *National Confidential Inquiry into Homicides and Suicides by People with Mental Illness* was established in 1996. This has a 5-year report cycle on avoidable deaths, and was first published in 2001, covering incidents of suicide for 1996–2000 and for homicide for 1996–1999, [57] and again in 2006,[51] covering incidents for 2000–2004 for suicide and 1999–2003 for homicide. Annual reports for England and Wales were published in 2009[58] and 2010,[59] and for England, Wales and Scotland in 2011.[60] The source of case-information is based on coroners' verdicts and data collected by completion of questionnaires from front-line consultant psychiatrists. This system has educated and engaged clinicians, and has an impressive 97% compliance of reporting. It has allowed comprehensive data on suicides in specialist mental health services to be analysed and themes for suicide reduction to be developed. However, the ability to accurately find the number of suicides, although improved, continues to present definitional and methodological dilemmas, with limitations due to the delay between incident, reporting and publication; and inconsistency between datasets and comparative data between service providers where permission to publish has not been forthcoming.

Continuing difficulties include that there is no agreement on the definitions of natural or unnatural deaths and suicides. Different datasets are used, as there is no clarity on whether to include all unnatural deaths or just suicides. The processes and reporting are not immediate; they are retrospective, rather than in real time. There is no national mandatory system for reporting, and finally there are major differences in coroner practice. The process by which a death is classified as suicide is complex, long and subject to local interpretation. Coroner verdicts may take many months or even years to become available, and a wider variety of verdicts is now used. There is no reliable national comparator for suicide rates in NHS trusts.

Scotland

In Scotland during the last two decades of the 20th century, there was a dramatic increase in suicide among young men aged 15–29 years, with a suicide rate of 42.5/100 000 in 1999. However, by the first decade of the 21st century, there had been a reduction of almost 40% in the suicide rate, to 24.5/100 000 in 2004. As with the UK national policy, a multifaceted policy programme was developed. Following devolution in 1999, the new Scottish Government set up a number of prevention initiatives, and these included tackling the high rates of social exclusion in deprived communities in Scotland, and the National Programme for Improving Mental

Wellbeing and Health. Other programmes established included Choose Life (the Scottish Suicide Prevention Strategy), the "see me" anti-stigma campaign, and Breathing Space (a confidential helpline targeted at young men). As part of the Choose Life Campaign, guidelines were set up on media reporting of suicide.[61]

Northern Ireland policy

In homicide and suicide generally, alcohol misuse is a more common feature in Northern Ireland than in the other UK countries,[26] and a broad public health approach, including better dual diagnosis of mental illness and alcohol or drug misuse, health education and alcohol pricing, are seen as key steps towards reducing the risk of both homicide and suicide. In particular, there needs to be a focus on developing new services for young people with problems of substance misuse.[26]

Suicide audit led by primary care commissioners: a whole-systems learning approach

Led by primary care commissioners, another helpful tool that has been developed is the annual suicide audit, seen as part of an overarching whole-systems approach to suicide prevention. The idea is that recommendations from local suicide audits within primary care populations (in partnership with other local agencies) and mental health trusts should feed into the local suicide-prevention and mental-health-promotion strategies.

Suicide prevention at the level of health-care providers

The Detroit suicide-prevention programme is an interesting example of the application of modern management techniques to deliver more effective services. The Henry Ford health-care providers in the USA have espoused the view that, as hard as an individual practitioner may try, it is very challenging to prevent harm at the level of suicide and that is exactly why the safety of the patient is more a system responsibility than an individual responsibility. The Henry Ford System is a not-for-profit integrated health system that provides full health-care coverage from primary care to specialist services and preventative health service for all its insured patients. It covers about 1 million of the population of southeast Michigan and has a varied insurance-plan population of self- and employer-financed health care.

The Detroit area in the USA has gone through a number of changes over the last 10 to 20 years with the decline of its local industry, car manufacturing, leading to areas with unemployment rates of 50–80%. This factor, combined with two other high-risk factors (the patient population has become older, and has more physical health comorbidities), increased the rates and risk of suicide. In a very committed and innovative programme, senior managers committed to the principles of excellent care,[62] which are that:

- care should be based on continuous healing relationships
- care is customized according to patient needs and values
- the patient is the source of control
- the patient's needs should be continually reviewed and anticipated
- knowledge is shared in partnership between all those likely to impact on care
- decision-making is evidence based
- safety is a top priority in the system
- transparency is embraced
- professionals cooperate with continual review and reduction in waste and inefficiency.

In order to "make suicide a zero event" in Detroit, the management team mapped their care pathway processes, to identify the areas where the organization's processes did not meet the principles of excellent care, or made it problematic for clinicians to deliver timely evidence-based care.[32]

Their approach was to develop the following service-improvement process, with an inclusive range of stakeholders:

- agree a vision of perfect care with patient, families, clinicians, funders

- process map the existing care pathways to identify factors that mitigate for and against the optimal care, and develop a programme plan for change
- develop an information strategy, which is critical to enable empowered users and families and support optimal clinician decision-making
- involve the whole community, and especially friends and families in supporting improved care
- build in a transparent evaluation cycle
- build in incentives in relation to reputation, care, outcomes, and finances.[32]

Clinicians found that, to prevent suicide, it was essential to understand that there is a *window of 10 minutes*, from the time when a person thinks about suicide to possible action, and therefore it is critical that there are well-publicized support access points during this time – for example, easy-to-read billboards with suicide helplines displayed. Interestingly, and empirically valid, was their approach of helping the patient, at the point of first assessment, to identify all of his/her potential support networks. This included family, friends, neighbours and social networks, and the person was supported to identify how these could offer ongoing support; the patient was also helped to identify and remove potential suicide methods, such as tablets or weapons. Another critical factor was the degree of communication between all practitioners from primary care to those caring for people with significant physical illnesses. The suicide rate declined by 75% among members receiving behavioural health care from the Henry Ford medical group, from 89 per 100 000 members at baseline in the year 2000, to 22 per 100 000 per year, on average, during the follow-up period 2002–2005. This was a significant drop in suicide rate, with a *P* value of 0.007. The team continued to improve on this success and have now had 10 successive quarters without a single suicide.

The role of primary care in prevention and reduction of suicide

The challenge in health care is to implement evidence obtained through research into routine practice. This section draws on the public health and policy evidence presented in the previous sections, and describes the more specific primary-care-focused research, to outline how primary care, in its many roles, can develop and deliver a suicide-reduction strategy. Many of the principles covered so far will have more relevance to high- and medium-income countries. Some principles may also be generalizable to low-income countries and these will be considered in more detail in the final section of this chapter.

Table 11.3 proposes an outline of how primary care can develop its health-care-delivery model to have the greatest impact on suicide reduction. General practitioners (GPs) and primary care teams in all countries have many roles. These include the roles as individual clinicians; the skill mix and training of the whole primary care team; new and innovative models for effective primary care mental health service; the structure of the practice organizational system; the role of specialist mental health and other services as commissioners; and the role of primary care as a leader in the community and a respected influence on public health focus. Table 11.3 delineates, how primary care leaders may translate the evidence-based international policy and practice strategies discussed into the routine practice and organization of their services.

Contact with primary care and specialist services

The role of primary care is critical to prevention and reduction of suicide. Luoma et al. undertook a review of 40 studies that reported information on the rates of contact with primary care and mental health-care professionals by individual suicide victims.[63] In the year prior to the suicide, roughly three-quarters of patients had contact with primary care clinicians, and approximately one-third had contact with mental health services. In the month prior to the suicide, about one in five suicide victims had contact with mental health services. In the same one-month time frame before suicide, using the methodologies of primary-care-based psychological autopsies and record reviews, studies found that 45% of suicide victims had contact with primary care providers.[63] These rates varied across age groups, with older adults having higher rates of primary care contact than younger adults in the month before their suicide.[63]

These findings are consistent with other work from the USA[64] and the UK.[65] In 1994, Gunnell and Frankel found that in the UK, approximately 25% of people who died by suicide had contact with a health-care

Table 11.3 The range of effective primary care mental health roles

Primary care role	Roles and responsibilities/strategies
GPs as individual clinicians	• Understanding of local rates of suicide and high-risk groups • Empathic and skilled communication and interview style • Use of evidence-based assessments for mental illness and substance misuse • Understanding of high-risk groups for early identification • Medication and psychological therapy, e.g. cognitive-behavioural therapy (CBT) and depression care guidelines • Alert to media portrayal/events likely to have an impact • Knowledge of local referral and care pathway arrangements • Knowledge of the range of local support services in all sectors
Primary care multidisciplinary team and new models from international best evidence	• Receptionists approach vulnerable people • Health visitors trained in identification of mental ill-health in young mothers and families • District nurses trained to identify depression in elderly, isolated people they visit for long-term physical conditions • Practice nurses working with people with severe mental illness (SMI) and long-term conditions – recording of depression in chronic illness as part of the Quality and Outcomes Framework (QOF) in the UK • Innovative primary-care-based depression case managers as per the American model • Outreach, especially for the vulnerable elderly • Tele-care and e-care • Intermediate care to support long-term conditions
Leadership and organization of the practice	• Establishment of care registers of high-risk groups, e.g. SMI, alcohol and drug dependence, long-term conditions, i.e. chronic disease registers in the UK • Practice protocol for suicide care pathway • Helpline numbers publicized in practice • Education on mental illness and information on how to seek help for depression is easily available • Practice-based, or access to, CBT therapists and counsellors • Alcohol and drug sessional experts available to do motivational interviewing and publicize peer support • Directory of available local services for mental health conditions and substance misuse
Primary care physicians as commissioners of services	• Data literacy with understanding of suicide rates • Local hot spots identified with reduction strategies • Commission outreach to high-risk groups • Contracted timely access to crisis referral and support from a local specialist • Commissioning of crisis home treatment team • Commissioning of outreach services for high-risk groups • Commissioning follow-up for those who have presented at an emergency department with deliberate self-harm
GPs as community leaders and public health contribution	• Education in schools • Support for employment and wider strategic social inclusion in the local area

professional, usually their GP, during the last week of life.[66] Appleby et al. found that the number of GP visits for people aged under 35 years increased significantly before death,[67] with both sexes having the same rate of GP visits before suicide. People suffering with mental health problems are therefore more likely to seek help from their primary care provider, rather than from specialist mental health services. The second key finding is that the rate of contact varies with age and sex. Persons aged 35 years and younger tend to have higher rates of contact with mental health services within a year of death, compared to persons dying of suicide aged 55 years and older. This age effect may be a cohort effect, since the younger group lived at a time when mental health issues became less stigmatized. Lifetime rates of contact with mental health services tended to be higher for women than for men.

Improving early identification through whole communities

One of the most fundamental premises in medicine is that the earlier the identification of a treatable illness, the better the outcome. Thus, early identification is essential. In an excellent review of suicide-prevention strategies in primary care, the evidence for how best to increase GP recognition and effective management was described.[68] The starting point is the *public health role of primary care*. Primary care does not work in isolation from community partners and in 1999, Aoun described a range of community agencies whose contact with potentially vulnerable populations provides an opportunity to identify at-risk individuals and direct them to appropriate assessment and treatment.[69] These "gatekeepers" include clergy, helpline and first responders, pharmacists, those caring for older adults, and those employed in institutional settings, such as schools, prisons, and the military. Components of effective programmes included: education covering awareness of risk factors, policy changes to encourage help-seeking, availability of resources, and efforts to reduce the stigma associated with help-seeking. In addition to gatekeeper training, these programmes also promoted organization-wide awareness of mental health and suicide and facilitated access to mental health services. Similar strategies were undertaken in the Detroit programme described earlier.[62]

Commissioning and providing outreach for high-risk groups

An increasing proportion of some high-risk groups, however, have help-seeking behaviours that mean primary care is not their point of first contact and it is vital that primary care considers how, within its structures, these groups are provided with information and care. National datasets, and a few research studies, have provided information on the rates of health-care contact for suicide victims from ethnic minorities. There are reports that minorities in the USA have lower levels of primary care and mental health-care usage,[64,65] and thus rates of contact with health services by those from ethnic and racial minorities who die from suicide may be lower than those reported for other groups. Similarly, in the UK, there is evidence that people from some high-risk black and minority ethnic communities do not seek help from primary care physicians, but come late to mental health services, often brought there by police in an advanced state of illness.[70] This finding applies to long-term physical conditions as well as mental health conditions and supports the need for primary care to commission and provide outreach to the most vulnerable groups who are less likely to seek help from GPs.

Once a practice has established its policies around suicide detection and identification of high-risk groups, there are major opportunities for suicide prevention in primary care through the practice of individual clinicians and wider practice-system organization.

Improving early identification in primary care

Prevention should be possible because most individuals who commit suicide have had contact with a primary care physician within a month before death. However, research consistently finds that depression and other psychiatric disorders are under-recognized and undertreated in the primary care setting.[71,72] Primary care physicians' lack of knowledge about, or failure to screen patients for, depression may contribute to the non-treatment seen in most suicides. Therefore, improving physician recognition of depression and evaluation of suicide risk is a component of suicide prevention. Research indicates that many older adults who visited a primary care physician within a month of dying by suicide had an undiagnosed mental illness associated with suicide, such as depression,[73] or had a common medical condition associated with an increased risk of suicide, such as congestive heart failure, chronic obstructive lung disease, urinary incontinence, anxiety disorders or moderate or severe pain.[74] Suicidal intent has been found to be a good predictor of a subsequent completed suicide. A 5-year follow-up study of more than 2500 patients showed that those who scored highly for suicidal intent at the time were at high risk of completed suicide, especially within the year after the attempt, so this is an important group to be identified as at high risk.

Women traditionally have higher consultation rates of attendance at GPs and have higher rates of diagnosed depression than men. In a case–control study in 1998, Haste et al. found that women at risk of suicide were more likely to have been diagnosed and treated for mental health problems than their male counterparts.[75] The conclusion was that GPs are underdiagnosing and undertreating men at risk, and that women are better placed to benefit from prevention activities aimed at primary care practices.

Effective training in primary care mental health

This interpretation is consistent with the influential Danish Gotland study,[76] in which an educational programme on the treatment of depression aimed at primary care appeared to mainly affect suicide rates in women. The benefit faded, as GPs were replaced by new doctors who were not trained, but there was some indication that it returned after a second education programme.[76] Another Swedish study, in Jamtland, also reported a decrease in the suicide rate after a GP education programme, compared with changes in the national suicide rate,[77] but the benefits of the programme were less pronounced than in Gotland.[76] The Jamtland study showed benefit of an education programme during a period when the Swedish national suicide rate decreased. While many studies across the UK,[78] Australia,[79] the USA,[80] and Northern Ireland[81] have demonstrated that programmes aimed at educating primary care physicians improved detection and increased treatment of depression, there are also studies that do not show improvement (United States,[82] Brazil,[83] and the UK[84]). These beg the questions: what are the critical components and methods in educational programmes that achieve best impact, and is an educational programme targeted at individual doctors enough, or what whole-systems change is needed to maximize outcomes and deliver a sustainable model of support to GPs and their primary care practices?

There is limited substantive research into the key components of effective training programmes for primary care suicide prevention. There is some evidence that education for GPs about depression, appropriate treatment and routine risk assessment may help to reduce the number of suicides.[67,85,86] Understanding the method is essential, as a later study in Hampshire failed to ascertain an increase in detection of depression or in patient recovery rates. This study used guidelines and education within a practice-based setting in a larger project.[84]

Studies examining the effect on suicidal behaviour of primary care physician education programmes mostly targeting depression recognition and treatment, in specific regions in Sweden,[87,88] Hungary,[89] Japan,[90] and Slovenia,[91] all reported increased rates of prescription for antidepressants and many also reported substantial declines in suicide rates. These studies represent the most striking known examples of a therapeutic intervention lowering suicide rates.

Whole-community approaches

Primary care does not work in a vacuum and some studies have demonstrated the better outcomes of wider community approaches. A Japanese community-based programme of improved depression management in the elderly population in a rural village reported a reduction in suicide rates compared with prior rates in the same village.[92] A recent German study of a depression education campaign (the Nuremberg Alliance Against Depression)[93] reported a reduction in non-fatal suicide attempts in an intervention region compared with a control region but no difference in effect on suicide rates. The strength of the German study is the use of a control region. Its limitation is that it used only 1 year of suicide data as a baseline for the control and intervention regions, and a low base rate makes change in suicide rates difficult to detect. The study did not report data on antidepressant use, leaving open the question as to why the rate of non-fatal suicide attempts declined. While the Japanese study suggested that a simple educational intervention could have an impact on suicide mortality,[92] unlike the German study,[93] it did not use a control region to control for local or national changes in suicide rates and treatment practice.

New and innovative redesign of primary mental health service teams

Across the world, new and effective service-delivery models of primary care mental health services are emerging. A programme in Hungary provided a training, systems redesign and whole-team sustainable approach.[94] Training was provided to 28 GPs servicing 73 000 people. The objective of the educational sessions was to determine the effectiveness of a depression-management educational programme for GPs on the suicide rate, and the effects were compared with a control region, the larger surrounding county, and Hungary. In addition to training individuals, services were reorganized and expertise commissioned to support primary care in a sustainable way. Thus, in addition to the 5-year depression-management educational programme for GPs, nurses were also trained, and a depression treatment clinic and psychiatrist telephone consultation service was established. The effectiveness was assessed by the outcome measure of annual suicide rate and the secondary outcome measure of antidepressant prescription use. The annual suicide rate in the intervention region decreased from the 5-year pre-intervention average of 59.7 per 100 000 to 49.9 per 100 000. The decrease was comparable with the control region, but greater than both the county and Hungary rates. In rural areas, the female suicide rate in the intervention region decreased by 34% and increased by 90% in the control region. The increase in antidepressant treatment was greater in the intervention region compared with the control region, the county, and Hungary and in women compared with men. The conclusion was that GP-based intervention produced a greater decline in suicide rates compared with the surrounding county and national rates. Increases in patients with depression treated and of dosing were modest. The key conclusion was that additional service reorganization such as depression case managers should be tried. The importance of alcoholism in local suicide was unanticipated and not addressed.

Innovation in primary care mental health services: depression case managers

Katon et al., early and consistent pioneers of effective primary care mental heath services, led the Improving Mood Promoting Access to Collaborative Treatment (IMPACT) study in 2005.[95] This study introduced depression care managers into primary care in the way that care coordinators have been introduced into specialist mental health services. The premise is that depression is a leading cause of functional impairment in elderly individuals and is associated with high medical costs, but there are large gaps in quality of access and treatment in primary care. The randomized controlled trial aimed to determine the incremental cost-effectiveness of a collaborative care management programme for late-life depression. The study was based in 18 primary care clinics from eight health-care organizations in five US states and recruited 1801 patients aged 60 years or older with major depression (17%), dysthymic disorder (30%), or both (53%). Patients were randomly assigned to the IMPACT intervention (n = 906) or to usual primary care (n = 895).

The IMPACT intervention was a 1-year, stepped, collaborative care approach that included either a nurse or psychologist care manager working in the participant's primary care clinic to support the patient's regular primary care physician. The depression care manager completed an initial biopsychosocial history and provided education about antidepressant medication and psychotherapy approaches to treatment. All patients were encouraged to engage in behavioural activation and were offered a choice of treatment with an antidepressant medication or problem-solving treatment in primary care (PST-PC). The latter was a 6–8-session psychotherapy programme designed for primary care patients, and was found to be as effective as antidepressant medication for treating major depression. The depression care manager received weekly supervision by a primary care physician with geriatric expertise, and a psychiatrist, to monitor the progress of cases and to adjust treatment plans according to a stepped-care treatment algorithm.[95] This algorithm guided short-term and continuation therapy and relapse-prevention recommendations over the 12-month treatment period. The depression care manager followed-up patients in person, or by telephone, approximately every 2 weeks during short-term treatment, and approximately monthly during the continuation phase. Depression care managers received training on pharmacotherapy and PST-PC during a 2-day workshop that included didactic training with a treatment manual and role-plays, and completed at least five videotaped training cases of PST-PC supervised by a psychologist. In the control arm of the study, physicians of patients assigned to usual care were notified of their diagnoses and these patients could receive all the treatments routinely provided for depression (antidepressant medication and supportive counselling by their physician, as well as self- or physician referral to specialty mental health care). The outcome measures were total outpatient costs, depression-free days, and quality-adjusted life-years. Relative to usual care, intervention patients experienced more depression-free days over 24 months. Results of a bootstrap analysis suggested a 25% probability that the IMPACT intervention was "dominant" (i.e. was associated with lower costs and greater effectiveness). The conclusion was that the IMPACT intervention is a high-value investment for older adults; it is associated with high clinical benefits at a low increment in health care.

Intervention

Innovative models of primary care teams

Nurse case management, collaborative care, or quality-improvement initiatives can further improve the recognition and management of depression,[96] and have application where education alone may be insufficient.

The future and the role of care pathways, managed care and payment by results

There are new emerging studies that include whole prescribed care pathways for the assessment and management of depression and other conditions that can be the precursors of suicide.

In the UK, the National Institute for Health and Clinical Excellence (NICE) has developed evidence-based clinical guidelines based on meta-analyses of international evidence, the assimilated experience of "experts by experience" and economists and statisticians.[97]

The stepped care pathway model for the care of people with depression has been an early priority and provides primary care with clear pathways guidance. This is discussed in detail in Chapter 17.

The IAPT (Improving Access to Psychological Therapies) programme in the UK has enabled some primary care mental health services to be provided in collaboration with other agencies such as employment and welfare benefits. It has prescribed assessment tools and sessional care pathways and has delivered unprecedented outcomes in terms of retention, engagement in employment and improved mental health.[98] This much more systematized approach is essential if the busy environment of primary care is to have embedded systems that support individual practitioners.

Individual clinician strategies

While many new and effective service-delivery models are emerging across the world, the fundamental need for each primary care clinician to be a skilled practitioner does not change. The WHO publication, *Preventing suicide. A resource for primary health care workers*,[99] already presents a succinct, comprehensive guide for individual primary care clinicians to support their assessment of suicide risk. Some of the key recommendations are presented next.

Recognizing the warning signs

Every GP needs to strengthen his/her own ability to recognize the warning signs of suicide and to make sure that the patient receives immediate and appropriate care for this life-threatening condition. The ability to get beneath what is often presented as a physical health concern requires a skilled interview technique. Warning signs are when the patient:

- talks about suicide or death
- gives direct verbal cues, such as "I wish I were dead" and "I'm going to end it all"
- gives less direct verbal cues, such as "what's the point of living?", "soon you won't have to worry about me" and "who cares if I'm dead, anyway?"
- isolates him or herself from friends and family
- expresses the belief that life is meaningless or hopeless
- gives away cherished possessions
- exhibits a sudden and unexplained improvement in mood after being depressed or withdrawn
- neglects his or her appearance and hygiene.

These signs are especially critical if the patient has a history or current diagnosis of a psychiatric disorder, such as depression, alcohol or drug abuse, bipolar disorder, or schizophrenia, and for older adult patients who are at an increased risk of dying by suicide.

Doctors will have a high risk group in mind and these include elderly patients who are physically ill and who exhibit warning signs of suicide such as:[100]

- stockpiling medications
- buying a gun
- giving away money or cherished personal possessions
- taking a sudden interest, or losing their interest, in religion
- failing to care for themselves in terms of the routine activities of daily living
- withdrawing from relationships
- experiencing a failure to thrive, even after appropriate medical treatment
- scheduling a medical appointment for vague symptoms.

Adolescents are also at an increased risk of dying by suicide, though their warning signs are different. GPs need to be alert for the following:

- volatile mood swings or sudden changes in their personality
- indications that they are in unhealthy, destructive, or abusive relationships, such as unexplained bruises, a swollen face, or other injuries, particularly those they refuse to explain
- a sudden deterioration in their personal appearance
- self-mutilation
- a fixation with death or violence
- eating disorders, especially combined with dramatic shifts in weight (other than those associated with a diet under medical supervision)
- gender-identity issues
- depression.

Responding to the warning signs

There are no hard and fast guidelines for determining a patient's risk of suicide. There are a number of well-validated, reliable standardized assessment tools. The most commonly used screening tools are for depression, i.e. the Patient Health Questionnaire (PHQ)[101] or the Hospital Anxiety and Depression Scale (HADS)[102] scores for depression as part of the QOF. The suggestion is not that a clinician uses a standardized measure in a time of crisis but that they assimilate the skilfully worded questions and incorporate these into their routine clinical practice. If there is a chance that a patient may be at risk, it is important to ask sometimes difficult questions that provide evidence about his or her state of mind and intentions, for example:

- do you ever wish you could go to sleep and never wake up?
- sometimes when people feel sad, they have thoughts of harming or killing themselves; have you had such thoughts?
- have you ever felt like harming yourself in any way?
- are you thinking about killing yourself?

A clinician should act immediately if there is any reason to believe that the patient is in imminent danger or poses a grave danger to him or herself. Immediate action should also be taken when warning signs are combined with any of the following risk factors:

- past incidents of suicidal behaviour or self-harm
- a family history of suicide
- a history of psychiatric disorders or abuse of alcohol and other drugs
- the patient's admission that he or she has considered suicide

- the patient's expressed wish to die
- any evidence of a current psychiatric disorder.

With the support of a well-organized practice system, GPs can best meet the needs of their patients by doing the following:

- referring the patient to a mental health professional who is better able to evaluate the patient's risk and recommend next steps
- helping the patient's family, friends, and caregivers develop a plan so that someone is with the patient at all times
- helping the patient's family, friends, and caregivers make sure that lethal means, especially firearms and medications, are not available to the patient
- hospitalizing the patient, if necessary.

Responding to a potential crisis is never easy and this is why well-organized practice timetables and rotas with ease of access to commissioned support from specialist mental heath care can be critical.

You may have to make arrangements for someone to remain at the side of the at-risk patient until family, friends, or a mental health professional arrives. It also takes extra effort not to violate the confidentiality of the at-risk patient or unduly alarm your staff and other patients. Every primary care office should have a crisis intervention plan and should train its staff for crisis intervention. If you have any suspicions that a patient is seriously considering harming him or herself, let your patient know that you care, that he or she is not alone and that you are there to help. You may have to work with the patient's family to ensure that he or she will be adequately supported until a mental health professional can provide an assessment.

The WHO guidance recommends that in some cases, the practice needs to have support available so that the patient can be accompanied to the emergency room at an area hospital or crisis centre.[108] If the person is uncooperative, combative, or otherwise unwilling to seek help, and if you sense that the person is in acute danger, it may be important to access support from those that can support legal detention under mental health legislation. Writing a practice policy on how to identify and practically manage potentially suicidal patients who attend, and discussing with all staff, would be beneficial.

When to refer

If the patient lives alone; has no protective factors (see Table 11.4); has had previous suicide attempts or mental health problems, etc; and shows suicidal intent while in surgery, it is important to refer immediately. Organize an appointment at an assessment centre before the patient leaves and ensure they have a relative or friend to accompany them.

If the patient is lower risk and has no intent but does have suicidal thoughts, arrange urgent assessment preferably within a few days and ensure monitoring by a relative or friend in the meantime.

If the patient is in any immediate danger, arrange admission to hospital.

Helping yourself and your colleagues

Along with recognizing warning signs in your patients, it is equally important to recognize warning signs among your colleagues and in yourself, and to take protective measures when necessary. Physicians are not immune to suicide. The culture among physicians often prohibits any complaints about the exhaustion and stress associated with long hours of work and minimal sleep. Gruelling schedules, coupled with the knowledge that a missed "cue" or clinical finding could lead to the illness, injury or death of a patient, places a great deal of stress on physicians. An American Foundation for Suicide Prevention consensus statement on depression and suicide among physicians cited a lack of attention in this area, and urged physicians, medical institutions, and health organizations to pay more attention to the treatment of depression and prevention of suicide among physicians.[103] The statement recommends a shift in professional attitudes and institutional policies – one that encourages physicians to seek help and obtain treatment for mental illness, if needed.

Table 11.4 Summary of risk factors to consider in the consultation

Static risk factors, baseline risk	Dynamic risk factors (why now?)	Protective factors
• History of self-harm: document all methods and functions for the patient • Seriousness of all previous suicide attempts, including the recent incident: perceived and actual lethality of method, attempts to avoid detection, final acts (e.g. leaving a suicide note) • Previous admissions to psychiatric unit • History of mental disorder: document multiaxial diagnosis • History of substance use disorder: what substances, what currently, any support? • Personality disorder/traits • Childhood adversity • Family history of suicide • Age, sex and marital status	• Suicidal ideation, intent and active plans • Hopelessness • Active psychological symptoms: insomnia, anorexia, low mood, negative cognitions; anergia, anhedonia, motivation, concentration, psychotic symptoms including delusional beliefs, command hallucinations • Treatment adherence: include any failure to attend appointments and level of engagement as well as considerations about medication • Substance use • Recent psychiatric admission and discharge • Psychosocial stress: relationships, employment, finances, family relationships, role changes; pay particular attention to recent loss, e.g. work, housing, relationship, bereavement • Recent life events and anniversaries • Physical health problems: especially those causing pain or insomnia • Problem-solving deficits	• Religious beliefs • Family/carer obligations (including pets) • Strong family and community supports • Good relationship with mental health service providers • Employment • Effective clinical care for mental, physical and substance use disorders

Special considerations for low-income countries and rural areas

Much of the research and principles of intervention described thus far are very useful for high- and medium-income countries with good coverage from secondary care accident and emergency and mental health services and an accessible network of primary care.

In many parts of Africa and other low-income nations, integrated mental health care is still a dream and not a reality and this book sets out how mental health can be better integrated into primary care.

A cornerstone of practice in any setting is the importance of good history-taking. Many mental health conditions are associated with significant comorbidity with physical health conditions and substance misuse. Good history-taking enables health-care workers to better identify all the conditions that carry a significant risk of suicide, so that they can provide earlier and more comprehensive interventions, thereby addressing and decreasing suicide risk.

Family doctors need to be patient advocates at all times, in order to harness the local resources available. In many religious and cultural settings, suicide is perceived as either a shameful or a sinful act.[104] The role of the family doctor in such settings is not only to treat but to advocate on behalf of such distressed patients, in order to address the stigma associated with suicidality by arguing for the full range of resources to be made available for people who are feeling suicidal, without such help-seeking being associated with unnecessary shame and taboo.

A key principle presented by this *Companion to Primary Care Mental Health* is to adopt a stepped care approach for the management of all mental health conditions and Chapter 33 "Multimorbidity in primary care mental health" provides a detailed account of how to best integrate the stepped care approach into day-to-day person-centred practice.

One of the key principles, "staffing up" proposes the provision of staff with a range of skills to address suicide risk assessment and management. We recommend that in low-income countries primary care doctors should prioritize the development of networks of all primary care doctors working in a specific area, so that they develop a collaborative network in order to mutually support one another and become a training resource for themselves. Such collaboratives are particularly useful in the management of suicidal patients because, when faced with the death of a patient by suicide, those working closest to that patient often require personal support. Such a collaborative network should also identify the nearest local psychiatric hospital or psychiatrist to support the stepped care approach, because it is often difficult to manage more complex patients solely in the primary care setting. Joint training between members of the collaborative network is a crucial element of this model.

In rural areas and low-income countries, local health workers should also recognize that the first point of contact for people suffering from distressing symptoms of suicidality may not be primary care as we traditionally know it. Local healers, elders, religious leaders and community workers may be the first people who are approached to provide help and support during such episodes of distress. Family doctors and GPs should identify those people in the community in their neighbourhood who may act as such a first contact and make themselves available to offer support to them so that they can be included in the management of suicidality using the stepped care model.

The role of family doctors cannot be completed until they adopt the role of true advocates; doctors constantly need to ensure that they are addressing the wider determinants of health as described in Chapters 2 and 3 of this book, and harnessing the opportunities provided by social interventions to prevent mental illness and promote good mental health.

In many areas, a place of safety for those suffering from suicidality is not yet available and family doctors can play a part by lobbying their governments to develop places of safety for the suicidal patient to be better assessed and managed while ensuring that human rights are not violated.

Where suicidal behaviour is associated with an underlying mental health condition, that condition should be treated appropriately, as described in Sections C and D of this book.

The management of suicidality in low-income countries and rural areas does not require high-level technology, it requires a caring empathic doctor who can take a good history, make an appropriate diagnosis, keep good records and use the resource of a collaborative network to apply the principles of management described in this book.

Conclusion

This chapter on suicide has brought together a series of principles that are necessary in high-, medium- and low-income countries to enable the family doctor to better manage the suicidal patient. We recognize the role of stigma and culture in the management of suicidality and believe that family doctors can play a major and important role in the recognition, assessment and treatment of suicidality.

Although written in four sections, many of the principles covered in each section are interrelated. The stepped care model is very important and useful in managing suicidality and the conditions that may give rise to suicidality. Primary care is unable to manage the problem of suicidality alone and needs to work collaboratively with the community and secondary and tertiary care, in order to prevent and reduce the risk of completed suicide. The role of family doctors is to advocate for their suicidal patients in places where places of safety and suicide prevention are not available.

References

1   Hawton K, van Heeringen K. Suicide. *The Lancet*, 2009, 373:1372–1381.

2   *The World Health Report 2001. Mental health: new understanding, new hope.* Geneva, World Health Organization, 2001.

3   Mental health. *Global charts.* Geneva, World Health Organization, 2012 (http://www.who.int/mental_health/prevention/suicide/charts/en/, accessed 30 January 2012).

4   Voracek M, Fisher ML, Marusic A. The Finno-Ugrian suicide hypothesis: variation in European suicide rates by latitude and longitude. *Perceptual and Motor Skills*, 2003, 97:401–406.

5   Centers for Disease Control and Prevention, National Center for Injury Prevention and Control. *Injury prevention and control. Data and statistics* (WISQARS™) (www.cdc.gov/ncipc/wisqars, accessed 30 January 2012).

6   Office for National Statistics. *Statistical suicide rates in the United Kingdom, 2000–2009.* Newport, Office for National Statistics, 2011.

7   CEMD (Confidential Enquiries into Maternal Deaths). *Why mothers die 1997–1999. London, Royal College of Obstetricians and Gynaecologists, 2001.*

8   Hoyert DL et al. Deaths. Final data for 2003. *National Vital Statistics Reports*, 2006, 54(13) (http://www.nber.org/perinatal/2003/docs/2003_Mortality_Final_Data.pdf, accessed 28 February 2012).

9   Hjern A. Suicide in first and second generation immigrants in Sweden: a comparative study. *Social Psychiatry and Psychiatric Epidemiology*, 2002, 37:423–429.

10 Bhui K, McKenzie K, Rasul F. Rates, risk factors and methods of self harm among minority ethnic groups in the UK: a systematic review. *BMC Public Health*, 2007, 7:336.

11 Cooper J et al. Ethnic differences in self-harm, rates, characteristics and service provision: three-city cohort study. *British Journal of Psychiatry*, 2010, 197:212–218.

12 Neelman J et al. Ethnic density and deliberate self harm; a small area study in south east London. *Journal of Epidemiology and Community Health*, 2001, 55:85–90.

13 Durkheim E. *Suicide: a study in sociology.* New York, Free Press, 1951.

14 Phillips MR, Li X, Zhang Y. Suicide rates in China, 1995–99. *The Lancet*, 2002, 359:835–840.

15 Conwell Y et al. Age differences in behaviors leading to completed suicide. *American Journal of Geriatric Psychiatry*, 1998, 6:122–126.

16 Harwood DMJ et al. Life problems and physical illness as risk factors for suicide in older people: a descriptive and case-control study. *Psychological Medicine*, 2006, 36:1265–1274.

17 National Center for Injury Prevention and Control (NCIPC) (http://www.cdc.gov/ncipc/wisqars/default.htm, accessed 30 January 2012).

18 Nadesan K. Pattern of suicide: a review of autopsies conducted at the University Hospital, Kuala Lumpur. *Malaysian Journal of Pathology*, 1999, 21:95–99.

19 Mellanby RJ. Incidence of suicide in the veterinary profession in England and Wales. *Veterinary Record*, 2005, 157:415–417.

20 Meltzer H et al. Patterns of suicide by occupation in England and Wales: 2001–2005. *British Journal of Psychiatry*, 2008, 193:73–76.

21 Lindeman S et al. A systematic review on gender-specific suicide mortality in medical doctors. *British Journal of Psychiatry*, 1996, 168:274–279.

22 Bertolote JM et al. Psychiatric diagnoses and suicide: revisiting the evidence. *Crisis*, 2004, 25:147–155.

23 Palmer BA, Pankratz VS, Bostwick JM. The lifetime risk of suicide in schizophrenia: a reexamination. *Archives of General Psychiatry*, 2005, 62:247–253.

24 Crumlish N et al. Early insight predicts depression and attempted suicide after 4 years in first-episode schizophrenia and schizophreniform disorder. *Acta Psychiatrica Scandinavica*, 2005, 112:449–455.

25 Appleby L et al. *Safer services. National Confidential Inquiry into Suicide and Homicide by People with Mental Illness.* London, Department of Health, 1999 (http://www.dh.gov.uk/en/Publicationsandstatistics/Publications/PublicationsPolicyAndGuidance/DH_4005479, accessed 30 January 2012).

26 Appleby L et al. *The National Confidential Inquiry into Suicide and Homicide by People with Mental Illness: Northern Ireland Report.* Manchester, the National Confidential Inquiry into Suicide and

Homicide by People with Mental Illness, 2011 (http://www.dhsspsni.gov.uk/suicideandhomicideni.pdf, accessed 30 January 2012).

27   Kõlves K et al. The role of alcohol in suicide: a case-control psychological autopsy, *Psychological Medicine*, 2006, 36:923–930.

28   Stack S. Media impacts on suicide: a quantitative review. *Social Science Quarterly*, 2000, 81:957–971.

29   Simkin S et al. Media influence on parasuicide, *British Journal of Psychiatry*, 1995, 167:754–759.

30   Hawton K et al. Effects of a drug overdose in a television drama on presentations to hospital for self poisoning. *BMJ*, 1999, 318:972–977.

31   Fekete S, Schmidtke A. Suicidal models. *Omega*, 1996, 33:233–241.

32   Stack S. Media coverage as a risk factor in suicide. *Journal of Epidemiology and Community Health*, 2003, 57:238–240.

33   Cheng A et al. The impact of media reporting on a celebrity suicide on suicidal behaviour in patients with a depressive disorder. *Journal of Affective Disorders*, 2007, 103:69–75.

34   Tousignant M et al. The impact of media coverage on the suicide of a well known Quebec reporter. *Social Science and Medicine*, 2005, 60:1919–1926.

35   Hawton K et al. UK legislation on analgesic packs: before and after study of long term effect on poisonings. *BMJ*, 2004, 329:1076.

36   Oliver RG, Hetzel BS. Rise and fall of suicide rates in Australia: relation to sedative availability. *Medical Journal of Australia*, 1972, 2:919–923.

37   Camidge DR, Wood RJ, Bateman DN. The epidemiology of self-poisoning in the UK. *British Journal of Clinical Pharmacology*, 2003, 56:613.

38   Ludwig J, Cook PJ. Homicide and suicide rates associated with implementation of the Brady Handgun Violence Prevention Act. *JAMA*. 2000, 284:585–591.

39   Ozanne-Smith J et al. Firearm related deaths: the impact of regulatory reform. *Injury Prevention*, 2004, 10:280–286.

40   Kapusta ND et al. Firearm legislation reform in the European Union: impact on firearm availability, firearm suicide and homicide rates in Austria. *British Journal of Psychiatry*, 2007, 191:253–257.

41   Gunnell D et al. The impact of pesticide regulations on suicide in Sri Lanka. *International Journal of Epidemiology*, 2007, 36:1235–1242.

42   Lester D. The effect of the detoxification of domestic gas in Switzerland on the suicide rate. *Acta Psychiatrica Scandinavica*, 1990, 82:383–384.

43   Kelly S, Bunting J. Trends in suicide in England and Wales, 1982–96. *Population Trends*, 1998, Summer:29–41.

44   Studdert DM et al. Relationship between vehicle emissions laws and incidence of suicide by motor vehicle exhaust gas in Australia, 2001–06: an ecological analysis. *PLos Medicine*, 2010, 7(1):e1000210.

45   Wasserman D, Värnik A. Suicide-preventive effects of *perestroika* in the former USSR: the role of alcohol restriction. *Acta Psychiatrica Scandinavica*, 1998, 98(Suppl. 394):1–44.

46   Lester D. Effect of changing alcohol laws in Iceland on suicide rates. *Psychological Reports*, 1999, 84(3 Pt 2):1158.

47   Dumesnil H, Verger P. Public awareness campaigns about depression and suicide: a review. *Psychiatric Services*, 2009, 60:1203–1213.

48   Bennewith O, Nowers M, Gunnell D. The effect of the barriers on the Clifton suspension bridge, England on local patterns of suicide: implications for prevention. *British Journal of Psychiatry*, 2007, 190:266–267.

49   Seiden RH. Where are they now? A follow-up study of suicide attempters from the Golden Gate Bridge. *Suicide and Life Threatening Behaviour*, 1978, 8:203–216.

50   *National Suicide Prevention Strategy in England*. London, Department of Health, 2002.

51   *National Confidential Inquiry into Homicides and Suicides by People with mental Illness*. Manchester: University of Manchester, 2006 (http://www.nmhdu.org.uk/silo/files/avoidable-deaths-five-year-report-.pdf, accessed 9 February 2012).

52   The World Health Organization and International Association for Suicide Prevention. *Preventing suicide: a resource for media professionals*. Geneva, World Health Organization, 2008.

53 Pirkis J et al. Reporting of suicide in the Australian media. *Australian and New Zealand Journal of Psychiatry*, 2002, 36:190–197.

54 *Saving lives: our healthier nation*. London, Department of Health, 1999.

55 *National Service Framework for Mental Health*. London, Department of Health, 1999.

56 *National Suicide Prevention Strategy in England*. London, Department of Health, 2002.

57 *Safety first: five-year report of the National Confidential Inquiry into Homicides and Suicides by People with Mental Illness*. London: Department of Health, 2001 (http://www.dh.gov.uk/prod_consum_dh/ groups/dh_digitalassets/@dh/@en/documents/digitalasset/dh_4058243.pdf, accessed 9 February 2012).

58 *National Confidential Inquiry into Homicides and Suicides by People with Mental Illness*. Annual report, England and Wales. Manchester: University of Manchester, 2009 (http://www.medicine.manchester. ac.uk/mentalhealth/research/suicide/prevention/nci/inquiryannualreports/AnnualReportJuly2009.pdf, accessed 9 February 2012).

59 *National Confidential Inquiry into Homicides and Suicides by People with Mental Illness*. Annual report, England and Wales. Manchester: University of Manchester, 2010 (http://www.medicine.manchester. ac.uk/mentalhealth/research/suicide/prevention/nci/inquiryannualreports/AnnualReportJuly2010.pdf, accessed 9 February 2012).

60 *National Confidential Inquiry into Homicides and Suicides by People with Mental Illness*. Annual report, England, Wales and Scotland. Manchester: University of Manchester, 2011 (http://www.medicine. manchester.ac.uk/mentalhealth/research/suicide/prevention/nci/inquiryannualreports/Annual_Report_ July_2011.pdf, accessed 9 February 2012).

61 Stark C, Stockton D, Henderson R. Reduction in young male suicide in Scotland. *BMC Public Health*, 2008, 8:80.

62 Coffey C, Edward J. Building a system of perfect depression care in behavioural health. *Joint Commission Journal on Quality and Patient Safety*, 2007, 33:193–199.

63 Luoma JB, Martin CE, Pearson JL. Contact with mental health and primary care providers before suicide: a review of the evidence. *American Journal of Psychiatry*, 2002, 159:909–916.

64 Regier DA, Goldberg ID, Taube CA. The de facto US mental health services system: a public health perspective. *Archives of General Psychiatry*, 1978, 35:685–693.

65 Kerwick SW, Jones RH. Educational interventions in primary care psychiatry: a review. *Primary care Psychiatry*, 1996, 2:107–117.

66 Gunnell D, Frankel S. Prevention of suicide: aspirations and evidence. *BMJ*, 1994, 308:1227–1233.

67 Appleby L et al. Aftercare and clinical characteristics of people with mental illness who commit suicide: a case–control study. *The Lancet*, 1999, 353:1397–1400.

68 Mann JJ et al. Suicide prevention strategies: a systematic review. *JAMA*, 2005, 294:2064–2074.

69 Aoun S. Deliberate self-harm in rural western Australia: results of an intervention study. *The Australian and New Zealand Journal of Mental Health Nursing*, 1999, 8:65–73.

70 Commander MJ et al. A comparison of the socio-demographic and clinical characteristics of private household and communal establishment residents in a multi-ethnic inner-city area. Social Psychiatry and Psychiatric Epidemiology, 1997, 32:421–427.

71 Hirchfield RMA et al. The National Depressive and Manic-depressive Association consensus statement on the undertreatment of depression. *JAMA*, 1997, 277:333.

72 Goldman LS, Nielsen NH. Awareness, diagnosis, and treatment of depression. *Journal of General Internal Medicine*, 1999, 14:56.

73 National Institute of Mental Health. *Older adults: depression and suicide facts*. Rockville, MD: National Institutes of Health, 2003 (NIH Publication No. 03-4593) (http://www.nimh.nih.gov/publicat/ elderlydepsuicide.cfm, accessed 30 January 2012).

74 Juurlink DN et al. Medical illness and the risk of suicide in the elderly. *Archives of Internal Medicine*, 2004, 164:1179–1184.

75 Haste F, Charlton J, Jenkins R. Potential for suicide prevention in primary care. An analysis of factors associated with suicide. *British Journal of General Practice*, 1998, 48:1759–1763.

76 Kerwick SW, Jones RH. Educational interventions in primary care psychiatry: a review (Gotland Study). *Primary Care Psychiatry*, 1996, 2:107–117.

77 Henriksson S, Isacsson G. Increased antidepressant use and fewer suicides in Jamtland county, Sweden, after a primary care educational programme on the treatment of depression. *Acta Psychiatrica Scandinavica*, 2006, 114:159–167.

78 Hannaford PC, Thompson C, Simpson M. Evaluation of an educational programme to improve the recognition of psychological illness by general practitioners. *British Journal of General Practice*, 1996, 46:333–337.

79 Naismith SL, Hickie IB, Scott EM, Davenport TA. Effects of mental health training and clinical audit on general practitioners' management of common mental disorders. *Medical Journal of Australia*, 2001, 175(Suppl.):S42–S47.

80 Pignone MP et al. Screening for depression in adults: a summary of the evidence for the US Preventive Services Task Force. *Annals of Internal Medicine*, 2002, 136:765–776.

81 Kelly C. The effects of depression awareness seminars on general practitioners knowledge of depressive illness. *Ulster Medical Journal*, 1998, 67:33–35.

82 Lin EH et al. Does physician education on depression management improve treatment in primary care? *Journal of General Internal Medicine*, 2001, 16:614–619.

83 Valentini W et al. An educational training program for physicians for diagnosis and treatment of depression [in Portuguese]. *Revista de Saúde Pública*, 2004, 38:522–528.

84 Thompson C et al. Effects of a clinical-practice guideline and practice based education on detection and outcome of depression in primary care: Hampshire Depression Project randomised controlled trial. *The Lancet* 2000, 355:185–191.

85 Rutz W et al. Prevention of depression and suicide by education and medication: impact on male suicidality: an update from the Gotland study 1997. *International Journal of Psychiatry in Clinical Practice*, 1997, 1:39–46.

86 Rihmer Z, Rutz W, Barsi J. Suicide rate, prevalence of diagnosed depression and prevalence of working physicians in Hungary. *Acta Psychiatrica Scandinavica*, 1993, 88:391–394.

87 Rutz W, Von Knorring L, Wålinder J. Frequency of suicide on Gotland after systematic postgraduate education of general practitioners. *Acta Psychiatrica Scandinavica*, 1989, 80:151–154.

88 Rutz W. Preventing suicide and premature death by education and treatment. *Journal of Affective Disorders*, 2001, 62:123–129.

89 Rihmer Z, Belso N, Kalmar S. Antidepressants and suicide prevention in Hungary. *Acta Psychiatrica Scandinavica*, 2001, 103:238–239.

90 Takahashi K et al. Suicide prevention for the elderly in Matsunoyama Town, Higashikubiki County, Niigata Prefecture: psychiatric care for elderly depression in the community [in Japanese]. *Seishin Shinkeigaku Zasshi* 1998, 100:469–485.

91 Marušič A et al. An attempt of suicide prevention: the Slovene Gotland Study. In: Program and abstracts of the 10th European Symposium on Suicide and Suicidal Behavior, August 2004, Copenhagen, Denmark.

92 Chiu HF, Takahashi Y, Suh GH. Elderly suicide prevention in East Asia. *International Journal of Geriatric Psychiatry*, 2003, 18:973–976.

93 Hegerl U, Althaus D, Schmidtke A, Niklewski G. The alliance against depression: 2-year evaluation of a community-based intervention to reduce suicidality. *Psychological Medicine*, 2006, 36:1225–1233.

94 Szanto K et al. A suicide prevention program in a region with a very high suicide rate. *Archives of General Psychiatry*, 2007, 64:914–920.

95 Katon WJ et al, for the IMPACT investigators. Cost-effectiveness of improving primary care treatment of late-life depression. *Archives of General Psychiatry*, 2005, 62:1313–1320.

96 Gilbody S, Whitty P, Grimshaw J, Thomas R. Educational and organizational interventions to improve the management of depression in primary care: a systematic review. *JAMA*, 2003, 289:3145–3151.

97 *Depression: management of depression in primary and secondary care.* London, National Institute for Health and Clinical Excellence, 2004 (CG23) (www.nice.org.uk/CG023, accessed 9 February 2012).

98 Clark DM et al. Improving access to psychological therapy: initial evaluation of two UK demonstration sites. *Behaviour Research and Therapy*, 2009, 47:910–920.

99 *Preventing suicide. A resource for primary health care workers.* Geneva, World Health Organization, 2000 (WHO/MNH/MBD/00.4).

100 Holkup P. *Evidence-based protocol-elderly suicide: secondary prevention*. Iowa City, IA, University of Iowa Gerontological Nursing Interventions Research Center, 2002.

101 Spitzer RL, Kroenke K, Williams JB. Validation and utility of a self report version of PRIME-MD: the PHQ primary care study. *JAMA*, 1999, 282:1737–1744.

102 Goldberg DP et al. *Manual of the General Health Questionnaire*. Windsor, NFER Publishing, 1978.

103 Center C et al. Confronting depression and suicide in physicians: a consensus statement. *JAMA*, 2003, 289:3161–3166.

104 Hartley D, Bird DC, Dempsey P. Rural mental health and substance abuse. In: Ricketts TC ed. *Rural health in the United States*. New York, NY: Oxford University Press Inc., 1999:159–178.

12 The principles of prescribing in primary care mental health

Shameem Mir and Carol Roberts

Key messages

- Prescribing principles underpin the safe and effective use of medicines.
- Safe and effective use of medicines in primary care can have a huge impact on the health economy but there are barriers to prescribing.
- The likely beneficial effect of the medicine should outweigh the extent of any potential harm, and, whenever possible, this judgement should be based on published evidence.
- It is important to communicate clearly with patients, their carers, and colleagues. Patients should be given important information about how to take the medicine. The more the patient knows about their treatment, the more likely they are to follow the treatment plan.
- Rationalization of psychotropic medicines is a simple and effective mechanism for managing side-effects and increasing concordance with the treatment plan.

Introduction

A prescription (℞) is a health-care programme implemented by a medical or non-medical prescriber. The prescription is a set of instructions that govern the accurate dispensing of medicines and the subsequent administration of the right medicine to the right patient, at the right dose, at the right time via the right route, by the patient.

Prescriptions have legal implications, as they may indicate that the prescriber takes responsibility for the clinical care of the patient and, in particular, for monitoring the efficacy and safety of the medicines prescribed.

The concept of prescriptions dates back to the beginning of history. So long as there were medicines and a writing system to capture directions for preparation by the pharmacist and usage by the patient, there were prescriptions.[1]

Prescribing is the main approach to the treatment and prevention of disease and illness. While medicines have the capacity to enhance health, they also have the potential to cause harm if used inappropriately. It is therefore essential that health-care professionals who prescribe medicines should do so based on certain prescribing principles, which underpin the safe and effective use of medicines.

Prescribing principles underpin the safe and effective use of medicines.

At any given time, approximately one in six adults will experience symptoms of mental illness. Mental illness is the largest single cause of disability in our society and costs the English economy at least £77 billion a year.[2]

The majority of people who have mental health problems initially seek help from their general practitioner (GP). Many continue to be treated in primary care, without ever being referred to specialist services. GPs and other health professionals working in primary care therefore need the skills to detect mental health problems and offer the best treatment.

The biopsychosocial model

Primary care health workers can manage mental illness by applying the biopsychosocial model. This is a general model or approach that posits that biological, psychological and social factors all play a significant role in human functioning in the context of disease or illness. Indeed, health is best understood in terms of a combination of biological, psychological and social factors rather than purely in biological terms.[3] This is in contrast to the traditional, reductionist biomedical model of medicine that suggests every disease process can be explained in terms of an underlying deviation from normal function such as a pathogen, genetic or developmental abnormality, or injury.

Complementary and alternative medicines

Complementary and alternative medicines (CAMs) can also be used to treat mental health problems.

These are ways of treating illness that have developed outside the mainstream of modern medicine. Many are traditional remedies that have developed in different cultures over the centuries. They include:

- herbal medicines
- foods
- nutritional supplements, such as vitamins and minerals.

Some of these treatments may work, but most have not been thoroughly tested. The studies have often been too small to give a clear answer. We know most about the treatments for depression, anxiety and insomnia.

Despite the lack of evidence, people all over the world take CAMs, and many report that they find them helpful. Ultimately, whether taking CAMs is a good idea depends on individual circumstances.

All these treatments can be used on their own, or in addition to conventional medicine. Care must be taken when co-prescribing CAMs with conventional medicine, as interactions between the two can occur. An example of this is St John's wort and antidepressants.

Relevance to the delivery of mental health in primary care

The safe and effective use of medicines in primary care could help to reduce the burden on the health economy. Early diagnosis and effective treatment of mental health disorders is likely to reduce the number of unnecessary admissions to hospital. In addition, the safer use of medicines could reduce unnecessary hospital admissions to acute hospitals that are a result of preventable adverse drug reactions.[4,5] The key, therefore, is to achieve the right balance between efficacy and safety of treatment in primary care.

Despite the obvious benefits of prescribing in primary care, there are certain factors that may prevent this from happening. These barriers include a lack of knowledge and experience in the assessment of mental health illnesses, and the use of psychotropic drugs.

Prescribers in primary care are more likely to initiate treatment for the less severe mental illnesses such as anxiety and depression. That said, up until recently, in the United Kingdom of Great Britain and Northern Ireland (UK), depression was often misdiagnosed, and when it was diagnosed, antidepressants (tricyclics) were often prescribed at subtherapeutic levels.[6] Now the situation has changed somewhat and GPs are much more likely to diagnose and effectively treat depression, using adequate doses of antidepressants.

In high-income countries, treatment of the more severe mental illnesses such as schizophrenia and bipolar disorder is more likely to be started in secondary care. However, prescribers in lower-income countries, who are usually primary care prescribers, are expected to initiate and continue treatment in the community and monitor for efficacy and safety.

Substance misuse can be managed effectively in primary care. People with addictions and chaotic lifestyles need easy access to care. High-income countries have government funding for clinics and "one-stop" shops for people with addictions, who more often than not do not have GPs. Low- and middle-income countries will have less funding. The stigma attached to this patient group and those with mental illnesses exists worldwide.

Barriers to prescribing in primary care include budgetary restrictions and formularies, although local formularies can also act as an aid to prescribing (see later). In low-income countries, where funding for medicines is limited, there is a need for international agreement on a limited formulary, for example, the World Health Organization (WHO) essential list of medicines.[7]

In higher-income countries, stigma is another barrier to treating mental illness in primary care. The stigma may lie with either the patient or their family, who are embarrassed to seek help, or with the prescriber who is not comfortable treating people with a mental illness.

In the UK, non-medical prescribing (NMP) can have a huge impact on the access to treatment in primary care. In low-income countries, NMP-led clinics could provide outreach assessment and treatment for people with mental health problems.

Safe and effective use of medicines in primary care can have a huge impact on the health economy but there are barriers to prescribing.

Principles of prescribing

In lower-income countries, health-care professionals other than qualified medical doctors may prescribe medicines routinely (even though they are not officially regarded as qualified prescribers). In higher-income countries, only qualified prescribers can prescribe medicines. Prescribers in the UK fall into two categories: medical prescribers, for example medical doctors with a 5–6-year medical training, and non-medical prescribers.

Non-medical prescribers

The Department of Health (DH) in the UK predicted that by October 2009, over 14 000 nurse independent prescribers, 1700 pharmacist independent and supplementary prescribers, many thousands of community practitioner nurse prescribers, and hundreds of allied health-care professional (AHP) prescribers would have qualified to prescribe within their competence.[8]

Enabling AHPs such as nurses, pharmacists, physiotherapists, radiographers, optometrists and podiatrists to become qualified non-medical prescribers (NMPs) allows patients improved access to medicines more quickly and efficiently.[9] The perceived benefits for patients have been defined as:[10]

- an avoidance of a delay in receiving medicines
- a reduction in the amount of unnecessary appointments
- reduced risk of hospitalization and faster recovery
- all leading to an increased level of value for money.

NMPs provides a means of promoting individual professional development as well as opportunities to develop innovative patient-focused services within health-providing organizations. In order to achieve the safe and effective development and implementation of NMP services, there is a need to have in place:

- governance structures/arrangements
- appropriate infrastructure
- stakeholder engagement
- adherence to national policy, professional body and legal standards of best practice
- continuous professional development.

Once NMP can be established in accordance with the above, this can then aid an organization in its ability to comply with the necessary patient safety standards and enhance service-delivery options.

The principles underpinning safe and effective prescribing fall into two broad categories: technical and clinical, which are discussed in the next sections.

Medicines can also be supplied via a *patient group direction* (PGD). In essence, a PGD is the supply or administration of a specified medicine(s), by named authorized health professionals, to a well-defined group of patients requiring treatment for the condition stated in the PGD. A PGD may be drawn up locally by doctors (or dentists), pharmacists and other health professionals but must meet certain legal criteria.[11]

Technical principles of prescribing

These principles can be applied to every prescription and are not influenced by patient factors.

- *Generic prescribing*: use generic drug names not trade names. This avoids confusion and decreases risk during the dispensing and administration processes. It also ensures economic prescribing, as branded medicines are likely to be more expensive.
- *Legible handwriting*: prescriptions, when handwritten, are notorious for often being illegible. Sloppy handwriting causes dispensing errors and can kill. Some countries have advocated the use of computer-generated prescriptions. Where this is not possible, prescriptions must be written in block capital letters, leaving no room for ambiguity.
- *Use of decimal points*: be careful when using decimal points:
  - avoid unnecessary decimal points: prescribe 5 ml instead of 5.0 ml, to avoid possible misinterpretation of 5.0 as 50.
  - always using zero prefix decimals: e.g. 0.5 instead of .5, to avoid misinterpretation of .5 as 5
  - avoiding trailing zeros on decimals: e.g. 0.5 instead of .50, to avoid misinterpretation of .50 as 50.
- *Volumes*: always use "ml" instead of "cc" even though they are technically equivalent, to avoid misinterpretation of "c" as "0". Avoid prescribing units such as "teaspoons" or "tablespoons".
- *Strengths*: prescribe units of strength clearly: mg, mcg, gram; always write "gram" in full.
- *Units*: when prescribing units of a drug, for example insulin, always write "units" in full. Abbreviations, such as "U" or "IU" should never be used, as they can be misread as a zero.
- *Abbreviations*: do not use abbreviations for names of medicines, as many are ambiguous and may be confused with something else. Abbreviations are commonly used for directions, and acceptable abbreviations are listed below:
  - ac – ante cibum (before food)
  - bd – bis die (twice daily)
  - od – omne die (once daily)
  - om – omni mane (every morning)
  - on – omni nocte (every night)
  - tds – ter die sumendus (to be taken three times daily
  - tid – ter in die (three times daily)
  - pc – post cibum (after food)
  - prn – pro re nata (when required)
  - qds – quater die sumendus (to be taken four times daily
  - stat – statim (immediately, at once).
- *Use permanent ink*: always use permanent indelible ink for prescriptions.
- *Sign and date prescriptions*: all prescriptions must be signed and dated by the prescriber.

Clinical principles of prescribing

The approach will be the same for every patient but choices will differ depending on each individual.

Reasons for prescribing

Establish an accurate diagnosis whenever possible (although this may often be difficult).

Be clear in what way the patient is likely to gain from the prescribed medicines. A prescribing decision does not always end in the prescription of a medicine. It may be a decision not to prescribe or to use non-drug interventions. Social prescribing is an example of this.[12] The most common examples of social prescribing are primary care-based projects that refer at-risk or vulnerable patients to a specific programme: for example, exercise on prescription, prescription for learning, and arts on prescription.

Medication history

Obtain an accurate list of current and recent medications (including over-the-counter and alternative medicines); prior adverse drug reactions; and drug allergies from the patient, their carers or colleagues. Establish reasons for stopping previous medicines; it is important to differentiate between discontinuing treatment because of a lack of efficacy or because of intolerable side-effects.

If an adequate response was not seen with a trial with a particular drug, there would be little benefit in restarting the same drug. Indeed, a different class of drugs should be considered. For example, a poor response to fluoxetine would indicate a probable poor response to another selective serotonin reuptake inhibitor (SSRI).

If a drug was discontinued due to "side-effects", it is essential to establish exactly what side-effects were experienced, before choosing another medicine. For example, if a patient previously on a typical antipsychotic drug stopped taking their medicine because they were experiencing impotence due to raised prolactin levels, it would be prudent to choose an antipsychotic that had less propensity to raise prolactin levels.

Current clinical status

Consider other individual factors that might influence the prescription, for example, physiological changes with age and pregnancy, or impaired kidney, liver, heart or thyroid function. Other special patients groups must also be considered, such as those with diabetes, epilepsy, Parkinson disease or dementia. Special consideration must also be given to those that are breastfeeding.

Before starting psychotropic medicines, a full blood count should be undertaken to establish baseline renal and liver function. Impaired liver or renal function may be an indication for using lower doses and choosing medicines with a shorter half-life. Other essential baseline tests include weight, blood pressure and blood glucose (depending on the choice of medicine).

Thyroid function should be assessed before starting lithium, and some antipsychotic drugs require a baseline electrocardiogram (ECG).

Select safe, effective and cost-effective medicines

The likely beneficial effect of the medicine should outweigh the extent of any potential harm, and, whenever possible, this judgement should be based on published evidence.

Higher-income countries will be more likely to have a wider range of available medicines, compared with middle- to lower-income countries. This may limit the application of evidence-based medicine. That said, even in higher-income countries, the availability of medicines can be limited and where "all things are equal", use of the cheapest available medicine is encouraged. This is usually implemented by the enforcement of local formularies. Primary care formularies are invaluable in ensuring similarities in cost-effective and evidence-based choice of medicines across the health economy. These should reflect prescribing choices in secondary care, so that medicines are not chopped and changed when people are admitted to or discharged from hospital.

Once the right medicine has been selected, choose the best formulation, dose, frequency, route of administration, and duration of treatment for that patient.

Medicines are sometimes prescribed outside of their product licence, "off-label", or outside standard practice. The prescriber must first be satisfied that an alternative medicine would not meet the patient's needs (this decision will be based on evidence and/or experience of their safety and efficacy).

Communicate and document prescribing decisions and the reasons for them

Communicate clearly with patients, their carers and colleagues. Give patients important information about how to take the medicine, what benefits might arise, adverse effects (especially those that will require urgent review), and any monitoring that is required. The more the patient knows about their treatment, the more likely they are to follow the treatment plan. Patients should be involved in the decision-making process about the choice of medicine. Seek to form a partnership with the patient when selecting treatments, making sure that they understand and agree with the reasons for taking the medicine.

All verbal information should be backed up by written information. For those that cannot read, information can be given in the form of drawings. Carers should also be given the information, to back up the knowledge of the patient.

Use the health record and other means to document prescribing decisions accurately. Poor documentation can lead to prescribing errors in the future. Prescribing and monitoring plans must be clear so that other healthcare professionals involved in the care of the patient can follow them.

Monitoring the beneficial and adverse effects of medicines

Initiating treatment

Once the correct medicine has been selected, the prescriber must have knowledge of how to initiate treatment safely. Most psychotropic drugs require titration so that initial adverse effects are minimized. Side-effects that commonly necessitate titration are sedation and hypotension.

Prescribers also need to know how long they should wait before increasing the dose. For example, in general, this is at least 2 weeks for oral antipsychotics and 2 months for depot antipsychotics. Knowledge around the time to response is also required, to inform decisions made around changing treatment due to inefficacy. This is also important when explaining to the patient when they might expect to feel better, so that patients' and carers' expectations are realistic and compliance encouraged.

The aim of any treatment is maximum benefit with minimum side-effects. The dose should not be increased too quickly, as one risks missing the minimum effective dose and causing unnecessary side-effects. This will be discussed in more detail later on.

Maintaining treatment

Once a maintenance dose is reached, the prescriber must identify how the beneficial and adverse effects of treatment can be assessed. For example, use rating scales to assess efficacy and side-effects. In addition to rating scales, appropriate physical health monitoring to assess safety of treatment will also have to be undertaken.

Monitoring the benefits

Recognized rating scales are available, and are a useful indicator to assess the efficacy of a particular drug. Some of these are listed in Table 12.1.

Monitoring the side-effects

Prescribers must have knowledge of adverse effects of medicines and report these using the available reporting mechanisms (in the UK via the Yellow Card scheme).

Table 12.1 Rating scales	
Diagnosis	**Rating scale**
Anxiety	Hamilton Anxiety Rating Scale (HAM-A)[13]
Depression	Montgomery Asperg Depression Rating Scale[14]
	Hamilton Rating Scale for Depression[15]
	The Beck Depression Inventory (BDI)[16] is a useful self-rating scale
Psychosis	Brief Psychiatric Rating Scale (BPRS)[17]
Mania	Young's Mania Rating Scale[18]

For side-effects of antipsychotic drugs, the following rating scales are well recognized:

- Glasgow Antipsychotic Side-effect Scale (GASS)[19]
- Side-Effects Scale/Checklist for Antipsychotic Medication (SESCAM)[20]
- Abnormal Involuntary Movement Scale (AIMS)[21]
- Barnes Akathisia Scale (BAS)[22]
- Liverpool University Neuroleptic Side-effect Rating Scale (LUNSERS).[23]

Therapeutic drug monitoring

Therapeutic drug monitoring is required for the safe use of lithium and to establish therapeutic doses of other drugs, such as clozapine and carbamazepine. Prescribers need to understand how to alter the prescription as a result of this information.

Avoid polypharmacy

For the purpose of this chapter, polypharmacy refers to the use of more than one drug for the same indication. Wherever possible, only one drug should be prescribed to treat an illness. This should be tried at a therapeutic dose for an appropriate length of time. If there is no response to the first drug, then a second drug should be selected, preferably from a different class. The second drug can often be started while the first drug is being withdrawn. In the majority of cases, very little benefit will be derived from using the two drugs at the same time, but the side-effects will almost definitely increase.

Rationalization of medicines

Rationalization of psychotropic medicines is a simple and effective mechanism for managing side-effects and increasing concordance with the treatment plan. Some examples are given below.

- Use once-daily dosing where possible. This simplifies medicines regimes and patients are less likely to miss a dose.
- For medicines with sedative properties, where daytime sedation is not desirable, wherever possible, prescribe as a single dose at night. This will reduce unwanted daytime sedation caused by sedative morning and lunch-time doses. If the patient is having trouble sleeping, giving a sedative medicine at night may prevent the need for prescribing a hypnotic and hence reduce the number of medicines prescribed.
- Prescribe morning doses for medicines that may have an effect on sleep, for example, SSRIs or anticholinergic drugs like procyclidine.
- Be aware of the additive side-effects of medicines. Many psychotropic drugs are hypotensive, sedative and anticholinergic. Prescribing more than one drug that has the same side-effect will cause additive side-effects.

Discontinuation of psychotropic drugs

Psychotropic drugs should not be discontinued abruptly; in general, the longer the treatment duration, the longer the time for discontinuation.

Discontinuation syndrome is well known when antidepressants are stopped suddenly. Symptoms can include anxiety, confusion and sweating.[24,25] It is more common with antidepressants with a short half-life, e.g. paroxetine. Fluoxetine is probably the only antidepressant that can be stopped abruptly, as it has a long half-life (4 weeks).

Withdrawal symptoms from antipsychotics may emerge during dosage reduction and discontinuation. Withdrawal symptoms can include nausea, emesis, anorexia, diarrhoea, rhinorrhoea, diaphoresis, myalgia, paresthesia, anxiety, agitation, restlessness and insomnia. The psychological withdrawal symptoms can include psychosis, and can be mistaken for a relapse of the underlying disorder. Conversely, the withdrawal syndrome may also be a trigger for relapse. Better management of the withdrawal syndrome may improve the ability of individuals to discontinue antipsychotic drugs.[26]

If lithium is discontinued abruptly, then the time to relapse is shorter than if it is gradually withdrawn.[27,28] Withdrawal of the different psychotropic drugs is discussed in more detail later in the chapter.

The above principles can be applied when prescribing any psychotropic drug. There are more specific principles underpinning the treatment of particular mental illnesses. Those for anxiety, depression, schizophrenia and bipolar disorder are discussed next.

Treatment of anxiety

General principles

Before prescribing, consider:

- age
- previous treatment response
- risks of deliberate self-harm or accidental overdose
- tolerability
- patient preference
- cost, where there is equal effectiveness.

Benzodiazepines

All guidelines and consensus statements recommend that this group of drugs should only be used to treat anxiety that is severe, disabling, or subjecting the individual to extreme distress. Because of their potential to cause physical dependence and withdrawal symptoms, these drugs should be used at the lowest effective dose for the shortest period of time (maximum 4 weeks), while medium-/long-term strategies are put in place. The National Institute for Health and Clinical Excellence (NICE) recommend that *benzodiazepines should not be used to treat panic disorder.*[29]

If benzodiazepines are prescribed for more than 4 weeks, they cannot be stopped immediately, as the patient may suffer withdrawal symptoms. Gradual withdrawal of benzodiazepines is prudent after long-term use. In general, short-acting benzodiazepines are replaced by longer-acting ones such as diazepam, and then the dose reduced gradually over weeks or months.

SSRIs – dose and duration of treatment

When used to treat generalized anxiety disorder (GAD) and panic disorder, SSRIs should initially be prescribed at half the normal starting dose for the treatment of depression. A response is usually seen within 6 weeks and continues to increase over time.

NICE (UK) guidance for the treatment of panic disorder and generalized anxiety[29]

Management of panic disorder

Following discussion with the patient and taking account of patient preference, offer (interventions are listed in descending order of evidence for the longest duration of effect):

- psychological therapy, or
- pharmacological therapy, or
- self-help.

Psychological therapy

- Cognitive-behavioural therapy (CBT) should be used. It should be delivered by trained and supervised people, closely adhering to empirically grounded treatment protocols. For most people, CBT should be in weekly sessions of 1–2 hours and be completed within 4 months.
- The optimal range is 7–14 hours in total. If offering briefer CBT, it should be about 7 hours, should be designed to integrate with structured self-help materials, and should be supplemented with appropriate

focused information and tasks. Sometimes, more intensive CBT over a very short period might be appropriate.

- Use short, self-complete questionnaires to monitor outcomes wherever possible.

Pharmacological therapy

- Offer an SSRI that is licensed for panic disorder, unless otherwise indicated. If an SSRI is not suitable or there is no improvement after a 12-week course, and if further medication is appropriate, consider imipramine or clomipramine. Although the latter two antidepressants are not licensed for the treatment of panic disorder, they have been shown to be effective in its management.
- Inform patients, at the time treatment is started about:
  - potential side-effects, including transient increase in anxiety at the start of treatment
  - possible discontinuation/withdrawal symptoms (see later)
  - the expected delay in onset of effect
  - the time course of treatment
  - the need to take medicines as prescribed, particularly with medicines with a short half-life, in order to avoid discontinuation/withdrawal symptoms.
- Review every 8–12 weeks if treatment is for more than 12 weeks.
- Written information appropriate for the patient's needs should be made available. Side-effects when starting may be minimized by starting at a low dose and slowly increasing the dose until a satisfactory response is achieved.
- Long-term treatment and doses at the upper end of the indicated dose range may be necessary.
- Benzodiazepines, sedating antihistamines or antipsychotics should not be prescribed for the treatment of panic disorder.

Self-help

- Offer bibliotherapy based on CBT principles.
- Offer information about support groups where available.
- Discuss the benefits of exercise as part of good general health.

Management of generalized anxiety

Psychological therapy

- CBT should be used.
- It should be delivered by trained and supervised people, closely adhering to empirically grounded treatment protocols:
  - for most people, CBT should be in weekly sessions of 1–2 hours and be completed within 4 months
  - the optimal range is 16–20 hours in total
  - if offering briefer CBT, it should be about 8–10 hours, should be designed to integrate with structured self-help materials, and should be supplemented with appropriate focused information and tasks.

Pharmacological therapy

- Offer an SSRI, unless otherwise indicated.
- If one SSRI is not suitable or there is no improvement after a 12-week course, and if further medication is appropriate, another SSRI should be offered.
- Inform patients, at the time treatment is initiated about:
  - potential side-effects (including transient increase in anxiety at the start of treatment)
  - possible discontinuation/withdrawal symptoms

- the expected delay in onset of effect
- the time-course of treatment
- the need to take medication as prescribed (this may be particularly important with short half-life medication, in order to avoid discontinuation/withdrawal symptoms).
  - Written information appropriate for the patient's needs should be made available.
  - Side-effects on initiation may be minimized by starting at a low dose and slowly increasing the dose until a satisfactory therapeutic response is achieved.
  - Long-term treatment and doses at the upper end of the indicated dose range may be necessary.

Self-help

- Offer bibliotherapy based on CBT principles.
- Consider large-group CBT.
- Offer information about support groups, where available.
- Discuss the benefits of exercise as part of good general health.
- Computerized CBT may be of value, but a NICE technology appraisal found the evidence was an insufficient basis on which to recommend its general introduction into the UK National Health Service (NHS).[30]

Treatment of depression

General principles

Which antidepressant?

Choose an antidepressant according to national or local guidance and initiate at the starting or minimum effective dose. All the main antidepressants appear to have a broadly similar efficacy, although there may be some differences, but there are differences in side-effect profile (see Table 12.2)[31] and therefore acceptability.

A meta-analysis by Cipriani et al. compared the efficacy of bupropion, citalopram, duloxetine, escitalopram, fluoxetine, fluvoxamine, milnacipran, mirtazapine, paroxetine, reboxetine, sertraline and venlafaxine for the acute treatment of unipolar depression. The authors concluded that (see Table 12.3):[32]

- escitalopram, mirtazapine, venlafaxine and sertraline were significantly more efficacious than duloxetine, fluoxetine, fluvoxamine, paroxetine and reboxetine
- escitalopram and sertraline showed the best profile of acceptability, leading to significantly fewer discontinuations than duloxetine, fluvoxamine, paroxetine, reboxetine and venlafaxine
- clinically important differences exist, both in efficacy and acceptability, in favour of escitalopram and sertraline. Sertraline, however, might be the best first choice because it has the most favourable balance between benefits, acceptability and cost.

Special patient characteristics

Sex

Note that women have a poorer toleration of imipramine.

Age

- For older adults with depression, give antidepressant treatment at an age-appropriate dose for a minimum of 6 weeks before considering that it is ineffective. If there is a partial response within this period, treatment should be continued for a further 6 weeks.
- When prescribing antidepressants for older adults, consider:
  - the increased risk of drug interactions
  - careful monitoring of side-effects, particularly with tricyclic antidepressants.

Table 12.2 Antidepressants – relative side-effects

Drug	Adult max dose mg/day	Elderly max dose mg/day	Anticholinergic	Cardiac	Nausea+	Sedation	Overdose	Proconvulsant	Sexual dysfunction
Amitriptyline	200	75	●●●	●●●	●●	●●●	●●●	●●	●●
Clomipramine	250	75	●●●	●●	●●	●●	●	●●	●●●
Dosulepin (dothiepin)	150	75	●●	●●	○	●●●	●●●	●●	●●
Doxepin	300	<Ad	●	●●	●	●●	●●	●●	●●
Imipramine	300	50	●●	●●	●●	●	●●●	●●	●●
Lofepramine	210	<Ad	●●	●	●	●	○	○	●
Nortriptyline	150	50	●●	●	●●	●	●●	●	●●
Trimipramine	300	<Ad	●●●	●●	●	●●	●●	●●	●●
SSRIs									
Citalopram	60	40	○	○	●●	○	●	○	●●
Escitalopram	20	<20	○	○	●●	○	○	○	●●
Fluoxetine	(20)	(80)	○	○	●●	○	○	○	●
Fluvoxamine	300	300	●	○	●●●	●	○	○	●●●
Paroxetine	50	40	○	○	●●	○	○	○	●●●
Sertraline	200	200	○	○	●●	○	○	○	●●
MAOIs									
Isocarboxazid	60	<Ad	●●	●●	●●	○	●●	○	●
Phenelzine	90	(90)	●	●	●●	●	●●●	○	●
Tranylcypromine	CA30	(30)	●	●	●●	●	●●●	○	●

continued overleaf

Table 12.2 Antidepressants – relative side-effects – *continued*

Others	Adult max dose mg/day	Elderly max dose mg/day	Anticholinergic	Cardiac	Nausea+	Sedation	Overdose	Proconvulsant	Sexual dysfunction
Agomelatine	50	50?	○	○	○	○	○	○	○
Bupropion/ amfebutamone (U)	–	–	●	○	●	○	●●	●●●	○
Duloxetine	120	Caution	○	○	●●	●	?	?	●●
Flupentixol	3	2	●●	○	○	●	●	?	●
Mianserin	90+	<Ad	●	○	○	●●●	○	○	●
Mirtazapine	45	45	○	○	○	●●	○	●●	●●
Moclobemide	600	600	●	○	●	○	○	?	●
Reboxetine	12	NR	●	●	●	○	○	○	○
Trazodone	600	+300	●	●	●●●	●●	●	○	●●
Tryptophan	6000 (6 g)	6000 (6 g)	○	○	●	●●	●	○	○
Venlafaxine	Plain 375 XL>225	Same	○	●●	●●	●	●●	●	●●

Reproduced, with permission from Bazire S. *Psychotropic drug directory*, Aberdeen, HealthComm UK, Ltd., 2010.[31]

●●● = marked effect

●● = moderate effect

● = mild effect

○ = little or minimal effect

? = no information or little reported

U = unlicensed in the UK for depression

+ = typical serotonergic side-effect

Ad = adult dose

CA = care above

MAOI = monoamine oxidase inhibitor.

Adult max dose = maximum adult oral antidepressant dose in UK summaries of product characteristics (SPCs).

Elderly max dose = maximum elderly oral antidepressant dose as stated in UK SPC. Most state that half the adult dose may be sufficient.

Overdose = based on the UK Fatal Toxicity Index.[33] For review of epidemiology and relative toxicity of antidepressant drugs in overdose see Henry 1997.[34]

Table 12.3 Rankings of the top antidepressants for efficacy and cost-effectiveness.

	Efficacy	Cost-effectiveness	
		Moderate depression	Severe depression
1	Mirtazapine	Mirtazapine	Mirtazapine
2	Escitalopram	Sertraline	Sertraline
3	Venlafaxine	Escitalopram	Escitalopram
4	Sertraline	Citalopram	Citalopram
5	Citalopram	Venlafaxine	Venlafaxine
6	Paroxetine	Paroxetine	Paroxetine
7	Fluoxetine	Fluoxetine	Fluoxetine
8	Duloxetine	Fluvoxamine	Duloxetine
9	Fluvoxamine	Duloxetine	Fluvoxamine
10	Reboxetine	Reboxetine	Reboxetine

Reproduced from Cipriani et al. Comparative efficacy and acceptability of 12 new-generation antidepressants: a multiple-treatments meta-analysis. *The Lancet*, 2009, 373:746–758, with permission from Elsevier.[32]

Patients with dementia

- Treat depression in people with dementia in the same way as depression in other older adults.

Patients with cardiovascular disease

- When initiating antidepressant treatment in patients with ischaemic heart disease, note that sertraline has the best evidence base.
- Consider the increased risks associated with tricyclic antidepressants in patients with cardiovascular disease.
- Perform an ECG before prescribing a tricyclic antidepressant for a depressed patient at significant risk of cardiovascular disease.
- Venlafaxine should not be prescribed for patients with pre-existing heart disease.

Partial or no response to initial antidepressant treatment

Pharmacological approaches

- If a patient fails to respond to the first antidepressant prescribed, check that the drug has been taken regularly and at the prescribed dose.
- If the response to a standard dose of an antidepressant is inadequate, and there are no significant side-effects, consider a gradual increase in dose in line with the schedule suggested by the SPC.
- Consider switching to another antidepressant if there has been no response after a month. If there has been a partial response, a decision to switch can be postponed until 6 weeks.
- If an antidepressant has not been effective or is poorly tolerated and, after considering a range of other treatment options, the decision is made to offer a further course of antidepressants, then switch to another single antidepressant.
- Choices for a second antidepressant include a different SSRI or mirtazapine; alternatives include moclobemide, reboxetine and tricyclic antidepressants (except dosulepin) (but see below).

- When switching from one antidepressant to another, be aware of the need for gradual and modest incremental increases of dose, of interactions between antidepressants, and the risk of serotonin syndrome when combinations of serotonergic antidepressants are prescribed. Features include confusion, delirium, shivering, sweating, changes in blood pressure and myoclonus.

Swapping and stopping antidepressants

- Inform patients about the possibility of discontinuation symptoms on stopping or missing doses or reducing the dose. These symptoms are usually mild and self-limiting but can occasionally be severe, particularly if the drug is stopped abruptly.
- Advise patients to take their drugs as prescribed, particularly drugs with a shorter half-life (such as paroxetine).
- Reduce doses gradually over a 4-week period; some people may require longer periods, and fluoxetine can usually be stopped over a shorter period.
- For mild discontinuation/withdrawal symptoms, reassure the patient and monitor symptoms.
- For severe symptoms, consider reintroducing the original antidepressant at the effective dose (or another antidepressant with a longer half-life from the same class) and reduce gradually while monitoring symptoms.
- Ask patients to seek advice from their medical practitioner if they experience significant discontinuation/withdrawal symptoms.
- Discontinuation symptoms are discussed in more detail in the next section "Discontinuation of antidepressant therapy".

Special considerations when switching to a new antidepressant other than a tricyclic

- If switching to mirtazapine, be aware that it can cause sedation and weight gain.
- If switching to moclobemide, be aware of the need to wash out previously prescribed antidepressants.
- If switching to reboxetine, be aware of its relative lack of data on side-effects, and monitor carefully.

Special considerations when switching to a new tricyclic antidepressant

- Consider their poorer tolerability compared with other equally effective antidepressants, and the increased risk of cardiotoxicity and toxicity in overdose.
- Start on a low dose and, if there is a clear clinical response, maintain on that dose with careful monitoring.
- Gradually increase the dose if there is a lack of efficacy and no major side-effects.
- Lofepramine is a reasonable choice because of its relative lack of cardiotoxicity.

For guidance on how to swap from one antidepressant to another, see Table 12.4.

Discontinuation of antidepressant therapy

When discontinuing therapy, the dose should be gradually reduced over a minimum of 4 weeks. Discontinuation syndromes have been reported for nearly all antidepressants, but in particular paroxetine and venlafaxine. Discontinuation symptoms usually appear within 1 to 5 days of stopping treatment, depending on the half-life of the antidepressant stopped – the shorter the half-life, the shorter the time to onset of symptoms. Discontinuation symptoms can improve within a week, although they can last longer.

Discontinuation symptoms may be entirely new or similar to some of the original symptoms of the illness, and can often be mistaken for the recurrence of depression, which begins after 3 weeks and continues to worsen.

Discontinuation symptoms can be broadly divided into five categories:

- affective, e.g. irritability
- gastrointestinal, e.g. nausea
- neuromotor, e.g. ataxia

Table 12.4 Antidepressants – swapping and stopping

To \ From	MAOIs – hydrazines	Tranyl-cypromine	Tricyclics	Citalopram/ Escitalopram	Paroxetine	Fluoxetine	Sertraline	Trazodone	Moclobemide	Reboxetine	Venlafaxine	Mirtazapine	Duloxetine	Agomelatine
MAOIs – hydrazines		Taper and stop then wait for 2 weeks	Taper and stop then wait for 2 weeks	Taper and stop then wait for 2 weeks	Taper and stop then wait for 2 weeks	Taper and stop then wait for 2 weeks	Taper and stop then wait for 2 weeks	Taper and stop then wait for 2 weeks	Taper and stop then wait for 2 weeks	Taper and stop then wait for 2 weeks	Taper and stop then wait for 2 weeks	Taper and stop then wait for 2 weeks	Taper and stop then wait for 2 weeks	Cross-taper cautiously
Tranylcypromine	Taper and stop then wait for 2 weeks		Taper and stop then wait for 2 weeks	Taper and stop then wait for 2 weeks	Taper and stop then wait for 2 weeks	Taper and stop then wait for 2 weeks	Taper and stop then wait for 2 weeks	Taper and stop then wait for 2 weeks	Taper and stop then wait for 2 weeks	Taper and stop then wait for 2 weeks	Taper and stop then wait for 2 weeks	Taper and stop then wait for 2 weeks	Taper and stop then wait for 2 weeks	Cross-taper cautiously
Tricyclics	Taper and stop then wait for 2 weeks	Taper and stop then wait for 2 weeks	Cross-taper cautiously	Halve dose and add citalopram, then slow withdrawal	Halve dose and add paroxetine then slow withdrawal	Halve dose and add fluoxetine then slow withdrawal	Halve dose and add sertraline, then slow withdrawal	Halve dose and add trazodone, then slow withdrawal	Taper and stop then wait for 1 week	Cross-taper cautiously	Cross-taper cautiously, starting with venlafaxine 37.5 mg/day	Cross-taper cautiously	Cross-taper cautiously, start at 30 mg/day. Increase very slowly	Cross-taper cautiously
Citalopram/ Escitalopram	Taper and stop then wait for 1 week	Taper and stop then wait for 1 week	Cross-taper cautiously			Taper and stop then start fluoxetine at 10 mg/day	Taper and stop then start sertraline at 25 mg/day	Cross-taper cautiously starting with low-dose trazodone	Taper and stop then wait for 1 week	Cross-taper cautiously	Cross-taper cautiously; starting with venlafaxine 37.5 mg/day and increase very slowly	Cross-taper cautiously	Abrupt switch possible. Start at 60 mg/day	Cross-taper cautiously
Paroxetine	Taper and stop then wait for 2 weeks	Taper and stop then wait for 1 week	Cross-taper cautiously with very low dose of tricyclic	Taper and stop then start citalopram at 10 mg/day		Taper and stop then start fluoxetine at 10 mg/day	Taper and stop then start sertraline at 25 mg/day	Cross-taper cautiously starting with low-dose trazodone	Taper and stop then wait for 1 week	Cross-taper cautiously	Cross-taper cautiously; start venlafaxine 37.5 mg/day and increase very slowly	Cross-taper cautiously	Abrupt switch possible; start at 60 mg/day	Cross-taper cautiously
Fluoxetine	Taper and stop then wait for 5–6 weeks	Taper and stop then wait for 5–6 weeks	Taper and stop fluoxetine. Wait 4–7 days. Start tricyclic at a very low dose and increase very slowly	Taper and stop fluoxetine; wait 4–7 days. Start citalopram at 10 mg/day and increase slowly	Taper and stop fluoxetine; wait 4–7 days. Start paroxetine at 10 mg/day and increase slowly		Taper and stop fluoxetine; wait 4–7 days. Start sertraline 25 mg/day and increase slowly	Cross-taper cautiously starting with low-dose trazodone	Taper and stop then wait at least 5 weeks	Cross-taper cautiously	Taper and stop. Start venlafaxine at 37.5 mg/day. Increase very slowly	Cross-taper cautiously. Start mirtazapine at 15 mg/day	Abrupt switch possible; start at 60 mg/day	Cross-taper cautiously

continued overleaf

Table 12.4 Antidepressants – swapping and stopping – *continued*

From / To	MAOIs – hydrazines	Tranyl-cypromine	Tricyclics	Citalopram/ Escitalopram	Paroxetine	Fluoxetine	Sertraline	Trazodone	Moclobemide	Reboxetine	Venlafaxine	Mirtazapine	Duloxetine	Agomelatine
Sertraline	Taper and stop then wait for 1 week.	Taper and stop then wait for 1 week	Cross-taper cautiously with very low dose of tricyclic	Taper and stop then start citalopram at 10 mg/day	Taper and stop then start paroxetine at 10 mg/day	Taper and stop then start fluoxetine at 10 mg/day		Cross-taper cautiously starting with low-dose trazodone	Taper and stop then wait for 1 week	Cross-taper cautiously	Cross-taper cautiously. Start venlafaxine at 37.5 mg/day. Increase very slowly	Cross-taper cautiously	Abrupt switch possible. Start at 60 mg/day	Cross-taper cautiously
Trazodone	Taper and stop then wait for at least 1 week	Taper and stop then wait at least 1 week	Cross-taper cautiously with very low dose of tricyclic	Cross-taper cautiously. Start citalopram at 10 mg/day	Cross-taper cautiously. Start paroxetine at 10 mg/day	Cross-taper cautiously. Start fluoxetine at 10 mg/day	Cross-taper cautiously. Start sertraline at 25 mg/day		Taper and stop then wait at least 1 week	Cross-taper cautiously	Cross-taper cautiously; start venlafaxine at 37.5 mg/day	Cross-taper cautiously	Cross-taper cautiously, start at 30 mg/day. Increase slowly	Cross-taper cautiously
Moclobemide	Taper and wait 24 hours	Taper and stop then wait 24 hours	Taper and stop then wait 24 hours	Taper and stop then wait 24 hours	Taper and stop then wait 24 hours	Taper and stop then wait 24 hours	Taper and stop then wait 24 hours	Taper and stop then wait 24 hours		Taper and stop then wait 24 hours	Taper and stop then wait 24 hours	Taper and stop then wait 24 hours	Taper and stop then wait 24 hours	Cross-taper cautiously
Reboxetine	Taper and wait for at least 1 week	Taper and stop then wait at least 1 week	Cross-taper cautiously	Cross-taper cautiously	Cross-taper cautiously	Cross-taper cautiously	Cross-taper cautiously	Cross-taper cautiously	Taper and stop then wait at least 1 week		Cross-taper cautiously	Cross-taper cautiously	Cross-taper cautiously	Cross-taper cautiously
Venlafaxine	Taper and stop and then wait at least 1 week	Taper and stop then wait at least 1 week	Cross-taper cautiously with very low dose of tricyclic	Cross-taper cautiously. Start citalopram at 10 mg/day	Cross-taper cautiously. Start paroxetine at 10 mg/day	Cross-taper cautiously. Start fluoxetine at 10 mg/day	Cross-taper cautiously. Start sertraline at 25 mg/day	Cross-taper cautiously	Taper and stop then wait at least 1 week	Cross-taper cautiously		Cross-taper cautiously	Taper and stop, start at 30 mg/day. Increase slowly	Cross-taper cautiously

Mirtazapine	Taper and stop then wait for 2 weeks	Taper and stop then wait for 2 weeks	Cross-taper cautiously with very low dose of tricyclic	Cross-taper cautiously	Cross-taper cautiously	Cross-taper cautiously	Cross-taper cautiously	Cross-taper cautiously	Taper and stop then wait for 1 week	Cross-taper cautiously	Cross-taper cautiously	Cross-taper cautiously	Cross-taper cautiously, start at 30 mg/day. Increase slowly	Cross-taper cautiously
Duloxetine	Taper and stop then wait at least 5 days	Taper and stop then wait at least 5 days	Cross-taper cautiously with very low dose of tricyclic	Cross-taper cautiously. Start citalopram at 10 mg/day	Taper and stop then start paroxetine	Taper and stop then start fluoxetine	Cross-taper cautiously. Start sertraline at 25 mg/day	Cross-taper cautiously starting with low-dose trazodone	Taper and stop then wait at least 5 days	Cross-taper cautiously	Taper and stop then start venlafaxine	Cross-taper cautiously		Cross-taper cautiously
Agomelatine	Stop agomelatine then start MAOI	Stop agomelatine then start tranylcypromine	Stop agomelatine then start tricyclic	Stop agomelatine then start citalopram	Stop agomelatine then start paroxetine	Stop agomelatine then start fluoxetine	Stop agomelatine then start sertraline	Stop agomelatine then start trazodone	Stop agomelatine then start moclobemide	Stop agomelatine then start reboxetine	Stop agomelatine then start venlafaxine	Stop agomelatine then start mirtazapine	Stop agomelatine then start duloxetine	Cross-taper cautiously
Stopping	Reduce over 4 weeks	Reduce over 4 weeks	Reduce over 4 weeks	Reduce over 4 weeks	Reduce over 4 weeks or longer if necessary	At 20 mg/day, just stop. At higher dose reduce over 2 weeks	Reduce over 4 weeks	Reduce over 4 weeks	Reduce over 4 weeks	Reduce over 4 weeks	Reduce over 4 weeks or longer if necessary	Reduce over 4 weeks or longer if necessary	Reduce over 4 weeks	Can be stopped abruptly

Reproduced, with permission, from Taylor D, Paton C, Kapur S. Maudsley prescribing guidelines in psychiatry. 11th ed. Chichester, Wiley Blackwell, 2012.[35].

- vasomotor, e.g. diaphoresis
- neurosensory, e.g paraesthesia.

Some symptoms are more likely with individual drugs (see Table 12.5).

NICE (UK) guidance for the treatment of depression (UK)[36]

Treatment of mild depression

NICE recommends the following stepwise approach:

- *watchful waiting*: in mild depression, if the patient does not want treatment or may recover with no intervention, arrange further assessment – normally within 2 weeks
- *sleep and anxiety management*: consider advice on sleep hygiene and anxiety management
- *exercise*: advise patients of all ages with mild depression of the benefits of following a structured and supervised exercise programme. The effective duration of such programmes is up to three sessions per week of moderate duration (45 minutes to 1 hour) for between 10 and 12 weeks

Table 12.5 Antidepressant discontinuation symptoms

Antidepressant class	Drugs most commonly associated with discontinuation symptoms	Common symptoms	Occasional symptoms
MAOIs	All Tranylcypromine is partly metabolized to amphetamine and is therefore associated with a true "withdrawal syndrome"	Agitation, irritability, ataxia, movement disorders, insomnia, somnolence, vivid dreams, cognitive impairment, slowed speech, pressured speech	Hallucinations, paranoid delusions
TCAs	Amitriptyline Imipramine	Flu-like symptoms, (chills, myalgia, excessive sweating, headache, nausea), insomnia, excessive dreaming	Movement disorders, mania, cardiac arrhythmia
SSRIs and SNRIs	Paroxetine Venlafaxine		
Bupropion		Flu-like symptoms, "shock-like" sensations, dizziness exacerbated by movement, insomnia, excessive (vivid) dreaming, irritability, crying spells	Movement disorders, problems with concentration and memory
Agomelatine		None	Few if any
Mirtazapine		Anxiety, insomnia, nausea	

MAOI, monoamine oxidase inhibitor; SNRI, serotonin and noradrenaline reuptake inhibitor; SSRI, selective serotonin reuptake inhibitor; TCA, tricyclic antidepressant.

Adapted, with permission, from Taylor D, Paton C, Kapur S. *Maudsley prescribing guidelines in psychiatry*, 11th ed. Chichester, Wiley Blackwell, 2012.[35]

Early data from one randomized controlled trial suggest that agomelatine is associated with low, if any, risk of discontinuation symptoms.

- *guided self-help*: for patients with mild depression, consider a guided self-help programme that consists of the provision of appropriate written materials and limited support over 6 to 9 weeks, including follow-up, from a professional who typically introduces the self-help programme and reviews progress and outcome
- *computerized CBT*: should be considered for the treatment of mild depression
- *psychological interventions*: in mild and moderate depression, consider psychological treatment specifically focused on depression (problem-solving therapy, brief CBT and counselling) of 6 to 8 sessions over 10 to 12 weeks. Offer the same range of treatments to older people as to younger people. In psychological interventions, therapist competence and therapeutic alliance have significant bearing on the outcome of intervention. Where significant comorbidity exists, consider extending the treatment duration or focusing specifically on comorbid problems
- *antidepressants*: are not recommended for the initial treatment of mild depression, because the risk–benefit ratio is poor. Where mild depression persists after other interventions, or is associated with psychosocial and medical problems, consider use of an antidepressant. If a patient with a history of moderate or severe depression presents with mild depression, consider use of an antidepressant
- *review in mild depression*: consider contacting all patients with mild depression who do not attend follow-up appointments.

Treatment of moderate to severe depression in primary care

Starting treatment

- In moderate depression, offer antidepressant medication to all patients routinely, before psychological interventions.
- Discuss the patient's fears of addiction or other concerns about medication. For example, explain that craving and tolerance do not occur.
- When starting treatment, tell patients about:
  - the risk of discontinuation/withdrawal symptoms
  - potential side-effects.
- Inform patients about the delay in onset of effect, the time course of treatment and the need to take medication as prescribed. Make available written information appropriate to the patient's needs.

Monitoring risk

- See patients who are considered to be at increased risk of suicide or who are younger than 30 years old, 1 week after starting treatment. Monitor frequently until the risk is no longer significant.
- If there is a high risk of suicide, prescribe a limited quantity of antidepressants.
- If there is a high risk of suicide, consider additional support such as more frequent contacts with primary care staff, or telephone contacts.
- Monitor for signs of akathisia, suicidal ideation, and increased anxiety and agitation, particularly in the early stages of treatment with an SSRI.
- Advise patients of the risk of these symptoms, and that they should seek help promptly if these are at all distressing.
- If a patient develops marked and/or prolonged akathisia or agitation while taking an antidepressant, review the use of the drug.

Continuing treatment

- See patients who are not considered to be at increased risk of suicide 2 weeks after starting treatment and regularly thereafter – for example, every 2–4 weeks in the first 3 months – reducing the frequency if response is good.
- For patients with a moderate or severe depressive episode, continue antidepressants for at least 6 months after remission.

- Once a patient has taken antidepressants for 6 months after remission, review the need for continued antidepressant treatment. This review may include consideration of the number of previous episodes, presence of residual symptoms, and concurrent psychosocial difficulties.

Choice of antidepressants

- For routine care, use an SSRI because they are as effective as tricyclic antidepressants and less likely to be discontinued because of side-effects.
- Consider using a generic form of SSRI. Fluoxetine or citalopram, for example, would be reasonable choices because they are generally associated with fewer discontinuation/withdrawal symptoms. Note the higher propensity of fluoxetine for drug interactions.
- Treatments such as dosulepin, phenelzine, combined antidepressants, and lithium augmentation of antidepressants should be routinely initiated only by specialist mental health-care professionals, including GPs with a special interest in mental health.
- Venlafaxine should be initiated only by specialist mental health-care professionals, including GPs with a special interest in mental health.
- Venlafaxine should be managed only under the supervision of specialist mental health medical practitioners, including GPs with a special interest in mental health.
- Consider toxicity in overdose; note that tricyclics (with the exception of lofepramine) are more dangerous in overdose.
- If increased agitation develops early in treatment with an SSRI, provide appropriate information and, if the patient prefers, either change to a different antidepressant or consider a brief period of concomitant treatment with a benzodiazepine followed by a clinical review within 2 weeks.
- St John's wort may be of benefit in mild or moderate depression, but its use should not be prescribed or advised because of uncertainty about appropriate doses, variation in the nature of preparations, and potential serious interactions with other drugs.
- Tell patients taking St John's wort about the different potencies of the preparations available and the uncertainty that arises from this, and about the interactions of St John's wort with other drugs (including oral contraceptives, anticoagulants and anticonvulsants).

Pharmacological treatment of atypical depression

- Treat patients with features of atypical depression with an SSRI.
- If there is no response to an SSRI and there is significant functional impairment, consider referral to a mental health specialist.

Treatment of schizophrenia

General principles

Choose an antipsychotic drug according to local guidance and patient factors and initiate at the starting or minimum effective dose. In general, it will take at least 2 weeks before there is any response and 4–6 weeks for a full response. If a partial response is seen at 4–6 weeks, then increase the dose further, if necessary, to the maximum dose and wait a further 4–6 weeks for full response. If there has been treatment failure with two antipsychotic drugs, then clozapine should be considered. This is not available in all countries and requires close monitoring, which may be difficult in low-income countries. Combinations of antipsychotics are not advised. The evidence base is poor, morbidity is high and hence the risks most often outweigh the benefits. Avoid using an atypical and a typical antipsychotic concurrently, except when switching, and avoid exceeding maximum doses of antipsychotics.

For a handful of patients that do benefit from combination or high-dose antipsychotic treatment, regular physical health monitoring is essential. Rating scales should be used at regular intervals to check the efficacy of the high-dose regime, and if the second drug or the higher dose has not proved beneficial, it should be withdrawn.

NICE (UK) guidance for the treatment of schizophrenia[37]

Initiating treatment (first episode)

Early referral

■ Urgently refer all people first presenting with psychotic symptoms in primary care to a local community-based secondary mental health service (early intervention services, crisis-resolution and home-treatment team, or community mental health team). Choose the appropriate team based on the stage and severity of illness and the local context.

■ Carry out a full assessment in secondary care, including assessment by a psychiatrist. Write a care plan with the service user as soon as possible. Send a copy to the referring primary health-care professional and the service user.

■ Include a crisis plan in the care plan, based on a full risk assessment. Define the roles of primary and secondary care in the crisis plan and include the key clinical contacts in case of emergency or impending crisis.

Early intervention services

■ Offer early intervention services to all people with a first episode or first presentation of psychosis, irrespective of age or duration of untreated psychosis. Refer from primary or secondary care.

■ Early intervention services should aim to provide the full range of interventions recommended in this guideline for people with psychosis.

Early treatment

■ If it is necessary for a GP to start antipsychotic medication, they should have experience in treating and managing schizophrenia (follow "Using oral antipsychotic medication" below).

Using oral antipsychotic medication

■ Offer oral antipsychotic medication to people with newly diagnosed schizophrenia.

■ Provide information on the benefits and side-effects of each antipsychotic drug and discuss these with the service user.

■ Decide which antipsychotic to use in partnership with the service user, and carer if appropriate.

■ When deciding on the most suitable medication, consider the relative potential of individual antipsychotics to cause extrapyramidal side-effects (such as akathisia), metabolic side-effects (such as weight gain), and other side-effects (including unpleasant subjective experiences). See Table 12.6.

■ Do not start regular combined antipsychotic medication, except for short periods (for example, when changing medication).

■ Before starting antipsychotic drugs, offer an ECG if:

  ● specified in the SPC

  ● physical examination shows specific cardiovascular risk (such as diagnosis of high blood pressure)

  ● there is personal history of cardiovascular disease, or

  ● the service user is being admitted as an inpatient.

■ Consider treatment with antipsychotic medication as an individual therapeutic trial:

  ● record the indications, expected benefits and risks, and expected time for a change in symptoms and for side-effects to occur

  ● start with a dose at the lower end of the licensed range and titrate upwards slowly within the dose range in the *British National Formulary* (BNF) or SPC

  ● justify and record the reasons for dosages outside the range specified in the BNF or SPC

  ● monitor and record the following regularly and systematically throughout treatment, but especially during titration:

    ■ efficacy, including changes in symptoms and behaviour

- side-effects of treatment, taking into account overlap with some of the clinical features of schizophrenia
  - adherence
  - physical health
- record the rationale for continuing, changing or stopping medication and the effects of such changes
- carry out a trial of the medication at optimum dosage for 4–6 weeks.

■ Discuss with the service user, and carer if appropriate, any non-prescribed therapies (including complementary therapies) the service user wishes to use. Also ask about alcohol, tobacco, prescription and non-prescription medication and illicit drugs.

■ Discuss their possible interference with the effects of prescribed medication and psychological treatments. Discuss the safety and efficacy of non-prescribed therapies.

■ When prescribing antipsychotic medication on an "as required" (prn) basis, review clinical indications, frequency of administration, therapeutic benefits and side-effects each week, or as appropriate. Check whether the dosage is above the maximum in the BNF or SPC.

■ Do not use a loading dose of antipsychotic medication ("rapid neuroleptization").

■ Warn of a potential photosensitive skin response with chlorpromazine and advise using sunscreen if necessary.

Treating the acute episode

Service-level interventions

■ Consider community mental health teams alongside other community-based teams as a way of providing services for people with schizophrenia.

■ Crisis-resolution and home-treatment teams should:
- be used to support people with schizophrenia during an acute episode in the community
- pay particular attention to risk monitoring as a high-priority routine activity
- be considered for people with schizophrenia who may benefit from early hospital discharge.

■ Acute day hospitals should be considered alongside crisis-resolution and home-treatment teams, instead of admission to inpatient care and to help early discharge from inpatient care.

Medication for the acute episode

Use oral antipsychotic medication.

■ Offer oral antipsychotic medication to people with an acute exacerbation or recurrence of schizophrenia.

■ When choosing a drug, look at the previous response and reiterate the side-effects (see Table 12.6).

■ Take into account the clinical response and side-effects of previous and current medication.

Rapid tranquillization

■ Consider rapid tranquillization for people who pose an immediate threat to themselves or others during an acute episode.

■ Follow the recommendations in "Violence" (NICE clinical guideline 25)[38] when managing immediate risk, facing imminent violence or considering rapid tranquillization.

■ After rapid tranquillization, offer the service user the opportunity to discuss and write an account of their experiences. Explain why the procedure was used. Record this and the account of their experiences in their notes.

■ Follow the NICE recommendations for "Self-harm"[39] when managing immediate risk and acts of self-harm.

Table 12.6 Antipsychotic drugs – relative side-effects

Drug	Adult max dose mg/day	Elderly max dose mg/day	Anticholinergic	Cardiac	EPSE	Hypotension	Sedation	Minor O/D	Weight gain	Prolactin	Proconvulsant
Phenothiazines											
Chlorpromazine	1000	<Ad	●●●	●●	●●	●●●	●●●	●●●	●●●	●●●?	●●●
Levomepromazine (methotrimeprazine)	1000	NR	●●	●●	●●?	●●●	●●●	●●	?	●●●?	●●?
Promazine	800	<Ad	●●	●●	●	●●	●●●	●●	?	●●●?	●●?
Pericyazine	(300)	<Ad	●	●●	●	●●	●●●	●●	?	●●●?	●●?
Thioridazine	600	<Ad	●●	●●●	●	●●	●●	●●	●●	●●●?	●
Fluphenazine	CA20	<Ad	●●	●●	●●●	●	●	●	●	●●●?	●●?
Perphenazine	24	<Ad	●	●	●●	●	●		●●	●●●?	●
Trifluoperazine	–	<Ad	○		●●	●	●		?	●●●	●●?
Others											
Benperidol	1.5	<Ad	?	?	?	●	●	?	?	●●●?	●?
Haloperidol	30	30	●	●●	●●●	●	●	●	●	●●●	●?
Flupentixol	18	<Ad	●●	○	●●	○	●	●	?	●●?	●●?
Zuclopenthixol	150	<Ad	●●	●	●●●	●	●●	●	○	●●?	○?
Pimozide	20	<Ad	○	●●	●	●	○	●	●	●●●	●●?
Amisulpride	1200	1200	●	○	●	○	●	●	●	●●●?	●●?
Sulpiride	2400	2400		○	●	●	●	●		●	○?
Depot and long-acting injections											
Fluphenazine decanoate	1–2/52	<Ad	●●	●●	●●●	●	●●	●	●	●●●?	●
Pipotiazine palmitate	200–4/52	<Ad	●●	●●	●●	●	●	?	?	●●●?	●●
Haloperidol decanoate	300–4/52	<Ad	●	●●	●●●	●	●	●	●	●●●	●
Flupentixol decanoate	400–1/52	<Ad	●●	○	●●	○	●	●	?	●●?	●
Zuclopentixol decanoate	600–1/52	<Ad	●●	●	●●●	●	●●	●●	?	●●?	●?
Fluspirilene	20–1/52	<Ad	●	○	●	●	●●	?	?	●●●?	●
Risperidone (Risperdal Consta®)	50–2/52	25–2/52	○	○	●	●●	●?	?	●		○
Olanzapine pamoate	300–2/52	See SPC	●	○	○	○	●●	○	●●●	●	●●

continued overleaf

Table 12.6 Antipsychotic drugs – relative side-effects – *continued*

Drug	Adult max dose mg/day	Elderly max dose mg/day	Anticholinergic	Cardiac	EPSE	Hypotension	Sedation	Minor O/D	Weight gain	Prolactin	Proconvulsant
Second-generation/ atypical antipsychotic drugs											
Aripiprazole	30	30	○	●	○	○	○	?	●	○	○
Asenapine	(10)	(20)	○?	?	●?	?	●?	?	?	?	?
Clozapine	900	(900)	●●●	●●	○	●	●●●	?	●●●	●	●●●
Olanzapine	20	20	●	○	○	○	●	○	●●●	●	●●
Paliperidone	12	12	○	○	●	●	●	○	●	●●	○
Quetiapine	800	<Ad	●	●	○	●	●●	●	●	●●	●
Risperidone	(16)	4	○	○	●	●	●?	?	●	●●	○
Sertindole	(20)	(20)	○	●●	○	●●	○	○	●●	○	○
Zotepine	300	150	●●	●●	●	●●	●●	?	●●●?	●●●?	●●●
Ziprasidone (U)	–	–	○		○	○	○	?	○	○	○

Reproduced, with permission from Bazire S. *Psychotropic drug directory*. Aberdeen, HealthComm UK, Ltd, 2010.[31]

●●● = marked effect

●● = moderate effect

● = mild effect

○ = little or minimal effect

? = no information or little reported

Ad = adult dose

CA = care above

EPSE = extrapyramidal side-effects

O/D = overdose

U = unlicensed in the UK

Adult max dose = maximum adult oral antidepressant dose in UK SPC or BNF

Elderly max dose = maximum elderly dose: half to a quarter of the adult dose should be adequate, with small dose increments

100–2/52 means 100 mg every 2 weeks; 400–1/52 means 400 mg every week, etc.

Treatment of bipolar disorder

General principles

A mood stabilizer is essential for those with bipolar disorder; the choice will depend on guidance and patient factors. The dose must be increased to achieve therapeutic doses and levels. Mood stabilizers are often used at subtherapeutic doses in primary care, leaving patients susceptible to hypomania and/or depression. Swings into highs and lows can still occur, even with therapeutic doses of a mood stabilizer, indicating the possible need for an antipsychotic and/or antidepressant. If antidepressant treatment is deemed necessary, it must not be started until and unless a therapeutic dose of a mood stabilizer has been achieved, as this is likely to cause a switch into mania.[40] Antipsychotics should only be used if and when attempts to use the mood stabilizer as an antimanic have failed, or the patient is experiencing psychotic symptoms.

In those with bipolar disorder, drug treatment is a case of fine tuning combinations of different groups of psychotropic medicines to obtain maximum stability with maximum effect and minimum adverse effects.

NICE (UK) guidance for the treatment of bipolar disorder[41]

Please note that in this section, drugs and treatments marked with a * do not have UK marketing authorization for the use in question at the time of publication of the guideline.

Managing acute episodes (see Figure 12.1)

- Decide treatment plans in collaboration with patients, considering the outcome of previous treatment(s) and the patient's preference.
- With all women of childbearing potential, discuss contraception and the risks of pregnancy (including relapse, damage to the fetus and risks associated with stopping and changing medication). Encourage women to discuss pregnancy plans with their doctor.
- See people having a manic episode or severe depressive symptoms again within a week of their first assessment. Continue to see them regularly – for example, every 2–4 weeks in the first 3 months, then less often if their response is good.

Managing depressive symptoms

Patients not taking antimanic medicines

- Patients who are prescribed an antidepressant should also be prescribed an antimanic drug. Base the choice of antimanic drug on:
  - decisions about future prophylactic treatment
  - likely side-effects
  - whether the patient is a woman of childbearing potential.
- When starting an antidepressant:
  - explain the risks of switching to mania and the benefits of taking an adjunctive antimanic agent
  - monitor carefully people who are unwilling to take an antimanic drug
  - start the antidepressant treatment at a low dose and increase gradually if necessary.

Patients taking antimanic medication

- Check the patient is taking the antimanic drug at the appropriate dose, and adjust it if necessary.

Patients with mild depressive symptoms

- Arrange a further assessment, normally within 2 weeks, if:
  - the patient's previous episodes of mild depression have not developed into chronic or more severe depression, or

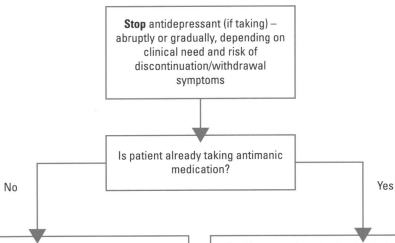

Stop antidepressant (if taking) – abruptly or gradually, depending on clinical need and risk of discontinuation/withdrawal symptoms

Is patient already taking antimanic medication?

No

Yes

No branch:

Consider, taking into account side-effects and future prophylaxis:

- an antipsychotic (normally olanzapine, quetiapine or risperidone), especially if symptoms are severe or behaviour disturbed
- valproate if symptoms have responded before (but avoid in women of childbearing potential)
- lithium if symptoms have responded before, and are not severe

If giving antipsychotic drugs:

- consider individual risk of side-effects (such as diabetes)
- start at low doses and titrate according to response
- consider adding valproate or lithium if response is inadequate
- be aware that older people are at higher risk of sudden onset of depression after recovery from mania

Consider adding short-term benzodiazepine (such as lorazepam*) for behavioural disturbance or agitation

Carbamazepine* should not be routinely used for acute mania

Gabapentin*, lamotrigine* and topiramate* are not recommended for acute mania

Yes branch:

If taking an antipsychotic, check the dose and increase if necessary. If the response is inadequate, consider adding lithium or valproate

If taking lithium, check plasma levels:

- if below 0.8 mmol/l, increase dose to a maximum blood level of 1.0 mmol/l
- if the response is not adequate, consider adding an antipsychotic

If taking valproate, increase the dose until:

- symptoms start to improve, or
- side-effects limit dose increases

If there is no improvement, consider adding olanzapine, quetiapine, or risperidone. Monitor carefully if the valproate dose is higher than 45 mg/kg

If taking lithium or valproate* and mania is severe, consider adding an antipsychotic while gradually increasing the dose of the original drug

If taking carbamazepine, do not routinely increase the dose. Consider adding an antipsychotic. Drug interactions are common with carbamazepine – adjust doses as needed

---

Advise all patients on:

- avoiding excessive stimulation – delaying important decisions
- calming activities – a structured routine with a lower activity level

Drugs marked with a * do not have UK marketing authorization for the use in question at the time of publication of the guideline.

Figure 12.1 Managing episodes of mania and hypomania. Adapted, with permission, from *Bipolar disorder: the management of bipolar disorder in adults, children and adolescents, in primary and secondary care*. London, National Institute for Health and Clinical Excellence, 2006 (CG38)[41]

- a more severe depression is not likely.
- If symptoms do not improve, follow the advice for moderate or severe depression.

Patients with moderate or severe depressive symptoms

- Consider:
  - prescribing an SSRI (but not paroxetine in pregnant women), or
  - adding quetiapine, if the patient is already taking an antimanic drug that is not an antipsychotic.
- For moderate depression, if there is no significant improvement after an adequate trial of drugs, consider a structured psychological therapy focused on depressive symptoms, problem-solving, improving social functioning, and medication concordance.
- Do not use routinely:
  - lamotrigine* as a single first-line drug in bipolar I disorder
  - transcranial magnetic stimulation*.

Antidepressant treatment and risk monitoring

- Avoid antidepressants for patients who have:
  - rapid-cycling bipolar disorder
  - a recent hypomanic episode
  - recent functionally impairing rapid mood fluctuations.
- Instead, consider increasing the dose of the antimanic drug or adding a second one (including lamotrigine*).

Starting antidepressants

- Address patients' concerns about taking antidepressants; for example, craving and tolerance do not occur.
- When starting antidepressant treatment, tell patients:
  - manic or hypomanic switching may occur
  - the onset of effect is not immediate, and improvement is gradual and fluctuating
  - about the need to take medication as prescribed and the risk of discontinuation/withdrawal symptoms
  - to look out for signs of akathisia, suicidal ideation (normally anyone under 30 years should be reviewed within 1 week of initiation of treatment), and increased anxiety and agitation (particularly at the beginning of treatment)
  - to seek help promptly if side-effects are distressing.
- If a patient develops marked and/or prolonged akathisia or agitation while taking an antidepressant, urgently review the use of the drug.
- Take care when prescribing SSRIs to people – particularly older people – taking medication that can cause intestinal bleeding, such as non-steroidal anti-inflammatory drugs (NSAIDs). Consider using a gastroprotective drug.

Stopping antidepressants after an episode

- If a patient is in remission from depressive symptoms, or symptoms have been significantly less for 8 weeks, consider stopping the antidepressant by reducing the dose gradually (particularly with paroxetine and venlafaxine) over several weeks, while maintaining the antimanic medication.

Incomplete response to treatment for acute depression

- If symptoms do not fully respond to an antidepressant, reassess for substance misuse, psychosocial stressors, physical health problems, comorbid disorders such as anxiety or severe obsessional symptoms, and poor adherence.

- Then consider:
  - increasing the dose of the antidepressant within "BNF" limits
  - individual psychological therapy focused on depressive symptoms
  - switching to a different antidepressant, such as mirtazapine or venlafaxine
  - adding quetiapine* or olanzapine, if the patient is not already taking them, or
  - adding lithium if the patient is not already taking it.
- If symptoms fail to respond to at least three adequate courses of antidepressant treatment, consider referring to (or seeking advice from) a specialist in bipolar disorder.
- For persistent depressive symptoms in patients with no recent history of rapid cycling (including those not taking an antidepressant), consider structured psychological therapy.

Concurrent depressive and psychotic symptoms

- For concurrent depressive and psychotic symptoms, consider augmenting treatment with an antipsychotic such as olanzapine, quetiapine or risperidone, or using electroconvulsive therapy (ECT, see below) if depression is severe.

The use of electroconvulsive therapy in manic and depressive disorders

- Consider ECT only for rapid and short-term improvement of severe symptoms after other treatments have proved ineffective or if the condition is life-threatening, in people with:
  - severe depressive illness
  - a prolonged or severe manic episode
  - catatonia.
- When making the decision, assess and document the risks and potential benefits, including:
  - the risks associated with anaesthetic
  - current comorbidities
  - anticipated adverse events, particularly cognitive impairment
  - the risks of not having treatment.
- When using ECT to treat bipolar disorder, consider:
  - stopping or reducing lithium or benzodiazepines before giving ECT
  - monitoring the length of fits carefully if the patient is taking anticonvulsants
  - monitoring the mental state for evidence of switching to the opposite pole.

Additional advice on managing depressive symptoms

- Advise about techniques such as structured exercise, activity scheduling, engaging in pleasurable and goal-directed activities, ensuring adequate diet and sleep, and seeking appropriate social support.
- Increase monitoring and formal support.

Managing acute mixed episodes

- Consider treating patients as if they had an acute manic episode, and avoid prescribing an antidepressant.
- Monitor patients at least weekly, particularly for suicide risk.

Preventing and managing behavioural disturbance

- When patients with bipolar disorder exhibit seriously disturbed behaviour, or are at risk of doing so:
  - place them in the least stimulating, most supportive environment available
  - review their safety and physical status, including hydration, and take appropriate action
  - consider using distraction techniques.

Pharmacological management of severe behavioural disturbance

Read this section in conjunction with the NICE clinical guideline *Violence: the short-term management of disturbed/violent behaviour in in-patient psychiatric settings and emergency departments.*[38]

- Use oral medication first – for example, lorazepam*, or an antipsychotic, or an antipsychotic and a benzodiazepine. Orodispersible formulations of risperidone and olanzapine are easier to take and more difficult to spit out.

- If rapid tranquillization is needed, consider intramuscular olanzapine (10 mg), lorazepam* (2 mg) or haloperidol (2–10 mg), wherever possible as a single agent. Take into account:
  - that olanzapine and lorazepam* are preferable to haloperidol because of the risk of movement disorders with haloperidol
  - olanzapine and benzodiazepines should not be given intramuscularly within 1 hour of each other
  - intramuscular doses can be repeated up to 20 mg per day (olanzapine), 4 mg per day (lorazepam*) or 18 mg per day (haloperidol), within "BNF" daily dose limits, including concurrent oral medication
  - the patient's previous response and tolerability, their current regular medication, and the availability of flumazenil.

- For behaviour disturbance, do not give routinely:
  - any psychotropic drug intravenously
  - diazepam* or chlorpromazine intramuscularly
  - paraldehyde*
  - zuclopenthixol acetate.

Long-term management of bipolar disorder

Drug treatment after recovery from an acute episode

Consider long-term treatment for bipolar disorder:

- after a manic episode involving significant risk and adverse consequences
- if a patient with bipolar I disorder has had two or more acute episodes
- if a patient with bipolar II disorder has significant functional impairment, is at significant risk of suicide or has frequent episodes.

Choice of drug

- Consider lithium, olanzapine or valproate* for long-term treatment of bipolar disorder, depending on:
  - the response to previous treatments
  - the relative risk, and precipitants, of manic versus depressive relapse
  - physical risk factors, particularly renal disease, obesity and diabetes
  - the patient's preference and history of adherence
  - sex (valproate* should not normally be prescribed for women of childbearing potential)
  - a brief assessment of cognitive state if appropriate, for example, for older people.

- If the patient has frequent relapses, or continuing functional impairment:
  - consider switching to a different prophylactic drug (lithium, olanzapine or valproate*)
  - adding a second drug; possible combinations are lithium with valproate*, lithium with olanzapine, valproate* with olanzapine
  - discuss with the patient (and document) the potential benefits and risks, and reasons for the choice
  - monitor closely the patient's clinical state, side-effects and, where relevant, blood levels.

- If a combination of prophylactic agents proves ineffective, consider:
  - consulting, or referring the patient to, a specialist
  - prescribing lamotrigine* (especially if the patient has bipolar II disorder) or carbamazepine.

- Do not use long-acting intramuscular injections of antipsychotic drugs routinely. However, they may be considered for people whose mania has responded to oral antipsychotic drugs, but have had a relapse because of poor adherence.

Length of treatment

- Normally, long-term pharmacological treatment should last for:
  - at least 2 years after an episode of bipolar disorder
  - up to 5 years if the person has risk factors for relapse, such as a history of frequent relapses or severe psychotic episodes, comorbid substance misuse, ongoing stressful life events, or poor social support.
- Discuss this with the patient and arrange regular reviews.
- Encourage patients to talk to their psychiatrist if they want to stop medication early.
- Offer regular contact and reassessment if, after careful discussion, a patient with bipolar disorder declines long-term medication.

After an acute depressive episode

- After successful treatment, patients should not normally continue on antidepressant treatment long term – there is no evidence that it reduces relapse rates, and it may increase the risk of switching.

Chronic and recurrent depressive symptoms

- For patients who are not taking prophylactic medication and have not had a recent manic or hypomanic episode, consider:
  - long-term treatment with SSRIs at the minimum therapeutic dose, and prophylactic medication
  - CBT (16–20 sessions) and prophylactic medication
  - quetiapine*, or
  - lamotrigine*.
- Consider lamotrigine* for patients with bipolar II disorder and recurrent depression.

Comorbid anxiety disorders

- For patients with significant comorbid anxiety disorders, consider psychological treatment focused on anxiety, or a drug such as an atypical antipsychotic.

Psychological therapy after an acute episode

- Consider individual structured psychological interventions, such as CBT, in addition to prophylactic medication for people who are relatively stable, but may have mild to moderate affective symptoms.
- The therapy should normally be at least 16 sessions over 6–9 months and:
  - include psychoeducation, the importance of a regular routine and concordance with medication
  - cover monitoring mood, detecting early warnings and strategies to prevent progression into full-blown episodes
  - enhance general coping strategies
  - be delivered by people who have experience of patients with bipolar disorder.
- Consider a focused family intervention if appropriate. This should last 6–9 months, and cover psychoeducation, ways to improve communication, and problem-solving.

Psychosocial support

- Consider offering befriending to people who would benefit from additional social support, particularly those with chronic depressive symptoms.
- This should be in addition to pharmacological and psychological treatments, and should be by trained volunteers providing, typically, at least weekly contact for between 2 and 6 months.

Promoting a healthy lifestyle and relapse prevention

- Give patients advice (including written information) on:
  - the importance of good sleep hygiene and a regular lifestyle
  - the risks of shift work, night flying and flying across time zones, and working long hours
  - ways to monitor their own physical and mental state.
- Provide extra support after life events such as loss of a job or a bereavement, and encourage patients to talk to family and friends.
- In collaboration with patients, identify the symptoms and indicators of an exacerbation, and make a plan of how to respond (including both psychosocial and pharmacological interventions).

Physical care of people with bipolar disorder

Physical monitoring

- People with bipolar disorder have higher levels of physical morbidity and mortality than the general population.
- Patients should have a schedule for physical monitoring, covering checks to be done as soon as practicable after initial presentation, at an annual check-up.
- *Give results of the annual check-up to the patient and health-care professionals in primary and secondary care (including whether the person refused any tests). A clear agreement should be made about responsibility for treating any problems.*

If a person gains weight during treatment

- Review their medication.
- Consider:
  - dietary advice from primary care and mental health services
  - advising regular aerobic exercise
  - referral to weight-management programmes in mental health services
  - referral to a dietician if there are comorbidities, such as coeliac disease.
- Drug treatments to promote weight loss are not recommended.

Long-term treatment: starting, stopping and risks

Antipsychotics

Starting

- If using quetiapine*, titrate the dose gradually to help maintain normal blood pressure.

Stopping

- Reduce the dose gradually:
  - over at least 4 weeks if the patient is continuing on other drugs
  - over up to 3 months if the patient is not continuing with other drugs, or has a history of manic relapse.

Risks

- Discuss with patients the risk of weight gain.
- Be aware of the possibility of worsening diabetes, malignant neuroleptic syndrome and diabetic ketoacidosis, particularly with patients with mania.

Lithium

Starting

- Do not start routinely in primary care.

- When starting lithium as long-term treatment:
  - tell patients that erratic compliance or stopping the drug suddenly may increase the risk of relapse
  - establish a shared-care protocol with the patient's GP for prescribing and monitoring
  - continue a trial for at least 6 months to establish effectiveness.

Monitoring

- Aim for:
  - 0.6–0.8 mmol/l normally, or
  - 0.8–1.0 mmol/l if the patient has relapsed previously on lithium or has subsyndromal symptoms.
- Monitor older adults carefully for symptoms of lithium toxicity.
- Do tests more often if there is clinical deterioration, abnormal results, a change in sodium intake, symptoms of abnormal renal or thyroid function, or other risk factors, such as starting angiotensin-converting enzyme (ACE) inhibitors, NSAIDs, or diuretics.
- Monitor the lithium dose and blood levels more closely if urea and creatinine levels rise, and assess the rate of deterioration of renal function. The decision on whether to continue the drug depends on clinical efficacy and the degree of renal impairment. Consider consulting a renal physician and specialist in bipolar disorder about this.
- Monitor for symptoms of neurotoxicity, including paraesthesia, ataxia, tremor and cognitive impairment.

Stopping

- Reduce the dose gradually over at least 4 weeks, and preferably over up to 3 months (even if the patient is taking another antimanic agent).
- If lithium treatment is stopped or is about to be stopped abruptly, consider changing to an atypical antipsychotic or valproate*, and monitor closely for early signs of mania and depression.

Risks

Advise patients:

- not to take over-the-counter NSAIDs (and monitor patients closely if these drugs are prescribed)
- to seek medical attention if they develop diarrhoea and/or vomiting
- to maintain their fluid intake, particularly after sweating, if they are immobile for long periods, or have a chest infection or pneumonia
- to consider stopping lithium for up to 7 days if they become severely ill with a metabolic or respiratory disturbance.

Valproate*

Starting

- Do not start routinely in primary care.
- Do not prescribe routinely for women of childbearing potential. If there is no alternative, ensure the woman is using adequate contraception, and explain the risks.
- Do not prescribe for women younger than 18 years because of the risk of polycystic ovary syndrome and unplanned pregnancy.

Stopping

- Reduce the dose gradually over at least 4 weeks.

Risks

- Explain the signs and symptoms of blood and liver disorders and advise patients to seek immediate medical help if these develop.
- Stop the drug if liver function is abnormal or blood dyscrasia is detected.

- Be aware of interactions with other anticonvulsants.
- Monitor sedation, tremor and gait disturbance in older people.

Lamotrigine*

Starting

- Do not start routinely in primary care.
- Titrate the dose gradually to minimize the risk of rashes, including Stevens–Johnson syndrome – more slowly in patients also taking valproate.
- Discuss alternatives to oral contraceptives with women. Reduce the dose of lamotrigine* by up to 50% if a woman stops taking an oral contraceptive.

Stopping

- Reduce the dose gradually over at least 4 weeks.

Risks

- Advise patients to make an urgent appointment if a rash develops. Stop the drug unless it is clear that the rash is not related to lamotrigine*.
- If an appointment cannot be arranged within a few days or the rash is worsening, advise patients to stop the drug and then restart it if the rash is not caused by lamotrigine*.

Carbamazepine

Starting

- Consult a specialist before using for long-term treatment.
- Increase the dose gradually to reduce the risk of ataxia.

Stopping

- Reduce the dose gradually over at least 4 weeks.

Risks

- Monitor possible interactions, including with oral contraceptives, because carbamazepine has a greater potential for drug interactions than other drugs used in bipolar disorder.

Smoking cessation

Nicotine replacement therapy

- Nicotine replacement therapy (NRT) is an effective aid to smoking cessation for those smoking more than 10 cigarettes a day. It is regarded as the pharmacological treatment of choice in the management of smoking cessation.
- In the UK there are many NRT products available, including patches, gum, lozenges, sublingual tablets, nasal sprays and inhalators. These products should be prescribed according to the individual's needs. For example, nicotine inhalators may be more appropriate for the patient who misses the physical act of smoking, while a patch may be more appropriate for the patient who doesn't.
- In many cases, combination therapy of two separate NRT products is most appropriate. For example, a patch may be combined with either an oral or nasal nicotine product. This is standard clinical practice throughout the UK and is associated with a higher success rate in smoking cessation.
- On some occasions, "preloading" may also be necessary. This technique involves the patient using NRT in conjunction with their normal tobacco intake for a specified period of time, prior to smoking cessation. This technique can be more useful in more resistant patients and is associated with a higher success rate in smoking cessation.

Bupropion

■ In the UK, NICE advocate the use of bupropion as a treatment option in those patients who require smoking cessation therapy. It should only be prescribed in combination with a programme of behavioural support.

■ The use of bupropion should be restricted to specialists in the smoking cessation area and preferably be prescribed in conjunction with the smoking cessation service.

■ Bupropion should only be prescribed as part of an abstinent-contingent treatment, in which the smoker makes a commitment to stop smoking on or before a particular date.

■ When prescribed, these treatments should be prescribed exclusively and not in combination with any other form of smoking cessation pharmacotherapy.

Varenicline

■ In the UK, NICE advocate the use of varenicline as a treatment option in those patients who require smoking cessation therapy.

■ It should only be prescribed in combination with a programme of behavioural support.

■ The use of varenicline should be restricted to specialists in the smoking cessation area and preferably be prescribed in conjunction with the smoking cessation service.

■ Varenicline should only be prescribed as part of an abstinent-contingent treatment, in which the smoker makes a commitment to stop smoking on or before a particular date.

■ When prescribed, these treatments should be prescribed exclusively and not in combination with any other form of smoking cessation pharmacotherapy.

Effect of smoking cessation on drug metabolism

■ Smoking cessation may alter the metabolism of a number of commonly used psychotropic drugs. Table 12.7 summarizes the effect of starting/stopping smoking on the metabolism of psychotropic drugs.

■ This effect is unrelated to nicotine and is caused by polycyclic aromatic hydrocarbons (PAHs) present in tobacco smoke. PAHs increase activity of the cytochrome P450 system that is responsible for the metabolism of a number of commonly used psychotropic drugs.

■ Following smoking cessation, the patient is no longer exposed to PAHs, and metabolism of these psychotropic agents decreases, resulting in increased plasma levels. Plasma levels will rise regardless of whether a patient is treated with NRT, bupropion or varenicline.

■ On prescribing smoking cessation pharmacotherapy, prescribers need to consider other prescribed medications and monitor for signs of increased plasma levels. In some cases, it may be possible to check plasma levels (for example clozapine).

■ Extreme caution should be taken in those patients taking theophylline. Smoking cessation may cause plasma levels of this drug, which has a narrow therapeutic index, to rise. Those taking theophylline should be supplied with NRT as appropriate, but the adviser must inform the client's doctor.

Workforce

The primary care workforce needs to include a health-care practitioner that can assess mental state, prescribe medicines and assess the efficacy and side-effects of the medicines, and is able to carry out physical observations such as temperature, blood pressure, pulse and blood glucose.

The prescriber could be either a medical or non-medical prescriber with knowledge of mental health and psychotropic medicines. In the UK, non-medical prescribers include nurses and pharmacists and they are very much used in secondary and primary care to assess and prescribe for patients, thus reducing the need for a medical doctor.

Table 12.7 The effect of starting and stopping smoking on metabolism of psychotropic drugs

Drug	Effect of smoking	Action on stopping smoking	Action on restarting smoking
Benzodiazepines[42,43]	Plasma levels reduced by 0–50% (depends on drug and smoking status)	Monitor closely; consider reducing dose by up to 25% over 1 week	Monitor closely, consider restarting "normal" smoking dose
Chlorpromazine[42,44]	Plasma levels reduced. Varied estimates of exact effect	Monitor closely; consider dose reduction	Monitor closely, consider restarting "normal" smoking dose
Clozapine[45,46]	Reduces plasma levels by up to 50% (depends on number/type of cigarettes smoked)	Take plasma level before stopping; on stopping reduce dose gradually (over 1 week) until around 75% dose is reached; repeat plasma level 1 week after stopping; consider further dose reductions	Take plasma level before restarting; increase dose to "normal" smoking dose over 1 week; repeat plasma level
Fluphenazine[47]	Reduces plasma levels by up to 50% (depends on number/type of cigarettes smoked)	On stopping, reduce dose by 25%; monitor carefully over the following 4–8 weeks. Consider further dose reductions	On restarting, increase dose to "normal" smoking dose
Fluvoxamine[48]	Drug metabolism is potently affected by smoking	Monitor closely; consider dose reduction	Monitor closely; consider restarting 'normal' smoking dose
Haloperidol[49,50]	Reduces plasma levels by around 20% (depends on number/type of cigarettes smoked)	Reduce dose by around 10%; monitor carefully; consider further dose reductions	On restarting, increase dose to 'normal' smoking dose
Lithium[31]	Smoking induces metabolism of caffeine, therefore theoretically smoking can reduce xanthine levels, which could reduce lithium excretion (raised plasma level)	Take plasma level before stopping; repeat plasma level 1 week after stopping and consider need for dose increase	Take plasma level before restarting; repeat plasma level 1 week after stopping and consider need for dose reduction
Olanzapine[51,52]	Reduces plasma levels by up to 50% (depends on number/type of cigarettes smoked); half-life can be 21% shorter in smokers[30]	Take plasma level before stopping; on stopping, reduce dose by 25%; after 1 week, repeat plasma level; consider further dose reductions	Take plasma level before restarting; increase dose to "normal" smoking dose over 1 week; repeat plasma level
Tricyclic antidepressants[42,43]	Plasma levels reduced by 25–50% (depends on drug and smoking status)	Monitor closely; consider reducing dose by 10–25% over 1 week; consider further dose reductions	Monitor closely; consider restarting "normal" smoking dose
Carbamazepine[42] Duloxetine[53] Flupentixol[44] Mirtazapine[54] Zuclopenthixol[55,56]	*May* be affected by smoking but effects on these drugs are usually clinically insignificant	"Caution" advised; monitor	"Caution" advised; monitor

In order to provide additional medicine supply and administration services via either PGDs or a non-medical prescriber, the following key primary care professionals are required to achieve the best outcomes:

- nurses (NHS, mental health, community, practice)
- optometrists (NHS, self-employed, private organization)
- pharmacists (NHS, self-employed, multiple organization)
- physiotherapists (NHS, self-employed, private organization, sport)
- podiatrists (NHS, self-employed, private practice)
- radiographers (NHS, private practice, etc.); the role fits well for therapeutic radiography.

In addition to the above general roles, primary care mental health (PCMH) services could be delivered by primary care mental health-care workers and Improving Access to Psychological Therapies (IAPT) high- and low-intensity therapists. Primary care mental health workers will be mental health professionals who have chosen to work in primary care. Trained staff will come from a range of backgrounds, including graduate primary care mental health workers, counsellors, mental health nurses, clinical psychologists, occupational therapists and psychotherapists. Mental health nurses and pharmacists are trained in the assessment of mental health and side-effects and physical observations.

References

1   Washington State University College of Pharmacy. *Pharmacy in Ancient Babylonia. History of pharmacy* (http://www.pharmacy.wsu.edu/History/history02.html, accessed 14 November, 2011).

2   Department of Health. Mental health and wellbeing (http://webarchive.nationalarchives.gov.uk/+/www.dh.gov.uk/en/Healthcare/Mentalhealth/index.htm, accessed 30 January 2012).

3   Santrock JW. *A topical approach to human life-span development*, 3rd ed. St Louis, MO, McGraw-Hill, 2007.

4   Peyriere H. Adverse drug events associated with hospital admission. *Annals of Pharmacotherapy*, 2003, 37:5–11.

5   McDonnell PJ, Jacobs MR. Hospital admissions resulting from preventable adverse drug reactions. *Annals of Pharmacotherapy*, 2002, 36:1331–1336.

6   Donoghue JM, Tylee A. The treatment of depression: prescribing patterns of antidepressants in primary care in the UK. *British Journal of Psychiatry*, 1996, 168:164–168.

7   *WHO model list of essential medicines*. Geneva, World Health Organization, 2011 (http://whqlibdoc.who.int/hq/2011/a95053_eng.pdf, accessed 11 November 2011).

8   *Non-medical prescribing by nurses, optometrists, pharmacists, physiotherapists, podiatrists and radiographers. A quick guide for commissioners*. Liverpool, National Prescribing Centre, 2010 (http://www.npc.nhs.uk/non_medical/resources/NMP_QuickGuide.pdf, accessed 30 January 2012).

9   *Non-medical prescribing by nurses, optometrists, pharmacists, physiotherapists, podiatrists and radiographers*. Leeds, National Prescribing Centre, 2010.

10   *Improving patients' access to medicines: a guide to implementing nurse and pharmacist independent prescribing within the NHS in England*. London, Department of Health, 2006.

11   National Electronic Library for Medicines. *Questions about PGDs and PCT commissioned NHS services – updated October 2010* (http://www.nelm.nhs.uk/en/Communities/NeLM/PGDs/FAQs/Questions-about-PGDs-and-PCT-commissioned-NHS-services/, accessed 14 November 2011).

12   Scottish Development Centre for Mental Health. *Developing social prescribing and community referrals for mental health in Scotland*. Edinburgh, Scottish Government, 2007 (http://www.scotland.gov.uk/Resource/Doc/924/0054752.pdf, accessed 14 November 2011).

13   Hamilton M. The assessment of anxiety states by rating. *British Journal of Medical Psychology*, 1959, 32:50–55.

14   Montgomery SA, Asberg M. A new depression scale designed to be sensitive to change. *British Journal of Psychiatry*, 1979, 134:382–389.

15   Hamilton, M. Rating depressive patients. *Journal of Clinical Psychiatry*, 1980, 41:21–24.

16 Beck AT. *Depression: causes and treatment*. Philadelphia, University of Pennsylvania Press, 2006.

17 Overall JE, Gorham DR. The brief psychiatric rating scale. *Psychological Reports*, 1962, 10:799–812.

18 Young RC et al. A rating scale for mania: reliability, validity and sensitivity. *British Journal of Psychiatry*, 1978, 133:429–435.

19 Waddell L, Taylor M. A new self-rating scale for detecting atypical or second-generation antipsychotic side effects. *Journal of Psychopharmacology*, 2008, 22:238–243.

20 Bennett J et al. (1995a). A rating scale/checklist for the assessment of the side-effects of antipsychotic drugs. In: Brooker C, White E, eds. *Community psychiatric nursing: a research perspective*, Vol. 3. London, Chapman and Hall, 1995:1–19.

21 Guy W. *ECDEU assessment manual for psychopharmacology*. Washington, DC, US Department of Health, Education and Welfare, 1976:534–537.

22 Barnes TR. A rating scale for drug-induced akathisia. *British Journal of Psychiatry*, 1989, 154:672–676.

23 Day et al. A self rating scale for measuring neuroleptic side effects. Validation in a group of schizophrenic patients. *British Journal of Psychiatry*, 1995, 166:650–653.

24 Warner CH et al. Antidepressant discontinuation syndrome. *American Family Physician*, 2006, 74:449–456.

25 Taylor D et al. Antidepressant withdrawal symptoms – telephone calls to a national telephone helpline. *Journal of Affective Disorders*, 2006, 95:129–133.

26 Ho B et al. Long-term antipsychotic treatment and brain volumes: a longtitudinal study of first-episode schizophrenia. *Archives of General Psychiatry*, 2011, 68:128–137.

27 Goodwin GM. Recurrence of mania after lithium withdrawal. Implications for the use of lithium in the treatment of bipolar affective disorder. *British Journal of Psychiatry*, 1994, 164:149–152.

28 Baldessarini RJ et al. Effects of the rate of discontinuing lithium maintenance treatment of bipolar disorders. *Journal of Clinical Psychiatry*, 1996, 57:441–448.

29 *Anxiety (amended): management of anxiety (panic disorder, with or without agoraphobia, and generalised anxiety disorder) in adults in primary, secondary and community care*. London, National Institute for Health and Clinical Excellence, 2002 (CG22).

30 *Computerised cognitive behaviour therapy for depression and anxiety. Review of Technology Appraisal 51*. Lonon, National Institute for Health and Clinical Excellence, 2005.

31 Bazire S. *Psychotropic drug directory*. Aberdeen, HealthComm UK, Ltd., 2010.

32 Cipriani et al. Comparative efficacy and acceptability of 12 new-generation antidepressants: a multiple-treatments meta-analysis. *The Lancet*, 2009, 373:746–758.

33 Henry JA, Alexander CA, Sener EK. Relative mortality from overdose of antidepressants. *BMJ*, 1995, 310:221–248.

34 Henry JA. Epidemiology and relative toxicity of antidepressant drugs in overdose. *Drug Safety*, 1997, 16:374–390.

35 Taylor D, Paton C, Kapur S. *Maudsley prescribing guidelines in psychiatry*, 11th ed. Chichester, Wiley Blackwell, 2012.

36 *Depression: management of depression in primary and secondary care*. London, National Institute for Health and Clinical Excellence, 2004 (CG23).

37 *Schizophrenia: core interventions in the treatment and management of schizophrenia in adults in primary and secondary care*. London, National Institute for Health and Clinical Excellence, 2009 (update of CG1).

38 *Violence: the short-term management of disturbed/violent behaviour in in-patient psychiatric settings and emergency departments*. London, National Institute for Health and Clinical Excellence, 2005 (CG25).

39 *The short term physical and psychological management and secondary prevention of self harm in primary and secondary care*. London, National Institute for Health and Clinical Excellence, 2006 (CG16).

40 Peet M. Induction of mania with selective serotonin re-uptake inhibitors and tricyclic antidepressants. *British Journal of Psychiatry*, 1994, 164:549–550.

41 *Bipolar disorder: the management of bipolar disorder in adults, children and adolescents, in primary and secondary care*. London, National Institute for Health and Clinical Excellence, 2006 (CG38).

42 Desai HD et al. Smoking in patients receiving psychotropic medications: a pharmacokinetic perspective. *CNS Drugs*, 2001, 15:469–494.

43 Miller LG. Recent developments in the study of the effects of cigarette smoking on clinical pharmacokinetics and clinical pharmacodynamics. *Clinical Pharmacokinetics*, 1989, 17:90–108.

44 Goff DC et al. Cigarette smoking in schizophrenia: relationship to psychopathology and medication side effects. *American Journal of Psychiatry*, 1992, 149:1189–1194.

45 Haring C et al. Influence of patient-related variables on clozapine plasma levels. *American Journal of Psychiatry*, 1990, 147:1471–1475.

46 Haring C et al. Dose-related plasma levels of clozapine: influence of smoking behaviour, sex and age. *Psychopharmacology*, 1989, 99(Suppl.):S38–S40.

47 Ereshefsky L et al. Effects of smoking on fluphenazine clearance in psychiatric inpatients. *Biological Psychiatry*, 1985, 20:329–332.

48 Spigset O et al. Effect of cigarette smoking on fluvoxamine pharmacokinetics in humans. *Clinical Pharmacology and Therapeutics*, 1995, 58:399–403.

49 Jann MW et al. Effects of smoking on haloperidol and reduced haloperidol plasma concentrations and haloperidol clearance. *Psychopharmacology*, 1986, 90:468–470.

50 Shimoda K et al. Lower plasma levels of haloperidol in smoking than in non-smoking schizophrenic patients. *Therapeutic Drug Monitoring*, 1999, 21:293–296.

51 Carrilo JA et al. Role of smoking-induced cytochrome P450 (CYP)1A2 and polymorphic CYP2D6 in steady-state concentration of olanzapine. *Journal of Clinical Psychopharmacology*, 2003, 23:119–127.

52 Gex-Fabry M et al. Therapeutic drug monitoring of olanzapine: the combined effect of age, gender, smoking, and co medication. *Therapeutic Drug Monitoring*, 2003, 25:46–53.

53 Eli Lilly and Company Limited. *Electronic medicines compendium. Cymbalta* (http://www.medicines. org.uk/EMC/searchresults.aspx?term=cymbalta&searchtype=QuickSearch, accessed 16 January 2012).

54 Grasmader K et al. Population pharmacokinetic analysis of mirtazapine. *European Journal of Clinical Pharmacology*, 2004, 60:473–480.

55 Jorgensen A et al. Zuclopenthixol decanoate in schizophrenia: serum levels and clinical state. *Psychopharmacology*, 1985, 87:364–367.

56 Jann MW et al. Clinical pharmacokinetics of the depot antipsychotics. *Clinical Pharmacokinetics*, 1985, 10:315–333.

13 Psychological interventions in primary care mental health

Tony Dowell, Caroline Morris, Tom Dodd and Brendan McLoughlin

> ## Key messages
>
> - Psychological interventions are an important component of primary mental health-care strategy and policy. They are effective in primary care settings.
> - Psychological therapies have potential applicability in every country. Disparities in access to therapies both between and within countries should be reduced.
> - Clarity is required by each country about the most effective way to deploy health professionals to deliver psychological therapies.
> - Stepped care models of provision should be encouraged and developed according to local resource and workforce opportunities and constraints.
> - The real value of psychological interventions in primary care will be seen through improvements in quality of life for patients and economic cost savings from increased productivity, rather than the impact on secondary services.

Introduction

The provision of psychological therapies in primary care clinics is an important theme in international mental health care. This is due to the high prevalence of common mental disorders (CMDs) in all countries, and the need for health systems to provide effective management of these conditions. While the overall effectiveness of psychological therapies in the management of these conditions is recognized, debate continues about any differences in effectiveness between therapies, the best way to deliver psychological therapies in primary care settings, the relative merits of psychological versus drug therapies and the overall costs of providing psychological therapies to large numbers of patients. This chapter reviews the overall evidence for the effectiveness of psychological therapies, discusses the delivery of therapy in primary care settings and provides a number of case-studies to position psychological therapies in an international context.

A key theme in psychological therapy provision relates to the prevalence of disorder, the number of potential patients who could be helped and the costs involved, given the relative intensity of "talking therapy" compared to a prescription for drugs.

In most countries, up to 50% of the population will meet the criteria for a mental disorder at some time in their lives, with up to 25% having had a disorder in the past 12 months.[1] The past-year prevalence of mental and substance abuse disorders in five countries (Canada, Chile, Germany, the Netherlands and the United States of America (USA)) has been estimated to range from 17% in Chile to almost 30% in the USA.[2] In addition, as many as 15% of the population may be affected by a CMD at any given point in time.[3] In those attending general practice clinics, up to one-third will be found to have one or more of the three most commonly presenting disorders: anxiety, depression or substance use disorder.[4]

Furthermore, recent estimates suggest that the cost of mental health problems in England increased from £77.4 billion in 2002/2003 to £105.2 billion in 2009/2010 (US$120.8 billion to US$164.2 billion), through health and social care costs, for output losses in the economy, and an imputed monetary valuation of the human cost of mental illness.[5] The London School of Economics calculated that "the total loss of output due to depression and chronic anxiety is some £12 billion a year – 1% of our total national income. Of this the cost to the taxpayer is some £7 billion – including incapacity benefits and lost tax receipts".[6]

If psychological intervention for common mental disorders is effective, then the challenge for health service planners is significant, due to both the increasing prevalence of these disorders,[7] and recognition of the fact that psychological disorders may contribute more to the overall burden of long-term chronic illness than other chronic illness conditions.[8]

As will be discussed in this chapter, the evidence base for the effectiveness of psychological intervention is more highly developed for depression than for other disorders, and for cognitive-behavioural therapy (CBT) than for other therapy. We suggest that the apparent prominence of both depression and CBT is likely to be due to a lack of research evidence rather than a lack of potential benefit for other conditions or a lack of benefit of other therapies. The key challenge is thus to develop and deploy a workforce that can deliver interventions that are financially realistic and culturally appropriate. Recent initiatives in many countries suggest that increasing access to psychological treatment is feasible and leads to improved outcomes.

In Australia, for example, the "Better Outcomes in Mental Health" initiative allowed general practitioners (GPs), following training, to refer service users to psychological treatments. Service-user and provider satisfaction with these programmes was high, and clinical data showed an improvement in patient outcomes. Flexibility in the structure of the programmes and adaptation to local need were found to be important features in that success.[9–11]

In England, the Improving Access to Psychological Therapies (IAPT) programme[12] is a National Health Service (NHS) initiative that seeks to establish services offering psychological therapies ("talking therapies") for the treatment of anxiety disorders and depression, as recommended by the National Institute for Health and Clinical Excellence (NICE).[13] The programme is delivered using a strategic health authority (SHA) regional infrastructure in which primary care trusts (PCTs) are the commissioners of health services, and manage the NHS budget exclusively at this time. In the future, responsibilities for commissioning may be given to a wider group of professionals, with a focus at primary care level.

Considerable costs are involved in these kinds of initiatives. In 2008 the government of the United Kingdom of Great Britain and Northern Ireland (UK) announced that an initial investment of almost £400 million would be made available to improve access to psychological therapies. The first phase would be conducted over a 3-year period and would finance the recruitment of 3600 new therapists and enable 900 000 people to access services, and 25 000 people to move off sick pay and benefits, with 50% recovery rates. Sites were to be established in half of the PCTs in England. The remainder of services were to be established in a second 3-year phase. A Department of Health document *Realising the benefits* describes a vision for the completed roll-out of the programme, providing access for 15% of those with anxiety disorders and/or depression.[14]

The most significant feature in health-sector spending is the cost of health-care workers, and psychological interventions are by their nature expensive. They have also been, until now, intensive, with therapy interventions spread over a number of sessions. Given that therapies have been developed from secondary care theoretical underpinnings, there is a need to determine the optimum duration of therapy for primary care settings. Given competing demands, resource constraints and uncertain diagnostic criteria, it is important that practitioners are given clear thresholds for both the duration and intensity of psychological therapy intervention.

In this chapter, we have deliberately tried to retain a focus on psychological therapy as it may be applied in an international context. While the majority of research evidence has been developed in Organization for Economic Co-operation and Development (OECD) countries, the main global burden of mental disorder falls on low- and middle-income countries. Therapy provision must be tailored to the context of each individual country, but with an ultimate responsibility to reduce international disparities in both service provision and mental health outcomes.

The context of mental disorders

This review encompasses the use of psychological interventions in the treatment of common mental disorders as a whole. It should be noted, however, that much of the contextual background information provided centres on the use of these therapies in the management of depression. Inevitably, this is where a substantial proportion of the literature lies. We suggest that the evidence base is likely to apply just as effectively to anxiety disorder and mixed anxious depression,[15] with some modifications to the management of substance use disorder.

Terminology

In this chapter, we use terminology that fits with an overall body of research evidence and a broad international context of common mental disorder.

Common mental disorder (CMD) refers to a grouping of high-prevalence mental disorders managed in primary care settings. They include anxiety, depression, the spectrum of mixed anxious depression, and substance use disorder. Psychotic and significant bipolar depression are not included.

Psychological interventions

The focus of this chapter is on the use of psychological interventions. However, it is important to recognize that these interventions should be considered as a therapy option alongside other possible options (e.g. social support, lifestyle interventions, pharmacological therapy). Furthermore, these different intervention approaches are complementary and sometimes usefully combined. An example of this is shown by the model of care described in the US case-study discussed later in this chapter.

In this section we provide a brief summary of the type of psychological interventions available and feasible for use in primary care mental health, together with the evidence for their use. The information has been drawn from the literature reviews that underpinned the development of three recently published national depression guidelines.[16–18] Comprehensive and systematic reviews of the literature that included an assessment of the place of psychological therapies in the treatment of depression were undertaken. These reviews were not restricted to the primary care setting. One guideline also included a health-economic perspective.[16]

Unless otherwise stated, the cited material relates to adult patients. It also needs to be borne in mind that in many cases the comparator used to assess the effectiveness of a specific intervention was "treatment as usual". This is something that is likely to vary widely across settings. Furthermore, research trials take place in a highly controlled environment that is unlikely to accurately reflect day-to-day clinical practice.

A wide range of psychological therapies potentially fall within the term "psychological interventions". They range from self-help support groups, through low-intensity psychosocial interventions to high-intensity psychological interventions.

Self-help support groups

Only one guideline specifically reviewed the evidence related to self-help support groups.[18] While there was no evidence to recommend such groups as a treatment option for depression, an extensive list of factors that practitioners should bear in mind in relation to their use was provided. This included the adequacy of training, supervision and support of group facilitators; the existence of appropriate links to groups able to offer the required resources and support; and the appropriateness and level of monitoring of the group.

Specific types of psychological therapy

Before summarizing the evidence for specific psychological therapies, a brief description of those commonly used is given.[17,18]

CBT, mindfulness-based cognitive therapy (MBCT), interpersonal therapy (IPT), behavioural activation (BA) and problem-solving therapy (PST) are all structured psychological interventions where the patient and the therapist work collaboratively. CBT aims to identify the thoughts, beliefs and interpretations that are at the root of the psychological problems, and help the patient develop the skills to recognize and overcome or cope with them. MBCT focuses on developing a patient's awareness of negative thoughts. The aim is for them to be "mindful" of these thoughts without responding to them. IPT focuses on reducing psychological symptoms by identifying and recognizing the effect of interpersonal problems (e.g. grief, role transition) and developing coping mechanisms, or working on ways to resolve the problem. The key approach in BA is the promotion of positivity by encouraging a patient to undertake satisfying activities instead of withdrawing. PST involves a practical, stepwise approach to enhance a patient's ability to cope with a problem. Steps include clarification and prioritization of problems and the development and implementation of possible solutions and coping strategies.

In psychodynamic psychotherapy, a focus is placed on the patient freely expressing and exploring with the therapist feelings related to both current conflicts and those from their past. Problems from the past may be being repeated in current relationships and may help the patient to better understand current difficulties.

Low-intensity psychosocial interventions

Psychological interventions that could be considered "low intensity" include guided or computerized self-help.[16]

In the UK context, guided self-help has been defined as an intervention administered by the patient, with limited professional contact in a supportive capacity.[16]

There is evidence for the clinical effectiveness of guided self-help based on the principles of CBT, and computerized CBT (CCBT) for the treatment of depression at the less-severe end of the scale. In addition, CCBT was considered cost effective compared to usual care for mild to moderate depression. No meaningful clinical or cost comparisons between these interventions could be drawn.[16] Both interventions have been recommended as treatment options for depression,[16,18] with the final choice determined by an individual patient's preference.[16]

High-intensity psychological interventions

Psychological interventions that have been considered "high intensity" are those based on cognitive-behavioural principles (CBTs including group therapy and MBCT), IPT, BA, couple (or couple-focused) therapy, PST, counselling and psychodynamic psychotherapy.[16]

Overall, the evidence suggests that high-intensity psychological interventions are effective for the treatment of depression. The volume of evidence relating to both clinical and cost-effectiveness varies considerably across these interventions, with most relating to CBT.[16]

The clinical effectiveness of individual *CBT* is approximately equivalent to pharmacological therapy.[17] Combination treatment has been shown to be more effective than pharmacological treatment alone. Health-economic modelling suggests that combined therapy is cost effective for moderate and severe depression. The final NICE guidance recommended that CBT alone should be one of several possible treatment options for patients with moderate depression.[16]

There is also evidence to suggest that CBT is effective in reducing relapse compared to pharmacological therapy. The strongest evidence base for relapse reduction relates to the use of group *MBCT* in those who have experienced at least three episodes of depression.[16]

While there is evidence to suggest that *IPT* is effective, there is none assessing its cost-effectiveness.[16]

Although there is a limited evidence base for the clinical effectiveness of *couple therapy*, it may have a role to play in very specific instances where the relationship is considered the cause of depression. Limited cost-effectiveness data exist for this therapy.[16]

Overall, there is some evidence to suggest that clinical effectiveness is approximately the same for IPT and couple therapy when compared to CBT.[16]

The evidence base for the clinical effectiveness for *BA* is less than for IPT and couple therapy, while no cost-effectiveness data exist.[16]

Although the evidence base for the clinical effectiveness of *PST* is limited, it has been considered reasonable that the use of this therapy as a part of brief "low-intensity" interventions will continue.[16] Furthermore, its use has been recommended as a treatment strategy for moderate depression.[17] It also aligns itself well to the consulting style of general practice in many countries.

Despite very widespread use in many countries, the evidence for the clinical effectiveness of both *counselling* and short-term *psychodynamic therapy* is inconsistent. In addition, no cost-effectiveness advantage has been demonstrated when these therapies are compared with usual care (both therapies) or pharmacological treatment (counselling). It has been suggested that these therapies should be considered for those people with mild to moderate depression who have refused treatment with an intervention for which there is greater evidence (e.g. CBT, IPT).[16]

These findings are reflected in the recommendations made in the recent Scottish Intercollegiate Guidelines Network (SIGN) guideline, where individual CBT, IPT and behavioural activation were treatment options for depression, and it was stated that PST and short-term psychodynamic psychotherapy could be considered as treatment options.[18] In addition, it was recommended that group MBCT could be considered as a relapse-reduction treatment in patients who have experienced at least three depressive episodes, and it should be viewed as best practice for couple therapy to be considered where the relationship is thought to be the cause of the depression. No recommendations were made around the place of counselling.[17]

Other therapies

A number of other high-intensity psychological interventions (art therapy, family therapy, hypnotherapy, music therapy, reminiscence therapy) were considered by SIGN.[18] There was no evidence (art therapy) or insufficient evidence (the remaining therapies) for recommendations to be made on the place of these therapies in the treatment of depression.

Psychological interventions in the primary care setting

Background

There is strong evidence that psychological therapies have a place in the management of depression, anxiety and other common mental disorders.[16,18] The treatment of mental health is increasingly being managed in primary care practice, and psychotherapy is a core part of that management and treatment. There is less evidence about exactly how these therapies should be used and integrated within a primary care setting. Indeed, Hegarty et al. identified that substantial limitations exist in the relevance to primary care of depression guidelines from seven high-income countries.[19] "Bringing psychotherapy to primary care" thus represents an important challenge.[20]

The evidence

Evidence regarding the use of the primary care setting comes from a number of different formats. Alexander et al. have produced a comprehensive narrative review of the international literature that considered psychotherapy interventions (across a range of mental disorders) that have been specifically adapted for use within primary care, or are compatible with the goals and ethos of primary care.[20] "High-intensity" psychological interventions in shortened, less-intense forms enables their use in a primary care setting. The majority of work conducted in this context to date relates to the use of PST. Guidelines have tended to provide commentary about individual disorders in primary care. The New Zealand guideline, for example, has focused specifically on the management of depression in the primary care setting.[17]

In primary care, a variety of brief structured psychological interventions have been identified as effective treatments for common mental disorders – PST and IPT for major depression, CBT for panic disorder. In addition, these therapies have shown potential for the treatment of other mental health problems (PST, IPT and CBT in dysthymia; PST in patients whose symptoms were not restricted to those of depression; CBT in generalized anxiety disorder, minor and major depression; IPT in minor depression).[20]

Adaptation of these therapies to enable manageable delivery in primary care generally entails fewer treatment sessions and/or briefer sessions (in length or intensity) than traditional therapy. It has been suggested that for the practical and useful application of psychological interventions in the primary care setting, "treatment length and intensity should be reduced, ideally to between four and six 30 minute sessions, and should include psychoeducation and self-management skill components".[20]

PST can be, and has been, adapted in some cases to largely meet these criteria, and is thus ideally suited to primary care delivery. Working towards the resolution of an existing problem can help "teach" patients problem-solving techniques that can be applied in the management of coexisting problems or new problems in the future. While "tailored" PST did not require delivery by a health-care worker with specialist mental health experience, training was necessary for those administering the therapy.[20] In contrast, the level of expertise needed to effectively deliver IPT and CBT within primary care was identified as potentially limiting their usefulness. Furthermore, patient response may ultimately depend upon both the therapist's expertise and the ability of the patient to engage with the therapy techniques. Although it may be more challenging to effectively deliver CBT in primary care within the suggested time frames, this is an intervention that particularly lends itself to delivery by a much wider variety of media (e.g. telephone, computer, Internet).[20] The use of CBT techniques in primary care patients from Europe and the USA is described in the case-studies later in this chapter.

While IPT has been reported as being delivered by telephone,[20] we later describe its adaptation for use in group therapy in an African community.

These findings reflect the recommendations from the New Zealand guideline.[17] This identified a lack of clear evidence from the primary care setting, endorsed the availability of brief psychological interventions including structured PST in primary care, and highlighted the need for more widespread access to these treatments.

Two small meta-analyses have recently added to the evidence base on the use of psychological therapies in patients from primary care.[15,21] The psychological treatment (ranging from guided self-help with therapist support, to face-to-face therapy) of adults from primary care with depression was found to be as effective as other settings – for example, patients recruited from specialized mental health services.[21] Brief CBT and PST (the therapies most frequently used in the included studies) administered within primary care for adults with anxiety, depression and mixed disorders were effective compared to treatment as usual.[15]

Innovations in delivery

Innovations in the media used for the delivery of psychological therapies have the potential to reduce some of the financial, social, and geographical barriers to access to therapy/therapists. These potentially include telephone, computer, Internet and text-messaging-based interventions. Alexander and co-workers have recently reviewed technological innovations in the delivery of psychological therapies, to which readers are referred for more detailed information.[20] Two more recent studies have confirmed their findings related to the effectiveness of online CBT,[22] and added to a limited information bank on patient acceptability of this medium.[23]

Online CBT delivered by a therapist, combined with usual care, appeared effective for the treatment of depression compared to usual GP care. However, delivery of therapy in this way is not necessarily acceptable to all patients.[23] While some patients felt comfortable with this delivery medium and considered the "anonymity" it brought helpful, some felt frustrated by the inability to develop a meaningful relationship with the therapist. Work on Internet-based psychotherapy interventions as a strategy for the prevention of depression has also been conducted.[24]

Utilizing electronic media for psychological interventions may be more convenient for some patients and has the potential to increase the accessibility of therapies for a greater proportion of the population, at both national and global levels.

As Alexander et al. identified, however, reducing one set of problems potentially creates a different set.[20] Access for therapies delivered in these ways will be unavailable to patients who do not possess, or prefer not to engage with, the technology. Furthermore, there may be challenging issues related to confidentiality, privacy, and the clinical and legal responsibility of the patients who access interventions in this way.[20]

Global challenges

A major challenge for the development and integration of psychological interventions into primary care across the globe stems from the substantial differences that exist in the structure, function and scope of primary care and psychological therapy services. Variability exists in how patients access primary care, the composition of the primary care workforce, the availability of training in psychological therapy techniques for members of the primary care team, the availability and training of the psychotherapist workforce, and the interface between primary care practice and secondary care mental health services.

Furthermore, patient and health-care practitioner perspectives on mental health disorders and their treatment will differ between cultures. In addition, the availability, cost and uptake of technological innovations will vary markedly across different populations.

Delivery of psychological therapy services

Models of care: contextual information

An overview of the literature describing primary care service-delivery systems and models of care is provided next. Although much of this information relates to mental health services in general, rather than to psychological therapies per se, it is relevant to that context. Box 13.1 summarizes the models identified in comprehensive reviews that were recently undertaken to underpin national guidelines for England and Wales,[16] and New Zealand.[17] This is followed by a brief synopsis of other relevant literature.

Box 13.1 Models of providing psychological therapies in primary care settings[16,17,a]

- Staff training:[16,17] upskilling of existing primary care staff to provide psychological interventions
- Consultation–liaison:[16,17] an ongoing educational relationship between mental health specialists and the primary care team to facilitate the care of specific patients
- Stepped care:[16,17] "A sequence of treatment options to offer simpler interventions first and more complex interventions if the patient has not benefited"[17]
- Collaborative care:[16,17] patient care is co-coordinated by a case manager, who actively engages with patients about care plans and ensures appropriate liaison between primary and secondary care and follow-up of patients.[16] This approach surfaced from the chronic care model of long-term condition management[17]
- Replacement/referral[17] (or attached professional[16]): a mental health specialist is responsible for the patient's presenting problem and its treatment (e.g. a course of psychotherapy)

a A degree of overlap is not uncommon, with some interventions displaying the features of more than one model.

Both reviews identified that much of this work was conducted in the USA, and its application globally is therefore potentially limited. Furthermore, apart from collaborative care, the evidence base is sparse. Both guidelines did, however, recommend that the stepped care approach be used, and acknowledged the potential importance of coordinated multidisciplinary care.[16,17] Of note, the evidence for collaborative care in depressed adults with a long-term physical health problem was deemed sufficiently strong that it was recommended that this model of care be considered in the NICE guideline on depression in adults with a chronic physical condition.[13] It is important to recognize that an existing member of the primary care team (e.g. GP/practice nurse) may be the case manager in collaborative care models and that Christensen et al. identified in a recent systematic review that the presence of a case manager was important for improvements in outcome when depression was managed in general practice.[25] A UK randomized controlled trial (RCT) that assesses both the clinical and cost-effectiveness of collaborative care compared to usual care in patients with moderate to severe depression is currently under way.[26] In this trial, case managers with a psychology or mental health background are responsible for the delivery of a low-intensity psychological therapy in primary care, based on CBT.

A Cochrane review has assessed the effects on primary care workload of primary care-based mental health workers delivering psychological interventions.[27] This identified significant reductions in consultations, prescribing and referral to specialist care. The reductions were modest, and no conclusions could be drawn on the overall clinical or economic impact.

Recently published papers have described further work from the UK[28] and USA[29] primary care that used complex interventions based on some of the concepts identified in Box 13.1 to improve the care of depression and anxiety disorders respectively. These concepts have also been applied in New Zealand Government-funded primary mental health initiatives.[30] Models of care in that setting were developed locally to address the needs of those with mild to moderate mental health disorders. Primary health organizations were given significant local autonomy and prioritized the organization of psychological therapies in their initiatives. Overall, the initiatives resulted in significant clinical improvements for patients and fulfilled the needs of the local population.

A recommended approach: stepped care

In this approach, the simplest and most effective intervention is offered first. If the patient fails to benefit from the initial intervention, or refuses that intervention, then a more complex intervention from the next "step" should be suggested.[16,17,31]

The place of psychological therapies ranging from low-intensity psychosocial interventions to complex/high-intensity psychological interventions is shown in Figure 13.1.

Although a firm evidence base for a stepped care approach is lacking, it is recommended in evidence-based guidelines as the approach to take in the management of depression in a number of high-income countries.[17,31] In addition, it is an intuitively sound and rational approach given the variability and sometimes scarcity of the necessary resources for the delivery of psychological interventions across the globe. Furthermore, examples of this approach have also been described in the treatment of depression and anxiety disorders in primary care in low- and middle-income countries, including India,[33] and Chile.[34]

Even in low-income countries where there is an absence of organized primary mental health-care provision, the model indicates that resources should be mobilized to provide a platform of self-help and community-based initiatives for mild and moderate disorders.

Psychological therapies lend themselves to a stepped care approach as they can be tailored to the availability of local resources. They can be delivered by different media and at differing levels of intensity. They can be used as self-guided therapy by the patient alone; self-guided therapy with limited support from a trained professional; stand-alone professionally delivered brief (low-intensity) or high-intensity interventions; or as an adjunct to pharmacological therapy. The precise way in which the therapy is delivered will govern the level of expertise (and hence training) required by the "therapist".

Potential models of care and issues

Which practitioner is responsible for the delivery of psychological interventions and whether or not this takes place within or outside the primary care practice will be dependent upon the resources, workforce and configuration of services within any given national setting. Possible delivery options include:[16,17]

- upskilling by primary care practitioners (within the practice)
- links with primary care practitioners outside the practice (e.g. counsellors, low-intensity psychotherapy workers)
- consultation–liaison (ongoing links with a mental health specialist)
- referral to secondary care.

This could therefore range from primary care practitioners offering psychological interventions within the practice, through primary care practitioners entering into a formal working relationship with a mental health specialist, to the specialist taking responsibility for the service. Any of these options are possible within a collaborative care model.

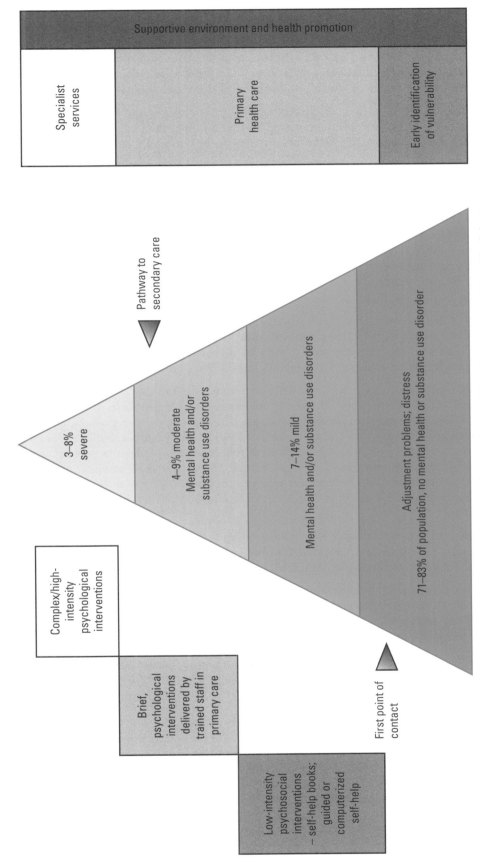

Figure 13.1 A stepped care approach to the use of psychological interventions ("talking therapies") in primary care mental health clinics[a]

Important notes:

[a] Psychological interventions should be considered as a therapy option alongside other possible options (e.g. social support, lifestyle interventions, pharmacological therapy).

A stepped care approach should not necessarily always mean progression in an "upward" direction. It is a structured, but fluid or dynamic approach – patients should be started at the most appropriate step when presenting or re-presenting, and transfer between steps (including moving down a step) as required.

Prevalence range figures cited are derived from a number of different countries and sources.[2,32]

Skill mix, workforce development and building capacity

A change in "skill mix" has a potentially important role to play in using the health-care workforce in the most effective way.[35] However, the challenges faced will vary across the globe. Variation in the relative availability of the different health-care professionals, national regulation of those professionals, and local cultures and customs will all have an impact to a degree on the development of primary care mental health services.[36]

Workforce imperatives include consideration of upskilling the existing primary care team versus the development of "new professional" roles (e.g. primary mental health coordinator, mental health nurse, primary care mental health worker) and identities. Decisions need to be made nationally, and regionally within a country, regarding service development, the appropriate use and maintenance of skills, the availability of appropriate training options including regular formalized supervision, addressing the level of demand, and future workforce additions or development. People taking up new positions in primary mental health should also be given the opportunity to meet regularly as a group for the purposes of problem-solving and information-sharing. It is obviously more efficient that, as primary mental health care develops, opportunities should be realized for the sharing of project-management resources, and for current staff to mentor those in the new initiatives. Furthermore, the therapy workforce (both intra- and internationally) is likely to be extremely varied in terms of qualifications, experience and type of treatment offered. Quality-assurance processes will therefore be essential.[30] In addition, the importance of cultural responsiveness and competence of the workforce should not be underestimated.

The increased use of psychological therapies and therapists represents a major potential change in the provision of primary mental health care in both high- and low-income countries. Workforce developments have already occurred in a number of high-income countries with a view to increasing access to them. The Australian "Better Outcomes in Mental Health" initiative,[9–11] and the UK's IAPT Programme[12] are two examples of this.

The drive in low- and middle-income countries has already been towards the training of primary care workers by mental health specialists for the "low-level" treatment of mental health problems ("scaling-up").[37] A collaborative project coordinated by a German university that aims to improve the psychosomatic knowledge and skills of doctors in China, Viet Nam and the Lao People's Democratic Republic has been described.[38] Doctors are taught to recognize, and treat, the most commonly occurring disorders in primary care, and work with specialists. Some doctors are trained as future teachers. In that initiative, it was acknowledged that differences in doctor–patient communication around, for example, discussion of emotions, between western and each of the eastern cultures needed to be openly discussed. Culture-specific beliefs could then be integrated into revised teaching material.

It is notable that high- and low-income countries are collaborating in the "Asia-Pacific Community Mental Health Development" project. This includes Australia, Cambodia, China (including Taiwan), Hong Kong, India, Indonesia, Japan, the Republic of Korea, Malaysia, Mongolia, Singapore, Thailand and Viet Nam and:

> . . . aims to illustrate and promote best practice in mental health care in the community through the use of information exchange, current evidence and practical experience in the region [this] exchange based on local practices will help enhance regional solutions to challenges in building capacity and structures for community-based mental health systems in the future.[39]

Indeed, there may be lessons to be learnt for high-income countries from the ways in which low-income countries have attempted to overcome the problem of poorly resourced and overburdened mental health services.[40]

Case-studies: examples of models of care that have been used for the delivery of psychological interventions across the globe

Five case-studies are provided next, summarizing models of care that have been used in the delivery of psychological interventions in low- and high-income countries.

The first, describes the world's largest national programme, the English initiative "Improving Access to Psychological Therapies" (IAPT) for delivering psychological interventions in primary care. This is followed by shorter summaries of initiatives from Africa, Australasia, continental Europe and North America.

These specific examples were chosen for a number of reasons. They reflect a range of approaches to care including individual, group, family-based and computer-delivered therapies. They cover a variety of mental disorders (depression, "mental health issues", addictions, anxiety) and age groups (youth, adults, older people) and also, in some instances, highlight the importance of management within the context of chronic illness. Importantly, they also all contain a focus on disadvantaged populations, or populations for whom access to services may be problematic, in primary or community care.

England: Improving Access to Psychological Therapies in London

Context

The model of care described is part of the IAPT programme as it applies in the capital city.

London, is one of 10 SHAs, and received £49 million (US$79 million) for the first 3-year phase of an initiative. This is directed towards training and employing 500 new workers, and aiming for 140 000 people to enter treatment, with 50% moving towards recovery, and 4000 people moving off sick pay and benefits. In the first 2 years of roll-out, an implementation team managed a competitive process involving PCT commissioners setting up new IAPT services, with matched funding offered by PCTs to establish services.

The London strategy was one of growth, involving a service to be established in each of 31 PCTs, targeting areas of greatest deprivation as a priority. In the first year (2008–2009), five sites were established – three full services and two as transition sites. In the second year (2009–2010), a further 10 sites were established, with two having transitional status. In wave 3 (2010–2011), a further 15 sites gained IAPT status, although many remained small requiring further expansion and investment to negate health inequalities across the region.

Location

Greater London, with a geographical area of 1572 km² (607 square miles) and serving a total population of approximately 7.7 million.

"Patient" group

The first phase of the IAPT programme was concerned with adults of working age. A wider scope of national outcomes was announced by the government in January 2011, which amounted to 2.6 million people expected to complete a course of therapy, 1.3 million moving to a measurable recovery, and 75 000 people to retain jobs, education or volunteering placements, with a further 2400 new therapists to be trained. The target population is now expanded beyond working-age adults to include children, older people, those with long-term physical health conditions, and those with a serious mental illness. Most importantly, the link between the increased presence of depression and anxiety disorders in some long-term conditions is made.

Services provided

Practitioners in the IAPT programme deliver low- and high-intensity evidence-based psychological interventions to people with depression or anxiety disorders, following the stepped care service model. Psychological well-being practitioners (PWPs) seek to meet the needs of those with milder problems. They deliver low-intensity interventions, including guided self-help; computer-assisted CBT, group therapy and assisted telephone therapy. High-intensity therapists work with those with moderate to severe problems. They primarily offer CBT for anxiety disorders and depression, but also some brief dynamic therapy, counselling for depression, behavioural couple therapy, or interpersonal therapy, for those experiencing depression, using evidence-based protocols and within a clear supervision structure.

All services collect a set of prescribed validated measures, with crucial clinical measures collected at each session to enable accurate measurement of outcomes for all who enter treatment – including those who drop out. These data have been used to produce national reports on the effectiveness of these services.[41]

Evidence for the benefits of employment support in primary care services is very limited. London pioneered a model based on individual placement and support, which is the main evidence-based model for secondary care mental health services. Evidence from services in London highlights the importance of integration of employment and clinical services to improve outcomes.[42] Employment is an important component of all IAPT services, and a concerted effort has been made to move towards clinical and employment support service integration. Employment support services provide support to those currently in work but struggling, and to those seeking to return to work. The majority of those with an employment issue who use IAPT services need help to retain their jobs.

IAPT has linked with other initiatives in London that are seeking to improve access in general, recognizing that those serving deprived populations would be likely to be meeting people experiencing anxiety disorders and depression. These have included health trainer services,[43] smoking cessation services,[44] long-term physical condition services,[13] debt advice services,[45] and children's centres.[46] Also, in England there are high rates of sickness absence due to stress and common mental health conditions.[47] Efforts were therefore also made to engage with employers. These included a "linked employer scheme", where active marketing of services to workforces took place.

The stigma associated with mental health conditions acts as a barrier to people seeking help from psychological therapy services. Information about where to find services and how to self-refer was posted on a specially developed web site,[48] together with information about where to find a range of sources of help and also a range of translated self-help materials. Funds were made available to services to explore ways of increasing the access to and use of such services. Some funded Internet-based services (such as the Big White Wall[49]), and others undertook specific marketing (for example, targeting local ethnic groups). An interesting finding occurred in one borough, where advertisements at bus stops increased self-referrals, which then reduced when those adverts ended.

The positive link between employment and mental health is firmly established.[50] Research demonstrates that work is good for people, and being unemployed is damaging to physical and mental health.[51] The proportion of unemployed people in need of psychological treatment is more than double that of those who are employed.[52] There is also a strong correlation between unemployment and higher mortality, higher medical consultation, higher health-care consumption and higher hospital admission rates.[51,53] After an individual has been absent from work for 6 months, there is only a 50% likelihood of the employee returning to work; this falls to 25% after a 12-month absence, and after 2 years it is virtually nil.[54]

Outcomes

Between 2008 and 2011, a total of 30 new services were established in London through a programme of recruitment, education and training. In the key performance areas defined through the national programme, London is on track to achieve the numbers of people entering treatment, to reach the 50% recovery rate expectation, and has already helped over 2500 individuals to either retain or find employment.

The title of the programme emphasizes the goal of "improving access". To this end, all services are expected to open up to self-referral. Initial concern from some that this may overwhelm services has not materialized. In fact, data from one of the pilot (demonstration) sites showed that by doing this, services saw a more ethnically representative population.[55] Services in London have followed this model and have succeeded in seeing a client group closely representing the regional population (see Figures 13.2 and 13.3). Given the historical underuse of psychological therapy services by those from ethnic minorities, this is significant. As part of the recruitment campaign for new therapists, successful additional advertising and profile raising was undertaken to seek an ethnically representative workforce. Some boroughs also specifically funded services delivered by local nongovernmental organizations (NGOs) that already worked with ethnic groups.

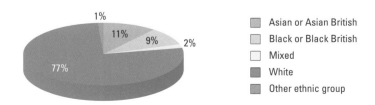

1%
11%
9%
2%
77%

Asian or Asian British
Black or Black British
Mixed
White
Other ethnic group

Figure 13.2 Ethnicity of the general population in London

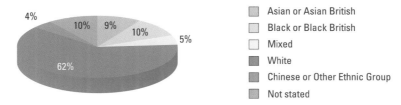

Asian or Asian British
Black or Black British
Mixed
White
Chinese or Other Ethnic Group
Not stated

Figure 13.3 Ethnicity of those who have entered treatment (waves 1 and 2)

Additional comments

Contributions to the future sustainability of these services include ongoing audit and evaluation, developing networks of cooperative working relationships, and establishing training courses in collaboration with services. There has been success in recruiting a balanced ethnically representative workforce, in line with the regional population, and the ethnicity of those accessing services is also broadly representative of that found in local communities.

Clinical-assurance programmes have ensured fidelity to evidence-based models delivering evidence-based interventions, with annual reviews at every site. The implementation team has supported clinical advisers to undertake this service, providing a basis for successful bidding to become an IAPT service, and supporting ongoing service development and performance management thereafter.

Agreed quality measures in this initiative include:

- a stepped care model is in place and operationalized
- a 60:40 ratio of high-intensity to low-intensity (PWP) therapists
- a 2:1 ratio of trainees to supervisors
- sessional data collection
- self-referral is advocated
- equity of access, by diagnosis, sex and ethnicity
- integrated employment services
- locally agreed, reasonable waiting times
- a range of NICE-recommended therapies is offered and clients receive the appropriate therapy for their diagnosis
- provisional International Classification of Diseases (ICD)-10 codes are to be obtained for all clients.

Services are not expected to have all of these things in place straight away but they are things that should be worked towards, and the clinical-assurance process has been instrumental in monitoring this. In addition, the team has maintained and supported clinical and commissioning networks and symposia, with objectives to maximize learning, ensure IAPT fidelity and promote positive practice.

As the programme moves into its second phase, the key components and the broad range of partnerships and initiatives to increase access will remain central to its ongoing success.

Africa: Uganda

Context

The model of care described formed part of an RCT conducted in rural sub-Saharan Africa.[56,57]

Location

Thirty randomly selected villages in south-west Uganda

"Patient" group

Three hundred and forty-one adults aged 18 years and over identified by themselves and other villagers as suffering from at least one of two local "depression-like" symptoms (self-loathing and self-pity), and meeting

Diagnostic and Statistical Manual of Mental Disorders (DSM-IV) criteria for depression or subthreshold depression.

Services provided

Group IPT sessions (between five and eight participants in single-sex groups) for 90 minutes per week for a total of 16 weeks; led by a local leader of the same sex who was bilingual in English and the local language; group leaders had no previous mental health or counselling experience, but were given 2 weeks' intensive training on group IPT. Participants were encouraged at these sessions to review their symptoms and mood in light of the week's events. Peer support from within the group was also encouraged.

Group IPT was the chosen psychological therapy, as it was thought to be the most culturally appropriate intervention for this group of people. Single-sex groups were used to ensure cultural acceptability. Participants were prioritized according to the severity of their symptoms; hence, when the number of eligible participants in a village exceeded the number of therapy "places", those with the most severe symptoms were included.

Outcomes

The depression section of a locally validated symptom checklist often used as a research instrument with non-western populations, and a locally valid functional impairment questionnaire were used as outcome measures. Group IPT was effective in reducing depression and dysfunction compared to treatment as usual; these benefits were maintained at 6 months post-treatment.

There was a high attendance rate at meetings during the intervention. Of note, it was identified at the 6-month follow-up that all but one of the groups had continued to meet in the absence of the group leaders after the formal intervention had finished. It is therefore possible that treatment benefit is sustained for 6 months and/ or that continuing with group meetings is beneficial.

Additional comments

This model of care relates to people within the community, rather than primary care patients per se.

As a result of this work, World Vision International (a humanitarian NGO) started to offer this treatment to those in the control group who needed support.

Australasia: New Zealand

Context

This model of care was one of the primary mental health initiatives developed in response to a New Zealand Government-funded request for proposals, and carried out with the support of locally based primary health organizations, or a district health board.[30] Across the country, 41 initiatives received funding of NZ$200 000 (US$161 000) per annum to support primary mental health service developments. Many initiatives funded a combination of increased GP consultation time, provision of psychological interventions by community-based counsellors, psychologists and other therapists, and infrastructure including a primary mental health coordinator. The project described next was the only initiative from this funding that had a focus on young people.

Location

A primary care organization in a low deprivation decile area of North Island, New Zealand where those aged less than 25 years formed the predominant patient group.

"Patient" group

Youth (aged 10–25 years) with mild to moderate mental health issues including addictions – youth in this area were of significant concern and considered a very "at-risk" population, due to a high incidence of alcohol and other addiction problems.

Services provided

Working within a nongovernmental disability support service, this model involved a youth liaison role that engaged with the wider community (schools, community groups, youth groups, and community and specialist mental health teams). It used a youth-friendly, family-based and strengths-based model.

A case-management and early-intervention approach provided risk and needs assessment for those referred, service coordination, family engagement/support, counselling (youth and their family), group sessions/ individual activity programmes (options were included to suit all New Zealanders including minority and disadvantaged populations), referral to an appropriate counselling/mental health specialist where necessary, and follow-up.

The service was delivered by three staff of mixed sex; a half-time service manager/youth mental health worker; a half-time youth mental health worker, and a 0.2 full-time equivalent youth worker. No health professional with a specific mental health services background was involved. The manager/youth worker had been previously involved in advising agencies on the best ways of working with indigenous Māori, while the youth mental health worker had a background in social work and had worked for "child, youth and family services" for some years.

Referrers to the service completed a referral form. Staff had a weekly intake meeting to decide if referrals were appropriate and to allocate referrals based on the needs identified and who possessed the best skill match. Service users were seen either at their school, in the centrally located office, or, occasionally, in their own home. The community-based premises were intended to encourage youth access and serve the needs of disadvantaged groups by being easily accessible and based in a non-medical environment.

Outcomes

Over 5 months, referrals were received for 29 service users. Most were referred by an education provider or a family member, or self-referred for either substance or behavioural issues ("behavioural issue" is a term more readily used by the education sector; it may mean a number of things within a health paradigm), or a combination of the two. Service users ranged in age from 12 to 20 years and were predominantly male. All service users identified as Māori.

Referrers to the service were generally very satisfied with the intervention received by service users. Data on the perspective of service users is necessarily limited due to the ethical issues associated with interviewing people aged under 16 years. The one service user interviewed (aged over 16 years) viewed the service provided favourably.

Additional comments

A key objective of this initiative was to coordinate services within the primary care team and to integrate the service in such a way as to function well with other youth mental health, and alcohol and drug, services without duplication.

It appeared to be working well with a number of other local agencies (e.g. schools). It is, however, a community-based intersectoral agency addressing alcohol, substance and behavioural issues, and takes a broader view of primary care mental health services. It is likely that it is also addressing mental health issues such as depression, but this has not been recorded in the available data. As the service is community based, rather than general practice based, the wider health needs of service users may remain hidden.

Referrals were predominantly taken from schools. It is hoped this will expand in the future to encompass general practice and other organizations such as youth justice and the police. While the initiative at this early stage had limited interaction with general practice, and no links had been established with primary care, it was hoped that the service would become more integrated with primary care over time.

Europe: the Netherlands

Context

The model of care described forms part of a multicentre RCT conducted in the Netherlands.[58–60]

Location

Recruitment was from 89 primary care practices (GP) in the southern region of the country.

"Patient" group

Adult primary care patients aged 60 years or more with a diagnosis of chronic obstructive pulmonary disease or type 2 diabetes, and meeting the Mini International Neuropsychiatric Interview criteria for one of the following conditions: minor depression, mild to moderate major depression or dysthymia.

Services provided

The DELTA study (Depression in Elderly with Long-Term Afflictions) compared a brief psychological intervention with usual care.

Community-based nurses with no additional training in mental health were responsible for delivering an intervention (in the patient's own home) that focused on patient self-management and CBT. They received training from a psychiatrist, GP and psychologist prior to commencement of the study intervention, and additional "booster" sessions at subsequent intervals throughout.

Completion of the programme required between two and ten intervention visits of approximately an hour's duration, over a maximum of 3 months.

Outcomes

Intervention patients had significantly fewer symptoms of depression (assessed using a validated measurement scale) at 3 months and 9 months following the intervention when compared to usual care. This appeared to be due, in part, to an improvement in symptoms in the intervention group and a deterioration of symptoms in the usual care group.

Although the intervention was identified to be highly acceptable to the majority of patients, an economic study showed no difference in cost-effectiveness compared to usual care.

Additional comments

This model of care relates to primary care patients treated within the community. It was, however, noted that this would be unlikely to occur outside of the trial setting due to the national configuration of primary care services.

North America: USA

Context

The model of care described forms part of a multicentre RCT conducted in the USA.[29,61,62]

Location

Diverse primary care clinics on the west coast of and in southern USA.

"Patient" group

English- or Spanish-speaking adult primary care patients aged between 18 and 75 years, meeting DSM-IV criteria for one of four included anxiety disorders: panic disorder, social anxiety disorder, generalized anxiety disorder or post-traumatic disorder.

Services provided

The CALM study (Coordinated Anxiety Learning and Management) provided a collaborative, stepped care model for the treatment of anxiety disorders that also accommodated the treatment of co-occurring depression and/or alcohol abuse. A focus was also placed on investigating the model's acceptability and effectiveness for minority groups including the African-American and Hispanic population.

Anxiety clinical specialists (ACSs) who had prior experience of patient care and primary care, but not necessarily mental health experience, were responsible for patient assessment, education provision, preparing patients for making decisions about therapy choice, and delivering CCBT. These on-site clinicians, from primarily nursing or social work backgrounds, received intensive and extensive training through workshops that included role play.

In consultation with the ACS, patients chose CBT and/or pharmacological therapy as part of the stepped care treatment model. Psychiatrist support was in place for dealing with patients who were not improving, and psychologist support was available if alterations to CBT therapy were needed. The expert professionals were able to track and clinically monitor patients through a "real-time" web site containing all patient information. This enabled them to focus their attention on patients who were not progressing appropriately.

The computer-assisted CBT programme contained some "core" components relevant to all the included anxiety disorders, while other parts focused on each specific disorder. It was available in both English and Spanish and was used in the primary care clinic by the patient and ACS together. It was deliberately developed to also "guide" the "novice clinician" (ACS) in the "delivery" of the psychotherapy intervention. Completion of the entire CBT programme required approximately eight sessions, each lasting around an hour.

Outcomes

The ACSs considered the computer-delivered CBT to be "user friendly", but identified that it could be improved by reducing the volume of text and simplifying the language used. Patients appeared able to understand the information provided and to "engage" with the programme.

CALM patients showed greater improvements in anxiety and depression symptoms, and functional status (assessed using validated measurement scales) during the 18-month follow-up period, when compared to usual primary care.

Additional comments

The computer delivery of CBT took place in the primary care clinic. Innovations currently being explored include CBT delivery through the Internet and by telephone, to facilitate its use in rural areas.

A key aim was to provide a workable and "user-friendly" evidence-based intervention for primary care, thereby helping to ensure its future sustainability outside of a trial setting.

An optimal model for a primary care psychological intervention initiative

The examples described above demonstrate the wide range of ways that psychological therapies are being introduced. It is clear that "one size does not fit all", and no single idea or initiative can address all service-delivery challenges worldwide. It is, however, possible to extract the elements from these examples and others that contribute to an optimal framework for the introduction of psychological services in primary care settings.

The key structural elements and service user pathways for such an optimal primary care psychological intervention initiative are shown in Figures 13.4 and 13.5 respectively.

Depending on the specific context and structural organization of health care within a country, a *primary care organization* (PCO) could be an individual general practice or family practice, or a collection of health-care providers that provide and/or commission primary health-care services for a specific population within a defined local geographical area.

Organizations at higher levels of the health sector could include umbrella organizations that are responsible for the governance and management of health-care services at a regional or national (government) level.

The structural elements are dependent on each other and all are important. Good training programmes will not improve mental health outcomes if the workforce is then placed in a health system where there are no clear inclusion or exclusion criteria for patient care, or where there are insufficient links with appropriate government agencies or secondary care. Indeed, the importance of the "social aspects" of the approach to care (e.g. the benefit of patients building social networks) should not be underestimated. Social aspects may also include identifying links, as necessary, with government agencies for social, welfare and education support, and links with NGOs including foodbanks and self-help groups.

Psychological therapy interventions must also be placed within a logical service user pathway that follows appropriate assessment and follow-up.

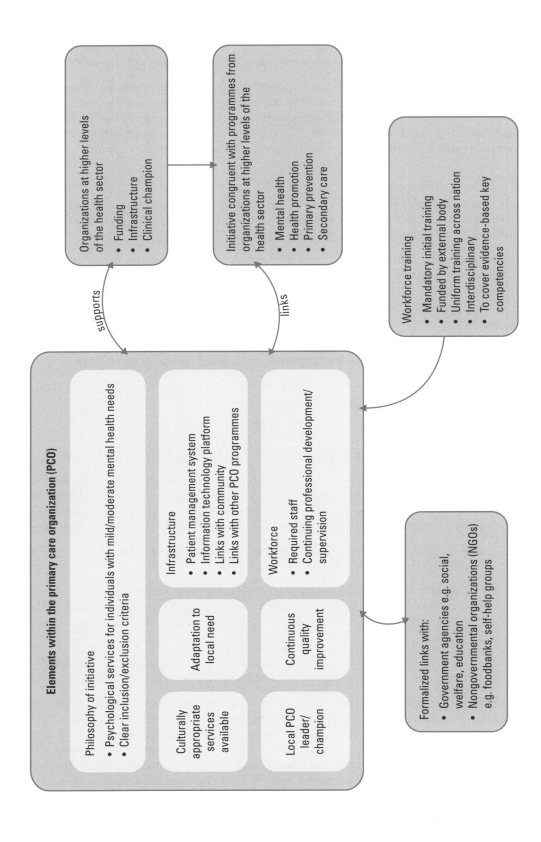

Figure 13.4 Key structural elements of a primary care psychological intervention initiative. Adapted, with permission, from Dowell A et al. *Evaluation of the primary mental health initatives: summary report 2008.* Wellington, Ministry of Health, 2009[30]

Companion to Primary Care Mental Health

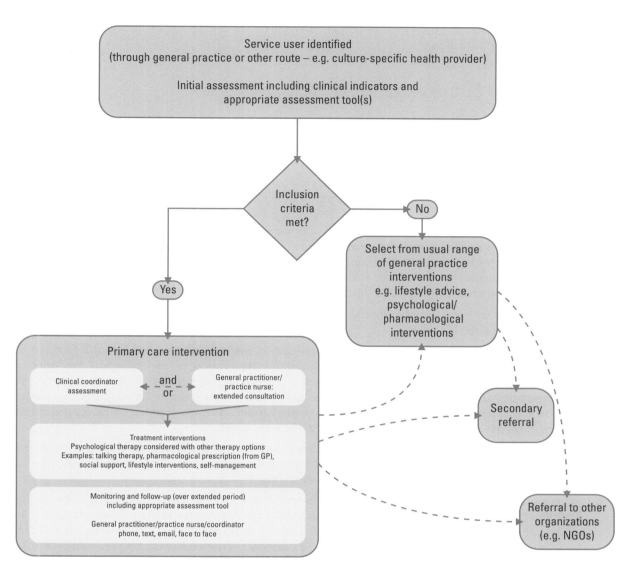

Figure 13.5 Service user pathway (in the context of the structure of Figure 13.4). Adapted, with permission, from Dowell A et al. *Evaluation of the primary mental health initatives: summary report 2008.* Wellington, Ministry of Health, 2009[30]

The place of psychological therapies in health promotion: their usefulness to help prevent mental health problems

The King's Fund has recently identified the importance of not only reacting appropriately to depressive illness, but also addressing the prevention of mental illness. Improving the mental health of younger members of society is likely to be key in this respect.[37] Psychological therapies have already shown some promise as a preventative intervention.[20]

The Internet has shown potential as a delivery medium for a psychological intervention for adolescents aimed at preventing depression;[24,63] "Project CATCH-IT" (Competent Adult-hood Transition with Cognitive-behavioral, Humanistic and Interpersonal Training) has three components based on behavioural activation, CBT and IPT. These techniques are designed to diminish behaviours linked to an increased likelihood for depression (e.g. avoidance, rumination) and promote protective behaviours (e.g. activating social networks). "Rewards" (e.g. a link to a games web site) are included as the participant completes each part.[24] Although this is a low-cost, socioculturally relevant intervention that has the potential to overcome the social stigma of accessing services, by default a certain level of literacy is required. Future developments may benefit from the use of online video and podcasting.[24]

Conclusions and future opportunities

This chapter provides an overview of the evidence surrounding psychological interventions in primary care settings, and uses case-studies to illustrate the variety of approaches being used. We have deliberately described a number of very different contexts to suggest that this is an area where many opportunities can lead to many appropriate solutions. There is an obligation on different countries and health systems to critically reflect on the present configuration of services and enhance and refine them. We hope the following list of conclusions and recommendations will underline the importance of psychological therapies in primary care and provide a checklist for future action.

- Psychological interventions are an important component of primary mental health-care strategy and policy, with an increasing evidence base for effectiveness and efficacy. In developing countries with severe shortages of mental health professionals and a lack of organized mental health services, the integration of mental health services within primary care is increasingly recognized as essential to the accessibility of treatment for mental illness.[64]

  Recommendation: every country should articulate the provision of psychological services as part of an overall mental health policy

- *A global perspective*: with the increasing provision of mental health services into primary care worldwide,[65] the challenge for the future will be the integration of psychological therapies into primary care settings that differ both culturally and operationally across the globe. It is important that the current disparities in access to psychological therapies are reduced both within and across different countries. The need is particularly acute for low- and middle-income countries where psychological interventions are unavailable for the majority of the population.[66]

  Recommendation: existing research and evidence base about psychological therapies in primary care should be made easily accessible to the international community. Future international research collaborations to tailor therapies to primary care contexts should be encouraged.

- *Workforce*: psychological therapies can be delivered in a variety of different ways, and by different health professionals. Existing primary care staff can be trained or upskilled to deliver therapies, and/or specialist mental health professionals can be utilized or trained to work in primary care settings. In addition, new posts and roles can be created; examples are the new graduate psychologists' role in the IAPT in the UK, or the creation of primary mental health coordinators in New Zealand. Evidence suggests that a wide range of employment options might provide equivalent outcomes. Creativity is likely to be required nationally in terms of delivery of services (e.g. making use of innovations in delivery media (computer/Internet based) in the face of the availability of professionally qualified psychotherapists in the workforce for the delivery of psychological interventions, or the availability of "experts" to train others in the primary care workforce. This, in turn, to some extent, will be dependent upon local information technology platforms and infrastructure.

  Recommendation: clarity is required by each country about the most effective way to deploy health professionals to deliver psychological therapies. The workload should be specified between existing primary care professionals and more specialist mental health workers.

- There has been a consistent focus on stepped care models within this chapter. Stepped care can lead to improvements in both the effectiveness and cost-efficiency of primary mental health delivery. Stepped care implies moving away from direct referral to more highly trained therapists and access to high-intensity therapies for disorders of mild to moderate severity.

  Recommendation: countries should investigate how best to implement stepped care models of provision according to local resource and workforce opportunities and constraints.

- *Targeting care*: much of the current delivery of psychological therapy in primary care settings has been targeted at young to mid-life adults with established disorders. Relatively few initiatives have been directed at either the young or the old, with services for those groups coming largely from specialist services.

Recommendation: the importance of psychological therapies in younger and elderly populations should be highlighted, and provision made for their delivery in primary care settings.

■ While CBT has the most highly developed evidence base, it is clear that other therapies such as PST and generic counselling are used widely in primary care settings.[67] There is a need to identify the most effective format and content for brief psychological interventions in primary care, taking into account appropriate cultural variation.

Recommendation: priority should be given to developing an evidence base for generic low-intensity psychological interventions based on problem-solving and cognitive change, suitable for adaptation in different countries.

■ The effectiveness of psychological interventions has traditionally been measured in terms of the impact on secondary care services. The interventions discussed in this chapter are unlikely to produce significant change in outcomes such as hospital admission or suicide, since these are very rare events in primary care settings.

Recommendation: the development of services to introduce psychological interventions in primary care should be guided by consideration of improvements in quality of life for patients and economic cost savings from increased productivity, rather than the impact on secondary services.

References

1 Oakley Browne MA, Wells JE, Scott KM, eds. *Te Rau Hinengaro: The New Zealand Mental Health Survey*. Wellington: Ministry of Health, 2006.

2 Bijl RV et al. The prevalence of treated and untreated mental disorders in five countries. *Health Affairs*, 2003, 22:122–133.

3 *Common mental health disorders. Identification and pathways to care*. London, National Institute for Health and Clinical Excellence, 2011 (CG 123).

4 MaGPIe Research Group. The nature and prevalence of psychological problems in New Zealand primary healthcare: a report on Mental Health and General Practice Investigation (MaGPIe). *New Zealand Medical Journal*, 2003, 116: U379.

5 Centre for Mental Health. *The economic and social costs of mental health problems in 2009/10*. London, Centre for Mental Health, 2010.

6 London School of Economics. *The depression report: a new deal for depression and anxiety disorders. The Centre for Economic Performance's Mental Health Policy Group*. London, London School of Economics, 2006.

7 Murray CJL, Lopez AD. Alternative projections of mortality and disability by cause 1990–2020: Global Burden of Disease Study. *The Lancet*, 1997, 349:1498–1504.

8 Moussavi S et al. Depression, chronic diseases, and decrements in health: results from the World Health Surveys. *The Lancet*, 2007, 370:851–858.

9 Winefield HR et al. Evaluating a program of psychological interventions in primary health care: consumer distress, disability and service usage. *Australian and New Zealand Journal of Public Health*, 2007, 31:264–269.

10 Vagholkar S et al. Better access to psychology services in primary mental health care: an evaluation. *Australian Health Review*, 2006, 30:195–202.

11 Thomas J, Jasper A, Rawlin M. Better outcomes in mental health care: a general practice perspective *Australian Health Review*, 2006, 30:148–157.

12 IAPT – Improving Access To Psychological Therapies (www.iapt.nhs.uk/, accessed 14 November 2011).

13 *Depression in adults with a chronic physical health problem: treatment and management*. London, National Institute for Health and Clinical Excellence, 2009 (CG91).

14 *Realising the benefits: IAPT at full roll out*. London, Department of Health, 2010.

15 Cape J et al. Brief psychological therapies for anxiety and depression in primary care: meta-analysis and meta-regression. *BMC Medicine*, 2010, 8:38.

16   National Collaborating Centre for Mental Health. *Depression. The NICE guideline on the treatment and management of depression in adults (updated edition)*. London, British Psychological Society and Royal College of Psychiatrists, 2010 (National Clinical Practice Guideline 90).

17   *Identification of common mental disorders and management of depression in primary care*. Wellington, New Zealand Guidelines Group, 2008.

18   *Non-pharmaceutical management of depression in adults. A national clinical guideline*. Edinburgh, Scottish Intercollegiate Guidelines Network, 2010 (SIGN114).

19   Hegarty K et al. How could depression guidelines be made more relevant and applicable to primary care? *British Journal of General Practice*, 2009, 59: e149–e156.

20   Alexander CL, Arnkoff DB, Glass CR. (2010). Bringing Psychotherapy to Primary Care: Innovations and Challenges. *Clinical Psychology: Science and Practice*, 2010, 17:191–214.

21   Cuijpers P et al. Psychological treatment of depression in primary care: a meta-analysis. *British Journal of General Practice*, 2009, 59:e51–e60.

22   Kessler D et al. Therapist-delivered internet psychotherapy for depression in primary care: a randomised controlled trial. *The Lancet*, 2009, 374:628–634.

23   Beattie A et al. Primary-care patients' expectations and experiences of online cognitive behavioural therapy for depression: a qualitative study. *Health Expectations*, 2009, 12:45–59.

24   Landback J et al. From Prototype to Product: Development of a Primary Care/Internet Based Depression Prevention Intervention for Adolescents (CATCH-IT). *Community Mental Health Journal*, 2009, 45:349–354.

25   Christensen H et al. Models in the delivery of depression care: A systematic review of randomised and controlled intervention trials. *BMC Family Practice*, 2008, 9:25.

26   Penisula Clinical Trials Unit. *Multi-centre randomised controlled trial of collaborative care for depression (CADET trial)* (http://penctu.pcmd.ac.uk/cadet/AboutCADET.aspx, accessed 14 November 2011).

27   Harkness E, Bower P. On-site mental health workers delivering psychological therapy and psychosocial interventions to patients in primary care: effects on the professional practice of primary care providers. *Cochrane Database of Systematic Reviews*, 2009, (1):CD000532.

28   Smith MJ et al. 'Doing well?': description of a complex intervention to improve depression care. *Primary Health Care Research and Development*, 2010, 11:326–338.

29   Craske MG et al. Treatment for anxiety disorders: Efficacy to effectiveness to implementation. *Behaviour Research and Therapy*, 2009, 47:931–937.

30   Dowell A et al. *Evaluation of the primary mental health initatives: summary report 2008*. Wellington, Ministry of Health, 2009.

31   *Depression. Treatment and management of depression in adults, including adults with a chronic physical health problem. NICE clinical guidelines 90 and 91. Quick reference guide*. London, National Institute for Health and Clinical Excellence, 2009.

32   *Primary solutions. An independent policy review on the development of primary care mental health services*. London, The Sainsbury Centre for Mental Health, 2003.

33   Chatterjee S et al. Integrating evidence-based treatments for common mental disorders in routine primary care: feasibility and acceptability of the MANAS intervention in Goa, India. *World Psychiatry*, 2008, 7:39–46.

34   Patel V et al. Treatment and prevention of mental disorders in low-income and middle-income countries. *The Lancet*, 2007, 370:991–1005.

35   Buchan J, Calman L. *Skill-mix and policy change in the health workforce: nurses in advanced roles. OECD Health Working Papers*. Paris, OECD, 2004.

36   Buchan J, Dal Poz MR. Skill mix in the health care workforce: reviewing the evidence. *Bulletin of the World Health Organization*, 2002, 80:575–580.

37   Naylor C, Bell A. *Mental health and the productivity challenge. Improving quality and value for money*. London, The King's Fund, 2010.

38   Fritzsche K et al. Improving the psychosomatic competence of medical doctors in China, Vietnam and Laos – The Asia-link Program. *International Journal of Psychiatry in Medicine*, 2008, 38:1.

39   Ng C et al. Mental Health Policy paper: Community mental health care in the Asia-Pacific region: using current best-practice models to inform future policy. *World Psychiatry*, 2009, 8:49–55.

40   McKenzie K, Patel V, Araya R. Learning from low income countries: mental health. *BMJ*, 2004, 329:1138–1140.

41   Clark DM, Layard R, Smithies R. *Improving access to psychological therapies; initial evaluation of the two demonstration sites*. 2008. London, LSE Centre for Economic Performance, 2008 (working paper 1648) (http://www.iapt.nhs.uk/silo/files/improving-access-to-psychological-therapy-initial-evaluation-of-the-two-demonstration-sites.pdf, accessed 14 November 2011).

42   Her Majesty's Government. *Work recovery and inclusion*. Norwich: TSO, 2009.

43   Department of Health. *Improving health: changing behaviour – NHS health trainer handbook*. London, Department of Health, 2008 (http://www.dh.gov.uk/en/Publicationsandstatistics/Publications/PublicationsPolicyAndGuidance/DH_085779, accessed 14 December 2011).

44   NHS Executive. *New NHS smoking cessation services*. Wetherby, Department of Health, 1999 (Health service circular 1999/087) (www.dh.gov.uk/en/Publicationsandstatistics/Lettersandcirculars/Healthservicecirculars/DH_4004990, accessed 14 November 2011).

45   Capitalise (www.capitalise.org.uk/, accessed 14 November 2011).

46   Department of Health. *SureStart children's centres* (www.direct.gov.uk/en/Parents/Preschooldevelopmentandlearning/NurseriesPlaygroupsReceptionClasses/DG_173054, accessed 14 November 2011).

47   *Absence management. Annual Survey report*. London, The Chartered Institute of Personnel and Development, 2010 (http://www.cipd.co.uk/hr-resources/survey-reports/absence-management-2010.aspx, accessed 14 December 2011).

48   Working for Wellness (www.workingforwellness.org.uk/, accessed 14 November 2011).

49   Big White Wall (www.bigwhitewall.com/my-account/login.aspx?ReturnUrl=%2f, accessed 14 November 2011).

50   Health Work and Wellbeing. *Working our way to better health*. Norwich, TSO, 2009.

51   Waddell G, Burton K. *Is work good for your health and wellbeing?* Norwich: TSO, 2006.

52   Paul KI, Moser K. Unemployment impairs mental health: meta-analyses. *Journal of Vocational Behavior*, 2009, 74:264–282.

53   Yuen P, Balarajan R. Unemployment and patterns of consultation with the general practitioner. *BMJ*, 1989, 298:1212–1214.

54   British Society of Rehabilitation Medicine. *Vocational rehabilitation: the way forward*. London, British Society of Rehabilitation Medicine, 2001.

55   Improving Access to Psychological Therapies. *Demonstration sites (Newham)* (http://www.iapt.nhs.uk/about-iapt/demonstration-sites/?keywords=newham, accessed 14 December 2011).

56   Bass J et al. Group interpersonal psychotherapy for depression in rural Uganda: 6-month outcomes: Randomised controlled trial. *The British Journal of Psychiatry*, 2006, 188:567–573.

57   Bolton P et al. Group interpersonal psychotherapy for depression in rural Uganda. *JAMA*, 2003, 289:3117–3124.

58   Jonkers C et al. Process evaluation of a minimal psychological intervention to reduce depression in chronically ill elderly persons. *Patient Education and Counseling*, 2007, 68:252–257.

59   Jonkers CCM et al. Economic evaluation of a minimal psychological intervention in chronically ill elderly patients with minor or mild to moderate depression: a randomized trial (the DELTA-study). *International Journal of Technology Assessment in Health Care*, 2009, 25:497–504.

60   Lamers F et al. A minimal psychological intervention in chronically ill elderly patients with depression: a randomized trial. *Psychotherapy and Psychosomatics*, 2010, 79:217–226.

61   Roy-Byrne P et al. Delivery of evidence-based treatment for multiple anxiety disorders in primary care. *JAMA*, 2010, 303:1921–1928.

62   Sullivan G et al. Design of the Coordinated Anxiety Learning and Management (CALM) study: innovations in collaborative care for anxiety disorders. *General Hospital Psychiatry*, 2007, 29:379–387.

63   Project CATCH-IT (http://catchit-public.bsd.uchicago.edu/, accessed 14 November 2011).

64 World Health Organization and World Organization of Family Doctors. *Integrating mental health into primary care: a global perspective.* Geneva, World Health Organization, 2008.

65 Kessler RC et al. Prevalence and treatment of mental disorders, 1990 to 2003. *New England Journal of Medicine*, 2005, 352:2515–2523.

66 Saxena S et al. Resources for mental health: scarcity, inequity, and inefficiency. *The Lancet*, 2007, 370:878–889.

67 Mynors-Wallis L. *Problem-solving treatment for anxiety and depression. A practical guide.* New York, Oxford University Press, 2005.

14 Social and environmental interventions in primary care mental health

Helen Rodenburg, Jill Benson and Filippo Zizzo

Key messages

- Holistic interventions that consider all social and relational aspects of the human being are required.
- Social problems must be addressed as part of the work of primary care mental health clinics.
- Culture and social change can impact on resilience; a cultural awareness tool can help assess this.
- Community-based interventions may be necessary, as well as individual interventions.
- Primary mental health clinics require access to a range of skills and interventions.

Introduction

Social and environmental factors are important in the development of mental distress and can have variable impact across the lifespan. At the macro level these are related to poverty, war and inequity. Urbanization, displacement, discrimination and economic instability are associated with poor mental health.[1] These are outside the direct influence of primary care mental health clinics but need to be considered in addressing the mental distress of individuals and communities. This is especially important in developing countries, to reduce the impact on primary care services.

While social and environmental factors can lead to specific problems that need addressing, they can also be part of the solution for people with mental distress.

It is important that a thorough biopsychosocial assessment is undertaken to enable appropriate interventions for people. The previous chapters have covered prescribing and psychological interventions; however, it is also essential to consider the impact of the person's environment and culture when taking a history. Practitioners with good communication and assessment skills, an understanding of the context and efficacy of available interventions and a multifaceted approach to patient safety, including good record keeping, can work with people (and communities) to improve mental health outcomes.

To support a comprehensive approach there is a need for psychological therapies that match different cultures and environments. Continuity of care supports the provision of a "package of interventions" to address the person's needs, including long-term follow-up.

The choice of which intervention to use depends on how the problem presents and the aetiology of that problem in the context of the local community. Community-based interventions may be necessary, as well as individual interventions.

If the problem presents as an environmental or social problem, then these parameters need to be part of the solution, whether this is a mild, moderate or severe mental health problem. The level of distress will determine the priority of interventions and the level of support required for the individual. There are often strong links with cultural issues, which must be considered in all situations, but especially when there is diversity between health practitioners and their patients.

Social and environmental factors are also key to the prevention of mental distress and mental health promotion.

In this chapter, we will consider social and environmental factors, with particular emphasis on assessment and interventions. Primary care mental health clinics with community links are well placed to do this.

Epidemiology

Epidemiological surveys study the differential frequency of symptoms or disorders in different populations, the distribution on the same population, and any specific qualitative or quantitative differences in populations or groups under comparison.[2] Epidemiological investigations use some benchmarks that are standardized for comparisons between several studies.[3] One of the main contributions of epidemiology in general practice/primary health care is the ability to identify risk factors with potential aetiologic significance for the different mental disorders in different populations. The hypothesis suggested by epidemiological data can be evaluated through a specific experimental programme design. Epidemiological investigations, on the other hand, can assess the reliability of interpretative models of aetiology of mental disorders when it is not possible to validate a specific model by clinical and experimental studies.[4] The presence of an inverse correlation between the incidence of psychiatric disorders and socioeconomic factors and social class, as emphasized at the beginning of the 20th century by the first studies on mental health, was confirmed by several contemporary studies.[5,6] The stability of this finding has implications not only at the level of knowledge of aetiopathogenetic mechanisms of the disease, but also in prevention, and perhaps in the therapeutic field. Consistent with the statement that was accepted by the World Health Organization (WHO), we can say that:

> The social determinants of health are the conditions in which people are born, grow, live, work and age, including the health system. These circumstances are shaped by the distribution of money, power and resources at global, national and local levels, which are themselves influenced by policy choices. The social determinants of health are mostly responsible for health inequities – the unfair and avoidable differences in health status seen within and between countries.[1]

These obvious inequities of social and cultural situations more easily determine psychiatric distress that can sometimes lead to real, disruptive and harmful diseases for an individual, and thereby to the social background that surrounds them.

Therefore, WHO has proposed three inevitable modes of intervention, defined as "overarching recommendations", presented below:

- improve daily living conditions
- tackle the inequitable distribution of power, money, and resources
- measure and understand the problem and assess the impact of action.[1]

These proposals are important, and the goals are difficult to reach in their entirety; however, it is possible to try to sensitize people so they can overcome the harmful aspects of inequality and social inadequacy.

Social factors to consider

Resilience

Resilience is the ability to recover from stress and adversity and to learn lessons from life's mistakes and mishaps. It is complex and multifactorial and will change at different times and in different circumstances for each person. There are some features of resilience that are moulded by seemingly "immutable" factors, such as genetic predisposition, culture, personality, religion, sense of humour, finances and early childhood history and relationships.[7] But these can also be transformed into learning experiences and resources if there is strong social support, good problem-solving skills, a positive outlook, perseverance, etc. Even the genetic and environmental predisposition to depression can be negated by strong social support.[8]

It is well known that physical health and psychological health influence each other, for better or for worse. This can be seen in the increased risk of depression with chronic disease, and the increased risk of cardiovascular disease in those with depression. The use of substances such as alcohol, and smoking, more prevalent in those with mental illness, will also have a major impact on physical health. Less well known is the trend for resilience to improve with better physical health. As personal care improves (as measured by parameters such as better nutrition, exercise, adequate sleep, fewer substances), so does a person's ability to problem-solve and "bounce back" from difficult situations. In addition, exercise has been shown to improve mood and decrease depression and anxiety.

Psychological stress will appear when personal resources are inadequate to deal with outside circumstances. Such stress can be addressed by problem-solving the "outside circumstances", such as changing jobs, building up better support systems, delegating difficult tasks or decreasing workload. Improvement in physical health will certainly improve personal resources but so will doing a course, learning more about a situation or discussing the situation with a friend.

A sense of humour is also a useful feature in developing resilience, as well as increasing the "endorphins" that "heal the brain". To laugh at a circumstance, one must stand apart from it and view it from a different angle, often with another trusted person. In the process of doing this, the problem loses its power and is unlikely to be so overwhelming. Children who learn that people are trustworthy, that the world is a safe place, that they are loved and the future is stable, and who develop a set of beliefs to guide their decisions and relationships, are more likely to grow up to be resilient adults. This is usually learnt in a nurturing family environment, mostly from a primary caregiver but also from the community, school, friends, etc. Those who have been psychologically, socially, sexually or physically abused, or exposed to neglect, malnutrition, violence or extreme uncertainty are likely to have unhealthy coping mechanisms and are much more likely to develop mental health problems as adults. Healing will take a long time and will be complex and multifaceted, as new connections will need to develop in the person's brain to replace the older dysfunctional ones. This may involve psychotherapy, but also positive support from a group or community and a pathway of good decisions about personal care, relationships and work.

A good psychotherapist will help a patient improve their resilience. Some of this will be by basic stress-reduction techniques such as relaxation and sleep hygiene, improving social supports and better physical health. But there are many other skills that can be learnt. Cognitive-behavioural therapy (CBT) assists a patient in challenging their learnt patterns, such as their negative view of themselves, their world and their future. A more positive outlook is likely to reap other benefits such as improving relationships, gaining more satisfaction from work and leisure, and engendering more hope and self-control. Problem-solving skills can be learnt and applied to many situations, both personal and in decision-making. Narrative therapy skills can help identify resources that have been used in other situations and help a patient have a more internal "locus of control".

Cultural and traditional factors

Cultural issues may also be part of a person's resilience. Some societies have good leaders who encourage safe, non-discriminatory and collaborative styles of relating within the community. In others, the status of women or children may not be conducive to resilience and well-being. Women may have no power to make their own decisions and have no access to education or the workforce. Children may have to abide by very strict rules and have no opportunities for self-expression or exploration. Domestic violence, early marriage and incest may be "normalized" in some cultures. Different cultures have different attitudes to relationships, extended family, humour, education, decision-making and many of the other parameters that influence how each person views the world and their place in it. Although many of these are impossible to challenge, going back to the basics of nutrition, exercise, social relationships, relaxation, a sense of meaning from work or leisure, and spirituality can improve psychological well-being.

The apparent security of a traditional collectivist culture and the individualism of a "western" culture may seem at odds with each other. But in every culture there are behaviours and beliefs that are accepted as normal that may be conducive to future resilience and good mental health, and others that may not. In all cultures, there are good parents who care for and respect their children, build up strong relationships and have a sense of connection, meaning and spirituality. Whereas a village lifestyle is more likely to encourage close relationships, mutual support and sharing of facilities, many in western cultures have favoured individual pursuits of career, leisure and technology. A sense of community, compassion and deeper purpose has been replaced with a fierce belief in individual rights, material gain and electronic communication. Children are spending more time on computers and in front of the television than with their families, or even their friends. Pain, suffering or mistakes are not viewed as "lessons to be learnt" or "problems to be worked through", but as abnormal occurrences where someone is to blame. Western cultures have seen a rise in substance abuse and suicide, as people struggle "without a sense of community, of caring for each other, of purpose that is beyond individual effort, of being connected to others no matter what has happened and of sharing hardship".[7]

When working with someone from a different culture, a health professional may be concerned that they do not fully understand the problem because of cultural differences. In many languages, there are no words for mood or mental health problems. People may understand psychological problems in spiritual or traditional ways, or may be more aware of physical than psychological symptoms. There may be stigma attached to mental health issues, or it may be that they do not view mental health problems as something that is "worthy" of a doctor's attention, and present with physical symptomatology. The "cultural awareness tool" (see Box 14.1) can assist in hearing the patient's story from their own perspective and can lead a health professional from a physical to a psychological or social problem.[9] It can also help the doctor to understand more about the patient's expectations of the consultation. Thus, if the basis of the problem is a traditional one, for instance if the person has broken a cultural taboo, it may be that a traditional healer or a community health worker will be needed to assist with the healing.

Box 14.1 Cultural awareness tool

- What do you think caused your problem?
- Why do you think it started when it did?
- What do you think illness does to you?
- What are the chief problems it has caused for you?
- How severe is your illness?
- What do you most fear about it?
- What kind of treatment/help do you think you should receive?
- Within your own culture, how would your illness be treated?
- How are your family and community helping you?
- What have you been doing so far?
- What are the most important results you hope to get from treatment?
- When would you like to come back?

Social change

Culture, community, family and society dictate how people make sense of their lives. Movement from one culture or one country to another, or major changes in society, are likely to cause problems in how a person sees their place in the world, relates to other people or views their future. If, in addition, there is political unrest, poverty or disruption to family and relationships, then people are more likely to develop mental health problems. Culture and community are part of what determines how each person unconsciously thinks, feels and acts, and how they make sense of their surroundings. Moving to another culture, or the culture around changing, can cause anxiety and depression as people are unsure of themselves, whether they are acting appropriately, whether people are disapproving of them and who they can relate to.

Those who move to a new country as refugees are more likely to have problems settling in the new country than those who have chosen to migrate for career, education or financial reasons. Added to this, they are likely to be suffering from poorer physical health, and the additional mental health problems such as post-traumatic stress disorder caused by violence, torture and trauma in their country of origin. If there is time to plan, to learn a new language, say goodbye to loved ones, settle accounts and to pack treasured items, the path is likely to be smoother. But even if there is a chance to do all this, there are still likely to be differences such as accent, food, dress, housing, education, skin colour and all those people, traditions and things that have been left behind. Acknowledging these differences and slowly working through how each one will be dealt with is part of beginning a new life. Each person should be encouraged to consciously choose what they will keep from their old culture and society and what they will "take on" from the new. Thus, a new "third culture" is formed. For many people, this process will involve challenging old beliefs and traditions and can be quite painful, for example – choosing marriage or a career, dress codes, contraception, discipline of children. For others, especially those from a more collectivist or indigenous culture, there is a deep sense of loss of culture and "country", related more to spirituality than to the material world.

Globalization, urbanization and rapid social change are part of a slowly worsening profile for mental health in many low- and middle-income countries.[10] In many countries that have previously had a collectivist worldview with a strong network of extended family, deep religious and traditional beliefs, an attachment to the land and communal decision-making, there is a move toward a more "westernized" individualistic culture. This has involved a decrease in village life, subsistence farming and traditional rules. For young people, this has meant more education, greater opportunities and more choices. But it has also meant a move to the city, unemployment, no social support, risk of substance abuse and sometimes interactions with the police and increased sexually transmitted infections. For older people, this has meant that they cannot pass on their traditions, they are lonely and may be alone in the village when they are sick or aged. There is an urgent need for the development of a primary health-care workforce trained in basic psychotherapeutic techniques to assist developing countries and indigenous populations in dealing with the increased mental health problems resulting from these changes.

Poverty, war, disaster and inequality

Marsella aptly says that mental health is "not only about biology and psychology, but also about education, economics, social structure, religion, and politics".[11] He goes on to say that the despair bred by powerlessness, the hopelessness bred by poverty, the anger and resentment bred by inequality, the low self-esteem and self-denigration bred by racism, and the confusion and conflict bred by cultural disintegration and destruction make mental health almost impossible in many places in today's world.

Issues such as politics, human rights and climate change are not usually the domains of health practitioners. But without food, safety and shelter, as well as a sense of personal power, hope, equality and political stability, the best medication and psychotherapy are unlikely to be of assistance. Mental health is not just about caring for patients at an individual level, but includes advocating for decreased stigma, more respect and better facilities in all countries. It is also about global efforts to decrease poverty, war and inequality, and sending aid to those countries that are struck by disaster of any type.

Human rights issues for those with severe mental health problems remain a huge problem in many countries. Rather than being an aid to healing, being locked up, shackled, starved, humiliated or "doped up" are inevitably going to cause further mental health problems. For those countries with limited mental health personnel, medication or facilities, it is very difficult to find humane ways of dealing with people with severe mental health problems such as schizophrenia or bipolar disorder. The stigma associated with these illnesses adds to the lifelong dysfunction experienced by many people, as they cannot access education, work or a normal social environment.

Religion and spirituality

Religion and spirituality are important features in the lives of many people. Religion gives structure and a cultural basis for many people's spirituality, providing them with a ritual and guidelines with which to lead a better life. For others, spirituality is about finding a purpose in their lives and connection with the world and other people, and finding hope or inner peace, without looking to organized religion. The "rules" of a religion may constrain a person or fill them with guilt, or, on the other hand, may give them guidance for decisions that would otherwise be difficult to make. Similarly, the deeply intuitive beliefs held by some may be impractical or illogical in everyday life.

Helping a patient find meaning and purpose in their life will often mean helping them plumb the depths of their spiritual beliefs and turning their religion into something supportive and practical. Many health professionals shy away from discussing religion, especially if the patient is of a different faith. However, this is denying access to what might be one of the causes of the mental health problems and/or to one of the sources of healing for those problems. Asking simple questions can help guide a patient to start the discussion, such as:[12]

- is faith (religion, spirituality) important to you?
- has faith (religion, spirituality) been important to you at other times in your life?
- do you have someone to talk to about religious matters?
- would you like to explore religious or spiritual matters with someone?

Opening up a respectful discussion can then lead to finding out about the importance of spirituality in the person's life, the "rules" of their religion, and how they relate to these, how they express their spirituality, etc. These are generic questions that can be asked whatever the patient's religion. Even if the patient and health professional are from the same religion, the patient's understanding, beliefs, practice and spirituality are likely to be different.

Assisting a patient to find the more helpful and meaningful side of their own religion, or to glean purpose and hope from their spiritual beliefs is not something most health professionals have been taught to do. However, it is a powerful intervention for many people with psychological problems.

Interventions that impact on individuals and communities

Environmental interventions

Where we live affects our health and chance of living flourishing lives. Last year saw, for the first time, the majority of human beings living in urban settings. At the moment, almost one billion live in slums. The daily conditions in which people live have a strong influence on health equity. Access to quality housing and clean water and sanitation are human rights. Therefore, greater availability of affordable housing by investment in urban slum upgrading, including, as a priority, provision of water, sanitation and electricity, is actually necessary.

Furthermore, "big cities" all over the world are characterized by social factors that can influence mental health and impact on the provision of mental health care. These factors include social inequalities, social marginalization and fragmentation, large-scale immigration, and a high proportion of mobile populations. Big cities tend to have higher levels of morbidity and higher costs of service provision than other parts of the same country. For example, in megalopolis London, services are provided by the National Health Service (NHS), with an emphasis on care in the community. While there have been large investments in mental health care and the establishment of a range of new teams with specialized functions over the last 10 years, funding has recently come under pressure and service provision may need to be reduced, which may affect the provision of care and increase risk. Bassi discusses the urban health penalty model, the urban sprawl model, the urban health advantage model and the urban living conditions model.[13] The urban health penalty model posits that urban areas, due to unhealthy environments, create the conditions for poor health. Thus, "penalty" represents higher rates of medical problems, mental illness and substance abuse.

A recent German study carried out by Dekker in 2008 found that higher levels of urbanization were linked to higher 12-month prevalence for almost all major psychiatric disorders (quoted by Bassi 2011[13]). Similarly, in the Netherlands, five levels of increasing urbanization were significantly associated with increasing prevalence of psychiatric disorders (Penn et al. 2007, quoted by Bassi 2009[14]). Life is increasingly related to issues that are critical for mental health, much more than in less urbanized areas. Such issues include a higher concentration of ethnic minorities and recent immigrants, a higher prevalence of poverty-related diseases, and a poorer outcome of care due to discrimination and limited access to mental health and social services. The study of mental health problems from this perspective makes it possible to gain a deeper understanding of many risk factors (see Box 14.2).

There is a perception of a strong need to expand collaborative efforts aimed at protecting and enhancing the mental health of populations, especially those living in big cities.[14]

- Higher concentration of ethnic minorities
- New immigrants
- Higher prevalence of poverty-related diseases
- Poorer outcome of care

WHO defines the "healthy city" as:

> one that is continually creating and improving those physical and social environments and expanding those community resources which enable people to mutually support each other in performing all the functions of life and in developing to their maximum potential.[15]

Mental health can be influenced by encouraging healthy eating and, above all, reducing violence and crime through good environmental design and regulatory controls, including control of alcohol outlets.

Social protection

In a period of severe social and economic crisis, we need to give utmost importance to employment and business continuity. Employment and working conditions have powerful effects on health equity. When these are good, they can provide financial security, social status, personal development, social relations and self-esteem, and protection from psychosocial illness. Everyone needs social protection throughout their lives, as young children, in working life, and in old age. People also need protection in case of specific shocks, such as illness, disability, and loss of income or work. Four out of five people worldwide lack the back-up of basic social security coverage. Extending social protection to all people, within countries and globally, will be a major step towards achieving health equity within a generation.

Community

The communities within which people live are an important part of the environment that influences mental well-being. Often groups will function as communities within the wider society, and, as such, these are important for health practitioners to understand.

Groups can strengthen communities, whether they are informal such as a local environmental clean-up group, or more formal representing a specific cultural grouping, for example immigrant groups. In some countries, nongovernmental organizations (NGOs) have arisen out of groups, and these receive funding and are more accountable for activities that can have significant impact on mental well-being.

It is important to understand the social and cultural contexts of groups, in order to work with them.

In working to promote positive social and environmental interventions, primary care mental health clinics may work with groups at different levels. By doing this, the clinic and its staff can help create an environment that improves the mental health of the community it serves. "Flourishing" is a measure, developed within the last decade, which has been used to determine the level of positive mental health in populations.[16] Clinics may wish to work with other groups to promote positive mental health and a "flourishing" community.

Culture in communities

In some communities where there are strong cultures, clinic staff may need to develop links with respected members or elders of a particular culture in order to establish credibility and effective interventions. It is important to work with a specific cultural group in relation to the way they view mental distress, and members of that cultural community may be part of the therapeutic response; for example, strengthening cultural ties and using cultural processes can have a positive impact for both individuals and communities.

Working with individuals

It is essential to know what is available within the wider community, so that at an individual level people can be linked in with appropriate groups for support and involvement in community activities. Engagement in community activities promotes self-esteem and the acquisition of skills.[17]

Working with groups

Primary care mental health clinics may also work at the organizational level with community groups on joint projects to improve mental well-being of both individuals and communities. This may be as simple as working with local church groups to promote mental health, being involved in promoting local festivals, or wider action to address specific problems.[18]

A community-development approach is a way of working that helps groups of people to change things for themselves, using the understanding and expertise that is often overlooked by people outside those communities, and this can lead to sustainable improvement in the mental health of those people.

In New Zealand, a new approach to mental health promotion has been developed. The approach adopted by *Building on strengths*[19] is to:

- start working towards a common understanding of mental health promotion
- recognize that different populations will have different needs
- recognize that the most effective programmes will take into account the context of the lives of different populations
- recognize that different models of service delivery will work in different circumstances.

The primary mental health initiatives in New Zealand have had a flexibility to work in different ways with different communities,[20] and this is still evolving. This is also important, in that different cultural groups have different concepts of mental health or distress and differing ways of dealing with them. In taking a flexible approach, it is possible to work with different communities to address individual and family needs as well as developing interventions to promote mental health across that community.

Teaching and caring for children

A healthy childhood, free from abuse and violence, improves the likelihood of developing into an adult with good mental health. Targeting at-risk families and children with behavioural disturbance who are at risk of developing future mental health problems is likely to have positive effects (see Box 14.3). It is important to review recent evidence before implementing any programmes.

Infancy and early childhood

In early childhood, home visiting for families at risk has a positive impact and should be part of primary health-care services.[20] Improving social support, parenting skills and early child–parent interactions are important inputs to these programmes and can reduce the rates of child abuse and neglect.

Children

If behavioural problems develop, then parenting programmes such as "Incredible Years" and the Positive Parenting Programme (PPP) have proven positive outcomes for supporting parents of young children to reduce future problems.[21]

Programmes that work to prevent violence and aggression with a whole-of-school approach have been shown to be effective.[22] This is particularly so if they take an approach that includes families and individual student skill development, as well as improved school ecology. An example of this comes from Hong Kong, where a health-promoting schools framework and healthy school's award has demonstrated improvements in health risk behaviour, self-reported health status and academic results.[23] This was more significant in primary school students than in secondary schools.

Infancy and early childhood

- Early childhood home visiting
- Parenting programmes for behavioural problems

Children

- Parenting programmes for behavioural problems
- Whole-of-school health-promotion programmes
- Comprehensive programmes to prevent violence and aggression, including family and student skill development

Youth

- Exposure to role models, "positive" people and experiences
- Troubled young people and those with parents who themselves have a mental illness may require specific programmes of mentoring
- Opportunities to learn and develop relationships and skills

Improvement in learning outcomes is a factor in positive mental and emotional health.[24] Improvements in health risk behaviours may not be reflected in depressive symptoms or social and school relationships.[25]

Youth

For young people, exposure to role models, "positive" people and experiences can facilitate the development of positive skills. There are four settings or environments in which young people naturally exist and where they can potentially access helpful people and have positive developmental experiences. These are:

- the family
- the community
- the school,[26] university, workplace or wider environment
- peers.

For positive youth development to occur, young people need a range of opportunities, including opportunities to:

- experience supportive adult relationships
- learn how to form close, durable human relationships with peers that support and reinforce healthy behaviours
- feel a sense of belonging and being valued
- develop a sense of mattering
- develop positive social values and norms
- build and master skills
- develop confidence in their abilities to master their environment (a sense of personal efficacy)
- make a contribution to their community.[27]

Troubled young people, and those with parents who themselves have a mental illness, may require specific programmes of mentoring and support, which can range from "buddies" who are community volunteers, to specific services including those working with individual young people with drug and alcohol problems.

Interventions to support individuals in caring for themselves

Self-management

Chronic care (long-term conditions) management includes self-management as a core element. This can be applied to mental illness directly, as people with mental health problems need to be able to self-manage to recover and prevent relapse.

It is also important in preventing depression in those with other long-term conditions, such as diabetes.

To promote self-management, individual education is important, but so is learning from others with the same condition and being able to support each other. Cultural outreach may also be necessary to support self-management.

Support groups

Peer support/groups have extensive research evidence. They are important for the spectrum of mental distress, with groups such as drop-in centres and user groups supporting a pathway to recovery for those with long-term problems such as schizophrenia, while groups such as Alcoholics Anonymous have a specific programme for people with alcoholism.

Primary care mental health clinics can work with existing groups and attempt to fill gaps by supporting the development of relevant support groups.

Peer support workers are part of many specialist mental health services and can also work with primary mental health clinics to provide support to individuals with long-term mental health problems. This may be formally in large services, or informally through networking.

Support for parenting

Home visiting has been shown to reduce the risk of future behavioural problems, and is important in supporting new parents. Social groups such as new mothers; support groups; and specific groups such as postnatal distress support groups have important roles to play in reducing the risk of poor mother–infant bonding and future problems.

Healthy behaviour

Physical activity

Healthy and safe behaviours have to be promoted equitably, including promotion of physical activity. Exercise is particularly important in treating mild to moderate depression and anxiety, as well as in improving self-esteem.[28] Opportunities for exercise need to be available in the environment, and individuals encouraged to exercise.

Relaxation

Stress arising from the environment in which people live and work is a factor in the development of mental distress. The ability to relax is important in effectively managing stress and anxiety. When we feel stressed, our bodies react with what is called the "fight or flight" response. Our muscles become tense, our heart and respiration rates increase, and other physiological systems become taxed. Without the ability to relax, chronic stress or anxiety can lead to burnout, anger, irritability, depression, medical problems, and more. Allowing yourself to deeply relax is the exact opposite of the "fight or flight" response.[29] Herbert Benson described what he referred to as the "relaxation response".[30] This is the body's ability to experience a decrease in heart rate, respiration rate, blood pressure, muscle tension, and oxygen consumption. The benefits of being able to induce the "relaxation response" in your own body include a reduction of generalized anxiety, prevention of cumulative stress, increased energy, improved concentration, reduction of some physical problems, and increased self-confidence.[31] Relaxation exercises can be a powerful weapon against stress (see Box 14.4). The following are some important facts about stress:

- 43% of adults have experienced adverse health effects from stress
- 75–90% of visits to a physician's office are for stress-related conditions and complaints
- stress has been linked to the six leading causes of death: heart disease, cancer, lung ailments, accidents, cirrhosis of the liver and suicide
- the Occupational Safety and Health Administration (OSHA) has declared stress a hazard of the workplace
- in the workplace, stress may be related to lost hours due to absenteeism, reduced productivity, and workers' compensation benefits. This costs the American industry more than $300 billion annually.[32]

- Diaphragmatic breathing
- Deep breathing
- Progressive muscle relaxation
- Guided imagery: the beach (take a mini-vacation as you are guided through the sights, sounds, smells, and sensations of a pleasant walk along the beach)
- Guided imagery: the forest (you are guided on a peaceful walk through a beautiful, lush forest near a trickling stream)
- Relaxing phrases: sometimes it is helpful to repeat certain phrases to yourself in order to deepen your state of relaxation
- Mindfulness meditations: much of the emotional distress people experience is the result of thinking about upsetting things that have already happened, or anticipating negative events that have yet to occur. Distressing emotions such as anger, anxiety, guilt, and sadness are much easier to bear if you only focus on the present – on each moment one at a time. These are exercises to increase your mindfulness of the present moment so that you can clear away thoughts about past and future events

Self-help using Internet-based tools

In the present society of global communication, various Internet-based tools can replace, at least partly, direct contacts with professionals and reach a high number of users of any social situation. It is important to note that the Internet is a support tool but does not replace in any way any health technician.

It is useful for staff working in primary care mental health clinics to understand self-help and which Internet tools are locally supported. Referring people to Internet sites can be a useful intervention but should be done in a situation where follow-up also occurs.

In the past, especially in Anglo-Saxon areas, a remarkable literature has been produced in self-help book form; currently the Internet provides these same tools but in a virtual form, by improving access to users and lowering costs. In short, we can say that self-help books are books written with the stated intention to instruct any readers on a number of personal problems. Self-improvement is a term that is a modernized version of self-help, and bookstores use both terms to classify these types of books in the store, like in Internet windows. Self-help books often focus on popular psychology or aspects of the mind and human behaviour, which believers in self-help feel can be controlled with effort. At various times in life, most people will be faced with one or more mental health, wellness or life issues that will cause them pain in one form or another and that they will want to rid themselves of. People faced with such issues and illnesses have three basic options for getting help:[33–35]

- they can seek help from medical or mental health professionals (or people who hold themselves out as teachers of one sort or another)
- they can choose to work on their problems themselves through a process of self-help
- they can combine professional/teacher and self-help approaches.[36,37]

There are many benefits to be had from professional helpers. In some cases and for some problems, the only real benefits that can be had are had through professional helpers. This is certainly the case with serious mental illnesses such as bipolar disorder or schizophrenia.[38,39] Nevertheless, professional helpers are expensive, seldom available as much as you might like, and limited in terms of what they can offer.

For these and other reasons which we will outline below, it is a very good idea for people dealing with painful issues and illnesses to learn methods for helping themselves. Self-help for mental health and wellness issues consists of learning about the nature of distressing issues, learning how to measure or assess those issues and how they can be resolved, and then choosing and following a course of action that will help to resolve those issues. A typical mental health self-help effort requires a person to pay attention, make an emotional investment in change, perform one or more self-assessments, educate about problem(s), consider multiple alternative possible actions for addressing problem(s), decide on a specific plan of action (selected from the alternatives available) that seems most likely to be helpful, and then finally commit and dedicate to executing that self-help plan.[40,41] Obviously, before people launch into a self-help process, they need to know that self-help is an appropriate means of addressing their issues. Self-help is not appropriate as a means of treatment when people are dealing with serious illness, or when they have reason to believe their judgement may be compromised. It is a more appropriate path to pursue when people are dealing with less serious, non-life-threatening conditions.

Internet-based tools can also be useful in dealing with problems of addiction, such as to alcohol and tobacco. To do this, one needs to understand the problem by identifying its nature: what might be causing that problem and why and how it has become an issue. Because mental health and life issues are usually troubling and anxiety provoking, there is a tendency to get emotional while thinking about them. It is easy to get distracted or fooled by self-defensive feelings when people get emotional, and also easy to act on mistaken perceptions. In "panic" to avoid dealing with a problem, it is possible to minimize it inappropriately (concluding that it is less of a problem than it really is), or exaggerate it (making a "mountain out of a molehill").[42] In order to have an appropriate evaluation process for the situation, the first logical tool to be used is to break the problem down into small parts. Then it is possible to make a plan for how it is possible to fix or address each part separately and choose the best solution for the real situation.

These processes make up a number of therapeutic techniques such as CBT, problem-solving and motivational interviewing. Internet-based tools can work to support this type of behaviour change.[43,44]

Implications for primary care workforce and clinics

In order to work effectively with the social and environmental aspects of mental distress, primary care mental health clinics will need to have staff with skill sets that extend beyond purely clinical care.

Clinical care is important in assessing individuals and using appropriate interventions that may include social and environmental factors. Clinical skill development will be linked with new service development and enhancing existing care.

Doctors will be part of a team providing primary mental health care. Their role will vary depending on the needs and resources available in the local community and the skills of other team members.

The "five star doctor" has been proposed as a model for general practitioners (GPs):[45]

- care provider, who considers the patient as an integral part of a family and the community and provides a high standard clinical care and personalizes preventive care within a long-term trusting relationship
- decision-maker, who chooses which technologies to apply ethically and cost-effectively while enhancing the care that he or she provides
- communicator, who is able to promote healthy lifestyles by emphatic explanation, thereby empowering individuals and groups to enhance and protect their health
- community leader, who, having won the trust of the people among whom he or she works, can reconcile individual and community health requirements and initiate action on behalf of the community
- team member, who can work harmoniously with individuals and organizations, within and without the health-care system, to meet his or her patients' and communities' needs.

Working with communities

In order to influence social and environmental impacts on mental distress, staff of primary mental health clinics will need skills that include building relationships with community groups, establishing groups and networks, and health promotion.

This will depend on the local circumstances, demands on the workforce and the existing skill mix. For example, health promotion may be part of the work of the clinical team, or be carried out by a trained health promoter working with the clinical team or by volunteers from the local community, or a combination.

The structure of the clinic needs to support teamwork and continuity of care, as well as providing easy access to information on community activities. There may be structured meetings between the clinic and groups in the community, or other mechanisms of communication.

Working with different cultures

In areas of cultural diversity, clinic staff will need to be aware of their own cultural perspectives in order to appreciate how that can differ from others'. The cultural awareness tool is one mechanism to start understanding different viewpoints. It is also important that staff have an overall understanding of what is culturally important for the people they are working with. It may be important that leaders or health workers from the local community are involved in the clinic, in either a governance, advisory or employment capacity. Cultural outreach can play a part in helping people become engaged in managing their health.

Working with families

Prevention is an important factor in working with families. Home visiting for families at risk should be part of the service provided, and workers can vary from nurses to trained community family support workers. Adequate training is essential, and evaluation of the effectiveness of different approaches should be considered.

Other stakeholders

It is essential, when planning primary mental health services, that the primary care philosophy is understood and respected and that practitioners from other disciplines, including public health, health promotion and secondary care, receive specific orientation to primary care. They will then be able to work effectively to support the primary mental health team and ensure that services are integrated and focused around the clinic and the community it serves.

Different resource implications

Low-, medium- and high-income countries will have communities with different mental health needs and priorities. In low-income countries, environmental issues such as nutrition or housing may be a priority for mental health, and this will imply that a different skill set will be required. In other places, an exercise expert may be required.

An understanding of community development and an ability to implement change will be important in reducing the demands on a primary mental health clinic in any environment; the level of training may vary from country to country.

Overall, it is important to match available workers with the mental health needs of local people and their communities.

Implications for mental health promotion and prevention

This chapter has outlined areas where mental health promotion and prevention are tools that can be used by primary mental health clinics to improve the mental health of their patients and communities. This will often involve working with other agencies in order to address the multiple determinants of mental distress. There is a need to take account of culture and local resources.

However, it is important that mental health clinics take an evidence-based approach and use their resources as effectively as possible. In different countries, there will be different organizations responsible for mental health prevention and promotion. It is important to work collaboratively to avoid duplication and to focus on local priorities.[1]

Mental health promotion aims to promote positive mental health by increasing psychological well-being, competence and resilience, and by creating supportive living conditions and environments. Prevention of mental disorder aims to reduce the symptoms and prevalence of mental disorders; mental health promotion is one tool in this that operates more at the social and community level than at the individual level.[1]

Specific areas of approach can include:

- building resilience
- supporting healthy families
- supporting healthy lifestyles
- working with communities, community development and focusing on "flourishing" communities
- taking an intersectoral approach
- working with comprehensive primary care services to reduce the impact of chronic disease and poor nutrition.

Conclusion

Social and environmental factors have a large impact on the development of mental distress, and primary mental health clinics will be working in communities that are subject to these influences. Overall, they can impact on daily living conditions and include the inequitable distribution of power, money and resources.

While social and environmental factors can lead to specific problems that need addressing, they can also be part of the solution for people with mental distress.

There are often strong links with cultural issues, which must be considered in all situations, but especially when there is diversity between health practitioners and their patients. Good history-taking, a comprehensive biopsychosocial approach and continuity of care in this context can ensure interventions are appropriate and lead to good outcomes.

The choice of which intervention to use depends on how the problem presents and the aetiology of that problem in the context of the local community. Community-based interventions may be necessary, as well as individual interventions.

References

1   World Health Organization Department of Mental Health and Substance Abuse, in collaboration with the Prevention Research Centre of the Universities of Nijmegen and Maastricht. *Prevention of mental disorders: effective interventions and policy options: summary report.* Geneva, World Health Organization, 2004.

2   Baron M et al. Modern research criteria and the genetics of schizophrenia. *American Journal of Psychiatry*, 1989, l146:697–701.

3   Baron M et al. A family study of schizophrenics and normal control probands: implications for the spectrum concept of schizophrenia *American Journal of Psychiatry*, 1985, 142:447–455.

4   Bergem M et al. Langfeldt's schizophreniform psychoses fifty years later. *British Journal of Psychiatry*, 1990, 157:351–354.

5   Coryell W, Tsuang M. DSM-III schizophreniform disorder. Comparison with schizophrenia and affective disorders. *Archives of General Psychiatry*, 1982, 39:66–69.

6   Coryell W, Tsuang M. Outcome after 40 years in DSM-III schizophreniform disorder. *American Journal of Psychiatry*, 1986, 1143:324–328.

7   Benson J, Thistlethwaite J. *Mental health across cultures: a practical guide for health professionals.* Oxford, Radcliffe, 2009.

8   Kaufman J et al. Brain-derived neurotrophic factor-5-HTTLPR gene interactions and environmental modifiers of depression in children. *Biological Psychiatry*, 2006, 59:673–680.

9   Seah E et al. *Cultural awareness tool: understanding cultural diversity in mental health.* Parramatta, West Australian Transcultural Mental Health Centre, The Royal Australian College of General Practitioners,

WA Research Unit, Commonwealth Department of Health and Ageing and Multicultural Mental Health, Australia, 2002 (http://www.mocmhc.org/documents/Cultural%20Awareness%20Tool.pdf, accessed 15 November 2011).

10 Patel V. Mental health in low- and middle-income countries. *British Medical Bulletin*, 2007, 81–82:81–96.

11 Marsella A, Yamada A. Culture and psychopathology. Foundations, issues, and directions. In: Kitayama S, Cohen D, eds. *Handbook of cultural psychology*. New York, Guilford Publications, Inc., 2007:797–818.

12 Lo B, Quill T, Tulsky J. Discussing palliative care with patients. *Annals of Internal Medicine*, 1999, 130:744–749.

13 Bassi M. Abstracts of the 19th European Congress of Psychiatry WPA International Congress Big Cities and Mental Health. Milan, Italy April 7–8, 2011 *European Psychiatry*, 2011, 26(Suppl.):2118.

14 Bassi M. Mental health and the European big cities *European Psychiatry*, 2009, 25:174.

15 World Health Organization. *Health promotion glossary*. Geneva, World Health Organization, 1998 (http://www.who.int/healthpromotion/about/HPR%20Glossary%201998.pdf, accessed 15 November 2011).

16 Norriss H. How can flourishing, positive mental health and wellbeing be increased? *Mindnet Newsletter*, 2010, 21.

17 Attree P et al. The experience of community engagement for individuals: a rapid review of evidence. *Health and Social Care in the Community*, 2011, 19:250–260.

18 McQueen-Thomson D, James P, Ziguras C. *Promoting mental health and wellbeing through community and cultural development: a review of literature focussing on community festivals and celebrations*. Melbourne, The Globalism Institute School of International and Community Studies RMIT University, 2004.

19 *Building on strengths – a new approach to promoting mental health in New Zealand*. Wellington, Ministry of Health, 2002.

20 Dowell AC et al. *Evaluation of the primary mental health initiatives: summary report 2008*. Wellington, University of Otago and Ministry of Health, 2009.

21 Doughty C. The effectiveness of mental health promotion, prevention and early intervention in children, adolescents and adults. *New Zealand Health Technology Assessment*, 2005, 8(2).

22 Stewart-Brown S. *What is the evidence on school health promotion in improving health or preventing disease and, specifically, what is the effectiveness of the health promoting schools approach?* Copenhagen, WHO Regional Office for Europe, 2006 (Health Evidence Network report).

23 Lee A et al. Can Health Promoting Schools contribute to the better health and well being of young people: Hong Kong experience? *Journal of Epidemiology and Community Health*, 2006, 60:530–536.

24 St Leger LH et al. *Promoting health in schools: from evidence to action*. Paris, International Union for Health Promotion and Education, 2009.

25 Gatehouse Project. Can a multilevel school intervention affect emotional well being and heath risk behaviours? *Journal of Epidemiology and Community Health*, 2004, 58:997–1003.

26 Fleming TM et al. Self-reported suicide attempts and associated risk and protective factors among secondary school students in New Zealand. *The Australian and New Zealand Journal of Psychiatry*, 2007, 41:213–221.

27 *Structured youth development programmes: a review of evidence*. Wellington, Ministry of Youth Development, 2009.

28 Taylor CB, Sallis JF, Needle R. The relation of physical activity and exercise to mental health. *Public Health Reports*, 1985, 100:195.

29 Linehan MM. *Skills training manual for treating borderline personality disorder*. New York, The Guilford Press, 1993.

30 Benson H. *The relaxation response*. New York, Morrow, 1975.

31 Bourne E. *The anxiety and phobia workbook*, 3rd ed. Oakland, CA, New Harbinger Publications, Inc., 2000.

32 Miller L, Smith AD, Rothstein L. *The stress solution: an action plan to manage the stress in your life*. New York, Pocket Books, 1994.

33 Andersson G et al. The use of the Internet in the treatment of anxiety disorders. *Current Opinions in Psychiatry*, 2005, 18:73–77.

34 Kenwright M, Marks IM. Computer-aided self-help for phobia/panic via internet at home: a pilot study. *British Journal of Psychiatry*, 2004, 184:448–449.

35 Carlbring P et al. Treatment of panic disorder: live therapy vs. self-help via the Internet. *Behaviour Research and Therapy*, 2005, 43:1321–1333.

36 Schneider AJ et al. Internet-guided self-help with or without exposure therapy for phobic and panic disorders. *Psychotherapy and Psychosomatics*, 2005, 74:154–164.

37 Farvolden P et al. Usage and longitudinal effectiveness of a Web-based self-help cognitive behavioral therapy program for panic disorder. *Journal of Medical Internet Research*, 2005, 7:e7.

38 Clarke G et al. Overcoming Depression on the Internet (ODIN) (2): a randomized trial of a self-help depression skills program with reminders. *Journal of Medical Internet Research*, 2000, 5:e16.

39 Christensen H, Griffiths KM, Jorm AF. Delivering interventions for depression by using the internet: randomised controlled trial. *BMJ*, 2004, 328:265.

40 Cunningham JA et al. Internet and paper self-help materials for problem drinking: is there an additive effect? *Addictive Behaviors*, 2005, 30:1517–1523.

41 Moore MJ, Soderquist J, Werch C. Feasibility and efficacy of a binge drinking prevention intervention for college students delivered via the Internet versus postal mail. *Journal of American College Health*, 2005, 54:38–44.

42 Cobb NK et al. Initial evaluation of a real-world Internet smoking cessation system. *Nicotine and Tobacco Research*, 2005, 7:207–216.

43 Etter JF. Comparing the efficacy of two internet-based, computer-tailored smoking cessation programs: a randomized trial. *Journal of Medical Internet Research*, 2005, 7:e2.

44 Kaldo-Sandstrom V, Larsen HC, Andersson G. Internet-based cognitive-behavioral self-help treatment of tinnitus: clinical effectiveness and predictors of outcome. *American Journal of Audiology*, 2004, 13:185–192.

45 Higgins R. From the President. *Wonca News*, 2000, 26:II.

Section D

Treatment in primary care mental health

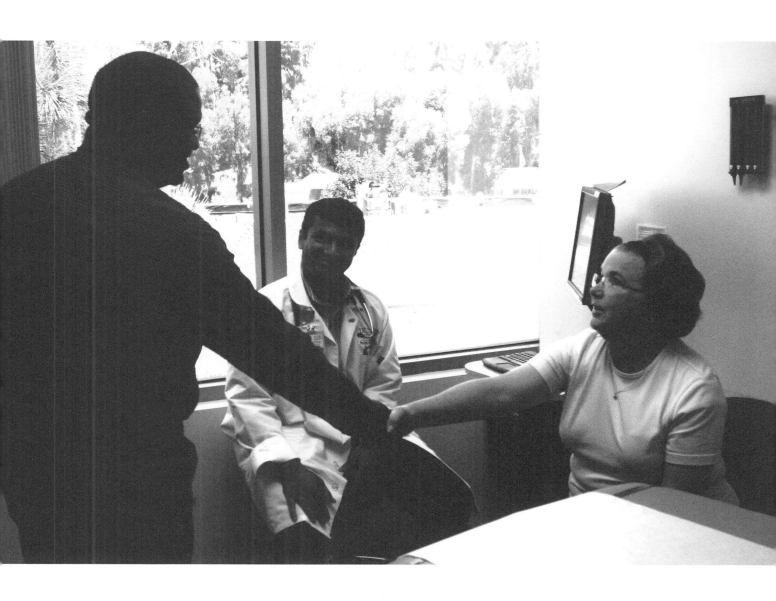

Part I

Dysphoric disorders in primary care mental health

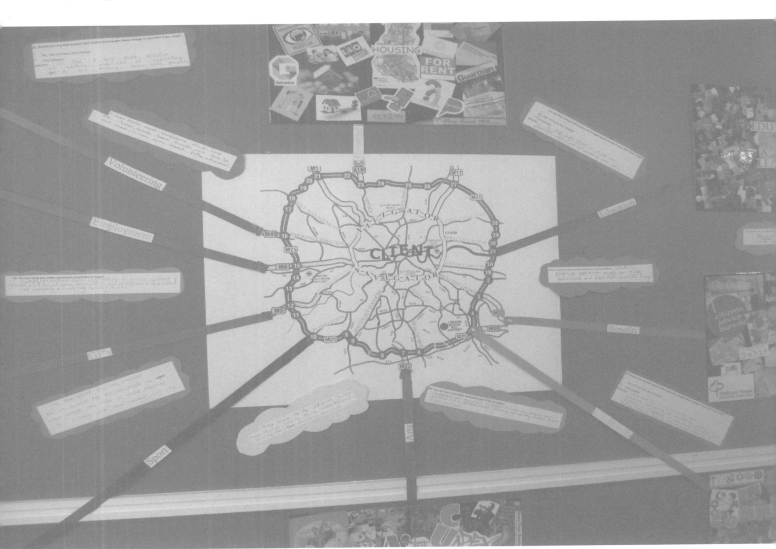

15 Anxiety in primary care mental health

Alberto Minoletti, Graciela Rojas and Irwin Nazareth

Key messages

- Individuals with anxiety disorders experience a significantly lower quality of life and functional impairments, leading in some cases to long-term disability and unemployment.

- Anxiety disorders are the most frequent of all mental disorders in the community and in primary care settings, and they are more prevalent among women than men.

- Anxiety disorders have a high rate of comorbidity with both mental and physical disorders.

- Early detection and treatment is possible, using a variety of instruments that have shown a relatively high sensitivity and specificity.

- It is necessary to rule out medical conditions in persons with anxiety disorders: anxiety disorders can present both psychological and physical manifestations, and several medical conditions and prescription medication can produce anxiety symptoms.

- General management, such as education about symptoms and treatment, active monitoring, self-help and support groups, bibliotherapy, and/or psycho-educational groups, can be effective to treat persons with mild to moderate anxiety disorders.

- Cognitive-behavioural therapy (CBT) or therapies based on CBT principles can be used effectively for the treatment of anxiety disorders in primary care.

- Antidepressants are the first choice for pharmacological treatment of anxiety disorders; benzodiazepines should not be offered as the evidence for their pharmacological effects on anxiety disorders remains inconclusive.

- A stepped care model for anxiety disorders in primary care is recommended.

Introduction

Anxiety is considered to be a healthy emotional response to a threat, and it helps human beings to deal adequately with a range of difficult situations. Workplace pressures, a newly born baby to look after, public speaking, highly demanding schedules, or sitting an exam can lead to a sense of worry, even fear, that moves people to cope more efficiently. However, these sensations can also become maladaptive if the severity or duration of anxiety is out of proportion to the level of threat, they occur in the absence of an identified stressor, they are accompanied by manifestations considered unacceptable and disruptive, and/or they lead to a deterioration of overall functioning.

Anxiety disorders are a group of clinical conditions characterized by different maladaptive manifestations of anxiety (see Box 15.1). They are usually the most common mental disorders in community settings and among people attending primary care facilities. Persons with anxiety disorders experience a significantly lower quality of life and functional impairments.[1] Furthermore, these disorders can be chronic, leading to long-term disability and unemployment. In spite of the high prevalence and burden of anxiety disorders, and the effectiveness of the treatments that have been developed over the last few years, they often go undiagnosed and untreated in primary care settings in most countries worldwide.

The three most important groups of factors that contribute to the aetiology of anxiety disorders are genetic predisposition, personality traits and stressful life events. Anxiety is the feeling a person gets when the body responds to a stressful situation (a frightening or threatening experience). It has been called the "fight or flight" response. The purpose of the physical manifestations of anxiety, therefore, is to prepare the organism to cope with a threat. When the stressful situation is highly threatening and/or lasts for a long period of time, there is a risk that the person develops an anxiety disorder, especially if there is a genetic predisposition and/or an anxious personality that tends to worry a lot.

Historically, anxiety disorders were described as early as the fourth century BC in the writings of Hippocrates, but their clinical importance was not fully appreciated until the end of the 19th century. Dr Jacob Mendez Da Costa wrote in 1871 about the "irritable heart syndrome" observed in soldiers suffering from shortness of breath, palpitations, respiratory problems and digestive disorders during the US Civil War. He believed it also occurred in civilians.[2] In 1895, Freud described, in a classical paper, a clinical syndrome that he called "anxiety neurosis" because all of its components could be grouped round the chief symptom of anxiety.[3] According to Freud, this syndrome may either exist in a chronic state or erupt in discrete attacks. The clinical concept of anxiety neurosis became universally used and was incorporated in the earlier versions of the *Diagnostic and Statistical Manual of Mental Disorders* (DSM) of the American Psychiatric Association (APA)[4] and the International Classification of Diseases (ICD)[5] of the World Health Organization (WHO), surviving for almost a century, to be finally replaced by the current concept of a group of anxiety disorders (see Box 15.1).

Box 15.1	Anxiety disorders according to the WHO ICD-10 diagnostic classification[5]	
F40	Phobic anxiety disorders	
F40.0	Agoraphobia	
	.00	Without panic disorder (PD)
	.01	With panic disorder (PD)
F40.1	Social phobias	
F40.2	Specific (isolated) phobias	
F41	Other anxiety disorders	
F41.0	Panic disorder	
F41.1	Generalized anxiety disorder (GAD)	
F41.2	Mixed anxiety and depressive disorder	
F42	Obsessive–compulsive disorder (OCD)	
F43	Reaction to severe stress	
F43.0	Acute stress reaction	
F43.1	Post-traumatic stress disorder (PTSD)	

Epidemiology

Anxiety disorders are very prevalent in the community and in primary care settings, and they are more prevalent among women than men. Epidemiological surveys of lifetime prevalence in the community have demonstrated that anxiety disorders overall are the most frequent of all mental disorders, that specific phobias are more prevalent than any other anxiety disorder (with a range of 6–12%), that OCD is consistently the least prevalent lifetime anxiety disorder, with estimates always less than 3%, and that the frequency of other anxiety disorders lies between these two figures.[6]

Many cases of specific phobia begin in childhood, and the vast majority have started by early adulthood, while social phobia and OCD have an age of onset somewhat later in life, with most cases starting by mid-life. Panic disorder, agoraphobia, and GAD have a median age of onset in the early to mid-20s, and PTSD has the latest age of onset but with a variable distribution in the life-course.[6]

One of the anxiety disorders with the highest amount of epidemiological research is GAD. General population surveys in the United States of America (USA) show an average current prevalence of between 1.5% and 3.0%, 1-year prevalence of 3–5%, and lifetime prevalence of 4–7%.[7] GAD is more common among women than men, and among people of low socioeconomic status (SES) than those of middle or high SES, as is the case for the majority of anxiety disorders.

Significant associations exist between early-onset anxiety disorders and the subsequent first episode of other mental and substance use disorders. For example, PD and social phobia are predictors of subsequent alcohol problems among adolescents and young adults.[8] Further studies are needed to evaluate the impact of early treatment of the anxiety disorders on prevention of alcohol problems in this population.

Although anxiety disorders have an early age of onset and have been demonstrated as significant risk factors for other mental and substance use disorders, the first treatment for this condition often occurs more than a decade after the onset of the disorder.[9] For this reason, some authors have suggested that adequate treatment of anxiety disorders in children and adolescents might be effective for the primary prevention of some mental and substance use disorders.[6]

In the mid-1990s, WHO conducted a very important epidemiological study in primary care services in 13 cities of different countries. The results of this survey demonstrated, according to the Composite International Diagnostic Interview (CIDI), that approximately 24% of all patients in primary care settings have a mental disorder, either as a single diagnosis or as a comorbidity of a physical disorder. The most common diagnoses were depression, anxiety disorders and substance abuse. This research did not find consistent differences between developed and developing countries.[10]

According to this WHO study, the highest prevalence rate of generalized anxiety was present in Rio de Janeiro, Brazil (22.6%) and the lowest prevalence was in Shangai, China (1.9%). Table 15.1 shows the prevalences for GAD and for all mental disorders in primary health-care services of the 13 cities participating in the study.

Anxiety disorders have a high comorbidity rate, with up to one-third of persons with these conditions in some studies meeting the diagnostic criteria for two or more anxiety disorders.[12] Furthermore, some surveys of the

Table 15.1 Prevalence of generalized anxiety and all mental disorders in primary care services in 13 cities of the world, according to the CIDI[11]

City, country	Generalized anxiety, %	All mental disorders, %
Rio de Janeiro, Brazil	22.6	35.5
Santiago, Chile	18.7	52.5
Paris, France	11.9	26.3
Berlin, Germany	9.0	18.3
Bangalore, India	8.5	22.4
Mainz, Germany	7.9	23.6
Manchester, UK	7.1	24.8
Groningen, The Netherlands	6.4	23.9
Nagasaki, Japan	5.0	9.4
Verona, Italy	3.7	9.8
Ibadan, Nigeria	2.9	9.5
Seattle, USA	2.1	11.9
Shangai, China	1.9	7.3
Total	7.9	24.0

prevalence of mental disorders in primary care have demonstrated that the frequency of comorbidity among people with anxiety is higher than among people with other disorders. This is true both for the comorbidity of two types of anxiety disorders and for one anxiety disorder with other mental and physical disorders.[13]

Depressive disorders (specifically major depression and dysthymia) are particularly common comorbidities with anxiety disorders; however, this combination is not often well recognized, despite its significant impact on increasing disability and disruption of normal functioning. Anxiety disorders are usually the primary disorder, occurring before the depressive disorder(s), and are associated with an increased risk for the subsequent onset and severity of depression.[7] Kessler et al. argue against the view expressed by some authors that GAD is better conceptualized as "a prodrome, residual, or severity marker of other disorders" (especially major depression) rather than as an independent disorder, and from their literature review, they concluded that the independent status of GAD is as strongly supported by available evidence as is that of other anxiety disorders.[7]

Relevance to the management of anxiety disorders in primary care

Since the Declaration of Alma-Ata on primary health care in 1978,[14] the importance of integrating mental health into primary care has been increasingly recognized as a public health strategy to decrease the enormous treatment gap for mental disorders worldwide. It is now widely recognized that primary care teams should screen and manage common mental disorders (anxiety and depressive clinical conditions) as part of their function.[15–17] Among the many advantages for managing mental disorders in primary care, WHO has stressed the holistic approach of meeting people's physical and mental health needs by the same team, with the enhancement of access to mental health services that are affordable and cost effective.[18]

The primary care team is in contact with the majority of persons who need help for anxiety disorders, and several studies have shown that primary care professionals can treat these conditions equally as well as specialists.[19–21] Furthermore, general practitioners (GPs) and all the members of the primary care team are in an ideal position to identify early symptoms and signs of anxiety disorders, and it is known that early identification can improve the prognosis of many mental health conditions and prevent the development of other mental disorders. Also, the stigma of attending specialist mental health services can be avoided if people are treated in primary care. People with mental problems or disorders prefer to go to a primary health centre rather than going to a psychiatric service.

The familiar faces of members of the primary care team can be a comfort to persons going through psychological problems, and the knowledge that these professionals have of their patients' backgrounds can contribute to a better understanding of the difficulties these individuals are facing, and to more effective management. Finally, there are greater opportunities for health education and follow-up in primary care than in specialist clinics, which is fundamental to the prevention of future episodes of anxiety disorders.[19]

Prevention of anxiety disorders

There is a growing research literature on the prevention of anxiety disorders, most of which shows promising results.[21–24] A number of investigations have focused on universal preventive interventions targeting entire school grades and have reported small reductions in the symptoms of anxiety in children undergoing active intervention. Slightly stronger effects have been demonstrated using the indicated interventions with schoolchildren presenting a high level of risk factors or early signs of anxiety disorders. Most school prevention programmes combine different cognitive-behavioural ingredients and include a limited number of group sessions with both children and their parents and/or carers.

Although most of the research in this field comes from high-income countries, there are also a few reports from middle- and low-income countries. In places as dissimilar as Chile, Iran and Nigeria, and with different populations (schoolchildren, nursing students and surgical patients), a significant reduction in the level of anxiety was observed after participation in a physical activity programme, educational counselling sessions, self-instructional training (SIT), or rational emotive therapy (RET).[25]

Notwithstanding the importance of the research done, anxiety-prevention studies are currently at the stage of testing and replicating interventions. As such, practical implications for the work of primary care teams are necessarily limited, and we have to wait for effectiveness trials before the implementation of large-scale preventive programmes for anxiety disorders in healthy populations.

Considering the characteristics of primary care work and the evidence available at present for prevention, it could be recommended to develop programmes for persons with early anxiety symptoms, although they may not meet all the diagnostic criteria for one of the anxiety disorders. Preventive approaches indicated with this kind of population should include both activities for screening anxiety symptoms among users of primary care facilities and a package of group interventions based on cognitive-behavioural techniques.

A variety of instruments have been developed to detect persons with anxiety disorders in primary care. Some of these tools include several questions to screen for both anxiety and depressive disorders,[26–31] while others are specific for anxiety and can be as short as only two questions.[32,33]

The Hospital Anxiety and Depression Scale (HADS) is a 14-item self-report screening scale that was originally developed to indicate the possible presence of anxiety and depressive states in the setting of a medical outpatient clinic. It contains two seven-item scales: one for anxiety and one for depression, both with a score range of 0–21.[26,28,34] Studies suggest that in primary care patients, HADS is also an adequate screening instrument.[16,35,36]

The Generalized Anxiety Disorder scale (GAD-7) is a seven-item validated diagnostic tool designed for use in the primary care setting for detecting GAD, but it is also fairly accurate for panic, social anxiety, and PTSD.[32,37] The first two questions of the GAD-7 make up the GAD-2, which can be used as an ultra-short diagnostic instrument. One approach would be to use the GAD-2 when screening for anxiety disorders in primary care, followed by the other five items of the GAD-7 for patients with positive results on screening. This is because the GAD-7 provides a broader score range to grade symptom severity and, consequently, may be useful in monitoring the response to treatment.

Most of the screening instruments have been proved to be valid to detect individuals with anxiety disorders, and they have shown a relatively high sensitivity and specificity. However, cultural differences in the language and meaning associated with anxiety disorders could decrease the reliability and validity of these instruments among different ethnic populations.[38] Consequently, although it seems highly convenient to utilize a brief tool to detect persons with anxiety disorders as early as possible, primary care teams should ensure that the tool they are going to use is validated with the different ethnic groups with whom they work.

According to resources and local evidence, a basic package of brief and time-limited group interventions can be designed for the management of persons with mild anxiety disorders of recent onset, or with subthreshold anxiety symptoms.[39,40] This package may include some of the following components:

- counselling on how to cope with current stressors
- education about how to prevent anxiety disorders and/or cope with early symptoms
- physical activity: 3–4 exercise sessions per week, with a duration of at least 20–30 minutes
- breathing and/or relaxation training
- self-help groups and support groups
- cognitive-behavioural therapy (CBT)-based bibliotherapy
- computerized cognitive-behavioural therapy (CCBT)
- CBT-based problem-solving treatment.

Another preventive approach to anxiety disorder is relapse prevention, oriented to decrease the frequency of recurrent episodes. In naturalistic longitudinal studies of persons with these disorders, the probability of experiencing new episodes is approximately 50%. Both antidepressant medication and CBT have been demonstrated to be effective at decreasing the rate of relapses.

Several double-blind, placebo-controlled studies, in which the therapy period has been extended to ≥12 weeks, have shown the efficacy of selective serotonin reuptake inhibitors (SSRIs, i.e. paroxetine, escitalopram) and serotonin and noradrenaline reuptake inhibitors (SNRIs; i.e. venlafaxine, duloxetine) for relapse prevention in anxiety disorders.[41–43] The current evidence supports the maintenance of one of these medications for at least 6 months after an acute trial of 3–6 months with significant reduction of symptoms. In individuals with two or more relapses, longer periods of treatment may be needed.

Relapse might be less frequent after stopping CBT than with drug treatments. Although there have been few long-term comparisons, some studies suggest that CBT has enduring effects that reduce the risk for subsequent episodes of anxiety disorders.[44] Booster therapy sessions have also been used to improve outcomes and decrease relapses. Six brief 15-minute booster phone contacts after CBT termination in primary care were shown to be effective in improving the symptomatic outcome for panic disorder after a 12-month follow-up.[45]

Evaluation and diagnosis of anxiety disorder

The baseline examination of a person suspected to have anxiety disorder should consider gathering relevant information about his/her psychosocial and physical conditions:

- main symptoms (see Box 15.2 for the clinical manifestations of anxiety disorders)
- recent stressful events
- past history of mental health problems
- current medical status and medication
- self-medication and/or abuse of alcohol or illicit drugs
- socioeconomic and cultural factors
- laboratory tests if a medical illness is suspected.

Several medical conditions can present with anxiety symptoms and should be ruled out:[46]

- thyrotoxicosis
- hypocapnia due to hyperventilation
- anaemia
- hypoglycaemia
- hypoxia or hypercapnia due to intermittent respiratory disorders
- poor pain control
- vertigo due to vestibular disorders.

Box 15.2 Clinical manifestations of anxiety disorders[4,5,46]

Physical manifestations

- Shakiness, trembling
- Muscle aches
- Sweating, cold or clammy hands
- Dizziness, vertigo
- Fatigue
- Racing or pounding heart
- Hyperventilation
- Sensation of lump in throat
- Choking sensation
- Dry mouth
- Numbness and tingling of hands, feet, etc.
- Upset stomach, nausea, vomiting
- Diarrhoea
- Decreased sexual desire
- Sleep disturbances

Psychological and social manifestations

- Jitteriness, tension
- Unrealistic or excessive worry
- Exaggerated startle reactions
- Fear of being away from home
- Irrational fears
- Avoidance of feared situations
- Recurrent disturbing dreams or nightmares
- Apprehension that something bad may happen to themselves or to their loved ones
- Impatience
- Irritability
- Distractibility
- Difficulty concentrating

Some prescription medication can also have side-effects that are similar to anxiety symptoms:[46,47]

- bronchodilators
- insulin and oral hypoglycaemic agents
- SSRI antidepressants
- corticosteroids
- nonsteroidal anti-inflammatory drugs (NSAIDs)
- thyroxine
- antihypertensive drugs
- sympathomimetics.

There is an extensive list of legal and illicit drugs that are suspected to cause anxiety when they are consumed or during withdrawal.[46] Drugs most frequently associated with anxiety include:

- alcohol
- caffeine
- amphetamine, methamphetamine
- cocaine
- lysergic acid diethylamide (LSD)
- 3,4-methylenedioxymethamphetamine (MDMA or ecstasy).

Many mental disorders may present secondary anxiety symptoms as part of their manifestations and they should also be considered in the differential diagnosis. Considering the high prevalence of depression among people attending primary care and the high frequency of anxiety symptoms in this condition, it is advisable to ask anxious patients a couple of questions to screen for depressive disorders. It should also be kept in mind that depressive and anxiety disorders often coexist, and they both need to be treated conjointly, if the intensity of the symptoms is similar, or sequentially, if one of them produces significantly more distress and disability than the other.

Figure 15.1 shows an algorithm to formulate the diagnosis of anxiety disorder after ruling out a medical illness, alcohol or drug use or withdrawal, and a depressive disorder.

Where resources available for mental health in primary care are scarce, the evaluation process could finish with a general diagnosis of "anxiety disorder" and an offer of a single basic therapeutic package regardless of the subtype of anxiety disorder. In places where this type of treatment is accessible for most people in need of it, and if mental health is scaling-up in primary care, a differential diagnosis between the different anxiety disorder subtypes should be attempted, in order to provide a more specific therapeutic approach for each subtype.

The main clinical features of the different anxiety disorder subtypes are discussed next.[4,5,46-49]

Post-traumatic stress disorder

PTSD arises after a person experiences, witnesses, or confronts a physical and/or psychological event that involves actual or threatened death or serious injury, or a threat to the physical integrity of oneself or others. Typical symptoms include reliving the trauma in intrusive memories (flashbacks), dreams or nightmares, a sense of numbness and emotional blunting, detachment from people, and a consistent pattern of avoidance of themes associated with the traumatic event. Other possible features of PTSD are hyperarousal and autonomic hyperactivities that may be manifested by difficulties with sleep or concentration, exaggerated startle reactions and, at times, anger outbursts. The onset usually follows a latency period of a few weeks.

Obsessive–compulsive disorder

Persons with OCD experience repetitive ideas (obsessions) that are distressing and provoke intense symptoms of anxiety. They often become involved in rituals and other repetitive behaviours (compulsions) to try to diminish their anxiety feelings. The compulsive behaviours can consume most of their time, and they can also

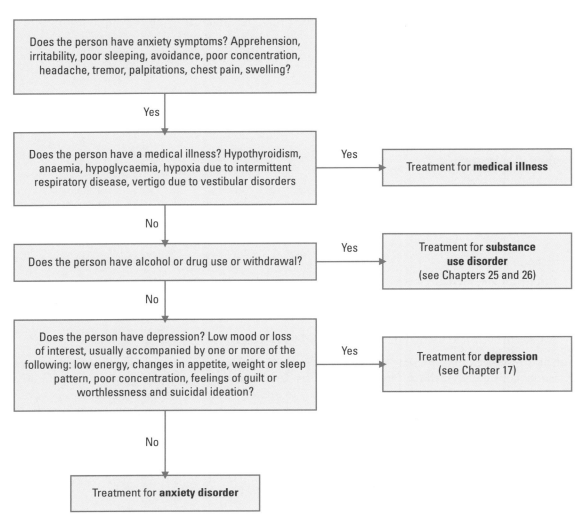

Figure 15.1 Diagnosis of anxiety disorder[48,49]

spend a lot of time avoiding situations with which the obsessions are associated, thus limiting their activities and range of behaviours. Despite patients' awareness of the irrational nature of their condition, they feel unable to control their obsessions or to prevent their compulsions. If untreated, OCD may lead to permanent disability because of the loss of meaningful interpersonal relations and employment.

Panic disorder

Persons with PD usually describe periods of intense fear or discomfort that develop abruptly with a peak in around 10 minutes. Very often, they seek medical treatment because they fear that their physical symptoms – which may include palpitations, pounding heart or tachycardia, sweating, chest pain, shortness of breath, dizziness, nausea, chills, trembling, and tingling sensations – are caused by a heart attack or another serious physical condition. Patients may worry about recurrent unexpected panic attacks. The anticipatory anxiety and intense fear of future attacks may lead to the development of phobic avoidance. The combination of panic symptoms and the phobic avoidance can impair the patient's work, social and familial functioning.

Agoraphobia

Persons with agoraphobia fear being in a situation in which escape might be difficult or embarrassing, or in which help will not be available if they experience anxiety or panic. As a result, they avoid situations that

Companion to Primary Care Mental Health

cause them these unpleasant emotions, like being outside the home alone, being in a crowd or standing in a line, being on a bridge, travelling in a bus, underground, or a plane, etc. This condition can be quite disabling. Agoraphobia can be accompanied by PD and panic attacks, or it can occur alone without a history of panic attacks.

Generalized anxiety disorder

Persons who experience GAD feel excessive nervousness most of the time, with exaggerated worry, tension, overarousal, and irritability that appear to have no cause or are more intense than the situation warrants. Physical signs – such as muscle tension, chest or back pain, headaches, restlessness, poor concentration, difficulty in falling or remaining asleep, being easily fatigued, trembling, twitching or sweating – often develop, which lead to further worries.

Social phobia

Persons with social anxiety have a persistent, intense, and ongoing fear of being extremely embarrassed or being watched, judged by others, or humiliated by their own actions, especially when they are with unfamiliar people or exposed to the scrutiny of others. The most common social phobia is fear of public speaking. Exposure to the feared social situations provokes anxiety that can sometimes reach panic proportions. The person recognizes that the fear is unreasonable but tries to avoid these situations whenever possible. The avoidant behaviour interferes considerably with the person's normal life.

Specific phobias

Phobias are irrational fears of specific objects or situations that trigger intense anxiety by their presence or just when the person sees or hears the name of the object, or sees pictures of the object. The most frequent phobias are related to flying, heights, animals, blood, darkness, injections, dentistry, and urinating or defecating in public places. The affected individual will totally or partially avoid all these specific things or situations. Sometimes they may faint when facing them, due to a vasovagal reaction. Persons with specific phobias seldom seek professional help because they cause little distress and interference with daily life.

See Figure 15.2 for a summary of the main features of the different anxiety disorders and an algorithm to facilitate the differential diagnosis between them.

General management

Information provision

Persons with anxiety disorders, their families and carers benefit from information about the nature, course and management of this condition. Information given in an understandable language can contribute to decreasing the fear associated with anxiety symptoms, especially those with bodily sensations, and to empower patients to participate actively in the management of their disorders.[48,49] The information can be given by the primary care professionals, directly face to face or through written materials. Self-help and support groups may also play a valuable role as a source of information. According to National Institute for Health and Clinical Excellence (NICE) guidelines, psycho-educational groups for people with GAD should be based on CBT principles, have an interactive design, include self-help manuals, have a ratio of one therapist to about 12 participants, and extend for six weekly sessions of 2 hours each.[49]

Shared decision-making

Health-care professionals should encourage individuals to make informed decisions during the process of diagnosis and in all phases of care.[47] Information on the use and likely side-effect profile of different medications is not only an ethical issue but also a help for patients to develop a sense of control over their treatment

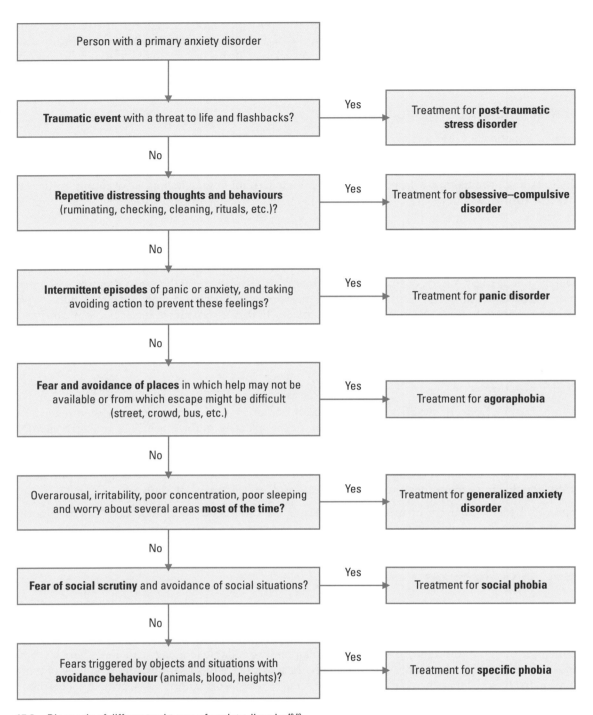

Figure 15.2 Diagnosis of different subtypes of anxiety disorder[48,49]

and symptoms. The participation of patients in the process of decision-making, and a relationship based on empathy and understanding increase their satisfaction with trust in the care and improve clinical results.[48]

Self-help groups and support groups

In high-income countries, there are usually a variety of offers from self-help groups and support groups for mental health, and professionals should encourage persons with anxiety disorders and their families to

Companion to Primary Care Mental Health

participate in them where appropriate.[47,49] However, in low- and middle-income countries, these groups are scarce or non-existent, and the role of professionals should be to facilitate the development of users' and families' organizations for mutual help and support.

Inclusion of the family in the general care

A significant burden placed on family members of individuals with anxiety disorders has been described. Living with or taking care of persons with these disorders appears to negatively impact the physical and mental health of family members.[50] Primary care professionals should acknowledge the impact of anxiety disorders on the family and provide information and support, as well as encouragement to participate in self-help groups and support groups to improve their quality of life.[49] If needed, family members should be offered assessment of their caring, physical and mental health needs, and, eventually, treatment to overcome their own mental health problems. It is also helpful for family members to receive contact numbers and information about what to do and who to contact in a crisis.[49]

Community support

Identification of the current psychosocial stressors and mobilization of possible sources of social support in the local area where the person with anxiety disorders lives can contribute to improving the effectiveness of the treatment.

Traditional health

Traditional and religious healers continue to play an important role in the management of anxiety disorders in low- and middle-income countries, especially in rural areas of Asia, Africa and Latin America. They provide care that is consistent with the culture of most people in those regions, and they are also more accessible and affordable than western medicine.[51] Whenever possible, primary care teams should establish a collaborative relationship with traditional and religious healers, and attempts should be made to build a system of mutual referrals. The development of this collaborative relationship is constrained by a lack of scientific knowledge about the efficacy and untoward effects of traditional and religious healing in different local communities.

Physical activity

There is growing evidence for positive effects of exercise and exercise training on anxiety and anxiety disorders.[52,53] From the clinical point of view, it should at least be included as an adjunct to established treatment approaches like psychological treatment or pharmacotherapy. Usually, 3–4 exercise sessions per week with a duration of at least 20–30 minutes are recommended.[53] However, further studies are needed to establish the details of the clinical effects of exercise, interaction with standard treatment approaches and the optimal type, intensity, frequency and duration. In addition, persons with anxiety disorders present special challenges for physical activity compliance, considering that the exercise setting itself can sometimes be an anxiety-inducing stimulus. Some may experience anxiety symptoms when in a group or an indoor facility, while exercising in the outdoors or in large spaces may be anxiety provoking for others. In these cases, gradual exposure to both exercise and the fear-inducing aspects of the exercise setting can help to overcome these barriers.[52]

Psychological treatment

Several psychological treatments have been demonstrated to be effective for anxiety disorders. Many principles and technical approaches function equally well for all the different subtypes, although there is some specific evidence related to each particular anxiety disorder.

Generalized anxiety disorder

There is a growing literature regarding the efficacy of CBT for the treatment of GAD, although most of the evidence comes from research carried out in secondary care services. CBT has been proved to have the longest duration of effect compared to pharmacotherapy. The overall goals of this approach are to help people to identify problematic beliefs and thought patterns, which are often irrational or unrealistic, and replace them with more rational and realistic views. CBT includes teaching:[54,55]

- coping skills to reduce physiological symptoms, such as relaxation training
- cognitive skills to restructure catastrophic thoughts associated with anxiety
- alternative responses to worry behaviour.

CBT should be delivered by trained, supervised and competent practitioners. The optimal range of duration is 12–15 weekly sessions, each lasting 1 hour. Briefer CBT can also be effective if supplemented with written or electronic materials, through a self-help programme, with 5–7 weekly or fortnightly face-to-face or telephone sessions, each lasting 20–30 minutes.[49]

Self-help written manuals based on CBT principles have been developed for primary care settings, and they are usually referred to as "bibliotherapy". These manuals have been designed to be used by the person himself/herself or in conjunction with limited therapist support.[56] Care models based on a computer-assisted CBT programme have also been developed, and the evaluations have shown that they are acceptable to clinicians and patients.[21,57]

Specific phobia

The simple or specific phobias have been effectively treated with a behaviour therapy called exposure therapy, which consists of exposing the affected person to the phobic stimulus in a safe and controlled setting as part of the therapeutic process. Different alternative methods can be used to confront a feared situation or object, namely exposure through imagination or exposure in real-life situations. Today, virtual reality offers interesting therapeutic potential in the treatment of phobias. This approach has been called virtual reality exposure and it offers a flexible and useful alternative for the treatment of phobias.[58]

Panic disorder

Controlled clinical trials evaluating cognitive-behavioural approaches for PD suggest substantial efficacy in the short and long term. These treatments assume that extinction of internal and external anxiogenic cues and reduction of catastrophic cognitions reduces panic symptoms. CBT protocols for the treatment of PD include several components like cognitive restructuring, psycho-education, relaxation, controlled breathing procedures, and exposure techniques. The optimal range of duration of CBT is 7–14 hours in total, but briefer CBT can be also effective if supplemented with appropriate focused information and tasks.[49] Bibliotherapy based on CBT principles and used like self-help therapy has also been developed for the treatment of PD in primary care.[56]

Obsessive–compulsive disorder

Research supports the effectiveness of CBT for the treatment of OCD. It includes exposure-based techniques and cognitive interventions. A typical CBT protocol for OCD is implemented in a time-limited format with 12–16 sessions.[59]

Post-traumatic stress disorder

Psychotherapy can reduce traumatic stress symptoms in people suffering PTSD. Trauma-focused CBT (TFCBT) and eye movement desensitization and reprocessing (EMDR) have the best evidence for efficacy.[60,61] There is some limited evidence that stress management can also be effective. TFCBT uses repeated exposure to the trauma memory and/or in vivo exposure to situations avoided since the traumatic event. The efficacy of the exposure therapy has been demonstrated in several specific trauma populations. The range of duration can be from 1 to 20 sessions.

EMDR utilizes dual-attention tasks to help the patient process the traumatic event, and involves him or her focusing on negative trauma-related memories, emotions, and thoughts, while engaging in a task involving some form of bilateral stimulation such as eye movements, hand tapping, or tones until distress is reduced and the person is able to focus on positive trauma-related thoughts. The duration of EMDR ranges from 1 to 12 sessions.

There is little evidence to support the use of psychological intervention for routine use following traumatic events. Not only are both multiple-sessions interventions and single-session interventions ineffective to prevent PTSD, but they may have an adverse effect on some individuals who have experienced a traumatic event.[62] In primary care settings, after the population has been exposed to an extreme stressor or trauma, psycho-education is very important to prevent the development of PTSD and other mental disorders. The key messages to deliver to these people are:[63]

- it is normal to have distressing symptoms after a traumatic experience
- it is important to talk with family and friends about the trauma and the feelings associated with it
- it is important to listen to people who have experienced a traumatic event and to have an attitude of support and acceptance towards them.

Multiple anxiety disorders

Psychological treatments for two or more types of anxiety disorder have also been developed for primary care. For example, a self-help manual based on cognitive-behavioural principles to be used by persons with GAD or PD with the support of trained and supervised GPs (five 20-minute sessions) has been shown to be equally as effective as CBT carried out by specialists (12 45-minute sessions).[64] The manual included explanations about anxiety, simple cognitive techniques and relaxation, and in vivo exposure exercises. In the first session, the GP informed the participants about the contents of the manual. Then the patients were told to practise self-help techniques for 3 hours each week. In all the subsequent sessions, the GP reinforced the patients' achievements and motivated them to continue with the use of the manual.

The Coordinated Anxiety Learning and Management (CALM) study demonstrated the effectiveness of a model of care that delivers evidence-based treatments – psychopharmacology and CBT – for PD with or without agoraphobia, GAD, social anxiety disorder, and PTSD in primary care.[21,65] The person affected and the clinician decided whether to use CBT, pharmacotherapy or both. The model used a computer-based system for supporting delivery of CBT for anxiety disorders by clinicians in primary care and also for guiding the patients in their learning process. The CBT treatment included five generic modules and three modules tailored to each specific anxiety disorder. Each module contained session goals, summaries of the main contents, educational information, review of homework, in-session practice of new skills, instructions for skills practice between sessions, and video demonstrations of specific CBT strategies for each anxiety disorder. At the end of each module, skill acquisition was assessed through self-ratings of understanding, multiple choice quizzes, and clinician ratings of patient skills. The contents learnt in a session were reinforced with individualized printed materials that are given to participants. The programme can be completed in six to eight sessions, but if additional care is needed, advanced modules are available. This programme requires the clinicians to be trained and supervised. CALM is available in English and Spanish.

Pharmacological treatment

Drugs have been used in the management of anxiety disorders for over 150 years. In the 19th century, physicians used bromides to treat "anxiety neurosis". This was later replaced by barbiturates in the early 20th century, until the advent of benzodiazepines in the 1960s. For the next 20 years, benzodiazepines became increasingly popular in the management of anxiety, with little concern for their potential for tolerance and dependence. Latterly, however, as these effects became more apparent and as the beneficial effects of antidepressant therapy for anxiety disorders became evident, benzodiazepine use for anxiety disorders declined.[66] Nevertheless, large numbers of people still continue to use benzodiazepines for anxiety disorders and other related psychological states. SSRIs, and to a lesser extent SNRIs (serotonin and noradrenaline reuptake inhibitors) and tricyclic antidepressants (TCAs), however, are now more widely used to treat GADs. Other drugs such as antihistamines (hydroxyzine), a $5HT_{1A}$ (hydroxytryptamine) receptor agonist (buspirone) and an anticonvulsant (pregabalin) have also been used or have shown promising results in people with GAD.

We will provide a detailed review of the drugs used for GAD, as there is perhaps the best available evidence for treatment of this condition. We will then provide an overview of the drug therapy for PD, PTSD and OCD. In most instances, as anxiety disorders often occur as mixed states with a general predominance of GAD or PD, the drugs used for these conditions can be appropriately used for many of these mixed anxiety states.

Generalized anxiety disorders

Some of the most recent evidence for the pharmacological treatment of GAD has been reviewed in the document published by NICE.[49] The pharmacological treatments discussed next are described in this document.

Antidepressant drug therapy

There remains limited research information on the efficacy of antidepressant therapy for the treatment of GAD when compared with placebo. NICE reviewed data on escitalopram (6 trials), sertraline (2 trials), paroxetine (8 trials), duloxetine (4 trials), venlafaxine (12 trials) and one trial each for imipramine and citalopram.[49] All antidepressants produced a small to moderate improvement of anxiety scores. Adverse events leading to discontinuation of treatment were greatest for paroxetine, duloxetine and venlafaxine.

Dose effects on GAD of various antidepressants

The evidence on dose effects is limited to merely three drugs: venlafaxine, escitalopram and duloxetine.[49] Venlafaxine at 75 mg daily produced a significant reduction in GAD anxiety score and fewer side-effects such as nausea and insomnia than higher doses of the drug. In the case of escitalopram, a significant reduction of anxiety occurred with 10 mg rather than 5 mg, with no increase in adverse events with the higher dose of medication. Lastly, there was a trend for daily dose of 60–120 mg of duloxetine to produce greater improvement in GAD outcomes.

Side-effects of antidepressants

The main adverse events that need to be monitored in people prescribed antidepressants are cardiovascular, gastrointestinal, bleeding, sexual dysfunction and weight change. SSRIs are not associated with an increased risk of cardiovascular events;[67,68] however, TCAs are associated with a higher risk of these adverse events.[67] SNRIs such as duloxetine and venlafaxine can produce increases in blood pressure,[67] and may have to be discontinued on this count. Duloxetine can also produce tachycardia and elevated cholesterol blood levels when compared with placebo,[69] and this limits its use in people with known cardiovascular risk.

A more serious adverse event with SSRIs is a threefold increased risk of bleeding.[70] This, however, is a relatively rare event, with approximately 4–5 events occurring every 1000 person-years. However, special care should be taken in people concomitantly using NSAIDs, as the risk of bleeding increases 15 fold.

Other, common side-effects associated with SSRIs include an increased risk of nausea, vomiting and diarrhoea. On the other hand, TCAs are associated with a higher risk of constipation when compared with fluoxetine. Many of these symptoms improve over a period of time while the patient is taking the drug. Adverse effects on sexual function can also prove to be a troublesome side-effect, particularly with SNRIs such as duloxetine and venlafaxine. Finally, although weight loss has been consistently reported early in treatment with fluoxetine,[71] longer-term data suggest that there is an overall weight gain from use of both paroxetine and fluoxetine.

Effects of antidepressant in comparison with each other and with other pharmacological agents

The six trials that have provided direct comparative data between various antidepressants (i.e. escitalopram versus paroxetine; sertraline versus paroxetine; escitalopram versus venlafaxine; and duloxetine versus venlafaxine) have demonstrated a small effect in favour of escitalopram in comparison with paroxetine, with a demonstrable trend towards greater discontinuation of paroxetine treatment due to adverse events.

Another set of trials that compared antidepressants with other pharmacological agents (i.e. venlafaxine versus pregabalin; venlafaxine versus buspirone; venlafaxine versus diazepam) showed no significant difference in reduction of GAD outcomes for venlafaxine in comparison with pregabalin, buspirone or diazepam. There was, however, an increased risk of discontinuation of venlafaxine on account of adverse side-effects when compared to other drugs.

Pregabalin therapy

NICE reviewed eight trials that examined the effect of pregabalin on GAD outcomes in comparison with placebo. There was moderate benefit in GAD as measured by reduction of mean anxiety scores, and only a borderline risk of discontinuation of treatment due to adverse events.[49]

Dose effects

The various comparisons made on doses ranging from 150 mg to 600 mg suggest that although a daily dose of 400–600 mg leads to greater reduction of anxiety than lower doses of 150 mg, this effect has to be balanced against the finding that 150 mg was associated with fewer adverse events, particularly dizziness and somnolence.

Pregabalin compared with other pharmacological agents

One trial made a direct comparison between pregabalin and alprazolam, and three trials compared pregabalin with lorazepam. All failed to show any difference in GAD outcomes between the various drugs. Moreover, the risk of discontinuation of therapy due to adverse events was no greater when compared with alprazolam, and the risk of discontinuation was reduced by half when compared with lorazepam.

Benzodiazepines

Despite the widespread use of benzodiazepines for GAD, there were only four randomized placebo trials for diazepam, alprazolam and lorazepam.[49] All reported inconsistent effects on GAD outcomes. The evidence for the pharmacological effects of all these drugs on GAD hence remains inconclusive, despite their widespread use. There was, however, no risk of discontinuation of benzodiazepines due to adverse effects, although trial data suggest an increased risk of experiencing sexual problems and an increased risk of symptoms of dizziness for all three drugs.

Other drugs

NICE identified five trials that compared buspirone to placebo, and these demonstrated a small benefit on GAD outcomes.[49] There was no risk of discontinuation of therapy due to adverse events, although people using the drug were reported to have experienced an increased risk of nausea and dizziness in comparison with placebo. The limited data from two trials showed no differences on GAD outcomes between buspirone and hydroxyzine, and buspirone and lorazepam. NICE reported three trials that compared hydroxyzine with placebo, with moderate effects on mean GAD scores and limited data on adverse events.

Complementary and alternative medicines

We include a brief overview of complementary and alternative therapies for anxiety, as they are commonly used by people seen in general practice. NICE found limited evidence on randomized placebo trials on chamomile, gingko biloa, combined plant extract (i.e. *Crataegus oxyacantha*, *Eschscholzia californica* and magnesium) and valerian extract.[49] These data showed that all but valerian extract had borderline to small effects on anxiety outcomes. However, in another study that made direct comparisons with benzodiazepines and herbal treatments, no differences were observed. All these studies were limited by small sample sizes and hence, based on current evidence, it would be premature to suggest that these treatments should be offered to people with GAD.

Maintenance therapy for GAD

NICE searched for trials that randomized people who had responded to pharmacological therapy for anxiety to maintenance therapy for longer periods of time. They found four trials that examined the effects of continuing pregabalin, duloxetine, escitalopram and paroxetine for at least 24 weeks after an initial response to treatment that was administered for at least 8 weeks.[47] There was good evidence for a beneficial effect on anxiety for all drugs (i.e. pregabalin, duloxetine, escitalopram and paroxetine) but all the trials were limited by high drop-out rates and variable lengths of follow-up. There was no difference between the drugs for the adverse events experienced with long-term therapy.

NICE recommendations for generalized anxiety disorder[49]

Using the evidence reported above, the recommendations on the drug management of GAD provided by NICE can be summarized as follows: if, after the diagnosis of GAD and the provision of simple education and active monitoring by the primary care practitioner, there continues to be a persistence of GAD symptoms, the patient must be offered either individual high-intensity psychological therapy or drug therapy with provision of verbal and written information on the likely benefits and disadvantages of each mode of treatment. The issues around the side-effects and possible withdrawal syndromes associated with drug treatments must be discussed. There is no current evidence that favours either psychological or drug therapy, and hence the final choice of treatment will be based on the personal preferences.

In the event of a person opting for drug treatment, the first choice should be an SSRI. The cost-effectiveness analysis models developed by NICE suggest that sertraline is the most cost-effective drug (even though it does not have marketing authorization for this indication in the UK). If sertraline is ineffective, the patient can then be offered an alternative SSRI or a SNRI (i.e. venlafaxine and duloxetine). The possibility of producing a withdrawal syndrome with drugs such as paroxetine and venlafaxine must be considered, in addition to other potential drug interactions and side-effects and the personal preferences for drugs. If the patient cannot tolerate SSRIs or SNRIs, they should be offered pregabalin. Benzodiazepine should not be offered for the treatment of GAD except as a very short-term measure, and antipsychotic drugs should not be offered at all.

Panic disorders

Evidence from the systematic reviews conducted by NICE suggest that SSRIs and TCAs are both effective in the management of panic disorder.[49] Higher doses of SSRIs are more effective than lower doses, and in general are as effective as TCAs. Benzodiazepines, on the other hand, are associated with poorer outcomes for panic disorders when compared with antidepressants. More evidence is required on the optimal duration of treatment with medication, the withdrawal or discontinuation effects of drugs used to treat panic disorders and the efficacy of these drugs in people who are older than 65 years.

Hence, NICE recommends that any SSRIs licensed for panic disorder should be considered as a first-line drug therapy. If an SSRI is not suitable, or if it fails to produce an effect after 12 weeks of continuous treatment, the primary care physician should then consider introducing either imipramine or clomipramine (however, neither of these drugs has been licensed for use in panic disorders). In order to minimize the adverse effects of the drug, physicians should consider prescribing the lowest possible dose before steadily increasing it until a satisfactory response has been achieved. If the panic symptoms improve with drug therapy, the treatment should be considered for at least 6 months. Longer-term therapy should be considered if necessary.

Post-traumatic stress disorder

NICE's review of drug treatments for PTSD provides disappointing results.[72] Only paroxetine showed a small positive effect for PTSD, and this was not observed for sertraline or any of the other drugs licensed for PTSD. NICE reports, however, that clinically important effects for mirtazapine, amitriptyline and the monoamine oxidase inhibitor (MAOI) antidepressants phenelzine and brofaromine were observed. But these findings are limited by research evidence emerging from small trials. Drug treatments for PTSD should therefore not be considered as a routine first-line treatment for adults in preference to trauma-focused psychological therapies. Drug therapy should only be considered in adults when the person expresses a preference not to engage in a trauma-focused psychological treatment; they cannot start psychological therapy due to ongoing violence; or there has been a poor response from trauma-focused therapy. The drugs of choice recommended by NICE are paroxetine or mirtazapine, which can be initiated in general practice, and amitriptyline or phenelzine, which NICE suggests are best initiated by a mental health specialist. When a person fails to respond to these treatment options even after increasing the dose of the antidepressant to the maximum approved limit, the physician may consider the use of adjunctive olanzapine. When drug therapy is started for PTSD, it should be continued for at least 12 months after the person has shown a good response to the treatment after a few weeks.

Obsessive–compulsive disorder

NICE recommends that for adults with OCD, the evidence for initiating SSRIs (namely fluoxamine, fluoxetine, paroxetine, sertraline or citalopram) based on randomized trial evidence is good.[73] Any of these drugs can be started as a first-line treatment and if there is lack of response after 4–6 weeks of taking the drug at standard doses, a gradual increase should be considered, while closely monitoring adverse effects. If the person responds to drug treatment, the drug should be continued for at least 12 months. After 12 months, the decision to continue drug therapy beyond this period can be decided based on the severity and duration of the initial illness, the number of previous episodes, the persistence of residual symptoms and concurrent psychological and social problems. If the drug is to be stopped after 12 months, it must be slowly tapered to minimize any side-effects from withdrawal. If there has been no response to one SSRI, a different one should be considered. Clomipramine can be started if the person does not respond following an adequate trial of at least one SSRI or if the person prefers clomipramine based on any previous experience of using the drug.

Phobias

Phobias often occur concurrently with GAD or panic states. In most instances, drug treatment for phobic states would focus on the treatment of concurrent anxiety syndromes or panic states and the guidance as described above for both these conditions would be the most appropriate therapeutic approach.

Stepped care approach

Most research about treatment of anxiety disorders has been carried out in secondary care services, and not all of the effective interventions demonstrated at this level can be easily applied to primary care. For example, although there is strong evidence that CBT is effective, it cannot be delivered on a large scale in primary care because it requires a high number of practitioners with specialized training and supervision. An alternative model that is recommended worldwide by most guidelines for anxiety disorders is the stepped care approach, where the treatment components are delivered in a sequential way and according to the needs of the different patients. The idea is that the interventions received by individuals should always be those that are effective, while burdening the health-care system as little as possible.[74]

A good example of a stepped care model is the one proposed by NICE in England, *Generalized anxiety disorder and panic disorder (with or without agoraphobia) in adults – management in primary, secondary and community care*,[49] which recommends the following steps:

- *step 1*: this step focuses on all suspected and confirmed cases of GAD, and the interventions are identification and assessment, education about GAD and treatment options, and active monitoring
- *step 2*: in this case, the focus is on people diagnosed with GAD that has not improved after education and active monitoring in primary care and the interventions are low-intensity psychological interventions, such as:
  - *individual non-facilitated self-help*: bibliotherapy with written or electronic materials, and minimal therapist contact
  - *individual guided self-help*: bibliotherapy and 5–7 sessions (20–30 minutes each)
  - *psycho-educational groups*: six weekly sessions (2 hours each)

- *step 3*: for people with GAD with an inadequate response to step 2 interventions or marked functional impairment. The person can choose between a high-intensity psychological intervention (12–15 weekly sessions of CBT/applied relaxation) or a drug treatment (a selective serotonin reuptake inhibitor)
- *step 4*: for persons with a complex treatment-refractory GAD and very marked functional impairment, such as self-neglect or a high risk of self-harm. Highly specialist treatment is required, such as complex drug and/or psychological treatment regimens, as well as input from multi-agency teams, crisis services, day hospitals or inpatient care.

The NICE stepped care model can probably be considered the gold standard approach to the management of anxiety disorders in high-income countries. Different stepped care models might be proposed for low- and middle-income countries according to their cultural backgrounds and resources available in primary care facilities. There is a need in countries with lower resources to explore alternative interventions that, being less expensive than CBT and antidepressants, can still contribute to decreasing the burden of anxiety disorders – for example, how traditional health can play a role in this sense, or how CBT principles can be used for self-help and support groups to improve anxiety symptoms.

Special issues for the management of anxiety disorders in primary care

Overlap between anxiety and depressive disorders

As mentioned earlier in this chapter, anxiety disorders have a high comorbidity rate with major depression and dysthymia. Anxiety and depressive disorders both share some similar symptoms (see Table 15.2) and they are frequently found together. There is even an argument that anxiety and depressive disorders are the same condition and any distinction between the two is merely artificial.[47] The coexistence between the two disorders may be cross-sectional, when the symptoms of both conditions appear together at the same time, or it may be longitudinal, when one clinical picture is followed closely in time by the other.[75]

According to NICE guidelines, "for people with GAD and a comorbid depressive or other anxiety disorder, treat the primary disorder first (that is, the one that is more severe and in which it is more likely that treatment will improve overall functioning)".[49] For the appropriate management of depressive disorders please refer to Chapter 17 in this book.

Table 15.2 Overlapping symptoms between anxiety and depressive disorders

Unique anxiety symptoms	Shared symptoms (anxiety and depression)	Unique depressive symptoms
• Exaggerated startle reactions	• Irrational fears	• Low mood
• Tension	• Unrealistic or excessive worry	• Anhedonia
• Shakiness, trembling	• Apprehension	• Weight gain/loss
• Avoidance of feared situations	• Irritability	• Loss of interest
• Compulsions	• Distractibility	• Suicidal ideation
	• Difficulty concentrating	
	• Decreased sexual desire	
	• Sleep disturbances	

Adapted, with permission, from Gask L et al. Diagnosis and classification of mental illness: a view from primary care. In: Gask L et al., eds. *Primary care mental health*. London, The Royal College of Psychiatrists, 2009:88–104.[75]

Assessing the risk of suicide

Assessment of the risk of suicide is indicated in persons with anxiety disorders if we consider that suicidal ideation and suicide attempts are significantly increased in this population, particularly in women, and still greater in the presence of risk factors such as:[76]

- comorbid major depression
- long-lasting severe anxiety symptoms
- previous self-harm
- suicidal plan and/or expressed intent
- access to lethal means of harm
- hopelessness and/or helplessness
- alcohol and/or drug abuse
- chronic physical illness and/or pain
- lack of social support
- separated/widowed/divorced
- male sex.

Suicide ideation and suicidal plans have to be actively explored in every person with anxiety disorder who has one or more of the above risk factors. The primary care worker needs to find the right words to lead into the topic gradually, in an empathic and non-judgemental manner. For this purpose, it is useful to prepare some sentences or questions that can be tailored to the particular circumstances of each individual.[76] For example:

- do you feel unhappy and hopeless?
- do you feel life is a burden?
- do you feel unable to cope with everyday life?
- do you feel that life is not worth living?

Insomnia[77]

Insomnia is one of the central symptoms of anxiety disorders, and it is often the presenting complaint to primary care for many people. In many cases, a careful history-taking can elicit excessive worry or other psychological symptoms of anxiety. Insomnia is a distressing and sometimes disabling condition that affects 20–30% of the general population. Between 25% and 30% of insomnia subjects also suffer from a concomitant mental disorder, mainly an anxiety or a depressive disorder, and about 25% have had a previous history of mental disorders.

Insomnia related to anxiety disorder does not need specific treatment, since it usually improves with the general psychological and pharmacological management for this condition. However, practitioners may consider the prescription of an antidepressant with more sedative effects at bedtime (i.e. TCA). A small proportion of persons treated with SSRIs and SNRIs experience activation, with symptoms such as increased anxiety, agitation and problems sleeping that may require stopping the medication.

Sexual dysfunction

Lack, or loss, of sexual desire, male erectile dysfunction and female sexual arousal dysfunction are frequent symptoms of anxiety disorders. On the other hand, antidepressants may affect sexual arousal and orgasm, in both men and women, and it is difficult to know whether the medication or the anxiety is impairing sexual responsiveness.[78] Sildenafil may be useful for men in both cases.[79]

Employment and anxiety disorders

Different studies have shown that anxiety disorders are associated with significant impairments in occupational and social functioning. For example, over 30% of people with GAD showed an annual reduction of work productivity of 10% or more compared to 8% of people with major depression.[49]

The fact that work-related stress may trigger or exacerbate anxiety disorders should be considered as part of the general management and psychological treatment of persons with these clinical conditions.

When to refer to specialists?

Most individuals with anxiety disorders can be treated by primary care professionals. According to the NICE guideline for GAD and PD, if there have been two interventions provided (any combination of psychological intervention, medication, or bibliotherapy) and the person still has significant symptoms, then referral to specialist mental health services should be offered.[49] This recommendation is probably adequate and feasible to implement in high-income countries. However, the insufficient number of mental health specialists in low- and middle-income countries makes this indication impossible to implement for most of them. The few specialists available in these countries could be utilized in a more efficient way if they focus on consulting with primary care teams to help them improve their competencies to treat persons with anxiety.

Placebo effect

Placebo-controlled double-blind studies of pharmacological treatment of anxiety disorders have demonstrated that a number of individuals with these conditions respond favourably to the prescription of placebo, reaching a clinically significant recovery rate as high as 28–46%.[80–83] Antidepressants, however, have demonstrated significantly better results in these studies, with a recovery rate of 50–80% of the persons undergoing treatment. A similar placebo effect in anxiety disorders has been described in studies comparing CBT with a non-specific psychological intervention.[84]

Conclusions

The prevalence of anxiety disorders is high in both community and primary care studies, and they are more frequent among women than men. Persons with anxiety disorders experience a significant lower quality of life and functional impairments, leading in some cases to long-term disability and unemployment. Up to one-third of persons with anxiety disorders meet the diagnostic criteria for two or more anxiety disorders, and a high proportion of them have also comorbidity with other mental and physical disorders.

A variety of instruments have been proved to be valid to detect individuals with anxiety disorders, and they have shown a relatively high sensitivity and specificity. According to resources and local evidence, a basic package of brief and time-limited group interventions can be designed for the management of persons with mild anxiety disorders of recent onset or with subthreshold anxiety symptoms, as a preventive approach.

Anxiety disorders can present both psychological and physical manifestations, and several medical conditions and prescription medications can produce anxiety symptoms. Consequently, a thorough biopsychosocial evaluation must be carried out in persons with anxiety symptoms.

General management – like education about symptoms and treatment, active monitoring, self-help and support groups, bibliotherapy and/or psycho-educational groups – can be effective to treat persons with mild to moderate anxiety disorders.

CBT or therapies based on CBT principles have proved to be effective for the treatment of moderate to severe anxiety disorders in primary care.

SSRIs, and to a lesser extent SNRIs and TCAs, are now widely recommended to treat anxiety disorders, and they are an alternative that is equally as effective as CBT. The evidence for the pharmacological effects of benzodiazepines on anxiety disorders remains inconclusive, despite their widespread use, and they should not be prescribed for these conditions.

Most guidelines for anxiety disorders recommend a stepped care approach, where the treatment components are delivered in a sequential way and according to the needs of the different persons. The idea is that the interventions received by the persons should always be those that are effective, while burdening the health-care system as little as possible.

References

1 Mendlowicz MV, Stein MB. Quality of life in individuals with anxiety disorders. *American Journal of Psychiatry*, 2000, 157:669–682.

2 Oglesby P. Da Costa's syndrome or neurocirculatory asthenia. *British Heart Journal*, 1987, 58:306–315.

3 Freud S. On the grounds for detaching a particular syndrome from neurasthenia under the description 'anxiety neurosis'. In: Strachey J. *The standard edition of the complete psychological works of Sigmund Freud, Volume III (1893–1899): early psycho-analytic publications*. London, Hogarth Press and the Institute of Psycho-Analysis, 1962:85–115.

4 *Diagnostic and statistical manual of mental disorders*, 4th ed, text revision (DSM-IV-TR). Washington, American Psychiatric Association, 2000.

5 *ICD-10 classification of mental and behavioral disorders*. Geneva, World Health Organization, 1996.

6 Kessler R, Ruscio A, Shear K, Wittchen H. Epidemiology of anxiety disorders. In: Stein M, Steckler T, eds. *Behavioral neurobiology of anxiety and its treatment, current topics in behavioral neurosciences*. Berlin, Heidelberg, Springer Verlag, 2010:21–35.

7 Kessler R, Keller MB, Wittchen HU. The epidemiology of generalized anxiety disorder. *The Psychiatric Clinics of North America*, 2001, 24:19–40.

8 Zimmermann P et al. Primary anxiety disorders and the development of subsequent alcohol use disorders: a 4-year community study of adolescents and young adults. *Psychological Medicine*, 2003, 33:1211–1222.

9 Christiana JM et al. Duration between onset and time of obtaining initial treatment among people with anxiety and mood disorders: an international survey of members of mental health patient advocate groups. *Psychological Medicine*, 2000, 30:693–703.

10 Üstun T, Sartorius N, eds. *Mental illness in general health care. An international study*. Chichester, John Wiley and Sons, 1995.

11 Goldberg DP, Lecrubier Y. Form and frequency of mental disorders across centers. In: Üstün TB, Sartorius N, eds. *Mental illness in general health care: an international study*. Chichester, John Wiley & Sons, on behalf of WHO, 1995:323–334.

12 Kessler RC. Epidemiology of psychiatric co morbidity. In: Tsuang MT, Tohen M, Zahner GEP, eds. *Textbook in psychiatric epidemiology*. New York, John Wiley & Sons, Inc., 1995:179–197.

13 Toft T et al. Mental disorders in primary care: prevalence and co-morbidity among disorders. Results from the functional illness in primary care (FIP) study. *Psychological Medicine*, 2005, 35:1175–1184.

14 *Declaration of Alma-Ata*. International Conference on Primary Health Care, Alma-Ata USSR, 6–12 September 1978 (http://www.who.int/hpr/NPH/docs/declaration_almaata.pdf, accessed 2 November 2011).

15 Olfson M et al. Prevalence of anxiety, depression, and substance use disorders in an urban general medicine practice. *Archives of Family Medicine*, 2000, 9:876–883.

16 Bunevicius A et al. Screening for depression and anxiety disorders in primary care patients. *Depression and Anxiety*, 2007, 24:455–460.

17 Prins MA et al. Primary care patients with anxiety and depression: need for care from the patient's perspective. *Journal of Affective Disorders*, 2009, 119:163–171.

18 World Health Organization and Wonca. *Integrating mental health into primary care. A global perspective*. Geneva, World Health Organization, 2008.

19 Kennerley H. The prevention of anxiety disorders. In: Kendrick T, Tylee A, Freeling P, eds. *The prevention of mental illness in primary care*. Cambridge, Cambridge University Press, 1996:188–206.

20 Boeijen CA et al. Treatment of anxiety disorders in primary care practice: a randomized controlled trial. *British Journal of General Practice*, 2005, 55:763–769.

21 Roy-Byrne P et al. Delivery of evidence-based treatment for multiple anxiety disorders in primary care: a randomized controlled trial. *JAMA*, 2010, 303:1921–1928.

22 Feldner MT, Zvolensky MJ, Schmidt NB. Prevention of anxiety psychopathology: a critical review of the empirical literature. *Clinical Psychology: Science and Practice*, 2004, 11:405–424.

23 Bienvenu OJ, Ginsburg GS. Prevention of anxiety disorders. *International Review of Psychiatry*, 2007, 19:647–654.

24   Rapee RM, Schniering CA, Hudson JL. Anxiety disorders during childhood and adolescence: origins and treatment. *Annual Review of Clinical Psychology*, 2009, 5:311–41.

25   Patel V et al. Treatment and prevention of mental disorders in low-income and middle-income countries. *The Lancet*, 2007, 370: 991–1005.

26   Zigmond AS, Snaith RP. The Hospital Anxiety and Depression Scale. *Acta Psychiatrica Scandinavica*, 1983, 67:361–370.

27   Hirschfeld RMA. The comorbidity of major depression and anxiety disorders: recognition and management in primary care. *Primary Care Companion Journal of Clinical Psychiatry*, 2001, 3:244–254.

28   Herrero MJ, Blanch J, Peri JM. A validation study of the hospital anxiety and depression scale (HADS) in a Spanish population. *General Hospital Psychiatry*, 2003, 25:277–283.

29   Farvolden P et al. A web based screening instrument for depression and anxiety disorders in primary care. *Journal of Medical Internet Research*, 2003, 5:e23.

30   Lang AJ et al. Abbreviated brief symptom inventory for use as an anxiety and depression screening instrument in primary care. *Depression and Anxiety*, 2009, 26:537–543.

31   Rickels MR et al. Assessment of anxiety and depression in primary care: value of a four-item questionnaire. *Journal of the American Osteopathic Association*, 2009, 109:216–219.

32   Kroenke K et al. Anxiety disorders in primary care: prevalence, impairment, comorbidity, and detection. *Annals of Internal Medicine*, 2007, 146:317–325.

33   Puddifoot S et al. A new case finding tool for anxiety: a pragmatic diagnostic validity study in primary care. *International Journal of Psychiatry in Medicine*, 2007, 37:371–381.

34   Wetherell JL et al. Screening for generalized anxiety disorders in geriatric primary care patients. *International Journal of Geriatric Psychiatry*, 2007, 22:115–123.

35   Spinhoven PH et al. Validation study of the Hospital Anxiety and Depression Scale (HADS) in different groups of Dutch subjects. *Psychological Medicine*, 1997, 27:363–370.

36   Bjellanda I et al. The validity of the Hospital Anxiety and Depression Scale: an updated literature review. Journal of Psychosomatic Research, 2002, 52:69–77.

37   Ebell MH. Diagnosis of anxiety disorders in primary care. *American Family Physician*, 2008, 78:501–502.

38   Johnson MR et al. Ethnic differences in the reliability and validity of a panic disorder screen. *Ethnicity and Health*, 2007, 12:283–296.

39   Van't Veer-Tazelaar PJ et al. Stepped care prevention of anxiety and depression in late life: a randomized controlled trial. *Archives of General Psychiatry*, 2009, 66:297–304.

40   Van't Veer-Tazelaar P et al. Cost-effectiveness of a stepped care intervention to prevent depression and anxiety in late life: randomised trial. *British Journal of Psychiatry*, 2010, 196:319–325.

41   Montgomery SA et al. A 24-week ramdomized, double-blind, placebo controlled study of escitalopram for the prevention of generalized social anxiety disorder. *Journal of Clinical Psychiatry*, 2005, 66:1270–1278.

42   Tyrer P, Baldwin D. Generalised anxiety disorder. *The Lancet*, 2006, 368:2156–2166.

43   Davidson JRT et al. Duloxetine treatment for relapse prevention in adults with generalized anxiety disorder: a double-blind placebo-controlled trial. *European Neuropsychopharmacology*, 2008, 18:673–681.

44   Hollon SD, Stewart MO, Strunk D. Enduring effects for cognitive behaviour therapy in the treatment of depression and anxiety. *Annual Review of Psychology*, 2006, 57:285–315.

45   Craske MG et al. CBT intensity and outcome for panic disorder in a primary care setting. *Behavior Therapy*, 2006, 37:112–119.

46   Khouzam HR. Anxiety disorders: guidelines for effective primary care, part 1, diagnosis. *Consultant*, 2009, 49(3) (http://www.consultant360.com/content/anxiety-disorders-guidelines-effective-primary-care-part-1-diagnosis, accessed 25 November 2011).

47   Arroll B, Kendrick T. Anxiety. In: Gask L et al., eds. *Primary care mental health*. London, The Royal College of Psychiatrists, 2009:145–155.

48   National Health Service of Spain Taskforce. *Clinical guideline for the management of patients with anxiety disorders in primary care* (in Spanish). Madrid, Government of Spain and Madrid Community, 2008.

49   *Generalised anxiety disorder and panic disorder (with or without agoraphobia) in adults – management in primary, secondary and community care.* London, National Institute for Health and Clinical Excellence, 2011 (CG113) (http://www.nice.org.uk/nicemedia/live/13314/52599/52599.pdf, accessed 16 November 2011).

50   Senaratne R et al. The burden of anxiety disorders on the family. *Journal of Nervous and Mental Disease*, 2010, 198:876–880.

51   Isaac M, Gureje O. Low and middle-income countries. In: Gask L et al., eds. *Primary care mental health*. London, The Royal College of Psychiatrists, 2009:72–87.

52   Martinsen EW. Physical activity in the prevention and treatment of anxiety and depression. *Nordic Journal of Psychiatry*, 2008, 62(Suppl. 47):25–29.

53   Ströhle A. Physical activity, exercise, depression and anxiety disorders. *Journal of Neural Transmission*, 2009, 116:777–784.

54   Newman MG, Borkovec TD. Cognitive-behavioral treatment of generalized anxiety disorder. *The Clinical Psychologist*, 1995, 48:5–7.

55   Beck AT, Emery G. *Anxiety disorders and phobias: a cognitive perspective*. New York, Basic Books, 1985.

56   Van Boeijen CA et al. Efficacy of self-help manuals for anxiety disorders in primary care: a review. *Family Practice*, 2005, 22:1–5.

57   McCrone P et al. Cost-effectiveness of computerised cognitive behavioural therapy for anxiety and depression in primary care: randomised controlled trial. *British Journal of Psychiatry*, 2004, 185:55–62.

58   Grös D, Antony M. The assessment and treatment of specific phobias: a review. *Current Psychiatry Reports*, 1996, 8:298–303.

59   Clark D. *Cognitive-behavioural therapy for OCD*. New York, The Guilford Press, 2004.

60   Bisson J, Andrew M. Psychological treatment of post-traumatic stress disorder (PTSD). *Cochrane Database of Systematic Reviews*, 2007, (3):CD003388.

61   Ponniah K, Hollon S. Empirically supported psychological treatments for adult acute stress disorder and posttraumatic stress disorder: a review. *Depression and Anxiety*, 2009, 26:1086–1099.

62   Roberts NP et al. Multiple session early psychological interventions for the prevention of post-traumatic stress disorder *Cochrane Database of Systematic Reviews*, 2009, (3):CD006869.

63   Foa EB, Davidson JRT, Frances A. The Expert Consensus Guideline Series: treatment of posttraumatic stress disorder. *Journal of Clinical Psychiatry*, 1999, 60(Suppl. 16):10–73.

64   Van Boeijen CA et al. Treatment of anxiety disorders in primary care practice: a randomised controlled trial. *British Journal of General Practice*, 2005, 55:763–769.

65   Roy-Byrne P et al. Brief intervention for anxiety in primary care patients. *Journal of the American Board of Family Medicine*, 2009, 22:175–186.

66   Davidson JRT, Feltner D, Dugar A. Management of generalised anxiety disorder in primary care: identifying the challenges and unmet needs. *Primary Care Companion of Clinical Psychiatry*, 2010, 12:1–13.

67   Swenson JR, Doucette S, Fergusson D. Adverse cardiovascular events in antidepressant trials involving high-risk patients: a systematic review of randomized trials. *Canadian Journal of Psychiatry*, 2006, 51:923–929.

68   Taylor D. Antidepressant drugs and cardiovascular pathology: a clinical overview of effectiveness and safety. *Acta Psychiatrica Scandinavica*, 2008, 118:434–442.

69   Duggan SE, Fuller MA. Duloxetine: a dual reuptake inhibitor. *Annals of Pharmacotherapy*, 2004, 38:2078–2085.

70   Yuan Y, Tsoi K, Hunt RH. Selective serotonin reuptake inhibitors and risk of upper GI bleeding: confusion or confounding? *American Journal of Medicine*, 2006, 119:719–727.

71   Demyttenaere K, Jaspers L. Bupropion and SSI-induced side effects. *Journal of Psychopharmacology*, 2008, 22:792–804.

72   *Post-traumatic stress disorder: the management of PTSD in adults and children in primary and secondary care.* London, National Institute for Health and Clinical Excellence, 2005 (CG26).

73   *Obsessive-compulsive disorder: core interventions in the treatment of obsessive-compulsive disorder and body dysmorphic disorder.* London, National Institute for Health and Clinical Excellence, 2005 (CG31).

74   Richards D, Bower P, Gilbody S. Collaborative care and stepped care: innovations for common mental disorders. In: Gask L et al., eds. *Primary care mental health*. London, The Royal College of Psychiatrists, 2009:395–408.

75   Gask L et al. Diagnosis and classification of mental illness: a view from primary care. In: Gask L et al., eds. *Primary care mental health*. London, The Royal College of Psychiatrists, 2009:88–104.

76   Dietrich S et al. Suicide and self-harm. In: Gask L et al., eds. *Primary care mental health*. London, The Royal College of Psychiatrists, 2009:125–144.

77   Ohayon MM, Roth T. Place of chronic insomnia in the course of depressive and anxiety disorders. *Journal of Psychiatry Research*, 2003, 37:9–15.

78   King M. Sexual problems. In: Gask L et al., eds. *Primary care mental health*. London, The Royal College of Psychiatrists, 2009:335–348.

79   Taylor MJ, Rudkin L, Hawton K. Strategies for managing antidepressant-induced sexual dysfunction: systematic review of randomised controlled trials. *Journal of Affective Disorders*, 2005, 88:241–254.

80   Allgulander C, Hackett D, Salinas E. Venlafaxine extended release (ER) in the treatment of generalised anxiety disorder: twenty-four-week placebo-controlled dose-ranging study. *The British Journal of Psychiatry*, 2001, 179:15–22.

81   Atul CP et al. Pregabalin in generalized anxiety disorder: a placebo-controlled study. *American Journal of Psychiatry*, 2003, 160:553–540.

82   Stahl SM, Gergel I, Li D. Escitalopram in the treatment of panic disorder: a randomized, double-blind, placebo controlled trial. *Journal of Clinical Psychiatry*, 2003, 64:1322–1327.

83   Rickels K et al. Paroxetine treatment of generalized anxiety disorder: a double-blind, placebo controlled study. *American Journal of Psychiatry*, 2003, 160:749–756.

84   Hofmann SG, Smits JAJ. Cognitive-behavioral therapy for adult anxiety disorders: a meta-analysis of randomized placebo-controlled trials. *Journal of Clinical Psychiatry*, 2008, 69:621–632.

16 Bereavement in primary care mental health

Bill Travers, Niloufer Ali and Lucja Kolkiewicz

Key messages

- Abnormal bereavement and distress disorders are prevalent and carry a significant rate of morbidity and mortality.
- Complicated grief treatment is more effective than standard interpersonal therapy, in terms of response rate and time to response for complicated grief.
- Health-care professionals are in an excellent position to help the individual with distress disorder or with abnormal bereavement, to prevent both physical and psychological morbidity.
- Counselling by minimally trained community workers in underprivileged communities has shown beneficial effect for anxiety and depression. It is recommended that skills for identification and counselling for distress disorders and abnormal bereavement should be incorporated in the training of community health workers in resource-constrained countries.

Introduction

Distress disorders are common in primary care and the previous chapter (Chapter 15) on anxiety describes the epidemiology, key symptoms and investigations necessary when dealing with distress disorders, including information-gathering, decision-making, self-help and treatment options.

Many family doctors are used to seeing patients who have experienced life events that lead to psychological disturbance. One such common life experience is that of bereavement, and all family doctors and their teams will come across patients who have experienced bereavement.

While the proposed new edition of the *International Classification of Diseases*, ICD-11 may not include bereavement as a distinct entity, because it shares so many features with other distress disorders,[1] we will use it as an example of a life transition that is followed by psychological disturbance.

What is bereavement?

Bereavement can be defined as the period of mourning and grief that follows the death of a loved one. Mourning consists of the rituals and symbolic behaviour that follow such a death. These features could, for example, include the funeral and the wearing of black clothing. The mourning rituals vary according to the culture and religion of the deceased and the bereaved.

Grief refers to the individual's experience of loss and comprises physical, psychological and spiritual responses.

Bereavement is an experience that virtually all individuals will experience at some point in their lives. It can be seen as a normal part of the life-cycle. Although it is a common phenomenon, it is usually not familiar as a personal experience to the person concerned and is associated with high levels of emotional distress and increased levels of morbidity and mortality.

Bowlby's work on attachment and its exploration of separation and loss has been highly influential in the understanding of grief.[2] His work on the development of the attachment between infants and their mothers highlighted the behaviours designed to bring about reunion after separation – crying and searching. Since such behaviours are so necessary for survival at the start of life, it is to be expected that the same behaviours, along with separation anxiety, will surface at a time of loss in later life.

There is a wide range of emotional and behavioural components within the grief response of the bereaved. The nature of the response is influenced by the individual characteristics of the bereaved, the nature of their relationship with the deceased, the circumstances of the death and the culture of the bereaved person.

Many authorities on bereavement, Parkes and Prigerson in particular,[3] have described well-recognized features that are usually present in the bereaved. These accounts describe the expected components, their sequence and their approximate timescale. Such models of understanding also rehearse a cycle of response that emphasizes the natural history of grief with expected phases and their eventual reduction in intensity. The majority of bereaved people come through their grief and resume their everyday functioning, albeit with an adapted psychological framework into which the death is integrated.

There is an acknowledgement that there is benefit through the grief process running its course and also that there are factors that can be associated with promoting this process. The blockage of such a process for whatever reason may leave the person stuck in responses and attitudes that are painful and not conducive to emerging from the bereavement in a healthy way. Complicated or prolonged grief is highly disabling and associated with high levels of suffering. Health-care staff have a vital role to play in supporting the bereaved; in identifying when a prolonged, complicated or abnormal bereavement has developed; and in providing or referring the person for appropriate treatment.

In descending order, the death of a child, a spouse or partner, or parent are said to be associated with the highest intensity of adult grief.[4] The loss of a loved one through suicide may also be recognized as having a particularly profound psychological impact. Bereavement is known to be associated with increased levels of morbidity and mortality.[2] It is therefore incumbent on health staff to pay careful attention to patients suffering such loss. There is considerable scope for interventions that can make a real difference to the level of suffering and the health, functional and social outcomes of the bereaved.

Key tasks for health-care professionals include the possession of good knowledge about the normal spectrum of bereavement reactions, skills in promoting grieving, and an ability to identify when a grief reaction has become abnormal, prolonged or complex, or when it has developed into a mental illness such as depression.

Additional skills include an ability to identify and know how to help children and those with communication difficulties to manage their grief.

An understanding of infant attachment is helpful in assisting bereaved children. Infants and toddlers react to the loss of an attachment figure by protesting vigorously, followed by the experience of despair and eventually detachment. By the age of 5 years, most children can understand the difference between a temporary separation and a permanent one as in death.[5]

Florid reactions do not tend to last longer than a few weeks but bereaved children have higher levels of emotional disturbance and symptoms than non-bereaved children. Early bereavement is associated with higher levels of childhood psychiatric disorder, and adults who lost a parent in childhood are more prone to psychiatric illness.

Stages of the bereavement process

Numbness/disbelief

There is a sense of disbelief and a failure to behave in a way that takes account of the loss of the loved one. The expectation that the bereaved person is about to see the person, that they will shortly walk through the door, makes for a recurrent feeling of alarm and intense distress when the reality of the death is repeatedly realized.

Yearning/pining

This is a phase of intense "pangs of grief" associated with anxiety representing separation distress. There is a feeling of emptiness coupled with a longing for the lost person. Searching behaviours are part of this phase and can entail the literal looking for the person, perhaps where they would have spent much of their time when alive, or alternatively it can mean a process of mental searching, or searching within to try to find a sense of connection with the lost person.

The bereaved person may find themselves identifying with the deceased's illness and experiencing their symptoms. They may also develop a strong sense of the presence of the dead person, typically by seeing or hearing the deceased in varying degrees of intensity but usually fleetingly.

Anger

It is not uncommon for there to be emotional responses that may be difficult to accept or understand. Anger is a relatively common response, most easily understood in terms of the bereaved person feeling they have been left or deserted to cope with not only their grief, but also whatever unresolved life situations have been left by the deceased. More complex motivations for feelings of anger may also develop in bereavements where the relationship between the dead person and the bereaved person was difficult, unhappy or ambivalent.

Sadness/depression

This phase of grief is one in which the full enormity of the loss is realized, and can entail a loss of all interest, enjoyment and motivation, weight loss, impaired concentration and short-term memory, disorganization and despair. Guilty feelings that the bereaved person could have in some way done something to prevent the death, alleviated the dead person's suffering or acted in any other way for a better outcome are extremely common. Again, such feelings can be more intense, persistent or difficult to deal with when the relationship with the dead person was problematic.

The most intense grief and peaks of distress usually begin to recede after 4 to 6 months.[4,6]

Resolution/acceptance

Over time, it is usual for the bereaved person to experience a gradual lessening in the intensity of their grief. The positive aspects of the dead person's personality and life are recalled with a mixture of both sadness and pleasure, and a more rounded view of the person is developed or regained.

While the sense of loss and pain does not disappear, the strength of the distress recedes and it is possible to begin to find meaning and enjoyment in life once again.

The bereaved person is able to recognize and hold on to a balanced view of the dead person, in which the positive and less positive features of the person are recalled; the sense of long-term psychological connection with the person is maintained; there is a return of an emotional equilibrium and the bereaved person can continue with their life.

Abnormal bereavement

A small proportion of the bereaved are known to undergo a more problematic, prolonged and complicated course. A number of studies have sought to characterize and differentiate those who develop what can be described as pathological grief from those that do not. Personality vulnerabilities leading to such relationship styles as avoidant and insecure attachments are likely risk factors.[7] A genetic marker of response to adversity may contribute.[8] Previous loss and adverse life experiences, such as those experienced by indigenous peoples losing land, culture and loved ones are described as further vulnerability features.[9]

Separation anxiety in childhood, previous psychiatric disorder, a history of family psychiatric disorder and substance misuse are all thought to increase vulnerability.[10]

Diagnoses of patients studied in such research fall into two categories, specific and non-specific.[3] The non-specific conditions include a range of psychiatric illness that can be triggered by a number of types of stressors as well as bereavement. The specific conditions are forms of complicated grief. In reality, bereaved people can sometimes show evidence of both non-specific disorder and specific disorder (pathological grief), i.e. a mixed picture.

Two main categories of abnormal grief have been described: prolonged grief disorder (PGD) and delayed or distorted forms of grief. PGD is now well established and the most frequent form of pathological grief, while the other category remains less well established.

There is no well-defined cut-off point between complicated and uncomplicated grief; they are thought to exist on a continuum.

Separate teams have carried out systematic studies on prolonged grief,[11,12] and subsequently reached agreement on the cluster of phenomena that are commonly present in those with PGD.

For PGD, Prigerson and colleagues have developed consensus criteria for a psychiatric disorder for provisional inclusion in DSM-V.[13] The proposed definition requires that the reaction to the loss includes not only the presence of prolonged grief but also a cluster of at least five of the following:

- sense of self as empty or confused since loss, or feeling that a part of oneself has died as a result of the loss
- trouble accepting the loss as real
- avoidance of reminders of the loss
- inability to trust others since the loss
- extreme bitterness or anger related to the loss
- extreme difficulty moving on with life (e.g. making new friends, pursuing interests)
- pervasive numbness or detachment since the loss
- feeling life is empty and the future bleak without the deceased
- feeling stunned, dazed or shocked by the loss.

The symptoms would need to have lasted at least 6 months, be associated with a significant level of functional impairment, not be due to the effects of a substance or a general medical condition and not be better accounted for by major depressive disorder, generalized anxiety disorder or post-traumatic stress disorder (PTSD).

Simple enquiry for key symptoms can likewise detect the presence of specific psychiatric illness such as depression. Grief measures can potentially offer a more structured means to clarify the presence of, and differentiate between, prolonged grief, depression, PTSD or other health problems.[14] Such structured measures are unlikely to be routinely necessary in primary care.

Prigerson and colleagues have developed a questionnaire called the Index of Complicated Grief (ICG),[15] since superseded by a simpler 13-item Prolonged Grief index (PG-13). In practice, the observation of intense levels of grief that last beyond 6 months, along with symptoms from the list of criteria suggested for inclusion in DSM-V would be indicative of a diagnosis of PGD.

Management of distress disorders including bereavement

The principles of assessment and management of anxiety disorder should be followed. These are presented in detail in Chapter 15.

Special considerations for the assessment and management of bereavement

For most bereaved people, counselling and specific treatment are not required. Assessment should be simple and carried out at the time of need, looking at the death itself, the circumstances, the nature of the relationship with the deceased and the bereaved person's experience since the death.

Assessment and initial management of the bereaved should be carried out in a sensitive, empathic and compassionate manner.

Just as in the case of distress disorder, where grief is particularly intense, complicated or prolonged, or where there are vulnerability factors, careful history-taking is important. It is then important to consider eliciting information in a systematic way about the effects of the death on the bereaved person and the progress of their grief. Suggested areas for focus include the presence and extent of symptoms associated with the known phases of grief:

- numbness and disbelief
- yearning and sadness
- anger
- guilt
- suicidal thoughts
- the meaning for the individual of their loss.

Evidence of particularly intense or prolonged reactions requires more detailed consideration. Vigilance for the presence of depression, anxiety disorder or PTSD is required.

Management of distress disorder and bereavement

Management of distress disorders including abnormal bereavement may depend on culture and resources, including the use of available social network and family support and can often be delivered in the primary care setting.

There is limited evidence for the effectiveness of specific treatments. The following guidance is based on suggested approaches from the literature, the authors' views drawn from practical experience, and the available research evidence base.

The role of primary care services

- Consider the diagnosis.
- Acknowledge the condition.
- Provide education and information about distress disorder and bereavement.
- Consider the provision of therapy that is supportive, active, flexible, goal directed, time limited, supportive of the patient's strengths and of a type that plays down past problems.[16-18]
- Consider brief therapies with three broad components:
  - enabling reduction or removal of the stressor
  - measures to facilitate adaptation
  - altering the response to the stressor; symptom reduction/behavioural change.

Therapeutic approaches that may be helpful include problem-solving, cognitive restructuring, mobilizing support such as the involvement of family members, relaxation techniques and dialectical behavioural therapy for deliberate self-harming behaviour.

Psychological therapies of a variety of modalities, including supportive, psycho-educational, cognitive and psychodynamic therapy, may all be of use. The evidence base for these approaches is limited.[19]

In distress disorder associated with bereavement, cognitive approaches can be useful, as described in the Dutch guidelines for the diagnosis and treatment of adjustment disorder.[20,21]

These guidelines are seen as best implemented within a scheme in which there are three phases:

- understanding and coping emotionally with what has happened, thereby gaining understanding and acceptance

- gaining insight into the relevant stressors and possible solutions and the acquisition of skills to implement solutions
- the application of skills and solutions.

A key principle within the implementation of this approach is active monitoring of the recovery process, seeking to ensure patients fulfil planned recovery tasks.

The limitations of these recommendations include the fact that they are mainly designed for work-related adjustment disorder and the physician (occupational health physician or general practitioner (GP)) requires specific training to provide the intervention.

Interventions in prolonged grief disorder

Systematic review of the current literature on bereavement intervention has revealed no consistent pattern of treatment benefit across well-designed experimental studies;[22] indeed, a universal treatment for complicated grief may not exist, as grief can be viewed as a multidimensional construct.[23]

Shear et al. conducted a randomized controlled trial that compared complicated grief treatment (CGT) with standard interpersonal psychotherapy (IPT) and found the former treatment to be more effective in terms of response rate and time to response.[24] The CGT protocol included an introductory, middle and termination phase. In the introductory phase, the therapist provided information about normal and complicated grief and described adaptive coping and adjustment to the loss. In addition, it included a focus on personal life goals. In the middle phase, the therapist addressed both processes in tandem. The termination phase focused on review of progress, plans for the future and feelings about ending treatment. IPT mainly focused on behaviours and relationships, whereas CGT focused on the dual problem areas of distress caused by the loss and the survivor's personal goals and restoration of a satisfying life. Basically, it is a two-pronged approach in which therapists simultaneously guide patients to focus both on the loss and on rebuilding their own lives.

CGT is a psychotherapeutic approach that includes cognitive-behavioural methods similar to those used for PTSD. In CGT, therapists guide patients as they narrate the story of the death, a process called "revisiting", and produce audio-recordings of the exercises that enable patients to listen to the story repeatedly and put aside the thoughts about the death, thereby lessening the effect of the pain. The patient is encouraged to make specific plans for pleasurable activities and to start to engage in situations that he or she has avoided following the loss of their loved one. The therapist also guides the patient through an imagined conversation regarding the person whom he or she has lost, which offers the opportunity to speak openly about the intense feelings that the two shared. At the same time, patients work on re-engaging in activities and relationships that promise satisfaction and work to define and achieve personal goals. Both patients and therapists evaluate the patient's symptoms throughout the course of the therapy.

The key findings from this study were that response rate and time to response were significantly better for CGT than IPT.[24] Also, those participants who were already taking an antidepressant drug at the time of their enrolment showed twice the response rate to IPT and slightly better results with CGT than those not on medications.

Recently, an Internet-based cognitive-behavioural intervention for complicated grief has been developed and evaluated by Wagner and Maercker.[25] This is a 5-week intervention that consists of two components: structured writing disclosure and cognitive-behavioural therapy. Results of this randomized controlled trial revealed that the treatment group experienced significant statistical and clinical reductions in various symptoms (e.g. intrusion, avoidance, failure to adapt) at post treatment and at 3-month follow-up. Wagner and Maercker also reported that the reduction in symptoms of complicated grief observed after treatment with an Internet-based cognitive-behavioural intervention was maintained at 1.5-year follow-up.[25] A recent meta-analysis conducted by Wittouck et al. concluded that treatment interventions can effectively diminish symptoms of complicated grief in both the short term and long term.[26]

Recommendations for primary care staff when responding to bereavement

The provision of empathic, sensitive and compassionate support is a key requirement in the initial stages. Guiding principles include acting in such a way as to do no harm, to seek to protect the patient's mental health and to anticipate and acknowledge the potential sequence of fluctuating and mixed emotional responses.

Answering questions about the deceased and their death, their illness or injuries and their suffering can be very important.

Support to enable the bereaved person to view the body, and guidance on practical matters to do with the funeral, are often of great value.

There is limited evidence to support guidance on how primary care staff should respond to bereaved patients. There is some evidence on how primary care doctors and nurses respond in the United Kingdom of Great Britain and Northern Ireland (UK).[27] Based on such work, it is considered desirable for GPs and practice nurses to offer support to all patients who are bereaved and to seek to proactively engage those who are judged to be at risk of an adverse bereavement outcome.

The aim of such intervention would be to provide support to the bereaved in a non-intrusive, responsive and practical way, highlighting the use of the patient's own resources and without interfering in a process that could be at risk of being over-medicalized.

Some of the main options available for primary care staff to consider are presented next.

The role of primary care services

- Establish contact with the bereaved. This may involve developing a system to alert the primary care team to this need when there is a death. The contact can be made by doctors or nurses, in person, by letter, appointment or home visit.
- Provide information about the death.
- Give information about bereavement and offer support. Remain available.
- Offer to listen/talk: show a willingness to hear the bereaved person's account and to acknowledge their grief.
- Consider the potential role for anxiolytic or hypnotic medication in the short term.
- Provide supportive counselling.
- Identify abnormal bereavement: if the timescale of intense distress exceeds 6 months and there is ongoing significant functional impairment, this would suggest a complicated grief reaction and/or the presence of a psychiatric disorder such as depressive illness, anxiety or PTSD.
- Identify depressive illness, PTSD and any other mental illness.
- Treat depressive illness with cognitive-behavioural psychotherapy and consider antidepressant medication, particularly where symptoms are severe.
- Bereavement counselling services: most acute hospitals in the UK have bereavement services attached to them. Patients can be referred by primary care staff and can also refer themselves.
- Give information about bereavement organizations such as Cruse Bereavement Care.
- Refer on to primary-care-based treatments or refer to secondary care mental health services if grief is intense, prolonged or complex.
- In the UK, consider referral to the local arrangements for improving access to psychological therapies (IAPT).
- Systematically review the progress of those who have risk factors and/or those who are known to be experiencing abnormal or prolonged reactions.

The role of mental health services

■ Mental health services such as practice-based/-linked psychology and counselling interventions may be available at a primary care level. Where the bereaved person is seeking further help and where distress levels are high, referral to such support is indicated.

■ Secondary care mental health services: primary care staff should consider referral to specialist psychiatry services when there is evidence of complicated grief that is not responding to primary-care-based psychological interventions; where depressive illness has not responded to initial treatment; where there is significant suicidal thinking; or where there is diagnostic or treatment uncertainty.

Conclusion

Distress disorders are part of the spectrum of dysphoric disorders. This chapter has specifically focused on bereavement, an example of a distress disorder that all family practitioners will encounter in their practice.

References

1   Goldberg D. A revised mental health classification for use in general medical settings: the ICD 11-PHC. *International Psychiatry*, 2011, 8:1–3.

2   Bowlby J. *Attachment and loss, Vol 1. Attachment.* London, Hogarth Press and Institute of Psychoanalysis, 1969.

3   Parkes C, Prigerson H. *Bereavement: studies of grief in adult life*, 4th ed. 2010, Harlow: Penguin Books, 2010.

4   Middleton W et al. A longitudinal study comparing bereavement phenomena in recently bereaved spouses, adult children and parents. *The Australian and New Zealand Journal of Psychiatry*, 1998, 32:235–241.

5   Black D. Bereavement in childhood. In: Parkes C, Markus A, eds. *Coping with loss.* London: BMA Books, 1998:28–35.

6   Byrne G, Raphael B. A longitudinal study of bereavement phenomena in recently widowed elderly men. *Psychological Medicine*, 1994, 24:411–421.

7   Stroebe M et al. The prediction of bereavement outcome: development of an integrative risk factor framework. *Social Science and Medicine*, 2006, 63:2446–2451.

8   Kaufman J et al. Social supports and serotonin transporter gene moderate depression in maltreated children. *Proceedings of the National Academy of Sciences of the United States of America*, 2004, 101:17316–17321.

9   Raphael B, Swan P, Martinek N. Intergeneration aspects of trauma for Australian Aboriginal people. In: Danieli Y, ed. *An international handbook of multigenerational legacies of trauma.* New York, Plenum Press, 1998:327–339.

10 Raphael B, Wooding S, Dunsmore J. Bereavement. In: Gelder M et al., eds. *New Oxford textbook of psychiatry*, 2nd ed, Vol 1. Oxford, Oxford University Press, 2009:724–728.

11 Horowitz M et al. Diagnostic criteria for complicated grief disorder. *American Journal of Psychiatry*, 1997, 154:904–910.

12 Prigerson H et al. Consensus criteria for traumatic grief: a preliminary empirical test. *British Journal of Psychiatry*, 1999, 174:67–73.

13 Prigerson HG, Vanderwerker LC, Maciejewski PK. A case for inclusion of prolonged grief disorder in DSM-V. In: Stroebe MS et al., eds. *Handbook of bereavement research and practice: advances in theory and intervention.* Washington DC, American Psychological Association, 2008:165–186.

14 Neimeyer R, Hogan N. Quantitative or qualitative? Measurement issues in the study of grief. In: Strobe M et al., eds. *Handbook of bereavement research: consequences, coping and care.* Washington DC, American Psychological Association, 2001:89–118.

15 Prigerson H et al. Inventory of Complicated Grief: a scale to measure maladaptive symptoms of loss. *Psychiatry Research*, 1995, 59:65–79.

16 Carlson J. Adjustment disorders and V codes. In: Sperry L, Carlson J, eds. *Psychopathology and psychotherapy: from DSM-IV diagnosis to treatment*. Washington, Taylor & Francis, 1996:267–278.

17 Maxmen J. *Essential psychopathology*. New York, WW Norton, 1986.

18 Sperry L, ed. Varieties of brief therapy. *Individual Psychology*, 1989, 45(1/2 special issue).

19 Van Der Klink J, Van Dijk F. Dutch practice guidelines for managing adjustment disorders in occupational and primary health care. *Scandinavian Journal of Work, Environment and Health*, 2003, 29:478–487.

20 Van der Klink J, ed. *Guideline for occupational physicians for mental disorders*. Eindhoven: NVAB (Dutch Association of Occupational Physicians), 2008.

21 Van der Klink J, ed. *Mental disorders and work: guideline for general practitioners and occupational physicians: test version*. Utrecht/Amsterdam, KNMG/SKB, 2000.

22 Forte AL et al. Bereavement care interventions: a systematic review. *BMC Palliative Care*, 2004, 3:3.

23 O'Connor M et al. Writing therapy for the bereaved: evaluation of an intervention. *Journal of Palliative Medicine*, 2003, 6:195–204.

24 Shear K et al. Treatment of complicated grief: a randomized controlled trial. *JAMA*, 2005, 293:2601–2608.

25 Wagner B, Maercker A. A 1.5 year follow-up of an internet-based intervention for complicated grief. *Journal of Traumatic Stress*, 2007, 20:625–629.

26 Wittouck C et al. The prevention and treatment of complicated grief: a meta-analysis. *Clinical Psychology Review*, 2011, 31:69–78.

27 Nagraj S, Barclay S. Bereavement care in primary care: a systematic literature and narrative synthesis. *British Journal of General Practice*, 2011, 61:53–58.

17 Depression in primary care mental health

Jane Gunn, Christopher Dowrick and Christos Lionis

Key messages

- There is a higher prevalence of depression in primary care than in the general population.

- Depression and physical illness commonly co-occur and depression is more common in those with a chronic condition.

- Many people miss out on adequate treatment for their depression: every year up to 30% of the population worldwide experiences a mental health problem, and at least two-thirds of those people receive no treatment, even in resource-rich countries.

- Subsyndromal, mild and moderate depression respond to non-pharmacological interventions; antidepressants should not be first-line treatment for these patients.

- For those with persistent subthreshold depressive symptoms or mild to moderate major depression, low-intensity psychosocial or psychological interventions should be considered. Behavioural activation and problem-solving approaches are recommended.

- Most selective serotonin reuptake inhibitors (SSRIs) are of similar efficacy. Escitalopram may be more effective for severe depression and sertraline may be the best choice for moderate to severe depression in adults.

- If there is no response to SSRIs in 3–4 weeks, the medication should be changed.

Introduction

Feeling sad and empty, lacking energy and interest in the activities of life and, for some, thinking dark thoughts of death or suicide, has been with humankind throughout documented history. Yet it is only in the past century that this mix of emotions and symptoms has been categorized and counted and come to be known as the "depression epidemic". The 1990s are a key decade in the recent history of depression: at the beginning of this decade, selective serotonin reuptake inhibitors (SSRIs) entered the global pharmaceutical market (fluoxetine launched in 1989 in the United Kingdom of Great Britain and Northern Ireland (UK));[1] in 1996 the World Bank published the *Global burden of disease* report,[2] predicting that by 2020 depression will be the biggest health burden in the world; and in 1997 The United States (US) Food and Drug Administration (FDA) relaxed the rules for direct-to-consumer advertising, allowing SSRIs and other medicines to be advertised in print and on television.[1] Depression and its consequences had been measured in terms of disability and put firmly into the public domain. The link between depression and disability, and depression and suicide, made the alarming predictions of the World Bank report ones that could not be ignored. Governments responded with public health campaigns, such as "Defeat Depression" in the UK (1992–1997) and those conducted by "Beyondblue" in Australia (1999 to present). Despite the public health campaigns and the emergence and uptake of the SSRIs, depression continues to cause suffering and disability and to place a huge demand upon health services across the world.

In this chapter we focus on the potential of the primary health-care clinic, where most people who are experiencing depression will make contact with the health-care system, to play an important role in managing depression as it presents in the community. The role of the primary health-care clinic is not a new one. Callahan and Berrios, in their careful documentation of the history of the treatment of depression in primary care, show that the prevalence rates and burden of emotional disorders in the mid-20th century are not significantly different from today.[3] In the late 1940s, however, a person presenting with emotional issues would be more likely to be labelled as experiencing a "nervous complaint" or a "psychoneurosis" rather than being diagnosed as depressed.

This raises the first challenge for the primary health-care clinic. Dealing with depression is difficult. The difficulties begin with diagnosis. Unfortunately, we have no gold standard biological test that can confirm or refute the diagnosis, and instead we rely upon symptom-based approaches such as used in the 4th edition of the *Diagnostic and Statistical Manual of Mental Disorders*, text revision (DSM-IV-TR)[4] and International Classification of Diseases (ICD)-10[5] (see Box 17.1). The uptake of these two diagnostic classification systems is highly variable in primary care clinics throughout the world. They are often difficult to apply in primary care. They do not adequately address comorbidity, the substantial prevalence of subthreshold disorders, or problems with cross-cultural applications.[6] A third classification system – the International Classification of Primary Care (ICPC) – represents a departure from the two classifications described above. The ICPC was designed to capture and code three essential elements of each clinical encounter: the patient's *reason for encounter*, the clinician's *diagnosis*, and the (diagnostic and therapeutic) *interventions*, all organized in an *episode of care* structure that links all encounters for the same clinical problem. This approach permits coding of 95% or more of primary care visits and enables the calculation of probabilities for important diseases.[7]

We also await the arrival of DSM-V and ICD-11, which are likely to have a different approach to the classification of mood disorders. It is hoped that they will prove more suited to use in primary care. In primary care, one should consider a diagnostic approach that takes into account the probabilities of common mental health problems encountered in primary care, with depression and anxiety being the two most commonly encountered problems, and they frequently coexist.

Increasingly, we are acknowledging the difficulties in distinguishing depression as a disease from depression as an experience. Horwitz and Wakefield, in their thought-provoking book *The loss of sadness*, warn us about the dangers of transforming normal human sadness into a medical disease labelled depression.[8] For the primary care practitioner, knowing when to apply a diagnostic label is probably one of the most challenging aspects of dealing with depression.[9] The area of diagnosis is still open to debate and Chapter 9 provides an account of the dilemmas that face primary care practice.

Box 17.1 Depressive disorders according to the two principal diagnostic classifications

DSM-IV-TR, American Psychiatric Association (APA)[4]

296.xx   Major depressive disorder

300.4   Dysthymic disorder

311   Depressive disorder NOS

ICD-10, World Health Organization (WHO)[5]

F32   Depression

F41.2   Chronic mixed anxiety and depression

Epidemiology of depression

Depression is more common in primary care settings than in the general population. A major international study on mental illness in general health care screened 25 916 people aged below 65 years, from 15 primary care centres across the world, using the General Health Questionnaire (GHQ). This was followed by a second-stage evaluation of a weighted sample using the Composite International Diagnostic Interview (CIDI). The overall prevalence of current depression was 10.4%, varying from 29.5% in Santiago, Chile; through 16.9% in Manchester, UK; 13.7% in Paris, France; 9.1% in Bangalore, India; 6.3% in Seattle, USA; 4.2% in Ibadan,

Nigeria; to 2.6% in Nagasaki, Japan.[10] In another large multicountry study (The Outcome of Depression International Network (ODIN) study), the prevalence rates for depression varied from 2.6% in urban Spain to 17.1% in urban UK.[11] In a nationwide study of 1896 patients from 191 family physicians in Italy, the prevalence of depression ranged from 7.8% to 9.0%, with increasing rates seen from north to south.[12] These findings show that depression is common, but that there are substantial social and cultural influences that shape the nature, understanding and prevalence of depression across the globe. Every year, up to 30% of the population worldwide experiences a mental health problem, and at least two-thirds of those people receive no treatment, even in resource-rich countries.[13] Overcoming this problem requires substantial investment,[13] and will only be possible if non-mental health professionals are engaged in a sustained response. The primary care clinic is well placed to play an integral role in meeting this challenge.

There is still much to learn about the aetiology of depression, but current research suggests gene–environment interactions. The stress-vulnerability hypothesis provides an explanatory model that is of particular relevance to primary care. This model states that developing symptoms of depression is the result of vulnerability factors (genetic risk, early life experiences, physical illness and lack of social support) interacting with exposure to stressful events such as grief and loss (of relationship, occupation, reputation, health).[14] This causal explanation can help to guide the optimal primary care response and we shall return to it later in the chapter. Box 17.2 shows the protective and risk factors for developing depression.

Box 17.2 Protective and risk factors for developing depression[15]

Protective factors
- Social and family support
- Self-esteem
- Physical health
- Active coping
- Self-efficacy
- Mastery

Risk factors
- Stressful life events: loss, unemployment, abuse, traumatic events, chronic stress, isolation
- Financial strain and low income
- Low educational attainment
- Comorbid mental health problems: anxiety, substance abuse, personality disorders
- Chronic physical conditions, especially painful and disabling conditions

---

For the primary care clinic, two key epidemiological questions emerge: "How many of the patients sitting in my waiting room are currently depressed?" and for those with a community-orientated approach to primary care, "How many of the patients in our community are currently depressed?". The prevalence rates for depression that the primary care clinic will discover will vary according to whether they use an instrument to diagnose depression (and again vary depending upon which instrument they choose),[16] or whether they use a clinical approach.

Depression and physical health conditions[17]

Depression and physical illness commonly co-occur and depression is more common in those with a chronic condition, as found in the large, worldwide WHO study.[17] In an Australian survey of 6738 primary care attendees, the proportion likely to be depressed ranged from 16.44% for those with no long-term physical conditions, through 23.44% for those with one long-term physical condition, to 40.88% for those with five or more long-term physical conditions.[18] It was also interesting to note that skin problems and back pain were as much associated with depression as diabetes and heart disease. In a large Canadian population study, having a long-term medical condition approximately doubled the risk of major depression, particularly for those reporting migraine headaches, sinusitis and back problems.[19] In the primary care clinic, managing depression is very likely to occur in the context of also managing a long-term physical health problem, and the primary care practitioner has to be just as alert in the context of migraine, back and skin problems as in diabetes and heart disease. There is also evidence to suggest that the mix of depression and long-term physical health problems carries with it a poor prognosis, as Lin and colleagues have documented that patients with diabetes and coexisting depression face substantially elevated mortality risks that are beyond what can be explained by cardiovascular deaths.[12]

An organized approach to managing depression in the primary health-care clinic[20]

Interestingly, most of the published literature has focused on the interaction between doctor and patient, with far less attention given to how depression care is actually organized at the practice level. Guidelines for depression exist, but there is room for improvement to ensure they are of relevance to the everyday work of primary care.[21]

Understanding the nature of usual care has received only a little attention. For example, Fickel et al. undertook a careful comparative case-study in 10 Veteran Affairs (VA) primary care clinics in the USA and found that screening was routine for new patients and carried out on an annual basis in all clinics, but that primary care practitioners did not routinely use a documented diagnostic classification system such as DSM-IV-TR. They also found that pharmacological treatment was the most common and that there were only ad hoc systems in place for monitoring treatment progress.[22] A practice-based participatory action project undertaken in six primary care organizations in Australia found that none of the practices had a routine approach to screening for depression, nor did they use a classification system such as the DSM-IV-TR or have documented, systematic approaches to monitoring or follow-up. In contrast to the USA study, non-pharmacological treatments were commonly used, often in combination with pharmacological treatments.[23]

Perhaps it is this lack of documented systematic approaches to depression care that has led to the considerable scrutiny of the ability of primary care practitioners to manage depression. In particular, researchers have focused on the diagnostic accuracy of general practitioners (GPs) in relation to depression. Depending upon the study quoted, GPs have been documented to underdiagnose depression,[24] or overdiagnose it,[25] or when they do detect it, to not treat it adequately.[26]

Identifying the group of patients with depression that might benefit from intervention is a key, but not simple, task for the primary care practitioner. The considerable current debate about appropriate classification systems, and the current evidence that suggests that screening alone will not impact upon health outcomes means that the primary care practitioner is faced with the difficult task of identification of depression, which must be followed by appropriate assessment, suitable intervention and follow-up.

Figure 17.1 shows a conceptual design for primary care depression care developed after an extensive consultation with 313 expert stakeholders from around the world and 576 patients from Australia with experience of depressive symptoms.[27] It documents three interrelated areas of importance: relational, competency and system domains. Organizing depression care requires attention to each of these domains. The longitudinal nature of primary care practice provides a unique opportunity to maximize the potential of the relational links, to develop "healing relationships", as proposed by Scott et al.[28]

Screening, case-finding and assessment

The first task for any primary care practitioner managing a clinical problem is to identify those with the condition of interest. One of the most controversial areas within the depression literature is determining the criteria for caseness. Gordon Parker, in Chapter 1 ("Diagnosis of depressive disorders") of the third edition of the World Psychiatric Association's *Depressive disorders*, gives a comprehensive and challenging account of the difficulties that we face in determining exactly who is depressed and who is not. He also notes that we

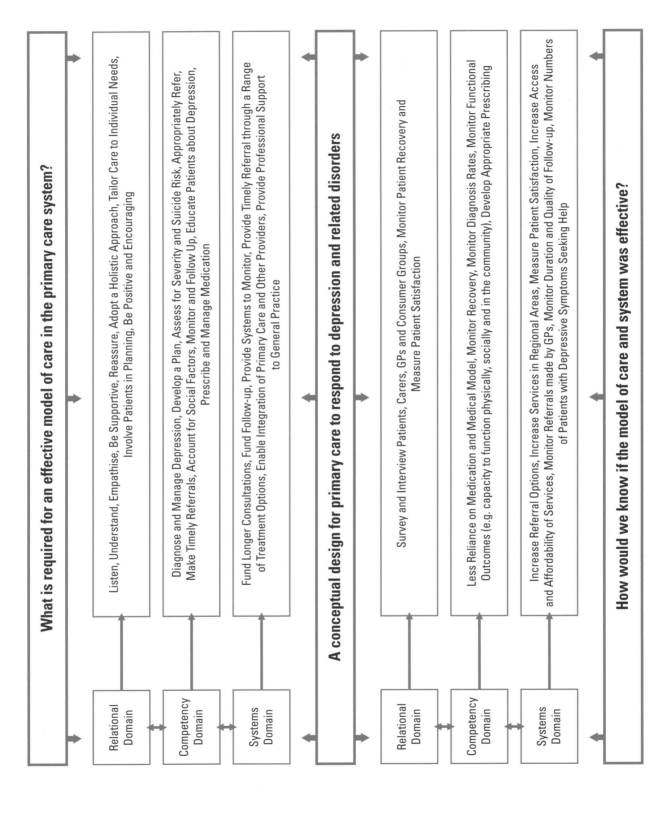

Figure 17.1 A conceptual design for the primary care response to depression. Reproduced, with permission from Oxford University Press, from Palmer V et al. Diverse voices, simple desires: a conceptual design for primary care to respond to depression and related disorders. *Family Practice*, 2010, 27:447–458[27]

are now at real risk of *overdiagnosing* depression and he calls for a rethink of how we make the diagnosis.[14] Meanwhile, as the researchers debate the diagnostic criteria, what is the primary care clinician to do?

Numerous survey instruments exist that can be used to screen for possible depression.[29] While screening for depression is routine within many primary care clinics in the USA, and routine for those with diabetes and heart disease in the UK, there is no evidence that screening alone will improve the health of patients.[30] Indeed, the evidence around the use of screening for depression has turned up the interesting finding that those for whom depression is undetected by their GP may have a better outlook than those who are diagnosed with depression.[9,31-33] This finding suggests either that GPs are using diagnostic skills that identify those at risk of a poorer prognosis, or that diagnosis leads to poorer outcomes; the former is more likely to be the case, but the latter cannot be ruled out.

As mentioned above, symptom-based criteria are available to help decide who is depressed and who is not. How these criteria are used in clinical practice will vary widely. Table 17.1, from Dowrick, presents the symptoms of depression and compares DSM with ICD criteria, to show that the ICD includes the lowering of self-esteem and lack of confidence as depressive symptoms, yet the DSM does not.[9]

Table 17.1 Summary of depressive symptoms in DSM-IV and ICD-10

	Symptoms of depression	DSM-IV	ICD-10
1	Depressed mood	+	+
2	Markedly diminished interest or pleasure in activities	+	+
3	Loss of energy or fatigue	+	+
4	Loss of confidence or self-esteem	–	+
5	Unreasonable self-reproach or guilt	+	+
6	Recurrent thoughts of death/suicide, or any suicidal behaviour	+	+
7	Diminished ability to think or concentrate, or indecisiveness	+	+
8	Psychomotor agitation or retardation	+	+
9	Insomnia or hypersomnia	+	+
10	Change in appetite	+	+

Reproduced, with permission from Oxford University Press, from Dowrick C. *Beyond depression: a new approach to understanding and management*, 2nd ed. Oxford, Oxford University Press, 2009[9]

When assessing a person for possible depression, the primary care practitioner should determine not only the number and severity of symptoms but also the degree to which the symptoms interfere with daily functioning, and the length of time the symptoms have been present. To begin with, the practitioner can use two questions designed around symptoms 1 and 2 from Table 17.1:

- "During the past month have you often been bothered by feeling down, depressed or hopeless?"
- "During the past month have you often been bothered by little interest or pleasure in doing things?"[34]

The addition of a third question increases the sensitivity and specificity of the two-question screening process and can be done by asking the patient who responds yes to one or both of the two questions:

- "Do you want help with this?"[35]

The patient who is identified via the above process, as possibly being depressed, should then be offered a full assessment for depression. Simply responding positively to a screening process does not constitute a diagnosis of depression. Considering the controversy around the diagnostic process, the prudent practitioner will ensure that a full assessment of each person is conducted and that they will confirm the diagnosis during a follow-up assessment 2–4 weeks following the initial diagnosis. This is especially important for those with mild to moderate symptoms.

It is important that the primary care practitioner undertaking a diagnostic assessment is equipped with the skills necessary to make the diagnosis. The practitioner needs to be confidently able to assess both physical health and mental health. In some settings, the use of self-completed symptom checklists may assist the primary care practitioner with this task. With increasing use of the World Wide Web and applications for iPhones and iPads, the use of automated screening and diagnostic technologies makes this a rapidly changing environment for the primary care practitioner. Many assessment technologies are available; few have been subject to the scrutiny of rigorous randomized controlled trials (RCTs). One could safely say that none of our current tools are perfect, so one approach is for the primary care practitioner to become familiar with a particular tool and understand its properties and hence its strengths and weaknesses (see Chapter 10).

The Patient Health Questionnaire (PHQ)-9 is a brief patient-completed questionnaire that is based upon the DSM-IV-TR and has been taken up in routine primary care use, especially in the USA, and more recently in the UK as a result of the implementation of the Quality and Outcomes Framework.[16] Research by Kendrick et al. in the UK showed that the PHQ-9 may overestimate the proportion of patients experiencing moderate to severe depression, especially when compared with a tool such as the Hospital Anxiety and Depression Scale (HADS).[16] They have called for the use of a cut-off score of 12 on the PHQ-9, rather than 10.

The DSM approach has been used in the latest (2009) update of the UK National Institute for Health and Clinical Excellence (NICE) guidelines for depression,[36] as it relies on more than a count of symptoms and takes account of functional impairment and disability. DSM criteria require that: (1) the patient reports either depressed mood or marked loss of interest or pleasure in activities; (2) the patient reports five or more of the nine DSM symptoms shown in the Table 17.1; (3) the symptoms have been present most days, most of the time for at least 2 weeks; (4) the symptoms are clinically significant and significantly impacting on the person's ability to perform their usual activities; (5) the symptoms are not able to be explained by a physical health condition or likely to be due to medication or illicit substance use; and (6) the person is not recently bereaved. The comprehensive DSM approach also includes a multi-axial assessment that assesses each patient across five important dimensions: the primary clinical disorder (e.g. bipolar disorder, depression, schizophrenia); their personality; their general medical conditions (e.g. heart failure, diabetes); psychosocial and environmental factors likely to affect their mental health; and finally the clinician's "global assessment of functioning" rated on a scale from 0 to 100.[4] The DSM approach as documented in the handbook is comprehensive and detailed and takes a view of the whole person in their context, yet it has not been taken up into routine primary care practice, even in the USA where it was developed.[22]

The spectrum of depression in primary care

Many people seen within primary care will not meet the full criteria for major depressive disorder, yet they will be experiencing significant distress and sometimes functional impairment that warrants a response from the practitioner. People with *subthreshold or minor depression* will report up to four depressive symptoms, including depressed mood or loss of interest or pleasure, and these symptoms will have been present for at least 2 weeks. Minor depression is very common in the primary care setting.

Dysthymia is a chronically depressed mood that is present for at least 2 years, with the person reporting that they feel down, depressed or hopeless for most of the day on more days than not. People with dysthymia will commonly report low interest in things and be filled with self-doubt and self-criticism. People with dysthymia are at an increased risk of developing an episode of major depressive disorder. Distinguishing between the various categories of depression can be problematic in primary care, and often a dimensional perspective is more useful.[37]

Understanding depression in the social and cultural context

Whenever the primary care practitioner suspects a diagnosis of depression, a full social and functional assessment should be conducted. Experiencing depression is often associated with significant social issues. People exist within a social network which comprises varying degrees and numbers of caring relationships and structural components like employment, finances, housing and the broader built environment. The structural and relational components of an individual's social world must be understood if we are to provide them with good depression care. For many, bringing about change in their social world will lead to change in their inner world, resulting in improvement of mood and, for some, resolution of depression. For example, the authors have encountered many examples in their clinical work, of women who, after leaving a violent and abusive relationship, are no longer depressed.

The experience of depression is also deeply influenced by cultural factors, which play an important role in the way an individual constructs their identity and their sense of meaning in life.[38] Depression, as constructed in western medicine and developed countries, is viewed very much as a problem at the level of the individual, but for cultures centred around a collective, this notion of depression as an individual illness is foreign and may be unhelpful.[39] The task for the practitioner is first to realize that their view of the world may well differ from that of the person seeking their care. They must seek to understand the various cultural backgrounds of the people who request their care, as well as being aware that the way depression presents will be affected by the cultural background. To fully understand may be way beyond the possibilities of the clinical encounter. But with careful listening and use of empathic responses, the primary care clinician will, hopefully, obtain some insight into how what they would diagnose as depressive symptoms may be viewed by the person experiencing them.

Assessment of functioning

It is important to assess the functional impairment that is present for each person experiencing depressive symptoms. The International Classification of Functioning, Disability and Health (ICF) is WHO's framework for measuring health and disability. This framework makes explicit that every individual can experience some degree of disability, and hence moves away from the idea that "disability" affects a minority of the population. Many people experiencing depressive symptoms will, to some degree, be experiencing a level of disability. The primary care practitioner should make an assessment of the level of functional impairment that the person is experiencing. The ICF domains assess disability from the body (functions: mental, sensory, voice, body systems and structures), individual (activity limitations and participation restrictions) and societal (environment, support and relationships, attitudes, services, systems and policies) perspectives. The ICF checklist may provide a useful guide for the clinician to assess functioning in a systematic way.[40] It requires the clinician to think systematically about the level of impairment, from mild (present less than 25% of the time, with an intensity a person can tolerate and that happens rarely over the past 30 days) through moderate and severe, to complete (present 95% of the time with an intensity that is totally disrupting life and that has been happening every day over the last 30 days).

This model, while too time consuming to conduct in full for every patient seen in primary care, does provide an excellent framework for thinking about the kind of assessment that needs to be made, even if the assessment is done over a series of visits. The framework will prompt the clinician to consider things such as vision and hearing problems and how these may be affecting mental health. For the elderly, in particular, these are commonly overlooked problems that can seriously affect their mental health.

Assessing suicide risk

Risk factors for suicide include not only depression but also post-traumatic stress disorder (PTSD), personality disorder, substance abuse, psychosis and some serious physical conditions such as neurological disorders, cancer and human immunodeficiency virus (HIV) infection, and belonging to a marginalized group or being incarcerated.

See Box 17.3 for points to consider when conducting a risk assessment for suicide.

General management

The goal of depression management in primary care should be the complete remission of symptoms.[41] The starting point for depression management should be the acknowledgement of suffering and the offer of hope.[8] The primary care practitioner must be well trained in active listening as well as in the diagnostic classification of depression and related disorders. As shown in Figure 17.1, the relational aspects of care form the foundation for management, and primary care is excellently suited to this task.

The NICE guidelines[36] are based upon a stepped care approach, whereby the least intrusive, most effective intervention is offered first and if the patient does not respond, care is intensified in a stepwise fashion until symptoms improve. The obvious exception is for the patient who is at risk of harming themselves or others, who is provided with maximal treatment at the outset.

The stepped care approach needs to be adapted to the setting in which it is to be delivered. In low-income countries, there may be a need to engage lay services and support in the management of depression, as formalized services may not be available. Specialized mental health services may be difficult to find, even in many developed countries. This makes it even more important for the primary care clinician to be confident in their ability to diagnose and manage depression and to assess suicide risk.

Step 1: support and education

Support and psycho-education form the foundation of depression management. Depression care needs to begin by fully hearing the story of the person in front of you. Despite the great similarities in the depression experience, each person's story is unique. Engaging with the person, acknowledging their suffering and offering to help them find a way out of their depression or distress can be a very therapeutic process in itself. Each practitioner must know their practice population, and needs access to culturally appropriate resources for patients that take account of the person's health literacy levels. The Internet is overloaded with depression-related material, much of which is not evidence based. We cannot provide an exhaustive list of resources here. At the time of writing, 153 000 000 hits were obtained when putting the words "depression information" into the Google search engine. A key role for the primary care practitioner is to assist each patient to find a source of information that is reliable and evidence based. Whether it is the South African Depression and Anxiety Group[42] or BluePages in Australia,[43] if you are going to recommend a web site to your patient, make sure you are familiar with the contents. Some patients will respond better to print-based materials such as: *The mindful way through depression: freeing yourself from chronic unhappiness*, by Williams et al.[44]

Spend time understanding the social and family context within which the depressive symptoms have emerged. Be aware that depression can arise when the individual is exposed to stressors such as family violence, sexual violence, community and workplace violence, financial hardship, loss of employment and housing insecurity. Consider social interventions that may be helpful (e.g. housing assistance, financial planning and assistance, friendship groups, volunteering, crisis intervention for those at risk of violence) and explore possibilities for joint intervention with other social and health-care practitioners. Knowing where the person lives, who they live with, and what their family circumstances are will assist in knowing how easy or appropriate it will be to mobilize their family supports.

It is important to remember to check with all patients about their sleep, diet, exercise and alcohol use. Encourage all patients to take regular exercise, ensure good sleep hygiene and a healthy diet and avoid alcohol excess or other substance use. Consider the life-stage at which depression is occurring, and how transitions from one life-stage to another are often accompanied by depressive symptoms. For the recent mother, make sure you enquire about how much practical help she is receiving to care for the baby and other children. Encouraging her to accept offers of help and to get some time to herself is a good starting point if she is experiencing mild to moderate symptoms.

Take time to review physical health and medication use. The elderly patient with arthritis may be experiencing increasing pain from their arthritic joints, and addressing this issue, by giving good pain relief and encouraging physical exercise, may be the most helpful starting point in dealing with their depression. Consider comorbidity and look at the extent to which chronic disabling physical conditions are well controlled. Most importantly, as a primary care practitioner, we can see the whole person and their life in perspective and can address both their physical and mental health needs; this is the strength of primary medical care. Pay attention to the protective and risk factors and make sure that you enquire about these and build upon the strengths for each particular patient. For example, for the person with good social networks, the primary care practitioner can encourage them to mobilize those supports, whereas for the person with a comorbid substance use problem, the best starting point may be to address their alcohol or drug problem. Much discussion has taken place on the role of a sense of coherence as a health asset that also protects from chronic physical illness.

All patients should be actively monitored for improvement in their symptoms. If no specific treatment has been initiated, it is important to ensure that you review the patient within 2 weeks to ensure that their symptoms are resolving. If the patient fails to return for review, the practitioner should make attempts to contact them.

Step 2: low-intensity psychosocial and psychological interventions or medication

For those with persistent subthreshold depressive symptoms, or those with mild to moderate major depression, who have not shown an adequate response to the approach outlined in step 1, the next step is to offer low-intensity psychosocial or psychological interventions based on the principles of cognitive-behavioural therapy (CBT). Behavioural activation and problem-solving approaches are key components, recommended by NICE.[36]

Problem-solving therapy (PST) is an approach that is easily learnt and can fit into the busy schedule of general practice.[45] It focuses on identifying the links between life problems (e.g. relationship or parenting problems, work stress, housing concerns, financial stress) and depression. It is a structured approach and can bring a sense of calm and hope to a primary care consultation, which can benefit the practitioner and the patient. The main focus is teaching the patient the skill of structured problem-solving, so they are able to apply it away from the consultation. *Most importantly, the GP has to refrain from giving advice.* It comprises six specific steps:

- define the problem(s) (e.g. feeling down and lacking exercise seen as problem)
- set specific, achievable goal(s) (e.g. I will walk outdoors for 20 minutes every lunch-time)
- brainstorm possible solutions – pros and cons
- decide on a solution
- implement the solution
- review progress.

Box 17.4 presents an example of this approach.

Recent evidence suggests that behavioural activation may be as effective as the more complicated CBT (which uses both behavioural activation and problem-solving techniques, as well as focusing on challenging negative thinking). Behavioural activation focuses on increasing behaviours that are likely to reduce depression (e.g. social contact, exercise, enjoyable activities) and decreasing behaviours that are likely to increase depression (e.g. excessive alcohol consumption, unhealthy food choices, certain social or work situations). A recent small trial (47 participants), undertaken in the UK and reported by Ekers et al., showed that behavioural activation when compared with usual care was an effective therapy for depression.[46] The behavioural activation was delivered by mental health nurses with no previous training in the technique.

Behavioural activation comprises the following basic techniques to increase positive behaviours.[47] From the list, you will see that it shares some features of PST:

- reinforcement, which is ideally immediate, consistent, appropriate, frequent and unmixed with criticism
- prompting or cueing

Box 17.4 A simple example of problem-solving therapy

Mateo was on edge and angry at home. He could not sleep. His work was very stressful; no matter what he tried, his supervisor complained that it was not good enough. He was dreading going to work but felt the pressure to provide for his young family. He was drifting apart from his wife. They had started arguing about small things. She suggested that he go and see the family GP. He had only visited the clinic on three occasions in the past – once for a sporting injury and twice for chest infections. He put off going to see the GP, thinking that he would be fine, things would improve. About 6 weeks later he woke up and just could not imagine going to work. He lay in bed crying – something he had never done in his life before. He felt so down and hopeless. He spoke to his wife and they both decided that he was depressed and needed help. He made an appointment to see the GP and told the GP that he was depressed and needed to do something. The GP assessed the depression to be of moderate severity, Mateo was not at immediate risk of harm, and the GP offered Mateo the option of trying PST. Mateo agreed, as he was not keen on taking medications and wanted to try another approach first.

Defining the problem

The GP and Mateo talked broadly about the problem. Mateo spoke about the depressive symptoms, being angry with his wife and how he could not get along at work. After a few minutes talking it through, Mateo noted that his real problem was also that he hated his work; it was not just the supervisor that was the problem. Mateo felt stuck but the GP encouraged him to just brainstorm all the possible solutions.

Brainstorming possible solutions

After some gentle prompting, Mateo stated that he could (1) work harder and try to please his current supervisor; (2) just put up with it and become more depressed; (3) complain about his supervisor to the senior management and try to get something changed; (4) look for another job; (5) leave the job without anything else to go to. The GP took each of these possibilities and asked Mateo to list the pros and cons of each option. For example, if he chose option (5), he decided he would have short-term relief because he would not have to cope with the supervisor that he did not like but he also stated that his savings would only last a few weeks and then his family would have nothing to live on. If he chose option (3), he would have to go through the stress of a lot of paper work and possibly negative consequences from his co-workers and the possibility that senior management would not see him in a favourable light.

Deciding on a solution

He decided that option (4) was the best thing to try. He felt that this option gave him some hope. He knew that it might take some time to find another job, but at least he could feel positive that he was taking active steps towards a positive solution.

Implementing the solution

He decided that he would make a list of all the possible places he could look for work and all the people that he knew who might be able to help him find a new workplace. He would also look in the newspapers, on the Internet and in the other places where jobs that suited him might be advertised.

Reviewing progress

Mateo returned to the GP one week later and was feeling positive about his future. He had spoken to a number of potential employers about work and he was hopeful that he would secure a new job in the not too distant future. He told the GP how helpful it had been to talk to him about his problems, and how this had put things in perspective in a way that he had not managed to do alone. At this visit, the GP assessed Mateo as having only mild depressive symptoms. They spoke about increasing his physical exercise and the GP gave him a written pamphlet on some simple ways to deal with anxiety. He agreed to return for follow-up in 2 weeks.

■ modelling and shaping: deciding the goal, breaking it down into specific small steps, identifying something in the patient's current way of doing things that is in the direction of the first step; this is reinforced

■ choosing the next appropriate step in the right direction; reinforcing; continuing this until the behaviour is obtained.

These techniques are easily learnt but practitioners who decide to deliver these therapies themselves will benefit from a high-quality training programme (these usually require a few days of training at least), and following that they need to have access to ongoing supervision to ensure that their skills are maintained. When working with patients and using these techniques, it is useful to begin with an agreement that the patient will attend six to eight sessions, and these should be supported by appropriate written materials.

Increasingly, computerized cognitive behaviourally based interventions are becoming available (for example see Moodgym[48]). Group-based CBT is also appropriate for this level of distress. Ideally, each primary care clinic would have access to the full suite of options for non-pharmacological interventions, yet we know this is rarely achieved anywhere in the world. Despite this, there is much that the primary care practitioner can do. Simple and active listening, offering hope and using the problem-solving or behavioural-activation techniques in addition to monitoring the patient over time can have dramatic effects, especially for those with milder levels of depression. Physical activity programmes should also be considered; NICE guidelines recommend they should be at least three times a week for 45-minutes' duration, for around 12 weeks.[36]

Use of medication should not be first line. It may be considered when the practitioner is not able to deliver cognitive- or behavioural-based therapies, or has no access to such interventions, and persistent symptoms are causing distressing disability for the patient (NICE guidelines do not recommend their routine use for persistent subthreshold or mild major depression).[36] NICE guidelines do not recommend the use of St John's wort, despite there being some RCT evidence that it is effective for mild to moderate depression;[49] this is because it is known to have potential serious interaction with some drugs (warfarin, oral contraceptives, anticonvulsants) and because there is poor quality control in the potency of available preparations. In some countries, however, St John's wort is used as an antidepressant for those with mild to moderate symptoms.

When using interventions outlined in step 2 of the stepped care approach, it is recommended that the patient is reviewed every 2–4 weeks.

Step 3: medication, high-intensity psychological treatments, combined treatments, collaborative care, referral

For those with moderate to severe major depression and for those with persistent subsyndromal depressive symptoms or mild to moderate depression that does not respond to step 2 interventions, more-intensive treatments are warranted. It is important to make a thorough assessment of each individual. Remember to assess them for their risk of self-harm and once again engage with them – acknowledging their distress and offering a real sense of hopefulness. At this stage of the treatment journey, the decision about whether to take medication, use high-intensity psychological treatments (CBT or interpersonal therapy (IPT)), or a combination of both, is a decision that is based upon the desires of the individual and the accessibility of the various treatments within the local context. In addition to individual preference and access to various treatments, other things that you should take into account include: the duration and trajectory of the symptoms, past history of depression and response to particular treatments, the likelihood of adherence to the treatment choice, and the likelihood of adverse effects.

When prescribing an antidepressant, NICE recommends SSRIs as first-line choice.[36] They increase the risk of bleeding and the use of a gastroprotective drug should be considered in older people and in those who are taking non-steroidal anti-inflammatory drugs (NSAIDs) or aspirin. Fluoxetine, fluvoxamine and paroxetine are more likely to cause drug interactions than other SSRIs.

In settings where SSRIs are not available, tricyclic antidepressants (TCAs) may be used. The prescriber must be aware of the risk of cardiotoxicity and death in overdose and be especially careful to assess each patient for their risk of self-harm. TCAs are also associated with dry mouth, drowsiness and constipation, and the user should be warned of these common side-effects and the prescriber should assess whether these pose particular problems for the workplace.

Most antidepressants demonstrate a flat "dose–response curve". To balance efficacy with tolerability, it is recommended that treatment is initiated at lower doses and increased only for those who do not respond. For example, sertraline should be commenced at 50 mg/day, with an optimal dose of 100 mg/day and a maximal dose of 200 mg/day. Fluoxetine, sertraline, paroxetine, citalopram and fluvoxamine all appear to have the same level of effectiveness, while escitalopram may be more effective for patients with severe depression. Sertraline may be the best choice when starting treatment for moderate to severe major depression in adults, because it has the most favourable balance between benefits, acceptability and acquisition cost.[50] Common side-effects include: nausea, sexual dysfunction, headache, insomnia, fatigue and jitteriness. Some people experience cognitive side-effects such as poor attention and feeling mentally slowed down. Weight gain can also be a problem, but evidence is conflicting. Abrupt cessation of SSRIs can cause adverse discontinuation events such as dizziness, insomnia, nervousness, irritability, nausea and agitation.[14] It is good practice to reduce antidepressants gradually to avoid these unpleasant experiences.

We lack good evidence on the long-term consequences of antidepressant use, and future research is needed into this area. We also lack information about the use of SSRIs in those with concurrent long-term physical conditions who are taking other long-term medications, or in those from different ethnic backgrounds. The developing field of pharmacogenetics may assist in guiding our use of medications; but other factors such as diet, use of herbal medicines, smoking, alcohol etc. may also impact the drug response.[14]

Once antidepressant treatment has been initiated, the patient should be monitored regularly until they reach remission. If they do not show any improvement over the first 3–4 weeks of using an antidepressant, they should switch to another antidepressant; if they still show no improvement, they should switch again following another 3–4 weeks of treatment. If they show some response to a particular treatment, then this can be increased in dose from the minimal starting dose to the optimal treatment dose. It is worth remembering that many people with depression will not respond to antidepressant treatment. In the well-known STAR*D project, participants began in an open-label trial of citalopram, which was followed by switching to other pharmacological treatments for non-responders (up to four switches over 48 weeks) until remission was achieved. Even in this regulated trial environment with excellent follow-up and support, 40% of participants were still depressed at the 48th week of follow-up.[14] For those who do respond to antidepressant treatment, NICE recommends that they continue on antidepressants for at least 6 months following remission.

Withdrawal of antidepressant treatment should be done in the context of a good relapse-prevention strategy and should be done slowly, over time, to avoid discontinuation syndromes (especially for paroxetine). For those who respond to antidepressant treatment and have had a number of relapses, long-term antidepressant treatment may be required. At present, we lack the studies to accurately inform patients of the potential adverse outcomes of very long-term use, particularly with respect to weight gain and the associated health consequences.[14]

For those who prefer, and have access to, high-intensity psychological treatments, NICE recommends that they commit to 16–20 sessions over 3–4 months of either IPT or CBT.[36] There is growing interest in group-delivered therapies and in mindfulness-based approaches.

Step 4: medication, high-intensity psychological interventions, electroconvulsive therapy, crisis intervention, combined treatments, multiprofessional and inpatient care

The primary health-care clinic needs to adapt to the needs of those with severe disabling depression and to those at risk of self-harm. For the patients that respond to the earlier approaches, the primary care clinic may well be able to meet all of their health-care needs. For those with more complicated paths, another approach is required. Firstly, we will deal with the needs of those at risk of self-harm. It should be noted that this risk can occur at any time for patients in any of the "steps" of the care. The primary care practitioner must always be alert and have a confident approach to assessing suicidal risk, which includes asking about suicidal thinking (see Box 17.3). Anyone at immediate risk of suicide should be kept safe until expert help can be arranged. This will vary from context to context. Many primary care practitioners express frustration at the lack of support for such mental health emergencies. Having a plan in place and knowing who to call when the emergency arises is essential for every primary care clinic.

For those who do not respond to the treatments already described, the next step of the stepped care model moves to a team-based approach based on the chronic care model.[51] This usually includes a model of care that requires a system-wide approach, to include:[52]

- a multiprofessional approach to patient care. Usually, a GP or family physician and at least one other health professional (e.g. nurse, psychologist, psychiatrist, pharmacist) are involved with patient care; each has a clearly defined role
- a structured management plan, which includes an organized approach and access to an evidence base. This is usually in the form of guidelines or protocols. Interventions usually include both pharmacological (e.g. antidepressant medication) and/or non-pharmacological interventions (e.g. patient screening and follow-up, patient and provider education, counselling, CBT)
- scheduled patient follow-ups: scheduled telephone or in-person follow-up appointments to provide specific interventions, facilitate treatment adherence, or monitor symptoms or adverse effects
- enhanced interprofessional communication: mechanisms to facilitate communication between professionals caring for the depressed person, such as team meetings, case conferences, individual consultation/supervision, shared medical records, and patient-specific written or verbal feedback between caregivers.

Interventions based on the chronic care model have been taken up and tested in many countries[53] throughout the world, with the expectation that they will be cost effective. Yet a recent systematic review shows that the evidence for this claim is still inconclusive and calls for a more thorough assessment of the costs and benefits of such approaches.[54]

When to refer to specialists?

Knowing when to refer will depend upon the skills of the primary care team, the complexity of the patients presenting to your clinic, and the availability of referral options. The following is based on the NICE guidelines for depression.[36]

Factors that favour general advice and active monitoring

- Four or fewer of the above symptoms with little associated disability
- Symptoms intermittent, or less than 2 weeks' duration
- Recent onset with identified stressor
- No past or family history of depression
- Social support available
- Lack of suicidal thoughts

Factors that favour more active treatment in primary care

- Five or more symptoms with associated disability
- Persistent or longstanding symptoms
- Personal or family history of depression
- Depression with a chronic physical health problem
- Low social support
- Occasional suicidal thoughts

Factors that favour referral to mental health professionals

- Inadequate or incomplete response to two or more interventions
- A recurrent episode within 1 year of the last one
- A history suggestive of bipolar disorder
- A patient with depression, or whose relatives request referral
- More persistent suicidal thoughts
- Self-neglect

Factors that favour urgent referral to specialist mental health services

- Actively suicidal ideas or plans
- Psychotic symptoms
- Severe agitation accompanying severe symptoms
- Severe self-neglect

What workforce do we need in the primary health-care clinic?

To implement the above approach, the primary health clinic needs a workforce that can:

- confidently engage with the patient in a professional way that includes providing psycho-education, acknowledges their degree of distress and offers them hope
- assess depression and suicide risk, while being aware of the complexities and debate around diagnosis
- monitor the progress over time, taking into account function in addition to symptoms
- prescribe with confidence, aware of the side-effect profile and potential for drug interactions and the need to consider switching antidepressants when there is no response. In addition, the prescriber must know how to taper and discontinue antidepressants to avoid adverse events
- deliver psychosocial and psychological interventions to those with persistent subsyndromal depressive symptoms and those with mild to moderate depression
- confidently know when to refer, and be able to match the patient to the appropriate service within the constraints of the context in which they work.

It is likely that in many countries, this workforce will comprise a primary care medical practitioner, a suitably trained nurse, and a health professional able to deliver psychological therapies (this may be a doctor, a nurse or a mental health professional).

Implications for mental health promotion

Preventing the negative impact of depression upon people's lives is another important task for the primary health-care clinic. Having a caring and welcoming environment in the clinic that encourages patients to tell their own story about how they are really feeling without fear of negative labels, negative consequences or unwelcome treatments is an important aim for primary care. Primary care is one place that a patient can attend without associated stigma, and many patients report how this is important to them.[55]

Relapse prevention should be the goal for those who are recovering from depression and it has a high importance, particularly in primary care systems where continuity is lacking. Ensuring that supports are mobilized and that physical and social functioning are optimized within the context in which the person lives is paramount. Assisting each individual to find meaning within their lives and to be engaged in living in a healthy and productive way is the long-term aim. For some, this will mean continued mental health care and may require longer-term psychological therapy, especially for those with recurrent or chronic depression.

Conclusions

Depression is a common problem that affects millions of people worldwide. In this chapter we have discussed how the spectrum of depression – from a self-limiting symptom to a disabling and long-term condition – requires a different approach. We have identified that the primary care clinic is best placed to use a stepped approach to manage the depression that presents within it. We have pointed out that there is still much controversy over when to apply the label of major clinical depression, and this is a controversy that is likely to continue for some time to come. We urge the primary care clinician to adopt a professional, caring approach when dealing with depression, and to be expert at the relational, technical and organizational levels of care. The NICE guidelines have been the prime source of clinical advice,[36] not because they are the only guidelines, but we note that they have been compiled recently and use a rigorous evidence-based approach, and that they echo, in the main, the guidelines in other countries.

References

1   Médawar C, Hardon A. *Medicines out of control? Antidepressants and the conspiracy of goodwill.* Amsterdam, Aksant Academic Publishers, 2004.

2   Scott J, Dickey B. Global burden of depression: the intersection of culture and medicine. *British Journal of Psychiatry*, 2003, 183:92–94.

3   Callahan CM, Berrios GE. *Reinventing depression: a history of the treatment of depression in primary care, 1940–2004.* New York, Oxford University Press, 2005.

4   *Diagnostic and statistical manual of mental disorders*, 4th ed, text revision (DSM-IV-TR). Washington, American Psychiatric Association, 2000.

5   *ICD-10 classification of mental and behavioral disorders.* Geneva, World Health Organization, 1996.

6   Gask L et al. Capturing complexity: the case for a new classification system for mental disorders in primary care. *European Psychiatry*, 2008, 23:469–476.

7   Lamberts H et al. The classification of mental disorders in primary care: a guide through a difficult terrain. *International Journal of Psychiatric Medicine*, 1998, 28:159–176.

8   Horwitz A, Wakefield JC. *The loss of sadness. How psychiatry turned normal sorrow into depressive disorder.* Oxford, New York, Oxford University Press, 2007.

9   Dowrick C. *Beyond depression: a new approach to understanding and management*, 2nd ed. Oxford, Oxford University Press, 2009.

10 Üstün TB, Sartorius N. *Mental illness in general health care: an international study.* Chichester, John Wiley and Sons, 1995.

11 Ayuso-Mateos JL et al. Depressive disorders in Europe: prevalence figures from the ODIN study. *British Journal of Psychiatry*, 2001, 179:308–316.

12 Lin EHB et al. Depression and increased mortality in diabetes: unexpected causes of death. *Annals of Family Medicine*, 2009, 7:414–421.

13 Chisholm D et al., Lancet Global Mental Health Group. Scale up services for mental disorders: a call for action. *The Lancet*, 2007, 370:1241–1252.

14 Herrman H, Maj M, Sartorius N, eds. *Depressive disorders*, 3rd ed. Chichester, John Wiley & Sons, 2009.

15 Colman I, Ataullahjan A. Life course perspectives on the epidemiology of depression. *Canadian Journal of Psychiatry*, 2010, 55:622–632.

16 Kendrick T et al. Management of depression in UK general practice in relation to scores on depression severity questionnaires: analysis of medical record data. *BMJ*, 2009, 338:b750.

17 Moussavi S et al. Depression, chronic diseases, and decrements in health: results from the World Health Surveys. *The Lancet*, 2007, 370:851–858.

18 Gunn J et al. The association between chronic illness, multimorbidity and depressive symptoms in an Australian primary care cohort. *Social Psychiatry and Psychiatric Epidemiology*, 2010, 25 December epub ahead of print.

19 Patten SB. Long-term medical conditions and major depression in a Canadian population study at waves 1 and 2. *Journal of Affective Disorders*, 2001, 63:35–41.

20 Johnson C, Gunn J, Kokanovic R. Depression recovery from the primary care patient's perspective: 'hear it in my voice and see it in my eyes'. *Mental Health in Family Medicine*, 2009, 6:49–55.

21 Hegarty K et al. How could depression guidelines be made more relevant and applicable to primary care? A quantitative and qualitative review of national guidelines. *British Journal of General Practice*, 2009, 59:e149–156.

22 Fickel JJ et al. Clinic-level process of care for depression in primary care settings. *Administration and Policy in Mental Health*, 2009, 36:144–158.

23 Gunn J et al. Embedding effective depression care: using theory for primary care organisational and systems change. *Implementation Science*, 2010, 5:62.

24 Zuithoff NPA et al. A clinical prediction rule for detecting major depressive disorder in primary care: the PREDICT-NL study. *Family Practice*, 2009, 26:241–250.

25 Aragones E, Pinol JL, Labad A. The overdiagnosis of depression in non-depressed patients in primary care. *Family Practice*, 2006, 23:363–368.

26 Von Korff M et al. Improving depression care: barriers, solutions, and research needs. *Journal of Family Practice*, 2001, 50:E1.

27 Palmer V et al. Diverse voices, simple desires: a conceptual design for primary care to respond to depression and related disorders. *Family Practice*, 2010, 27:447–458.

28 Scott JG et al. Understanding healing relationships in primary care. *Annals of Family Medicine*, 2008, 6:315–322.

29 Lam RW, Michalak EE, Swinson RP. *Assessment scales in depression, mania, and anxiety*. Oxford, Taylor & Francis, 2005.

30 Gilbody S, House AO, Sheldon TA. Screening and case finding instruments for depression. *Cochrane Database of Systematic Reviews*, 2005, (4):CD002792.

31 Posternak MA et al. The naturalistic course of unipolar major depression in the absence of somatic therapy. *Journal of Nervous and Mental Disease*, 2006, 194:324–329.

32 Dowrick C, Buchan I. Twelve month outcome of depression in general practice: does detection or disclosure make a difference? *BMJ*, 1995, 311:1274–1276.

33 Goldberg D et al. The effects of detection and treatment on the outcome of major depression in primary care: a naturalistic study in 15 cities. *British Journal of General Practice*, 1998, 48:1840–1844.

34 Arroll B, Khin N, Kerse N. Screening for depression in primary care with two verbally asked questions: cross sectional study. [see comment] *BMJ*, 2003, 327:1144–1146.

35 Arroll B et al. Effect of the addition of a "help" question to two screening questions on specificity for diagnosis of depression in general practice: diagnostic validity study. *BMJ*, 2005, 331:884.

36 *Depression: the treatment and management of depression in adults*. London, National Institute for Health and Clinical Excellence, 2009 (CG90).

37 Thompson C et al. Dimensional perspective on the recognition of depressive symptoms in primary care: The Hampshire Depression Project 3. *British Journal of Psychiatry*, 2001, 179:317–323.

38 Kirmayer LJ. Cultural variations in the clinical presentation of depression and anxiety: implications for diagnosis and treatment. *Journal of Clinical Psychiatry*, 2001, 62(Suppl. 13):22–30.

39 Kokanovic R et al. Lay accounts of depression amongst Anglo-Australian residents and East African refugees. *Social Science and Medicine*, 2008, 66:454–466.

40 ICF checklist (http://www.who.int/classifications/icf/training/icfchecklist.pdf, accessed 17 November 2011).

41 *The guidelines manual*. London, National Institute for Health and Clinical Excellence, 2009.

42 The South African Depression and Anxiety Group (http://www.sadag.org/, accessed 17 November 2011).

43 BluePages (http://bluepages.anu.edu.au/home/, accessed 17 November 2011).

44 Williams JMG et al. *The mindful way through depression: freeing yourself from chronic unhappiness*. Guilford, Guilford Press, 2007.

45 Pierce D, Gunn J. Using problem solving therapy in general practice. *Australian Family Physician*, 2007, 36:230–233.

46 Ekers D et al. Behavioural activation delivered by the non-specialist: phase II randomised controlled trial. *The British Journal of Psychiatry*, 2011, 198:66–72.

47 France R, Robson M. *Behaviour therapy in primary care: a practical guide*. Beckenham, Croom Helm, 1986.

48 The MoodGYM Training Program (http://www.moodgym.com.au/welcome, accessed 17 November 2011).

49 Linde K, Berner MM, Kriston L. St John's wort for major depression. *Cochrane Database of Systematic Reviews*, 2008, (4):CD000448.

50 Cipriani A et al. Comparative efficacy and acceptability of 12 new-generation antidepressants: a multiple-treatments meta-analysis. *The Lancet*, 2009, 373:746–758.

51 Wagner EH, Austin BT, Von Korff M. Organizing care for patients with chronic illness. *Milbank Quarterly*, 1996, 74:511–544.

52 Gunn J et al. A systematic review of complex system interventions designed to increase recovery from depression in primary care. *BMC Health Services Research*, 2006, 6:88.

53 Richards DA et al. Collaborative care for depression in UK primary care: a randomized controlled trial. *Psychological Medicine*, 2008, 38:279–287.

54 de Bruin SR et al. Impact of disease management programs on healthcare expenditures for patients with diabetes, depression, heart failure or chronic obstructive pulmonary disease: A systematic review of the literature. *Health Policy*, 2011, 101:105–121.

55 Boardman F et al. Resilience as a response to the stigma of depression: a mixed methods analysis. *Journal of Affective Disorders*, 2011, 135:267–276.

Part II

Psychotic disorders in primary care mental health

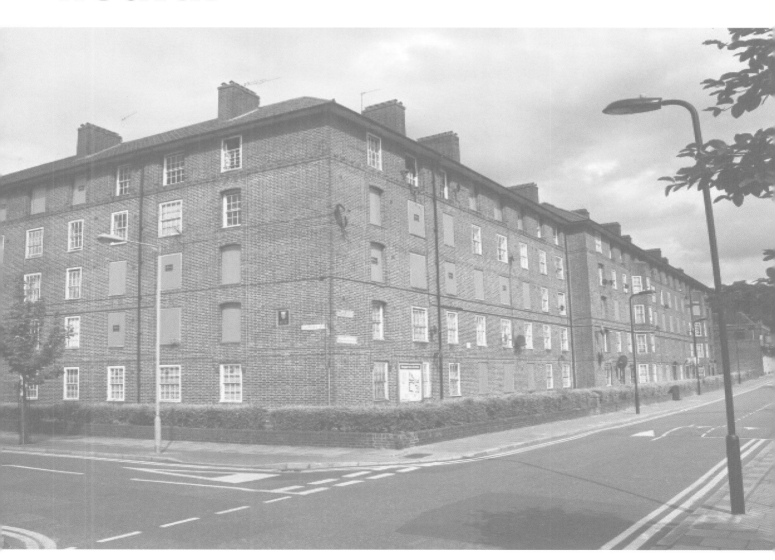

18 Bipolar disorder in primary care mental health

Joseph Deltito, Christos Lionis and Juan M Mendive

Key messages

- In primary care, when there is a history of a manic/hypomanic episode, even if it is very remote in time to a current depressive episode, a bipolar spectrum diagnosis should be considered.

- However, in many primary care practices, and unfortunately even in psychiatric practices, patients presenting with severe depression are regularly treated with standard antidepressants without inquiry into these other indications of potential bipolarity.

- Patients with an underlying genetic vulnerability to depression or bipolar disorder may be more likely than the general population to show symptoms of mood disorder in the face of comorbidity.

- Some medical conditions and some medications that are regularly used by primary care physicians may result in symptoms that are similar to bipolar disorder.

- There is evidence of effectiveness for several agents in treating the various phases of bipolar disorder, including lithium, anticonvulsant mood stabilizers, atypical antipsychotics, high-intensity light therapy, sleep deprivation therapy and electroconvulsive therapy.

Introduction

One of the most elusive clinical challenges to primary care physicians who evaluate and treat psychiatric disorders remains the appropriate recognition of bipolar disorder.

It is of utmost importance to immediately control any abnormal mood states associated with acute bipolar episodes and to then prepare a plan that will minimize the possibility of future relapse. Acute episodes of depression, mania or hypomania may have severe consequences – medical, social and occupational. Obviously, our main concern during depression is to avoid potential suicide. We also know that there appears to be an excess mortality in bipolar patients due to other medical conditions, as patients may remain non-compliant with medical treatments they need (such as taking antihypertensives or attending to chronic comorbid conditions such as diabetes). In hypomania or mania, such patients may engage in high-risk behaviours that they would ordinarily have the prudence to avoid. Such patients, frequently disinhibited, are at risk for contraction of human immunodeficiency virus (HIV) and other infections associated with sexual excesses. Family and occupational relationships are often destroyed due to odd or aggressive behaviours. Primary care physicians are well placed to work with families to oversee potential patients for identification of early warning signs of an episode, to help them comply with treatment and to maintain activities that overall promote health and avoid potential harm. Patients with bipolar disorder often develop problems with the legal system, based on spending money they do not have or leaving important bills unpaid. They may also engage in erratic behaviours that may result in their arrest. A primary care physician who knows the patient over time as a reasonable and law-abiding citizen can be a potent advocate with law enforcement, to help disentangle patients from any problems that may develop. The primary care physician becomes the de facto protector of the individual with bipolar disorder.

Bipolar disorder is a mood disorder, frequently known as manic depressive illness or manic depression, which involves cycles of depression and episodes of irritability or the elation of mania. Clinicians often find it valuable to subdivide the bipolar grouping of patients into specific categories. The term bipolar I disorder is generally reserved for those patients with a history of depression as well as episodes of frank mania with intervening periods of wellness. Bipolar II disorder refers to similar patients who, instead of meeting the full criteria or severity for mania, are seen as having variants of hypomania (a milder form of the disorder). Cyclothymia is a term reserved for patients who have few intervening episodes of full wellness and seem to alternate through milder, but persistent episodes of increased or decreased mood, which fall short of a definition of full depression, hypomania or mania. Nevertheless, such patients show some form of distress or disability due to their disorder.[1]

The rate of bipolar disorder in the general populations of countries around the world is highest in the United States of America (USA), at 4.4%, and lowest in India, at 0.1%. It is unclear from global studies how much these numbers represent true base rates or, as is more likely, the results of enhanced awareness and differences in the methods employed for diagnosis. Certainly genetic or social differences among countries could account for true variability. Worldwide, the incidence is put at 2.4% of the population.[2] Obviously, this number depends on how broad or restricted a definition of bipolar disorder is used. Various studies and polls have shown that a majority of patients with bipolar disorder have received misdiagnoses of their condition for 10 years or longer before being properly diagnosed.[3] In the developed world, the role of the primary care physician is mainly to identify the disorder and then transfer the patient to a psychiatric specialist who is well versed in the sophisticated biological and psychosocial management of this often difficult to manage condition. In low- and middle-income countries, primary care physicians are likely to be the main, or sole, caregivers and unlikely to have the luxury of referral to specialists. Current investigation supports the central role of general practitioners (GPs)/family physicians in facilitating diagnoses, referring appropriate patients to specialist care, providing continuity of care, and monitoring patients, particularly in identifying any early warning signs of relapse.[4] Primary care physicians treating bipolar patients with other serious medical conditions (such as HIV, diabetes or hypertension) need to address the stability of these patients in relation to their bipolar disorder, so the patient will remain fully cooperative and comply with the treatment for these other medical conditions. One of the most important tasks for GPs/family physicians is to enhance and promote adherence to mood-stabilizing and antipsychotic medication.[5] It is known that the more episodes one has of mania or depression, the natural history of the disorder is to increase in intensity and frequency into older age groups.

Another challenge for GPs/family physicians is the high correlation of bipolar disorder with substance abuse disorders. According to the hypothesis of Maremmani et al.:[6]

> cyclothymic, and to a lesser extent irritable traits could represent the temperamental profile of heroin addicts, largely irrespective of comorbidity . . . and tend to cohere to previous conceptualizations hypothesizing "sensation-seeking" (and "novelty-seeking") as the main personality characteristics of addiction.

The foremost clinical challenge in the management of bipolar disorder is the avoidance of misdiagnoses[7] with such conditions as unipolar depression, schizophrenia, attention deficit disorder, anxiety disorders and *Diagnostic and Statistical Manual of Mental Disorders* (DSM)-IV cluster B personality disorders (borderline, sociopathic, histrionic and narcissistic), as well as drug and alcohol dependence and eating disorders.[5] Certain physical disorders, including thyroid diseases, cerebrovascular disease and dementia, may confuse the primary care physician when bipolar disorders are considered.

The missed and confused diagnoses with unipolar depression and attention deficit disorder may lead to particularly noxious outcomes, as standard pharmacological treatments for these disorders (e.g. standard antidepressants and psychostimulants) may not just fail to improve patients' clinical condition but may dramatically worsen their disorder by inducing agitation, insomnia, psychosis, frank mania and/or rapid cycling.[8] There is reason to believe that when these negative developments are iatrogenically drug induced, they may be more difficult to control than when they appear apparently spontaneously during the course of a patient's illness. The roles of drug and alcohol dependence and eating disorders pose particular diagnostic challenges.[5]

The DSM 4th edition (DSM-IV) defines a depressive episode as a distinct period of at least 2 weeks during which there is either depressed mood or loss of interest or pleasure in nearly all activities, causing a marked impairment in occupational or social functioning.[8] For the diagnosis of bipolar disorder, the DSM-IV requires one single mania or mixed episode. According to the International Classification of Diseases (ICD)-10,[10] the diagnosis of bipolar disorder in adults requires at least two episodes, one of which must be mania or hypomania.

Currently DSM-IV and ICD-10 definitions of bipolar disorders provide a certain degree of reliability for the selection of prototypical subjects for research study, but, as with most major psychiatric illnesses, they do so at the expense of excluding too many patients who may in reality have the disorder. Because of atypical or mixed presentations, many patients are therefore not captured by the clinician as bipolar, if he or she relies on these tools alone for making a correct diagnosis. There are diagnostic indicators not included in the DSM-IV or ICD-10 definitions, which may bring more sensitivity and validity to the identification of bipolar conditions. These include data on family history, age of onset, previous response – both positive and negative – to pharmacological treatments, and the influence of environmental factors such as responses to sleep deprivation, jet lag and seasonality. Realistically, the DSM-IV and ICD-10 are not manuals of diagnostics geared to determine a choice of therapies. They primarily identify pure prototypical cases (mostly for research purposes), that are often not readily recognizable as the ordinary patients seen by treating clinicians in their clinical offices. Certainly, the DSM-IV and ICD-10 systems represent a reasonable starting point for clinicians, but they are a beginning and not an end for the establishment of diagnoses.

Another challenge for primary care physicians is the establishment of a working relationship with their patients and family that will facilitate the reporting of symptoms and identification of early warning signs of relapse.

In spite of the well-known classification criteria, there is a current undertaking to update both the ICD-10 and DSM-IV for the new ICD-11 and DSM-V. The working groups in both classifications committees have made good progress, and we are close to having new refined diagnostic criteria. As far as bipolar disorder is concerned, it seems that no major changes affecting primary care management are expected in the new classifications.[11]

Undoubtedly, bipolar disorder represents a spectrum of disorders with a tenuous agreement as to the definitions of these various overt variations.[12] Even when a consensus can be agreed concerning certain subsets with some reasonable inter-rater agreement (e.g. bipolar I, bipolar II, bipolar III, cyclothymia, hyperthymic and cyclothymic temperamental disorders), it should be remembered that virtually all treatment studies have focused exclusively on bipolar I disorder, which probably represents at most 20% of all patients belonging to the bipolar spectrum. Therefore, one is guided mostly through analogy and anecdotal evidence when selecting the correct treatment for these non-bipolar I patients. In many psychotherapeutic/psychoanalytical treatment centres, a conceptualization of cluster B personality disorders as conditions that should not be clinically treated pharmacologically (only psychotherapeutically) persists, despite research studies demonstrating that perhaps more than 50% of these patients suffer from underlying bipolar conditions, and many of these would presumably benefit from standard pharmacotherapy.[13]

Epidemiology and clinical manifestations

Although bipolar disorder remains frequently undiagnosed in primary care, it is estimated that 3.3–21.6% of primary care patients diagnosed with unipolar depression may, in reality, have a bipolar disorder.[14]

Bipolar disorder is a chronic illness manifested by episodes of mania (usually associated with severe consequences or a lack of appreciation of reality) or hypomania (an attenuated disorder usually not associated with severe consequences or breaks with reality). Although there is usually a history of episodic or chronic depressions, these are not necessary for making a diagnosis of bipolar disorder. Epidemiological studies suggest that when considering the whole spectrum of bipolar illnesses, as much as 5% of the general population is afflicted. When GP–patient encounters are evaluated, the prevalence of bipolar disorders accounts for 1.1% of their practice.[15]

This makes bipolar disorder one of the most common serious illnesses presenting for medical treatment. Patients will typically seek initial evaluation and treatment for depressive rather than manic or hypomanic episodes. Depressive episodes tend to predate patients' episodes of mania/hypomania and, in most cases, depressive episodes will outnumber manic/hypomanic episodes over a patient's lifetime. The assignment of an acute depressive episode as representing part of either a unipolar or bipolar condition is undoubtedly the most frequently encountered challenge facing primary care physicians treating depression. Frequently, the true condition is misdiagnosed.

It is of the utmost importance to remember that there is no specific symptom or sign of a severe depressive episode that is unique to a unipolar or bipolar disorder.[16] When there is a history of a manic/hypomanic episode, even if very remote in time to the current depressive episode, a diagnosis of bipolar spectrum should be considered. Nevertheless, there will be patients, truly afflicted with bipolar disorder, who are currently depressed, but who may not yet have shown obvious clinical signs of mania/hypomania. This is of particular importance when evaluating children or adolescents with a first episode of depression. There are, however, aspects of a patient's longitudinal history that may strongly suggest that he or she suffers from a bipolar rather than a unipolar disorder.[16]

These features would include, but are not limited to, the following:

- a strong family history for bipolar disorder
- an initial presentation of severe depression in childhood or adolescence
- a cyclicity to the appearance of depressive episodes (if multiple)
- a more abrupt rather than slowly insidious onset of depression
- mood destabilization with sleep deprivation or jet lag
- destabilization under previous treatments with antidepressants or psychostimulants
- resolution of previous depressions when treated with lithium, atypical antipsychotics or anticonvulsant mood stabilizers (e.g. valproate, carbamazepine, lamotrigine, gabapentin and others)
- reversed vegetative signs of depression (increased sleep and appetite)
- a baseline history of high intelligence, marked creativity, interpersonal popularity, and/or marked promiscuity
- comorbity with DSM-IV cluster B personality disorders: borderline, sociopathic, histrionic or narcissistic.

Although none of these lifetime features in a currently depressed patient are confirmatory of a bipolar condition, they increase the likelihood that a depressed patient does not validly have a unipolar condition. Yet in many primary care practices, and unfortunately even in psychiatric practices, patients presenting with severe depression are regularly treated with standard antidepressants (e.g. fluoxetine, imipramine, sertraline, venlafaxine) without inquiry into these other indications of potential bipolarity. In dealing with a first episode of depression, it is preferable to err on the side of making a bipolar diagnosis rather than a unipolar diagnosis (obviously it is best to make a correct diagnosis). This is because if tricyclic antidepressants (TCAs), selective serotonin reuptake inhibitors (SSRI) or other antidepressants are given to a truly bipolar patient erroneously diagnosed as a unipolar patient (the so-called pseudo-unipolar bipolar patient), this will frequently result in worsening of their clinical condition.[17] This occurs through the induction of rapid cycling, mania, agitation, suicidal ideation or completed suicide. Conversely, should a clinician erroneously treat a truly unipolar patient, or a patient with a personality disorder, as bipolar and give treatment with lithium, atypical antipsychotics, anticonvulsant mood stabilizers or electroconvulsive therapy (ECT), the chance of iatrogenically worsening the condition is minimal (understanding that the patient may not improve, but is at least not made worse by the treatment). Logic would appear to dictate that in a patient with depression, especially a younger patient with a first episode, the burden on the diagnosing physician is to rule out bipolarity and not assume unipolarity.

There are many medical conditions that may produce symptoms similar to bipolar disorder (see Box 18.1 for some of the most commonly encountered). A primary care physician needs to be aware that any of these may be present in apparently depressed, hypomanic or manic patients. The clinical issue is further complicated by the fact that patients with an underlying genetic vulnerability to depression or bipolar disorder may be more likely than the general population to show mood disorder symptoms in the face of comorbidity. For example, patients with a previous history or family history of severe depression are more likely to show depressive symptoms if they develop hypothyroidism or systemic lupus erythematosus later in life.

There are also some medications that are regularly used by primary care physicians that may result in symptoms similar to bipolar disorder (see Box 18.2).

Assessment tools for screening and monitoring

There is ample information about the utility of assessment tools for screening and monitoring bipolar disorder. One of them is the Mood Disorder Questionnaire, a self-report, single-page paper and pencil inventory that

Box 18.1 Medical conditions that may produce symptoms similar to bipolar disorder

- Hypothyroidism
- Hyperthyroidism
- Cushing's disease
- Addison's disease
- Systemic lupus erythematosus
- Pellagra
- Vitamin B_{12} deficiency
- Uraemia
- Drug intoxications (amphetamines, alcohol, cocaine, hallucinogens)

Box 18.2 Frequently used medicines that may produce symptoms similar to bipolar disorder

- Antidepressants
- Levodopa
- Theophylline
- Anticholinergics
- Digoxin
- Opioids
- Steroids
- Psychostimulants

can be completed under the guidance of a medical doctor, nurse or trained assistant.[18] Other commonly used screening instruments for bipolar disorder are the Hypermania Checklist (HCL-32) and Bipolar Spectrum Diagnostic Scale (BSDS); both have been used in primary care settings, but they show a low positive predictive value and they are recommended for detecting broader definitions of bipolar disorder than those defined by DSM-IV.[14] A review article by Baldassano in 2005 concluded that while there are many rating scales for the assessment of various clinical aspects of bipolar depression, there is only a limited number of assessment tools that are suitable for use in routine clinical practice.[19] This does not decrease the value of brief self-reported assessment tools but it underlines the utility of daily visual analogue scales or daily mood graphs. These seem to be very helpful tools, not only to monitor the course of bipolar depression but as key instruments for patient and family education. These are also useful tools when psychological therapies, including cognitive-behavioural therapy (CBT) are selected as an addition to pharmacotherapy.

Treatment of established bipolar spectrum disorders

Once a clinician has made a firm or provisional diagnosis of a bipolar spectrum disorder, a comprehensive treatment plan should be put into place. Bipolar disorder shows varied phenotypes, presumably having, at least in part, a shared genotype underlying the disorder. One can only talk about treating bipolar disorder according to a given targeted phase. The major phases to be considered are acute bipolar depression, acute mania or hypomania, and long-term prophylactic maintenance. These phases can then be subdivided into those that have features of particular therapeutic concern, such as the presence of rapid cycling, psychoses, seasonality and subtypes of bipolar disorder that blend into personality, anxiety and temperamental disorders.

When treating an individual with a bipolar course that is primarily episodic, that is, they have episodes of mania/hypomania, depression or mixed states with long periods of well-being (euthymia) in between, it is important not only to take into account the acute episodes but also to include a strategy that will decrease the frequency of future episodes. Agents that are used for prophylaxis will decrease the frequency, severity and duration of future episodes. As these agents are used long term, or perhaps given for a lifetime, issues of safety and tolerability are of particular importance. One always needs to follow the dictates of balancing risks against potential benefits. As untreated bipolar disorder is associated with a high degree of morbidity and mortality, a treating clinician must be prepared to accept a relatively high degree of risk (collateral effects) in acute and long-term treatment strategies. There are ways to mitigate potential unwanted side-effects through close clinical and laboratory monitoring and the use, when possible, of less potentially toxic agents for shorter periods.

For the primary care physician, the clinical issue related to bipolar disorder that is most commonly encountered will be the treatment of acute depression. As noted previously, the treatment of an individual with an acute depressive episode who is bipolar is considerably different from the treatment of someone who is unipolar. In bipolar depression, the use of standard antidepressants should be rigorously avoided, and if a decision is made to use such agents because of particular clinical issues encountered in a given patient, they should be used only while the patient is on a therapeutic dose of a mood-stabilizing medication such as lithium, valproate or carbamazepine. There is some evidence to suggest that, of all the standard antidepressants, bupropion may be the safest to use in bipolar depressed patients. The best first-line options for treating bipolar depression is lamotrigine, lithium or an atypical antipsychotic (particularly aripiprazole). ECT should be considered for the profoundly depressed patient, particularly if there is a significant concern about suicide.

Several agents have evidence of effectiveness in treating the various phases of bipolar disorder.[20] These are lithium, anticonvulsant mood stabilizers (particularly lamotrigine when treating depression), atypical antipsychotics, high-intensity light therapy (particularly for those with regularly cyclic wintertime depressions), sleep-deprivation therapy and ECT. Often the use of combinations of these therapies may be helpful.

Lithium

Lithium has potential use in the treatment of acute mania/hypomania, acute depression and for chronic prophylaxis. In acute mania it can be quite beneficial but the full effectiveness is generally not achieved for 10 to 20 days. Therefore, one would usually treat full-blown mania initially with a more rapidly acting antipsychotic medicine (e.g. olanzapine, risperdal, aripiprazole), while also initiating an increasing titration with lithium. Hopefully, when euthymia is achieved and a patient has been on lithium for 2–3 weeks, the antipsychotic medicine can be weaned and discontinued. In milder forms of hypomania, one may rely on lithium treatment alone, as long as there is adequate surveillance of the patient to determine that they do not show escalation of their condition.

In general, lithium treatment is initiated with 300 mg bd (twice daily), and increased by 300 mg every day until the desired clinical effect is achieved or a blood level of 1.1–1.4 mEq/l is obtained. This will generally occur at dosage levels between 900 and 1500 mg/day. Serum levels are generally monitored about 12 hours after a patient's evening dosage and before they take their morning medicines. During long-term prophylaxis, lithium levels, renal function (blood urea nitrogen (BUN), creatinine, urine concentration) and thyroid function (thyroid-stimulating hormone (TSH), free thyroxine (T_4), tri-iodothyronine (T_3) uptake) should be monitored every 4–6 months. The side-effects and toxicity of lithium can be rather high.

Serious complications are usually diminished by maintaining serum levels below 1.5 mEq/l. At lower dosages, one may encounter hand tremors, nausea, diarrhoea, drowsiness and weight gain. At moderate dosages, one might encounter disturbed higher cognitive functions (e.g. memory, attention), ataxia and dysarthria. At very high dosages (as when a patient might attempt suicide with the ingestion of massive amounts of lithium), convulsions and death might occur. In addition to these dose-related side-effects, there are other side-effects more associated with the long-term exposure of organ systems to the effects of lithium. Most notable are effects upon kidney and thyroid functioning. When these problems develop, they generally occur slowly and insidiously, so, as mentioned above, routine blood testing is usually adequate to ensure that a trend towards kidney or thyroid disease is not developing. If a patient has an underlying disease (e.g. diabetes mellitus, systemic lupus erythematosus) that may present with kidney damage over time, it is probably best to avoid the use of lithium and choose another mood-stabilizing agent (e.g. valproate).

Lithium has been associated with fetal abnormalities and should be avoided during pregnancy and lactation if at all possible.

Anticonvulsant mood stabilizers

There are a number of medications originally developed for the treatment of epilepsy, that enjoy widespread use in the treatment of various phases of bipolar disorder. Among the most commonly used are valproate, carbamazepine, lamotrigine, gabapentin and topiramate. Some of these have a large body of research evidence supporting their use (e.g. valproate, carbamazepine and lamotrigine). Others have less rigorous scientific evidence to support their use but have much anecdotal evidence and opinion from expert consensus analyses maintaining their usefulness (gabapentin, topiramate). Each of these medications has some particular benefit in at least some phase of bipolar disorder and each may also show some potential difficulties with their use. A rational selection of which of these agents to use depends on the particular issues encountered in a given patient at a given phase of their illness.

Each of the above medications is used by clinicians in all phases of bipolar disorder. While all of the anticonvulsant mood stabilizers can be used for the up or down phases of the disorder, it appears that all but lamotrigine have a more reliable effect on the up rather than down phases of the illness. Lamotrigine appears to uniquely have more of a robust effect on depressive rather than manic/hypomanic episodes. Therefore, of this category of medicines, lamotrigine should be considered the drug of choice when dealing with acute depression or for prophylaxis in patients who have a history significant for predominantly depressive episodes. In fact, the treatment strategy that appears most beneficial for the majority of bipolar patients is the use of lamotrigine in combination with another mood-stabilizing drug with increased usefulness for the prevention or attenuation of manic/hypomanic episodes, such as lithium.

Valproate

Valproate appears to be as effective as lithium for the treatment of acute mania and, like lithium, might take several days before clinical control can be attained using this medication alone. Studies have suggested superiority of valproate in mixed states and rapid cycling. A blood level of 50 mcg/ml to 100 mcg/ml is considered the usual therapeutic range. It can be quite helpful for prophylaxis as well as for acute phases.[21] This medication is sometime limited by its side-effect profile, particularly the ability to induce hair loss and weight gain. In rare cases, hepatic failure and thrombocytopenia have been reported. In addition, a number of clinically important drug–drug interactions may occur, and any concomitantly used medication must be explored for potential interactions. Of particular note may be interactions with erythromycin, lamotrigine and carbamazepine.

The most common form of valproate used is as an enteric-coated sustained-release tablets known as divalproex sodium. Dosing usually begins at 250 mg bd, with upward dosage adjustment until a desired clinical outcome is achieved. For prophylaxis, a blood level of 80–150 mcg/ml is sought. As in treatment for acute mania with lithium, it may be wise in most cases to initiate treatment concomitantly with an atypical antipsychotic agent, while increasing the level of divalproex until clinical remission is achieved. After a few weeks of euthymia, the antipsychotic can be removed, leaving the patient on a substantial amount of divalproex sodium. Divalproex sodium also seems to have effects on mood in patients beyond those who suffer from obvious bipolar disorder.[22] There seems to be a use in patients who suffer from aggression, agitation, low frustration tolerance and impulsivity regardless of diagnosis. Therefore, divalproex sodium appears to be an excellent medication for use with individuals with cluster B personality disorders, many of whom arguably properly belong to a bipolar spectrum of disorders.

Carbamazepine

Carbamazepine appears to be an effective treatment for both the acute and maintenance phases of bipolar disorder. The onset of its clinical effect may be shorter than for lithium or valproate. Its clinical profile suggests it may be a particularly good choice for more severe forms of mania, mixed states with dysphoria associated with mania, and rapid cycling. In most cases of acute mania, treatment would be started concomitantly with initial use of an atypical antipsychotic. Usually the clinician attempts to lower the long-term exposure to atypical antipsychotics and hopefully will transition to prophylaxis with carbamazepine alone.

Although a drug with good efficacy in many patients, its use is attenuated by potential side-effects and drug–drug interactions. In rare cases, it can be associated with bone marrow suppression and possible full agranulocytosis or aplastic anaemia. The greatest risk for this appears to be within the first 6 months of treatment. There may also be transient leucopenia or thrombocytopenia. Elevated liver function tests may also occur, but full liver failure is rare. Therefore, in order to increase safety, it is best to obtain at baseline, before starting carbamazepine, a complete blood count, with differential and platelet count along with standard liver function tests. After the initiation of treatment, these should be repeated every 2 weeks for the first 2 months and then every 2 months while the patient is maintained on carbamazepine.

Carbamazepine use may cause several important drug–drug interactions. When used in combination with valproate, the valproate levels may decrease over time, with an increase of carbamazepine levels. When given with lamotrigine, there can be a decrease in lamotrigine levels such that dosage can be started at lower levels and raised more rapidly for both preparations. Carbamazepine can induce its own metabolism, as well as metabolism of anticoagulants, oral contraceptives and benzodiazepines. SSRI and tricyclic antidepressants have been known to increase carbamazepine levels and lead to toxicity. Therefore, appropriate monitoring of blood levels and clinical effectiveness of all these medications is recommended.

Gabapentin

Large-scale controlled studies of gabapentin in the treatment of bipolar disorder have, for the most part, failed to show a robust clinical effect in bipolar populations. There is reason to believe that some of these larger studies have been methodologically flawed. Erroneously, some have concluded that there is evidence that gabapentin does not have efficacy in the treatment of bipolar disorder. Yet we know this conclusion to be invalid, and the absence of clinical evidence from a given trial is not evidence that there is an absence of clinical usefulness. Gabapentin, potentially, is one of the more useful medications within the armamentarium of our potential treatments for various phases of bipolar illness. What makes it so potentially attractive, especially to the primary care physician, is the exceptionally low risk and side-effect profile, combined with virtually no drug–drug interactions or potential organ system toxicity. It is therefore an excellent first-line treatment choice, especially in patients with attenuated forms of the disorder such as hypomania or cyclothymia, or those milder bipolar conditions that tend to blend into personality disorders (e.g. borderline personality disorder) or anxiety disorders (obsessive–compulsive disorder or panic disorder). For more severe forms of frank mania, the use of valproate or carbamazepine as first-line mood stabilizers is preferred. Gabapentin can be given to patients with marked hepatic compromise. It is excreted essentially unmetabolized.

Gabapentin has some intrinsic anti-anxiety properties that can also make it a useful medication for agitated/anxious patients, whether or not they suffer from a bipolar spectrum disorder. This medication can also be used successfully for long-term prophylaxis.

There appears to be a rather large therapeutic range at which this medication will be optimized (usually using 300 mg three times a day (tds) to 1000 mg tds). Generally, treatment is initiated with 100 mg tds and raised by 100–200 mg per day until a desired clinical effect is achieved, with a maximum dose of 3 g/day. For prophylactic use in bipolar I patients, doses in the range of 2100 mg/day to 3000mg (divided into three daily doses) are usually used.

Topiramate

This medication is primarily used for the milder presentations of bipolar spectrum disorders. It poses an interesting "niche" among the anticonvulsant mood stabilizers, as in many patients (approximately 35–50%) it can be a potent appetite suppressant. This is of particular importance for those bipolar patients who have already gained weight due to previous or current use of other medication that tends to promote weight gain (e.g. olanzapine or valproate). It can sometimes be used in a strategy to control weight gain when stimulated by another agent, by adding in a small amount to the existing regimen of medications. At times one might not want a medication that is associated with appetite suppression, and topiramate should be avoided (e.g. patients undergoing chemotherapy for cancer, patients with comorbid eating disorders). Side-effects include the development of episodic paraesthesias (which are benign but may be annoying to some patients) and some acute memory problems (usually in patients taking >100 mg/day). It is usually given in divided dosages starting at 25 mg bd. This can be raised over a week to 100 mg/day. Like gabapentin, it may be best not to rely on topiramate for treatment of severe mania but to reserve it for milder forms of the bipolar spectrum. It can be quite useful in treating the personality disorders (e.g. borderline personality disorder) that show an association with bipolar disorder.

Important note regarding the use of multiple mood stabilizers and/or lithium concurrently

In cases of long-term prophylaxis of bipolar patients in particular, dosages of mood stabilizers that are considered to be therapeutic are not always tolerated, due to the profile of side-effects of a given agent. Lithium may be associated with an intolerable hand tremor, valproate with hair loss, carbamazepine with thrombocytopenia and topiramate with acute memory problems. Should this be the case, an interesting clinical strategy may be the combination of lower dosages of mood-stabilizing agents, such that there is no addition of side-effects (as these have differing collateral effects) while attaining an addition of their clinical usefulness. Obvious issues of any given drug–drug interactions need be observed.

Atypical antipsychotic medications

Whereas older-generation antipsychotic drugs may be quite useful in the acute treatment of mania, they have been for the most part replaced by the use of the newer-generation atypical antipsychotics because of an overall more favourable safety/side-effect profile. While the newer-generation antipsychotic drugs (e.g. aripiprazole, ziprasidone, olanzapine, risperdal, quetiapine and asenapine) are for the most part an advance over older antipsychotics (e.g. haloperidol, chlorpromazine, thiothixine), these older medications are also effective and have the benefit of generally being markedly less expensive. The atypical antipsychotics are not without problematic side-effect/safety issues. When used in very high dosages (when either large dosages are taken or more normal dosages are taken in conjunction with medications that may lead to undesirably increased blood levels), they start to assume side-effect profiles and safety issues that are more in keeping with the older typical antipsychotics.

A commonly encountered example of poor treatment might follow this hypothetical scenario. A patient presents to a primary care physician's office with an acute depressive syndrome and, whether or not a diagnosis of bipolar or unipolar depression is made, that patient is treated with a standard antidepressant, in this case 20 mg/day of paroxetine. Ten days later, the patient reports he is feeling somewhat less depressed but now has newly developed marked insomnia and agitation. His treating physician places him on 2 mg at bedtime (qhs) of risperdal. In a few days, he is sleeping better but feels his depression to be worsening. The doctor now increases the paroxetine to 40 mg/day. The patient then develops fidgetiness, inability to sit still or concentrate for any sustained period – a state of marked restlessness (akathisia). That night he has a severe muscle spasm in his neck, requiring an emergency visit to the hospital (an acute dystonic reaction).

What happened? The concomitant use of a relatively high dose of paroxetine led to competitive metabolism with the risperdal, which was no longer being metabolized efficiently. Although the patient remained on only 2 mg/day of risperdal, it became as if he was effectively taking the equivalent of 10 mg/day. The side-effect profile for the 2 mg/day of risperdal, usually being quite favourable, was no longer so risk-free, as it behaved as if it was a high dose of a typical antipsychotic (e.g. haloperidol).

What should have been done? At initial presentation, the primary care physician should have determined if the depressive episode represented a unipolar or bipolar variant. If unipolar, 20 mg of paroxetine would have been a reasonable choice for initial treatment. It would have been highly unlikely that the patient would have then developed the agitation/insomnia noted in our hypothetical case. In this case, the patient suffered from a bipolar variant and treatment with a standard antidepressant (which flipped this patient into a mixed state, and then the eventual problems with the paroxetine/risperdal combination) should have never been initiated. Proper treatment may have been (assuming the patient was judged to be of no danger to himself or others, therefore not requiring inpatient treatment) a starting treatment of 25 mg/day of lamotrigine, to be increased by 25 mg/day on each subsequent week until a dosage of 200 mg/day or clinical remission was achieved. If the patient has agitation or insomnia as part of the original clinical presentation, or does not reach remission at 200 mg/day, a small dose of an atypical antipsychotic may prove helpful, such as 25 mg at bedtime of quetiapine or 2 mg qds of aripiprazole.

The main concerns with typical antipsychotics are extrapyramidal side-effects. These include acute dystonic reactions (which can even be life threatening, as in the case of an acute laryngospasm), akathisia and, most importantly, tardive dyskinesia (TD). TD is a chronic movement disorder, usually afflicting the muscles of the head and neck, which does not always subside with the termination of antipsychotic medicines. It can be most debilitating. TD is usually seen in the context of long-term, high-dose use of typical antipsychotics over many years. It is therefore more commonly encountered in clinical populations with chronic schizophrenia than those with bipolar disorder. There is some suggestion that patients with bipolar disorder may be at risk of developing TD with a smaller dosage and fewer years of exposure. Atypical antipsychotics also have the potential to cause TD, but apparently at a greatly reduced rate. For this reason, as well as others, it is preferable, when using any antipsychotic medication with patients with bipolar disorder, to use it sparingly, at low dosages and for brief amounts of time. There will be some patients who might require high dosages over long periods, but they are in the minority. Limiting the exposure of patients with bipolar disorder to antipsychotics can be maximized through the use of mood-stabilizing drugs with a more favourable long-term risk profile.

In recent years, it has become increasingly apparent that the whole group of atypical antipsychotics has the potential to cause various metabolic syndromes, some of which may be life threatening. An increased base rate of cases of adult-onset diabetes, unfavourable lipid profiles and hypercholesterolaemia can develop under treatment with atypical antipsychotics. Whereas the majority of these problems occur in those patients with acute and significant weight gain, these difficulties have also been encountered in patients of normal weight, and those who have not shown significant weight gain. Most patients who are going to show a significant weight gain will show signs of this early in treatment. Strong consideration should be given to switching those showing a weight gain of greater than 10% of their baseline body weight in the first 6–10 weeks of treatment to treatment with another agent. It is unclear to what extent each atypical antipsychotic may be more prone than the others to cause these problems. Generally speaking, olanzapine seems to pose the largest risk. Patients treated with atypical antipsychotics should have their weight noted on a regular basis, and laboratory tests should be carried out for fasting blood sugar, lipid profile and serum cholesterol every 4–6 months if patients are maintained on these agents long term. Every effort should be made not to maintain bipolar patients on antipsychotic medicines for more than a couple of months (unless demonstrated to be necessary).

These medications should also be avoided in elderly patients with dementia who also have psychoses, due to an increase in cardiovascular deaths in this population. An increase in suicidal ideation has been reported in adolescents, and there may be an increase in suicide attempts in some patients treated with atypical antipsychotics.

Due to dopamine blockade, some patients develop hyperprolactinaemia, which may present as menstrual difficulties, galactorrhoea or sexual inhibitions (particularly when treated with risperdal). These events should be inquired about during follow-up visits.

Some patients have shown cardiovascular problems, particularly orthostatic hypotension, dizziness and prolongation of the QT interval on electrocardiographic (ECG) monitoring. Ziprasidone may pose particular risk in this regard and should be used with caution in susceptible patients.

Standard dosage ranges for atypical antipsychotic drugs in the treatment of bipolar disorder

The therapeutic dose is the dose that resolves the clinical issue under treatment (with the physician taking care not to cause toxicity and generally maintaining the lower end of recommended dosage schedules). Prolonged exposure should be limited in most cases. In general when dealing with the spectrum of mild hypomania to severe mania, the more severe the condition, the more of an atypical antipsychotic is needed. Typical daily dose ranges in mg/day may include the following:

- aripiprazole 2–30
- asenapine 10–20
- olanzapine 5–20
- quetiapine 100–800
- risperdal 1–6
- ziprasidone 80–160.

High-intensity light therapy

Undoubtedly, seasonal affective disorder (SAD) forms part of the bipolar and not unipolar spectrum of disorders. These patients suffer from regular wintertime depression, usually demonstrating hypomania and sometimes mania during the summer months. During the winter, they characteristically feel fatigue, increased need to sleep, weight gain with carbohydrate craving and cognitive dulling. This is of particular importance to primary care physicians, as each of these symptoms are common complaints for which patients seek evaluation. A typical patient with SAD might come to his primary care physician not complaining of depression but complaining of tiredness, or unexplained weight gain, or cognitive difficulties. The differential diagnoses considered should include SAD as a possible underlying cause of these complaints, particularly in the wintertime. Once recognized, most of these patients are easily treatable with high-intensity light therapy delivered through a specially designed "light box".[23]

Patients should be instructed not to use normal lamps and light bulbs for their treatment, as retinal damage can occur. Light boxes are specifically made to block out the spectrum of light associated with potential ocular harm. Patients usually use the light box in the morning within an hour of their normal waking time. In general, 45 minutes of light therapy with an intensity of 10 000 LUX or greater will lead to resolution of the depression within 4–8 days. Patients then generally continue light therapy throughout the period of wintertime when they traditionally have suffered depression.

There is also evidence that high-intensity light therapy is helpful in the treatment of bipolar depressions presenting in the wintertime that do not follow a regular repeating seasonality. Therefore, in treating refractory bipolar depressed patients, particularly during periods of limited ambient light, high-intensity light therapy should be considered as a primary or adjunctive treatment modality.

Sleep deprivation therapy

Sleep deprivation may prove to be a potent agent in treating the depressed phase of bipolar disorder. The required frequency of administration has not been well studied, but a clinician may start by keeping a patient awake for 24 hours every 4 days until clinical remission is obtained.

Electroconvulsive therapy

ECT is generally reserved for those patients with particularly severe presentations or when patients have not shown a response to other established treatments. In these cases, ECT has been demonstrated to be often quite useful and, at times, life saving, due to reducing suicide or enabling compromised patients to care for themselves. Many otherwise long hospitalizations can be shortened with ECT. Due to issues of exposing the patient to genera anaesthesia and the availability of properly trained and equipped psychiatric centres, ECT is used sparingly.

Early warning signs of relapse

One of the most important tasks for the primary care physician is to identify early signs and symptoms that indicate relapse or onset of a manic or depressive episode. The ability to do so is strongly related to the continuity of care and the physician's capacity to closely monitor the course of bipolar disorder. The use of daily mood graphs and a close relationship with the family of a patient is crucial. Mitchell et al. have demonstrated that both the patient and his or her family can identify the behavioural changes leading to a transitional phase of a patient's condition.[4] They suggest possibly early warning signs for hypomanic or manic episodes: increased activity and busyness, reduced need for sleep, impulsive behaviour, speaking in a caustic manner and telephoning friends indiscriminately, while in depressive episodes, we see patients feeling tearful, moody, withdrawn, snappy, slowed down, negative, stubborn, pessimistic, hopeless or excessively self-doubting. The BMJ publishing group has issued some guidance on "how can I avoid a relapse in a bipolar disorder" in its series of patients leaflets.[24] Primary care physicians seem to be effective in providing psycho-educational approaches that might include provision of videos to both patients and parents or partners, and recommendations of appropriate web sites[25] that can inform them about the early warning signs of relapse.

Common pitfalls for primary care physicians

The evaluation and treatment of patients with bipolar disorders consist of many potential pitfalls and challenges; primary care physicians should be aware that:

- the patients frequently do not report their symptoms or comply with physicians' recommendations, especially in noting early warning signs or their symptomatic experiences
- the patients frequently stop medications for a range of reasons, many of which seem illogical or idiosyncratic
- the parents or partners of bipolar patients are sometimes not informed about the natural course of bipolar disorders (treated or untreated). This is most common in countries where primary care is not well developed.

Issues of integrated care and management of comorbidity

The management of bipolar disorders is usually enhanced through the services of nurses, social workers and psychologists, who are indispensable for integrated health-care services – an effective cooperation between primary and mental health care for both patients and their families.[25] An integrated primary care team can jointly look at increasingly complex family, social and economic issues that are associated with a patient's health problems.

Referral of the patient to other specialists and practitioners is also critical; the role of primary care physicians is to share with them any relevant information available in their medical records, including the episodes of care, medication and medication changes, as well as issues regarding the patient's family involvement.[5]

Another important task for the primary care physician is to treat other clinical entities that may coexist with bipolar disorders – either psychological or physical. The European Psychiatric Association, supported by the European Association for the Study of Diabetes and the European Society of Cardiology published a position statement where the excess of cardiovascular mortality associated with bipolar disorder is partly attributed to an increased risk of the modifiable coronary heart disease risk factors including obesity, smoking, diabetes mellitus, hypertension and dyslipidaemia.[26] It suggests that an additional task for family physicians is to look at the prevalence of abdominal obesity, hypertriglyceridaemia, low high-density lipoprotein cholesterol, high blood pressure and fasting hyperglycaemia. This is clearly reflected in the above-mentioned position paper, which states:[26]

> The intention is to initiate cooperation and shared care between the different healthcare professionals and to increase the awareness of psychiatrists and primary care physicians caring for patients with severe mental illness to screen and treat cardiovascular risk factors and diabetes.

Psychosocial management strategies for bipolar disorder

Psychological and social interventions are most important in the overall management of this disorder. Psychosocial support consists of a union of pharmacological treatment and psychological therapy, which needs to be maintained even after recovery from an acute episode. This is particularly important to those with chronic depressive symptoms.[27] It begins with education of the patients about the nature of their disease (*psycho-education*). In particular, patients need to have some reasonable expectation regarding the natural course of their disease, both treated and untreated. They will often maintain good health for longer periods of time if they follow some basic behavioural suggestions. In particular, they should avoid sleep deprivation and not use recreational drugs, particularly psychostimulants and cocaine. Maintaining a regular routine in their daily activities may also prove useful.

A clinician should involve family members who might live with the patient for psycho-education, and recruit them into a partnership to help with the surveillance and therapy of the patient (*family therapy*). They are in the best position to recognize subtle changes in behaviour, activity or speech suggesting the beginning of an episode. They should then prompt the afflicted individual to return to his or her physician for further evaluation and treatment adjustments. Families may inadvertently have interactive styles that contribute to relapse, such as creating an environment that is full of interpersonal tension and pathological drama. These features should be addressed in family therapy. Psychotherapy of a cognitive-behavioural variety, challenging the worldview, interpretation of events and decision-making of patients with bipolar disorder can also prove to be invaluable (*CBT*). In Europe, increasing numbers of primary care practitioners and family physicians have been exposed to CBT; in a popular book by David Lee,[28] a method of using CBT within a busy GP's office is presented. It includes approaches to overcome depression in general practice by using CBT, and offers certain examples of how a GP can change behaviour in depression by scheduling weekly activities and discussing activity charts. However, sophisticated CBT is best delivered by trained clinicians. In addition to basic pharmacotherapy, CBT leads to reframing the negative thoughts that are common in the negative/pessimistic episodes of a bipolar patient.

Social workers can also play an important role in both screening and management of patients with bipolar disorders.

Two key factors that are not always taken into account fully when considering the management of patients with bipolar disorder are the roles of family and community.

The family of the patient suffering from bipolar disorder plays a particularly key role in the exchange of information with the family physician, who generally has more family interaction and information than physicians from other disciplines.

The ability of patients with bipolar disorder to actively get involved in community activities (nongovernmental organizations, voluntary work, etc.) has frequently provided excellent clinical outcomes.

Conclusions

In conclusion, bipolar disorders are relatively common in primary care but frequently underdiagnosed. There are many issues that current clinical research in primary care should address. Among them, of key interest, is early recognition of the complex presentations of bipolar disorders, the use of suitable screening tools, and effective long-term management in the primary care setting.

An integrated team approach in primary care settings should be shared among all the involved professionals working in concert. Of utmost importance is the screening role that primary care nurses can provide to guarantee early diagnoses, as soon as possible. This can be particularly crucial for populations attending clinics for chronic medical conditions under the management of primary care nurses (e.g. hypertension, diabetes, asthma), where bipolar disorder and other psychiatric conditions can be detected at any moment in their management. Such identification not only helps a patient in relation to their underlying mood disorder, but undoubtedly leads to better outcomes regarding their chronic medical diseases under treatment. Therefore, better overall outcomes regarding quality of life, morbidity and mortality can be expected.

Finally, the family physician is often the most important caregiver in a community for the recognition and treatment of severe psychiatric disorders. His or her abilities are enhanced when working with other professionals with complementary skills to his own for detection and treatment. Family members and community resources can greatly contribute to patients' acute and chronic well-being.

In low-income countries, the ability for a family practitioner to enjoy the resources of helpful colleagues or have at his disposal a full array of useful pharmacological agents or clinical laboratory facilities may, unfortunately, be absent. Support and education for such individuals are sorely needed. One resource that can be accessed worldwide is the *World Federation of Societies of Biological Psychiatry*.[29]

References

1   MedicineNet.com. Definition of bipolar disorder (http://www.medterms.com/script/main/art.asp?articlekey=2468, accessed 17 November 2011).
2   Esch J. Bipolar rates highest in the US. *Third Age Media*, 8 March 2011.

3   Merikangas KR et al. Lifetime and 12 month prevalence of bipolar spectrum disorder in the National Comorbidity Survey replication. *Archives of General Psychiatry*, 2007, 64:1039.

4   Mitchell PhB, Loo CK, Gould BM. Diagnosing and monitoring of bipolar disorder in general practice. *Medical Journal of Australia*, 2010, 193:S10–S13.

5   Piterman L Jones KM, Castle DK. Bipolar disorder in general practice: challenges and opportunities. Medical Journal of Australia, 2010, 193:S14–17.

6   Maremmani I et al. Affective temperament in heroin addiction. *Journal of Affective Disorders*, 2009, 117:186–192.

7   Mendive JM. *Trastorno bipolar*. Siete Días Medicos, 2009, 789:88–94.

8   Kukopulos A et al. Rapid cyclers, temperament, and antidepressants. *Comprehensive Psychiatry*, 1983, 24:249–258.

9   *Diagnostic and statistical manual of mental disorders*, 4th ed, text revision (DSM-IV-TR). Washington, American Psychiatric Association, 2000.

10   *ICD-10 classification of mental and behavioral disorders*. Geneva, World Health Organization, 1996.

11   American Psychiatric Association DSM-5 Development. *Bipolar disorders* (http://www.dsm5.org/ proposedrevision/Pages/BipolarandRelatedDisorders.aspx, accessed 17 November 2011).

12   Perugi G et al. Clinical subtypes of bipolar mixed states: validating a broader European definition in 143 cases. *Journal of Affective Disorders*, 1997, 43:169–180.

13   Deltito J et al. Do patients with borderline personality disorder belong to the bipolar spectrum? Journal of Affective Disorders, 2001, 67:221–228.

14   Smith DJ et al. Unrecognised bipolar disorder in primary care patients with depression. *British Journal of Psychiatry*, 2011, 199:49–56.

15   Britt H et al. *General practice activity in Australia, 2008–09*. Canberra, Australian Institute of Health and Welfare, 2009 (General practice series no. 25; Cat. no. GEP 25).

16   McIntyre RS (2011). Differential diagnosis of bipolar disorder. In: bipolar disorder: differential diagnosis and evidence based treatment strategies. *Current Psychiatry*, 2011, Suppl.:3–22.

17   Ghaemi SN et al. Diagnosing bipolar disorder and the effects of antidepressants: a naturalistic study. *Journal of Clinical Psychiatry*, 2000, 61:804–808.

18   Hirschfeld RMA et al. Development and validation of a screening instrument for bipolar spectrum disorder: the Mood Disorder Questionnaire. *American Journal of Psychiatry*, 2000, 157:1873–1875.

19   Baldassano CF. Assessment tools for screening and monitoring bipolar disorder. *Bipolar Disorders*, 2005, 7(Suppl. I):8–15.

20   Nemeroff CB, Schatzberg A. *Recognition and treatment of psychiatric disorders: a psychopharmacology handbook for primary care*. Washington DC, Americal Psychiatric Press, 1999.

21   Deltito JA et al. Naturalistic experience with the use of divalproex sodium on an inpatient unit for adolescent psychiatric patients. *Acta Psychiatrica Scandinavica*, 1998, 97:236–240.

22   Deltito JA. The effect of valproate on bipolar spectrum temperamental disorders. *The Journal of Clinical Psychiatry*, 1993, 54:300–304.

23   Deltito JA et al. Non-seasonal unipolar and bipolar depressive spectrum disorders. *Journal of Affective Disorders*, 1991, 12:231–237.

24   BMJ Group. *Bipolar disorder: how can I avoid a relapse?* London, BMJ Publishing Group Limited, 2009 (Patients leaflets from BMJ Group).

25   Black Dog Institute (www.blackdoginstitute.org.au, accessed 18 November 2011).

26   De Hert M et al. Cardiovascular disease and diabetes in people with severe mental illness position statement from the European Psychiatric Association (EPA), supported by the European Association for the Study of Diabetes (EASD) and the European Society of Cardiology (ESC). *European Psychiatry*, 2009, 24:412–424.

27   *Bipolar disorder: the management of bipolar disorder in adults, children and adolescents, in primary and secondary care*. London, National Institute for Health and Clinical Excellence, 2006 (CG38).

28   Lee D. Using CBT in general practice: the 10 minute consultation. Bloxham, Scion Publishing Ltd, 2006.

29   World Federation of Societies of Biological Psychiatry (http://www.wfsbp.org/, accessed 17 November 2011).

19 Schizophrenia in primary care mental health

David Goldberg, Gabriel Ivbijaro, Lucja Kolkiewicz and Sammy Ohene

Key messages

- Schizophrenia is a treatable disorder and some patients are able to maintain employment despite persisting symptoms and/or disability.
- Although it is often necessary to admit these patients to hospital, care in the community should be arranged where possible, with close collaboration with the mental health service.
- Antipsychotic drugs should suppress the positive symptoms of the disorder, and should be offered to all patients. No single drug is clearly preferable to others.
- Patients who fail to respond to conventional treatments should be offered treatment with clozapine after two other drugs have been tried.
- Family interventions reduce the risk of relapse and reduce the level of symptoms. Other effective interventions include cognitive-behavioural therapy modified for psychosis (CBTp), and arts therapy.
- Those caring for these patients in the community should pay special attention to their social adjustment, and ensure that they live in a social context that is as normal as possible.

Introduction

Schizophrenia is the name given to a group of mental disorders in which delusions and hallucinations predominate, and there are alterations in a person's perception, thoughts, feelings and behaviour. Each person with the disorder will have a unique combination of symptoms and experiences. Typically, there is a *prodromal period*, often characterized by some deterioration in personal functioning. This period may include memory and concentration problems, unusual behaviour and ideas and disturbed communication and affect.

Schizophrenia affects approximately 7 per 1000 people from adolescence onwards. It is an illness with low incidence and high prevalence, due to the effects of chronicity, and is of importance to primary care because of a shortage of mental health specialists globally, especially in low- and middle-income countries.[1] In most countries, whatever their income, primary care will be the first contact for many people who suffer from mental health conditions.[2]

Historical background

Schizophrenia has been noted in all cultures throughout recorded history. In the 19th century, the French psychiatrist Benedict Morel, who observed rapid intellectual deterioration in a young teenage boy from a good student to one with confused thoughts and grossly disorganized behaviour over a few months, named the disorder *demence précoce*.[3] In 1893, the fourth edition of Emil Kraepelin's textbook *Psychiatrie* introduced dementia praecox under the heading of "Psychic degenerative processes".[4]

In 1911, Eugene Bleuler replaced the term "dementia praecox" with "schizophrenia", because he believed the cognitive impairment associated with the disorder arose from splitting of psychic function.[5] Bleuler identified four disturbances, known as "the four As", as fundamental to the disorder. These were **A**ffective blunting, loosening of **A**ssociation, **A**utism and **A**mbivalence. He considered hallucinations and delusions as non-specific to the diagnosis of schizophrenia, since they occurred in patients with other conditions such as manic-depressive (bipolar) illness.

In 1959 Kurt Schneider, a German psychiatrist, drew attention to the importance of psychotic symptoms in the diagnosis of schizophrenia and identified certain "first rank" psychotic symptoms as diagnostic, thus introducing greater objectivity and specificity into the diagnostic process.[6] First-rank symptoms included thought insertion, thought withdrawal, thought broadcasting, delusions of control, audible thoughts, voices arguing about the subject, voices commenting on actions in the third person and delusional perception.

Epidemiology of schizophrenia

Schizophrenia is an illness with an unclear aetiology, which is likely to be both complex and multifactorial and to involve gene–environment(s) interaction. The best way to consider this in a primary care setting is by adopting a life-course approach, which begins from genetics, obstetric complications, childhood adversity, adolescent adversity and other life events of adulthood.

There is an association between schizophrenia and family history, as having a first-degree relative with schizophrenia increases a person's likelihood of experiencing schizophrenia 10-fold, while having two affected parents or an affected twin confers a likelihood of 50%.[7] There is also evidence that prenatal infections can be associated with schizophrenia; these include rubella,[8] influenza[9] and toxoplasmosis.[10] One of the theories proposed to explain this association is the role of cytokine and chemokines as mediators of the host response to infection.[11] In addition to obstetric infections, other obstetric complications may be associated with an increased incidence of schizophrenia.[12] There is evidence that childhood trauma may be associated with psychosis;[13] however, Morgan and Fisher are of the opinion that a number of conceptual and methodological issues need to be addressed before a definite conclusion can be reached.[14]

Adolescent and adult psychosocial stressors, including first- and second-generation migration,[15,16] and inner-city environment,[17–19] and, in some cases, substance misuse,[20–22] are all associated with onset, maintenance and relapse of schizophrenia.

The incidence of schizophrenia is higher in men than in women.[23,24]

Key lessons for primary care are summarized in Box 19.1.

Box 19.1   Lessons for primary care

- There is a need for a biopsychosocial approach to the management of schizophrenia.
- Prevention starts with:
  - genetic counselling for those parents who have a high genetic risk
  - prevention of infections in the prenatal period
  - good obstetric care during delivery
  - prevention of childhood trauma and deprivation
  - support for migrants
  - good environmental planning to decrease the stress of living in inner cities.

Positive and negative symptoms

There are two main groups of symptoms, and both may be present simultaneously or each can occur on their own. The prodromal period is usually followed by an acute episode marked by *positive symptoms* such as hallucinations, delusions and behavioural disturbances, accompanied by agitation and distress. *Negative symptoms* may take the form of social withdrawal, apathy and reduced interest in daily activities. In those with prolonged illnesses, there may be some cognitive decline over many years.

Acute episodes and persistent states

The *International Classification of Diseases* (ICD)-11 for primary health care (ICD11-PHC) is due to be released by the World Health Organization (WHO) in 2014. It distinguishes between acute episodes of psychosis and persistent psychotic states, where the illness has not resolved fully and may display both positive and negative features. The concept of "acute psychosis" includes transient psychotic states that last less than one month, as well as schizophrenia, which is the name given to illnesses that have lasted more than one month. For primary care purposes, the broader concept is preferable, as an individual primary care clinician is more likely to see cases of transient psychotic states than first onset of schizophrenia. Since schizophrenia is often a long-lasting disorder, primary care clinicians are most likely to see cases of persistent psychotic illness.

Acute psychotic disorder

Presenting symptoms and complaints

Patients can present with sudden onset of severe disturbance, characterized by strange beliefs and grossly abnormal behaviour. They may be apprehensive, confused or extremely suspicious. Acute psychosis can be very transient in nature, lasting for a few hours to a few days, or can last for a few weeks. Complete recovery is the norm. *Schizophrenia should not be diagnosed until the disorder is still present after 4 weeks.* It is often very difficult to know the extent to which drugs may be responsible for psychotic experiences, and patients should always be asked what drugs they have used in recent weeks.

Diagnostic features

Acute psychotic disorder is a diagnostic label given to patients with unusual symptoms of sudden onset, usually with florid disturbance and lasting from a few days to a few weeks. While complete recovery is the norm, a minority of patients can have a relapse with similar presentations.

The unusual experiences, abnormal beliefs and behaviours may include:

- *required symptoms*:
  - delusions (strange beliefs may involve being persecuted or poisoned, of special powers, of one's spouse's infidelity, of being controlled or of being talked about by strangers)
  - hallucinations (hearing voices or seeing visions)
- *other common symptoms*
  - withdrawal
  - agitation
  - restlessness or disorganized behaviour
  - muddled thinking
  - incoherent or irrelevant speech
  - labile emotional states.

Differential diagnosis

- Bipolar disorder – the manic phase and psychotic forms of depression may have many similar features; patients may develop symptoms of classical mania and depression or may go on to become chronic, mandating a change in diagnosis over time
- Drug-induced psychotic states
- Exacerbations of a persistent psychosis, with a total duration of illness of more than 3 months
- Medical conditions such as delirium, with systemic or cerebral infections, and epilepsy

Persistent psychotic disorder

Presenting symptoms and complaints

The presentations include abnormal beliefs, hearing voices or seeing visions and may involve abnormal behaviour. Patients can also present with lack of energy for daily chores, lack of motivation to work, difficulty in concentrating, apathy and withdrawal from family, friends and colleagues.

Diagnostic features

Acute exacerbations include:

- delusions (strange beliefs of being persecuted or poisoned, of special powers, of one's spouse's infidelity, of being controlled or of being talked about by strangers)
- hallucinations (hearing voices and seeing things that others cannot see)
- restlessness and agitation
- grossly abnormal behaviour.

Persistent problems include:

- lack of energy or motivation to carry out daily chores and work
- apathy and social withdrawal
- strange and abnormal speech
- poor personal care or neglect.

Differential diagnosis

- Bipolar disorder – the manic phase may have many similar features
- Psychosis can also be associated with medical illnesses (e.g. infections and tumours of the brain, head injury, epilepsy, thyroid disorder)
- Dementia – organic psychoses (e.g. dementia) can have similar features
- Substance use – e.g. alcohol, cannabis, opioids, etc.

Interviewing and assessing a psychotic patient

Time is always short in primary care, and you may have to speed up your assessment. Some basic strategies follow.

The patient must perceive you as their own doctor, rather than the agent of their parents. If the patient is accompanied, start your interview with the patient, and only take a history from others with the patient's consent. Listen to the patient's account of the present problem, with sympathy and encouragement. If the patient is not sure why he or she has come, ask what has worried other people and suggested that they visit. If you are still not making much progress, ask whether the patient has had any experiences they could not account for, or has had any recurrent thoughts that troubled them.

If odd experiences are described, ask if they were taking any drugs at the time, or whether they have experimented with them in the last few weeks. If you are still making little progress and they are accompanied, ask if they mind asking the person with them what they have noticed that worries them.

In any case, you will need to take control of the interview and do a quick *mental state examination*. How are they feeling at present? Are they worried about themselves? Have they felt that life isn't worth living? (*If so, have they had thoughts about harming themselves?*) Have they found that they can hear things that other people don't seem to hear? Or have they seen things that they couldn't account for? (*Have they had auditory or visual hallucinations: can they describe what they have heard/seen?*) Have they had any problems with their thinking (*thoughts inserted, or controlled by others*)? Can they tell you where they are, what date/day of week it is, and who you are (*orientation*)?

Management of schizophrenia in primary care

The management of schizophrenia requires an integrated approach that recognizes the central importance of the patient, their family and carers, is holistic, and focuses on developing patient strengths and promoting recovery.

Management of schizophrenia requires a recognition that the person with schizophrenia is an individual who should be treated with respect and empowered to manage the illness, so that they can maintain hope and obtain treatment in the least restrictive environment possible, and live a satisfying, hopeful and contributing life, despite the limitations caused by illness.[25]

As with all other mental health conditions, it is important to invest in manpower to improve patient access to treatment, so that mental and physical health needs are addressed in an integrated way that can deliver the best possible outcomes.

It is known that not all people with schizophrenia will visit primary care, as illustrated by Goldberg and Huxley;[26] therefore, a systematic approach to the management of schizophrenia that takes into account prevention, the subtype of schizophrenia and its course is necessary.

Low- and middle-income countries

In *middle-income countries* where secondary care mental health services are less well developed, general practitioners and family physicians should form an alliance with their local psychiatrist so that they can readily elicit support and advice to help them better manage early-onset cases of schizophrenia and those who have not responded to the usual treatment interventions. This approach can be better supported where locally agreed management guidelines have been jointly developed by primary care physicians and secondary care psychiatrists, as this will provide a clear guideline on when it is appropriate to ask for extra help or refer to the local mental health service. Liaison with mental health services can be further enhanced by organizing regular meetings between primary care staff and the local psychiatrist at the primary care clinic, where complex cases can be brought and discussed. Many middle-income countries have a network of local district general hospitals that provide a range of services. General practitioners and family physicians should negotiate admission rights for psychiatric patients requiring inpatient care, supported by a clear admission guideline and treatment protocol. In such circumstances, the role of the psychiatrist is to assist in developing evidence-based treatment protocols and guidelines, regular educational support and ongoing coaching to medical staff who are managing people with schizophrenia.

In *low-income countries*, where primary care services and secondary care mental health services are poorly developed, the roles of the general practitioner or family physician are different, as, not only are they the first point of contact, they also have to take on the role of local specialist for a range of mental health disorders. In such situations, it is even more important for primary care to develop very detailed schizophrenia protocols and guidelines to follow. If there are other general practitioners or family physicians in the area, they should form an alliance of mutual support or cooperation, including co-mentoring and peer support. They should develop the role of health-care workers to support their mental health interventions, and work with local opinion leaders and advocates to address stigma and promote access. In some countries where traditional healers play a role, general practitioners and other health professionals working in primary care should work with their local health boards to generate a list of local traditional healers, so that they can provide them with mental health education and support, and their usefulness can be harnessed as part of the extended primary health-care team.

In all countries, there is a need to develop a local formulary of a range of medications that are affordable, and of proven benefit in the treatment of schizophrenia, so that access to pharmacological interventions can be guaranteed.

The key to delivering good health is to keep the patient and their family or carer at the centre of the service.

Specific interventions for the treatment of schizophrenia

Once a history has been taken and a diagnosis made, an intervention plan should be developed using the following headings.

General

The person presenting with schizophrenia should be provided with a diagnosis and explanation of the disorder in a form that they can easily understand.

All people with schizophrenia should be assessed for risk to self and others. (For more details, please refer to Chapter 11 "Risk assessment and the management of suicidality in primary care mental health".)

The prodromal phase

In many parts of the world, specialized early-intervention services are not available, and primary care staff must use their own judgement in deciding what assistance to offer the person in a prodromal phase. If there is access to a local mental health service, it may sometimes be helpful to refer the patient, provided that he or she agrees to this. Where available, there are three components to the assistance a mental health service provides: firstly, early identification and therapeutic engagement of people in the prodromal phase; second, provision of specialized pharmacological and psychosocial interventions during or immediately following a first episode of psychosis; and third, education of the patient and his or her family and the wider community to reduce obstacles to early engagement in treatment.

An acute episode of psychosis

- For people with newly diagnosed schizophrenia presenting with positive symptoms, offer *oral antipsychotic medication*. Provide information and discuss with the service user the benefits and side-effect profile of any drug you intend to use, bearing in mind the relative potential of individual antipsychotic drugs to cause extrapyramidal side-effects (including akathisia), metabolic side-effects (including weight gain) and other side-effects (including unpleasant subjective experiences). In nine randomized controlled trials (RCTs) with a total of 1801 participants with first-episode or early schizophrenia (including people with a recent onset of schizophrenia and people who had never been treated with antipsychotic medication), the evidence suggested there were no clinically significant differences in efficacy between the antipsychotic drugs examined.[27] These medications are effective in reducing all florid symptoms, and in reducing excited behaviour.

- Referral to a specialized *mental health service* will depend upon local availability of such a service. Patients with grossly disturbed behaviour, or where there is thought to be a danger to either the patient or to others, are usually referred. If possible, all first episodes of acute psychosis should be referred to the specialist service.

- If patients are to be *managed in the community*, it is advisable for them to be visited by a mental health nurse who is able to give advice and support to carers. Interface with the local mental health service is facilitated if there is a *written care plan* that has been agreed between the two services and the service user and his or her family. Such care plans typically include details of symptoms both in relapse and admission, the usual medication and an acceptable alternative, details of any mental health nurse allocated to the case, and information on how to arrange readmission if this becomes necessary. There should be opportunities to have *case discussions* between primary care and mental health staff, especially at times of crisis.

- When the crisis of an acute episode is resolved, offer *family intervention* to all families of people with schizophrenia who live with or are in close contact with the service user. This is a specialized procedure best carried out by someone who has been trained to deliver such interventions. Family interventions aim to reduce the level of expressed emotion in the family and to decrease critical comments towards the patient, as well as to help carers deal with problems and to improve knowledge about the illness in both the service user and his or her family. Therapists are most likely to be a mental health professional. In 32 RCTs including 2429 participants, there was robust and consistent evidence for the efficacy of family intervention.[27] When compared with standard care family interventions have been shown to reduce the risk of relapse and to produce a lower level of active symptoms for up to 2 years after the intervention.[28,29]

- The National Institute for Health and Clinical Excellence (NICE) recommends that general practitioners and other primary health-care professionals should *monitor the physical health* of people with schizophrenia at least once a year. You should focus on cardiovascular disease risk assessment as described in the NICE guideline, *Lipid modification*, but bear in mind that people with schizophrenia are at higher risk of cardiovascular disease than the general population. A copy of the results should be sent to the care coordinator and/or psychiatrist, and put in the secondary care notes.[30]

- *Do not* initiate regular combined antipsychotic medication, except for short periods (for example, when changing medication).

Interventions for people with schizophrenia whose illness has not responded adequately to treatment

- First, review the diagnosis. Other possible explanations for symptoms include intoxications with drugs or alcohol and organic brain disease.

- Next, try to establish whether there has been adherence to antipsychotic medication, prescribed at an adequate dose and for the correct duration.

- Review engagement with and use of psychological treatments and ensure that these have been offered.

- If there is access to a specialist mental health service, ask for an opinion on which drug to try next. At least one of the drugs should be a non-clozapine second-generation antipsychotic.

- If trained staff are locally available to administer *cognitive-behavioural therapy adapted for schizophrenia* (CBTp), suggest this as next step. When compared with standard care, CBTp was effective in reducing both the rate of re-admissions to hospital and the duration of admissions. Negative symptoms were reduced at one-year follow-up.[31] Early CBT trials tended to be particularly symptom focused, helping service users develop coping strategies to manage hallucinations.[31] Since then, however, CBTp has evolved and now tends to be based on a manual. It should take place over a series of sessions, and establish links between the patient's thoughts, feelings or actions and their current or past level of functioning, and allow the patient to re-evaluate how their perceptions, beliefs or reasoning relate to the target symptoms.

- Offer *clozapine* to people with schizophrenia whose illness has not responded adequately to treatment despite sequential use of adequate doses of at least two different antipsychotic drugs. In 18 RCTs including 2554 participants whose illness had not responded adequately to treatment, clozapine had the most consistent evidence for efficacy over the first-generation antipsychotics included in the trials.[32] A number of patient-related factors have been reported to increase the variability of plasma clozapine concentrations, with sex, age and smoking behaviour being the most important.

Patients with persistent psychotic states

Patients may reach a relatively stable state, with some residual positive symptoms in addition to some negative symptoms. Positive symptoms may reappear when the patient has experienced a stressful life event, or when they have stopped taking their medication. The advice given above will apply to management of the positive symptoms.

The use of depot medication

Consider this only where there is clear evidence that antipsychotic drugs are effective in controlling symptoms, and where there is evidence that the patient repeatedly relapses when medication is not taken, and agrees to receiving depot medication.

Combining clozapine with another antipsychotic

In six RCTs including 252 participants with schizophrenia whose illness had not responded adequately to clozapine treatment, there was some evidence that clozapine augmentation with a second antipsychotic might improve both total and negative symptoms if administered for an adequate duration.[33,34]

Negative symptoms

There is no consistent evidence that one antipsychotic drug is any better at relieving negative symptoms than the others. In 10 RCTs including 1200 participants with persistent negative symptoms, there was no evidence of clinically significant differences in efficacy between any of the antipsychotic drugs examined.[27] Careful clinical assessment is warranted, to determine whether such persistent features are primary or secondary, and may identify relevant treatment targets, such as drug-induced Parkinsonism, depressive features or certain positive symptoms.[32] However, if clozapine is augmented with another antipsychotic drug, there is some evidence of efficacy, as discussed above.

There are also social and psychological treatments that are effective to some extent. *Arts therapies*, which allow expression of emotions, whether by drama, by pottery or by painting, have been shown to have such an effect. There is consistent evidence that arts therapies are effective in reducing negative symptoms when compared with any other control.[32] There is some evidence indicating that the medium to large effects found at the end of treatment were sustained at up to 6 months' follow-up.[32] *CBTp* may also reduce negative symptoms.

Social care and rehabilitation

A *social assessment* is necessary to ensure that an individual is obtaining whatever social benefits are available, and has somewhere to live that provides shelter from adverse weather and adequate food. Social interventions for schizophrenia should include supported employment, including opportunities for volunteering,[35] access to education and leisure activities and appropriate housing. Supported employment programmes may provide assistance to people with schizophrenia who wish to return to work or gain employment. However, they should not be the only work-related activity offered when individuals are unable to work or are unsuccessful in their attempts to find employment. Patients with persistent psychotic disorders need to *structure their time* usefully, and gain help and support from regular social contacts, perhaps in a group setting.

Re-referral to the specialist mental health services

For a person with schizophrenia being cared for in primary care, consider referral to secondary care again if there is a poor response to treatment, non-adherence to medication, intolerable side-effects from medication, coexisting substance misuse, or risk to self or others.

Reducing the risk of relapse and the promotion of recovery

The NICE guideline showed that in 17 RCTs including 3535 participants with schizophrenia, the evidence suggested that, when compared with placebo, all of the antipsychotics examined reduced the risk of relapse or overall treatment failure.[27] Although some second-generation antipsychotic drugs show a modest benefit over haloperidol, there is insufficient evidence to choose between antipsychotics in terms of relapse prevention.

Conclusions, prognosis and future developments

It cannot be emphasized enough that the schizophrenic cluster of psychoses are by no means always chronic disorders. In the WHO 10-country study, it was found that, even in high-income countries, of those satisfying criteria for schizophrenia, about 37% may expect to have a remitting course and eventually to recover. In low- and middle-income countries, the outlook is much more positive, with 63% having such a favourable course.[36] This is despite the fact that the former patients were on antipsychotic drugs for more than 75% of the 2-year follow-up, while in the latter the corresponding figure was 16%. Primary care staff are therefore urged to take a positive, even modestly optimistic view of the prognosis, and this is especially true for transient psychotic disorders.

Indicators of a poor outlook are a slow, gradual onset over months or years, a long duration of untreated psychosis, a poor premorbid adjustment, and a schizoid personality. One or more of Schneider's "first rank" symptoms (see earlier, "Historical background") mean that the patient will have a three-fold increased risk of relapse.[36] The best predictor of relapse is failure to continue to take antipsychotic medication,[37] and those using cannabis are also at greatly increased risk of relapse.[38]

In contrast, a sudden onset, a severe precipitating life event, and a good adjustment during adolescence, being married, having close friends and avoiding street drugs all indicate a more favourable course.[39]

Future developments include a continuing tendency to avoid caring for these patients in large institutions, and instead to look after them in as normal as possible a social context. Negative symptoms accumulate in unstimulating environments, and they are strikingly less evident in those cared for in the community. It is likely that further advances will be made in identifying the genetic basis for schizophrenia, and, in particular, in our understanding of the social environments that interact with these genes.

References

1   *Mental health atlas*, revised edition. Geneva, World Health Organization, 2005.

2   World Health Organization and Wonca. *Integrating mental health into primary care. A global perspective.* Geneva, World Health Organization, 2008.

3   Morel BA (1860). *Traité de maladies mentales.* Paris: Victir Masson, 1860.

4   Kraepelin E. *Psychiatrie*, 4th ed. Liepzig, JA Barth, 1893.

5   Bleuler E. *Dementia praecox or the group of schizophrenias* (translated by Zinkin L). New York, International Universities Press, 1911.

6   Schneider K. *Clinical psychopathology.* New York: Grune & Stratton, 1959.

7   Kendler KS, Diehl SR. The genetics of schizophrenia: A current, genetic epidemiological perspective. *Schizophrenia Bulletin*, 1993, 19:261–285.

8   Brown AS et al. Pre-natal rubella, premorbid abnormalities and adult schizophrenia. *Biological Psychiatry*, 2001, 49:473–486.

9   Brown AS et al. Serologic evidence for prenatal influenza in the aetiology of schizophrenia. *Archives of General Psychiatry*, 2004, 61:774–780.

10 Brown AS et al. Maternal exposure to toxoplasmosis and risk of schizophrenia in adult offspring. *American Journal of Psychiatry*, 2005, 167:767–773.

11 Buka SL et al. Maternal cytokine levels during pregnancy and adult psychosis. *Brain Behaviour and Immunity*, 2001, 15:411–420.

12 Crow T. Obstetric complications and schizophrenia. *American Journal of Psychiatry*, 2003, 135:1011–1012.

13 Read J et al. Childhood trauma, psychosis and schizophrenia: a literature review with theoretical and clinical implications. *Acta Psychiatrica Scandinavica*, 2005, 112:330–350.

14 Morgan C, Fisher H. Environmental factors in schizophrenia: childhood trauma – a critical review. *Schizophrenia Bulletin*, 2007, 33:3–10.

15 Cantor-Graae E, Selten JP. Schizophrenia and migration: a meta-analysis and review. *American Journal of Psychiatry*, 2005, 162:12–24.

16 Coid JW et al. Raised incidence of all psychoses among migrant groups. *Archives of General Psychiatry*, 2008, 65:1250–1258.

17 van Os J et al. Neighbourhood variations in incidence of schizophrenia. Evidence for person-environment interaction. *British Journal of Psychiatry*, 2000, 176:243–248.

18 van Os J et al. Prevalence of psychotic disorder and community level of psychotic symptoms: an urban – rural comparison. *Archives of General Psychiatry*, 2001, 58:663–668.

19 Sundquist K et al. Urbanisation and incidence of psychosis and depression. Follow up study of 4.4 million women and men in Sweden. *British Journal of Psychiatry*, 2004, 184:293–298.

20 Andréasson S et al. Cannabis and schizophrenia. A longitudinal study of Swedish conscripts. *The Lancet*, 1987, 330:1483–1486.

21 Phillips P, Johnson S. How does drug and alcohol misuse develop among people with psychotic disorder? A literature review. *Social Psychiatry and Psychiatric Epidemiology*, 2001, 36:269–276.

22 Batel P. Addiction and schizophrenia. *European Psychiatry*, 2000, 15:115–122.

23 Castle DJ, Wessley S, Murray RM. Sex and schizophrenia: Effects of diagnostic stringency, and associations with premorbid variables. *British Journal of Psychiatry*, 1993, 162:658–664.

24 Iacono WG, Beiser M. Are males more likely than females to develop schizophrenia? *American Journal of Psychiatry*, 1992, 149:1070–1074.

25 Anthony WA. Recovery from mental illness: the guiding vision of the mental health service system in the 1990s. *Psychosocial Rehabilitation Journal*, 1993, 17:169–170.

26 Goldberg DP, Huxley PJ. *Common mental disorders – a biosocial model.* London, Routledge, 1992.

27 National Collaborating Centre for Mental Health. *Schizophrenia. The NICE guideline on core interventions in the treatment and management of schizophrenia in adults in primary and secondary care (update edition)*. London, Royal College of Psychiatrists and British Psychological Society, 2010.

28 Pilling S et al. Psychological treatments in schizophrenia: i. Meta analysis of family intervention and cognitive behaviour therapy. *Psychological Medicine*, 2002, 32:763–782.

29 McGill CW et al. Family education intervention in the treatment of schizophrenia. *Hospital and Community Psychiatry*, 1983, 34:934–938.

30 *Lipid modification: cardiovascular risk assessment and the modification of blood lipids for the primary and secondary prevention of cardiovascular disease*. London, National Institute for Health and Clinical Excellence, 2008 (CG67).

31 Tarrier N et al. The community management of schizophrenia: a controlled trial of a behavioural intervention with families to reduce relapse. *British Journal of Psychiatry*, 1988, 153:532–542.

32 *Schizophrenia: core interventions in the treatment and management of schizophrenia in adults in primary and secondary care* (update). London, National Institute for Health and Clinical Excellence, 2009 (CG82).

33 Buckley P et al. When symptoms persist: clozapine augmentation strategies. *Schizophrenia Bulletin*, 2001, 27:615–628.

34 Potter WZ et al. Clozapine in China: a review and preview of US/PRC collaboration. *Psychopharmacology*, 99:S87–S91.

35 Becker D et al. A long term follow up of adults with psychiatric disabilities who receive supported employment. *Psychiatric Services*, 2007, 58:922–928.

36 Jablensky A, Schwarz R, Tomov T. WHO Collaborative Study of impairments and disability associated with schizophrenic disorders. *Psychological Medicine Monograph Supplement*, 285, 62:152–163.

37 Dencker SJ, Malm U, Lepp M. Schizophrenic relapse after drug withdrawal is predictable. *Acta Psychiatrica Scandinavica*, 1986, 73:181–185.

38 Linszen DH, Dingemans PM, Lenior ME. Cannabis abuse and the course of recent onset schizophrenic disorders. *Archives of General Psychiatry*, 1994, 51:273–279.

39 Strauss JS, Carpenter WT Jr. Relationships between predictor and outcome variables: a report from the WHO international pilot study of schizophrenia. *Archives of General Psychiatry*, 1974, 31:37–42.

Part III

Perinatal disorders in primary care mental health

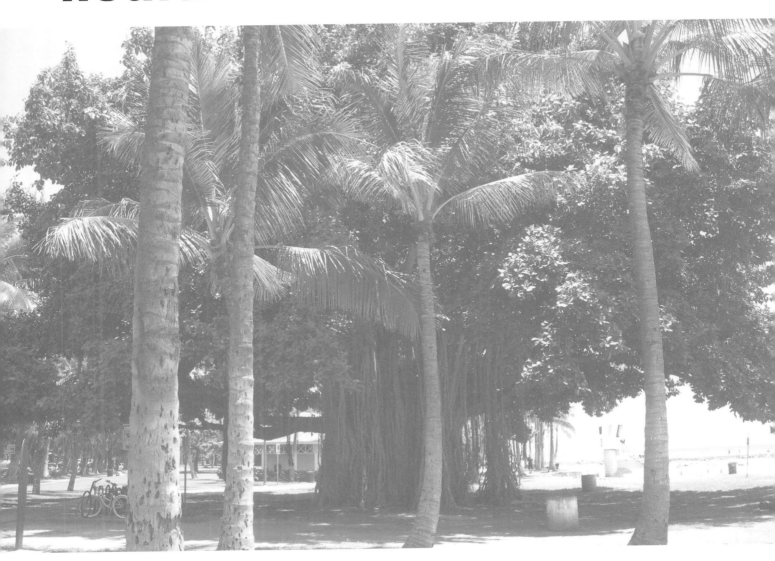

20 Perinatal mental health in primary care: an overview of current models across the globe

Maria Muzik, Susan Hamilton, Tamsen Jean Rochat, Jane RW Fishe, Bryanne Barnett, Prabha Chandra, Carol Henshaw and Vesna Pirec, with contributions from Geetha Desai, Somashekhar Bijjal and Michelle Haling

Key messages

- Perinatal mental illness is common across the world, yet often unrecognized and undertreated. Worldwide, the prevalence of perinatal mental illness is highest among the most economically stressed women living in rural areas of the world.

- Prevention, early detection and treatment of perinatal mental illness are crucial to avert negative consequences for the mother, the developing child and the whole family. Yet access to professional health-care workers is limited in many parts of the world, particularly in countries with low to medium resources.

- Lay and professional health-care workers in primary care settings can be effectively trained to screen for, detect and deliver treatments to women with perinatal mental illness.

- Brief screening tools and structured manualized interventions need to be adapted to make them culturally acceptable and appropriate for use in such primary health-care settings across the world.

- More complex cases of perinatal mental illness need treatment delivered by specialized personnel in a mental health-care setting. High-income countries have developed algorithms with the goal of delivering a stepped care model of service dependent on patient needs; low-income countries are still in need of building regional networks of specialized mental health-care services to address this demand.

Introduction

Pregnancy and motherhood are often portrayed as happy and fulfilling experiences for women and their families. In reality, experiences of pregnancy and motherhood are highly contextualized and can be strongly influenced by situations of adversity. High rates of unplanned pregnancies, challenging social circumstances, low social support, poverty or illness can all significantly influence a women's psychological health during the perinatal period, defined as conception to 12 months postpartum.[1] In addition, the perinatal period is a vulnerable time, associated with exposure to a multitude of physiological, social and psychological risks. Serious consequences of untreated mental illness in the context of low treatment rates among affected women across the globe have led to worldwide efforts to develop methods of preventing, recognizing and treating perinatal psychiatric conditions. Primary health-care systems across the globe need to be sensitized to the risk of depression for women throughout the life-course, particularly during the perinatal period, as a vulnerable stage of life, and serve as key structures around which systems of care are organized.

Mental health itself is broadly defined, not simply as the absence of diagnosable mental illness, but as psychological, social, cultural and spiritual well-being. Therefore, the perinatal stage should be seen as an opportunity to promote health for the family and community as well as to identify and manage parent and infant risk factors and illness. Women are most likely to seek health services and be motivated to improve their well-being during pregnancy and the early postpartum period, and this opportunity needs to be seized. Increased contact with health-care providers during pregnancy and postpartum may provide unique opportunities for screening, prevention and early treatment. The Edinburgh Postnatal Depression Scale (EPDS-10)[2] is the most widely used screening tool for the detection of depression during pregnancy and postpartum,[3,4] and has been validated for use in many countries. Many obstetric groups have noted the high risk of perinatal depression and anxiety disorders and recommended extension of preconception planning to assess and address the known risks and enhance resilience.[5]

As attachment theory emphasizes, early life experiences are crucial for social and emotional development. Because severe mental illness almost systematically results in disabilities in social interaction skills and activities of daily living, the parenting skills of mentally ill parents are a crucial issue for the child. Children with an unstable early foundation are thus left more vulnerable to normative stress and the development of psychiatric disorders over time, because their early childhood experiences dramatically influence their capacity for healthy social and emotional development.[5-7] In order to support families with young children, where a caregiver is struggling with depression, it is essential that community-based interventions are readily available without stigma.[8]

Perinatal mental health: needs and resources across high-, medium- and low-income countries

The World Bank classifies countries on the basis of average gross national income per capita into low-, lower-middle-, upper-middle- and high-income groups.[9] The Human Development Index (HDI) is a composite measure of progress in three dimensions:[10] length of healthy life, access to knowledge, and standard of living. It is calculated as an algorithm of average life expectancy, years of completed formal education and per capita income, on which countries can be ranked and are classified as having high, medium or low development.

In high-income and high-development countries,[9] there has been substantial research since the 1960s about the nature, incidence, prevalence and determinants of mental health problems in women during pregnancy and in the postnatal year, and of interventions to address these. Systematic reviews conclude that in these countries, about 10% of pregnant women and 13% of women who have recently given birth have significant mental health problems, of which depression and anxiety are the most common.[11-14] High-income countries are generally well resourced, including with technologically sophisticated health services provided in a comprehensive health system. In contrast, in most low-income settings, non-psychotic common mental disorders, including depression and anxiety during the perinatal period, are rarely recognized, and there are few services to address them. In addition, low-income countries face additional challenges such as malnourishment, vulnerability to disease and poor access to quality medical care, all of which are competing burdens for perinatal care and interfere with a focus on mental health.[15,16]

In high-income countries, women have universal access to schooling, and there is commitment in most school curricula to education about sexual health, reproductive rights and interpersonal skills. Most women participate in income-generating work and have access to social protection including maternity leave and state benefits. The political environment promotes individual autonomy and endorses and protects women's rights to safety, equality and full social and economic participation. Importantly, they have ready access to comprehensive family planning services, technically sophisticated antenatal care, well-resourced hospitals in which to give birth, skilled multidisciplinary teams of birth attendants and access to specialized and primary health care. There is now general recognition that perinatal mental disorders in women are a public health problem and warrant systematic responses, including as a component of routine antenatal and postnatal screening.[17] Primary health-care practitioners are trained to recognize common mental health problems in women, to provide first-line treatments for those with mild to moderate problems, and referral to specialist psychiatric care for those with more severe problems.[1]

However, most women live in the world's 112 often densely populated, resource-constrained low- and lower-middle-income and low-development countries.[9] Many girls in these settings lack access to primary and secondary education and have limited opportunities to learn about their sexual and reproductive health. Many women live in crowded housing, undertake hard physical work, and are malnourished and vulnerable to communicable diseases. Their lives are often constrained by rigid gender stereotypes about women's roles and responsibilities, including opportunities to earn money, and make financial decisions. Gender-based violence occurs in all societies, but especially in cultures in which women have low status and their rights are not respected. Women in these settings often lack access to family planning services, skilled birth attendants, health-care facilities in which to give birth, and basic and emergency obstetric care. In these settings, there is little awareness of mental health as a determinant of maternal mortality and morbidity.[18,19]

Research about the perinatal mental health of women living in resource-constrained countries has only been conducted more recently, with most studies being published since 2000. This is in part because of competing health priorities, including high rates of maternal deaths from obstetric emergencies, and limited local research resources and capacity. However, research attention has also been slowed by beliefs that traditional confinement and postpartum practices, including social seclusion, prescribed rest, increased practical support from female family members, provision of specific foods and herbal preparations, gift giving and an honoured status were protective of mental health and that perinatal mental health problems are only observable in high-income countries.[19] More recent literature on the study of postnatal depression in cross-cultural contexts raises two concerns: (1) that the contextual factors (risk and protective) that frame a women's experience of depression in different cultures may differ, and (2) the methodological approaches to the measurement of depression, which use diagnostic tools that have been validated predominantly in developed settings, may not be valid in less-developed contexts, and in contexts with greater cultural diversity. There is growing evidence that postnatal depression is not the culture-bound phenomenon purported by Stern and colleagues;[20] instead Posmontier and Horowitz[21] argue that many of the risks and protections hypothesized by traditional practices are operationalized through social support, which is often lacking in modernized societies, particularly in adverse socioeconomic settings, regardless of culture. Reports of culture-bound manifestations of maternal depression are highly variable and uncommon, and an expanding global literature has demonstrated that maternal depression occurs in a variety of countries, in a more similar than a different way, and that it can be effectively measured. In a review of the impact of cultural variables on the experience and recovery from postnatal depression,[22] Bina found that while many studies emphasize the impact of culture on the diagnosis and identification of depression, very few examine the possible impact culture may have on alleviating depression. This review found that five studies, one from Kenya, three from Asia and one from the United States of America (USA) reported an alleviating impact of cultural practices, in particular practices involving mandatory postnatal rest periods. However, many studies in this review showed a neutral effect, or demonstrated that cultural factors such as gender inequality and infant gender bias played a negative role in recovery from postnatal depression. Likewise, Patel[23] showed that as much support can be found for similarities (an etic approach) as for differences (an emic approach) in the international epidemiology of depression. This is because the clinical presentation of depression in all cultures is associated with multiple somatic symptoms of chronic duration. Psychological symptoms are also equally important to the diagnosis of depression, and can be easily elicited in most settings. Overemphasis on the role of culture in postnatal depression may draw attention away from the urgent need for public health investments to prevent, detect and treat postnatal depression for all women, regardless of culture or context.[24]

In the subsequent sections, we will provide exemplary accounts of perinatal mental health-care needs and practices, specifically relating to standard of care and integration in primary care, across low-, medium- and high-income countries worldwide. These contributions have been written by clinicians working in their respective country or geographic area and are meant to demonstrate more specifically the unique challenges in perinatal care across these locations.

Perinatal mental illness through its life-course

Throughout the perinatal period, women can experience the negative effects of mental illness during three stages: *pregnancy* (conception to birth), *early postpartum* (up to 6 weeks after birth) and *late postpartum* (6 weeks to 1 year after birth). While many of these problems are shared by women across the globe, the clinical presentation, and therefore interventions, differ among low-income, medium-income and high-income countries. Ideally, intervention should begin as soon as a woman presents for prenatal care, but most of the interventions described next can be useful during any stage of the perinatal period.

Common contextual factors affecting perinatal well-being

Pregnancy

Pregnancy is a time of role transition for all women. Throughout pregnancy, a woman may be dealing with emotions ranging from terror and anger to joy and excitement. She may be very young, unable to work outside the home, have an abusive or absent partner, be overwhelmed with caring for several other children, fear being ostracized from her community, feel under enormous pressure to have a healthy child, especially after previous pregnancy losses, or be fighting co-occurring illnesses such as diabetes or human immunodeficiency virus (HIV).[25-27] The pregnancy may have been unplanned or unwanted or a result of sexual assault. As the pregnancy progresses and stressors persist, her risk of developing perinatal mental illness increases. Gender-based violence, including both emotional and physical abuse, exerts adverse effects on women's mental health, which can be even more destructive during pregnancy when a woman's dependence is increased.[27-30] Most women who struggle with mental illness prior to or during pregnancy are more likely to continue to struggle later in the postpartum period as well. Thus, early detection and intervention during pregnancy is crucial to positive health outcomes for the mother and her child.[31]

Early postpartum period

In the early postpartum period, a woman is faced with the responsibility of caring for a helpless infant while managing her own physical and mental health needs. She may have increased social support, but attention is now focused on the baby instead of the mother. Having a baby profoundly alters a woman's role as a self-reliant individual and her relationship with her partner, as well as her role within her family and community. In some countries, gender-based factors play a strong role. For example, the birth of a male child may be preferred, whereas baby girls are devalued and fetal sex determination is attributed to women. Role restrictions including responsibilities for household work and infant care and excessive unpaid workloads, especially in multigeneration households in which a daughter-in-law has little autonomy, are also commonly encountered experiences. Some women are forced to resume work shortly after birth, out of financial or social necessity. The experience of labour and delivery may have been invasive and terrifying and can trigger trauma-related anxiety symptoms such as hyperarousal, nightmares and agitation. In addition, the sudden drop in oestrogen that occurs soon after birth may trigger mood swings, irritability, trouble with sleeping, and sadness. This phenomenon, called the "baby blues", is considered a normal part of the early postpartum period and usually subsides within the first few weeks after birth. By contrast, new mothers experiencing hallucinations, periods of confusion, and/or paranoia suffer from a rare but serious disorder called postpartum psychosis and require immediate treatment. A woman with postpartum psychosis is experiencing a break in reality, and often engages in irrational judgement and delusional thinking, which may cause harm to herself or her baby. Few women who suffer from postpartum mental health problems seek help in the early weeks or months after labour, in part because of the burden of leaving the home to access health care, and in part because of the depressive symptoms of amotivation, low energy and social withdrawal. These women benefit from routine home visits to screen for common problems.

Later postpartum period

In the later postpartum period, health care and social support often decrease, leaving both mother and baby vulnerable and sometimes isolated. If the "baby blues" have persisted beyond the first few weeks after birth, true postpartum depression may have developed, but may go undetected and untreated. If women in middle- to high-income countries seek treatment for postpartum depression, they may be reluctant to initiate antidepressant use because they are breastfeeding. Women may become increasingly preoccupied with the baby's health and becoming a capable parent. These preoccupations may become obsessions, and occasionally deteriorate to psychotic thinking. By the time a baby is 6 weeks old, many women are expected to fully resume their normal work responsibilities, whether paid or unpaid. If a mother works outside the home, she must seek childcare for her baby, which can add a financial and emotional burden. Some women may welcome the restored autonomy of not needing to care for the baby during working hours, while others are devastated that they cannot care for the baby full time, and some women experience both emotions simultaneously. At this stage, new mothers can benefit from interventions that connect them and their babies to ongoing sources of social support, as well as education about mental health, mother–infant bonding, nutrition and child development.

Intervention models: low-income countries

In resource-constrained countries, many poor, rural women lack access to basic medical and prenatal care, which means that mental health care often takes a back seat to reducing infant and maternal mortality.[32-35] Overall, the prevalence of perinatal depression is up to 2–3 times higher in low-income than in high-income settings,[6] particularly among the poorest rural-dwelling women who have the least access to primary health-care services.[36]

In *Africa*, the burden of depression and poor maternal mental health most likely relates to women's exposure to multiple depression-related risk factors such as extreme poverty, violence, displacement, migration and the increasing threat of HIV and acquired immunodeficiency syndrome (AIDS).[4,37,38] In addition, since many African women will test for HIV for the first time during their pregnancy, high HIV prevalence has also raised concern about women's psychological health during pregnancy.[25,39-42]

In *south-east Asia*, risk appears to be increased among those who have less access to the protective factors of education, who cannot participate in income-generating work, are denied access to sexual and reproductive health services to promote fertility management, and lack supportive, non-judgemental family relationships.[24,42-44] There is growing evidence over the past decade that, along with other physiological and poverty-related risk factors and the threat of HIV, perinatal depression introduces significant risk for maternal morbidity in low- and middle-income country contexts, and subsequently threatens healthy development in the offspring of affected women.[33,45]

Governments of resource-constrained countries have the complex obligation of providing comprehensive health care to very large populations, with most living in rural or remote areas and experiencing much higher rates of communicable diseases than the populations of high-income countries. However, primary health-care systems vary in structure and reach. Primary health care centres (PHCCs) are staffed by health workers with diverse levels of training, including doctors, nurses and midwives, and country-specific health-care providers with more limited training. Primary health-care services are less likely to be accessible to those who live in remote rural areas,[8,34,46] and mortality and severe morbidities associated with childbirth are much higher in many of these countries than in high-income settings.[47] In Africa, evidence suggests that the task shifting of primary care and prevention functions to community health-care workers (CHWs) improves the health outcomes of populations at a reasonable cost.[48] Limited resources favour a collective clinic-centred care model as compared to the client-centred models frequently seen in well-resourced private settings.[34,49] Harnessing the potential of CHWs to deliver client-centred approaches to prevention and treatment in public health settings requires short, effective and user-friendly screening approaches.[41] Challenges to the detection of depression in pregnancy include inadequate training for health professionals and inadequate time and resource allocation within primary health care, but one of the biggest issues facing clinicians and policy-makers is the stigmatization of psychological problems, which prevents both symptom reporting and delivery of care. Screening within routine care enhances detection, as compared to screening through parallel mental health services, which are often more stigmatized and poorly attended by pregnant women.[50]

No research to date has examined the effectiveness of brief versions of the EPDS in Africa and other countries, creating a lack of routine and efficient screening tools.[39] Further research is required to establish and adapt appropriate CHW-level interventions,[51] and to evaluate treatment and referral algorithms.[52,53]

In order to facilitate such screening, the following is necessary:

- primary health-care nurses must be sensitized to the special risk of mental illness during pregnancy and trained to conduct mental health screening as a routine part of first antenatal care visits

- within primary health-care settings, nurses require treatment guidelines and training to respond to depression when identified
- every primary health-care facility requires at least one mental health trained or psychiatric nurse
- CHWs and prevention of mother-to-child transmission (of HIV) (PMTCT) counsellors should be trained to deliver mental health interventions in clinic or community settings.

In Africa, public health interventions, particularly those linked to the scaling-up of HIV-treatment services will hopefully begin to result in increasing numbers of women attending an increasing number of antenatal sessions during pregnancy.[41] Unfortunately in Africa, most women present late in pregnancy, and women presenting later in pregnancy are often at increased mental health risk.[54,55] Significant efforts need to be made to increase the number of antenatal care visits and to encourage the earlier initiation of care, in line with revised guidelines.[41] In resource-poor settings, mothers may test for pregnancy at 10–14 weeks' gestation, but not receive antenatal care until later in the pregnancy, with many women only initiating antenatal care between 24 and 28 weeks. Initiation of antiviral treatment for HIV from 14 weeks, as in the revised guidelines,[56] presents opportunities to address mental health screening during pregnancy as well if it is effectively integrated with PMTCT and HIV-treatment and -prevention services. All women, regardless of whether they test positive or negative, find HIV testing during pregnancy stressful, and women who test negative but have difficulties with infidelity in their partnerships during the window period for HIV, have been found to be equally at risk of antenatal depression as women who are HIV positive.[39,57] Within a vulnerability–stress framework of depression, HIV must also be viewed as a possible tipping point stressor that may elicit strong emotional responses, reducing resilience and worsening the severity of an existing depression. Finally, risk factors for depression are similar to those for HIV, and women may be exposed to multiple risk factors, including partnership conflict and violence, suggesting that counselling for HIV testing and prevention should include a broader set of mental health interventions.[58–60]

The development of better integration of HIV and mental health care is required to address the following important issues:[41]

- HIV counselling and testing approaches during pregnancy should take a longer-term perspective, given that this is the perspective from which childbearing is experienced
- depressed pregnant woman may be less likely or able to engage with HIV-prevention activities and information, requiring added support and guidance
- testing HIV positive may further motivate women who were already depressed and suicidal, and who perceive HIV as a death sentence, to pursue suicide as a possible resolution, not only for themselves but also for their baby, given their own HIV infection
- PMTCT counsellors need guidance to distinguish between counselling needs and their capacity to intervene with severe mental illness, referring to a nurse or mental health professional when required
- since information about treatment brings hope to HIV-positive women, which is critical to recovery from depression, information during pregnancy should not only focus on prevention but also provide information on maternal health and future treatment options
- women with unplanned and unwanted pregnancies, and those who test HIV positive, may benefit from the opportunity to consider termination of pregnancy, requiring that contact and counselling occur early, ideally prior to routine antenatal care.

Many women in Africa present with minor depression or distress, which can be equally concerning in terms of disability and health functioning.[12,17,62] This phenomenon is not limited to Africa but has also been reported in other low-income countries.[17,62] A variety of interventions are helpful in preventing the risk of onset of depression and reducing the severity of current symptomatology. However, recent evidence continues to suggest that social interventions alone, and in particular interventions focused only on income relief, have less impact on mental health than expected.[30] Instead, services and community-level interventions are urgently needed.[33]

This broader set of interventions may include:

- family psycho-educational activities, helping families support the mental health of pregnant women[41,62]
- fatherhood interventions aimed at encouraging men to take an active role in emotional and practical support towards the pregnancy, despite the context of poverty[26,63]

- interventions focused on social support, which would be equally beneficial to both HIV-positive and HIV-negative women.[64,65]

In communities that are heavily affected by conflict, HIV and poverty, family-centred and community-level interventions can play a moderating role for women who are facing stressful life events and difficult partnerships during pregnancy.[25,60,62,63,65–67] These interventions may focus on:

- community-level reproductive health planning awareness campaigns, which encourage young women and communities to reduce unwanted pregnancies
- family support, which is one of the strongest mediating factors in coping with depression and could have a similar impact on coping with HIV
- social support programmes that increase women's financial security, including basic income support in communities heavily affected by HIV; these have a preventative effect for depression among women who are not depressed[63]
- family-strengthening activities to ensure that families are better able to practically respond to and recover from unplanned pregnancies.

A significant amount of depression seen in primary health-care contexts will be severe and chronic, suggesting that most cases may warrant individual or group psychotherapy interventions and would not respond to social support interventions alone.[68] While interventions may be less expensive within the primary health-care setting, depressive symptoms may hinder compliance with treatment. Where possible, therapeutic interventions should be supported by home-based care to ensure improved compliance and reduce the effect of functional disability on both mother and child. In Africa, using CHWs to deliver interventions for depression in home-based settings is an effective model.[53,69–71]

Unfortunately, group therapy interventions,[53,72] although effective, occur in isolation of the socioeconomic and family stressors that may have precipitated the depression, possibly reducing the positive impact and placing women at risk for relapse.[27] A broader set of psychosocial interventions may be appropriate, alongside therapeutic interventions for severe depression, including:

- improved family planning interventions to strengthen women's autonomy to make reproductive health choices in rural settings
- relationship interventions to improve communication and autonomy within partnerships and encourage partnership support for the pregnancy and the child
- cognitive-skills-based interventions focused on management of interpersonal and social conflict.

Similarly, given guidelines around psychopharmacological treatment for difficult-to-treat populations,[75] including pregnant women,[74] and increasing delivery of complex medical regimes, including antiretroviral therapies[75] and mental health interventions,[76] by community health-care workers in Africa,[77] in cases where warranted, innovation around delivery of minimum care in poorly resourced settings is required.

In Asia, there are only a few randomized controlled trials (RCTs) of primary health-care interventions to reduce maternal mental health problems in resource-constrained settings, but the findings are very promising. Pakistan's Thinking Healthy Program (THP) is a manualized intervention incorporating cognitive and behavioural techniques of active listening, problem-solving, collaboration with the family, non-threatening inquiry into the family's health beliefs and substitution of alternative information when required, and intersession practice activities.[70] It was implemented by lady health workers (LHWs), community-based primary health workers with some secondary education and further training in maternal and child health education and general health information, but none in mental health. The study was conducted in union councils in a rural area 65 km south-east of Rawalpindi city in Pakistan. Union councils each have a population of 15 000 to 20 000 people and are served by a basic health unit (BHU). Each BHU has a multidisciplinary staff including LHWs who are responsible for 100 households in their local villages. The intervention group received: one THP session per week for the last month of pregnancy, three sessions in the first postpartum month and one session per month for the subsequent 9 months (a total of 16 sessions) and the control group received the same number and schedule of home visits, but from an untrained LHW. Study participants were married women aged between 16 and 45 years, in the third trimester of pregnancy, who had been diagnosed by a local psychiatrist, using a structured clinical interview, as experiencing a major depressive episode. After adjusting for covariates, mothers in the intervention group were less likely to be depressed and experiencing functional disability and had better global functioning and perceived social support at 6 and 12 months after the intervention ($P < 0.0001$). Infants of mothers in the intervention group had fewer episodes of diarrhoea at 12 months ($P = 0.04$) and were more likely to be fully immunized ($P = 0.001$).

This structured intervention delivered by non-specialized, briefly trained and supervised local primary health-care workers provides a clear model for other resource-constrained countries that have an equivalent workforce, but would require adaptation in countries that do not. There are potential barriers, for example to home visiting by male community health workers in many settings, but the programme could be modified for use in a group-based format and implemented by non-health workers, including women's organizations.

Intervention models: medium-income countries

In medium-income countries like *India*, perinatal care currently focuses on prevention and treatment of anaemia, recognizing high-risk pregnancy, preventing infections, and ensuring institutional deliveries by trained health workers rather than home deliveries. There are no specific programmes on perinatal mental health issues, and maternal and child health workers are not specifically trained in mental health issues. There are only 4500 psychiatrists, 1500 psychiatric nurses and 300 clinical psychologists for a population of one billion. Mental health professionals have an important role in working closely with maternal and child health workers by offering consultative and training services in early detection and referral. Despite low resources for some mental health facilities, newer antipsychotics, mood stabilizers and antidepressants are available at reasonable cost. Parenting assessments and family planning issues need to be integrated into the routine care of women with severe mental illness, as many will be on psychotropic medication and need special services for preconception counselling, requiring special training of mental health personnel.[77] Joint admissions in specialized mother and baby units are the preferred context for handling postpartum women with severe mental illness, with their babies. However, due to limited resources, there is only one dedicated perinatal psychiatry outpatient service and one mother and baby inpatient unit in the entire country. While tertiary centres can offer specialized services for a very few, they can focus on research, training and evolving innovative ways of delivering mental health services for mothers, including domiciliary care by trained nurses, volunteers, peers or even supervised female relatives.

In countries like India, where maternal health services are fairly well established but there are no programmes for perinatal mental health care, training of health workers and traditional birth attendants is important. Perinatal mental health care needs to be addressed with creative solutions that are cost effective and keep the social, economic and cultural issues in mind. For example, spiritual leaders, such as temple, church and/or Dargah (Muslim) priests are often the first port of call for treatment of mental illness. In addition, nongovernmental organizations (NGOs) and Stree Shakthi (self-help empowerment groups for women) work on increasing health awareness in villages to aid in prevention of perinatal mental illness. Health-care workers are from the community and are more aware of the practices that are present during pregnancy and delivery. The first step towards providing perinatal mental health services is to train these health workers, as well as general practitioners (GPs), to identify signs and symptoms of mental illness in pregnant and postpartum women and bring them for early treatment. In addition, health workers can play a major role in increasing awareness about perinatal mental health issues in the community. Brief leaflets and posters need to be made available in antenatal and paediatric clinics, so that women can self-identify mental health problems. This information should also be available to practitioners of traditional medicine, temple priests and informal healers, so that they can provide the correct advice. Finally, in this era of technology, it is possible to provide support and training to the health-care service providers from any distance. Several centres in India have telemedicine services, which need to be utilized for perinatal mental health. The Internet and mobile technology are other methods that can be used to provide services and follow-up for perinatal mental health services, in order to overcome the human resource shortage.

Intervention models: high-income countries

In the *United Kingdom of Great Britain and Northern Ireland (UK)*, as an example of a high-income country with long history of established national health-care infrastructure, a variety of professionals relate to pregnant and postpartum women, but the GP alone holds the entire medical record. Women with low-risk pregnancies are managed by midwife-led services in primary care. They will probably undertake only one or two hospital antenatal visits, e.g. for ultrasound scans, or none at all. In contrast, those whose pregnancies are deemed high risk receive the majority of their antenatal care in hospital settings, with more input from obstetricians. Referral to antenatal booking *must* include the psychiatric history, including drug or alcohol use, as recommended by the Centre for Maternal and Child Enquiries (CMACE),[78,79] to enable those at high risk of recurrence, e.g. women with bipolar disorder or those with existing serious mental illness, to be identified and referred to a psychiatric service for advice and/or management.

Maternity services are required to train their staff to routinely ask about current and previous mental health problems and use of prescribed and non-prescribed drugs, including illicit drugs and alcohol, and to sensitively enquire about the severity of any problems. Markers of severity are previous treatment by or admission to psychiatric services, or a family history of serious mental illness or suicide. Midwives check on their patients' mental health during pregnancy and during postpartum care. Psychiatric teams caring for pregnant and postpartum women accept a referral directly from midwives if a problem arises requiring their input. Pregnant women with substance abuse/dependence should not be managed solely by GPs and midwives, but be referred to a specialist service within maternity services.

GPs are advised to refer women with pre-existing serious mental illness for preconceptual counselling in relation to risks relating to their illness and psychotropic medication. Ideally, women are seen by a specialist perinatal psychiatry service, but these teams are not universal, so a referral to a more distant service might be required.

The majority of pregnant women with mental health problems will have mild to moderate disorders that can be managed within primary care. National Institute for Health and Clinical Excellence (NICE) guidelines recommend guided self-help, e.g. using books, and brief computerized cognitive- behavioural therapy (CBT).[80] An awareness of local support groups in non-stigmatizing settings, such as children's centres, can help in meeting their needs. The use of health visitors (HVs), mainly community nurses, trained in non-directive counselling (listening visits) delivered at home is an effective intervention,[81] as is cognitive-behavioural counselling delivered by HVs.[82,83] However, although many have been trained to deliver listening visits and some in CBT skills, this is not universal, and refresher training and supervision are very variable. If such skills are not available via HVs, then a referral to the local Improving Access to Psychological Therapies (IAPT) service or equivalent is initiated. The IAPT service in the UK is mandated to prioritize pregnant and postpartum women, although waiting lists can still be long in some areas.[84]

Postpartum care in the community is delivered by community midwives, who, in the majority of cases, will hand over to the HVs at around 10 days postpartum. Most women have their postnatal check carried out by their GP at around 6 weeks after delivery. A small number of women whose deliveries were complicated will have their postnatal check done by their obstetrician.

The NICE guidelines propose that at a woman's first contact with primary care, at her booking visit and postnatally (usually at 4 to 6 weeks and 3 to 4 months), health-care professionals (including midwives, HVs and GPs) should ask two questions to identify possible depression:[85]

- during the past month, have you often been bothered by feeling down, depressed or hopeless?
- during the past month, have you often been bothered by having little interest or pleasure in doing things?

If the woman answers "yes" to both of the initial questions, then she should be asked:

- is this something you feel you need or want help with?

Some areas of the UK are using these questions, but many are using the EPDS.[86,87]

In pregnancy, many women may suffer from short-lived, mild anxiety or depression lasting 2 weeks or less. The recommendation is to monitor for early signs of a more serious affective disorder,[79] by conducting frequent review sessions and referring to mental health services if symptoms persist or worsen, or if the woman already has a personal or family history of serious affective disorder. Some women presenting with perinatal depression or anxiety may actually have physical illness, which, if undetected, may lead to maternal death;[78] GPs screen for somatic symptoms such as fever, elevated heart rate, blood pressure or respiration rate, to screen for medical comorbidity. Women who do not respond to psychological therapy or who have a more severe disorder require augmentation with pharmacotherapy. Those who have recurrent depressive disorder may require long-term antidepressant therapy and this should only be discontinued if the patient is planning a pregnancy or is currently pregnant again, after a full risk–benefit analysis, given the high rate of recurrence on discontinuation.[87]

Severe or treatment-resistant depression, mania or psychosis are referred to secondary mental health services – to a perinatal mental health service if there is one. Unfortunately, these are not equitably distributed across the UK and are concentrated in the south-east, so the woman may have to be referred to general psychiatric services that have little expertise in managing pregnant or recently delivered women and their infants.

To fully meet the needs of women with perinatal mental health problems, a specialist service should be available to the primary care professionals treating them. However, when last surveyed, less than half of the trusts in England provided any specialist perinatal service. Fifty-eight per cent had protocols and documents related to the management of perinatal psychiatric disorders but over half were inadequate or outdated.[88] The number of dedicated inpatient mother and baby beds has fallen since the early 1990s, leaving 75% of trusts without a mother and baby unit, and women who need admission are still being admitted to beds in general adult wards without their infants. Fewer than 25% provide the full range of inpatient and community perinatal mental health services. In Scotland, admission to a mother and baby unit when required is mandated in the Mental Health Act.[89]

In the current economic climate, funds for training of primary care staff have been cut, and reduced staffing numbers mean less time for training. In many areas, HVs have been moved into teams and are no longer based in GP practices, making continuity of care and communication more difficult.

Australia is another example of a high-income perinatal context; however, a nationwide perinatal infrastructure has been established only recently. In Australia, many early childhood nurses working in the community routinely screen for postnatal depression and facilitate self-help and postnatal depression groups, and a few psychiatric inpatient units, public and private, offer beds for admission of mothers and babies together. A critical player in this process has been *beyondblue*, the national depression initiative.[90] Established in 2000, beyondblue is a national, independent, not-for-profit organization working to raise community awareness and literacy about depression and anxiety, reducing stigma, training and supporting the workforce to recognize and manage the problems effectively, and supporting relevant research. With funding and support from beyondblue, research on perinatal mental illness was completed,[91,92] resulting in the National Perinatal Depression Initiative,[93] and guidelines for improving care, such as support for perinatal workforce training and development programmes (including cultural awareness and respect), and identification of appropriate pathways to support and treatment (self-help, community based and inpatient).

Several initiatives addressing psychological assessment and/or depression screening were trialled around Australia from 1990 onwards. Most had the limited goal of identifying major depression or risk factors associated with that diagnosis. The development of one of these programmes, known as Integrated Perinatal Care or IPC,[94] will be described in detail to illustrate the complexities involved.

IPC aims to comprehensively combine physical and mental health aspects for both the mother and infant, and includes husbands or partners and other family members, as appropriate, in the care. Comprehensive care is provided by a suite of collaborating health professionals (e.g. medical, nursing, allied health) and other relevant organizations (e.g. child protection, housing).

Rather than simply identifying or predicting mental *illness* in the mother and then providing psychiatric treatment for her as an individual, IPC focuses on prevention and early intervention for the parents, child and family. Interventions aim to acknowledge all levels of risk and offer information, additional appointments or referral to appropriate health or other services, including, but by no means restricted to, mental health services. IPC was established in a large, stressed, disadvantaged, multicultural area in Sydney. The population included small, but significant, communities of Aboriginal and Torres Strait Islander peoples, with high birth rates and limited resources. The first and most significant level of intervention here is the provision, at primary care level, of care through an appropriately trained and supported professional.

Universal, routine comprehensive consultation is the mode of delivery, to avoid both stigma and missed opportunities, and this occurs at least twice during pregnancy and twice during the first 12 months postpartum, with the first assessment by a trained midwife occurring at the time of the initial visit at the mother's selected hospital, and the first postnatal assessment by a trained early childhood nurse occurring within 2–3 weeks postpartum during a home visit. Where appropriate, the results of the assessment are conveyed to the woman's GP. Thoughtful, competent assessment is critical. These fields of inquiry are familiar to professionals working in child and family psychiatry, but may be outside the comfort zone of many midwives or early childhood nurses. Not only is the integrated consultation longer, but a more sensitive, counselling-oriented stance is required. Staff are expected to engage with the woman, and any other relatives or friends who may be present, conveying a message that the service cares about her personally. Many obstetric and mental health questions are intrusive, so sensitivity as well as competence is required of the interviewer. Basic training starts with four 3-hour modules, comprising workshops on the importance of perinatal mental health, ways to address it with patients and which resources to offer, if needed. This is followed by advanced training modules, on attachment theory and its application to perinatal health, managing anxious clients, basic counselling skills, promoting couples communication, dealing with loss and grief, and any other aspect requested by the staff themselves, such as self-care.

The actual assessment includes collecting general medical and obstetric history, screening for depressive symptoms using the EPDS, and additional psychological and social questions to assess strengths and vulnerabilities in the family (see Box 20.1). These factors are translated into simple, user-friendly questions that are understandable and acceptable to local workers and the differing populations being assessed. The aim of the expanded clinical assessment is to identify a much broader range of problems (or their antecedents) than depression or anxiety per se, whether antenatal or postnatal. The semi-standardized procedure is intended to ascertain whether vulnerability is present or possible, not to assess the details of the problem in depth. Unless further action is urgently required, a weekly multidisciplinary discussion occurs, in which referral and resource availability are determined and formal notes made regarding recommendations.

Box 20.1 Variables associated with reduced maternal (and child) well-being

- *Age*: "too young"; "too old"
- *Obstetric history*: current and past problems, including infertility
- *Health care*: attendance late or minimal, poor diet, exercise, lifestyle
- *Pregnancy*: unplanned and/or unwanted, termination contemplated
- *Drug use*: alcohol, cigarettes, other – past or present (woman or partner)
- *Social support*: perceived lack of availability of practical *and* emotional support from partner, mother, other family, friends (including no partner, abuse, violence)
- *Personality*: low self-esteem, high trait anxiety
- *Mental health*: current and/or previous problems of any kind, e.g. stress, anxiety or depression, especially if pregnancy related or linked with the menstrual cycle or oral contraceptive use
- *Family mental health*: current or past problems or illness
- *Bereavements* (recent or otherwise significant), including miscarriages, terminations, stillbirth, sudden infant death
- *Childhood experiences*: major separations, neglect, witnessing or experiencing physical, emotional or sexual abuse, including harsh, coercive parental discipline
- *Refugee or recent migrant*
- *Community status*: member of a minority group
- *Life events*: recent or longstanding stressors, including cultural, health, housing, financial, employment, language, isolation and related difficulties

---

As the staff gradually gained confidence in their own skills, fewer women were referred to mental health services. Evaluation studies were positive, e.g. the midwives and the women believed the expanded assessment offered better care,[95] and women designated "low risk" fared better at follow-up.[96]

After the initial consultation, if the woman or the midwife has any concerns, and if the woman wishes, further appointments are set up with the midwife, social worker or other appropriate service, e.g. the perinatal and infant mental health service. A letter is sent to the woman's GP, reporting her EPDS score and whether there are any psychosocial aspects of concern. Eventually, the IPC programme was extended into non-English-speaking and indigenous communities. Education modules have been provided for interpreter services. Many translations of the EPDS are now available, including some specifically modified in consultation with Aboriginal and Torres Strait Islander women.

This and related programmes now form an essential part of the infrastructure for Families NSW, the New South Wales Government's strategy to support parents in giving their children, from conception to 8 years, a good start in life. See the web site for more details.[97] Government departments work in partnership with parents, community organizations and local government to provide support and linkage to services according to level of need (stepped care management model; see Figure 20.1). For example, all families will receive at least one postnatal home visit, but high-risk families may be provided with professional home visitation, beginning antenatally and sustained over the following two years.

Antenatal and postnatal health clinic consultations provide many opportunities for prevention, early intervention and health promotion. For best results, these clinics need to be physically and psychologically accessible and user friendly. For those who need care but cannot attend, home visits should be offered and women linked to community resources, including other mothers. Experienced mothers can be trained to provide perinatal care and support for troubled women. Much of the help and support needed by pregnant women and those with young children can be obtained by facilitating group interaction, i.e. self-help. Other resources for self-help that are currently widely used are available using the Internet. These offer self-diagnosis, self-help by working through a training programme based on CBT or other therapies, and online contact with both professionals and fellow sufferers.

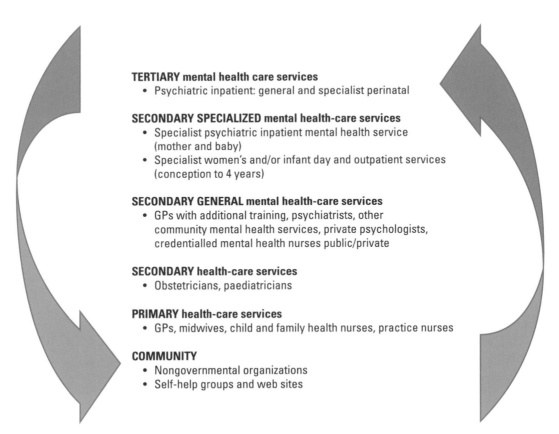

TERTIARY mental health care services
- Psychiatric inpatient: general and specialist perinatal

SECONDARY SPECIALIZED mental health-care services
- Specialist psychiatric inpatient mental health service (mother and baby)
- Specialist women's and/or infant day and outpatient services (conception to 4 years)

SECONDARY GENERAL mental health-care services
- GPs with additional training, psychiatrists, other community mental health services, private psychologists, credentialled mental health nurses public/private

SECONDARY health-care services
- Obstetricians, paediatricians

PRIMARY health-care services
- GPs, midwives, child and family health nurses, practice nurses

COMMUNITY
- Nongovernmental organizations
- Self-help groups and web sites

Figure 20.1 Stepped model of care (Australia). Patients do not necessarily progress in an orderly fashion from one tier to the next – in either direction

Finally, the *United States of America* is the last example of a high-income country, yet standards for perinatal services are not nationwide but state and community dependent. What follows is the description for an "ideal standard" prototype, which may hold up only in more urban communities connected to large university-based teaching hospitals and outpatient clinics. Overall, while pregnant women have increased contact with health-care providers, depression has been under-recognized and undertreated in obstetric practices.[98] Typically, one of the validated screening tools for perinatal depression such as the Patient Health Questionnaire (PHQ-9) or EPDS is administered. Current practice in most primary settings is to screen during the first visit, around 28 weeks of gestation and at 6 weeks postpartum. The recommendation is that screening for depression should continue throughout the first year after delivery, which would ideally occur in the paediatric offices during well-child visits.

Women who screen positive (≥9 on the PHQ and/or EPDS, any suicidality) discuss the results with the primary care provider and are then referred for a comprehensive psychiatric assessment. Unfortunately, referral to outside clinics reduces the likelihood for women to be properly evaluated and treated, as women get "lost in transition". Barriers such as transportation, mental health providers with different cultural backgrounds, lack of available mental health providers, and stigma often stand in the way of appropriate treatment.

All reproductive health-care providers should be educated about perinatal mental health symptoms and disorders and normal thought patterns and behaviours, so that if any concerns are raised, feelings and thoughts can be discussed and normalized prior to making the next step. Since perinatal depression has been associated with psychosocial stressors, preventive psycho-education for women and their partners, as well as other family members, should be offered. Information and education provided in the primary settings could include nutrition, exercise, bonding with a child, typical and problematic perinatal mood patterns, and simple coping strategies.

Perinatal depression screening does not improve treatment entry or clinical outcome.[99] Therefore, a model in which assessment and treatment of mild to moderate cases would occur in the primary setting has been proposed and studied. In the stepped care disease management model, a full psychiatric assessment is completed by a behavioural specialist who is physically located at the primary care site. Mild to moderate perinatal depression is further treated at the primary care site by offering psychotherapy, medication management or both. More severe cases of perinatal unipolar depression, bipolar mood disorder and psychosis are referred out to be treated in mental health clinics. The stepped care model has not been widely implemented,[100] but could significantly improve the frequency of treatment engagement and overall outcome. An illustration of the management model implemented in Illinois, USA follows.

Summary of a stepped care management model in Illinois, USA

- Women are screened for perinatal depression by their primary care provider.
- A validated tool is used (EPDS or PHQ-9).
- Screening occurs on several occasions during pregnancy and postpartum.
- When screening is positive, findings should be normalized and discussed with the patient, i.e. PHQ-9 symptoms may sometimes overlap with physical symptoms of pregnancy.
- If screening is above the cut-off score, concern for perinatal depression is raised and a full mental health assessment is necessary. Ideally, the assessment would occur in the primary setting; otherwise a referral is made to a mental health clinic.

Treatment algorithms

If mild to moderate unipolar depression is detected

- Refer to individual therapy, usually cognitive-behavioural or interpersonal techniques, or group therapy, either supportive or therapeutic structured, if available.
- Symptoms requiring medication management could be prescribed by the woman's primary care physician.

If severe unipolar depression, bipolar mood disorder and/or psychosis is detected

- Severe symptoms, such as psychosis or suicidality, require referral to a mental health clinic or psychiatric hospital for further assessment and treatment.

- Various medications can be used, depending on symptoms. Antidepressants, antipsychotics, mood stabilizers, hypnotics, anti-anxiety medication and electroconvulsive therapy can be considered. During pregnancy and breastfeeding, risks versus benefits are carefully evaluated and the patient and family are educated about the choices and potential consequences of both treatment and lack of treatment of a perinatal mental health disorder.

Summary and recommendations

- The focus of maternal health in most developing countries has been mainly on reducing maternal and infant mortality. It will be important to expand it to also include maternal mental health.

- The strongest predictor of perinatal depression is the presence of a previous history of depression.

- Despite limited research, the prevalence of perinatal mental illness appears to be highest in the poorest women who live in rural areas. The presumption that culturally prescribed postnatal care is welcome and available to all does not reflect reality for many women.[101]

- Women face multiple and cumulative risks, including poverty and human immunodeficiency virus (HIV) infection, that significantly increase their risk of depression during the perinatal period. Despite the availability of effective treatment, perinatal depression frequently remains undetected and untreated, due to a powerful stigma in many countries.

- Increased contact with health-care providers during pregnancy and the postpartum period may provide unique opportunities for screening, prevention and early treatment. However, in resource-constrained countries, early detection and prevention of depression during pregnancy and the postpartum period is limited by critical shortages of health-care professionals.

- With structured training and supervision, community-based primary health-care workers can learn to recognize and respond helpfully to women experiencing perinatal mental illness.

- Since treatment for depression can effectively be delivered by lay professionals and community health-care workers, developing brief screening methods is an important step in optimizing prevention and treatment during pregnancy and the postpartum period.

- There is a need in all countries for local evidence about the nature, prevalence and risks for perinatal mental illness.

- Structured manualized interventions need to be adapted to make them culturally acceptable and appropriate for use in primary health-care settings in resource-constrained countries.

- Successfully translating evidence-based strategies from research into clinical practice is neither simple nor straightforward.

- Basic and ongoing training, support and supervision options for staff are essential. Flexible basic and advanced training modules need to be developed to suit local needs. These may be in written, manualized, online and similar formats, but should include some face-to-face training time. Staff unaccustomed to participating in reflective work or clinical supervision may need encouragement to participate. A well-trained clinician constitutes a significant intervention.

- In high-income countries, a significant portion of women suffering from perinatal mental health disorders can be managed in a primary care setting.

- All providers in primary care settings should be sensitive to potential issues in the perinatal period, know how to administer and interpret screening tools, and understand that positive screening is not a diagnostic tool, but a signal that the woman requires a full assessment, which should ideally be completed in a primary care setting as well.

- All prescribers in primary care settings should have some knowledge regarding medication (mostly antidepressant/anti-anxiety) use during pregnancy and breastfeeding. Occasionally, a primary care provider could refer a woman for a second opinion with a reproductive psychiatrist, after which the treatment can resume in a primary care setting.

- More complex cases should be referred out and treated in a mental health-care setting by specialized personnel.
- Different centres and clinics providing evaluations and treatment for women with perinatal mental health disorders should develop a regional network.

Conclusions

Ensuring that women in need of perinatal mental health care receive adequate services is a challenge across the globe. The prevalence of perinatal mental illness is high, especially among poorer women living in rural areas or in cities with more barriers to care, such as lack of transportation or money to cover the costs of treatment. In many resource-constrained countries, even emergency health care is lacking. Many people go without basic services like immunizations and antibiotics for infections, and the focus of perinatal health has been mainly on reducing maternal and infant mortality. It is difficult to provide routine obstetric care, and even more difficult to assess for and offer perinatal mental health-care services. Professional health-care workers are scarce, but trained community workers often successfully provide the bulk of services. Even in wealthier countries, health care during pregnancy is often focused on evaluating and maintaining physical health. Taking mental health-care needs into consideration is sometimes viewed as an unnecessary burden on staff, despite the clearly negative effects of untreated mental illness on mother and child.

In resource-constrained countries, such as found in Africa, large parts of India, or south/south-east Asia, far less research has been done to assess the mental health-care needs of pregnant and postpartum women, which means that fewer services are available and negative health outcomes are more common. In order to assess and deliver care to women in these countries, health-care workers have employed a variety of innovative, culturally sensitive and community-specific techniques, including training community health workers to offer interventions for depression in home-based settings, and combining perinatal visits with HIV treatment. Pakistan's successful Thinking Healthy Program, which was implemented by non-specialized, briefly trained local health-care workers, can be adapted to fit many communities in resource-constrained countries. Stigmatization of psychological problems is a barrier to reporting symptoms and receiving treatment across the world, but is a particular challenge in resource-constrained countries. In these countries, training workers to go into local communities to deliver mental health-care services to each individual woman alongside routine health care is essential to the reduction of negative health outcomes. Increased contact with health-care workers during pregnancy, combining psychological services with less-stigmatized health care, developing brief depression-screening methods and considering cultural adaptations of traditional psychiatric techniques, will contribute to more women receiving care during this vulnerable time.

In order to gain a true perspective on the needs of high-risk women and deliver adequate care, perinatal mental illness must first be acknowledged as a serious problem affecting women everywhere. Then, steps need to be taken to assess the needs of women in each country, using screening tools that have been widely culturally validated with the goal to conduct large- or small-scale research on the risk factors for developing perinatal mental illness, as well as the barriers to receiving mental health care in each community across the globe. Once needs have been assessed, each community is better equipped to develop culturally sensitive services that will be accepted by the population.

In high- and medium-income countries such as Australia, the UK, the USA and parts of India, ample research has provided a wealth of information about perinatal mental illness, and more resources are available to implement programmes that meet the needs of the population, thus decreasing the likelihood of negative health outcomes. Research in these countries has demonstrated that physical health can significantly impact mental health during pregnancy, and treating both is crucial. Fewer women live in remote, rural areas, and government programmes offer financial assistance, making health-care centres a practical option. In addition, awareness of perinatal mental illness is increased with education, stigma is decreased and psychopharmacology is more available to women in these countries. The establishment of psychiatric mother and baby units in the UK and Australia (and other European locations such as France and Germany) took perinatal mental health care one step further by promoting strong relationships between mother and child, along with psychotherapy, parenting education and increased support. Overall, more resources, detailed research, accurate screening tools, awareness of the problem by both the community and government officials, and trained medical and psychiatric professionals, combined with fewer barriers, contribute to more effective delivery of care.

References

1   Muzik M, Borovska S. Perinatal depression: implications for child mental health. *Mental Health in Family Medicine*, 2010, 7:1–10.

2   Cox JL, Holden JM, Sagovsky R. Detection of postnatal depression. Development of the 10-item Edinburgh Postnatal Depression Scale. *British Journal of Psychiatry*, 1987, 150:782–786.

3   Halbreich U, Karkun S: Cross-cultural and social diversity of prevalence of postpartum depression and depressive symptoms. *Journal of Affective Disorders*, 2006, 91:97–111.

4   Sawyer A, Ayers S, Smith H. Pre- and postnatal psychological wellbeing in Africa: a systematic review. *Journal of Affective Disorders*, 2010, 123(1–3):17–29.

5   Stein A et al. The influence of postnatal psychiatric disorder on child development. *Psychopathology*, 2009, 42:11–21.

6   Parsons CE et al. Postnatal depression and its effects on child development: a review of evidence from low- and middle-income countries. *British Medical Bulletin*, 2011, 3 December epub ahead of print.

7   Muzik M, Thelen K, Rosenblum K. Perinatal depression: detection and treatment. Invited review. *Neuropsychiatry*, 2011, 1:179–195.

8   Patel V et al. Improving access to psychological treatments: lessons from developing countries. *Behaviour Research and Therapy*, 2011, 49:523–528.

9   World Bank Development Indicators (http://data.worldbank.org/about/world-development-indicators-data, accessed 18 November 2011).

10 *Human Development Report 2010 – 20th anniversary edition. The real wealth of nations: pathways to human development*. New York, United Nations Development Programme, 2010.

11 Bennett HA et al. Prevalence of depression during pregnancy: systematic review. *Obstetrics and Gynecology*, 2004, 103:698–709.

12 O'Hara M, Swain A. Rates and risks of postpartum depression – a meta-analysis. *International Review of Psychiatry*, 1996, 8:37–54.

13 Gavin NI et al. Perinatal depression: a systematic review of prevalence and incidence. *Obstetrics and Gynecology*, 2005, 106:1071–1083.

14 Robertson E et al. Antenatal risk factors for postpartum depression: a synthesis of recent literature. *General Hospital Psychiatry*, 2004, 26:289–295.

15 Patel V et al. Prioritizing health problems in women in developing countries: comparing the financial burden of reproductive tract infections, anaemia and depressive disorders in a community survey in India. *Tropical Medicine and International Health*, 2007, 12:130–139.

16 Rahman A et al. The neglected 'm' in MCH programmes – why mental health of mothers is important for child nutrition. *Tropical Medicine and International Health*, 2008, 13:579–583.

17 Muzik M et al. When depression complicates childbearing: guidelines for screening and treatment during antenatal and postpartum obstetric care. *Obstetrics and Gynecology Clinics of North America*, 2009, 36:771–88, ix–x.

18 Eustace RW, Ilagan PR. HIV disclosure among HIV positive individuals: a concept analysis. *Journal of Advanced Nursing*, 2010, 66:2094–2103.

19 Patel V et al. Treatment and prevention of mental disorders in low-income and middle-income countries. *The Lancet*, 2007, 370:991–1005.

20 Stern G, Kruckman L. Multi-disciplinary perspectives on post-partum depression: an anthropological critique. *Social Science and Medicine*, 1983, 17:1027–1041.

21 Posmontier B, Horowitz JA. Postpartum practices and depression prevalences: technocentric and ethnokinship cultural perspectives. *Journal of Transcultural Nursing*, 2004, 15:34–43.

22 Bina R. The impact of cultural factors upon postpartum depression: a literature review. *Health Care for Women International*, 2008, 29:568–592.

23 Patel V. Cultural factors and international epidemiology. *British Medical Bulletin*, 2001. 57:33–45.

24 Patel V, Rodrigues M, DeSouza N. Gender, poverty, and postnatal depression: a study of mothers in Goa, India. *American Journal of Psychiatry*, 2002, 159:43–47.

25 Stein A et al. Babies of a pandemic. *Archives of Diseases of Childhood*, 2005, 90:116–118.

26 Ramchandani P, Psychogiou L. Paternal psychiatric disorders and children's psychosocial development. *The Lancet*, 2009, 374:646–653.

27 Pereira M, Canavarro MC. Relational contexts in adjustment to pregnancy of HIV-positive women: relationships, social support and personal adjustment. *AIDS Care*, 2009, 21:301–308.

28 *Women's mental health: an evidence based review, in mental health determinants and populations department of mental health and substance dependence.* Geneva, World Health Organization, 2000.

29 Lund C et al. Poverty and common mental disorders in low and middle income countries: A systematic review. *Social Science and Medicine*, 2010, 71:517–528.

30 Nasreen HE et al. Prevalence and associated factors of depressive and anxiety symptoms during pregnancy: a population based study in rural Bangladesh. *BMC Women's Health*, 2011, 11:22.

31 Muzik M et al. Depression in pregnancy: detection, comorbidity and treatment. *Asia-Pacific Psychiatry*, 2010, 2:7–18.

32 Kieling C et al. Child and adolescent mental health worldwide: evidence for action. *The Lancet*, 2011, 378:1515–1525.

33 Walker SP et al. Child development: risk factors for adverse outcomes in developing countries. *The Lancet*, 2007, 369:145–157.

34 Patel V et al. Reducing the treatment gap for mental disorders: a WPA survey. *World Psychiatry*, 2010, 9:169–176.

35 Walker SP et al. Inequality in early childhood: risk and protective factors for early child development. *The Lancet*, 2011, 378:1325–1338.

36 *Mental health aspects of women's reproductive health: a global review of literature.* Geneva, World Health Organization, 2009.

37 Broadhead JC, Abas MA. Life events, difficulties and depression among women in an urban setting in Zimbabwe. *Psychological Medicine*, 1998, 28:29–38.

38 Brandt R. Putting mental health on the agenda for HIV+ women: a review of evidence from sub-Saharan Africa. *Women and Health*, 2009, 49:215–228.

39 Rochat TJ et al. Depression among pregnant rural South African women undergoing HIV testing. *JAMA*, 2006, 295:1376–1378.

40 Rochat T, Richter L, Shisana O. 'What now, what next': reflecting on the vulnerability of children and youth in the context of human immunodeficiency virus and acquired immunodeficiency syndrome. *Vulnerable Children and Youth Studies*, 2008, 3: p. 85–91.

41 Rochat TJ et al. Towards a family-centered approach to HIV treatment and care for HIV-exposed children, their mothers and their families in poorly resourced settings. *Future Virology*, 2011, 6:687–696.

42 Rahman A, Iqbal Z, Harrington R. Life events, social support and depression in childbirth: perspectives from a rural community in the developing world. *Psychological Medicine*, 2003, 33:1161–1167.

43 Gausia K et al. Antenatal depression and suicidal ideation among rural Bangladeshi women: a community-based study. *Archives of Women's Mental Health*, 2009, 12:351–358.

44 Fisher J et al. Common perinatal mental disorders in northern Viet Nam: community prevalence and health care use. *Bulletin of the World Health Organization*, 2010, 88:737–745.

45 Minkovitz CS et al. Maternal depressive symptoms and children's receipt of health care in the first 3 years of life. *Pediatrics*, 2005, 115:306–314.

46 Patel V et al. Effect of maternal mental health on infant growth in low income countries: new evidence from South Asia. *BMJ*, 2004, 328:820–823.

47 *Country profiles on maternal and newborn health.* Geneva, World Health Organization, 2011.

48 McPake B, Mensah K. Task shifting in health care in resource-poor countries. *The Lancet*, 2008, 372:870–871.

49 Patel V et al. Effectiveness of an intervention led by lay health counsellors for depressive and anxiety disorders in primary care in Goa, India (MANAS): a cluster randomised controlled trial. *The Lancet*, 2010, 376:2086–2095.

50 Lusskin SI, Pundiak TM, Habib SM. Perinatal depression: hiding in plain sight. *Canadian Journal of Psychiatry*, 2007, 52:479–488.

51 Patel VL et al. Cognitive and learning sciences in biomedical and health instructional design: A review with lessons for biomedical informatics education. *Journal of Biomedical Informatics*, 2009, 42:176–197.

52 Global Health Workforce Alliance. *Integrating community health workers in national health workforce plans. Community health workers – key messages.* Geneva, World Health Organization, 2010 (http://www.who.int/workforcealliance/knowledge/resources/CHW_KeyMessages_English.pdf, accessed 18 November 2011).

53 Murray LK et al. Building capacity in mental health interventions in low resource countries: an apprenticeship model for training local providers. *International Journal of Mental Health Systems*, 2011, 5:30.

54 Elul B et al. Pregnancy desires, and contraceptive knowledge and use among prevention of mother-to-child transmission clients in Rwanda. *AIDS*, 2009, 23(Suppl. 1):S19–26.

55 Leigh B, Milgrom J. Risk factors for antenatal depression, postnatal depression and parenting stress. *BMC Psychiatry*, 2008, 8:24.

56 *Rapid advice: use of antiretroviral drugs for treating pregnancy in women and preventing HIV infection in infants.* Geneva, World Health Organization, 2010.

57 Rochat TJ et al. The prevalence and clinical presentation of antenatal depression in rural South Africa. *Journal of Affective Disorders*, 2011, 135:362–373.

58 Dunkle KL et al. Gender-based violence, relationship power, and risk of HIV infection in women attending antenatal clinics in South Africa. *The Lancet*, 2004, 363:1415–1421.

59 Jewkes RK et al. Intimate partner violence, relationship power inequity, and incidence of HIV infection in young women in South Africa: a cohort study. *The Lancet*, 2010, 376:41–48.

60 Ketchen B, Armistead L, Cook S. HIV infection, stressful life events, and intimate relationship power: the moderating role of community resources for black South African women. *Women and Health*, 2009, 49:197–214.

61 Rahman A, Creed F. Outcome of prenatal depression and risk factors associated with persistence in the first postnatal year: prospective study from Rawalpindi, Pakistan. *Journal of Affective Disorders*, 2007, 100:115–121.

62 Betancourt TS et al. Family-centred approaches to the prevention of mother to child transmission of HIV. *Journal of the International AIDS Society*, 2010, 13(Suppl. 2):S2.

63 Ramchandani PG et al. Predictors of postnatal depression in an urban South African cohort. *Journal of Affective Disorders*, 2009, 113:279–284.

64 King E et al. Interventions for improving the psychosocial well-being of children affected by HIV and AIDS. *Cochrane Database of Systematic Reviews*, 2009, (2):CD006733.

65 Richter L, Rochat T. Foundations of human development: maternal care in the early years. In: Chandra PS et al., eds. *Contemporary topics in women's mental health*. Chichester, John Wiley & Sons, Ltd, 2009:559–579.

66 Pequegnat W, Bell CC, Allison S. The role of families among orphans and vulnerable children in confronting HIV/AIDS in sub-Saharan Africa. In: Pequegnat W, Bell CC, eds. *Family and HIV/AIDS*. New York, Springer, 2012, 173–194.

67 Richter LM et al. Strengthening families to support children affected by HIV and AIDS. *AIDS Care*, 2009, 21(S1):3–12.

68 McKee MD et al. Health-related functional status in pregnancy: relationship to depression and social support in a multi-ethnic population. *Obstetrics and Gynecology*, 2001, 97:988–993.

69 Patel V, Kirkwood B. Perinatal depression treated by community health workers. *The Lancet*, 2008, 372:868–869.

70 Rahman A et al. Cognitive behaviour therapy-based intervention by community health workers for mothers with depression and their infants in rural Pakistan: a cluster-randomised controlled trial. *The Lancet*, 2008, 372:902–909.

71 Rahman A et al. Cluster randomized trial of a parent-based intervention to support early development of children in a low-income country. *Child Care Health and Development*, 2009, 35:56–62.

72 Bolton P et al. Group interpersonal psychotherapy for depression in rural Uganda: a randomized controlled trial. *JAMA*, 2003, 289:3117–3124.

73 American Psychiatric Association and the American College of Obstetricians and Gynecologists. The management of depression during pregnancy: a Report from the American Psychiatric Association and the American College of Obstetricians and Gynecologists. *Obstetrics and Gynecology*, 2009, 114:703–713.

74 Kuehn BM. Depression guideline highlights choices, care for hard-to-treat or pregnant patients. *JAMA*, 2010, 304:2465.

75 Selke HM et al. Task-shifting of antiretroviral delivery from health care workers to persons living with HIV/AIDS: clinical outcomes of a community-based program in Kenya. *Journal of Acquired Immune Deficiency Syndromes*, 2010, 55:483–490.

76 Petersen I et al. A task shifting approach to primary mental health care for adults in South Africa: human resource requirements and costs for rural settings. *Health Policy and Planning*, 2011, 15 February epub ahead of print.

77 Chandra PS. Post-partum psychiatric care in India: the need for integration and innovation. *World Psychiatry* 2004, 3:99–100.

78 Lewis G. *Saving mothers' lives: reviewing maternal deaths to make motherhood safer – 2003–2005. The Seventh Report on Confidential Enquiries into Maternal Deaths in the United Kingdom.* London, The Confidential Enquiry into Maternal and Child Health (CEMACH), 2007.

79 Wilkinson H; Trustees and Medical Advisers. Saving mothers' lives. Reviewing maternal deaths to make motherhood safer: 2006–2008. *British Journal of Obstetrics and Gynaecology*, 2011, 118:1402–1403.

80 Hairon N. NICE guidance on antenatal and postnatal mental health. *Nursing Times*, 2007, 103:25–26.

81 Holden JM, Sagovsky R, Cox JL. Counselling in a general practice setting: controlled study of health visitor intervention in treatment of postnatal depression. *BMJ*, 1989, 298:223–226.

82 Appleby L et al. A controlled study of fluoxetine and cognitive-behavioural counselling in the treatment of postnatal depression. *BMJ*, 1997, 314:932–936.

83 Morrell CJ et al. Clinical effectiveness of health visitor training in psychologically informed approaches for depression in postnatal women: pragmatic cluster randomised trial in primary care. *BMJ*, 2009, 338:a3045.

84 Improving Access to Psychological Therapies. *Perinatal positive practice guide.* London, Department of Health, 2009.

85 *Antenatal and postnatal mental health: clinical management and service guidance.* London: National Institute for Health and Clinical Excellence, 2007 (CG45) (http://www.nice.org.uk/nicemedia/live/11004/30433/30433.pdf, accessed 2 December 2011).

86 Summers AL, Logsdon MC. Web sites for postpartum depression: convenient, frustrating, incomplete, and misleading. *MCN. The American Journal of Maternal Child Nursing*, 2005, 30:88–94; quiz 95–86.

87 Einarson A, Selby P, Koren G. Abrupt discontinuation of psychotropic drugs during pregnancy: fear of teratogenic risk and impact of counselling. *Journal of Psychiatry and Neuroscience*, 2001, 26:44–48.

88 Oluwatayo O, Friedman T. A survey of specialist perinatal mental health services in England. *Psychiatric Bulletin*, 2005, 29:177–179.

89 Alder EM et al. Policy and practice in the management of postnatal depression in Scotland. *Archives of Women's Mental Health*, 2008, 11:213–219.

90 beyondblue (www.beyondblue.org.au, accessed 18 November 2011).

91 Buist A et al. Acceptability of routine screening for perinatal depression. *Journal of Affective Disorders*, 2006, 93:233–237.

92 Buist A, Bliszta J. *The* beyondblue *national postnatal screening program. Prevention and early intervention 2001–2005. Final report.* Volume 1. Melbourne: beyondblue: the national depression initiative, 2006 (http://www.beyondblue.org.au/index.aspx?link_id=4.665&tmp=FileDownload&fid=348, accessed 2 December 2011).

93 Austin M-P and the Guidelines Expert Advisory Committee. *Clinical practice guidelines. Depression and related disorders – anxiety, bipolar disorder and puerperal psychosis – in the perinatal period. A guideline for primary care health professionals.* Melbourne, beyondblue: the national depression initiative, 2011.

94 Henshaw C, Elliott S. *Screening for perinatal depression.* London, Philadelphia, Jessica Kingsley, 2005.

95 Matthey S et al. *Evaluation of the routine psychosocial assessment at Liverpool Hospital antenatal clinic: June 2002.* Sydney, WAPMHU Publications, 2002.

96 Karatas JC, Matthey S, Barnett B. Antenatal psychosocial assessment: how accurate are we in determining 'low-risk' status? A pilot study. *Archives of Women's Mental Health*, 2009, 12:97–103.

97 Families NSW (www.families.nsw.gov.au, accessed 18 November 2011).

98 Coates AO, Schaefer CA, Alexander JL. Detection of postpartum depression and anxiety in a large health plan. *Journal of Behavioral Health Services and Research*, 2004, 31:117–133.

99 Gilbody S, Sheldon T, House A. Screening and case-finding instruments for depression: a meta-analysis. *Canadian Medical Association Journal*, 2008, 178:997–1003.

100 Miller L, Shade M, Vasireddy V. Beyond screening: assessment of perinatal depression in a perinatal care setting. *Archives of Women's Mental Health*, 2009, 12:329–334.

101 Fisher JR et al. Prevalence, nature, severity and correlates of postpartum depressive symptoms in Vietnam. *British Journal of Obstetrics and Gynaecology*, 2004, 111:1353–1360.

Part IV

Bodily distress disorders in primary care mental health

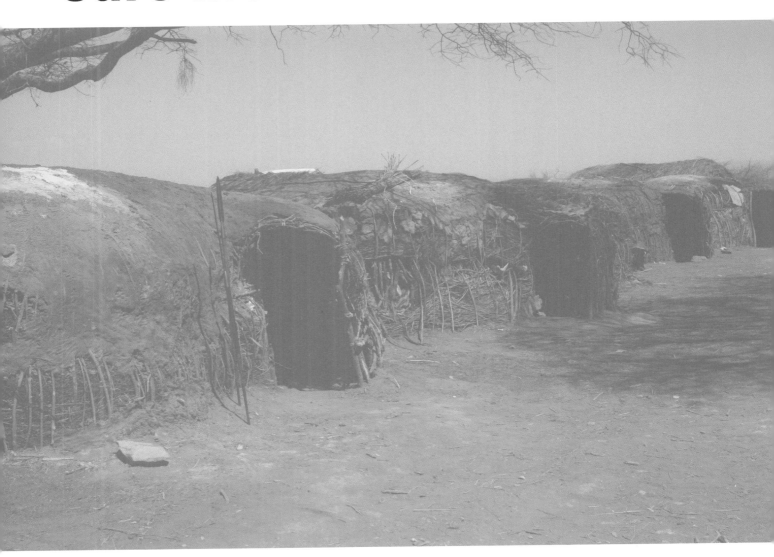

21 Bodily distress syndrome in primary care mental health

Norman H Rasmussen and David C Agerter

Key messages

- The World Health Organization has proposed the term "bodily distress syndrome" should be used instead of "medically unexplained symptoms" (MUS) but the literature to date uses MUS.
- Bodily distress syndrome is common and presents a challenging condition in primary care.
- The presentation of bodily distress syndrome in the primary care clinic may vary from country to country and may take new forms as cultures evolve and medical paradigms shift.
- The relevance of bodily distress syndrome to primary care health services delivery is related to patient suffering, functional disability and cost to the health-care system.
- Conventional wisdom for understanding the onset and course of bodily distress syndrome is embedded in a multifactorial explanatory model.
- Gold standard assessment is based on patient self-report tests that are compatible with the time constraints in the routine office visit.
- Cognitive-behavioural interventions delivered in specialty mental settings and selective serotonin reuptake inhibitor antidepressant medication prescribed in primary care settings have the greatest empirical support for treatment effectiveness.

Introduction

Bodily distress syndrome, also known as "medically unexplained symptoms" (MUS), presents a clinical challenge in primary health care because of patient suffering, the often poor response to intervention and subsequent functional disability, and the high use of medical services and associated costs.[1-3] *Bodily distress syndrome*[4] is the new term proposed by the World Health Organization (WHO), which moves us from the therapeutic nihilism suggested by the terminology *medically unexplained symptoms* and, furthermore, better supports patient engagement.[5] It should be noted, however, that this syndrome has been classically described in the literature as "medically unexplained symptoms" and most of the scholarly work in the field is referenced using these key terms. Interest in patients with medically unexplained syndromes is on the rise, which is understandable considering it is the most common disorder seen in primary care, especially when including the abridged form of MUS.[6] While recognizing the value of the proposed new term, "bodily distress syndrome", this chapter uses "MUS" when discussing published work, as it is the term most frequently used in the literature discussed.

This chapter particularly addresses providers in the primary care setting (e.g. family physicians, internists, nurse practitioners, case and care managers, nurses, psychologists, psychiatrists, social workers) but may also be of interest to a broader audience in tertiary internal medicine. Important topics relevant to primary care in understanding, identifying, and treating bodily distress syndrome are covered: emergence and the developmental course; epidemiologic factors; cross-cultural differences; relevance to the delivery of mental health in primary care; the role of symptoms; comorbidities; biological, cognitive-perceptual, developmental and personality explanatory mechanisms; assessment and management; and key stakeholders. The chapter emphasizes equipping the family physician (and care team) with knowledge and implementation skills for brief and user-friendly dispensed interventions that are empirically supported best practices.[7–9]

Approximately 50% of all outpatient medical visits are related to somatic concerns, of which at least one-third to one-half are medically unexplained.[10] Many are individual physical reports, such as pain (e.g. low back pain, headache), but others are clusters of somatic symptoms referred to as *functional somatic syndrome* (e.g. fibromyalgia, irritable bowel syndrome). The functional somatic syndromes have overlapping symptoms and are comparable in terms of psychiatric comorbidity, functional impairment and medical service use.[11] For an in-depth recent review of the four most common functional syndromes – fibromyalgia, irritable bowel, chronic fatigue and multiple chemical sensitivity – Susan K Johnson's textbook (2008) is recommended.[12]

Patients who present with physical symptoms that cannot be explained with pathologically defined disease are commonly seen in primary care.[13,14] Their symptoms represent a spectrum of conditions ranging from mild and self-limiting to severe and disabling.[15] Kroenke et al.[16] and Rasmussen et al.[17] demonstrated that as the number and severity of symptoms increase, so do the level of disability, prevalence of psychiatric disorder, and dysfunctional illness beliefs. A British descriptor of the physician's reaction to a patient with bodily distress syndrome is the "heartsink experience",[18] which reflects the challenging and often chronic nature of this condition.

Lipowski described persistent somatization as the experience and communication of psychological distress through physical symptoms.[19] Furthermore, the patient with persistent bodily distress syndrome has a maladaptive and largely unconsciously motivated coping strategy in struggling with life's demands and frustrations. This persistent form of bodily distress syndrome is of most concern to the primary care provider.

Evidence-based treatment of patients who have bodily distress syndrome or somatoform disorders has been established for cognitive-behavioural therapy (CBT)[20,21] and antidepressants.[22] Comprehensive reviews of these treatments are available.[23–26]

The brief and valid interventions proposed in this chapter are presented in a stepped care manner, to be delivered directly by the primary care provider independent of the type of collaborative or integrated primary care medical–behavioural health-care model (or solo practice) that might characterize the primary care provider's current practice.[27] Furthermore, the brief, stepped interventions are designed to construct a solution to the patient's vexing problem, with minimal, if any, historical analysis, and to promote patient autonomy, self-efficacy, self-management, and emotion regulation.

Before the advent of empirically supported brief interventions designed for use by the family physician and the physician's care team, the standard best practice medical care visit for a patient with MUS was often grounded in a contingency-based behavioural management model.[28] This model was a rudimentary stepped care approach that, at the first level, emphasized validating the patient's symptoms as real, performing a brief and focused physical examination, and scheduling increasingly spaced follow-up visits, rather than patient-initiated office appointments, which are usually triggered by new or exacerbated symptoms and associated illness distress. The second level of care involved a conjoint family physician–mental health specialist reflecting interview with the patient (and family members if the patient chose to invite them) that focused on family-of-origin dynamics and current biopsychosocial stressors. This second care level was aimed at changing the medical visit agenda from symptoms only to symptom–life event conjunctive possibilities (i.e. making the case for a link between physical symptoms and psychological factors). The final care step involved a mental health specialty referral if the first two levels of intervention did not result in the desired outcomes, such as diminished illness worry, improved functional status and increased self-efficacy and self-management of MUS.[28] Later, Rief and associates provided empirical evidence for the effectiveness of this model upon the family physician completing a 1-day training package, "How to manage patients with unexplained physical symptoms".[29]

Although the present chapter focuses on adult bodily distress syndrome, somatization in the paediatric population is pertinent to the primary care provider because the prevalence ranges from 5% to more than 20% in children and adolescents.[30] Silber pointed out that MUS have a sex disparity in favour of girls and the rate of somatization is highest among lower socioeconomic groups.[30]

Epidemiologic data in high-, medium- and low-income countries

The prevalence of bodily distress syndrome in adults varies with the classification systems and measures used to define it and the context from which study samples were drawn. A WHO epidemiologic study reported that cross-cultural prevalence rates range from 0.03% to 19.7%.[31] A German study of prevalence in primary care concluded that two-thirds of all reported symptoms in women and younger persons were medically unexplained.[32] Immigrants, especially those from less industrialized countries, are often assumed to express distress through somatization more than people from western countries do, who express it through psychological symptoms.[33] Such differences could seriously complicate western health-care systems for immigrants, as these systems tend to focus on either physical or psychological symptoms.

Studies around the world, and particularly in Europe and the United States of America (USA), indicate that 25% to 50% of primary care patients present with bodily distress syndrome/MUS.[33] Fabiao and colleagues recently conducted a systematic review of studies in primary care from 1998 to 2009 and found considerable prevalence variability, depending on the sample studied and the identification method used.[34] A prevalence between 12% and 58% was reported for patients identified as having MUS through multiple diagnostic classification systems. Somatization disorder with characteristics that followed more restrictive WHO criteria produced a prevalence between 0.5% and 16.1%,[35] with the American Psychiatric Association (APA) criteria giving a lifetime prevalence from 0.2% to 2.0%.[36] When abridged criteria, specifically the Somatic Symptom Index (Somatic Symptom Index$_{4,6}$),[37] constituted the definition of somatization, the majority of studies found prevalence rates of approximately 20%. In a consecutive sample of primary care patients at Walter Reed Army Medical Center in the USA, Jackson and Passamonti found that one-third of initially presented symptoms at the index visit were MUS.[38] Furthermore, these symptoms persisted as unexplained in 35% of the patients at 5 years.

To summarize, the prevalence of somatization reported in a study depends on the classification method and measurement tools used to define the parameters, in addition to the sampling context from which the data are extracted. During the past decade, a group of studies, particularly in Europe and the USA, has allowed better understanding of the extent of somatization in primary care, and this information must now be used to assess service needs across the world. Of particular concern in relation to the noteworthy prevalence of bodily distress syndrome/MUS and other mental health disorders is the WHO finding that more than 75% of people living in developing countries do not receive any mental health treatment or care.[39]

Cross-cultural considerations

Patients with bodily distress syndrome present for medical consultation with one or more conceptually distinct clinical problems. Kirmayer and Sartorius described three distinct clinical presentations that occur in isolation or co-occur across cultures.[40] These presentations are (1) excessive bodily preoccupation, illness worry, or unjustified conviction that one is ill; (2) MUS clusters or functional somatic syndromes, such as fibromyalgia, irritable bowel, chronic fatigue, or multiple chemical sensitivity; and (3) somatic symptoms accounted for by another disorder (e.g. depression). A worldwide view is that culture involves the flow of information, roles and institutions that offer patients and providers multiple models for understanding illness in general and bodily distress syndrome/MUS specifically. More detailed reviews are available of cross-cultural explanations[41,42] and the impact of varying ethnicities among western and non-western groups.[43]

Cross-cultural patient relational preference style

Efficient, effective treatment depends on a positive and comfortable communication style between the family physician and patient. The family physician has the responsibility to tailor the communication approach and delivery of health-care services in a patient-centred manner because most patients across cultures and ethnicities prefer care that engages them as an expert partner in a collaborative path.[44] Mulvaney-Day et al. reported on empirical evidence that a relational style that addresses the preference of diverse cultural groups is associated with patient engagement in treatment, increased treatment adherence and improved care outcomes.[45] Thus, diverse racial and ethnic expectations in communication and relational style do impact disparities in health-care access, health service delivery and health outcomes. An effective relationship is facilitated when the family physician encourages a patient to describe his or her unique cultural communication and boundary aspects.[46]

However, initial caution or hesitation should be anticipated because frank discussion of issues of mistrust or misunderstanding is often difficult for patients, regardless of race and ethnicity.

What follows is a brief summary of findings from a comparative qualitative explanation of relational style preference in African American, Latino, and non-Latino white patients in northeastern USA.[45] Of significance, these racial ethnic groups did not differ in their most important contextual subthemes in a physician–patient office visit or encounter – listening, understanding, managing social difference and spending time. However, racial ethnic differences did exist within the subtheme identification. The authors identified the following subthemes as most important to health care:

- *listening*: African American patients valued the "listening to who I am" because the patient is the expert on herself or himself, in contrast to Latino patients, who see merit in attentive listening as an expression of the quality of the relationship. The non-Latino white patients assigned significance to listening as evidence of a safe and "comfortable" context to talk and express feelings

- *understanding*: understanding aspects of self that cannot be seen is important to African American patients, whereas understanding feelings and being empathic were critical for Latino patients. Non-Latino white patients valued understanding the complexity of the patient's choices and life circumstances

- *managing social difference*: African American patients accept that differences will surface but expect that the physician will take the initiative to bridge these differences in order to connect. Latino patients welcome a direct and authoritative stance on the part of the physician, compared with non-Latino white patients, who show a preference for the absence of power dynamics

- *spending time*: this subtheme did not emerge as a relevant issue for African American patients. Latino patients wanted sufficient time to reach a deep level of connection, to ensure a more complete and open communication, whereas non-Latino white patients wanted a non-rushed pace to express the patient's needs without feeling ashamed.

Relevance to the delivery of mental health in primary care

Patients with bodily distress syndrome and illness are a clinical challenge in relation to emotional and physical suffering, an often poor response to treatment, functional disability socially and in the workplace, and high use of medical services.[3] Bodily distress syndrome is the most common disorder seen in primary care practice, particularly when the frequency assessment includes the abridged form of MUS.[6] A review of US studies and studies around the world[47] indicated that 25% to 50% of primary care patients present with MUS and, subsequently, are often given the label *frequent clinic attendee*.[48]

Multiple labels have appeared in the published literature referencing MUS. Johnson, in her informative book on unexplained medical illness (p.4),[12] listed the following characteristics as representative of these conditions: chronic dysfunctional illness, functional stress syndrome, chronic multisymptom illness, affective spectrum disorder, multisomatoform disorder, antidepressant-responsive disorder, and unexplained illness. Notwithstanding the confusion surrounding the nomenclature, common factors among all medically unexplained illnesses are insufficient biopathophysiologic findings to explain the symptoms; functional impairment; and female predominance.[12,36]

Revision in diagnostic labelling is at the planning stage for the fifth edition of the American Psychiatric Association's *Diagnostic and Statistical Manual of Mental Disorders* (DSM-V),[49] scheduled for publication in 2012. The DSM-V Somatic Symptom Disorder Work Group is recommending that the section "Somatoform disorders" be renamed "Somatic symptom disorders". Furthermore, the work group is proposing that the existing diagnoses of somatization disorder, undifferentiated somatoform disorder, hypochondriasis, pain disorder associated with psychological factors and a general medical condition, and pain disorder associated with psychological disorders be subsumed under the newly minted unitary diagnostic label *complex somatic symptom disorder*. This suggestion is made because of the overlapping symptoms and unreliability of the existing diagnostic disorders. The DSM-V work group proposal is supported by a recent Danish investigation that showed that most MUS and functional syndromes were "covered" by the authors' empirically established diagnosis of bodily distress syndrome.[4]

Relevance is also related to the chronic illness course of patients with bodily distress syndrome/MUS. Recovery rates or significant symptom improvement reported in a recent systematic review of the literature for predominately primary care patients in the Netherlands, United Kingdom of Great Britain and Northern Ireland (UK), USA, Spain, Africa and Germany varied from 30% to 50% in follow-up periods ranging from 6 months to 5 years.[50] Patients with newly presented unexplained physical symptoms recruited from general practice clinics in the southern and western parts of the Netherlands showed that 57% of the original unexplained reports continued to be unexplained.[51] Furthermore, 43% of the patients still reported suffering from their initial physical concerns.

Consecutive adults presenting to the primary care walk-in clinic at the Walter Reed Army Medical Center, USA, were studied for initial symptom recovery.[38] The investigators concluded that for more than half of the patients, the presenting physical concern is resolved at 5 years, but for one-third, the concern continues to be medically unexplained. Smits et al. studied the rate of persistence beyond the 1-year frequent attender pattern (attendance rate ranked nearest the top 10th percentile for age and sex) in five primary health-care centres in Amsterdam.[48] They determined that 15% of the 1-year frequent attenders became persistent frequent attenders, defined as patients continuing this pattern for at least 3 more years. Taken as a whole, these studies document the chronicity of MUS in a sizeable proportion of primary care adult patients who are frequent clinic attenders.

In sum, and notwithstanding the confusion surrounding nomenclature, the common factors among all medically unexplained illnesses are (1) insufficient biopathophysiologic findings to explain the symptoms; (2) functional impairment; and (3) female predominance.[12,36]

The role of symptoms

Family physicians are oriented and trained to ask about and determine the meaning of patient symptoms. In the context of a busy practice and numerous interruptions during the working day, it is tempting to focus narrowly on only the biological and medical aspects of the patient's presenting concern. However, this focus is a mistake with patients who have bodily distress syndrome, because frequent attenders are likely to have psychiatric disorders, social difficulty and emotional distress.[48,52]

Furthermore, an estimated 35% to 43% of index bodily distress syndrome/MUS persists as unexplained at 1- and 5-year follow-up, respectively.[38] Rasmussen et al. investigated a large sample of primary care patients and found a robust relationship between the number of physical concerns and mental distress.[17] Headache, chest pain, dizziness, sleep problem, shortness of breath, fatigue and fainting spells were valid triggers for suspecting a psychiatric disorder. However, the most powerful predictor of psychiatric disorder in their study was the total number of physical symptoms, particularly those symptoms judged by the family physician as medically unexplained (somatoform).

Consistent evidence for greater physical symptom reporting in women across cultures has been found. Representative examples of the presence of more physical symptoms reported by women than men in primary care samples has been established in Qatar,[53] the USA,[54] and the Netherlands.[55] The investigation by Gijsbers van Wijk et al.[55] is particularly impressive because patient health diaries were used. In a representative sample of the general German population, Rief et al. showed a small sex effect in physical symptom reporting, in favour of women.[56] An interesting study of adolescent athletes participating in echocardiographic screening at a cardiology clinic found that the girls reported significantly more physical symptoms than the boys, independent of cardiac abnormalities.[57] In a Finnish population, data from all 31-year-old medical public outpatient records showed greater physical symptom reporting in females than males.[58] Although the reasons for female predominance in physical symptom reporting have not been fully elucidated, Johnson cites evidence for a strong link to higher rates of depression and anxiety and thus an increased likelihood of somatization.[12]

Psychiatric comorbidity

In a recent population-based study in Norway, Leiknes et al. reported that 44% of participants with MUS also had concurrent depression or anxiety disorder.[59] The investigators found a two- to three-fold increase in depression and anxiety disorders in patients with distressing somatic symptoms, especially among older adult patients. Furthermore, the evidence suggests increased disability when bodily distress syndrome/MUS is comorbid with psychiatric disorders, particularly depression and anxiety, in primary care.[60] In a case-control study of five general practices in Edinburgh, UK, patients with MUS and current depression, anxiety or panic disorder were more than twice as likely to be referred to hospital specialists than those who did not meet the diagnostic criteria for a psychiatric disorder.[61]

Pre-eminence of the biopsychosocial explanatory model

A biopsychosocial explanatory model represents the confluence of multifactorial aetiologic mechanisms and subsequent sustaining factors in the origin and course of bodily distress syndrome. The complexity of bodily distress syndrome/MUS is represented in an organizational chart (see Figure 21.1) that appeared in the literature more than a decade ago,[62] and continues to be relevant today.

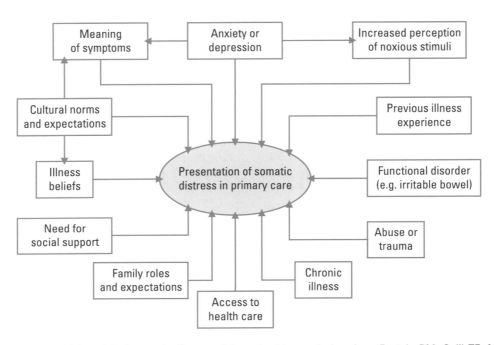

Figure 21.1 Biopsychosocial model of somatic distress. Adapted, with permission, from Epstein RM, Quill TE, McWhinney IR. Somatization reconsidered: incorporating the patient's experience of illness. *Archives of Internal Medicine*, 1999, 159:215–222. Copyright © 1999 American Medical Association. All rights reserved[62]

Johnson made a significant contribution to the biopsychosocial explanatory model by blending sex into the discussion and reviewing specific psychological mechanisms that correlate with the aetiologic factors, developmental course and response to treatment in patients with MUS.[12] The sex contribution addresses a long-overdue foundational imperative for any comprehensive understanding of the origin and course of bodily distress syndrome/MUS. The confluence of physical, psychological and sociocultural variables that explain the preponderant female prevalence across the spectrum of bodily distress syndrome and medically unexplained syndromes was reviewed and empirically substantiated. Factors that occur more often in women – neglect, abuse, role strain and greater reliance on an emotion-based coping style versus problem-focused coping strategies – were meticulously woven into a discussion on the precipitation and chronic nature of medically unexplained illness in females. The WHO has detailed the issues of women and mental health, particularly the disparity in services.[63]

Mediating mechanisms: predisposing, precipitating, and sustaining factors

This biopsychosocial concept is the foundational model for understanding the pathogenesis and course of bodily distress syndrome, but several cogent and more specific biological, social and developmental, cognitive, and personality factors are essential mediating mechanisms with explanatory value.[12] Our intention is to present the complex and dynamic interaction of numerous factors and avoid reductionism or biological primacy, by focusing on the contributions of interdependent mechanisms across the physiologic, psychosocial and cultural continua.

Multiple overlapping mechanisms mediate and moderate the emergence and course of bodily distress syndrome. No single mechanism fully accounts for or explains the predisposing, precipitating and sustaining factors associated with bodily distress syndrome. Sorting out the mediating and moderating mechanisms involves identifying and accepting a patient's culturally based explanation for the symptoms. When the primary care provider validates the cultural meaning of the symptoms and suffering, most patients acknowledge that stress, social conditions and emotions have an effect on their physical condition.[64]

We describe briefly the common, empirically supported mediating mechanisms based on developmental, cognitive-perceptual, biological or personality processes and linked with the emergence and course of bodily distress syndrome. More detailed information on mediating mechanisms is available.[12,65] The state of the current knowledge base suggests the need for new and revised research models to better apportion the variance among the many factors that interact dynamically and in a bidirectional manner to explain medically unexplained illness.

Biological mechanisms

Rief and Barsky provided a signal-filter process that is fundamental for understanding biological mechanisms associated with bodily distress syndrome/MUS.[66] Their model assumes a continuous flow of sensory information sent from internal organs and other body parts, including the skin, that is forwarded to higher cortical structures. A healthy nervous system filters this "sensory noise", preventing overstimulation (and associated exaggerated symptom interpretation) of the cortical structures with irrelevant and often ambiguous information. This mechanism, called *gate control*, was defined nearly 50 years ago to explain variability in pain experience,[67] but more recently it has been adapted for bodily distress syndrome/MUS. A physiological disturbance in the signal-filter process is believed to initiate a cascade of sensory amplification and emotional overarousal or excitability, an increase in the probability of misattribution of the sensation–illness relationship, catastrophic disease predictions, illness worry, and, as the final pathway in this progression, medical-service seeking.

Physiological abnormalities such as lowered cerebral metabolism[68] or activated T-cell inflammatory response,[69] have been implicated in the development of MUS. Cornerstone physiological structures are the sympathetic nervous system, and adrenal-medullary and hypothalamopituitary-adrenal (HPA) axes.

Johnson describes the stress physiology associated with MUS.[12] The sympathetic nervous system produces adrenaline (epinephrine) and noradrenaline (norepinephrine), and the HPA produces glucocorticoids. The hypothalamus synthesizes corticotropin-releasing hormone (CRH), which prompts the pituitary to release adrenocorticotropic hormone (corticotropin; ACTH). In turn, ACTH acts on the adrenal gland cortex, which releases stress hormones, such as cortisol, into the bloodstream. The HPA possesses a capacity to regulate various constituent elements in the sympathetic nervous system, either positively or negatively. For instance, the adrenal cortex releases cortisol, which downregulates adrenal cortex secretion through signals sent to the hypothalamus and anterior pituitary. Through such action, synthesis of CRH and ACTH pauses and, in turn, cortisol levels decrease.

Of interest, Tak and Rosmalen reviewed 20 years of research and concluded that hypocortisolism may be essential in the aetiology of MUS subgroups.[70] Although the HPA axis is self-regulating, chronic hyperarousal, as precipitated by internal or external stressors, may cause a permanent change in hormone release.[12]

Neuroimaging investigations of functional somatic symptoms are in the inceptive stage and so are limited. Garcia-Campayo et al. provide a brief, but comprehensive, review of the preliminary research and the limitations of neuroimaging techniques and the comparatively low level, to date, of interest in investigating bodily distress syndrome/MUS compared with such disorders as depression, schizophrenia or Alzheimer's disease.[71] Additionally, genetic research has produced only modest and inconclusive findings.[72,73]

Cognitive-perceptual mechanisms

Two patient cognitive processes in particular are crucial in understanding bodily distress syndrome – a catastrophizing interpretation of physical symptoms, and distorted causal attributions in their explanation for somatic symptoms. Dysfunctional symptom beliefs and attributions have a central role in the formation and maintenance of bodily distress syndrome, especially for those patients who have characteristics of the hypochondriac or "health worrier" type.

Fulton et al. summarized four dysfunctional beliefs and attributions triggered by bodily symptoms:[74] (1) serious illnesses are more prevalent than they actually are; (2) ambiguous or vague symptoms are likely indicative of serious, or even life-threatening, illness; (3) if an illness is not diagnosed and treated immediately, the results will be disastrous; and (4) to be healthy, a person must be free of symptoms. These dysfunctional attributions reflect the patient's overestimation of probabilities, catastrophic thinking, overinterpretation, and unrealistic perceptions of the health state.

The final pathway is intolerance of ambiguous symptoms, often in the context of an anxious or depressed mood, or both, prompting frequent use of medical services in search of a diagnosis and treatment. These magnifications and misattributions of normal bodily symptoms are reflective of the somatosensory amplification mechanism introduced by Barsky and Wyshak in 1990,[75] and later elaborated by Rief and Barsky[66] using a signal-filter model. Primary care patients with higher levels of somatoform symptoms attributed the symptoms to organic illness beliefs.[76] In this mechanism, normal bodily symptoms are amplified and misinterpreted, resulting in alarm or worry, or both, out of proportion to the objective somatic disturbance.

Developmental and social mechanisms

In the USA, 10% to 30% of children and adolescents are found to have functional somatic symptoms.[77] Multiple risk factors or protective factors of the social, environmental and familial type interact in the final pathway that expresses bodily distress syndrome, with parent attention versus distraction being a primary construct studied.[78] Epidemiologic research found no evidence for sex differences in the presentation of MUS before puberty.[79] However, Berntsson and Kohler reported twice as many functional somatic symptoms in adolescent girls as in adolescent boys.[79]

In a developmental report on functional somatic symptoms, parent illness and psychological distress, and especially the mother's exposure to childhood adversity, were associated with an increased preponderance of functional somatic symptoms in the child.[80,81] The potential mechanism explaining familial bodily distress syndrome/MUS is exposure to family adversity during childhood, which interferes with attachment development and self-efficacy.[82] High self-esteem, social competence, stable family environment, and male sex appear to be the most probable protective factors, as reported by Beck.[81]

Perhaps the strongest evidence for a social and developmental association with the emergence of bodily distress syndrome is a history of sexual, emotional or physical abuse and trauma, or a combination.[83–85] Dissociation, conversion, and cognitive mechanisms have been postulated as triggers for the presentation of unexplained physical symptoms in childhood or a delayed onset in early adulthood. Paras et al. have published a systematic review and meta-analysis on the relationship between sexual abuse and lifetime diagnosis of common functional somatic disorders.[86]

Personality mechanisms

Consistent with personality mechanisms,[87] bodily distress syndrome and associated suffering serve as a defence in resolving conflicting emotions, such as dependency versus autonomy or the need for, but fear of, interpersonal intimacy. Individuals possessing such personality traits as neuroticism and negative emotionality are predisposed to somatic symptom reporting, because these emotionally reactive individuals are highly self-attentive and sensitive to bodily sensations.[88] This sensitivity prompts hypervigilant body scanning and a high level of symptom awareness and reporting.

Alexithymia has often, but not always, been correlated with symptom reporting and health-care seeking, and is particularly associated with reports of MUS.[89,90] The term "alexithymia", which literally means "no words for feelings", was introduced in the psychosomatic literature by Sifneos in 1973.[91] It refers to a cognitive-affective personality trait that influences the capacity to regulate affects, particularly in stressful situations. The affect regulation problems in alexithymia are difficulty in identifying or describing feelings, diminished capacity for distinguishing between feelings and bodily sensations, constricted imaginal processes as evidenced by a paucity of fantasies, and a concrete externally oriented thinking style. Since alexithymic persons have difficulty expressing emotions or distinguishing between emotion and bodily sensations, the associated physiological arousal is thought to be misinterpreted as somatic symptoms that are perhaps indicative of medical illness. Thus, alexithymia is an emotion-dysregulation risk factor for bodily distress syndrome/MUS and often interacts with cognitive factors, such as distorted causal attributions.[65]

The role of attachment style in the aetiologic characteristics and maintenance of bodily distress syndrome has empirical support. The specific risk factor is an insecure attachment style,[92] defined as being overly dependent, feeling discomfort with emotional intimacy, and fear of abandonment in interpersonal relationships. Noyes et al. also reported a high correlation between scores on a fear-of-death scale and measures of hypochondriasis, health anxiety and somatization in a sample group of primary care patients.[92] Additional support for an association between attachment style and MUS has been reported in primary care patients.[93,94]

Taken together, these studies suggest that bodily distress syndrome results from a multifactorial interplay among biological, cognitive, personality and social factors. Figure 21.2 summarizes common mediating and moderating mechanisms, as portrayed in dynamic and bidirectional relationships.

Gold standard identification and assessment practices

Standardized testing should consist of brief, but valid and reliable, self-report instruments that are compatible with the routine office visit in a busy primary care clinic. Front desk personnel or the rooming nurse can

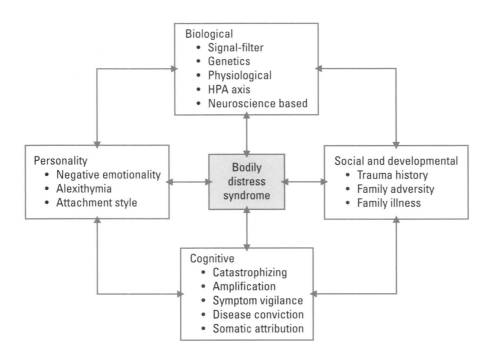

Figure 21.2 Mechanisms associated with the emergence and course of bodily distress syndrome. HPA = hypothalamopituitary adrenal

be trained to score and enter the results in the medical record, preferably an electronic medical record, for longitudinal display and analysis. The scope of assessment, at a minimum, should include evaluation of depression, anxiety, alcohol use or abuse, drug use or abuse, and somatoform symptoms.[95]

Instruments that conform to the validity, reliability and briefness criteria and also cover the scope of what needs to be assessed include the Alcohol Use Disorders Identification Test (AUDIT);[96] the seven-item Generalized Anxiety Disorder test (GAD-7);[97,98] the complete Patient Health Questionnaire (PHQ),[99,100] which assesses somatoform, depressive, anxiety, alcohol and eating symptoms; the nine depression items from the PHQ (PHQ-9);[100] and the 13 physical symptoms items plus two depression items from the PHQ for detecting somatoform status (PHQ-15).[101] Table 21.1 details select characteristics of each assessment tool. Additional information on testing for somatization and best practices for assessment is available.[102]

Table 21.1 Basic assessment tools

Assessment tool	Domain measured	Number of test items	Administration type (time in minutes)	Approximate scoring time (minutes)
AUDIT	Alcohol use disorders	10	Self-report (5) or clinician interview (15–20)	5
GAD-7	General anxiety symptoms (e.g. nervousness, excessive worry)	7	Self-report or clinician interview (5)	5
PHQ	Somatoform, mild and major depression, panic and generalized anxiety, alcohol use, and eating disorders	58	Self-report (10)	10
PHQ-9	Major and minor depression	9	Self-report (5) or clinician interview (10)	5
PHQ-15	Physical symptoms (e.g. back pain), dizziness, fainting spells, shortness of breath, nausea, and two depression items	15	Self-report (5) or clinician interview (10)	5

AUDIT = Alcohol Use Disorders Identification Test; GAD = Generalized Anxiety Disorder; PHQ = Patient Health Questionnaire.

Gold standard treatment and first-line interventions in primary care

The purpose of this section is to present brief, empirically supported, and cost-effective stepped interventions easily applied by family physicians or other primary care providers (e.g. care managers) in a 15- to 30-minute routine patient visit. The objectives of intervention for the patient with bodily distress syndrome are increased symptom tolerance and reduction, enhanced functional performance related to interpersonal and family relationships and work, and increased sense of self-efficacy or personal agency – not a complete cure. A complete recovery to normal functioning is not the objective for most patients with this chronic condition. However, important outcomes are the development of proactive strategies to facilitate pre-emptive action that prevents or minimizes the potential impact of a detected stressor, and the formulation of an effective, problem-based coping style.[103]

We propose an interventional "six-pack" for the family physician's toolkit. Each of the six proposed interventions respects the research finding that patients with MUS are less likely to talk about psychological symptoms or psychosocial stressors than other primary care patients.[104] The interventions we propose are based on empirically supported treatment (EST) evidence rather than the more restrictive gold standard of randomized controlled treatment trials that characterize evidence-based medicine. EST is state of the art with regard to family physician implementation of psychosocial interventions,[105] and compellingly indicates that more EST research is needed.

With the importance of family physician independence in applying brief and empirically supported interventions, the second aim is for family physicians to create a gold standard system of behavioural health-care delivery, or the most feasible approximation given their resources. In our view, the gold standard therapy for patients with MUS is the disease management practice model as described by Collins et al. in their Millbank Memorial Fund report (pp.26–29).[27] The disease management model emphasizes first the early identification in primary care populations of those patients at risk for the costly and chronic nature of bodily distress syndrome/MUS. Second, the disease management practice model stresses the provision of education, self-management, and evidence-based interventional algorithms[106] that can be effectively delivered by primary care staff, and particularly family physicians and care managers. A hallmark of the disease management approach is the creation and use of a patient registry. Randomized controlled trials (RCTs) have shown that the disease management model with a care manager in close communication with the family physician is clinically effective and cost effective.[107] This model has shown a cost offset between 20% and 40% for primary care patients receiving behavioural health services.

Resources are available of brief and user-friendly psychosocial interventions designed to be implemented by the family physician, that are likely to be of interest. The *Recovering mental health in Scotland* document,[108] which details very good outcomes from interventions that promoted narrative therapy principles, is a useful read. Stuart and Lieberman's (1986) seminal book,[109] which has been revised three times,[110–112] outlines strategies that can be effectively implemented in the standard 15-minute office visit. The authors' "15-minute hour" office visit is consistent with the belief that psychosocial interventions are most effective when delivered in brief and frequent "spoonfuls" by family physicians, which is compatible with continuity of care. Also, a book on brief interventions for the family physician on a wide range of psychosocial problems that present in primary care, particularly the "high-utilizing" patient with MUS, will likely be of interest (pp.61–74).[113]

The foundation for effective intervention

A strong therapeutic alliance is the foundation for an effective technical and interpersonal exchange in the physician–patient relationship. The quality of the therapeutic alliance and the communication therein have been associated with health outcomes, health-care satisfaction, health status change, treatment adherence, and malpractice claims.[114–117] Specifically, an effective relationship alliance is based on empathy, non-verbal congruence, unambiguous transmission of information, collaborative exploration of informed choice, and patient involvement in decision-making. Interventional outcomes are especially positive when collaborative decision-making is explicitly encouraged by the physician, rather than simply allowed.[118] In the Netherlands, Heijmans and colleagues recently published their findings from a systematic review of the literature, combined by conducting a focus group with MUS experts, and concluded that an essential element in treatment is the creation of a safe therapeutic environment in which the patient feels comfortable in openly sharing problematic symptoms and concerns.[119] The listening, talking, and relating that occur between the patient and physician are a focal point of the teaching and research agenda in family medicine.[120] In 2002, the Society of Teachers of Family Medicine devoted the entire May issue of *Family Medicine* to physician–patient communication.[121] In summary, Mendoza and associates referred to the physician–patient relationship as the "seventh element of quality" (p.83).[122]

Core facilitative ingredients

Contextual ingredients, or common factors, are the core facilitative elements in effective intervention and cannot be overstated. Overlapping and communal facilitative factors that have been empirically established are (1) a confiding and emotionally charged relationship that is collaborative but with one person identified as the helper; (2) provider empathy, genuineness, positive regard, and compassionate feedback; (3) a collaboratively developed explanatory framework that accounts for the patient's symptoms and life story or narrative; and (4) a belief on the parts of the provider and patient that the healing process can work and requires effort and participation from both persons.[8,123,124] These contextual factors are central to all change interventions and maximal treatment outcome. The common factors maximize treatment effect because of their positive contribution in creating a sufficiently safe and emotionally supportive healing climate that allows the patient to be introspective and self-reflective and to contemplate alternative choices and a course of action.

Targeting and tracking intervention outcomes

Interventional outcomes are of two broad types – patient centred and system focused (see Table 21.2). The dichotomization of outcomes is arbitrary because of the bidirectional and dynamic interaction of the measurement and tracking of variables. An important provider task is to select one or more outcomes to measure and track with concentrated preference on patient-centred variables. Tracking outcomes with the measuring, monitoring, and feedback approach developed by Lambert[125] will guide the collaborative provider–patient decision-making (e.g. persisting with a chosen intervention, changing the intervention, initiating a specialty mental health referral). The point is that collaborative decision-making should be based on data and collaboratively pursued.

Table 21.2 Patient and system outcomes of care

Patient-centred outcomes	System-centred outcomes
Increase tolerance for unexplained symptoms	Decrease the number of emergency department visits
Strengthen emotion-focused and problem-focused coping skills	Reduce inpatient episodes of care
Improve work satisfaction and/or performance	Diminish laboratory testing and imaging studies
Identify and treat psychiatric comorbidity (e.g. depression, anxiety)	Decrease office visit frequency
Enhance psychological insight	Decrease the number of "urgent" phone calls

A uniquely important, but seldom constructed, treatment target that is cross-culturally relevant to a chronic illness condition such as bodily distress syndrome is the expressed emotion (EE) concept.[126] EE is the emotion expressed by family members and close relatives in reaction to the onset and course of an illness state that often becomes a chronic condition. Cheng pointed out that the original concept of EE consists of positive and negative emotions,[127] but research in western and non-western countries has focused on three negative components: criticism, hostility and emotional over-involvement. All of these negative components are a matter of cultural definition. For example, among relatives with schizophrenia, a high level of EE was found in 8% in rural India compared with 67% in urban USA. In view of the evidence for cross-culture variation in family response to the sick role, a provider might choose to collaborate with the patient in constructing an EE-related treatment goal, to reduce the risk of weakening the therapeutic alliance or alienating family members in a systemic family intervention. Endley and Berry demonstrated that a single training session can produce a significant increase in professional staff knowledge of EE and an increase in confidence in engaging patients and their families.[128]

Realistic treatment goal setting is obviously an important issue. Convention among experts in treatment outcome is often in terms of the "five Rs" suggested by Hollon et al.:[129] response, typically defined as a 50% reduction in symptoms; remission or virtually a return to normal; recovery that involves being in remission for at least 6 months; relapse or a return of the symptoms at a level consistent with the original illness episode; and recurrence construed as a new episode. Generally, the end-of-treatment outcome goal is response and, possibly, remission, but relapse must be expected, given the highly fluctuating course that is frequently characteristic of bodily distress syndrome.

In summary, treatment targets for patients with bodily distress syndrome are not restricted to a decrease in unexplained symptoms. Rather, treatment goal allocation often combines a patient-centred focus – such as increasing tolerance for unexplained symptoms and an improving functional status relative to work or family relationships – with system-centred goals (e.g. decreasing the number of emergency department visits or of inpatient episodes of care).[28,130]

The stepped care delivery model: general principles

We propose that behavioural health interventions be cast in an integrated, stepped care model. Integration typically entails interdisciplinary care teams comprising a physician, nurse practitioner, care manager and mental health specialist, but it also might include a pharmacist, triage nurse, or chronic-disease social worker.[130,131] Stepped care is predicated on implementing resources no earlier or more intense than necessary but no later or less intense than needed.[132] Seekles and associates suggested a stepped care model consisting of four steps:[132] first, watchful waiting with 4 weeks of observation, but no intervention, to identify the patients who recover spontaneously; second, guided self-help based on a one-to-one patient session with a care manager for discussion of psycho-educational materials, offering advice and lifestyle change suggestions; third, problem-solving treatment that is brief (~5 sessions) provided by the care manager; and fourth, pharmacotherapy or specialized mental health treatment, or both. However, any proposed model of stepped care must be sufficiently flexible to accommodate the interaction of the family physician's knowledge of the patient and the patient's treatment preference.[133] Therefore, although a stepped care model is outlined in a sequential manner guided by time- and resource-intensive principles, the integrated care team can begin at any of the intervention levels and move up and down the hierarchy.

Of note, the stepped care interventions outlined herein are designed to be implemented by the family physician without direct assistance or involvement from specialty mental health personnel. The specific intention is to outline the key steps in implementing brief interventions that can be independently delivered without assistance from specialty mental health services, to accommodate the family physician in low- or medium-income countries and not solely high-income geographic sites where there are generally ample mental health specialists available.

Before implementing any one, or combination, of the proposed interventions (see below), suicidal risk and a safety plan, if needed, must be addressed. It is best to periodically assess self-harm risk in the patient with bodily distress syndrome,[134] on the basis of a combination of patient report and clinician observation. Ivbijaro and colleagues developed the guideline strategy "look, listen, and test" for depression in primary care, which can be used to do the periodic assessment of the patient's self-harm risk.[135]

To conclude, an integrated, stepped model of health-care delivery must address issues related to access; disjointed silos of care; escalating costs; an ageing population; the impact of social and family determinants on health, provider and caregiver burnout; the risks and benefits of Internet use; rapidly changing technology; and determination of the best fit regarding available interventions and patient preference.

Interventions for bodily distress syndrome: a six-pack toolkit

The proposed interventional, six-level stepped approach, referred to as a *six-pack toolkit*, is based in part on the transtheoretical model of behaviour change.[136] That is, behaviour change is viewed as a process that unfolds over time and progresses through predictable stages. Interwoven among all of the proposed interventions is the importance of both creating patient ambivalence about the status quo and resolving that ambivalence in committed behavioural action is a good match between the patient's choice of solution and his or her personal limitations. A specific intention is to outline the key steps in implementing brief interventions that can be delivered by the family physician independently, without assistance from specialty mental health personnel, to accommodate providers not only in low- or medium-income countries where mental health services are scarce, but also in high-income geographic sites where there are probably ample mental health specialists available.

The stepped care interventions described here flow progressively from non-directive physician behaviour that emphasizes problem awareness and insight (levels 1 to 3) to more directive, physician-implemented strategies that stress the co-construction of specific solutions (levels 4 to 6) (see Table 21.3). Table 21.3 categorizes the level of research support for each intervention when it is implemented in primary care by a family physician as either EST or evidence-based treatment (EBT), verified by conventional definition.[7] *EST* indicates probable treatment effectiveness but validation of the intervention is an ongoing work in progress. In contrast, *EBTs* have stronger support for treatment efficacy, as supported by several RCTs (Table 21.3).

It should be noted that our rationale for ordering the interventions, beginning with the engagement session and ending with pharmacotherapy or referral to a mental health specialist, or both, is predicated on the interaction of numerous variables. These variables are patient problem severity, patient insight or problem awareness, and an estimate of the implementation time and effort – all of which are initially gauged by the family physician. With mindfulness of these variables, each succeeding intervention is designed to address a more complex patient problem and generally involves a greater expenditure of family physician time and effort. Although parsimony of effort is suggested, the family physician must be cautious because poor outcomes from an initial

Table 21.3 Levels of stepped care in the direct–indirect, awareness–action, and treatment effectiveness spectra

Level of stepped care	Direct–indirect continuum	Awareness–action continuum	Treatment effectiveness
1 Engagement session	Indirect	Awareness	EST
2 Reflecting interview	Indirect	Awareness	EST
3 Linking and reattribution encounter	Indirect	Awareness	EST
4 Motivational interviewing	Direct	Action	EST
5 Solution-focused problem-solving	Direct	Action	EST
6 Pharmacotherapy and/or speciality mental health referral	Direct	Action	EBT

EBT = evidence-based treatment; EST = empirically supported treatment.

intervention (e.g. implementing a single reflecting interview instead of several motivational interviewing sessions) may have a negative impact on patient confidence, receptivity and adherence to future interventions. The point is that there is flexibility in the family physician's initial choice for intervention.

In summary, it is suggested that the family physician's mindset for implementing any of the interventions discussed herein includes the following guidelines:

- personalize the goals and values to ensure that the solutions fit the patient, not the problem.[137] That fit, in large part, depends on the patient's resources and personal strengths and limitations
- guide the patient in constructing solutions, with little, if any, analysis of the patient's family background or psychodynamic underpinnings
- understanding the cause of the problem is not essential or even helpful in most cases, because searching for causes often leads only to self-blame, blaming others, or self-justifying attitudes and behaviour, which may escalate the problem rather than solve it
- view patients with multiple problems as persons with multiple solutions
- the past is something to learn from, but the principal focus is on constructing solutions in the patient's present and near future.

Level 1: engagement session

The difficult-to-engage patient is at risk for being underserved in the primary care clinic and often is in need of an interjection of hope.[138] We recommend a single-session engagement encounter, described by Zuckoff et al.,[46] as the first level of intervening with a patient with bodily distress syndrome who is reluctant to consider any symptom explanation other than a complete biological version. The easing-in type of session is intended to diminish the initial hesitation or marginal motivation of, for example, the distrustful, alexithymic,[90] demoralized,[139] or psychologically naive patient.[104] It is critical that the family physician communicates to the patient that he or she believes the patient's bodily distress syndrome is real, results from a physiological process, and is potentially linked to unrecognized stress or psychosocial problems whose impact may not be fully appreciated. Introducing the symptom–stress link early and empathically in the provider–patient conversation changes the agenda from a symptoms-only approach to one of symptom–life event conjunctive possibilities. When the patient surrenders, or at least loosens the grip on the framework of symptom–biological disease only, then acceptance of and insight into the symptom–stress link begins. In turn, the acceptance and insight open the conversation for psychosocial explanation and intervention.

The engagement conversation is typically a single session that concentrates on communicating the family physician's understanding of potential barriers related to self-disclosure discomfort, trust or shame and the potential benefits, such as awakening hope or problem resolution. The sequential intervention steps for an engagement session outlined in Box 21.1 represent a hybrid of procedures, suggested by Zuckoff et al.[46] and Rollnick et al.[140]

1. Elicit the story

Begin with a question, such as "What has been going on in your life that is troubling you?" It is critical that the patient feels understood. Suggest potential value in behavioural or attitudinal change in the patient's distressed emotional state and situation.

2. Provide feedback and psycho-education

In this step, the goal is to offer the patient a different perspective on the "situation" or distressful problem. State, "I can understand how this problem is challenging and distressful but, I think, also potentially solvable or at least improvable". This step is not intended to minimize the problem but to interject hope. Usually, it is beneficial to reframe the distressing, and sometimes hopeless, situation as a "dilemma" worthy of collaborative conversation and problem-solving. Conclude with a *crystallizing* summary of the dilemma and the patient's wish to escape from the distress (e.g. "You are experiencing an emotionally painful isolation and sense of abandonment in your marriage, and your most immediate need is to obtain relief from the suffering"). The family physician might want to provide his/her favourite patient education material on the effects of persistent stress.

3. Explore the history of coping and prior treatment outcomes

Ask, "What have you tried on your own to fix this problem?" Be sure to reward the patient for effort and creativity, even though the patient has not been able to satisfactorily solve the problem or obtain emotional relief. Then ask, "Have you talked with a mental health specialist about the current concerns or past problems?" If the answer is yes, then ask, "Did that help – were those conversations beneficial?"

4. Identify barriers to recommended treatment

Be aware that the patient's first impulse might be to deny any barriers. If this happens, offer examples that other patients have shared with you. Examples of barriers are cost, trust, time away from work, and fear of significant-other reactions. Conversely, if the patient expresses a barrier, address the barrier through a series of reflecting questions ranging from "What do think will happen if you address that barrier or obtain help from a mental health professional?" to "How might you go about coping with that reaction or challenge?"

5. Summarize and clarify the treatment commitment

Conclude with a brief recapitulation of the patient's dilemma, past efforts to resolve the problem, possible ways to cope with currently perceived barriers, your recommendation (e.g. any one of the stepped care interventions), and your perception of the patient's commitment to further intervention, if any at all. After the recapitulation, seek closure on this engagement session by asking such questions as "How does this sound to you?" and "Is this what you want to do?" The final task is to make a follow-up statement that includes the logistics for the patient's interventional preference and your role in nurturing the process. It is suggested that whatever is collaboratively agreed on, your final statement can be the following: "I look forward to seeing you again and working together to provide you with the best medical care possible".

If the family physician is finding it difficult to get started or to "elicit the story" (step 1), it may be useful to employ the BATHE questions[111] to explicitly isolate the patient-identified stress-related issue that needs intervention. Briefly, BATHE consists of four sequenced questions followed by an empathic statement:

- **B**ackground question: "What do you think is the most stressful current issue?"
- **A**ffect question: "How do you feel about this problem?"
- **T**rouble question: "What about this situation troubles you?"
- **H**andling question: "How are you coping with this stressful situation?"
- **E**mpathy statement: "This must be very difficult for you".

The four questions respectively elicit the context of the patient's stressful situation, probe the initial affect, clarify the subjective meaning attached to the problem, and identify currently used coping strategies, most of which ostensibly are not working.

In summary, the engagement session is designed to explore the value and barriers of investing time and energy in the process of behavioural change. If the patient is ready to move forward, the family physician offers the initial intervention, names it (e.g. *reflecting interview*), and briefly outlines the what and the why. For the patient who does not commit to moving forward by agreeing to intervention, a waiting period of a few weeks followed by a second engagement session is suggested.

Level 2: reflecting interview

The reflecting interview intervention is a scripted interview developed by Rasmussen et al.[130] that combines elements of Launer's[141] narrative-based creation of a new patient story and the contingency behavioural contracting approach suggested by Rasmussen and Avant[28] and validated by Rief et al.[29] The salient ingredients are non-judgemental and empathic listening, construction of a three-generational genogram, and a shared reflective process that encourages collaborative rethinking, revising and reinterpreting of the MUS, aimed at creating a new patient story that captures a more useful reframing of the illness beliefs, illness behaviour and medical care decision-making. The reflecting interview is best implemented in one 60- to 75-minute conversation with the patient and may need repeating at 3- to 6-month intervals to sustain treatment gains.

The flow of this intervention proceeds as follows: establishing trust, creating a climate for introspection, introducing new meaning possibilities for the symptoms, exploring likely consequences for the patient and his or her family if nothing changes, and collaboratively developing a follow-up plan that reflects change behaviour consistent with a new meaning or reinterpretation of the symptoms. The reflecting interview implementation steps are summarized in Box 21.2.

Box 21.2   Reflecting interview: step-by-step implementation

1. Introduction and purpose statement

State, "The plan for today is to have a conversation about your life narrative (or life story) that will help us to provide you with the best medical care possible".

2. Establishment of the focus

State, "The hope is that we gain new insights and a new perspective on your medical condition and health care. I'm going to ask several questions, but I hope that you also will pose questions". The intention is to sharpen the patient's awareness that prior and current action plans have not produced the hoped-for or desired results and that it is time to rethink individual (both patient and provider) and conjoint positions on pathways to improve medical and/or psychological outcomes.

3. Reflection on the critical mass of provocative questions

The family physician poses several predetermined questions. During this reflective process, periodically summarize the patient's reactions and offer him/her the opportunity to restate or elaborate on your synopsis. Ask and process the following questions in sequence:

■ "What perplexing medical problems have members of your family, such as your parents or siblings or your spouse, recently experienced or have occurred in the more distant past, even as far back as when you were a child?"

■ "How did family members react to these medical problems, and was your reaction the same as or different from theirs?"

■ "Which family reactions seemed to help you cope best with the medical problem and which reactions or actions appeared to worsen it?"

4. Shoot for the bull's-eye

Ask, "As a result of our talking today, have you become aware of a new or different explanation or belief about your medical symptoms that makes more sense than what we have concluded in the past?" The objective is to determine whether new beliefs or perceptions might be penetrating prior illness distortion or denial.

5. Hypothesize health outcomes

Ask, "What do you think will happen if your symptoms do not get better?" This question is intended to elicit the patient's hopes, fears and uncertainties.

6. Closure statement and follow-up plan

Ask, "What did we learn today that may be beneficial moving forward in providing you the best medical care possible?" Finally, summarize the follow-up plan that reflects hopeful self-help strategies, such as diaphragmatic breathing control, exercise and pleasant visualization imagery and that promotes increased symptom tolerance and a more parsimonious approach to office visits, laboratory testing or emergency department episodes.

Level 3: reattribution and linking encounter

In the reattribution and linking encounter, the family physician directly requests psychosocial information and uses that information to explain bodily distress syndrome. This intervention addresses the problem that family physicians often ignore psychosocial and psychological cues offered by the patient with bodily distress syndrome/MUS,[142] but if the patient and the health-care provider discuss psychosocial issues, then the somatic interventions, such as prescriptions, laboratory testing, and specialty referrals, decline. A recent study showed that after 6 hours of family physician reattribution training, patients with MUS were more likely to disclose and discuss psychosocial problems and even propose psychosocial explanations for their symptoms.[143] It was reported that 25% of the patients in the study discussed psychosocial issues "extensively". To date, the effect of reattribution and linking interventions on health and physical symptoms of patients with bodily distress syndrome/MUS has been small,[144] but cost effective due to reductions in somatic testing, additional somatic intervention, or specialty referral. Box 21.3 outlines the step-by-step implementation of the reattribution and linking encounter.

Box 21.3 Reattribution and linking encounter: step-by-step implementation

1. Provide empathic listening

The critical physician response at this step is to clearly communicate acceptance of the validity of the patient's symptoms and a desire to be of help. While listening empathically, do the following:

- conduct a brief, focused physical examination
- normalize the symptom(s) whenever possible
- do not interrupt the patient. This action virtually guarantees that the patient knows he/she is being heard or listened to.

2. Change the agenda from symptoms only to symptom–life event conjunctive possibilities

The critical physician response at this step is to link the symptoms to life events on the basis of prior and current knowledge of the patient's psychosocial life. Do the following:

- emphasize the negative physical examination findings
- continue to validate the patient's reality of the symptoms and associated pain and/or distress
- probe the patient's mood state with questions such as "What's stressful in your life?" and "How are you coping with that?"
- explore the patient's illness beliefs and explanatory model with questions such as "What do you think is causing your symptoms?"

3. Make the link!

The critical physician response is to use constructions such as "perhaps", "I wonder if", or "do you suppose it is possible that", rather than assertions stated in an authoritative style. Use one or more of the following strategies:

- explanation: anxiety (e.g. stress, nervousness) activates the HPA axis, causing physical symptoms

- explanation: depression (e.g. sadness, hopelessness, fatigue) lowers the threshold for pain
- practical demonstration: for example, demonstrate how holding one's arms out at shoulder height for an extended period of time creates tension, fatigue, and even mild pain, which is similar to how stress affects multiple body sites and processes often outside the conscious awareness when one is experiencing duress or is worried
- demonstration: life events (e.g. how stressful events can cause us to "tighten up" external muscles in our forehead or neck (and perhaps elicit a headache)) and/or internal (smooth) muscles in the digestive tract can create symptoms, such as nausea, constipation, or loose stools.

4. Establish closure and collaboratively set the follow-up plan

Do the following:

- ask the patient for his/her summary of the discussion by asking questions such as "What might be helpful from our talk today?" or "What might you want to change going forward, and what do you wish to keep the same?"
- comment on the patient's summary with clarifying statements of your own and offer your own conclusions by stating one or two key outcomes from the talk
- collaboratively decide on the patient's tasks or "behavioural homework" between office visits, aimed at tolerating or lessening ambiguous or distressful physical symptoms (e.g. relaxation training, exercise, reading patient education materials).

Gask and Usherwood have published a brief but detailed outline that is useful to the family physician who would like more specifics on the implementation of a reattribution-type medical interview.[145]

Level 4: motivational interviewing

Motivational interviewing (MI) is a quasi-Socratic style of questioning that confers a prominent role to patient ambivalence in the personal change process.[146] It is certainly a counterpoint to the highly confrontational counselling style. Problem types that especially match well with MI are alcohol use or abuse, smoking cessation, medication adherence, weight control and exercise planning. Of note, a recently published book validates the use of MI in addressing a much broader range of clinical problems, including obsessive-compulsive disorder, depression and eating disorders.[147] MI has great potential for intervening with bodily distress syndrome but it is in need of empirically validating studies. The family physician who practises MI has four basic tasks: establishing a supportive collaboration; highlighting a discrepancy between the patient's health risk behaviour and a strong competing personal value; avoiding arguing or lecturing the patient; and, finally, focusing on the patient's effort and strengths in the change process (see Box 21.4).

Box 21.4 Motivational interviewing: step-by-step implementation

1. Ask permission

The aim is to establish a collaborative and supportive relationship and to increase awareness of a provider-identified problem avoided or denied by the patient (e.g. reluctance to acknowledge psychosocial factors) in understanding the medically unexplained symptoms. Start by asking the question:

- "I'm concerned about the medically unexplained symptoms that we have been talking about for some time but with little helpful progress. Would it be okay for us to talk about this now?"

2. Elicit change talk

The aim is to evoke thoughts about the disadvantages of the status quo, the advantages of change, specific change possibilities, and taking the first step toward change. Proceed by asking the following type of questions:

- "What do you think will happen if these symptoms do not get better?"
- "What could work for you if you decided to change something that might help you to better tolerate these symptoms or possibly decrease their frequency or intensity?"
- "What might be some good things about trying these changes?"
- "What would you be willing to try as a first step?"

3. Importance check

The aim is to have the patient self-rate readiness and motivation as related to cherished personal values and embrace behaviour change and to have the family physician reinforce change talk. The following is an example:

- "On a scale of 1 to 10, with 1 being the lowest and 10 being the highest, how important is it for you to make changes or experiment with a fresh approach to the problems?"

4. Ability check

The aim is to assess confidence in personal ability to change and to overcome barriers to change. The following are examples of questions to ask:

- "How confident are you that you will succeed in making a behaviour change? Again, use the 1-to-10 scale"
- "What do you see as barriers to independently making new choices, and how might you overcome these obstacles?"

5. Provide a statement to obtain session closure

The aim is to summarize the main discussion points, the patient's commitment to a first change step, and the follow-up plan. It is important for the physician to state what the patient has agreed to but also what he/she has not agreed to. The following are examples of statements:

- "If I may summarize our discussion, you are willing to make changes that are likely to help you with your symptoms and specifically you are going to [state the specific change or changes]"
- "You have ultimate and final control over your decision-making about these changes. I can be only your helper"
- "Let's talk about this again in a couple of weeks to check on progress, to assess how you are coping with barriers to change, and to modify the solution(s) a bit if necessary".

More detailed information on implementing MI across the spectrum of psychological and medical disorders that present in primary care is contained in publications by Rollnick et al.[146] and Arkowitz et al.[147]

Level 5: solution-focused problem-solving

Solution-focused problem-solving (SFPS) is aimed at helping patients achieve their preferred outcome by evoking and implementing a collaboratively constructed solution based on a practical evaluation of available options.[148–150] Greenberg et al. have provided a useful summary of the core assumptions that underlie the SFPS techniques:[151] (1) change is constant, inevitable and contagious; (2) patients are experts on their lives; (3) the use of presuppositional language that change will occur thus creates a climate of "when" versus "if"; (4) patients come with at least some coping skills and resources to drive change; and (5) solution-focused conversation has been undervalued in the past. The multiple variants of SFPS intervention are referred to as *the DIG technique*[152] (Dream the miracle that the problem has been solved and notice the change that occurred; Inititate the first small problem-solving step in the desired change direction; Get going and persist in the problem-solving action) or *MECSTAT* (Miracle questions; Exception questions; Coping questions; Scaling questions; Time out; Accolades; Task).[151] Box 21.5 lists step-by-step implementation of SFPS.

During the initial step of problem identification when implementing SFPS intervention, the patient is often unaware of or reluctant to talk about underlying factors (e.g. child abuse, underlying depression or anxiety) that may be eliciting the unexplained somatic presentation. The family physician has an obligation to initiate a sensitive exploration using questions such as "Were you under stress as a child? This can have a role in illness

---

Box 21.5   Problem-solving: step-by-step implementation

1. Identify the problem

Identify a specific problem that is interfering with the patient's well-being and/or medical care. The patient with bodily distress syndrome will often state that the problem is MUS and often avoids talking about trauma from the past, such as child abuse. The goal in this first step is to get a clear description of one problem to work on. Ask questions like the following:

- "What is the problem that is keeping you from feeling better?"
- "What do you think needs fixing?"
- "Were you under stress as a child?"

2. Consider multiple potential solutions

The aim is to collaboratively consider and brainstorm about the alternative solutions to the agreed-on problem. Ask questions like the following:

- "What options do you see as possibly helping with this problem?" Assist the patient in constructing at least two possible solutions that are different from current or past failed actions
- "What are the advantages and disadvantages of each option that was identified in our brainstorming discussion?"

3. Seek patient commitment

The aim is to get a commitment from the patient to try a new and preferred solution, to state a clear action goal, and to set a starting time. Ask questions like the following:

- "Which new solution of the ones we discussed are you willing to try?" (commitment)
- "Please review for me exactly what you are going to do." (clear and achievable goal or action plan)
- "When are you willing to start?" (counter procrastination).

4. Provide a summary statement and follow-up

The family physician summarizes the main points of the solution-focused, problem-solving collaborative discussion and recommends a follow-up plan for assessing outcomes so that the patient is not put off if the first solution does not work. Barriers that may have arisen are addressed. Consistent application of the solution is encouraged, and positive self-reinforcement for small initial success is modelled. Ask questions like the following:

- "If I may summarize our discussion, the problem is . . . , you are committed to an action plan by specifically doing . . . starting . . . . Does this fairly summarize the plan?"
- "Let's talk about this again in a couple of weeks to check on your progress, to discuss what is working or not helping, and to modify the solution a bit if necessary".

---

in adults". More detailed information is available on the nuances of implementing SFPS in publications by O'Connell and Palmer,[149] Searight,[153] and De Jong and Berg.[154]

Level 6: pharmacotherapy or referral to a mental health specialist, or both

While implementing any one of the above interventions, the family physician might simultaneously prescribe medication. When mental health specialty assistance is desired, the family physician will either consult with or refer the patient to a psychiatrist or behavioural psychologist. Tricyclic antidepressants[24] and CBT as provided by a mental health specialist[21] are the mainstay of EBT. The most common reason for pharmacologic treatment of patients with MUS is treatment of their comorbid or underlying depression or anxiety, or both. Antidepressant medication effects an independent improvement on mood or anxiety symptoms and attenuates the severity of pain, which in turn decreases the somatic complaints.

Adherence to treatment

An estimated 55% and 60% of primary care patients do not follow through with mental health recommendations.[155] Furthermore, 25% of patients in a Spanish sample who had requested a mental health referral did not attend their scheduled appointment.[156] Adherence to any of the proposed stepped care treatments outlined herein will result from a myriad of unique and interactive factors. Martin et al., in their book on treatment adherence,[157] classified those factors into the following broad categories: intrapersonal (e.g. personal beliefs, personality traits), interpersonal (e.g. social support), structural (e.g. access to treatment) and disease related (e.g. severity of symptoms, stage of illness, medication adverse effects, medication regimen demand).

Preventing treatment failure

When there is poor patient response to the interventions used, a first course of action is to assess the patient's readiness for change, using the Prochaska and DiClemente transtheoretical stages of change model.[158] In this model, behaviour change is viewed as a process that unfolds over time and progresses through a series of five stages: precontemplation, contemplation, preparation, action and maintenance. Table 21.4 summarizes the five stages as outlined by Norcross et al.[136]

Table 21.4 Stages of change[136]		
Stage	**Description**	**Patient state**
1 Precontemplation	Having no intention to change behaviour in the foreseeable future	Unaware or underaware of the problem
2 Contemplation	Thinking about change to overcome a problem but taking no committed action	Aware that a problem exists but struggles with the effort and energy needed to change
3 Preparation	Reporting very small behavioural changes but has not reached a criterion for effective change	Intends to take criterion-level action in the next month for solving the problem
4 Action	Taking criterion-type action that involves a modification in behaviour and the environment to overcome a problem	Has transformed intention into committed action
5 Maintenance	Engaging in behaviour to prevent relapse and to consolidate gains during the action stage that lasts for ≥6 months	Is consistent and committed to sustaining the gains

The suggested guideline is to use one or more of the stepped care interventions at levels 1 to 3, when the patient is at the precontemplation or contemplation stage, because these methods contain awareness-building strategies. Interventions of levels 4 to 6 match with the action and maintenance stages of change, because these strategies provide the greatest degree of applied behavioural change mapping. Furthermore, if a patient seems stuck at precontemplation or contemplation, it is recommended that the two-by-two decisional worksheet[159] be used to assist in creating and resolving change ambivalence by collaboratively exploring the pros and cons of changing versus not changing. As a final point, the physician needs to facilitate the patient through the stages in sequence. For example, he or she should not make the mistake of trying to move the patient from the precontemplation stage to the action stage in a single step.

A systematic review of enhanced care by family physicians or general medical practitioners for functional somatic symptoms and disorders is available in the Cochrane database.[105,160]

Key stakeholders for delivering the gold standard identification and treatment

There are multiple key stakeholders related to integrated behavioural health-care services for patients with MUS: the patient and his or her family, the family physician and the health-care team, and the payers. Payers' interest is heightened by the direct financial costs associated with MUS and the related somatoform disorders. Health-care expenditures in the USA in 2008, for example, were about $7681 per resident, surpassing $3.2 trillion in total, and accounted for 16.2% of the gross domestic product.[161]

Important recent developments of interest to stakeholders are the accountable care organizations[162] and patient-centred medical home (PCMH) literature.[163–166] Accountable care organizations are vertically integrated organizations of care, which at minimum are composed of primary care physicians, a hospital and specialists, aimed at working together to both improve quality of care and slow spending growth in designated medical populations. Fisher and Shortell noted that the concept of accountable care has broad appeal,[162] but only a robust, comprehensive, and transparent performance measurement system can bring the organizations' objective to fruition and satisfy both those who deliver care and the payers. A policy brief recently published by the Berkeley Center details a set of recommendations for establishing and implementing an accountable care organization.[167]

Emotional and physical suffering and the caregiver burden associated with MUS create high interest, with both patient and family investments in treatment possibilities and associated costs.[26] The PCMH offers the greatest possibility for effectively and efficiently merging and delivering integrated primary care and behavioural health services,[165] mainly because of its emphasis on centring care around the patient and the patient's family, improving access to care, and coordinating care between providers and community resources. For a review of extensive information on the PCMH, including evidence-based outcomes, access the Patient-Centered Primary Care Collaborative web site.[168] Shared decision-making[169] is an important element in establishing and effectively using a PCMH.

The primary care workforce needed to achieve best outcomes

Although the 2010 National Resident Matching Program in the USA noted a 3.1% increase in the number of family resident positions filled compared with 2009, a substantial shortage of primary care physicians continues in the country.[170]

The recently enacted US health-care reform legislation, which calls for eliminating financial barriers for preventive services, will likely create increased demand for these services and give physicians a better opportunity to provide preventive care.[171] In turn, this response will create the need for even greater use of health-care teams composed of nurse practitioners, physician assistants, care managers, social workers, pharmacists and mental health personnel. Clearly, the new workforce model must recognize the impact of genomics.[172]

Implications for mental health promotion and prevention in primary care

The multiple challenges that face primary care in the 21st century, such as access to services, quality of care and cost-effectiveness, highlight the importance of new and refined models of care. The new model of care must be grounded in medicine's timeless values of personalized, patient-centred care coupled with the application of new technologies and systems.[170,173] It is worth noting that the May/June 2011 issue of *Annals of Family Medicine* was devoted to the topic "personalizing health care".[137] It is essential that care modelling emphasizes core human values and the potential for improving the health care of all nations in the world community.

Family practice needs to continue improving integrated behavioural health care, because the vast majority of patients in primary care have either a physical problem that is affected by stress, problems maintaining healthy lifestyles, or a psychological disorder. This approach is clinically effective and cost effective.[174] Persons in leadership positions must have a vision for the future that includes planning for the changes and developments in primary care that are virtually certain to occur in the next 5 to 10 years, and must prepare contingency plans for developments that might catch health-care providers by surprise.

Other relevant issues

Global health

Global health represents the interrelationship between the family physician's local practice setting and the global community. The Declaration of Alma-Ata in 1978 emerged from the International Conference on Primary Health Care.[175] This declaration became a major milestone of the 20th century in the field of public health, and it identified primary health care as the key to the attainment of the goal of health for all. Health promotion and disease prevention are the hallmarks.[176] In condensed form, the basic tenets expressed by Alma-Ata are as follows:[176]

- health is not simply the absence of disease. Health is a state of physical, mental and social well-being, and is a fundamental human right
- the inequality among developed and developing countries in population health status is politically, socially and economically unacceptable
- planning and implementing their health care is the right and obligation of the patients
- primary health care is essential to individuals and families in the community at an affordable and sustainable cost to the community and country. It is the first level of health-care access for individuals and the family, and should be as close as possible to where people live and work
- basic health care for all the people of the world by the year 2000 can be attained through more effective use of the world's resources. A genuine policy of independence, peace, détente and disarmament around the world could and should create sufficient health resources.

The reality is that 30-plus years later, the intent of the Declaration of Alma-Ata has not been realized. Hall and Taylor reported on the sobering finding that many people in resource-poor countries, and even in wealthy sovereign nations, still do not have equitable access to even basic services, especially in rural areas.[177] Almost as soon as the Alma-Ata conference concluded, politicians and care experts from developed countries attacked the primary health-care principle that communities in developing countries would have responsibility for planning and implementing their own health-care services. Critics driven by political and economic ideology advocated for only interventions that reduce child mortality rates and declared the health care for all as unrealistic because of market forces and unacceptable national debt implications. The authors concluded that the time has come to abandon economic and political ideology and reorganize and revitalize nongovernmental oraganizations, academics, and patients in the community to accomplish the first step – access to the most basic of health services for all.[177]

Malpractice

Patients with bodily distress syndrome often request, or even demand, medical testing and specialty consultations related to their concern and anxiety about illness. Legal liability can lead a family physician to practise so-called defensive medicine in fear of being sued by the patient. A claim of malpractice is predicated on four elements often referred to as the "4 Ds".[178] First, a plaintiff must establish "duty", which means proving that a physician–patient relationship existed. Second, "dereliction," or a breach of that duty, must be shown. "Direct" harm to the patient is the third condition that must be established to make a case for malpractice. Fourth, "damages" from breach of duty must be proven.

Although defendants prevail in the majority of malpractice litigations,[179] it is not uncommon that physician worry affects medical decision-making. Several factors are associated with malpractice risk reduction: (1) clear and empathic communication with the patient; (2) honest communication of unexpected adverse outcomes from a test or procedure;[180] (3) consultation with medical colleagues; and (4) detailed documentation. Therefore, it is highly desirable that the family physician establishes a favourable physician–patient relationship based on clear and empathic communication and collaborative decision-making, consulting with colleagues to promote effective care, carefully document care, and maintain detailed clinical records.

Issues affecting bodily distress syndrome research

Jackson and Kroenke outlined critical factors that are currently complicating or confounding MUS research.[181] Those crucial investigative considerations include imperfect dichotomization, an often unclear locus of therapy, salient outcomes and multicomponent or layered interventions.

Conclusions and future opportunities

The most prevalent patient with bodily distress syndrome in primary care tends to be female, has attained a low education level, and may possess psychiatric comorbidity. The MUS condition will be characterized by medically unexplained or underexplained symptoms. Patient presentation can be dichotomized as monosymptomatic, consisting of a single symptom – often low back pain or headache – or polysymptomatic, consisting of multiple different symptoms across biological systems. Bodily distress syndrome should be considered as subjectively real and distressing and beyond deliberate control and thus distinct from factitious disorders or intentional production for secondary gain.

Multiple biological, cognitive, personality, cultural, spiritual and social mechanisms interact dynamically to explain the predisposing, precipitating and sustaining course of bodily distress syndrome. The biopsychosocial model illuminates the contextual matrix that contains these dynamic interactions and is the substance of our perception of symptom generation, disease or illness attributions, and health-care-seeking behaviour. To complicate matters, the directionality of the relationship between psychological and somatic symptoms is often indeterminate. At present, the state of our models and explanations can best be described as a work in progress.

Cognitive-behavioural psychological interventions and antidepressant medications have the strongest evidence-based support for treatment effectiveness. Current treatments described in the published literature are typically bundled interventions, making it difficult to disentangle the incidental elements from the essential ingredients that yield positive patient outcomes. Psychological and pharmacological interventions currently dominate the treatment landscape. Being mindful of the challenges faced by low-income countries, it is imperative that the next wave of newly minted validated strategies includes self-directed lifestyle approaches that are not time and resource intensive.

Future research on bodily distress syndrome should focus on multifactorial, bidirectional designs that will disentangle the aetiologic variance and isolate the essential treatment components. An example would be combining genetic, neuroendocrine and psychological constructs related to distress tolerance or emotion regulation.

Providing the best possible health care to patients with bodily distress syndrome is inextricably interwoven with producing salient outcomes for the many who are suffering. Perhaps this issue was best stated by Jackson and Kroenke:[181]

> Although death is an unlikely consequence, other D's relevant to MUS include disability, discomfort, dissatisfaction, and destitution, i.e. the considerable medical costs resulting from somatization. For these reasons, medically unexplained symptoms should not be synonymous with medically ignored.

References

1   Kisely S, Simon G. An international study comparing the effect of medically explained and unexplained somatic symptoms on psychosocial outcome. *Journal of Psychosomatic Research*, 2006, 60:125–130.

2   Lowe B et al. Depression, anxiety and somatization in primary care: syndrome overlap and functional impairment. *General Hospital Psychiatry*, 2008, 30:191–199.

3   Kroenke K et al. Multisomatoform disorder: an alternative to undifferentiated somatoform disorder for the somatizing patient in primary care. *Archives of General Psychiatry*, 1997, 54:352–358.

4   Fink P, Schroder A. One single diagnosis, bodily distress syndrome, succeeded to capture 10 diagnostic categories of functional somatic syndromes and somatoform disorders. *Journal of Psychosomatic Research*, 2010, 68:415–426.

5   Goldberg D. A revised mental health classification for use in general medical settings: the ICD11-PHC (editorial). *International Psychiatry*, 2011, 8:1–2.

6   Dickinson WP et al. The somatization in primary care study: a tale of three diagnoses. *General Hospital Psychiatry*, 2003, 25:1–7.

7   Messer SB. Evidenced-based practice: beyond empirically supported treatments. *Professional Psychology: Research and Practice*, 2004, 35:580–588.

8   Norcross JC, Hill CE. Empirically supported therapy relationships. *Clinical Psychology*, 2004, 47:19–24.

9   Fraser JS, Solovey AD. *Second-order change in psychotherapy: the golden thread that unifies effective treatments*. Washington, American Psychological Association, 2007.

10 Kroenke K. Patients presenting with somatic complaints: epidemiology, psychiatric comorbidity and management. *International Journal of Methods in Psychiatry Research*, 2003, 12:34–43.

11 Kroenke K, Rosmalen JG. Symptoms, syndromes, and the value of psychiatric diagnostics in patients who have functional somatic disorders. *Medical Clinics of North America*, 2006, 90:603–626.

12 Johnson SK. *Medically unexplained illness: gender and biopsychosocial implications*. Washington, DC, American Psychological Association, 2008.

13 Toft T et al. Mental disorders in primary care: prevalence and co-morbidity among disorders: results from the functional illness in primary care (FIP) study. *Psychological Medicine*, 2005, 35:1175–1184.

14 Verhaak PF et al. Persistent presentation of medically unexplained symptoms in general practice. *Family Practice*, 2006, 23:414–420.

15 Rosendal M et al. Improving the classification of medically unexplained symptoms in primary care. *European Journal of Psychiatry*, 2007, 21:25–36.

16 Kroenke K et al. Physical symptoms in primary care: predictors of psychiatric disorders and functional impairment. *Archives of Family Medicine*, 1994, 3:774–779.

17 Rasmussen NH, Bernard ME, Harmsen WS. Physical symptoms that predict psychiatric disorders in rural primary care adults. *Journal of Evaluation in Clinical Practice*, 2008, 14:399–406.

18 Mathers NJ, Gask L. Surviving the 'heartsink' experience. *Family Practice*, 1995, 12:176–183.

19 Lipowski ZJ. Somatization: the concept and its clinical application. *American Journal of Psychiatry*, 1988, 145:1358–1368.

20 Jackson JL, O'Malley PG, Kroenke K. Antidepressants and cognitive-behavioral therapy for symptom syndromes. *CNS Spectrums*, 2006, 11:212–222.

21 Woolfolk RL, Allen LA. *Treating somatization: a cognitive-behavioral approach*. New York, Guilford Press, 2007.

22 Abbass A, Kisely S, Kroenke K. Short-term psychodynamic psychotherapy for somatic disorders: systematic review and meta-analysis of clinical trials. *Psychotherapy and Psychosomatics*, 2009, 78:265–274.

23 Allen LA et al. Psychosocial treatments for multiple unexplained physical symptoms: a review of the literature. *Psychosomatic Medicine*, 2002, 64:939–950.

24 Kroenke K. Efficacy of treatment for somatoform disorders: a review of randomized controlled trials. *Psychosomatic Medicine*, 2007, 69:881–888.

25 Sumathipala A. What is the evidence for the efficacy of treatments for somatoform disorders? A critical review of previous intervention studies. *Psychosomatic Medicine*, 2007, 69:889–900.

26 Witthoft M, Hiller W. Psychological approaches to origins and treatments of somatoform disorders. *Annual Review of Clinical Psychology*, 2010, 6:257–283.

27 Collins C et al. *Evolving models of behavioral health integration in primary care.* New York (NY) Milbank Memorial Fund, 2010 (http://www.milbank.org/reports/10430EvolvingCare/EvolvingCare.pdf, accessed 22 November 2011).

28 Rasmussen NH, Avant RF. Somatization disorder in family practice. *American Family Physician*, 1989, 40:206–214.

29 Rief W et al. Evaluation of general practitioners' training: how to manage patients with unexplained physical symptoms. *Psychosomatics*, 2006, 47:304–311.

30 Silber TJ. Somatization disorders: diagnosis, treatment, and prognosis. *Pediatrics in Review*, 2011, 32:56–63.

31 Gureje O et al. Somatization in cross-cultural perspective: a World Health Organization study in primary care. *American Journal of Psychiatry*, 1997, 154:989–995.

32 Steinbrecher N et al. The prevalence of medically unexplained symptoms in primary care. *Psychosomatics*, 2011, 52:263–271.

33 Kirmayer LJ. Cultural variations in the clinical presentation of depression and anxiety: implications for diagnosis and treatment. *Journal of Clinical Psychiatry*, 2001, 62(Suppl. 13):22–28.

34 Fabiao C, Silva MC, Fleming M, Barbosa A. [Somatoform disorders: a revision of the epidemiology in primary health care]. *Acta Médica Portuguesa*, 2010, 23:865–772 [in Portuguese].

35 *International statistical classification of diseases and related health problems*, 10th revision, 2nd edition. Geneva, World Health Organization, 2007.

36 *Diagnostic and statistical manual of mental disorders*, 4th ed, text revision (DSM-IV-TR). Washington, American Psychiatric Association, 2000.

37 Escobar JI et al. Somatic symptom index (SSI): a new and abridged somatization construct. Prevalence and epidemiological correlates in two large community samples. *Journal of Nervous and Mental Disease*, 1989, 177:140–146.

38 Jackson JL, Passamonti M. The outcomes among patients presenting in primary care with a physical symptom at 5 years. *Journal of General Internal Medicine*, 2005, 20:1032–1037.

39 World Health Organization. *Mental health intervention guide to make care more accessible* [internet; podcast]   (http://www.who.int/mediacentre/multimedia/podcasts/2010/mentalhealth_20101018/en/index.html, accessed 22 November 2011).

40 Kirmayer LJ, Sartorius N. Cultural models and somatic syndromes. *Psychosomatic Medicine*, 2007, 69:832–840.

41 Escobar JI, Gureje O. Influence of cultural and social factors on the epidemiology of idiopathic somatic complaints and syndromes. *Psychosomatic Medicine*, 2007, 69:841–845.

42 Baarnhielm S, Ekblad S. Introducing a psychological agenda for understanding somatic symptoms: an area of conflict for clinicians in relation to patients in a multicultural community. *Culture, Medicine and Psychiatry*, 2008, 32:386–405.

43 Bekker MHJ, Schepman R. Somatization and psychological awareness of ethnic minority clients in Western-European mental health care: a pilot study. *European Journal of Psychiatry*, 2009, 23:135–139.

44 Beck BJ, Gordon C. An approach to collaborative care and consultation: interviewing, cultural competence, and enhancing rapport and adherence. *Medical Clinics of North America*, 2010, 94:1075–1088.

45 Mulvaney-Day NE et al. Preferences for relational style with mental health clinicians: a qualitative comparison of African American, Latino and Non-Latino White patients. *Journal of Clinical Psychology*, 2011, 67:31–44.

46 Zuckoff A, Swartz HA, Grote NK. Motivational interviewing as a prelude to psychotherapy of depression. In: Arkowitz H et al., eds. *Motivational interviewing in the treatment of psychological problems.* New York, Guilford Press, 2008:109–144.

47 Burton C. Beyond somatisation: a review of the understanding and treatment of medically unexplained physical symptoms (MUPS). *British Journal of General Practice*, 2003, 53:231–239.

48 Smits FT et al. Epidemiology of frequent attenders: a 3-year historic cohort study comparing attendance, morbidity and prescriptions of one-year and persistent frequent attenders. *BMC Public Health*, 2009, 9:36.

49 *Somatoform disorders*. Arlington, American Psychiatric Association, 2010 (http://www.dsm5.org/PROPOSEDREVISIONS/Pages/SomatoformDisorders.aspx, accessed 22 November 2011).

50 olde Hartman TC et al. Medically unexplained symptoms, somatisation disorder and hypochondriasis: course and prognosis: a systematic review. *Journal of Psychosomatic Research*, 2009, 66:363–377.

51 Koch H et al. The course of newly presented unexplained complaints in general practice patients: a prospective cohort study. *Family Practice*, 2009, 26:455–465.

52 de Waal MW et al. Follow-up study on health care use of patients with somatoform, anxiety and depressive disorders in primary care. *BMC Family Practice*, 2008, 9:5.

53 Bener A, Ghuloum S, Burgut FT. Gender differences in prevalence of somatoform disorders in patients visiting primary care centers. *Journal of Primary Care Community Health*, 2010, 1:37–42.

54 Kroenke K, Spitzer RL. Gender differences in the reporting of physical and somatoform symptoms. *Psychosomatic Medicine*, 1998, 60:150–155.

55 Gijsbers van Wijk CM, Huisman H, Kolk AM. Gender differences in physical symptoms and illness behavior: a health diary study. *Social Science and Medicine*, 1999, 49:1061–1074.

56 Rief W, Hessel A, Braehler E. Somatization symptoms and hypochondriacal features in the general population. *Psychosomatic Medicine*, 2001, 63:595–602.

57 Movahed MR et al. Differences according to gender in reporting physical symptoms during echocardiographic screening in healthy teenage athletes. *Cardiology in the Young*, 2008, 18:303–306.

58 Karvonen JT et al. Somatization symptoms in young adult Finnish population: associations with sex, educational level and mental health. *Nordic Journal of Psychiatry*, 2007, 61:219–224.

59 Leiknes KA et al. Overlap, comorbidity, and stability of somatoform disorders and the use of current versus lifetime criteria. *Psychosomatics*, 2008, 49:152–162.

60 Hanel G et al. Depression, anxiety, and somatoform disorders: vague or distinct categories in primary care? Results from a large cross-sectional study. *Journal of Psychosomatic Research*, 2009, 67:189–197.

61 Burton C et al. Depression and anxiety in patients repeatedly referred to secondary care with medically unexplained symptoms: a case-control study. *Psychological Medicine*, 2011, 41:555–563.

62 Epstein RM, Quill TE, McWhinney IR. Somatization reconsidered: incorporating the patient's experience of illness. *Archives of Internal Medicine*, 1999, 159:215–222.

63 World Health Organization. 2010. *Gender and women's mental health* (http://www.who.int/mental_health/prevention/genderwomen/en/, accessed 22 November 2011).

64 Kirmayer LJ, Groleau D, Looper KJ, Dao MD. Explaining medically unexplained symptoms. *Canadian Journal of Psychiatry*, 2004, 49:663–672.

65 Rief W, Broadbent E. Explaining medically unexplained symptoms: models and mechanisms. *Clinical Psychology Review*, 2007, 27:821–841.

66 Rief W, Barsky AJ. Psychobiological perspectives on somatoform disorders. *Psychoneuroendocrinology*, 2005, 30:996–1002.

67 Melzack R, Wall PD. Pain mechanisms: a new theory. *Science*, 1965, 150:971–979.

68 Hakala M et al. Severe somatization in women is associated with altered cerebral glucose metabolism. *Psychologie Médicale*, 2002, 32:1379–1385.

69 Rief W et al. Immunological differences between patients with major depression and somatization syndrome. *Psychiatry Research*, 2001, 105:165–174.

70 Tak LM, Rosmalen JG. Dysfunction of stress responsive systems as a risk factor for functional somatic syndromes. *Journal of Psychosomatic Research*, 2010, 68:461–468.

71 Garcia-Campayo J et al. Brain dysfunction behind functional symptoms: neuroimaging and somatoform, conversive, and dissociative disorders. *Current Opinion in Psychiatry*, 2009, 22:224–231.

72 Henningsen P, Creed F. The genetic, physiological and psychological mechanisms underlying disabling medically unexplained symptoms and somatisation. *Journal of Psychosomatic Research*, 2010, 68:395–397.

73 Holliday KL et al. Genetic variation in neuroendocrine genes associates with somatic symptoms in the general population: results from the EPIFUND study. *Journal of Psychosomatic Research*, 2010, 68:469–474.

74 Fulton JJ, Marcus DK, Merkey T. Irrational health beliefs and health anxiety. *Journal of Clinical Psychology*, 2011, 67:527–538.

75 Barsky AJ, Wyshak G. Hypochondriasis and somatosensory amplification. *British Journal of Psychiatry*, 1990, 157:404–409.

76 Rief W, Nanke A. Somatoform disorders in primary care and inpatient settings. *Advances in Psychosomatic Medicine*, 2004, 26:144–158.

77 Campo JV, Fritsch SL. Somatization in children and adolescents. *Journal of the American Academy of Child and Adolescent Psychiatry*, 1994, 33:1223–1235.

78 Walker LS et al. Parent attention versus distraction: impact on symptom complaints by children with and without chronic functional abdominal pain. *Pain*, 2006, 122:43–52.

79 Berntsson LT, Kohler L. Long-term illness and psychosomatic complaints in children aged 2–17 years in the five Nordic countries: comparison between 1984 and 1996. *European Journal of Public Health*, 2001, 11:35–42.

80 Fiddler M et al. Childhood adversity and frequent medical consultations. *General Hospital Psychiatry*, 2004, 26:367–377.

81 Beck JE. A developmental perspective on functional somatic symptoms. *Journal of Pediatric Psychology*, 2008, 33:547–562.

82 Stuart S, Noyes R Jr. Attachment and interpersonal communication in somatization. *Psychosomatics*, 1999, 40:34–43.

83 Waldinger RJ et al. Mapping the road from childhood trauma to adult somatization: the role of attachment. *Psychosomatic Medicine*, 2006, 68:129–135.

84 Brown RJ. Introduction to the special issue on medically unexplained symptoms: background and future directions. *Clinical Psychology Review*, 2007, 27:769–780.

85 Roelofs K, Spinhoven P. Trauma and medically unexplained symptoms towards an integration of cognitive and neuro-biological accounts. *Clinical Psychology Review*, 2007, 27:798–820.

86 Paras ML et al. Sexual abuse and lifetime diagnosis of somatic disorders: a systematic review and meta-analysis. *JAMA*, 2009, 302:550–561.

87 Clark LA. Stability and change in personality disorder. *Current Directions in Psychological Science*, 2009, 18:27–31.

88 Aronson KR, Barrett LF, Quigley K. Emotional reactivity and the overreport of somatic symptoms: somatic sensitivity or negative reporting style? *Journal of Psychosomatic Research*, 2006, 60:521–530.

89 Wearden AJ et al. Adult attachment, alexithymia, and symptom reporting: an extension to the four category model of attachment. *Journal of Psychosomatic Research*, 2005, 58:279–288.

90 Rasmussen NH et al. Somatisation and alexithymia in patients with high use of medical care and medically unexplained symptoms. *Mental Health in Family Medicine*, 2008, 5:139–148.

91 Sifneos PE. The prevalence of 'alexithymic' characteristics in psychosomatic patients. *Psychotherapy and Psychosomatics*, 1973, 22:255–262.

92 Noyes R Jr et al. Hypochondriasis and fear of death. *Journal of Nervous and Mental Disease*, 2002, 190:503–509.

93 Taylor RE et al. Attachment style in patients with unexplained physical complaints. *Psychological Medicine*, 2000, 30:931–941.

94 Ciechanowski PS et al. Association of attachment style to lifetime medically unexplained symptoms in patients with hepatitis C. *Psychosomatics*, 2002, 43:206–212.

95 Hatcher S, Arroll B. Assessment and management of medically unexplained symptoms. *BMJ*, 2008, 336:1124–1128.

96 Babor TF et al. *The alcohol use disorders identification test (AUDIT): guidelines for use in primary care*, 2nd ed. Geneva, Department of Mental Health and Substance Dependence, World Health Organization, 2001 (http://whqlibdoc.who.int/hq/2001/who_msd_msb_01.6a.pdf, accessed 22 November 2011).

97 Spitzer RL et al. A brief measure for assessing generalized anxiety disorder: the GAD-7. *Archives of Internal Medicine*, 2006, 166:1092–1097.

98 Ruiz MA et al. Validity of the GAD-7 scale as an outcome measure of disability in patients with generalized anxiety disorders in primary care. *Journal of Affective Disorders*, 2011, 128:277–286.

99 Spitzer RL, Kroenke K, Williams JB. Validation and utility of a self-report version of PRIME-MD: the PHQ primary care study. Primary Care Evaluation of Mental Disorders. Patient Health Questionnaire. *JAMA*, 1999, 282:1737–1744.

100 Kroenke K et al. The Patient Health Questionnaire Somatic, Anxiety, and Depressive Symptom Scales: a systematic review. *General Hospital Psychiatry*, 2010, 32:345–359.

101 van Ravesteijn H et al. Detecting somatoform disorders in primary care with the PHQ-15. *Annals of Family Medicine*, 2009, 7:232–238.

102 Wrong Diagnosis. *Diagnostic tests for somatization disorder* (http://www.wrongdiagnosis.com/s/somatization_disorder/tests.htm, accessed 22 November 2011).

103 Rasmussen NH et al. Coping style in primary care adult patients with abridged somatoform disorders. *Mental Health in Family Medicine*, 2010, 7:197–207.

104 Kirmayer LJ, Robbins JM. Patients who somatize in primary care: a longitudinal study of cognitive and social characteristics. *Psychological Medicine*, 1996, 26:937–951.

105 Huibers MJH et al. Psychosocial interventions by general practitioners. *Cochrane Database of Systematic Reviews*, 2007, (3):CD003494 (http://onlinelibrary.wiley.com/doi/10.1002/14651858.CD003494.pub2/pdf, accessed 22 November 2011).

106 Mauer BJ. *Background paper: behavioral health/primary care integration models, competencies, and infrastructure.* Rockville MD, National Council for Community Behavioral Healthcare, 2002 (http://www.thenationalcouncil.org/galleries/business-practice%20files/PC-BH%20Models-Competencies.pdf, accessed 22 November 2011).

107 Blount A et al. The economics of behavioral health services in medical settings: a summary of the evidence. *Professional Psychology: Research and Practice*, 2007, 38:290–297.

108 Brown W, Kandirikirira N. *Recovering mental health in Scotland: report on narrative investigation of mental health recovery.* Glasgow, Scottish Recovery Network, 2007.

109 Stuart MR, Lieberman JA 3rd. *The fifteen minute hour: applied psychotherapy for the primary care physician.* New York, Praeger, 1986.

110 Stuart MR, Lieberman JA 3rd. *The fifteen minute hour: applied psychotherapy for the primary care physician*, 2nd ed. Westport, CT, Praeger, 1993.

111 Stuart MR, Lieberman JA 3rd. *The fifteen minute hour: practical therapeutic interventions in primary care*, 3rd ed. Philadelphia, Saunders, 2002.

112 Stuart MR, Lieberman JA 3rd. *The fifteen minute hour: therapeutic talk in primary care*, 4th ed. New York, Radcliffe Publishing, 2008.

113 Bloom MV, Smith DA. *Brief mental health interventions for the family physician.* New York, Springer, 2001.

114 Levinson W et al. Physician–patient communication: the relationship with malpractice claims among primary care physicians and surgeons. *JAMA*, 1997, 277:553–559.

115 Haskard KB et al. Physician and patient communication training in primary care: effects on participation and satisfaction. *Health Psychology*, 2008, 27:513–522.

116 Street RL Jr et al. Patient participation in medical consultations: why some patients are more involved than others. *Medical Care*, 2005, 43:960–969.

117 Street RL Jr et al. How does communication heal? Pathways linking clinician–patient communication to health outcomes. *Patient Education and Counseling*, 2009, 74:295–301.

118 Haywood K, Marshall S, Fitzpatrick R. Patient participation in the consultation process: a structured review of intervention strategies. *Patient Education and Counseling*, 2006, 63:12–23.

119 Heijmans M et al. Experts' opinions on the management of medically unexplained symptoms in primary care: a qualitative analysis of narrative reviews and scientific editorials. *Family Practice*, 2011, 28:444–455.

120 Steele DJ, Marvel K. Listening, talking, relating: the state of the art and science of the doctor–patient relationship in family medicine education. *Family Medicine*, 2002, 34:310–311.

121 Official Journal of World Organization of Family Doctors (Wonca). *Family Medicine*, 2002, 34(5).

122 Mendoza MD et al. The seventh element of quality: the doctor–patient relationship. *Family Medicine*, 2011, 43:83–89.

123 Frank JD, Frank JB. *Persuasion and healing: a comparative study of psychotherapy*, 3rd ed. Baltimore, Johns Hopkins University Press, 1991.

124 Lambert MJ, Barley DE. 2001. Research summary on the therapeutic relationship and psychotherapy outcome. *Psychotherapy: Theory Research Practice Training*, 2001, 38:357–611.

125 Lambert MJ. *Prevention of treatment failure: the use of measuring, monitoring, and feedback in clinical practice*. Washington DC, American Psychological Association, 2010.

126 Bhugra D, McKenzie K. Expressed emotion across cultures. *Advances in Psychiatric Treatment*, 2003, 9:342–348.

127 Cheng AT. Expressed emotion: a cross-culturally valid concept? *British Journal of Psychiatry*, 2002, 181:466–467.

128 Endley L, Berry K. Increasing awareness of expressed emotion in schizophrenia: an evaluation of a staff training session. *Journal of Psychiatric and Mental Health Nursing*, 2011, 18:277–280.

129 Hollon SD, Thase ME, Markowitz JC. Treatment and prevention of depression. *Psychological Science in the Public Interest*, 2002, 3:39–77.

130 Rasmussen NH et al. Innovative reflecting interview: effect on high-utilizing patients with medically unexplained symptoms. *Disease Management*, 2006, 9:349–359.

131 Adam P et al. Effects of team care of frequent attenders on patients and physicians. *Family Systems and Health*, 2010, 28:247–257.

132 Seekles W et al. Stepped care for depression and anxiety: from primary care to specialized mental health care: a randomised controlled trial testing the effectiveness of a stepped care program among primary care patients with mood or anxiety disorders. *BMC Health Services Research*, 2009, 9:90.

133 Mergl R et al. Are treatment preferences relevant in response to serotonergic antidepressants and cognitive-behavioral therapy in depressed primary care patients? Results from a randomized controlled trial including a patients' choice arm. *Psychotherapy and Psychosomatics*, 2011, 80:39–47.

134 Gask L, Morriss R. Assessment and immediate management of people at risk of harming themselves. *Foundation Years*, 2008, 4:64–68.

135 Ivbijaro GO et al. Look, listen and test: mental health assessment: the Wonca Culturally Sensitive Depression Guideline. *Primary Care Mental Health*, 2005, 3:145–147.

136 Norcross JC, Krebs PM, Prochaska JO. Stages of change. *Journal of Clinical Psychology*, 2011, 67:143–154.

137 Stange KC. Personalizing health care [editorial]. *Annals of Family Medicine*, 2011, 9:194–195.

138 Scioli A et al. Hope: its nature and measurement. *Psychology of Religion and Spirituality*, 2011, 3:78–97.

139 Sansone RA, Sansone LA. Demoralization in patients with medical illness. *Psychiatry*, 2010, 7:42–45.

140 Rollnick S, Mason P, Butler C. *Health behavior change: a guide for practitioners*. New York, Churchill Livingstone, 1999.

141 Launer J. *Narrative-based primary care: a practical guide*. Abingdon, Radcliffe Medical Press, 2002.

142 Salmon P et al. Why do primary care physicians propose medical care to patients with medically unexplained symptoms? A new method of sequence analysis to test theories of patient pressure. *Psychosomatic Medicine*, 2006, 68:570–577.

143 Morriss R et al. Randomized trial of reattribution on psychosocial talk between doctors and patients with medically unexplained symptoms. *Psychological Medicine*, 2010, 40:325–333.

144 Larisch A et al. Psychosocial interventions for somatizing patients by the general practitioner: a randomized controlled trial. *Journal of Psychosomatic Research*, 2004, 57:507–514.

145 Gask L, Usherwood T. ABC of psychological medicine: the consultation. *BMJ*, 2002, 324:1567–1569.

146 Rollnick S, Miller WR, Butler CC. *Motivational interviewing in health care: helping patients change behavior*. New York, Guilford Press, 2008.

147 Arkowitz H et al. *Motivational interviewing in the treatment of psychological problems*. New York, Guilford Press, 2008.

148 Bell AC, D'Zurilla TJ. Problem-solving therapy for depression: a meta-analysis. *Clinical Psychology Review*, 2009, 29:348–353.

149 O'Connell B, Palmer S. Solution focused coaching. In: Palmer S, Whybrow A, eds. *Handbook of coaching psychology: a guide for practitioners*. New York, Routledge, 2007:278–292.

150 Oxman TE et al. Problem-solving treatment and coping styles in primary care for minor depression. *Journal of Consulting and Clinical Psychology*, 2008, 76:933–943.

151 Greenberg G, Ganshorn K, Danilkewich A. Solution-focused therapy: counseling model for busy family physicians. *Canadian Family Physician*, 2001, 47:2289–2295.

152 Poon VH. Short counseling techniques for busy family doctors. *Canadian Family Physician*, 1997, 43:705–708.

153 Searight HR. Efficient counseling techniques for the primary care physician. *Primary Care*, 2007, 34:551–570.

154 De Jong P, Berg IK. *Interviewing for solutions*, 3rd ed. Belmond, Thomson Higher Education, 2008.

155 Gonzalez J et al. Adherence to mental health treatment in a primary care clinic. *Journal of the American Board of Family Practice*, 2005, 18:87–96.

156 Livianos-Aldana L et al. Patients who miss initial appointments in community psychiatry: a Spanish community analysis. *International Journal of Social Psychiatry*, 1999, 45:198–206.

157 Martin LR, Haskard-Zolnierek KB, DiMatteo MR. *Health behavior change and treatment adherence: evidence-based guidelines for improving healthcare*. New York, Oxford University Press, 2010.

158 Prochaska JO, DiClemente CC. Stages and processes of self-change of smoking: toward an integrative model of change. *Journal of Consulting and Clinical Psychology*, 1983, 51:390–395.

159 Miller WR, Rollnick S. *Motivational interviewing: preparing people for change*, 2nd ed. New York, Guilford Press, 2002.

160 Rosendal M et al. Enhanced care by generalists for functional somatic symptoms and disorders in primary care. *Cochrane Database of Systematic Reviews*, 2009, (4):CD008142.

161 US Department of Health and Human Services. Centers for Medicare and Medicaid Services. *NHE fact sheet* (http://www.cms.gov/NationalHealthExpendData/25_NHE_Fact_Sheet.asp, accessed 22 November 2011).

162 Fisher ES, Shortell SM. Accountable care organizations: accountable for what, to whom, and how. *JAMA*, 2010, 304:1715–1716.

163 Kessler R, Stafford D, Messier R. The problem of integrating behavioral health in the medical home and the questions it leads to. *Journal of Clinical Psychology in Medical Settings*, 2009, 16:4–12.

164 Kessler R. What we need to know about behavioral health and psychology in the patient-centered medical home. *Clinical Psychology: Science and Practice*, 2010, 17:215–217.

165 Scherger JE. Future vision: is family medicine ready for patient-directed care? *Family Medicine*, 2009, 41:285–288.

166 *Blueprint for the medical home: transforming primary care to improve practice economics, care coordination, and patient engagement*. Washington DC, The Advisory Board Company, 2009 (http://www.alliantmanagement.com/file_uploads/Medical%20Home%20-%20Motzer.pdf, accessed 22 November 2011).

167 Shortell SM, Casalino LP, Fisher E. *Implementing accountable care organizations. Advancing national health reform*. Berkeley, Berkeley Center on Health, Economic and Family Security, 2010 (http://www.mdpso.com/documents/2010_05_Implementing_Accountable_Care_Organizations.pdf, accessed 22 November 2011).

168 Patient-Centered Primary Care Collaborative (http://www.pcpcc.net/, accessed 22 November 2011).

169 Mayo Foundation for Medical Education and Research, *Shared decision making national resource center* (http://shareddecisions.mayoclinic.org/, accessed 22 November 2011).

170 American Academy of Family Physicians. *Critical challenges for family medicine: delivering emergency medical care: "equipping family physicians for the 21 century"* (http://www.aafp.org/online/en/home/policy/policies/e/emposition.html, accessed 22 November 2011).

171 Arvantes J. *Health care reform law will increase demand for preventive services, say experts*. Leawood KS, American Academy of Family Physicians, 2010 (http://www.aafp.org/online/en/home/publications/news/news-now/government-medicine/20100728hcreformprevent.html, accessed 22 November 2011).

172 Fickenscher K. *The Fickenscher list on "the next 10 things to do" in healthcare* (http://www.justmeans.com/blogs/The-Fickenscher-List-on-The-Next-10-Things-to-Do-in-Healthcare/303.html, accessed 22 November 2011).

173 Collaborative Family Healthcare Association (CFHA) (http://www.cfha.net, accessed 22 November 2011).

174 Blount A. Integrated primary care: organizing the evidence. *Families, Systems and Health*, 2003, 21:121–134.

175 *Declaration of Alma-Ata*. International Conference on Primary Health Care, Alma-Ata USSR, 6–12 September 1978 (http://www.who.int/hpr/NPH/docs/declaration_almaata.pdf, accessed 2 November 2011).

176 Lawn JE et al. Alma-Ata 30 years on: revolutionary, relevant, and time to revitalise. *The Lancet*, 2008, 372:917–927.

177 Hall JJ, Taylor R. Health for all beyond 2000: the demise of the Alma-Ata Declaration and primary health care in developing countries. *Medical Journal of Australia*, 2003, 178:17–20.

178 Brendel RW et al. An approach to selected legal issues: confidentiality, mandatory reporting, abuse and neglect, informed consent, capacity decisions, boundary issues, and malpractice claims. *Medical Clinics of North America*, 2010, 94:1229–1240.

179 King JS, Moulton BW. Rethinking informed consent: the case for shared medical decision-making. *American Journal of Law and Medicine*, 2006, 32:429–501.

180 Gallagher TH, Studdert D, Levinson W. Disclosing harmful medical errors to patients. *New England Journal of Medicine*, 2007, 356:2713–2719.

181 Jackson JL, Kroenke K. Managing somatization: medically unexplained should not mean medically ignored. *Journal of General Internal Medicine*, 2006, 21:797–799.

Part V

Bodily function disorders in primary care mental health

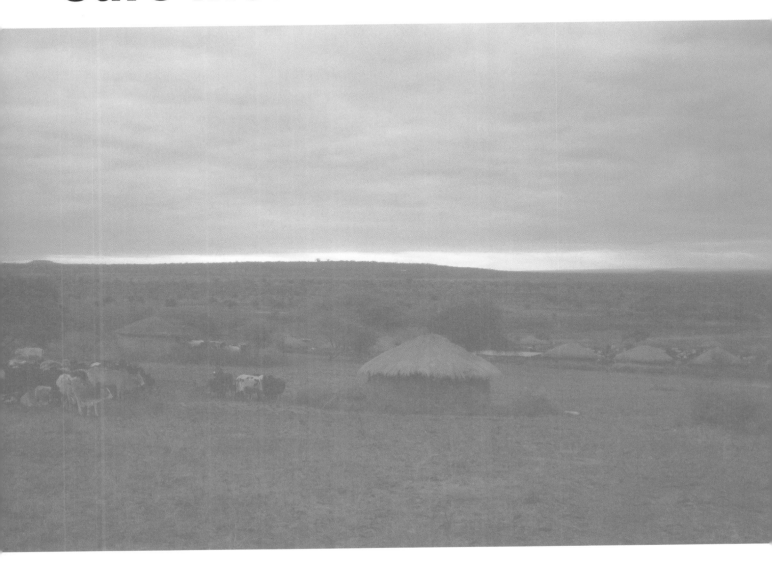

22 Eating disorders in primary care mental health

Allan S Kaplan, and Zeynep Yilmaz

> ## Key messages
>
> - There are three recognized eating disorders: anorexia nervosa (AN), bulimia nervosa (BN) and binge eating disorder (BED). AN is characterized by an underweight state with or without binge eating and purging, bulimia nervosa by binge eating and purging at a normal weight, and binge eating disorder by binge eating and no purging, usually in the context of an overweight/obese state.
>
> - There are effective evidence-based treatments: psychotherapy and pharmacotherapy for BN and BED; for AN there are effective evidence-based treatments for children and adolescents (family therapy) but not for adults.
>
> - Primary care health providers have an important role to play in the recognition, assessment and, with proper training, treatment of patients with eating disorders. For BN and BED, this includes the provision of evidence-based pharmacotherapy and psychotherapy, and for AN the important role of medical monitoring.
>
> - Early identification and intervention is a very important role for primary care physicians, specifically the recognition of high-risk groups of patients who include young women with weight loss and undue weight and shape concerns; and young women who have been sexually abused, have menstrual irregularities, have diabetes, present with vague gastrointestinal complaints or present with mood and anxiety disturbances.
>
> - As is the case with many medical illnesses, there is a group of patients with eating disorder who are treatment resistant and run a chronic course. Primary care physicians have an important role to play in providing medical monitoring and psychological support for this group of ill patients.

Introduction

Eating disorders are characterized by the presence of disordered eating behaviour as well as characteristic psychological disturbance. The *Diagnostic and Statistical Manual of Mental Disorders* fourth edition (DSM-IV)[1] currently recognizes two eating disorders: anorexia nervosa (AN) and bulimia nervosa (BN). Another eating disorder, binge eating disorder (BED), has not yet been officially recognized by the DSM-IV, but has gained research interest and increasing validity as a serious clinical problem, and the DSM-5 Eating Disorders Work Group has recommended that BED be included as a new eating disorder in the new DSM-5, scheduled to be published in 2013.[2] This chapter will focus primarily on the diagnosis, prevalence, assessment and treatment of AN, BN and BED in adults, although the principles enunciated here are generally also applicable to the assessment of children and adolescents with eating disorders.

The name anorexia nervosa comes from the Greek word *orexis* ("appetite"), and the term meaning "lack of appetite" is a misnomer. The first documented case in the medical literature of loss of appetite and extreme wasting without any evidence of known disease was described by the English physician Richard Morton as "nervous atrophy, or consumption" and appeared in his book *Treatise of consumptions*, published in 1689. However, the term AN was first described independently by two separate physicians. Charles Lasegue, a French physician, published a detailed report in 1873 based on his case-studies of young women suffering from *l'anorexie hysterique*. The English physician Sir William Gull also described this syndrome in an address published in *The Lancet* around the same time, coining the current term anorexia nervosa for this illness.[3]

Some historians argue that the fasting saints of the Middle Ages such as Catherine of Siena, rumoured to have survived on very little food and a spoonful of herbs each day, were the first high-profile cases of AN; however, the validity of these claims is hard to determine.[4] AN was featured in the original DSM published in 1952,[5] and has been in the media spotlight since the 1970s.

Although binge eating and purging behaviours date back to Roman times, BN as a psychiatric syndrome can be classified as more of a modern illness, first named and described by Gerald Russell in 1979[6] and featured for the first time as *bulimia* (meaning "ox hunger" in Greek) in the DSM-III in 1980,[7] and changed to bulimia nervosa in the DSM-III-R.[8] Finally, binge eating without any compensatory behaviours (as in BED) was categorized as a mental health disorder in need of research and validation in 1994 as part of the DSM-IV.[1]

For many decades, eating disorders were thought to occur exclusively in young Caucasian women with upper middle-class upbringing,[9] but this theory has been seriously challenged in the past few decades, as eating disorders now cross ethnic and racial lines as well as all social classes. Although they are much more commonly observed in western cultures, they also occur in non-westernized societies.

Diagnosis

Anorexia nervosa

The pathognomonic feature of AN is low weight. The current DSM-IV[1] criteria for AN are:

    A   refusal to maintain body weight at or above a minimally normal weight for age and height (weight loss leading to maintenance of body weight less than 85% of that expected; or failure to make expected weight gain during a period of growth, leading to a body weight less than 85% of that expected)

    B   intense fear of gaining weight or becoming fat even though underweight

    C   disturbance in the way in which one's body weight is experienced, undue influence of body weight or shape on self-evaluation, or denial of the seriousness of the current low body weight

    D   in post-menarchal females, amenorrhoea (the absence of three consecutive menstrual cycles)

subtypes:

    1   *restricting type*: during the current episode of anorexia nervosa, the person has not regularly engaged in binge-eating or purging behaviour

    2   *binge-eating/purging type*: during the current episode of anorexia nervosa, the person has regularly engaged in binge-eating or purging behaviour.

Proposed changes to anorexia nervosa criteria in the DSM-5

The DSM-5 Eating Disorders Work Group has proposed several changes to the diagnosis of AN for the DSM-5, expected to be published in 2013:[10–13]

    A   restriction of energy intake relative to requirements leading to a significantly low body weight in the context of age, sex, developmental trajectory, and physical health. Significantly low weight is defined as a weight that is less than minimally normal, or, for children and adolescents, less than that minimally expected

    B   intense fear of gaining weight or becoming fat, or persistent behaviour that interferes with weight gain, even though at a significantly low weight

    C   disturbance in the way in which one's body weight or shape is experienced, undue influence of body weight or shape on self-evaluation, or persistent lack of recognition of the seriousness of the current low body weight

subtypes:

    1   *restricting type*: during the last 3 months, the person has not engaged in recurrent episodes of binge-eating or purging behaviour (i.e. self-induced vomiting or the misuse of laxatives, diuretics or enemas)

2   *binge-eating/purging type*: during the last 3 months, the person has engaged in recurrent episodes of binge-eating or purging behaviour (i.e. self-induced vomiting or the misuse of laxatives, diuretics or enemas).

For the Criterion A, the word *refusal* is likely to be removed, as it may be confusing and difficult to assess, and replaced with a more detailed description of the syndrome.[10,11] Criterion B has been changed to reflect the fact that some patients with AN deny fear of weight gain; the new criterion includes the behavioural correlates as well.[10,11] Complete elimination of the amenorrhoea criterion has been proposed for several reasons. Amenorrhoea cannot be applied to men, premenarchal patients or female patients taking oral contraceptives. There are also many descriptions of patients with AN who are still menstruating at a very low weight. In addition, research has shown that patients with and without amenorrhoea do not differ in terms of various clinical measures, suggesting that amenorrhoea may be more useful as a severity indicator as opposed to a diagnostic criterion.[12] Finally, it has been recommended that the subtype classification should be limited only to the last 3 months, due to the high rate of crossover from restriction to binge/purge and vice versa.[13]

Bulimia nervosa

The pathognomonic clinical feature of BN is binge eating with compensation. The current DSM-IV criteria for BN are:[1]

A   recurrent binge eating: an episode of binge eating is characterized by eating, in a discrete period of time, an amount of food that is definitely larger than most people would eat during a similar period of time or under similar circumstances. It also consists of a sense of lack of control over eating during the episode (for example, a feeling that one cannot stop eating or control how much one is eating)

B   recurrent inappropriate compensatory behaviour to prevent weight gain, such as self-induced vomiting, misuse of laxatives, diuretics, enemas or other medications; fasting or excessive exercise

C   the binge-eating and compensatory behaviour in order to prevent weight gain both occur, on average, at least twice a week for 3 months

D   self-evaluation is unduly influenced by body weight and shape

E   the disturbance does not occur exclusively during episodes of anorexia nervosa

subtypes:

1   *the purging type*: during the current episode of BN, a person has regularly engaged in self-induced vomiting or the misuse of laxatives, diuretics or enemas

2   *the non-purging type*: the person has used other inappropriate compensatory behaviours, such as fasting or excessive exercise, but has not regularly engaged in the purging methods.

Proposed changes to bulimia nervosa in the DSM-5

An updated version for the diagnosis of BN recommended by the DSM-5 Eating Disorders Work Group is as follows:[14,15]

A   recurrent episodes of binge eating: an episode of binge eating is characterized by eating an amount of food that is definitely larger than most people would eat during a similar period of time and under similar circumstances in a discrete period of time (for example, within any 2-hour period). It also consists of a sense of lack of control over eating during the episode (for example, a feeling that one cannot stop eating or control what or how much one is eating)

B   recurrent inappropriate compensatory behaviour in order to prevent weight gain, such as self-induced vomiting; misuse of laxatives, diuretics, or other medications, fasting; or excessive exercise

C   the binge eating and inappropriate compensatory behaviours both occur, on average, at least once a week for 3 months

D   self-evaluation is unduly influenced by body shape and weight

E   the disturbance does not occur exclusively during episodes of anorexia nervosa.

Recent research has shown that clinical characteristics of individuals reporting a lower frequency of binge eating and purging (i.e. once a week) are similar to those who binge/purge twice or more per week.[14] As a result of this, the binge eating/purging frequency threshold in Criterion C is likely to be decreased from twice a week to once a week. In addition, the non-purging subtype is likely to be removed, as bulimic patients who do not engage in purging behaviours have been shown to be more similar to those with BED than purging subtype BN.[15]

Binge eating disorder

BED involves recurrent episodes of binge eating in the absence of regular use of the inappropriate compensatory behaviours characteristic of BN. Patients with BED are usually overweight or obese because of the regular binge eating that occurs without compensation (purging, exercise or fasting). Obesity in the absence of disordered eating and psychological disturbance is not considered an eating disorder but rather a metabolic disturbance. As many as 30–40% of obese individuals have BED.

Currently, in the DSM-IV,[1] BED is included in the residual category "eating disorder not otherwise specified" (EDNOS; see below) and is described in the DSM-IV Appendix with the following diagnostic criteria, primarily for research and validation purposes. These include:

A   recurrent episodes of binge eating. An episode of binge eating is characterized by eating an amount of food that is definitely larger than most people would eat in a similar period of time under similar circumstances in a discrete period of time. It also consists of a sense of lack of control over eating during the episode

B   the binge-eating episodes are associated with three (or more) of the following: eating much more rapidly than normal; eating until feeling uncomfortably full; eating large amounts of food when not feeling physically hungry; eating alone because of being embarrassed by how much one is eating; feeling disgusted with oneself, depressed, or very guilty after overeating

C   marked distress regarding binge eating present

D   the binge eating occurs, on average, at least 2 days a week for 6 months

E   the binge eating is not associated with the regular use of inappropriate compensatory behaviours and does not occur exclusively during the course of anorexia nervosa or bulimia nervosa.

Proposed changes to binge eating disorder in the DSM-5

It is expected that the BED will be moved out of EDNOS and achieve official diagnostic status in the DSM-5.[16] The criteria are likely to stay the same as the DSM-IV Appendix criteria, with the exception of changing days to episodes, as is the case with BN, and lowering the frequency of binge eating from at least 2 days per week to at least one binge episode a week (similar to the proposed changes to BN). Because the non-purging subtype BN is likely to be removed from the DSM-5 and grouped with BED, the frequency of BED diagnoses is likely to increase significantly with the proposed changes.

Eating disorder not otherwise specified

This is a residual category of individuals who have significant disturbed eating behaviour and psychopathology and who do not fulfil the full criteria for AN, BN or BED. This category is expected to decline significantly in the DSM-5,[17] as BED will be taken out of EDNOS and moved to full diagnostic status and there will also be broadening of the weight criteria for AN and lowering of the frequency criteria for BN.

Epidemiology

Prevalence rates in western cultures

AN has a lifetime prevalence rate of 0.5–1%,[18–20] and 90% of the patients are female. A recent nationwide survey conducted in the United States of America (USA) found the prevalence rate of AN to be about 0.3%

among adolescents between the ages of 13 and 18 years.[21] The onset of illness often occurs in adolescence and it affects mostly young women; however, prepubescent onset is not uncommon, and stressful life events may result in the development of AN later in life as well.

Binge-eating behaviour is relatively common in the general population.[18] However, binge eating at a regular frequency associated with characteristic psychopathology, with or without purging is less prevalent and requires psychiatric attention. BN has been reported to affect 2–3% of young adult women and, similar to AN, about 90% of those afflicted are female. BED has an estimated prevalence rate of 3–5%, which is likely to increase slightly with its inclusion in the DSM-5.[22] Unlike the pattern observed in AN and BN, the sex distribution is roughly equal. BED is also highly prevalent among people seeking help for obesity.[23]

Prevalence rates in non-western cultures and low-income countries

Although initially thought to occur only in western cultures, eating disorders are seen in non-western societies as well. Lifetime prevalence rates for eating disorders have been reported to be 1.4% among teenagers in Brazil,[24] 1% among female university students in Turkey,[25] and 1.25% among children and adolescents in India.[26] The prevalence rates of eating disorders in Hong Kong, Japan and Taiwan have been shown to be comparable to those in western societies,[27,28] and a similar pattern is observed in the middle eastern nations such as Iran.[29]

Prevalence rates of specific eating disorder diagnoses may also vary from culture to culture. For example, although the rates of AN are comparable to those observed in western cultures, BN has been reported to be relatively rare in Turkey.[25] Hispanic and African-American women in the USA may have higher prevalence rates of BED compared to Caucasian women.[30] In addition, treatment seeking and mental health service utilization rates may be lower in low-income countries and among ethnic minorities living in high-income countries. Research has shown that although the rates of eating disorders are roughly comparable among African-American and Hispanic-American individuals in the USA, they are much less likely to seek treatment for their eating disorder.[30]

It is important to note that the presentation of symptoms of eating disorder may be culture bound, as there may be variations even in core symptoms based on culture. Fear of fatness, body image distortion, and obsession with weight and shape have been believed to be the *sine qua non* of eating disorders for many years, but these key symptoms may be missing or verbalized differently in individuals from non-western cultures.[31] Indeed, many patients with eating disorders in non-western societies focus on somatic complaints such as bloating, abdominal discomfort and distaste for food, rather than cognitive symptoms such as fear of weight gain and distortion of body image.[32,33] Absence of fat phobia in AN has been consistently described in Hong Kong, mainland China, Singapore, Japan, Malaysia and India.[34] Similarly, Filipino and Omani populations have been reported as having much lower rates of fat phobia and higher reported rates of somatic complaints compared to their European and American counterparts.[35] In Ghana, patients with AN deny the fear of becoming fat and view their symptoms positively, based on religious attitudes towards restraint.[36] Among Chinese adolescents, facial appearance and acne, not the fear of becoming fat, have been identified as possible causes of AN.[37] On the other hand, numerous studies have also reported eating disorders with weight preoccupation and fat phobia in both Hong Kong and mainland China, which may be due to the influence and internalization of western norms.[37] In summary, it is important for clinicians to consider the cultural background of the patient and assess symptoms of eating disorder accordingly.

Aetiology

Genetics

Our understanding of the aetiology of eating disorders has changed drastically over the past few decades. For many years, eating disorders were thought to be almost entirely caused by environmental factors, including the objectification of women and idealization of thinness by society, as well as due to dysfunctional family dynamics. It was believed that these factors led to a sense of a lack of control in one's life, resulting in the need to control an aspect of life such as weight and eating. It has also been proposed that sexual abuse, and characteristic traits such as perfectionism, may further contribute to these feelings of ineffectiveness.

Over the last three decades, the knowledge of genetics and heritability in psychiatric disorders has greatly increased and with the development of more sophisticated tools, researchers are now able to make more meaningful connections between complex disorders and genes. It is now understood that eating disorders have sociocultural, psychological and neurobiological risk factors that contribute to their aetiology. This section will specifically examine the role of genetics in the development of eating disorders.

Heritability

Eating disorders are highly heritable. The heritability index obtained from identical twin studies is up to 0.71 for AN (meaning that 71% of phenotypic variation can be explained by genetic factors),[38] 0.50–0.60 for BN,[39] and 0.29–0.43 for BED.[40] Although all three eating disorders tend to run in families, the familial component and heritability are more significant in the case of AN.

Eating disorders are complex traits with biological, psychological, and sociocultural factors contributing to their development, which makes it challenging for genetic researchers to pinpoint the exact genetic cause and contribution to these disorders. However, their complex aetiology does not discredit the role that genetic factors may play in an individual's predisposition to developing these disorders. Like most other psychiatric illnesses, it can be concluded that the heritability of eating disorders follows a non-Mendelian pattern, with many genes making a small contribution to their development.

Dopaminergic genes

Involvement of the dopaminergic genes in eating disorders has been extensively studied. Dopamine is involved in a large variety of brain functions, including feeding behaviour and reward systems. Dopamine dysfunction may predispose to eating disorders by disturbing reward association with food intake. For example, the hypofunctional 7-repeat allele of the dopamine receptor D4 (DRD4) gene's 48-bp VNTR (variable number of tandem repeats) polymorphism on exon III has been associated with a higher lifetime maximum body mass index (BMI) in BN.[41]

The dopamine transporter (DAT1; official symbol LMO3) gene has been another candidate for the association studies of eating disorders, particularly for binge eating. Individuals in the general population who binge eat may be more likely to carry the 9-repeat allele of the DAT1 gene.[42] Although this has not yet been replicated in patients with BN, this preliminary finding suggests a possible association between the DAT1 VNTR and binge-eating behaviour.

Finally, variations in the dopamine receptor D2 (DRD2) gene have been associated with increased reward sensitivity in BED patients,[43] and patients with eating disorder who have the hypofunctional genetic variant report higher levels of drive for thinness and of ineffectiveness.[44] In addition, specific variants of the DRD2 gene may be more common in patients with AN compared to healthy individuals, and individuals with AN are more likely to have inherited these variants from their parents, pointing to a possible preferential transmission.[45]

Serotonergic genes

Because of the important role serotonin plays in eating behaviour, serotonergic genes and their involvement in eating disorders have been studied extensively. The serotonin 2A receptor (HTR2A) gene has been associated with AN and low body weight in both healthy populations and those with eating disorder.[46-48] Furthermore, the same variant of this gene is associated with lower dietary fat intake in healthy children and adolescents,[49] suggesting that the HTR2A gene plays an important role in feeding behaviour and weight regulation.

As for the other serotonergic genes, the polymorphisms in the serotonin 1B receptor (HTR1B) gene may predict minimum lifetime BMI in patients with BN.[50] Similarly, some variants of the serotonin 2C receptor (HTR2C) gene may be more likely to be passed on to an individual with AN,[51] and has been correlated with low weight in AN as well as in healthy controls.[52] In summary, there is substantial evidence for the involvement of a number of serotonergic genes in weight regulation in both healthy populations and patients with eating disorders.

Other gene systems

Brain-derived neurotrophic factor (BDNF) is a protein responsible for neural growth and assigned function of neurons, and it may also be important for appetite and weight regulation. The BDNF gene has been repeatedly associated with AN,[53-55] and variants of this gene may also play a role in determining the higher end of the weight spectrum in BN.[41]

The release of endogenous opioids plays at least a partial role in the positive reinforcing effects of food; hence, it is important to examine the role of the genes that regulate the opioid system in eating disorders. The opioid delta 1 receptor (OPRD1) gene has been associated with AN, whereas specific variants of the opioid mu 1 receptor (OPRM1) gene may be more common in patients with BED compared to healthy controls.[56] Considering the important role endogenous opioids play in high-caloric food consumption to regulate negative affect, there is need for more research to explore the role of opioid gene polymorphisms in BN.

Stimulation of brain melanocortin results in a decrease in food intake and weight,[57] and mutations in the melanocortin 4 receptor (MC4R) gene are responsible for 6% of all obesity cases.[58] MC4R haploinsufficiency has been associated with maximum lifetime BMI in BN,[59] and it has been proposed that MC4R genetic mutations may also be an important aetiological factor in BED.[60] In light of the recent genome-wide association study findings on the role of MC4R in obesity, more research is needed to understand the MC4R gene's potential role in the aetiology of eating disorders.

Sociocultural factors

Eating disorders in general are most prevalent in western culture where the female beauty ideal is tied to thinness,[61] and cultural messages about dieting and thinness are proposed to play a major role in the development of weight and shape dissatisfaction. These cultural preferences are communicated through a complex and multidimensional set of channels, such as the media, fashion, popular culture, economic structures and values, and expectations.[62]

It is important to note that not every woman living in western culture suffers from an eating disorder. As reviewed in the previous section, genetic susceptibility is key in the aetiology of eating disorders. Similarly, a person with genetic vulnerability to disordered eating may not go on to develop an eating disorder if the environmental triggers are not present. This interaction is the foundation of the biopsychosocial model of disease: *the genes load the gun, and the environment pulls the trigger.*

Environmental factors also play an important role in the development of eating disorders. Growing up in a family that is overly preoccupied with weight and shape is associated with increased risk for disordered eating.[63,64] In addition, professions that focus unduly on weight and shape can also act as triggers for problems with body image and eating disorders. Up to 83% of ballet dancers may meet lifetime diagnostic criteria for an eating disorder,[65] and fashion models are much more likely to report full or partial symptoms of eating disorder compared to the general population.[66]

Early traumatic events may also act as a trigger for eating disorders; up to 35% of individuals report a history of trauma, especially in the form of sexual abuse.[67] It is possible that traumatic events encountered in earlier life act as a vulnerability factor for eating disorders, possibly resulting in a dissociative experience that blunts negative emotions. Indeed, women with a history of trauma are much more likely to cope with negative affect through binge eating and purging.[68]

Assessment

Differences in the presentation of anorexia nervosa and bulimia nervosa

There are differences in the presentation of AN compared to BN. The symptoms of an anorexic individual are ego-syntonic; that is, the patient is not usually disturbed by the symptoms, especially weight loss. The individual typically minimizes the medical complications resulting from weight loss or attributes them to other difficulties. They do not see why the people around them are concerned, and secretly feel proud of the accomplishment of weight loss. If the individual does agree to treatment, it is often for the purposes of appeasing concerned individuals or because they desire treatment for a depressed mood or similar psychiatric or medical difficulty associated with the eating disorder. Patients with AN do not usually come seeking help of their own accord; concerned people around them usually coerce them to seek care. Individuals with BN on the other hand, are different, because although they do not wish to gain weight, they are distressed by their binging and purging. They are usually embarrassed that they engage in these behaviours and wish to eliminate them. It is not clearly evident to others that individuals with BN have an eating problem, as they often appear to be of normal weight and tend to keep the symptoms to themselves because of the shame and embarrassment associated with the binge eating and purging. The individual with AN tends to see their weight loss as an accomplishment and tends to feel proud of it and therefore tenaciously holds on to it, whereas the individual with BN wishes to be rid of the disordered eating. Many patients with BN feel like "failed anorexics" because they would like to have the self-control to restrict their food intake, but are unable to and end up binging instead. Both AN and BN patients tend to try and hide their bodies and to dress in baggy clothes, but for different reasons. Patients with AN may try to hide their weight loss because of the obvious negative attention their emaciation brings and their fear of demands for weight gain by parents and clinicians. Patients with BN tend to be normal or slightly overweight and to be ashamed of their bodies and their weight and shape. A significant challenge for parents and clinicians in assessing and treating these disorders is that the end goal for both AN and BN individuals – a thin body shape – is something society promotes as worthwhile and desirable. As a result, there are powerful forces that reinforce the pathologic ideas and behaviours seen in patients with eating disorder. For a vulnerable individual with low self-worth, little self-confidence and a feeling of ineffectiveness, this pursuit of thinness becomes an all-consuming endeavour in the pursuit of external validation.[69]

Engaging patients in the interview

Assessment of eating disorders presents challenges in engaging patients.[70] These are primarily related to their lack of trust in authority and the intense need to feel in control. Patients can experience fears of weight gain, of overeating and/or binging, of hospitalization and confinement and of loss of control of their lives. Their symptoms may also serve very powerful functions in their lives, which can include the need to keep a family together, attention seeking, the modulation of negative mood states, a fear of psychological and physical maturity and a fear of sexuality.

The engagement process can be facilitated by explaining to patients that anxiety and apprehension are understandable and expected given the nature of their problem, by being empathic, gentle, validating and non-judgemental while not colluding with their denial of illness. The clinician's being aware of and monitoring the patients' counter-transference is very important in dealing with these individuals, as they often invoke anger, frustration and helplessness in caregivers. The patient with an eating disorder is very sensitive to and aware of such reactions, having evoked similar reactions in members of their family. It is critical to be completely honest with patients about the need for nutritional rehabilitation and weight gain, as well as to take a matter-of-fact stance about the realities of the illness and not collude with the individual in their denial of symptoms and the risks associated with their pathologic behaviours. Individuals with eating disorder will not engage with clinicians if they do not feel that the clinician is knowledgeable about eating disorders in general and if the clinician does not demonstrate in the interview specific expertise about their problems.

For patients over the age of consent, it is essential they are interviewed alone without family members present. In the absence of clear suicidal risk, for adult patients, any contact with family should occur only with the patient's consent and only in the patient's presence. For younger patients, involvement of the family in the assessment process is critical, and whenever possible should occur with the patient present.

Differences in interviewing adults and children with eating disorders

The interview and assessment of a child or a young adolescent with an eating disorder has some unique features. There is increased urgency when assessing children because they become medically compromised more quickly than adults, as they do not have the same physiological energy reserves. The effects of weight loss and malnutrition are more critical when the individual is in a growth and development phase, which can be permanently affected by weight and nutritional compromise. It is also much more challenging to assess for mood and anxiety in younger individuals. Involvement of the family in the assessment is critical; in addition, assessment of the child and adolescent with eating disorder needs to involve the school and the child's primary care physician or paediatrician. After nutritional and weight stabilization, one of the primary modalities of treatment is family therapy, especially when the child is under the age of consent and still living at home.

Proper assessment of an adult patient with an eating disorder is critical to the development of an appropriate treatment approach. Such an assessment should consist of: (1) clinical interview, including mental status examination; (2) physical examination; (3) investigations; and (4) differential diagnoses.[71]

Clinical interview

The clinical interview should include information about age, marital status, whether the patient has children, living situation including with whom the individual lives (parents, siblings, children, etc.), education, employment and financial status, and religious affiliation. It is important to enquire about the individual's religious or cultural background because they may have food restrictions and cultural rituals around eating related to cultural or religious practice. The patient should state in their own words what brought them in for an assessment. It is important to note how much insight the patient has into their problem: do they recognize that there is a psychological basis to their difficulties, or do they only see it as a behavioural problem?

Weight

In reviewing the history of the chief complaint, a detailed weight history should be obtained. The patient should be weighed without shoes and if possible in a hospital gown. Patients with eating disorders are notoriously unreliable in their self-estimation of their weight. The patient's current weight, height, and corresponding BMI should be noted. This is calculated as the weight in kilograms divided by the height in metres squared. A healthy BMI is between 20 and 25 kg/m^2. The patient's highest and lowest weights in their teenage or adult lives and when these weights occurred, for how long and what the patient's eating patterns was like at the time should be recorded. An attempt should be made to establish the weight that tends to be the most stable for the patient without dieting. This may have to be elicited from family, as the patient may tell you a lower weight than is realistic. This is an important weight, as it allows the clinician to determine the weight associated with the best chance of curbing disordered eating behaviours such as binge eating. The clinician should also ask the patient how they feel about their weight and body image.

Body image

The importance of assessing body image cannot be overemphasized. Many individuals will tell you that they have lost weight or are trying to control their weight for reasons such as health or fitness. It is important to point out to patients that typically the more weight they lose, the more disturbed their body image becomes and the stronger their drive for thinness. Does the patient see certain body parts as overweight and, if so, which parts? These individuals often see specific body parts as unrealistically large or feel that after eating their body parts are "growing".

It is important to establish when the patient first became concerned with their weight and shape, and what their weight was like as a young child and as a teenager. Were they ever involved in activities promoting a thin body image or weight, such as competitive sports, ballet, gymnastics or modelling? The individual should be asked gently about any relationship between significant life events and weight status. This can help to make them aware of the connection between emotions and feelings about weight and shape by identifying upsetting life events that contributed to dissatisfaction with weight and shape.

Eating behaviour

The clinician should enquire in detail about a history of eating-disordered behaviours, as the patient is unlikely to reveal these behaviours voluntarily without the clinician asking about them. The presence of such behaviours may give clues as to potential medical complications, diagnostic information and prognosis. Furthermore, it is important to ask specifically about the frequency and duration of the following behaviours:

- food restriction and food rituals; vegetarianism in the context of an eating disorder is almost always driven by a fear of fat; patients may believe they have food intolerances or allergies to certain foods that they use to justify why they cannot eat certain foods
- self-induced vomiting
- laxative abuse (number taken)

- diuretic or diet pill use (number taken)
- use of herbal weight-loss products
- thyroid medication abuse or ipecacuanha use
- if the patient has diabetes, manipulation of insulin to lose weight
- use of illicit substances to control weight, such as amphetamines or cocaine
- level of exercise.

It is important to determine the patient's type and frequency of exercise, particularly in the presence of a compromised medical state. Exercising in the context of an eating disorder should always be considered as illness behaviour. Such exercise is characteristically done alone, in a rigid, repetitive and compulsive manner that is rarely pleasurable and seldom has any goal other than burning calories.

Binge eating, defined as eating a very large amount of food (over 1000 calories, and usually many more), in a short period of time (under one hour), accompanied by a sense of loss of control, occurs in all patients with BN and roughly half of patients with AN. Clinicians should enquire as to when the binge eating began, the current frequency and timing (usually night time) of episodes, and triggers for binge eating, (usually hunger or emotional upset). It is helpful to suggest that the patient records in writing what they eat each day for a one-week period, to be reviewed with the patient at another interview. Although such dietary self-reports can be helpful, the clinician should keep in mind that the accuracy of self-reporting of dietary intake decreases dramatically after 24 hours.

Psychiatric comorbidities

The clinical interview should also review other psychiatric symptoms: comorbidity is the rule rather than the exception in patients with eating disorders. Knowledge of psychiatric comorbidities is necessary, as these should be treated concurrently with the eating disorder in order to optimize the chance of full recovery from the eating disorder.

Depression and anxiety

Many patients with eating disorders suffer from comorbid depression. The prevalence rate of major depression is estimated to be around 86% for AN and 63% for BN.[72] Suicide risk is up to 23-fold elevated among patients with eating disorders compared to the general population, with the rates being much higher for patients who engage in purging behaviours.[73]

Anxiety disorders also frequently co-occur with eating disorders. Studies have revealed that 55–83% of patients with AN and 68–71% of patients with BN report having a lifetime history of at least one anxiety disorder.[74,75] Obsessive–compulsive disorder (OCD) is one of the most commonly diagnosed anxiety disorders; up to one-third of individuals with eating disorders also suffer from OCD,[72] and the rates for OCD are generally higher among patients with AN compared to those with BN or BED. Social phobia and generalized anxiety disorder are also highly comorbid with eating disorders.

Substance use/abuse

Patients with eating disorders (especially those who engage in binge eating) have higher rates of substance use – both alcohol and street drugs – compared to the general population. Up to 35% of teenagers with eating disorders have substance abuse problems, and substance use is often associated with poorer outcome and increased severity of eating disorder.[76] Patients will often seek out street drugs that result in weight loss, including amphetamine-containing substances and other stimulants. Abuse of prescription drugs given for other conditions is also common among individuals with eating disorders, especially if these drugs lead to weight loss. Some of these prescription drugs include methylphenidate (Ritalin®) and thyroid preparations. Patients will also use a variety of over-the-counter diet pills, diuretics and supplements such as ephedrine to lose weight or maintain low weight.

Personality and temperament

Individuals with AN differ in terms of their personality from individuals with BN and BED. AN patients are more likely to be compulsive, over-controlled, socially avoidant, conflict-averse, passive and fearful. In contrast, BN and BED patients tend to be more impulsive and thrill seeking, and they are more likely to engage in impulsive behaviours such as self-harm, stealing, substance abuse and promiscuity.[65]

Attention-deficit hyperactivity disorder

As much as one-third of patients who regularly binge eat report classical symptoms of attention-deficit hyperactivity disorder (ADHD).[77] In a recent study, a history of childhood ADHD was present in close to 24% of individuals with BN.[78] In addition, impulsivity may be an important factor in determining the severity of BN.[79] On the other side of the coin, females with ADHD appear to be at 6-fold higher risk for developing eating disorders than female controls who do not have ADHD.[79,80] Individuals who regularly binge eat may be inattentive to their internal sense of hunger, satiety and amount of food consumed on a daily basis, which is a phenomenon also observed in individuals with ADHD.[77] Thus, impulsivity and lack of inhibition may play a large role in triggering binges.[81]

Medical comorbidities

Patients with eating disorders can have medical complications related either to starvation, low weight or the effects of binge eating or purging that affect every organ system. A full description of the medical complications associated with eating disorders is beyond the scope of this chapter; the reader is referred to the descriptions below related to physical examination, to investigations, and to Kaplan and Garfinkel (1993).[82] It is important to note that many of the medical complications are the result of starvation, which is continuous in AN and intermittent in BN, and the body's attempt to conserve energy in the face of decreasing energy intake and supply. This results in downregulation of the autonomic nervous system and a metabolic adaptation to conserve energy. These are, for the most part, reversible once nutrition improves and the starvation state is alleviated.

Briefly, the commonest medical complications found in patients with AN and BN relate to the starvation state described above and to fluid and electrolyte imbalance (secondary to purging) leading to hypokalaemia, hypochloraemia, and metabolic alkalosis. Low weight and starvation not uncommonly lead to hypotension, bradycardia and cardiac arrhythmias, including QT prolongation, and, on occasion, can lead to sudden death. Renal function can be impaired and prerenal failure can occur as a result of dehydration due to purging and/or fluid restriction. Gastrointestinal disturbances are very common, including gastro-oesophageal reflux, pancreatitis and gastroparesis leading to constipation, parotid gland enlargement and oesophagitis, as well as oesophageal tears and even Boerhaave's syndrome, which is rare but often fatal. Dental complications include erosion of enamel secondary to the acidic gastric contents in the mouth after repeated vomiting, as well as severe gum disease.

There are many endocrine abnormalities found in patients with eating disorders, most of which are secondary to the effects of starvation and are reversible. Thyroid abnormalities in particular are common and resemble a "euthyroid sick syndrome", characterized by low tri-iodothyronine (T_3) and thyroxine (T_4) but normal thyroid-stimulating hormone (TSH) levels. It is important not to treat these laboratory abnormalities with exogenous thyroid replacement, which only increases metabolic rate and interferes with weight gain.

Two common and potentially serious complications that occur are osteopenia/osteoporosis and cerebral atrophy, the effects of which may not be reversible. Bone abnormalities occur in up to 90% of patients with AN.[83] Osteopenia and osteoporosis can result in stunted growth in adolescents and eventually lead to pathologic fractures and non-union of fractures. Treatment with supplemental oestrogen, either as hormone therapy or oral contraceptives, has not been found to be helpful in the treatment of osteoporosis in patients with AN and should not be prescribed for this purpose in these patients. This relates in part to the fact that the bone abnormalities found in AN are due not only to poor new bone formation secondary to low oestrogen, but also to accelerated bone breakdown secondary to hypercortisolism, which occurs in starvation. The only effective treatment of osteopenia and osteoporosis in patients with eating disorders is weight restoration to a level that enables normal menses. The use of bisphosphanates in patients with AN is not recommended due to concerns about long-term safety and efficacy in this patient population.

Cerebral atrophy commonly occurs, with loss of both white and grey matter, and may lead to cerebral atrophy, ventricular enlargement and neurocognitive deficits. There is evidence that these changes and resulting deficits in cognitive functioning may not be reversible with refeeding.

There is some evidence that patients with BED and obesity are at greater risk for medical complications, including type 2 diabetes, than obese patients without BED.[84] Having said that, obese patients with BED should be monitored, as with any obese patient, for the presence of hypertriglyceridaemia, decreased levels of high-density lipoprotein cholesterol, and increased levels of low-density lipoprotein cholesterol. Obesity is also associated with gallbladder disease and some forms of cancer, as well as sleep apnoea, chronic hypoxia and hypercapnia, and degenerative joint disease. Obesity is an independent risk factor for death from coronary heart disease.

Medical history

It is important to review the patient's medical history to rule out the other medical conditions that may be associated with weight loss or abnormal eating, as well as to be aware of ongoing medical complications associated with the eating disorder.

Questions in the medical assessment should include:

- any significant past medical illnesses
- history of head injuries or seizures
- surgery, and particularly any plastic surgery
- a history of bone pain or bone fractures
- any history of abnormal laboratory findings that are common in people with eating disorders; these include abnormal electrolytes such as potassium, anaemia and/or evidence of dehydration
- age of menarche, weight at that time, present menstrual function, a history of absence of regular periods, and length of time of any abnormalities; the presence and history of any pregnancies
- any other medical diagnoses the patient has been given by a physician to explain their symptoms. Patients with eating disorders present to their physician with physical symptoms that often get misdiagnosed and whose treatment often exacerbates their eating disorder. Examples of this include hypoglycaemia, which is common in starved individuals, and irritable bowel syndrome or lactose intolerance. In patients who conceal laxative abuse, cramps, diarrhoea and abdominal pain can occur and these symptoms mimic those associated with irritable bowel syndrome or lactose intolerance. It is, however, important to be aware that laxative abuse can, in fact, often lead to a temporary state of lactose intolerance. Treatment should be aimed at ceasing laxative use rather than restricting lactose in the diet. In addition, patients are often misdiagnosed with hypothyroidism and then given thyroid hormone, which they use to increase their metabolism and lose weight. In the face of starvation, it is common to have low normal thyroid indices, which should not be treated by thyroid replacement but by refeeding.

It is important to ask about the current medications that the patient is taking, as well as any allergies to any medications.

Past psychiatric treatment or treatment for eating disorder

It is important to know whether there has been previous specialized medical or psychiatric treatment for an eating disorder and, if so, whether it was as an outpatient or inpatient. Information about the nature of the treatment (psychotherapy, medication) and its duration and effectiveness is important. Similarly, it is important to know the nature of any treatment received for any other psychiatric disorder.

Family history

As with any psychiatric interview, it is important to ascertain a detailed family history. Specifically, this should include the disorders that commonly run in families of patients with eating disorders, including eating disorders, substance abuse or dependence, mood disorder and suicide, or anxiety disorders, especially OCD.

In terms of family relationships, the clinician should ask how the individual would describe their relationship with their parents and siblings and what involvement they have with each, as well as whether weight preoccupation and dieting are emphasized in the family.

Personal history

Developmental history

- Pregnancy and birth history: for the newborn and during infancy, ask about the pattern of feeding and growth.
- In the toddler period, the key questions include: temperament, developmental delays, and attachment issues.
- In childhood, note any separation difficulties (i.e. going to school), ability to make friends and major stressful events. The clinician should also ask about weight status and growth as a child in comparison to siblings and children of similar age.
- Family environment: who was the individual closest to and why? Did both parents take an equal part in parenting?
- Eating patterns at home, sit-down meals, regularity of eating, and fanaticism around food or dieting.

School/occupational history

- School history and how the individual fared academically.
- Occupational history such as the number of different jobs, reason for ending jobs and specifically jobs or activities that focused on weight and shape (i.e. modelling, dance, gymnastics) or food (waitressing, chef).

Relationship history

- Review both platonic and intimate relationships. This should include assessing difficulty in making friends, and comfort in relationships with others. How many girlfriends or boyfriends has the individual had, how long did the relationships last and what was/were the reason(s) for the relationships ending? Does the patient's current partner know about the eating disorder and how does he or she try to help the patient?
- Sexual activity, including the age of first intercourse and degree of consensuality, emotional reaction to sexual intimacy, and any homosexual relationships.
- Abuse history, including physical, sexual or emotional abuse. The clinician should ask in a direct but gentle way if there ever was a time in the individual's life when they were victimized or abused. If so, what occurred, how often, what was the identity of the perpetrator(s) and what was the reaction if the individual told family, friends or the police?
- Major life events, such as significant losses, moves, etc.

At the end of the interview, the clinician should ask the patient why they think they have an eating disorder and how they think it started. The clinician should also explore the patient's motivation for treatment. This can be done, in part, by asking the patient how they feel about the illness, how it has impacted on their life and how they see it playing out in the future. These questions can help to uncover the patient's level of denial, and can also challenge patients to think about what benefits or detriments are associated with recovering or staying ill.

Mental status examination

The mental status examination is similar to what is determined for other psychiatric illnesses with a few exceptions. The core requirements are:

- *appearance*: type of dress, grooming, cleanliness, eye contact and cooperativeness. Does the patient look their age, what is their weight status, and how medically ill do they appear? It is also important to note characteristic visible physical sequelae of the patient's disordered eating and purging, which are mentioned below
- *speech*: rate and tone of the patient's speech
- *motor activity*: any abnormal motor activity but also excessive activity, which is either used to burn calories or is a sign of anxiety. Some patients may be fidgety due to discomfort in answering questions; others even stand and pace throughout the interview in order to facilitate burning calories

- *mood*: ask about current mood on a scale of one to ten, with one being the worst the patient has ever felt. What is the patient's mood at the time of the interview?
- the patient should be asked about *suicidal and homicidal thoughts*. Patients with eating disorder often do become suicidal, which tends to be more pronounced at very low weights, with chaotic eating, and on approaching more normal weights with treatment. Thoughts about self-harm (overdosing, cutting, burning) are quite common in patients with eating disorder and should be asked about and noted
- *thought form and content*: patients do not usually have a disorder of thought form, although the content is often near delusional regarding their body image. The presence of obsessions and compulsive rituals that are not food related should be explored and noted
- *perceptual abnormalities*: patients often see certain parts of their bodies as too big, or they may focus on a specific body part, believing it is in some way abnormal without as much of a focus on its size. Intellect should be explored informally by assessing the response to questions in the interview
- *memory and concentration*: short- and long-term memory and concentration can be adversely affected by weight loss, dehydration and starvation and should be assessed through standardized tests (recall of three words that the interviewer gives to the patient to remember, ability to count backwards from 100 by 7s)
- *judgement*: assessing the patient's judgement, specifically as it relates to their medical and nutritional state, is important. In severe cases, this can be markedly impaired and may be grounds to involuntarily impose treatment if the patient's life is threatened by the illness
- *insight*: does the patient recognize that they are ill and do they recognize the need for treatment?

Physical examination

Eating-disordered behaviour, whether it is starvation or any of the forms of purging, can result in physiological abnormalities that need to be investigated as part of the assessment. A comprehensive physical examination is an important component of the assessment of a patient with eating disorder and is also important as it can demonstrate to the patient the negative health effects resulting from their illness.

Many of the physical symptoms patients complain of are the result of downregulation of the autonomic nervous system secondary to starvation and subsequent lowering of basal metabolism. However, the physical and emotional effects are not specific to the eating disorder itself, as the same effects are seen in starved individuals who do not have an eating disorder. This was first demonstrated in a study conducted in 1944 by the US military, in which conscientious objectors were voluntarily starved for several months in order to ascertain the effects of starvation on eating behaviour.[85] The US military was mystified by the bizarre eating behaviour that freed prisoners of war in Japan and survivors of the concentration camps in Europe demonstrated when they were liberated and given food to eat. Many of these individuals began to binge eat, in some instances to the point of death, when they were refed. The subjects in this study following 3 months of semi-starvation showed very definite changes in their eating behaviour, mood and cognitions. These subjects became apathetic, lost interest in life, and had impaired concentration. Many suffered insomnia, intense food cravings and preoccupation with food, including hoarding of food, dreaming about food and wanting to become chefs. When the study was stopped and they were given as much food as they wished, they experienced episodes of binge eating. They reported that they had lost all sense of satiety, i.e., knowing when they were full after eating. Even when their weight was restored, they had problems with satiety. They also complained of physical symptoms such as weakness, fatigue, dizziness, reduced libido, constipation, bloating and indigestion with eating, headaches and cold intolerance. All these symptoms resulted from a lowering of their metabolism to conserve energy (calories), resulting in lowered blood pressure and pulse, contributing to their dizziness; lowered basal body temperature resulting in their feeling cold; reduced levels of testosterone, leading to their reduced libido; and reduced intestinal movement, resulting in bloating and constipation. All these symptoms are common in patients with eating disorders and require nutritional rehabilitation and weight gain to reverse.

A physical examination should include the following:
- *examination of the skin*: often it is pale or sallow and the patient may have scars on the dorsum of their hand from vomiting (Russell's sign). Blue fingers and toes are not uncommon due to reduced peripheral blood flow in order to conserve heat. As a result, the skin will be cold peripherally and

dry. The skin may look slightly orange due to carotenaemia (excessive carotene levels in the blood). Specific signs attributable to the effects of vomiting include sores and rash around the mouth due to irritation of the skin from the acid contents of vomitus, salivary or parotid gland swelling, and periorbital (around the eyes) petechiae from vomiting

- *examination of the mouth*: of note are dry lips and tongue (dehydration), dental erosion, caries and mouth sores. The patient's breath may have a sweet acetone smell, indicative of ketosis, which occurs in starvation
- *a check for thinning hair and lanugo hair*
- *measurement of temperature*, lying and standing, *and blood pressure and pulse rate*; postural drops of blood pressure are common
- *height and weight*: calculate the BMI – mass (kg) divided by height squared (m^2)
- *examination of cardiovascular status* including peripheral pulses, evidence of dependent or generalized oedema, and pulse rate. Bradycardia or a slow heart rate (usually defined as below 60 beats per minute) and an irregular heart rhythm are common
- *examination of gastrointestinal function* by conducting an abdominal examination, including noting the presence or absence of bowel sounds or abnormal masses or tenderness. Patients with eating disorders can develop subclinical pancreatitis and would demonstrate tenderness and an abnormal mass as a result
- *neurological examination*: patients with eating disorders can develop peripheral neuropathies and seizures. Prolonged starvation can contribute to the development of headaches, and reflexes may be diminished with electrolyte abnormalities, or hyperactive with mineral deficiencies.

Investigations

There are certain tests that should always be completed to screen for imminent medical risk. These include a complete blood count and differential, electrolytes, and renal function, which include creatinine and blood urea nitrogen (BUN) and an electrocardiogram (ECG). There are other tests that should be completed if other abnormalities are found or the patient complains of certain physical symptoms. These include thyroid indices (TSH, T_3, T_4), serum phosphate, magnesium and calcium, blood glucose, liver function tests, serum amylase and a urinalysis. A stool examination may be necessary if gastrointestinal bleeding, abdominal complaints and anaemia are present.

Bone densitometry can be considered but its routine usefulness is questionable, other than to help the patient realize the ongoing physical damage the eating disorder is causing. It is only reasonable to do this if the individual has a history of unexplained bone fractures or bone pain and has been amenorrhoeic for a long period of time. However, there is no known effective treatment for the osteopenia/osteoporosis that occurs in patients with AN, other than treatment of the disorder itself, which requires nutritional rehabilitation and weight gain. Exogenous hormones (i.e. oral contraceptives) should not be given, as they are ineffective for treatment of the osteopenia/osteoporosis that occurs in AN.[86] This is because the nature of the osteoporosis that occurs in AN is different from that which occurs in postmenopausal women. As already discussed, in addition to reduced new bone formation due to decreased oestrogen in AN, there is also increased bone destruction due to the hormone changes that result from starvation, and this is not corrected by exogenous hormones.

Medical signs potentially necessitating admission to a hospital include:

- *electrolyte abnormalities*: symptoms associated with electrolyte abnormalities include palpitations, fatigue, muscle weakness and spasms, diminished reflexes, irritability, and convulsions. If the blood potassium is below 2.5 mmol/l, this usually requires intravenous treatment and cardiac monitoring in hospital
- *weight loss that is rapid* or greater than 25% loss of total body weight
- *cardiovascular abnormalities* such as cardiac arrhythmias on an ECG, severe bradycardia, oedema or severe hypotension
- *seizures and/or delirium*

- *acute gastrointestinal conditions* such as bowel obstruction, pancreatitis or oesophageal or gastric tears or rupture.

The patient with highest-risk for serious medical complications is purging, anorexic, and has significant acute weight loss. The primary psychiatric reason for an emergency admission to hospital is acute suicidality.

Differential diagnoses

Medical disorders

The commonest medical conditions associated with weight loss that therefore may be misdiagnosed as AN include thyroid disease, inflammatory bowel disease, a hypothalamic tumour and rare forms of malabsorption. However, in none of these conditions does the patient actively pursue thinness and engage in self-starvation. Medical causes of overeating are extremely rare and usually involve brain abnormalities such as rare tumours or degenerative disorders.

Psychiatric disorders

The weight loss associated with AN needs to be distinguished from other psychiatric conditions associated with weight loss.[87] These include:

- *mood disorders*, especially depression. However, in depression, the patient is usually distressed by their weight loss and attributes it to a true loss of appetite and disinterest in eating. This is completely different from the patient with AN, who is obsessively preoccupied with food and shockingly unconcerned about weight loss
- *anxiety disorders*, such as specific food phobias not associated with caloric content. OCD can also be accompanied by weight loss if the patient is so consumed by ritualistic behaviours that they cannot eat properly. The obsessions in OCD are not food related, but rather are related to fears of contamination or anxiety around the need for checking or counting rituals
- *substance abuse*: certain substances, such as amphetamines or cocaine, reduce appetite through their effects on brain function and can therefore be associated with considerable weight loss
- *conversion disorders* such as psychogenic vomiting can be accompanied by significant weight loss. In this condition, the patient denies vomiting to get rid of calories but vomits because of abdominal pain, or is unaware of the reasons
- *schizophrenia, or delusional disorder*: in psychotic states such as occur in schizophrenia, a patient can believe that their food is being poisoned and they therefore stop eating. This can lead to dramatic weight loss, the cause of which is clearly very different than in AN
- *dementia, or delirium*: in organic brain conditions such as dementia or delirium, patients can lose a tremendous amount of weight because they are cognitively impaired and are unable to care for themselves, which would include inability to feed themselves.

There are few other psychiatric conditions where binge eating is a prominent feature and where patients do not have weight and shape concerns. Some patients who have impulse-control difficulties, like those with borderline personality disorder, may binge eat as one of many impulsive behaviours in which they engage.

Treatment

The primary goals of treatment for AN are nutritional rehabilitation associated with weight gain, for BN a cessation of binge eating and purging and the regular intake of adequate calories, and for BED a cessation of binge eating and some degree of weight loss if obese. Treatment usually requires regular medical monitoring and treatment of medical complications, nutritional therapy, some form of psychotherapy and, in some cases, medication.[88] Treatment in a structured, intensive specialized programme is necessary in cases that are more severe, especially for AN. The evidence-based treatments for each of the three eating disorders will be reviewed in this section, followed by a stepped care approach to care and then a brief discussion of the role of primary care in the treatment of eating disorders.

Anorexia nervosa

There are no clear evidence-based treatments for adults with AN. Any effective treatment should be focused on the core disturbances in AN, which are manifested symptomatically by disordered eating behaviour, weight loss and characteristic psychopathology. These core disturbances include a disturbance in cognition, a disturbance in enteroceptive awareness manifested by a profoundly disturbed body image which phenomenologically is considered an overvalue idea bordering on delusional, a disturbance in affect regulation, a disturbance in activity, and a pervasive sense of anhedonia. Any treatment, whether psychological or pharmacological, needs to address these underlying core disturbances to be truly effective. With the lack of empirical evidence for psychological or drug treatments, approaches to the treatment of AN as recommended in established treatment guidelines (American Psychiatric Association in the USA and National Institute for Health and Clinical Excellence in the United Kingdom of Great Britain and Northern Ireland) rely on uncontrolled trials and generally accepted clinical practice.[89,90]

Cognitive-behavioural therapy (CBT) is the psychological treatment with the most evidence of efficacy in adults with AN, albeit with only modest results.[91,92] There is good evidence for the effectiveness of family-based therapy for AN in young adolescent patients.[93] For a comprehensive review of psychological treatments for AN, see Kaplan (2002).[94]

There is no conclusive evidence that pharmacotherapy is effective in the acute stage of the illness when the patient is underweight. Many different classes of drugs have been studied in AN, with the primary aim of increasing appetite (a somewhat faulty paradigm as AN is more a disorder of satiety than of hunger), increasing weight, reducing pre- and postprandial anxiety, or drugs aimed at treating comorbid conditions such as OCD or depression, in the hope that this will alleviate some of the core symptoms of AN. Selective serotonin reuptake inhibitors (SSRIs) have been studied in acutely ill AN patients,[95,96] with little evidence of efficacy. It has been hypothesized that one reason for this lack of efficacy may be related to the effect of starvation on the levels of serotonin produced in the brain in AN patients. Starvation results in lower levels of tryptophan, an essential amino acid and a necessary precursor to serotonin, which is ingested in the diet. The low levels of serotonin produced in the brains of patients with AN mitigate the effectiveness of SSRIs, which work by blocking the reuptake of serotonin produced in vivo in the brain. This has led to studies that have evaluated the effectiveness of SSRIs, specifically fluoxetine, in preventing relapse in weight-restored patients, based on the rationale that levels of serotonin would normalize in these patients. However, evidence for the efficacy of SSRIs in reducing relapse in weight-restored patients is conflicting. One small randomized controlled trial found fluoxetine to be more effective than placebo in reducing relapse,[97] while a larger more rigorous trial showed no difference between placebo and fluoxetine in reducing relapse over one year of treatment.[98]

More recent attention has focused on atypical antipsychotics, as these drugs, through their effects on neurotransmitter systems like dopamine, impact many of the disturbances described above. Several recent small, randomized clinical trials have shown promise for olanzapine when compared to placebo in reducing obsessiveness and anxiety and facilitating weight gain in AN subjects.[99,100] Larger multisite trials are needed to definitively answer whether olanzapine has a role in the treatment of acutely ill patients with AN.

Bulimia nervosa

In contrast to AN, there are well-validated psychotherapeutic[101] and pharmacologic treatments for BN. There are good evidence-based psychotherapies for BN. CBT is the treatment of first choice.[102] This structured, manualized relatively short-term treatment delivered over 16 weeks has been found to lead to abstinence in over 50% of patients and to an 80% reduction in symptoms in those who do not reach abstinence. There is also evidence for the effectiveness of interpersonal therapy for BN.[103,104] In a very recent study that examined a stepped care approach to the treatment of BN,[105] individual CBT followed by fluoxetine for those who were not responding to CBT by 6 weeks, was compared to a stepped care approach that began with self-help, followed by up to 60 mg/day fluoxetine for those who did not respond to self-help, followed by CBT for those who were not abstinent with self-help and fluoxetine. The stepped care sequence of self-help, fluoxetine and CBT was more effective at 1-year follow-up than CBT alone and should be the approach taken by clinicians in actual practice.

There are close to 15 randomized, placebo-controlled trials evaluating antidepressants for the treatment of BN.[106] The majority of these demonstrate the effectiveness of drug over placebo, but with only 30% of patients achieving abstinence after a therapeutic trial of antidepressants. The largest studies conducted utilized the SSRI fluoxetine,[94] which is the only drug with Food and Drug Administration (FDA) approval for use in BN in the USA.[87] The gold standard in clinical practice for pharmacotherapy is to begin treatment with fluoxetine, and to use higher doses than those used in the treatment of major depression, up to 60–80 mg/day. Other SSRIs such as sertraline, citalopram and fluvoxamine have been evaluated in the treatment of BN, with equal effectiveness.[107,108] Generally, the choice of which SSRI to use should depend on anticipated side-effects and the clinical state of the patient. A BN patient with a comorbid anxiety disorder may be better served by using a more sedating SSRI (citalopram) than one that is more activating (fluoxetine). Bupropion, despite its demonstrated effectiveness in one large randomized trial in BN, is contraindicated in patients who are actively symptomatic, because of its propensity to cause seizures in such patients. In clinical practice, SSRIs should be used in BN patients for whom CBT is not available, or for those patients who have shown a partial response to CBT, as the combination is more effective than either alone, especially in the presence of comorbid depression. The use of psychostimulants in patients with BN (or AN) is not recommended because of their appetite-suppressing effects and potential to exacerbate restrictive eating in patients with eating disorder.

Binge eating disorder

Similar to the situation for BN, there are evidence-based psychotherapies for BED. It is important to note that most patients with BED are obese, so the goals for treatment are not only a reduction of binge eating and related psychopathology but also some degree of weight loss. The evidence-based psychotherapies include CBT,[109] and interpersonal therapy, specifically delivered in group format.[110] Both of these psychotherapies could be considered first-line treatments for BED; however, neither results in significant weight loss despite being effective in reducing binge eating. There is also preliminary evidence for the effectiveness of dialectical behaviour therapy for BED.[111]

There is evidence to support pharmacotherapy for BED; for a review of this literature, see Reas and Grilo (2008).[112] SSRIs such as fluoxetine and sertraline[113] and anti-obesity drugs such as topiramate,[114] have been studied in the treatment of BED, with close to 50% abstinence rates from binging following treatment. However, there is little evidence to suggest that pharmacotherapy treats the psychological disturbances that accompany BED, or that significant weight loss occurs with SSRI treatment of BED. In one study, orlistat led to weight loss in BED but not a significant reduction in binge eating.[109]

Stepped care approach to treatment

Anorexia nervosa

A stepped care approach for patients with AN is not usually possible or useful, because the majority of these patients need refeeding in an intensive setting, either a day/partial hospital programme (weight between 75% and 85% of ideal body weight, or BMI 17–18.5 kg/m²) or a specialized inpatient programme (less than 75% of ideal body weight or BMI < 17 kg/m²) at some point in the course of their illness. Family therapy for patients aged under 16 years and ill for less than 3 years, delivered in an intensive treatment setting, is the treatment of choice for younger patients. Other than family therapy, no outpatient treatment approach has been shown to be effective in the treatment of AN.

Bulimia nervosa and binge eating disorder

Most patients with BN and BED can be effectively treated as outpatients and will not need to be hospitalized. Evidence-based stepped care approaches to these disorders, from most cost effective, least intensive to most expensive most specialized/intensive would include:

1 guided self-help
2 psycho-education
3 group outpatient CBT
4 individual outpatient CBT with nutritional counselling

5 individual outpatient CBT with nutritional counselling, with the addition of SSRIs

6 individual outpatient interpersonal psychotherapy, with or without SSRIs

7 individual outpatient dialectic behaviour therapy for multi-impulsive patients

8 day hospital/partial day programme for treatment-resistant patients or those with complex comorbidities (diabetes, borderline personality disorder).

The vast majority of patients with BN or BED (approximately 80%) will experience a clinically significant improvement of behavioural symptoms (a reduction in binge eating/purging) after utilizing the outpatient interventions listed above. Patients with BED can also benefit from behavioural weight-loss programmes following generally accepted medical guidelines, in addition to the above interventions.

The role of primary care clinicians

Screening and early intervention

Screening and early identification of patients with eating disorders is an important role for primary care physicians and other non-mental health clinicians. Examples of specific high-risk target groups for screening and early intervention should include:

- low-weight adolescent girls and young women (BMI < 17 kg/m^2)
- adolescent girls and young women who present with significant weight and shape concerns despite being at a normal healthy weight
- young women who have unexplained menstrual disturbances or amenorrhoea
- young women with vague, non-specific gastrointestinal complaints in the absence of any physical findings; think purging behaviours (vomiting; laxative abuse)
- young women with mood disturbance, anxiety and/or substance abuse
- children and adolescents who have been sexually abused
- young adolescents or even children who present with poor growth and development
- young women with type 1 diabetes mellitus in poor diabetic control and who may be overusing insulin to lose weight.

Screening can best be done by asking the appropriate questions of every adolescent and young woman related to symptoms of an eating disorder, as detailed previously. In addition, there are screening instruments that can be used, including the Eating Attitudes Test (EAT),[88] where appropriate cut-offs have been validated in community samples that suggest the presence of an eating disorder.

Medical monitoring

Patients who are actively symptomatic with eating disorders should be seen by primary care physicians at least once a month for weighing, laboratory investigations (at a minimum, complete blood count, electrolytes, BUN and creatinine) and an ECG.

The high-risk patient requiring hospitalization for medical stabilization is severely underweight (BMI < 15 kg m^2), is binge eating and purging frequently, has demonstrable fluid and electrolyte abnormalities with ECG changes, and is hypotensive and bradycardic.

Psychosocial support

Patients with eating disorders require much psychological support and often respond to non-specific support as well as specific interventions such as CBT, interpersonal psychotherapy or family therapy, which, with specialized training, can be delivered successfully by the primary care physician. Training and supervising primary care clinicians in such specialized psychotherapies provides an opportunity for a shared care approach.

Pharmacotherapy monitoring

Patients with BN and BED often respond to the antibulimic effects of antidepressants, as well as the effects of these drugs on their comorbid mood and anxiety disorders. The same is only sometimes true for patients with

AN. Primary care physicians have an important role to play in initiating and monitoring these medications. Once again, training and supervising primary care clinicians in the pharmacotherapy of eating disorders provides an opportunity for a shared care approach.

Conclusions

The eating disorders are relatively common, serious illnesses with a complex biopsychosocial aetiology. Effective treatments for BN and BED are available but not widely disseminated to primary care clinicians. AN remains largely a treatment-resistant illness with disturbingly high morbidity and mortality. Going forward, research needs to focus on innovative evidence-based treatments for AN that improve the quality of life of patients who suffer from AN and reduce the mortality and morbidity of this serious disorder. Dissemination of the evidence-based treatments for BN and BED should be a high priority for the field. Primary care clinicians play an important role in the provision of care for patients with eating disorders, including in terms of screening, early detection, assessment and treatment.

References

1   *Diagnostic and statistical manual of mental disorders*, 4th ed. Washington, American Psychiatric Association, 2000.

2   Oldham J. DSM-5: a work in progress. *Journal of Psychiatric Practice*, 2010, 16:371.

3   Brumberg JJ. *Fasting girls: the history of anorexia nervosa*. New York, Vintage Press, 2000.

4   Vandereyken W, van Deth R. *From fasting girls to anorexic girls: the history of self-starvation*. New York, New York University Press, 1994.

5   *Diagnostic and statistical manual of mental disorders*, 1st ed. Washington, American Psychiatric Association, 1952.

6   Russell G. Bulimia nervosa: an ominous variant of anorexia nervosa. *Psychological Medicine*, 1979, 9:429–448.

7   *Diagnostic and statistical manual of mental disorders*, 3rd ed. Washington, American Psychiatric Association, 1980.

8   *Diagnostic and statistical manual of mental disorders*, 3rd ed revised. Washington, American Psychiatric Association, 1987.

9   Bruch H. *The golden cage: the enigma of anorexia nervosa*. Cambridge, MA, Harvard University Press, 1978.

10 Becker AE, Eddy KT, Perloe A. Clarifying criteria for cognitive signs and symptoms for eating disorders in DSM-V. *International Journal of Eating Disorders*, 2009, 42:611–619.

11 Bravender T et al. Classification of child and adolescent eating disturbances. Workgroup for Classification of Eating Disorders in Children and Adolescents (WCEDCA). *International Journal of Eating Disorders*, 2007, 40(Suppl.):S117–S122.

12 Attia E, Roberto CA. Should amenorrhea be a diagnostic criterion for anorexia nervosa? *International Journal of Eating Disorders*, 2009, 42:581–589.

13 Peat C et al. Validity and utility of subtyping anorexia nervosa. *International Journal of Eating Disorders*, 2009, 42:590–594.

14 Wilson GT, Sysko R. Frequency of binge eating episodes in bulimia nervosa and binge eating disorder: Diagnostic considerations. *International Journal of Eating Disorders*, 2009, 42:603–610.

15 van Hoeken D et al. The validity and utility of subtyping bulimia nervosa. *International Journal of Eating Disorders*, 2009, 42:595–602.

16 Wonderlich SA et al. The validity and clinical utility of binge eating disorder. *International Journal of Eating Disorders*, 2009, 42:687–705.

17 Sysko R, Walsh BT. Does the broad categories for the diagnosis of eating disorders (BCD-ED) scheme reduce the frequency of eating disorder not otherwise specified? *International Journal of Eating Disorders*, 2011, 44:625–629.

18 Hudson JI et al. The prevalence and correlates of eating disorders in the national comorbidity survey replication. *Biological Psychiatry*, 2007, 61:348–358.

19 Agras WS, Gotestam KG. General population-based epidemiological study of eating disorders in Norway. *International Journal of Eating Disorders*, 1995, 18:119–126.

20 Hoek HW. Review of the epidemiological studies of eating disorders. *International Journal of Eating Disorders*, 1993, 5:61–74.

21 Swanson SA et al. Prevalence and correlates of eating disorders in adolescents: results from the National Comorbidity Survey Replication Adolescent Supplement. *Archives of General Psychiatry*, 2011, 68:714–723.

22 Hudson JI et al. By how much will the proposed new DSM-5 criteria increase the prevalence of binge eating disorder? *International Journal of Eating Disorders*, 2012, 45:139–141.

23 Latner JD, Clyne C. The diagnostic validity of the criteria for binge eating disorder. *International Journal of Eating Disorders*, 2008, 41:1–14.

24 Moya T, Fleitlich-Bilyk B, Goodman R. Brief report: young people at risk for eating disorders in Southeast Brazil. *Journal of Adolescent Health*, 2006, 29:313–317.

25 Uzun O et al. Screening disordered eating attitudes and eating disorders in a sample of Turkish female college students. *Comprehensive Psychiatry*, 2006, 47:123–126.

26 Mammen P, Russell S, Russell PS. Prevalence of eating disorders and psychiatric comorbidity among children and adolescents. *Indian Pediatrics*, 2007, 44:357–359.

27 Stark-Wroblewski K, Yanico BJ, Lupe S. Acculturation, internalization of Western appearance norms, and eating pathology. *Psychology of Women Quarterly*, 2005, 29:38–46.

28 Lee S et al. The changing profile of eating disorders at a tertiary psychiatric clinic in Hong Kong (1987–2007). *International Journal of Eating Disorders*, 2010, 43:307–314.

29 Nobakht M, Dezhkam M. An epidemiological study of eating disorders in Iran. *International Journal of Eating Disorders*, 2000, 28:265–271.

30 Marques L et al. Comparative prevalence, correlates of impairment, and service utilization for eating disorders across US ethnic groups: implications for reducing ethnic disparities in health care access for eating disorders. *International Journal of Eating Disorders*, 2010, 44:412–420.

31 Pike KM, Borovoy A. The rise of eating disorders in Japan: issues of culture and limitations of the model of "Westernization". *Culture, Medicine, and Psychiatry*, 2004, 28:493–531.

32 Cummins LH, Lehman J. Eating disorders and body image concerns in Asian American women: Assessment and treatment from a multicultural and feminist perspective. *Eating Disorders*, 2007, 15:217–230.

33 Rieger E et al. Cross-cultural research on anorexia nervosa: assumptions regarding the role of body weight. *International Journal of Eating Disorders*, 2001, 29:205–215.

34 Becker AE. Culture and eating disorder classification. *International Journal of Eating Disorders*, 2007, 40(Suppl.):S111–116.

35 Viernes N et al. Tendency toward deliberate food restriction, fear of fatness and somatic attribution in cross-cultural samples. *Eating Behaviors*, 2007, 8:407–417.

36 Bennett D et al. Anorexia nervosa among female secondary school students in Ghana. *British Journal of Psychiatry*, 2004, 185:312–317.

37 Jackson T, Chen H. Identifying the eating disorder symptomatic in China: the role of sociocultural factors and culturally defined appearance concerns. *Journal of Psychosomatic Research*, 2007, 62:241–249.

38 Kipman A et al. Genetic factors in anorexia nervosa. *European Psychiatry*, 1999, 14:189–198.

39 Bulik CM et al. Understanding the relation between anorexia nervosa and bulimia nervosa in a Swedish national twin sample. *Biological Psychiatry*, 2010, 67:71–77.

40 Mitchell KS et al. Binge eating disorder: a symptom-level investigation of genetic and environmental influences on liability. *Psychological Medicine*, 2010, 40:1899–1906.

41 Kaplan AS et al. A DRD4/BDNF gene–gene interaction associated with maximum BMI in women with bulimia nervosa. *International Journal of Eating Disorders*, 2008, 41:22–28.

42 Shinohara M et al. Eating disorders with binge-eating behaviour are associated with the s allele of the 3'-UTR VNTR polymorphism of the dopamine transporter gene. *Journal of Psychiatry and Neuroscience*, 2004, 29:134–137.

43 Davis C et al. Reward sensitivity and the D2 dopamine receptor gene: a case-control study of binge eating disorder. *Progress in Neuro-Psychopharmacology and Biological Psychiatry*, 2008, 32:620–628.

44 Nisoli E et al. D2 dopamine receptor (DRD2) gene Taq1A polymorphism and the eating-related psychological traits in eating disorders (anorexia nervosa and bulimia) and obesity. *Eating and Weight Disorders*, 2007, 12:91–96.

45 Bergen AW et al. Association of multiple DRD2 polymorphisms with anorexia nervosa. *Neuropsychopharmacology*, 2005, 30:1703–1710.

46 Martaskova D et al. Polymorphism in serotonin-related genes in anorexia nervosa: The first study in Czech population and meta-analyses with previously performed studies. *Folia Biologica (Praha)*, 2009, 55:192–197.

47 Ricca V et al. Psychopathological traits and 5-HT2A receptor promoter polymorphism (-1438G/A) in patients suffering from anorexia nervosa and bulimia nervosa. *Neuroscience Letters*, 2004, 365:92–6.

48 Sorli J et al. Impact of the -1438G>A polymorphism in the serotonin 2A receptor gene on anthropometric profile and obesity risk: a case-control study in a Spanish Mediterranean population. *Appetite*, 2008, 50:260–265.

49 Herbert B et al. Polymorphism of the 5-HT2A receptor gene and food intakes in children and adolescents: the Stanislas Family Study. *American Journal of Clinical Nutrition*, 2005, 82:467–470.

50 Levitan RD et al. Polymorphism of the serotonin 5-HT1B receptor gene (HTR1B) associated with minimum lifetime body mass index in women with bulimia nervosa. *Biological Psychiatry*, 2001, 50:640–643.

51 Hu X, Giotakis O et al. Association of the 5-HT2C gene with susceptibility and minimum body mass index in anorexia nervosa. *NeuroReport*, 2003, 14:781–783.

52 Westberg L et al. Association between a polymorphism of the 5-HT2C receptor and weight loss in teenage girls. *Neuropsychopharmacology*, 2002, 26:789–793.

53 Dmitrzak-Weglarz M et al. BDNF Met66 allele is associated with anorexia nervosa in the Polish population. *Psychiatric Genetics*, 2007, 17:245–246.

54 Ribases M et al. Met66 in the brain-derived neurotrophic factor (BDNF) precursor is associated with anorexia nervosa restrictive subtype. *Molecular Psychiatry*, 2003, 8:745–751.

55 Ribases M et al. Association of BDNF with restricting anorexia nervosa and minimum body mass index: a family-based association study of eight European populations. *European Journal of Human Genetics*, 2005, 13:428–434.

56 Davis CA et al. Dopamine for "wanting" and opioids for "liking": a comparison of obese adults with and without binge eating. *Obesity*, 2009, 17:1220–1225.

57 Adan RA, Vink T. Drug target discovery by pharmacogenetics: mutations in the melanocortin system and eating disorders. *European Neuropsychopharmacology*, 2001, 11:483–490.

58 Farooqi IS et al. Clinical spectrum of obesity and mutations in the melanocortin 4 receptor gene. *New England Journal of Medicine*, 2003, 348:1085–1095.

59 Hebebrand J et al. Genetic predisposition to obesity in bulimia nervosa: a mutation screen of the melanocortin-4 receptor gene. *Molecular Psychiatry*, 2002, 7:647–651.

60 Branson R et al. Binge eating as a major phenotype of melanocortin 4 receptor gene mutations. *New England Journal of Medicine*, 2003, 384:1096–103.

61 Eddy KT, Hennessey M, Thompson-Brenner H. Eating pathology in East African women: the role of media exposure and globalization. *The Journal of Nervous and Mental Disease*, 2007, 195:196–202.

62 Jung J, Forbes GB. Body dissatisfaction and disordered eating among college women in China, South Korea, and the United States: contrasting predictions from sociocultural and feminist theories. *Psychology of Women Quarterly*, 2007, 31:381–393.

63 Francis LA, Birch LL. Maternal influences on daughters' restrained eating behavior. *Health Psychology*, 2005, 24:548–554.

64 Neumark-Sztainer D et al. Family weight talk and dieting: how much do they matter for body dissatisfaction and disordered eating behaviors in adolescent girls? *Journal of Adolescent Health*, 2010, 47:270–276.

65 Ringham R et al. Eating disorder symptomatology among ballet dancers. *International Journal of Eating Disorders*, 2006, 39:503–508.

66 Preti A et al. Eating disorders among professional fashion models. *Psychiatry Research*, 2008, 159:86–94.

67 Federici A, Kaplan AS. Anorexia nervosa: overview of evidence on the underpinnings of anorexia nervosa. In: Dancyger I, Fornari V, eds. *Evidence-based treatments for eating disorders: children, adolescents and adults* (pp.1–18). New York, Nova Science Publishers, 2009:1–18.

68 Stewart SH et al. Why do women with alcohol problems binge eat? Exploring connections between binge eating and heavy drinking in women receiving treatment for alcohol problems. *Journal of Health Psychology*, 2006, 11:409–425.

69 Vitousek K, Watson S, Wilson GT. Enhancing motivation for change in treatment-resistant eating disorders. *Clinical Psychology Review*, 1998, 18:391–420.

70 Kaplan AS, Garfinkel PE. Difficulties in treating patients with eating disorders: a review of patient and clinician variables. *Canadian Journal of Psychiatry*, 1999, 44:665–670.

71 Kaplan AS. Medical and nutritional assessment of eating disorders. In Kaplan AS, Garfinkel PG, eds. *Medical issues and the eating disorders: the interface*. New York, Brunner Mazel, 1993:1–16.

72 O'Brien KM, Vincent NK. Psychiatric comorbidity in anorexia and bulimia nervosa: nature, prevalence, and causal relationships. *Clinical Psychology Review*, 2003, 23:57–74.

73 Foulon C et al. Switching to the bingeing/purging subtype of anorexia nervosa is frequently associated with suicidal attempts. *European Psychiatry*, 2007, 22:513–519.

74 Godart NT et al. Anxiety disorders in anorexia nervosa and bulimia nervosa: co-morbidity and chronology of appearance. *European Psychiatry*, 2000, 15:38–45.

75 Kaye WH et al. Comorbidity of anxiety disorders with anorexia and bulimia nervosa. *American Journal of Psychiatry*, 2004, 161:2215–2221.

76 Castro-Fornieles J et al. Prevalence and factors related to substance use among adolescents with eating disorders. *European Addiction Research*, 2010, 16:61–68.

77 Fleming J, Levy L. Eating disorders in women with AD/HD. In: Quinn PO, Nadeau KG, eds. *Gender issues and AD/HD: research, diagnosis, and treatment*. Silver Spring, MD, Advantage Books, 2002:411–426.

78 Yilmaz Z et al. COMT Val158met variant and functional haplotypes associated with childhood ADHD history in women with bulimia nervosa. *Progress in Neuro-Psychopharmacology and Biological Psychiatry*, 2011, 35:948–952.

79 Surman CB, Randall ET, Biederman J. Association between attention-deficit/hyperactivity disorder and bulimia nervosa: analysis of 4 case-control studies. *Journal of Clinical Psychiatry*, 2006, 67:351–354.

80 Biederman J et al. Are girls with ADHD at risk for eating disorders? Results from a controlled, five-year prospective study. *Journal of Developmental & Behavioral Pediatrics*, 2007, 28:302–307.

81 Schweickert LA, Strober M, Moskowitz A. Efficacy of methylphenidate in bulimia nervosa comorbid with attention-deficit hyperactivity disorder: a case report. *International Journal of Eating Disorders*, 1997, 21:299–301.

82 Kaplan AS, Garfinkel PG, eds. *Medical issues and the eating disorders: the interface*. New York, Brunner Mazel, 1993.

83 Grinspoon S et al. Prevalence and predictive factors for regional osteopenia in women with anorexia nervosa. *Annals of Internal Medicine*, 2000, 133:790–794.

84 Johnson JG, Spitzer RL, Williams JB. Health problems, impairment and illnesses associated with bulimia nervosa and binge eating disorder among primary care and obstetric gynaecology patients. *Psychological Medicine*, 2001, 31:1455–1466.

85 Keys A et al. *The biology of human starvation*. Minneapolis, MN, The University of Minnesota Press, 1950.

86 Klibanski A et al. The effects of estrogen administration on trabecular bone loss in young women with anorexia nervosa. *Journal of Clinical Endocrinology and Metabolism*, 1995, 80:898–904.

87 Garfinkel PE et al. Differential diagnoses of emotional disorders that cause weight loss. *Canadian Medical Association Journal*, 1983, 129:939–945.

88 Garner DM, Garfinkel PE. *Handbook of treatments for the eating disorders*, 2nd ed. New York, Guilford Press, 1997.

89   American Psychiatric Association. Treatment of patients with eating disorders, third edition. *American Journal of Psychiatry*, 2006, 163(7 Suppl.):4–54.

90   *Eating disorders: core interventions in the treatment and management of anorexia nervosa, bulimia nervosa and related eating disorders.* London, National Institute for Health and Clinical Excellence, 2004 (CG9).

91   Pike KM et al. Cognitive behavior therapy in the posthospitalization treatment of anorexia nervosa. *American Journal of Psychiatry*, 2003, 160:2046–2049.

92   McIntosh VW et al. Three psychotherapies for anorexia nervosa: A randomized controlled trial. *American Journal of Psychiatry*, 2005, 162:741–747.

93   Lock J et al. *Treatment manual for anorexia nervosa: a family-based approach.* New York, The Guilford Press, 2001.

94   Kaplan AS. Psychological treatments for anorexia nervosa: a review of published studies and promising new directions. *The Canadian Journal of Psychiatry*, 2002, 47:235–242.

95   Attia E et al. Does fluoxetine augment the inpatient treatment of anorexia nervosa? *American Journal of Psychiatry*, 1998, 155:548–551.

96   Brambilla F et al. Combined cognitive-behavioral, psychopharmacological and nutritional therapy in eating disorders: 1. Anorexia nervosa-restricted type. *Neuropsychobiology*, 1995, 32:59–63.

97   Kaye WH et al. Double-blind placebo-controlled administration of fluoxetine in restricting- and restricting-purging-type anorexia nervosa. *Biological Psychiatry*, 2001, 49:644–652.

98   Walsh BT et al. Fluoxetine after weight restoration in anorexia nervosa. *JAMA*, 2006, 295:2605–2612.

99   Bissada H et al. Olanzapine in the treatment of low body weight and obsessive thinking in women with anorexia nervosa: a randomized, double-blind, placebo-controlled trial. *American Journal of Psychiatry*, 2008, 165:1281–1288.

100 Attia E et al. Olanzapine versus placebo for out-patients with anorexia nervosa. *Psychological Medicine*, 2011, 22:1–6.

101 Wilson GT, Grilo C, Vitousek K. Psychological treatment of eating disorders. *American Psychologist*, 2007, 62:199–216.

102 Fairburn CG. *Cognitive behavior therapy and eating disorders.* New York, Guilford Press, 2008.

103 Agras WS et al. Outcome predictors for the cognitive behavior treatment of bulimia nervosa: data from a multisite study. *American Journal of Psychiatry*, 2000, 157:1302–1308.

104 Agras WS et al. A multicenter comparison of cognitive-behavioral therapy and interpersonal psychotherapy for bulimia nervosa. *Archives of General Psychiatry*, 2000, 57:459–466.

105 Mitchell JE et al. Stepped care and cognitive-behavioural therapy for bulimia nervosa: randomised trial. *The British Journal of Psychiatry*, 2011, 198:391–397.

106 Bacaltchuk J, Hap P. Antidepressants versus placebo for people with bulimia nervosa. *Cochrane Database of Systematic Reviews*, 2003, (4):CD003391.

107 Milano W et al. Treatment of bulimia nervosa with sertraline: a randomized controlled trial. *Advances in Therapy*, 2004, 21:232–237.

108 Sloan DM et al. Efficacy of sertraline for bulimia nervosa. *International Journal of Eating Disorders*, 2004, 36:48–54.

109 Grilo CM, Masheb RM, Wilson GT. Efficacy of cognitive behavioral therapy and fluoxetine for the treatment of binge eating disorder: a randomized double-blind placebo-controlled comparison. *Biological Psychiatry*, 2005, 57:301–309.

110 Wilfley DE et al. *Interpersonal psychotherapy for group.* New York, Basic Books, 2000.

111 Telch CF, Agras WS, Linehan MM. Dialectical behavior therapy for binge eating disorder. *Journal of Consulting and Clinical Psychology*, 2001, 69:1061–1065.

112 Reas DL, Grilo CM. Review and meta-analysis of pharmacotherapy for binge-eating disorder. *Obesity*, 2008, 16:2024–2038.

113 McElroy SL et al. Placebo-controlled trial of sertraline in the treatment of binge eating disorder. *American Journal of Psychiatry*, 2000, 157:1004–1006.

114 Claudino AM et al. Randomized, double-blind, placebo controlled trial of topiramate plus cognitive-behavior therapy in binge eating disorder. *Journal of Clinical Psychiatry*, 2007, 68:1324–1332.

23 Gender dysphoria in primary care mental health

Kevan Wylie, Gabriel Ivbijaro, Jane Thornton and Elizabeth Wainwright

---

Key messages

- Gender dysphoria is uncommon but not a lifestyle choice.
- The diagnosis is often self-made, alongside exclusion of any mental health disorder.
- The role of the general practitioner and specialist gender team is to assess, advise and support individuals through the gender transition.
- Careful monitoring of prescriptions of cross-gender hormones can be undertaken under shared care arrangements.
- A multidisciplinary team can provide tailor-made interventions to ensure successful gender transition.

Introduction

Gender dysphoria is relatively uncommon but general practitioners (GPs) may come across trans people in their practice, although it is very rare. When patients present to their family doctor with dysphoria such as this, the GP must be in a position to offer some assistance and know how to proceed. This chapter is designed to equip GPs to deal with this problem that they may encounter once in a while.

Presentation

Individuals with gender dysphoria make up a very small proportion of the community, so many GPs may never encounter a patient with this condition in the course of their working life. However, as society becomes more accepting of gender diversity and people with transgender issues, including the recognized syndromes of gender identity disorder and transsexualism (more commonly referred to as gender dysphoria), it is more likely that these individuals will seek help from primary care clinicians.

A patient with gender dysphoria has a psychological experience of themself as male or female that is incongruent with their external sexual characteristics. It is estimated that there may be up to 15 000 people in the UK receiving some form of medical intervention for gender dysphoria. A study in Scotland identified that the proportion in the general population is one in 12 225.[1] There is some evidence that the ratio of trans men to trans women may be closer than previously noted.[2]

Aetiology

Gender dysphoria was initially attributed to insanity/psychopathology,[3] and it was not until the 1960s that Harry Benjamin, in his book *The transsexual phenomenon*, first described gender dysphoria as an endocrinological and sexual disorder and explained the affirmative treatment path he pioneered.[4] The *Diagnostic and Statistical Manual of Mental Disorders* (DSM) first described transsexualism in 1980,[5] and this diagnosis has subsequently been modified (see Box 23.1).

Box 23.1 Diagnostic criteria for gender dysphoria

DSM-IV-TR[6] diagnostic criteria for gender identity disorder

A   A strong and persistent cross-gender identification (not merely a desire for any perceived cultural advantages of being the other sex). In children, the disturbance is manifested by four (or more) of the following:

   1   repeatedly stated desire to be, or insistence that he or she is, the other sex

   2   in boys, preference for cross-dressing or simulating female attire; in girls, insistence on wearing only stereotypical masculine clothing

   3   strong and persistent preferences for cross-sex roles in make-believe play, or persistent fantasies of being the other sex

   4   intense desire to participate in the stereotypical games and pastimes of the other sex

   5   strong preference for playmates of the other sex

B   Persistent discomfort with his or her sex, or sense of inappropriateness in the gender role of that sex

C   The disturbance is not concurrent with a physical intersex condition

D   The disturbance causes clinically significant distress or impairment in social, occupational, or other important areas of functioning

The International Classification of Diseases (ICD)-10[6]

Transsexualism (F64.0) has three criteria:

- the desire to live and be accepted as a member of the opposite sex, usually accompanied by the wish to make his or her body as congruent as possible with the preferred sex through surgery and hormone treatment
- the transsexual identity has been present persistently for at least 2 years
- the disorder is not a symptom of another mental disorder or a chromosomal abnormality.

Dual-role transvestism (F64.1) has three criteria:

- the individual wears clothes of the opposite sex, in order to experience temporary membership in the opposite sex
- there is no sexual motivation for the cross-dressing
- the individual has no desire for a permanent change to the opposite sex.

Gender identity disorder of childhood (64.2) has separate criteria for girls and for boys.

For girls:

- the individual shows persistent and intense distress about being a girl, and has a stated desire to be a boy (not merely a desire for any perceived cultural advantages to being a boy), or insists that she is a boy
- either of the following must be present:
  - persistent marked aversion to normative feminine clothing and insistence on wearing stereotypical masculine clothing
  - persistent repudiation of female anatomical structures, as evidenced by at least one of the following:
    - an assertion that she has, or will grow, a penis
    - rejection of urination in a sitting position
    - assertion that she does not want to grow breasts or menstruate
- the girl has not yet reached puberty
- the disorder must have been present for at least 6 months.

For boys:

- the individual shows persistent and intense distress about being a boy, and has a desire to be a girl, or, more rarely, insists that he is a girl
- either of the following must be present:
  - preoccupation with stereotypic female activities, as shown by a preference for either cross-dressing or simulating female attire, or by an intense desire to participate in the games and pastimes of girls and rejection of stereotypical male toys, games, and activities
  - persistent repudiation of male anatomical structures, as evidenced by at least one of the following repeated assertions:
    - that he will grow up to become a woman (not merely in the role)
    - that his penis or testes are disgusting or will disappear
    - that it would be better not to have a penis or testes
- the boy has not yet reached puberty
- the disorder must have been present for at least 6 months.

Other gender identity disorders (F64.8) has no specific criteria.

Gender identity disorder, unspecified has no specific criteria.

Either of the previous two diagnoses could be used for those with an intersexed condition.

Psychological, social and cultural factors are important,[8–10] while it must also be recognized that there may be some biological contribution towards the condition.[11–14] The consequences of cultural determination of gender are described in a recent review of the exclusion of hijra people in Bangladesh,[15] which also considers transgender communities historically within other cultural contexts.

Standards of care

In 1979, the Harry Benjamin International Gender Dysphoria Association (HBIGDA) first introduced standards of care to articulate the international associations' professional consensus about the psychiatric, psychological, medical and surgical management of gender identity disorders. These were subsequently modified in 1980, 1981, 1990, 1998 and 2001, and the current revised standards of care (version 7) were issued in 2011.[16] The World Professional Association for Transgender Health is the new successor association to HBIGDA as the body representing both clinicians and advocates.

The principles of good practice continue to evolve and this includes moving away from viewing the care of patients with gender dysphoria as wholly the province of psychiatry to a much more mixed model, with a number of professional disciplines potentially involved in care.

While the condition of gender dysphoria is uncommon, the model of management where patients must be seen within specialist tertiary services has led to an unfortunate clash between service users and clinicians, particularly from an advocacy standpoint. Long waiting times and poor resourcing of clinics for patients with this condition has made working relationships difficult on many occasions. It is now recognized by health-care providers and service users that a negotiated position of support and facilitation through gender transition is likely to be more productive in terms of professional relationships with physicians and the primary care team. It also ensures that the individual going through transition is able to seek maximum benefit from those providing or facilitating care.

There is considerable comorbidity between gender dysphoria and other mental health problems (see below). However, it is argued that much of this is because of the stigma associated with the condition, and the often poor support that patients receive during their transition. A recent review has identified additional needs where patients are unable to seek support.[17] Increasingly, with subspecialization of primary health-care physicians, the overall management of patients with gender dysphoria can be more usefully seen as being best placed within the province of primary health care rather than within the traditional hospital clinic service. This is exemplified by the financial constraints in cities such as Vancouver and Sydney resulting in a need for services to change.[18]

Diagnosis

The diagnosis of gender dysphoria is primarily made by the individual who experiences a number of symptoms and, with appropriate awareness and education, would be able to identify themselves as having gender dysphoria. The diagnosis is essentially confirmed by the clinician. As mental health problems may present with symptoms of gender dysphoria, and as there are also occasionally other undeclared factors that may lead to a determination for gender transition, it is imperative that a mental health assessment be carried out by a general psychiatrist at an early stage in the assessment process. The role of the psychiatrist has been well described by Gorin-Lazard et al.[19] It is important to confirm the diagnosis and establish the differential diagnosis around psychiatric pathology such as delirium, sexual ambiguity, fetishistic transvestism and dysmorphophobia, as well as the more traditional identified states that may involve delusional ideas such as severe depression, schizophrenia and other organic states. A successful transformation, with global satisfaction and psychosocial adaptation, is the primary focus for the psychiatrist, or other clinician, leading the support through the transition. Regret after surgery is low (2%) and temporary regret is also low (8–10%);[20,21] nevertheless, it is important to carefully consider appropriate decisions along the care pathway.[22]

Psychological comorbidity

For many individuals, comorbid psychiatric states may have only minimal impact on gender transition. However, some authors have sought to demonstrate considerable risk of comorbidity. In a recent review of comorbid diagnostic patterns of 10 consecutive patients interviewed in a gender identity clinic, Levine and Solomon found that 90% of these diverse patients had a least one other significant form of psychopathology.[23] These findings seem to be a marked contrast to the rhetoric of many who advocate for transgender adults. Psychopathologies included problems of mood and anxiety regulation and adapting to the world. In the report by Levine and Solomon,[23] two of the ten patients interviewed had persistent significant regrets about previous transitions. The authors note that the distressing experience of some of the patients interviewed illustrates the disadvantage of discussing professional concepts with a lay audience. Emphasis on the patient's civil rights is not a substitute for recognition and treatment of associated psychopathology. Gender identity specialists, unlike the media, need to be concerned about all their patients and not just those who are apparently functioning well in transition. The applicability of these findings to the general population is still being considered by the profession and serves as a point of caution to ensure adequate mental health review.

The role of psychotherapy: the "real-life experience"

The role of psychotherapy both in the lead up and during the "real-life experience" (see below) is an area of controversy. Although it is not an absolute requirement for the real-life experience to have begun before commencing hormonal therapy or indeed genital reconstructive surgery, psychotherapy is often helpful.[24] Individuals are encouraged to explore options with their clinician without either the patient or clinician pre-judging the direction of any therapy or progression to attempt to resolve the dysphoria.

Applicants for genital reconstructive surgery are required to live at least one year full time in the preferred gender role, which is named the "real-life experience" (previously the "real-life test"). This prepares the patient as well as possible to make an informed decision about irreversible surgery. Psychotherapy can play an important role in planning the real-life experience and in developing resilience to cope with the inevitable psychosocial challenges that follow.

Use of questionnaires

During the preliminary assessment, it is worth considering whether the use of questionnaires can assist in the diagnostic process, particularly where access to psychological care and a psychologist is not possible. A recent review of the use of scales found that questionnaires would not impact on overall health care, whereas patient-led diagnosis of gender dysphoria was more influential.[25]

Preparation of the patient for hormonal treatment is another part of the preliminary assessment and will require taking a full medical and prescribed medication history. This is described in more detail by Manieri et al.[26]

Management

Counselling

Counselling of patients about storage of gametes to preserve their reproductive potential should always be considered on an individual basis and recorded in the clinical notes. Funding for such procedures, as well as subsequent fertility interventions, is often dependent on local policy or individual affordability.

Planning treatment

For a trans woman (that is a biological male transitioning to the female role), the principal treatment is feminizing hormones. For a trans man (a biological woman transitioning to the male role), masculinization with testosterone is the principal treatment. The different preparations for both feminization and masculinization have been described more recently by a consensus group at the Endocrine Society of America.[27] A review of the use of gonadotrophin-releasing hormone (GnRH) analogues has also been published recently.[28]

A number of contraindications to hormone therapy are recognized and should be considered carefully before initiating therapy. Individuals who are suffering with cardiovascular disease or are predisposed to strokes, thromboembolism or have a hormone-dependent cancer should be evaluated with care. Where necessary, advice from an endocrinologist can be helpful in establishing safety and an appropriate, yet adequate, dosing regime for hormone medication. Given the increased risk of thromboembolism, patients who smoke should be encouraged to stop before commencing hormone therapy. Similarly, patients who are overweight should be given advice on dietary intake, restriction of calories and exercise, which are important both for reducing the risk of side-effects from hormonal therapy, and for increasing the opportunity for safe surgical interventions at a later stage. Many surgeons are now placing weight restrictions for patients wanting to have genital confirmation surgery, and so adequate forewarning and management of diet and weight is an important early intervention.

Speech and language therapy

The role of other professionals during the transition is extremely valuable and varies by individual circumstances. Most patients will find consultations with a speech and language therapist are valuable for working with the transgender voice. Peer-agreed practice and research findings that relate mainly to English-speaking populations have recently been reviewed and described by Thornton.[29] Addressing non-verbal communication, linguistic and phonetic features in addition to pitch change enables the individual who presents well physically to "complete the package" and achieve a more gender-specific communication style.

All those undergoing transition to their preferred gender may consult a speech and language therapist to discuss their voice, speech and communication style. For some, particularly those who transition very early or late in their adult life, their communication skills may be gender appropriate but most trans people feel that while they may look passable, as soon as they speak, they are "read" in their original gender. Speech and language therapy facilitates safe development and habitualization of a gender-appropriate voice and communication style that is comfortable for the person to use on a daily basis without causing vocal fatigue or damage. It should also be age appropriate and in congruence with their physique and culture. Any existing voice disorder that may have arisen as the individual tried to change their voice should be investigated and treated before embarking on specific trans voice therapy.

It is usual, although not always the case, that communication and voice therapy coincide with transition, as it is often easier to practise the new skills while living full time in the new gender role. Specific areas of therapy will focus on pitch and intonation, resonance, articulation, use of language, prosody, rate of speech and non-verbal communication, e.g. eye contact, proxemics, etc. These aspects have been shown to influence the listener's judgement of speaker gender[30] and should be explored in both trans men and women. Different styles of communication and voice use will be addressed in order that the person develops a natural and flexible use of voice and communication.

It is often assumed that taking androgens will deepen the trans man's voice, by adding mass to the vocal cords, to create a passable male voice. This can be sufficient for some, but for others the pitch change may be limited and the person will need therapeutic direction to both stabilize the laryngeal mechanism and maximize pitch change and address the other aspects of verbal and non-verbal communication outlined above. Direction and monitoring can be given in the therapy sessions but the majority of change will occur through regular practice by the individual. The goal for pitch change in trans women is to raise the pitch to a "gender-ambiguous" level, between 145 Hz and 165 Hz or above, without vocal strain. Those individuals with good perceptual skills, a "musical ear" and sheer determination usually progress steadily to achieve a satisfactory communication style. This may, however, take many months/years to achieve. Some trans women have a naturally deep pitch to their voice and, because of laryngeal anatomical constraints, minimal pitch change will be possible. In this situation there is the option of pitch-change surgery using thyroplasty techniques (described later). In this case, therapy is advisable both before and after surgery, to maximize potential.

Voice change often continues following discharge as the person becomes more "settled" in their core gender, with increasing acceptance of the new voice enabling more vocal flexibility and confidence in communication. The amount of change is specific to the individual and some may decide not to alter their voice/communication. Ultimately, it is the individual's perception of satisfaction with their communication in different situations, rather than a single communication style, that will determine successful functioning in their lives. Speech and language therapists work with the trans person to experiment with varying degrees of change, to enable the individual to decide how and when to use these new skills.

Psychosocial issues

For some patients, there are considerable psychosocial and interfamily issues. The value of an occupational therapist in the team has recently been evaluated (Johnson and Wylie, personal communication 2010). Similarly, the role of support for the family and relatives has been described in detail by Reed et al.[31] In terms of the impact of transition on daily occupations, patients undertaking a transition encounter significant changes and stresses. As already discussed, adopting a new or evolving gender role in everyday life is known as the "real-life experience",[16] and is predominantly acquired through a social process involving clothing, mannerisms, grooming, voice inflection, social interests[32] and career activities. Changing one's gender presentation has an immediate effect on personal and social aspects of life, as well as on interpersonal relationships and vocational, educational, economic and legal aspects.

Personal appearance

Personal appearance is an important feature of being accepted in the acquired gender. This can become all-consuming to patients and a significant part of therapeutic work.[31] An image consultant within gender clinics provides valuable support and constructive opinions on clothing, style and general visual appearance, including hair style, make-up and deportment. Some patients may utilize advice from supportive family members or friends who can provide suggestions and assistance. The Internet also has a vast array of information for trans people.

A common complaint made by trans women in the process of transition, is difficulty with obvious facial hair. There is increasing recognition of the need to support individuals with hair-removal therapy as soon as possible, either before or during the "real-life experience". A number of options are available to the individual, including laser hair removal and pulse-wave-light removal. For those individuals where these methods are not indicated, for example those who are fair skinned or have blonde or grey hair, electrolysis remains the treatment choice.

Removal of body hair, including hair on the torso and back, is another procedure that is often required for patients. Removal of scrotal and other genital hair is advocated by some surgeons prior to creation of a vaginoplasty (see below), as it may reduce the likelihood of hair ball formation within the vaginoplasty. It is important to identify with the patient which surgery will be selected, as skin trauma is commonplace with laser hair removal, but some procedures require a total absence of any trauma to the skin prior to surgery.

Work and leisure

Transitioning at work is a key area of stress outlined by both trans men and trans women. Having supportive work colleagues and managers is important to a successful transition, as is the maintenance of continued employment. However, there have been instances where transgendered people have been fired, demoted or pressurized to resign when their gender variance is discovered.[33] This inevitably has consequences for personal finances and results in additional daily pressures. Many trans people resort to prostitution to support the costs of transition (particularly hormones and surgery), and many are also subject to violence, slavery and increased risk of infection (including sexually transmitted infection and human immunodeficiency virus) associated with financial dependence.[15,34]

The main barrier to continuing to carry out leisure pursuits is commonly reported to be fear surrounding changing facilities, particularly those without private cubicles, due to consciousness of body image and how others may react to them (Johnson and Wylie, personal communication 2010). Recent legislation in the Equality Act 2010 now provides an extended legally accessible framework of discrimination law. This protects individuals from unfair treatment within the workplace and in the use of goods and services across the voluntary, community, or public sectors, promoting a fair and more equal society.

Psychosocial adaptation

The "real-life experience" produces a temporary imbalance of daily occupations as people's lives begin to proceed in a different direction. The occupational therapist can provide assessment and intervention during the real-life experience of daily activities to facilitate transition and support the parameters described in Box 23.2.

Box 23.2 Parameters of the 'real-life experience'

When clinicians assess the quality of a person's "real life experience" in the desired gender, the following abilities are reviewed:

1 to maintain full- or part-time employment
2 to function as a student
3 to function in community-based volunteer activity
4 to undertake some combination of items 1–3
5 to acquire a (legal) gender-identity-appropriate first name
6 to provide documentation that persons other than the therapist know that the patient functions in the desired gender role.

For successful psychosocial adaptation, the aim is to support social inclusion and maintain meaningful activities that sustain the patient's evolving personal identity. This can be done through the use of individual or group contact. Groups can be run by a range of clinicians experienced in group behaviour and group leadership.[34] Various activities are incorporated to address a range of significant issues. They provide a space for reflection and empowerment through the expression of individual identity and choice. In addition, involvement in groups provides support between group members and increases skills and knowledge through education.

The role of small group work, either facilitated by a clinician or self-led, should not be underestimated. A number of self-help groups and support networks are available for individuals undergoing transition. Access to information on the Internet will often allow networks to develop. Sharing of experiences and ideas and the opportunity to share positive and negative health advice should be encouraged.

Hormone therapy and surgery

A number of factors are important in making decisions about both eligibility and readiness to proceed to both commencing hormones and seeking second opinions for surgery. The eligibility and readiness criteria for commencing hormone therapy are described in Box 23.3. It is important that assessment is made by a number of clinicians rather than decisions being made by an individual alone. This can be achieved by the development of clinical networks where patients are offered a range of services by different clinicians who will communicate with each other and meet on occasions to consider and discuss progress. They will also work as a team to consider individual patient needs that may be causing particular concern, especially when the presenting need(s) is/are complex.

After a minimum period of one year in the "real-life experience", eligibility and readiness need to be considered again, before progression to surgery should this be a decision that the patient wishes to make. The eligibility and readiness criteria are described in Box 23.3. If the patient is sufficiently able to make a decision with adequate consent, they should be referred for a second opinion to a clinician with experience in gender dysphoria.

Once two positive opinions for surgery have been obtained, the process is then to refer to a surgeon who has expertise in gender confirmation surgery. Information about individual surgeons, their method and type of surgical procedure, as well as the outcome is extremely helpful and valued by patients. Genital reassignment surgery for transsexual people has been described recently by Sohn and Exner.[35] Postoperative care is also important both during the recovery period in hospital, which may be 8 days or more, and thereafter in the community.

The following procedures are common for trans women:

- *orchidectomy* – removal of the testes
- *penectomy* – removal of the penis
- *vaginoplasty* – creation of a vagina.

Eligibility criteria

The administration of hormones is not to be lightly undertaken because of their medical and social risks. There are three criteria:

1   age 18 years

2   demonstrable knowledge of what hormones can and cannot do medically and their social benefits and risks

3   either:
   - a documented real-life experience of at least 3 months prior to the administration of hormones, or
   - a period of psychotherapy of a duration specified by the mental health professional after the initial evaluation (usually a minimum of 3 months).

In selected circumstances, it can be acceptable to provide hormones to patients who have not fulfilled criterion 3 above, for example to facilitate the provision of monitored therapy using hormones of known quality, as an alternative to black-market or unsupervised hormone use.

Readiness criteria

There are three criteria:

1   the patient has had further consolidation of gender identity during the "real-life experience" or psychotherapy

2   the patient has made some progress in mastering other identified problems leading to improving or continuing stable mental health (this implies satisfactory control of problems such as sociopathy, substance abuse, psychosis and suicidality)

3   the patient is likely to take hormones in a responsible manner.

In addition, creation of a clitoris (*clitoroplasty*) and labia (*labiaplasty*) is carried out. In those cases where breast development is inadequate after 18–24 months of hormone therapy, breast augmentation takes place in patients where adequate levels of oestrogenization can be demonstrated through biochemical measures. Specific details about surgery for trans women is available elsewhere.[36]

For trans men, the first surgical procedure is often *chest reconstruction* with *bilateral mastectomy*, which is carried out by surgeons with experience in performing surgery for trans men or for gynaecomastia in men. This often predates lower surgery, and for many trans men there is a reluctance to proceed with lower surgery, given the procedures required to undertake such surgery as well as the limitation of surgery in both cosmetic and functional terms. In some patients, this may be limited to *hysterectomy* (removal of the uterus) and *vaginectomy* (removal of the vagina) alongside *salpingo-oophorectomy* (removal of the ovaries and Fallopian tubes). Although many women will have cessation of the menses with adequate prescription of testosterone with or without a GnRH analogue, the longer-term consequences of testosterone stimulation on both the uterine lining and the ovaries would lead to a recommendation of hysterectomy and oophorectomy regardless of whether male confirmation surgery was accepted. For some patients, *metoidioplasty* (creation of a micro penis) is sufficient following adequate masculinization. For those who seek a phallus and the desire to micturate standing up, *phalloplasty* (creation of a phallus), *urethroplasty* (creation of the urethra), *scrotoplasty* (creation of a scrotum) with *placement of a testicular prosthesis* and *implantation of a penile prosthesis* can all be offered. This is often a three-stage process and may be complicated by skin necrosis, fistulae and infections. Details of the various procedures for trans men have been described elsewhere.[37]

Additional surgery is sometimes important in ensuring good acceptance in society. Trans women may opt for a *chondrolaryngoplasty* to reduce the prominence of the thyroid cartilage (Adam's apple), and/or a *cricothyroid approximation*, which increases the tension of the vocal cords, i.e. raises overall pitch by closing the gap between the cricoid and thyroid cartilages.[38] Laryngeal framework surgery is rarely undertaken by trans men. A more controversial procedure is facial feminization surgery, which is useful for some patients and has been described by van de Ven.[39] Preparation for surgery is crucial, and providers should ensure information is made available in advance of admission. Appropriate follow-up appointments must be made to address the patient's postoperative needs for hormonal prescriptions and check their psychological adaptations to the new gender.

References

1   Wilson P, Sharp C, Carr S. Prevalence of gender dysphoria in Scotland: a primary care study. *British Journal of General Practice*, 1999, 49:991–992.

2   De Cuypere G et al. Prevalence and demography of transsexualism in Belgium. *European Psychiatry*, 2007, 22:137–141.

3   von-Krafft-Ebing R. *Psychopathia sexualis*, 10th ed. London, Rebman, 1901.

4   Benjamin H. *The transsexual phenomenon*. New York, The Julian Press, Inc., 1966.

5   *Diagnostic and statistical manual of mental disorders*, 3rd ed. Washington, American Psychiatric Association, 2000.

6   *Diagnostic and statistical manual of mental disorders*, 4th ed, text revision (DSM-IV-TR). Washington, American Psychiatric Association, 2000.

7   *ICD-10 classification of mental and behavioral disorders*. Geneva, World Health Organization, 1996.

8   Barrett J. *Transsexual and other disorders of gender identity*. Oxford, Radcliffe Publishing, 2007.

9   Cohens-Kettenis PT, Gooren LJG. Transsexualism: a review of etiology, diagnosis and treatment. *Journal of Psychosomatic Research*, 1999, 46:315–333.

10 Lev AI. *Transgender emergence: counselling gender-variant people and their families*. Binghamton, NY, Haworth Press, 2004.

11 Chung WCJ et al. Sexual differentiation of the bed nucleus of the stria terminalis in humans may extend into adulthood. *Journal of Neuroscience*, 2002, 22:1027–1033.

12 Hare L et al. Androgen receptor repeat length polymorphism associated with male to female transsexualism. *Biological Psychiatry*, 2009, 65:93–96.

13 Kruigver FPM. *Sex in the brain*. Amsterdam, Netherlands Institute of Brain Research, 2004.

14 Zhou JN et al. A sex difference in the human brain and its relation to transsexuality. *Nature*, 1995, 378:68–70.

15 Khan SI et al. Living on the extreme margin: social exclusion of the transgender population (hijra) in Bangladesh. *Journal of Health, Population and Nutrition*, 2009, 27:441–451.

16 World Professional Association for Transgender Health. *Standards of care version 7* (http://www.wpath.org, accessed 17 February 2012).

17 Hainsworth K, Wylie KR, Ryles S. Support needs of people on a wait list for GD assessment. *International Journal of Transgenderism*, 2007, 10:91–98.

18 Bockting W, Knudson G, Goldberg J. *Counselling and mental health care of transgender adults and loved ones*. Vancouver, Transgender Health Program, 2006 (http://transhealth.vch.ca/resources/library/tcpdocs/guidelines-mentalhealth.pdf, accessed 17 February 2012).

19 Gorin-Lazard A et al. Gender identity disorder: what is the role of a psychiatrist. *Sexologies*, 2008, 17:225–237.

20 Tsoi WF. Follow-up study of transsexuals after sex-reassignment surgery. *Singapore Medical Journal*, 1993, 34:515–517.

21 Baranyi A, Piber D, Rothenhäusler HB. [Male-to-female transsexualism. Sex reassignment surgery from a biopsychosocial perspective.] *Wien medizinische Wochenschrift*, 2009, 159:548–557.

22 Smith YLS et al. Sex reassignment: outcomes and predictors of treatment for adolescent and adult transsexuals. *Psychological Medicine*, 2005, 35:89–99.

23 Levine SB, Solomon A. Meanings and political implications of "psychopathology" in a gender identity clinic: a report of 10 cases. *Journal of Sex and Marital Therapy*, 2009, 35:40–57.

24 Bockting WO. Psychotherapy and the real-life experience: from gender dichotomy to gender diversity. *Sexologies*, 2008, 17:211–224.

25 Gillott S, Wylie K. The clinical value and cost effectiveness of using psychometric-rating scales in the assessment of patients with gender dysphoria. *Sexologies*, 2008, 17:238–244.

26 Manieri C et al. Hormone treatment in gender dysphoria. *Sexologies*, 2008, 17:265–270.

27 Hembree WC et al. Endocrine treatment of transsexual persons: an Endocrine Society Clinic Practice Guideline. *Journal of Clinical Endocrinology and Metabolism*, 2009, 94:3132–3154.

28 Wylie KR et al. Recommendations of endocrine treatment for patients with gender dysphoria. *Sexual and Relationship Therapy*, 2009, 24:175–187.

29 Thornton J. Working with the transgender voice: the role of the speech and language therapist. *Sexologies*, 2008, 17:271–276.

30 Adler RK, Hirsch S, Mordant M. *Voice and communication therapy for the transgender/transsexual client: a comprehensive clinical guide*. San Diego CA: Plural Publishing.

31 Reed B et al. Medical care for gender variant young people: dealing with practical problems. *Sexologies*, 2008; 17:258–264.

32 Istar Lev A. *Transgender emergence*. Binghamton, NY, The Haworth Press Inc., 2004.

33 Gagne P, Tewsbury R, McGaughey D. Coming out and crossing over: identity formation and proclamation in a transgender community. *Gender and Society*, 1997, 11:478–508.

34 Finlay L. *Groupwork in occupational therapy*. Cheltenham, Nelson Thornes Ltd, 1993.

35 Sohn MHH, Exner K. Genital reassignment surgery for transsexual people. *Sexologies*, 2008, 17:283–290.

36 Goddard JC, Vickery RM, Terry TR. Development of feminizing genitoplasty for gender dysphoria. *Journal of Sexual Medicine*, 2007, 4:981–989.

37 Ralph D et al. Trauma, gender reassignment and penile augmentation. *Journal of Sexual Medicine*, 2010, 7:1657–1667.

38 Parker AJ. Aspects of transgender laryngeal surgery. *Sexologies*, 2008, 17:277–282.

39 van de Ven BFML. Facial feminisation, why and how? *Sexologies*, 2008, 17:291–298.

Part VI

Substance use disorders in primary care mental health

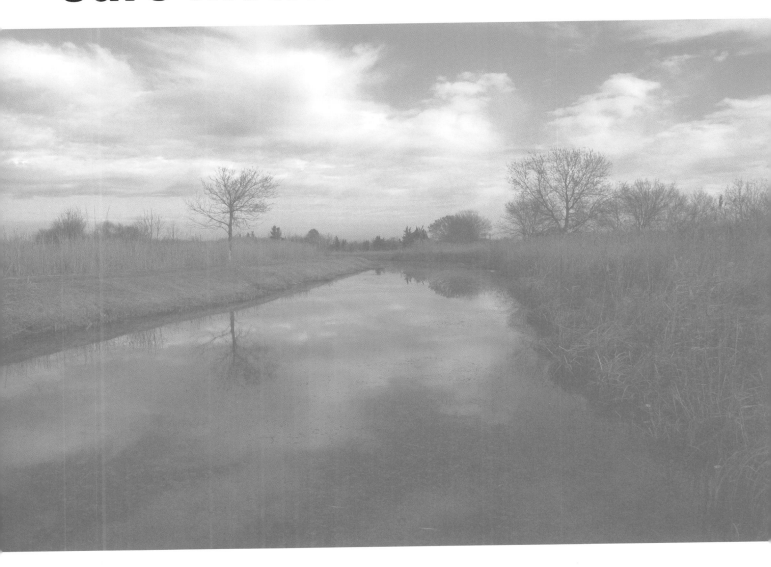

24 Tobacco use disorder in primary care mental health

Christine Runyan and James Anderson

Key messages

- Prevalence rates for tobacco use remain unacceptably high and continue to rise in many areas of the world, making routine inquiry about smoking status and offering treatment in primary care a health-care imperative.

- Primary care providers can greatly impact tobacco cessation attempts and success rates, using brief, specific interventions informed by motivational interviewing strategies.

- Interventions for smoking cessation are most effective when pharmacotherapy and behavioural interventions are combined, and cessation rates rise with higher intensity and duration of treatment.

- All patients, unless contraindicated, should be offered pharmacotherapy options to improve long-term abstinence rates.

- Adjunctive supportive therapy, practical counselling, rapid follow-up after a projected quit date, and telephonic quit line counselling are core components of effective interventions.

Introduction

Tobacco use is the unequivocal leading cause of preventable death worldwide, accounting for one in every ten adult deaths.[1,2] It is a substantial risk factor for six of the eight leading causes of death, making it directly responsible for nearly 6 million deaths per year.[3] Sadly, a disproportionately higher number of the world's smokers live in low- and middle-income countries, and death rates secondary to tobacco use are much higher in these countries.[2] If current trends continue, by 2030 tobacco will kill more than 8 million people worldwide each year.[4]

Although there are many geographical areas where prevalence rates have either levelled or been dropping in the past few years, there are also epicentres of comparatively high and rising prevalence rates. Worldwide, not only are more people smoking, but smokers are consuming more cigarettes. Almost one billion men in the world smoke: about 35% of men in developed countries and 50% of men in developing countries. Roughly 250 million women in the world are daily smokers: about 22% of women in developed countries and 9% of women in developing countries smoke tobacco.[2] Prevalence rates among women are either remaining steady or even rising in many European countries. Initiation of tobacco use is also a public health problem among youth – United States of America (USA), over 80% of smokers begin prior to the age of 18 years and the addictive potential of smoking is extremely high.[5] Most teenage smokers are already addicted to nicotine while in adolescence. The highest youth smoking rates can be found in central and eastern Europe, sections of India and some of the western Pacific islands.[2]

Even if prevalence rates fall, the absolute number of smokers will increase due to population growth and the increase in female smoking rates, especially in developing countries. Table 24.1 presents a snapshot of current international prevalence estimates. Per region, the countries with the highest and lowest prevalence rates are included.[4]

Table 24.1 Age- and sex-standardized adult smoking prevalence

Region	Highest	Lowest
Africa	Sierra Leone: 22%	Ethiopia and Niger: both at 3%
The Americas	Chile: 34%	Belize and Guatemala: both at 4%
South-East Asia	Indonesia: 29%	Sri Lanka: 11%
Europe	Greece: 49%	Uzbekistan: 10%
Eastern Mediterranean	Lebanon: 37%	Oman: 4%
Western Pacific	Kiribati: 55%	Fiji: 8%

Additionally, China, Russia, Turkey, Japan, Mexico, Viet Nam, and the Ukraine have rates of smoking among males that exceed 50% of the population. Norway, France, Germany and Argentina are among the countries with comparatively higher rates of smoking for women. Age- and sex-standardized smoking prevalence among adults in the USA is 16%.

A combination of population-based and individually targeted approaches of prevention, policy and intervention will be needed to adequately combat the epidemic of preventable deaths due to tobacco use. Population-based tobacco control policies are credited with a least some measure of decreased prevalence rates; however, policies that are routine in the USA (e.g. smoke-free environments, health warnings and labelling, taxation) are not widely implemented in most countries. Even where these do exist, compliance with the policies is highly variable.[4] The vast majority of the world continues to be inundated with tobacco advertising – aggressive marketing and promotional campaigns, creating the imperative for aggressive and effective smoking cessation interventions to be delivered at the individual level as well as within the context of routine health care.

Tobacco use disorders have a natural course of addiction that is characterized not only by physiological addiction and dependence but also by behavioural aspects. For example, operant conditioning contributes every time someone experiences reinforcing and pleasurable effects from smoking, or alternatively, if they experience the removal of negative symptoms that may be related to cravings, urges, or nicotine dependence once they take another puff. The negative sequelae of smoking are substantially delayed in comparison to the immediate rewards experienced from smoking, which are both powerful and immediate, thereby increasing the likelihood of continued use. Moreover, principles of classical conditioning also contribute to tobacco use and dependence when someone repeatedly pairs smoking with other activities, such as drinking coffee or following a meal. Over time, as these activities are paired with one another, the occurrence of one becomes a highly influential cue to trigger the urge for the other. To the extent that some of the behavioural pairings are with activities that are unavoidable, such as ending a meal for example, a process of extinction is needed to reduce the saliency of cues to return to smoking. Educating patients about both of these phenomena can increase their understanding about urges and help to create effective quit plans that take into account their particular reinforcements, cues to smoking and paired behaviours.

The impact of smoking cessation

While the negative health impacts of smoking are unequivocal and widely documented, it can be more difficult to describe the specific benefits and reductions in risks associated with quitting smoking tobacco. Yet, it is critical to do this, because the perceived benefits of change can sometimes serve as a greater incentive for change.[7,8] Quitting smoking can lead to improved health status, decreased health-care utilization over time, improved quality of life and decreased morbidity and mortality. Moreover, the benefits of smoking cessation are almost immediate. For example, measurable improvements in blood pressure and cardiac functioning occur within a day of quitting; improved circulation, less phlegm production, and a reduction in coughing occur within a week.[2] In addition, a more favourable lipid profile begins to develop within weeks of quitting, including an increase in high-density lipoprotein (HDL), an increase in the HDL/LDL (low-density lipoprotein) ratio and a decrease in LDL[9,10] Within one year, the excess risk of coronary heart disease is half that of a current smoker.[2,11] Cessation is especially effective for those with established cardiovascular disease. A recent systematic review provided strong evidence that quitting smoking after acute myocardial infarction or cardiac surgery can decrease a person's risk of death by at least a third.[9,12] Although the relative risks decline considerably with age, the absolute excess mortality caused by smoking rises progressively with age. Therefore, it is important for clinicians to promote smoking cessation even in elderly smokers.

Smoking cessation interventions

Decades of research on smoking cessation have yielded a plethora of data, with the most recent guidelines on smoking cessation interventions benefiting from well over 50 meta-analyses completed to date. The gold standard approach for smoking cessation includes a combination of pharmacotherapy tailored to the individual, brief counselling, and follow-up support (telephone or in person but not necessarily with the primary care physician (PCP)) – with more intensive interventions consistently yielding higher quite rates (i.e. a dose–response relationship).[3] However, it should be noted that a considerable translation gap continues to exist in the routine implementation of evidence-based smoking cessation interventions within the clinic setting. Fortunately, many medical practitioners ask about smoking status, and estimates in the USA suggest over 50% of medical providers give some advice about quitting. The less encouraging data are that fewer than 20% of practitioners provide any *specific* assessment or assistance for smoking cessation, leaving many missed opportunities.[13,14] The reasons for this are undoubtedly many and varied, but the implications are such that no single clinic-based intervention has emerged as a clear gold standard *based on a population perspective*. Although some of the interventions are highly efficacious, they tend not to be easily scalable. For example, this is the case with some types of pharmacotherapy for smoking cessation. Since 2002, nicotine replacement therapy (NRT) has been available over the counter in many countries; however, parts of South America, Asia, most of Africa and portions of the Middle East are still lacking readily available, low-cost NRT. Moreover, some highly efficacious brief counselling interventions using motivational interviewing (MI) strategies are also not yet highly scalable, since these techniques are not standard education and training for medical providers worldwide. Thus, the impact of even the most effective interventions wanes when its implementation is too complex and resource intensive to be easily maintained or it is not feasible based on the workforce resources.

Pharmacological treatments

Pharmacotherapy for smoking cessation consistently yields the highest short- and long-term quit rates, with cessation rates nearly double those of usual care.[15] There are several types of pharmacotherapy, each associated with its own risks and benefits.

Bupropion

Bupropion inhibits the reuptake of serotonin, noradrenaline (norepinephrine) and dopamine, acts as a nicotine receptor antagonist, and at high concentrations inhibits the firing of noradrenergic neurons in the locus coeruleus.[16] It is approved by the US Food and Drug Administration (FDA) as a treatment for major depression, but typically not used as an antidepressant in other countries. It has not been definitively demonstrated which of these effects is the mechanism of action in bupropion's role in smoking cessation, though it seems likely that it helps by lessening the reduction of dopamine and noradrenaline that occur during nicotine withdrawal.

Sustained-release bupropion (bupropion SR) has repeatedly demonstrated efficacy in helping individuals quit smoking. Mills and colleagues analysed 31 studies and concluded that participants who received bupropion were more than twice as likely as control participants to be abstinent from nicotine at 4 weeks, almost all of whom received a placebo control.[17] Hayford and colleagues investigated whether or not a regimen of bupropion initiated 1 week prior to the target quit date increased rates of smoking cessation.[18] Participants were randomized to receiving doses of 100 mg, 150 mg or 300 mg of bupropion SR, or placebo. These researchers found that individuals who received active treatment were significantly more likely to be abstinent than those who received placebo, both at post-treatment and at 1-year follow-up. A significant dose effect was detected at both time points ($P < 0.001$ at post-treatment; $P = 0.020$ at 1 year), indicating that higher doses of bupropion were associated with higher quit rates. Hayford and colleagues concluded that treatment for smoking cessation with bupropion increased rates of successful cessation for people with or without a history of depression or alcoholism.[18]

Despite the mounting evidence supporting the efficacy of bupropion in increasing rates of smoking cessation, it is not without drawbacks. In the USA, the FDA has issued a "black-box" warning for Zyban® and its generic equivalents (i.e. bupropion). In 2009, it issued a public health advisory announcing that bupropion has been associated with serious adverse effects such as aggression, hostility, irritability and suicidal thoughts or actions.[19] Individuals using the medication are strongly encouraged to tell their prescribing physicians should any such effects emerge. Providers who are considering the use of bupropion must also be aware of these risks, and be willing and able to provide the follow-up monitoring necessary to assess for the emergence of such adverse events, as well as the care to manage them if they present.

Nicotine replacement therapy

Nicotine replacement therapy has been available as a means of facilitating smoking cessation for approximately 30 years.[20] It works by stimulating nicotine receptors, leading to the release of dopamine and a reduction in symptoms of nicotine withdrawal. NRT is available in a number of different forms, including gum, transdermal patches, lozenges, sublingual tablets, inhalers and nasal spray. While nicotine from cigarettes is delivered to the brain in high doses within seconds of inhalation, nicotine from the systems described above is delivered in smaller doses over a matter minutes, or hours in the case of the patch. As is the case with other drugs, a shorter duration of onset of effects, as occurs with smoking, followed by rapid de-escalation of effects is associated with onset of dependence and corresponding withdrawal.

NRT has been evaluated as a tool to encourage smoking cessation in dozens of studies over more than three decades. As part of the Cochrane Collaboration, Silagy and colleagues reviewed 123 trials of the efficacy of NRT as a smoking cessation aid.[21] These researchers concluded that use of NRT nearly doubles the rate of successful cessation compared to no treatment. Although some smokers who use NRT do relapse, individuals who quit using NRT are also more likely to remain abstinent than those who attempt to quit without assistance.

Across the trials reviewed by these researchers, nicotine gum, nicotine patches, nicotine inhalers, nicotine spray and nicotine lozenges were all evaluated, and all demonstrated efficacy compared to no treatment or placebo. In choosing which mode of NRT to offer, providers may consider patient preference, cost and the intensity of smoking. There is little evidence that use of NRT significantly increases the probability of abstinence in smokers who smoke fewer than 10 cigarettes per day. On the other end of the spectrum, providers may consider increasing the intensity of NRT interventions for heavy smokers. This may include augmenting the use of a nicotine patch with nicotine gum, as needed, for "break-through" cravings, or offering 4 mg gum rather than 2 mg gum.

The adverse effects associated with NRT are relatively mild. The patch appears to have the fewest adverse effects, with skin irritation at the site of use being the only one that seems to deter its use.[22] Although up to 54% of users may experience some degree of irritation, it is rarely severe enough to lead users to stop using the patch. Nicotine gum is associated with more potential negative side-effects than the patch, including hiccups, stomach discomfort, discomfort of the jaw and dental problems. Other modes of NRT may lead to a runny nose, sore throat, or irritation at the site of administration.

Varenicline

Varenicline (Chantix®, Champix®) is a non-nicotine pharmaceutical agent developed specifically for facilitation of smoking cessation. It is a selective partial agonist of nicotinic acetylcholine receptors that reduces the rewarding effects of nicotine.[23] It has been available in the USA and Europe since 2006, and has quickly established itself as an effective treatment for smoking cessation. In direct comparisons using randomized clinical trials of 1 mg of varenicline twice daily and bupropion SR 150 mg twice daily, approximately 50% of those who received varenicline were abstinent for seven consecutive days after 12 weeks of treatment, compared to 36% of those who received bupropion and 21% of those who received placebo.[24,25] In both studies, varenicline demonstrated superiority over placebo at one year but it was only significantly better than bupropion in one of the studies.[24]

In a convenience sample of 412 participants, those who received varenicline were between one and a half and two times more likely to be abstinent at one month than those who received NRT.[26] In a randomized, open-label study, continuous abstinence rates for those receiving varenicline were significantly better than for those using the patch (56% versus 43%) during the final 4 weeks of treatment.[27] While these initial studies suggest that varenicline may be more efficacious than NRT, further study with tighter control and longer follow-up is necessary to draw more firm conclusions. Nonetheless, it is now a first-line intervention strategy for smoking cessation.[3]

Significant adverse effects associated with the use of varenicline

The FDA's "black-box" warning includes rare but severe potential side-effects such as agitation, depressed mood, suicidal ideation and behaviour, and worsening of pre-existing psychiatric illness. Between 30% and 50% of those who take varenicline may experience nausea, although this is typically mild.[28] Other commonly reported negative side-effects include insomnia, abnormal dreams and gastrointestinal effects. Most of these adverse events seem to be dose dependent, and reducing the dose may reduce or abolish these symptoms. In a recent meta-analysis of 14 double-blind studies that included a total of 8216 participants, smokers who took varenicline faced significantly elevated risk for serious cardiovascular events compared to those who took placebo (1.06% versus 0.82%).[29] Insufficient data prevented meaningful comparisons for mortality rates. Prescribers should work with their patients to balance the benefits obtained from the medication with potential unpleasant side-effects, which can be assessed in a relatively quick follow-up (1–2 weeks) after the patient's target quit date.

Other agents

Bupropion, NRT, and varenicline have all been classified as first-line pharmacological smoking cessation aids in the 2008 revision of the *Treating tobacco use and dependence clinical practice guidelines*.[22] Two other pharmacotherapies have also demonstrated some promise in helping smokers quit: clonidine and nortriptyline. However, neither has been studied as extensively as the first-line strategies described above and both have more significant side-effect profiles. For more information on the extant research regarding the use of clonidine and nortriptyline for tobacco cessation, please see the guidelines referenced above.[22]

Combining medications

Although data are sparse, there is some evidence to suggest a beneficial effect, as compared to placebo, of combining bupropion and the NRT patch, with both used at standard dosage, as well as for combining the NRT patch and nicotine inhaler. A few studies have examined whether adding either nicotine gum or nasal spray for "break-through" cravings may increase efficacy over either alone, but data are not sufficient for definitive conclusions. Varenicline should not be combined with NRT treatments.[3] Clinicians should bear in mind that while combining medications may be helpful for some patients, it also increases the cost and the risks of side-effects. Table 24.2 provides a summary of pharmacotherapy recommendations.

Behavioural interventions for smoking cessation

Behavioural interventions for tobacco use disorders maximize long-term abstinence rates and have very few risks. Behavioural therapy encompasses a broad range of techniques, ranging from strong, personalized, empathetic messages from a primary care provider to more elaborate and programmatic interventions delivered over weeks or months. Although the literature is sparse regarding the relative benefits of one specific behavioural technique compared to another, there are some behavioural approaches for smoking cessation with unequivocal efficacy. These include implementation of the "5As" model (see below) to help patients quit (National Cancer Institute),[3] MI techniques to assess and increase readiness to quit, and using intervention strategies matched to a patient's stage of change.

Table 24.2 Factors to consider in selecting medication for smoking cessation: first-line interventions with high and well-established efficacy and FDA approval for tobacco cessation

	Risk factors	Side-effects (partial list)	Dosing guidelines	Clinical notes
Varenicline (Chantix®, Champix®)	• Pregnancy (*contraindicated*) • Significant psychiatric history • Carries FDA "black-box" warning	• Strange dreams • Nausea • Insomnia	• 0.5 mg once/day for 3 days • 0.5 mg twice/day for 4 days • 1.0 mg twice/day for 3 months • Approved for maintenance for up to 6 months	• Quit date should be 8th day of medication • Most expensive cessation option • Availability may be limited in some areas • Prescribers should monitor for changes in mood/behaviour
Bupropion (Zyban®, Welbutrin®)	• Pregnancy • MAO inhibitors within 14 days (*contraindicated*) • History of anorexia or bulimia (*contraindicated*) • History of seizures (*contraindicated*) • Carries FDA "black-box" warning	• Dry mouth • Insomnia • Weight change • Nausea	• 150 mg/day for 3 days • 150 mg twice/day for 7–12 weeks • May be used for up to 6 months for maintenance	• Quit date should be 1–2 weeks after initiation of treatment • May also be helpful in managing symptoms of depression • Alcohol use should be monitored while on this medication
NRT: patch	• Pregnancy • Within 2 weeks of myocardial infarction period • Serious arrhythmia • Unstable angina periods	• Skin irritation • Insomnia • Vivid dreams	• 21 mg/24 hours for 4 weeks, then • 14 mg/24 hours for 2 weeks, then • 7 mg/24 hours for 2 weeks This is just a sample regimen. Many variations are available	• Should be placed at a location with minimal hair • Rotate location to minimize irritation
NRT: oral	• Pregnancy (*contraindicated*) • Within 2 weeks of myocardial infarction period • Serious arrhythmia • Unstable angina periods	• Nasal irritation (nasal spray) • Nausea • Hiccups • Heartburn • Coughing (inhaler)	Varies based on type	• Available over the counter in some forms (e.g., gum) • Patients may have an idiosyncratic preference for a particular form • Gum, lozenge, inhaler and nasal spray all appropriate as first-line intervention • Nasal spray has the highest addiction potential

MAO = monoamine oxidase.

Behavioural counselling should always be included in treatment, with telephone or other similar support. More intensive interventions yield higher quit rates but, at a minimum, brief interventions are indicated for every smoker. Follow-up 1–2 weeks after targeted quit date with at least four sessions ≥10 minutes by the PCP or other clinician.

The "5As" include:

- *Ask* every patient about their current smoking status and desire to quit
- *Assess* the patient's willingness to quit within the next month
- *Advise* all smokers to quit
- *Assist* in the quit attempt
- *Arrange* follow-up.

Ask

Smokers tend to have a more positive view of providers who assess smoking status, and up to 60% of smokers are at least thinking about quitting.[30] Although formal assessment instruments exist (e.g. the Fagerstrom Nicotine Dependence Scale),[31] simply asking patients if they currently smoke is sufficient. However, this question alone will not decipher the patient's level of nicotine dependence or other clinical data needed to select the most appropriate pharmacotherapy interventions. Follow-up inquiry may thus be needed, and Box 24.1, adapted from Anczak and colleagues[32] offers a relatively simple but adequate series of questions that additionally assesses the level of nicotine dependence as well as whether there are other smokers in the home, which are both relative predictors of success.

Box 24.1   A tool to ask about smoking status

- Do you now smoke cigarettes?
  - Yes
  - No
- Does the person(s) you live with or the person(s) closest to you smoke?
  - Yes
  - No
- How many cigarettes do you smoke each day?
- How soon after you wake up do you smoke your first cigarette?
  - Less than 30 minutes
  - More than 30 minutes
- How interested are you in stopping smoking?
  - Not at all
  - A little
  - Somewhat
  - A lot
  - Very

Assess

Assessing readiness to quit can be determined in one simple question "How likely (or ready) are you to make a quit attempt in the next 6 months?" Further assessment can elucidate the patient's stage of readiness in more detail, allowing the clinician to gauge the next logical intervention. Importance and confidence rulers are commonly used techniques based on MI principles:

1   On a scale of 1–10, how important is it to you to quit smoking?

2   On a scale of 1–10, how confident are you that you could quit smoking?

As shown in Figure 24.1, when patients express a high degree of importance and confidence, they are ready for active assistance with smoking cessation, to ideally include a combination of pharmacotherapy, behavioural counselling, and support. When importance ratings are high, but confidence ratings are low, assistance with building self-efficacy is needed prior to active cessation interventions. When importance is low and confidence is high, further discussion about the pros and cons of smoking versus quitting, and other MI strategies are indicated (e.g. the "5Rs", discussed later in this chapter).

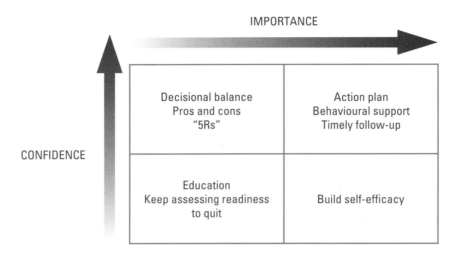

Figure 24.1 Readiness assessment guides intervention

Advise

A follow-up statement regarding the importance of quitting as the single best action someone can take to improve his or her health *is always indicated* for current smokers. Brief advice has been shown to significantly increase quit rates by 1–3%.[33] Although the magnitude of the effect is small, if health-care providers universally and systematically talk with their patients at every opportunity about their smoking, even for 3–5 minutes, this small effect will represent a considerable population impact. Moreover, brief discussions about smoking cessation, using techniques informed by motivational interviewing, can be over five times more effective than simply delivering a message about the harms of smoking and advice to quit.[34]

Assist

When patients express a willingness to quit, PCPs should always offer pharmacotherapy unless it is unavailable, cost prohibitive or contraindicated. In addition, PCPs or ancillary clinical staff can quickly implement the STAR approach, which entails: having the patient *set* a quit date (S); *tell* family and friends to enlist adequate support (T); *anticipate* and problem-solve potential challenges, such as withdrawal symptoms or triggers to smoke (A); and *remove* all tobacco products, such as ashtrays and lighters prior to or on their quit date (R). Although the evidence is marginal supporting the use of self-help materials, such as patient handouts and web sites, these are unlikely to cause any harm and can be used adjunctively. However, telephone quit lines are effective, and whenever possible should be offered and encouraged, especially when there is uncertainly about other adequate social supports.[35]

Depending on available resources, PCPs or other personnel (effectiveness is similar across disciplines) can further assist patients by providing specific counselling strategies, including problem-solving training and skills training to manage urges and high-risk situations for relapse. Assisting patients to actively use their social supports while quitting is also associated with a significant increase in abstinence rates. Table 24.3, largely excerpted from the Public Health Service clinical guidelines, highlights elemental behavioural counselling strategies.[36]

Arrange

When arranging follow-up, PCPs should be aware of a clear dose–response relationship between the intensity of behavioural interventions and cessation rates. Individual, group and telephone counselling are all effective

Companion to Primary Care Mental Health

Table 24.3 Strategies for brief smoking cessation interventions. Adapted from Fiore MC et al. *Tobacco use and dependence: 2008 update*. Rockville MD, US Department of Health and Human Services, 2008[37]

Counselling component	Examples
Psychoeducation • About smoking • About quitting	• Any smoking (even a single puff) increases the likelihood of a full relapse • Cutting down does not have demonstrable health benefits • Withdrawal symptoms typically peak within 1–2 weeks after quitting but may persist for months. These symptoms include negative mood, urges to smoke, and difficulty concentrating • The addictive nature of smoking – why it is so hard to quit • Keeping track of cigarettes before quitting can help identify your pattern before quitting
Developing coping skills • Identify coping skills • Build new skills as needed • Practise implementing skills	• Learning to anticipate and avoid temptation and trigger situations • Learning cognitive strategies that will reduce negative moods • Accomplishing lifestyle changes that reduce stress, improve quality of life, and reduce exposure to smoking cues • Learning cognitive and behavioural activities to cope with smoking urges (e.g. distracting attention; changing routines)
Practise problem-solving high-risk situations • Recognize danger situations • Identify high-risk events/activities • Identify and recognize high-risk internal states • Practise new skills	• Negative affect and stress • Being around other tobacco users • Drinking alcohol • Experiencing urges • Smoking cues (conditioned links with smoking such as coffee or after meals; some people stop coffee for a while while quitting) • Availability of cigarettes • The nature of cravings – they wax and wane; they will peak and then stop; use distraction or chew gum or hard vegetables

treatment modalities to enhance treatment intensity. The goal is multiple contacts with a patient during the beginning period of smoking cessation, and the initial follow-up should occur soon after the quit date, preferably during the first or second week.

When the smoker is not ready to quit

The initial assessment and brief behavioural interventions delineated above are feasible for most PCPs, and in most clinics, once adequate knowledge and skills are developed. More challenging for the PCP is the current smoker who is not interested in quitting. In this case, PCPs are encouraged to use MI techniques in an effort to enhance the patient's readiness to change, a strategy with consistent evidence of its impact as compared to advice alone. MI is a patient-centred approach of guiding the patient towards change by exploring and resolving their ambivalence. A 2010 meta-analysis of MI in 31 studies reported an odds ratio (OR) of 1.45 (95% confidence interval (CI) = 1.14 to 1.83), compared to usual treatment.[38]

For example, asking affect-arousing questions and encouraging patients to re-evaluate themselves as smokers are interventions physicians can use to help patients who are not prepared to quit smoking. Exploring the personalized disadvantages of smoking, in addition to what the patient likes most about smoking can also be a useful discussion (i.e. a decisional balance exercise). Most patients know they should quit smoking to improve their health and most have been told this by one or more health-care professionals. What they may not have been asked, however, are the reasons they continue to smoke despite the negative health effects. Understanding what maintains smoking (beyond the nicotine dependence) can help PCPs know what types of interventions and tactics might yield the most benefit, and avoid highlighting more barriers for the patient. Matching interventions according to someone's readiness to change is critical, as behavioural interventions, such as providing substitutes for cigarettes and removing or altering cues for smoking, are most helpful for patients who are ready to take action. However, when such interventions are delivered to a patient who is not currently interested in quitting, this approach will not only be completely ineffective but is likely to leave both the patient and PCP highly frustrated. The use of stage-matched, patient-centred counselling can help PCPs and patients feel less frustrated and allow PCPs to be more effective in their efforts to help a broad range of their patients.

More specifically, when patients are unwilling to quit, a discussion based on the "5Rs" is recommended.

- *Relevance to health*: this involves delivering highly personalized messages linking a patient's current visit or health status with their smoking and highlighting what might change if the patient quits. In one intervention, patients were told their "lung age" (i.e. the age of the average nonsmoker with the same FEV_1 (forced expiratory volume in 1 s) as the patient), which was found to increase rates of sustained cessation for those who were not interested in quitting. Based on this intervention alone, quit rates were 6.4% of the control group and 13.6% in the intervention group ($P = 0.005$).[39]

- *Risk of smoking*: try to have the patient describe potential short- and longer-term risks associated with smoking that are personally relevant; these might include shortness of breath, asthma, impotence, infertility, pregnancy complications, heartburn or frequent respiratory infections.

- *Rewards of quitting*: inquire about whether the patient can identify any potential benefits of quitting such as saving money, food tastes better, setting a good example to children, less hassle given the current restrictions on smoking.

- *Roadblocks to quitting*: patients are typically able to recite the barriers to quitting, which might include fear of withdrawal, or failure, weight gain, lack of support, or feeling like they would be losing their best friend. Often patients feel it is their main coping strategy and way to calm down. Invite patients to express these barriers while reducing the reflexive impetus to challenge or problem-solve the barriers. When patients are given the opportunity to express these feelings without pressure to change, it often has a seemingly paradoxical effect of increasing change talk, which leads to quit attempts.

- *Repetition of this discussion* at each visit, with a reminder to patients that most people make repeated quit attempts before succeeding.

Well-resourced primary care clinics can rely on universal screening for tobacco use, brief assessments to determine stage of readiness, and brief interventions by physicians, as well as referrals to behaviour change experts within the clinic to further personalize the quit plan. Behaviour change experts might be nurses, mental health professionals or other trained clinical staff. They would work individually with patients to help set a quit date, schedule regular and frequent follow-ups relative to the quit date, and establish individually tailored plans to prepare for quitting, as well as relapse-preventions plans. In an ideal scenario, proactive telephone outreach would be available to all patients expressing a desire or intention to quit, and certainly every patient to whom pharmacotherapy for smoking cessation was prescribed.

Providers and clinics with fewer resources might use similar strategies but decrease the intervention intensity, especially if a nurse or behavioural health experts are not available. As noted earlier, however, primary care providers can still deliver brief but highly effective behavioural counselling. Once PCPs can hone in on the most effective behavioural change techniques described above and begin to experience the significant impact of brief, behavioural interventions on the smoking cessation rates within their patient population, commonly cited constraints of PCPs (e.g. lack of time and training) become less formidable barriers to implementation.

As the reductionist biomedical model of medicine and health care too often relied upon in the USA is not universally accepted, alternative and complementary medicine approaches for smoking cessation are also being evaluated, although not as rigorously. Perhaps due to the lack of scientific rigor, the consensus is that most alternative therapies examined to date, such as acupuncture and hypnosis, are not as effective as more traditional approaches for smoking cessation.[40] However, these approaches often have few side-effects and little potential for harm. Providers should not routinely recommend such interventions, but they may have a placebo effect so should not be discouraged among patients who are trying these techniques on their own.

Making it happen: translating research into practice

A recent meta-analysis of 37 unique studies to evaluate the strategies for increasing the delivery of smoking cessation interventions in primary care clinics found multicomponent approaches tended to yield the most promising results of increasing the implementation of the "5As".[22,41] Beyond this conclusion, the provision of adjunctive counselling for smokers trying to quit, real-time prompts for providers to initiate counselling for smoking cessation (e.g. through the use of embedded prompts in an electronic medical record), and specific feedback to practitioners and practices, were also found to be effective.[5,22,42] As a single component strategy, adjunctive counselling yielded the most consistent pattern of positive findings from multiple well-designed randomized controlled trials. This is encouraging, as the other approaches are significantly more resource intensive, whereas simply linking patients to adjunctive support that is either internal or external to the clinic will have greater public health impact.

Special populations

Pregnant women

Due to the serious deleterious health effects of smoking on both mother and fetus, pregnant smokers should be offered person-to-person psychosocial interventions. Although brief interventions and using the "5As" model are also recommended, more aggressive interventions are warranted for this population. Moreover, quitting early in pregnancy is ideal but the health benefits exist if the mother quits at any point during her pregnancy.[43] Behavioural and supportive interventions are the gold standard for this population.

Patients with low education

Pharmacotherapy for smoking cessation is indicated for this patient population. A 2008 meta-analysis of five studies compared the effectiveness of counselling versus usual care on smoking cessation rates among individuals with low socioeconomic status and limited formal education. The results showed that behavioural counselling is also effective in treating smokers from this population (OR = 1.42; 95% CI = 1.04 to 1.92).[3]

Patients with comorbid mental illness

Although there are few studies, the same smoking cessation interventions used among a general population (i.e. pharmacotherapy, behavioural counselling and supportive therapy) appear to be equally effective when used with patients who suffer from serious mental illness.[44]

Conclusions

Prevalence rates for tobacco use remain unacceptably high. Although smoking rates may be declining in some areas of the world, some geographical areas are experiencing increases in prevalence, especially among women. Public health and policy-level initiatives for tobacco control are improving but cannot combat this epidemic alone. Routine inquiry about smoking status and offering some type of evidence-supported treatment in all primary care settings is a health-care imperative. Primary care providers can greatly impact tobacco cessation attempts and success rates. All patients interested in making a quit attempt should be offered one of the effective pharmacotherapy options to improve long-term abstinence rates, unless contraindicated or unavailable. Interventions for smoking cessation are most effective when pharmacotherapy and behavioural interventions are combined. Thus, adjunctive supportive therapy, practical counselling, telephone quit line counselling, and timely follow-up after a projected quit date are also core components of the most effective interventions. The evidence to date is consistent in reporting that short- and long-term cessation rates rise with treatments of higher intensity and longer duration. Finally, multicomponent system-level changes will also be required to make tobacco cessation a routine practice in primary care clinics worldwide. Bridging the translation gap from evidence to implementation remains a work in progress. Barriers such as developing an adequately trained workforce to prescribe optimal pharmacotherapy and deliver brief counselling interventions using MI strategies are formidable but surmountable. Every setting will encounter unique resource constraints; however, the richness of the available data on the effectiveness of various approaches for smoking cessation make it possible for virtually every primary care clinic to implement one or more of the key smoking cessation recommendations and thus improve on existing practice. The option of doing nothing more than current practice seems indefensible given the consequences of inaction, whereas the collective impact of even small changes will surely be substantial and save lives.

References

1   Mokdad AH et al. Actual causes of death in the United States, 2000. *JAMA*, 2004, 291:1238–1245.

2   WHO atlas maps global tobacco epidemic. *Public Health Reports*, 2002, 117:479.

3   Clinical Practice Guideline Treating Tobacco Use and Dependence 2008 Update Panel, Liaisons and Staff. A clinical practice guideline for treating tobacco use and dependence: 2008 update. A US Public Health Service report. *American Journal of Preventive Medicine*, 2008, 35:158–176.

4   *WHO report on the global tobacco epidemic, 2011: warning about the dangers of tobacco*. Geneva, World Health Organization, 2011.

5   Elders MJ et al. The report of the Surgeon General: preventing tobacco use among young people. *American Journal of Public Health*, 1994, 84:543–547.

6   *WHO report on the global tobacco epidemic, 2009: implementing smoke-free environments*. Geneva, World Health Organization, 2009.

7   Becker MH. The health belief model and sick role behaviour. In: Becker MH, ed. *The health belief model and personal behaviour*. Thorofare NJ, Charles S Black Inc., 1974:82–92.

8   Rosenstock IM. Why people use health services. *The Milbank Memorial Fund Quarterly*, 1966, 44(3 Suppl.):94–127.

9   Thomas D. Cardiovascular benefits of smoking cessation. *Presse Medicale*, 2009, 38:946–952.

10   Gastaldelli A, Folli F, Maffei S. Impact of tobacco smoking on lipid metabolism, body weight and cardiometabolic risk. *Current Pharmaceutical Design*, 2010, 16:2526–2530.

11   Mikhailidis DP, Papadakis JA, Ganotakis ES. Smoking, diabetes and hyperlipidaemia. *Journal of the Royal Society of Health*, 1998, 118:91–93.

12   Campbell SC, Moffatt RJ, Stamford BA. Smoking and smoking cessation: the relationship between cardiovascular disease and lipoprotein metabolism: a review. *Atherosclerosis*, 2008, 201:225–235.

13   Katz DA et al. and the AHRQ Smoking Cessation Guideline Study Group. Effectiveness of implementing the agency for healthcare research and quality smoking cessation clinical practice guideline: a randomized, controlled trial. *Journal of the National Cancer Institute*, 2004, 96:594–603.

14   Chase EC, McMenamin SB, Halpin HA. Medicaid provider delivery of the 5As for smoking cessation counseling. *Nicotine and Tobacco Research*, 2007, 9:1095–1101.

15   Stead LF et al. Nicotine replacement therapy for smoking cessation. *Cochrane Database of Systematic Reviews*, 2008, (1): CD000146.

16   Roddy E. Bupropion and other non-nicotine pharmacotherapies. *BMJ*, 2004, 328:509–511.

17   Mills E et al. Smoking cessation reduces postoperative complications: a systematic review and meta-analysis. *The American Journal of Medicine*, 2011, 124:144–154.e8.

18   Hayford KE et al. Efficacy of bupropion for smoking cessation in smokers with a former history of major depression or alcoholism. *British Journal of Psychiatry*, 1999, 174:173–178.

19   Food and Drug Administration. *Drug Safety Newsletter*, 2009, 2(1).

20   Molyneux A. Nicotine replacement therapy. *BMJ*, 2004, 328:454–456.

21   Silagy C et al. Nicotine replacement therapy for smoking cessation. *Cochrane Database of Systematic Reviews*, 2004, (3):CD000146.

22   Fiore MC, Keller PA, Curry SJ. Health system changes to facilitate the delivery of tobacco-dependence treatment. *American Journal of Preventive Medicine*, 2007, 33(6 Suppl.):S349–356.

23 Nides M et al. Smoking cessation with varenicline, a selective alpha4beta2 nicotinic receptor partial agonist: results from a 7-week, randomized, placebo- and bupropion-controlled trial with 1-year follow-up. *Archives of Internal Medicine*, 2006, 166:1561–1568.

24 Jorenby DE et al. and the Varenicline Phase 3 Study Group. Efficacy of varenicline, an alpha4beta2 nicotinic acetylcholine receptor partial agonist, vs placebo or sustained-release bupropion for smoking cessation: a randomized controlled trial. *JAMA*, 2006, 296:56–63.

25 Gonzales D et al. and the Varenicline Phase 3 Study Group. Varenicline, an alpha4beta2 nicotinic acetylcholine receptor partial agonist, vs sustained-release bupropion and placebo for smoking cessation: a randomized controlled trial. *JAMA*, 2006, 296:47–55.

26 Stapleton JA et al. Varenicline in the routine treatment of tobacco dependence: a pre-post comparison with nicotine replacement therapy and an evaluation in those with mental illness. *Addiction*, 2008, 103:146–154.

27 Aubin HJ et al. Varenicline versus transdermal nicotine patch for smoking cessation: results from a randomised open-label trial. *Thorax*, 2008, 63:717–724.

28 Hays JT, Ebbert JO. Varenicline for tobacco dependence. *The New England Journal of Medicine*, 2008, 359:2018–2024.

29 Singh S et al. Risk of serious adverse cardiovascular events associated with varenicline: a systematic review and meta-analysis. *Canadian Medical Association Journal*, 2011, 183:1359–1356.

30 Quinn VP et al. Tobacco-cessation services and patient satisfaction in nine nonprofit HMOs. *American Journal of Preventive Medicine*, 2005, 29:77–84.

31 Heatherton T et al. The Fagerstrom Test for Nicotine Dependence: a revision of the Fagerstrom Tolerance Questionnaire. *British Journal of Addiction*, 1991, 86:1119–1127.

32 Anczak JD, Nogler RA, 2nd. Tobacco cessation in primary care: maximizing intervention strategies. *Clinical Medicine and Research*, 2003, 1:201–216.

33 Stead LF, Bergson G, Lancaster T. Physician advice for smoking cessation. *Cochrane Database of Systematic Reviews*, 2008, (2):CD000165.

34 Lai DT et al. Motivational interviewing for smoking cessation. *Cochrane Database of Systematic Reviews*, 2010, (1):CD006936.

35 Stead LF, Perera R, Lancaster T. Telephone counseling for smoking cessation. *Cochrane Database of Systematic Reviews*, 2006, (3):CD002850.

36 Cabezas C et al. and ISTAPS Study Group. Effectiveness of a stepped primary care smoking cessation intervention: cluster randomized clinical trial (ISTAPS study). *Addiction*, 2011, 106:1696–1706.

37 Fiore MC et al. *Tobacco use and dependence: 2008 update.* Rockville MD, US Department of Health and Human Services, 2008.

38 McCaul KD et al. Motivation to quit using cigarettes: a review. *Addictive Behaviors*, 2006, 31(1): 42–56.

39 Parks SJ et al., eds. *Morbidity and mortality in people with serious mental illness.* Alexandria, National Association of State Mental Health Program Directors (NASMHPD) Medical Directors Council, 2006.

40 White AR et al. Acupuncture and related interventions for smoking cessation. *Cochrane Database of Systematic Reviews*, 2011, (1):CD000009.

41 Glasgow RE, Emont S, Miller DC. Assessing delivery of the five 'As' for patient-centered counseling. *Health Promotion International*, 2006, 21:245–255.

42 Boyle RG, Solberg LI, Fiore MC. Electronic medical records to increase the clinical treatment of tobacco dependence: a systematic review. *American Journal of Preventive Medicine*, 2010, 39(6 Suppl. 1):S77–82.

43 Murin S, Rafii R, Bilello K. Smoking and smoking cessation in pregnancy. *Clinics in Chest Medicine*, 2011, 32:75–91, viii.

44 Banham L, Gilbody S. Smoking cessation in severe mental illness: what works? *Addiction*, 2010, 105:1176–1189.

25 Alcohol use disorder in primary care mental health

Pratima Singh, Pedro Camacho, Peter Selby, Raúl Martín del Campo and Himanshu Tyagi

---

Key messages

- There is strong evidence to suggest that screening for alcohol use disorder and early intervention in primary care settings are highly effective.
- Primary care physicians should opportunistically identify alcohol use disorders and harmful drinking and deliver a brief intervention.
- Motivational interviewing techniques should be considered when delivering brief interventions for harmful drinking in primary care.
- The principles of stepped care should be followed for patients with alcohol problems and dependence.
- Unlike most withdrawals from other chemical agents, alcohol withdrawal syndrome can be fatal and should be managed carefully with appropriate help from acute and specialist services.

Introduction

Use of alcohol is a global phenomenon that is widely accepted and has been associated with relaxation and pleasure across cultures and all sections of society since historical times. Alcohol use affects the brain, and therefore behaviour, in a variety of ways. These effects are influenced by a number of variables, including biological, social and psychological factors. Harmful drinking patterns and alcohol dependence are common conditions that contribute considerably to morbidity, mortality and burden to health-care systems and society. Alcohol remains a leading cause of death in industrialized countries. A significant proportion of these deaths are due to an increased risk of suicide as a result of alcohol use. A person with an alcohol-related problem is more likely to consult a primary care physician than a person without alcohol-related problems. As most of these deleterious effects can be managed cost effectively at an earlier stage, the role of primary care in treatment of alcohol use disorders is vitally important. Patients presenting with alcohol-related problems frequently suffer from comorbid mental health problems. From a broader perspective, patients with a comorbid situation between an addiction and a psychiatric trouble are at risk of being under-diagnosed for one of the two diseases. This chapter outlines the relevant issues in diagnosis and management of alcohol-related health problems in primary care settings.

Definitions

Alcohol use disorders have been recognized as mental health disorders by the World Health Organization since 1992.[1] In this chapter, the term "alcohol use disorder" is used in place of the widely used term "alcoholism", as the latter lacks the clear definition necessary to be useful for diagnostic purposes. Definitions and explanations for some of the terms that are frequently used in the literature on alcohol use disorder follow.

Unit of alcohol

Units of alcohol are a measure of the volume of pure alcohol in alcoholic beverages. This is useful for measuring and monitoring alcohol consumption at individual or community levels. In the United Kingdom of Great Britain and Northern Ireland, one unit of alcohol is defined as 10 ml, and in Australia it is 10 g (12.7 ml).

An average healthy adult can metabolize about 9.5 ml of pure alcohol or 95% of a UK unit of alcohol, in about one hour.[2]

Harmful alcohol use

Research has demonstrated that harmful alcohol use is conceptually and statistically distinct from alcohol dependence.[3] Harmful alcohol use is defined by the *International Classification of Diseases* (ICD-10) as:[1]

> A pattern of psychoactive substance use that is causing damage to health. The damage may be physical (e.g. hepatitis) or mental (e.g. depressive episodes secondary to heavy alcohol intake).

The ICD-10 diagnosis of harmful alcohol use requires the presence of one or more symptoms of physical or psychological damage secondary to alcohol use. Adverse social consequences, although acknowledged, are not required to make a diagnosis.

The closest corresponding category to "harmful alcohol use" in DSM-IV is "alcohol abuse".

Hazardous alcohol use

The term "hazardous drinking" is widely used. Hazardous use of alcohol is defined as the pattern of alcohol use that increases the risk of harmful consequences for the user. It is not a diagnostic term recognized by any major classification systems, including ICD-10[1] and the *Diagnostic and Statistical Manual of Mental Disorders* (DSM-IV),[4] but is mainly used by the World Health OrganizationWHO[5,6] and various governments in their public health programmes. It is synonymous with "at-risk drinking". For operational purposes, it is usually defined as the regular consumption of:

- over 40 g of pure ethanol (5 UK units) per day for men
- over 24 g of pure ethanol (3 UK units) per day for women.

These figures are derived from population studies showing the relationship of self-reported levels of drinking to risk of harm. It is arbitrary; i.e. it is the point on the risk curve that is deemed to merit a warning about continuing alcohol use.

Many authorities, including the UK Government, have quoted recommended upper limits for alcohol consumption of 21 units per week for men and 14 units per week for women.

Consuming over 40 g alcohol per day on average doubles a man's risk for liver disease, raised blood pressure, some cancers (for which smoking is a confounding factor) and violent death (because some people who have this average alcohol consumption drink heavily on some days). For women, over 24 g per day average alcohol consumption increases their risk for developing liver disease and breast cancer.

The term "hazardous drinking" is also used to loosely cover those who have experienced minimal harm with alcohol use, as opposed to serious harm.

Alcohol dependence

Both the ICD-10[1] and DSM-IV[4] recognize alcohol dependence as a category of mental disorder. Alcohol dependence is defined as a cluster of physiological, behavioural and cognitive phenomena in which the use of alcohol takes on a much higher priority for a given individual than other behaviours that previously had greater value. A central characteristic of alcohol dependence syndrome is the desire (often strong, sometimes perceived as overpowering) to drink alcohol. Return to drinking after a period of abstinence is often associated with rapid reappearance of the features of the syndrome (priming). In 1976, Edwards and Gross established seven core features for alcohol dependence syndrome (summarized in Box 25.1), which later formed the basis for the diagnostic criteria in ICD-10.[7]

Box 25.1 Provisional criteria for alcohol dependence syndrome[7]

- Narrowing of the drinking repertoire
- Salience of drink-seeking behaviour
- Increased tolerance to alcohol
- Repeated withdrawal symptoms
- Relief or avoidance of withdrawal symptoms by further drinking
- Subjective awareness of compulsion to drink
- Reinstatement after abstinence

According to the ICD-10,[1] a definitive diagnosis of dependence should usually only be made if three or more of the following have been present together at some time during the previous year:

- a strong desire or sense of compulsion to take alcohol
- difficulty in controlling drinking in terms of its onset, termination or level of use
- a physiological withdrawal state when drinking has ceased or been reduced (e.g. tremor, sweating, rapid heart rate, anxiety, insomnia, or, less commonly, seizures, disorientation or hallucinations) or drinking to relieve or avoid withdrawal symptoms
- evidence of tolerance, such that increased doses of alcohol are required in order to achieve effects originally produced by lower doses (clear examples of this are found in drinkers who may take daily doses sufficient to incapacitate or kill non-tolerant users)
- progressive neglect of alternative pleasures or interests because of drinking, and increased amount of time necessary to obtain or take alcohol or to recover from its effects (salience of drinking)
- persisting with alcohol use despite awareness of overtly harmful consequences, such as harm to the liver, depressive mood states consequent to periods of heavy drinking, or alcohol-related impairment of cognitive functioning.

A note on differences between the ICD-10[1] and DSM-IV[4]

As compared to the ICD, which is an international diagnostic and classification system, DSM diagnostic criteria for alcohol use disorders are primarily used in the United States of America (USA). Because of the poor correlation between the diagnostic criteria dealing with alcohol abuse and dependence between these two major classification systems in their earlier editions,[8] they have been revised in a coordinated worldwide effort to make them consistent with one another as much as possible.[8,9] However, there still are some differences between these two major diagnostic criteria.

Epidemiology

An estimated 3.8% of all global deaths and 4.6% of disability-adjusted life-years (DALYs) are attributable to alcohol.[10] Most of these deaths are associated with injury, cancer, cardiovascular disease and liver cirrhosis. WHO has maintained a Global Information System on Alcohol and Health database (GISAH) since 1997,[11] which indicates that overall 4.6% of the global burden of disease and injury is attributable to alcohol; 33.6% of all alcohol-attributable DALYs are in the age group 18–29 years, followed by 30–44 years (31.3%) and 45–59 years (22.0%). Alcohol use disorders are among the top five leading causes of years lost due to disability (YLD) in low-/middle- (4th place) and high-income countries (3rd place). On average, the global male burden for alcohol is almost seven times higher than for females. It should be noted that these data only include the direct burden of alcohol use disorders. The total attributable burden of disability due to alcohol use is much larger.[12]

The burden of disease is closely related to average volume of alcohol consumption.[12] On average, in a single year, an adult consumes 6.2 litres of pure alcohol (100% ethanol).[11] However 45% of men and 66% of women worldwide remain abstinent throughout their lifetime.[11] Men consume more alcohol than women.[11] Women in high-income countries consume more than those in low-income countries.[10] The burden of disease for every unit of alcohol has been found to be strongest in poor or marginalized people.[10] In high- to middle-income countries, the costs associated with alcohol are more than 1% of the gross national product.[10]

Epidemiology of alcohol use disorders in mental health

Alcohol use disorder is more common in mental illness than with the general population. Forty-seven per cent of patients with a lifetime diagnosis of schizophrenia or schizophreniform disorder, 83.6% of patients with antisocial personality disorder, 23.7% of patients with anxiety disorders, and 32% of patients with affective disorders meet criteria for some form of substance abuse, including alcohol use disorder.[13] In addition, alcohol has a strong association with a wide range of mental health problems, such as anxiety, depression, substance abuse and self-harm. Research has found psychiatric comorbidity in up to 85% of patients attending specialized alcohol treatment centres.[14] Comorbidity with affective and anxiety disorders was noted to be present in more than three-quarters of such patients; just over half had a diagnosis of a personality disorder; and one-fifth suffered with a psychotic disorder.[14] Evidence also suggests that up to 41% of suicides can be attributed to alcohol and up to a quarter of people who engage in deliberate self-harm are alcohol dependent.[15,16] Up to 26% of mental health patients under community treatment can be hazardous or harmful drinkers.[14] One study showed that hazardous and harmful alcohol use increases the risk of a suicidal presentation by a factor of three in adults admitted to inpatient mental health units.[17] The same study demonstrated an eight-fold increase in the same risk in an alcohol-dependent individual. Screening for alcohol use disorder in this population is vitally important, as unrecognized concomitant alcohol use disorder makes it very difficult to treat mental illness.

Relevance to the management of alcohol use disorder in primary care

Worldwide, there is a large gap between the need for alcohol treatment and actual access to treatment.[18] The main reason appears to be a lack of early detection and intervention. There is strong evidence to suggest that screening and early intervention in primary care settings is highly cost effective.[19,20] Therefore, detection of risky alcohol consumption through routine screening should be conducted in all primary health-care settings. Typically, opportunities for early detection and brief intervention in primary care are implicit in nature. This is because people with alcohol-related problems do not seek treatment purposefully. These patients may approach the primary health-care professional for other health needs, which in most cases might be secondary to alcohol use. However, some may voluntarily seek advice or treatment at an addiction clinic or mental health department. Moreover, patients who seek help in primary care are not necessarily aware of the risky nature of their alcohol consumption style. Therefore, provision of systematic screening in primary care settings could lead to early detection of those who may in future develop alcohol use disorder.

Strategies are needed to encourage people who drink in a hazardous way to consume alcohol in a moderate way, thereby enhancing its health indices. Due to the broad consequences to individual health, family and social life, as well as associated costs, it becomes essential that the route of treatment that best suits the patient needs and the seriousness of his or her consumption is easily accessible.

In terms of resources, screening and brief intervention should be delivered in the course of routine clinical practice. Screening and interpretation with typical questionnaires requires only a few minutes. Only a small proportion (5–20%) of primary care patients will require a brief intervention, which can be delivered within five minutes for most patients. A small minority will require a slightly longer intervention, which can be delivered within 15 minutes.[21]

Prevention of alcohol use disorder

Early intervention is important in the prevention of alcohol use disorder. The likelihood of disordered alcohol use depends on various factors, including parental influence, peer pressure, susceptibility to advertising, age of onset for alcohol consumption, and psychological and genetic factors. Alcohol use disorder cannot be prevented by the health-care sector in isolation, and close collaboration with a range of social and government agencies at various levels is required.

Evaluation and diagnosis of alcohol use disorder

Characteristics of treatment seeking

Less than a quarter of people with drinking problems will seek help from a health-care professional.[22–24] A large proportion of individuals with an alcohol use disorder will not use treatment services until they are required to do so by a family member, employer or a court.[25] But it is important to note that up to three-quarters of all risky drinkers do make positive changes on their own and this can include stable moderation and abstinence.[26,27] Denial of the alcohol problem does not appear to be the primary reason for not seeking treatment.[28] There are numerous social, cultural, political and economic barriers to treatment. Some of these are social stigma, belief that the problem is not serious,[29,30] worries about privacy, financial problems, and problems in making or keeping appointments. The social consequences of heavy drinking drive people to seek help in different ways.[24] Cultures where heavy drinking is discouraged promote treatment-seeking behaviours in individuals with alcohol problems, while help-seeking behaviour is more likely to be seen in individuals belonging to a culture accepting heavy drinking.[31–33]

Screening

Screening tests are a first-line defence in the prevention of disease. Screening for alcohol problems can take place in a wide variety of populations and settings. Detecting alcohol abuse and dependence early in the course of disease enables clinicians to get people the help they need, either by initiating a brief intervention or by referring the patient to treatment. Even patients who do not have an alcohol disorder, but who are drinking in ways that are harmful, can benefit from screening and brief intervention.

Routine screening for alcohol use disorder is a relatively recent practice. In the last two decades, enough research evidence has been gathered to justify its use in all medical settings.[34] It is important to note that alcohol use disorder may be missed in patients who do not look like "typical substance users". Research evidence suggests that there is no typical substance user, and problem alcohol use occurs in people across sexes, age groups and ethnic backgrounds.[35] Therefore, it is important that clinicians evaluate all patients on a routine basis. Questions about current and past alcohol use, including the quantity and frequency of drinking, can be asked while taking a medical history.[36] Exploration of the circumstances of any previous accidents and injuries can elicit clues to a potential alcohol problem.[37] Laboratory tests for the liver enzyme gamma-glutamyltransferase (GGT) may also reveal the presence of unsuspected alcohol problems,[36] although it would be impractical to use these on a routine basis in primary care. However, use of an appropriate standardized screening questionnaire appears to be the simplest and most reliable and cost-effective method in primary care settings.

Screening tools for alcohol use disorder can vary from a single question to the use of multiple questionnaires. As there are several standardized screening questionnaires to choose from, the primary care physician can select the most appropriate method depending on the clinical setting or presentation, patient characteristics, comorbid mental health or medical problems and available resources (see Box 25.2).

Screening questions can be incorporated in the patient check-in process at primary care centres, or can use used as a part of annual physical health check-ups. Most of the common screening questionnaires can be used in conjunction with other health-assessment questionnaires without a problem. Wherever possible, the questions should be asked in response to problems that might indicate a possible alcohol use disorder.[38] Specific questions or extended questionnaires should be used to better determine the nature and severity of the problem if the individual:

- appears to be at risk for alcohol-related medical problems
- appears to minimize or hide the use of alcohol.

- Agitation or restlessness
- Sweating
- Multiple bruises (recent or healed)
- Scratch marks
- Tremor
- Hepatic flap
- Palmar erythema
- Duptuyren's contracture
- Clubbing
- Koilonychia
- Nicotine stains
- Nystagmus
- Tachycardia
- Jaundice
- Pallor
- Fetor hepaticus
- Spider naevi/spider angiomas
- Gynaecomastia
- Loss of body hair
- Caput medusae
- Eversion or inversion of the umbilicus
- Hepatomegaly
- Hardened liver
- Splenomegaly
- Ascites
- Testicular atrophy
- Hyperreflexia or hyporeflexia
- Decrease in motor strength
- Peripheral neuropathy
- Proximal myopathy
- Dysdiadokinesia
- Gait abnormalities

Note: significant physical findings are usually not found in the early stages of alcohol use disorders.

Because alcohol and drug dependence are likely to co-occur, this should also be explored in individuals who test positive for alcohol misuse.

In a busy outpatient setting, even asking a single question about alcohol consumption can help identify the patients meeting criteria for harmful drinking. Taj et al. suggested a single question:[39]

- "On any single occasion during the past 3 months, have you had more than five drinks containing alcohol?"

The simple and easy to remember CAGE questionnaire[40] is a popular screening instrument with reliable results.[41] The four questions in the CAGE questionnaire (see Box 25.3) can be used to screen for problem drinking and alcohol-related health problems. The CAGE questions must precede any other alcohol-related question during a consultation, as its sensitivity is dramatically enhanced by an open-ended enquiry.

Box 25.3 The CAGE questionnaire[40]

C: have you ever felt you should **C**ut down on your drinking?

A: have people **A**nnoyed you by criticizing your drinking?

G: have you ever felt bad or **G**uilty about your drinking?

E: **E**ye opener: Have you ever had a drink first thing in the morning to steady your nerves or to get rid of a hangover?

Two or more positive answers are considered a positive test, with a sensitivity of 93% and a specificity of 76% for the identification of problem drinking. In comparison, a GGT liver function test detects only one-third of patients having more than 16 "drinks" per day. A positive response to one or more questions on the CAGE questionnaire may indicate at-risk alcohol use. *Problem* alcohol use is defined as one or more positive responses to the CAGE questionnaire and evidence of alcohol-related medical or behavioural problems. *Dependent* use is defined as either three or four positive responses to the CAGE questionnaire and/or evidence of one or more symptoms of alcohol dependence (i.e. compulsion to drink, impaired control over drinking, withdrawal symptoms, drinking to relieve withdrawal, and increased tolerance to alcohol).

Longer tests, such as the 10-question Alcohol Use Disorders Identification Test (AUDIT),[42] may be used to obtain more detailed information about an individual's alcohol consumption. The AUDIT includes questions about the quantity and frequency of alcohol use, as well as binge drinking, dependence symptoms and alcohol-related problems (see Box 25.4). This test is particularly useful in identifying individuals with problem drinking who are not yet dependent on alcohol.[41] It is also useful when screening women, minorities, adolescents and young adults.[43,44] However, it appears to be less accurate in older patients.[43,45] Quick screening is possible by using the computerized versions of the AUDIT and other screening instruments.

The Michigan Alcoholism Screening Test (MAST) includes 25 questions,[46] and this and its derivative "brief MAST"[47] were widely used for in-depth assessment of alcohol use disorders before the introduction of the AUDIT questionnaire. The MAST is particularly useful for identifying alcohol dependence.[48]

A note on sex differences

Traditional screening questionnaires (e.g. MAST, CAGE) are less effective in identifying drinking problems among women, as they have different patterns of alcohol consumption and different thresholds for problem drinking.[9] In addition, alcohol dependence is relatively uncommon among pregnant women.[49] The same quantity of alcohol consumed over the same time period produces higher blood alcohol levels in women than in men.[50] Alcohol-related organ damage, such as cardiomyopathy and myopathy, also appear to be more common in women.[51,52] Therefore, the cut-off scores for most alcohol screening measures need to be set differently for women.[53]

Other screening instruments

Other potentially useful instruments for screening and assessment of problematic alcohol use in primary care are:

- *the Severity of Alcohol Dependence Questionnaire* (SADQ-C): this is a short, easy-to-complete, self-administered, 20-item questionnaire designed to measure the severity of dependence on alcohol as formulated by Edwards and Gross.[7] It has been adapted from the original SADQ for use in general health settings. It is free to use and takes less than a minute to interpret
- *the Leeds Dependence Questionnaire* (LDQ): this measures dependence in abstinent patients. The instrument is sensitive to mild and moderate levels of dependence and so can be helpful in determining treatment goals. It is also useful in detecting dependence in patients with mental illness problems who have dual diagnoses. It is copyright free and easily available online
- *the Clinical Institute Withdrawal Assessment of Alcohol Scale, revised* (CIWA-Ar): this is a shortened version of the best known scale for alcohol withdrawal i.e. CIWA-A. This scale has well-documented reliability, reproducibility and validity.[54–56] It consists of 10 items and is easy to use in a variety of clinical settings including primary care settings. High scores indicate severe withdrawal and are predictive of the development of seizures and delirium.[57,58] It is also used to guide symptom-triggered loading protocols with diazepam for acute withdrawal
- *the Alcohol Problems Questionnaire* (APQ): this was designed as a clinical instrument for measuring alcohol-related problems. It is reliable and simple to administer in primary care settings.[3]

Screening during pregnancy

Prenatal alcohol exposure, even at very low levels, can negatively affect the developing fetus.[59–62] Such effects can range from subtle developmental problems and birth defects to a full-blown fetal alcohol syndrome. In addition, certain neurobehavioural sequelae of prenatal alcohol exposure can persist into adolescence[63] and adulthood.[64] There is no universally safe level of alcohol consumption during pregnancy,[65] and abstinence is generally recommended from the preconception period to delivery.[49,65] However, a significant proportion of women will drink during pregnancy and unfortunately this figure is on the rise.[49] Research has demonstrated

Box 25.4 The Alcohol Use Disorders Identification Test (AUDIT)[43]

Please circle the answer that is correct for you.

1 How often do you have a drink containing alcohol?

| Never | Monthly or less | Two to four times a month | Two to three times per week | Four or more times per week |

2 How many drinks containing alcohol do you have on a typical day when you are drinking?

| 1 or 2 | 3 or 4 | 5 or 6 | 7 to 9 | 10 or more |

3 How often do you have six or more drinks on one occasion?

| Never | Less than monthly | Monthly | Two to three times per week | Four or more times per week |

4 How often during the last year have you found that you were not able to stop drinking once you had started?

| Never | Less than monthly | Monthly | Two to three times per week | Four or more times per week |

5 How often during the last year have you failed to do what was normally expected from you because of drinking?

| Never | Less than monthly | Monthly | Two to three times per week | Four or more times per week |

6 How often during the last year have you needed a first drink in the morning to get yourself going after a heavy drinking session?

| Never | Less than monthly | Monthly | Two to three times per week | Four or more times per week |

7 How often during the last year have you had a feeling of guilt or remorse after drinking?

| Never | Less than monthly | Monthly | Two to three times per week | Four or more times per week |

8 How often during the last year have you been unable to remember what happened the night before because you had been drinking?

| Never | Less than monthly | Monthly | Two to three times per week | Four or more times per week |

9 Have you or someone else been injured as a result of your drinking?

| No | Yes, but not in the last year | Yes, during the last year |

10 Has a relative or friend, or a doctor or other health worker, been concerned about your drinking or suggested you cut down?

| No | Yes, but not in the last year | Yes, during the last year |

The Alcohol Use Disorders Identification Test (AUDIT) can detect alcohol problems experienced in the last year. A score of 8+ on the AUDIT generally indicates harmful or hazardous drinking. Questions 1–8 = 0, 1, 2, 3, or 4 points. Questions 9 and 10 are scored 0, 2 or 4 only.

that having more than three drinks per week significantly increases the risk of a spontaneous abortion in the first trimester of pregnancy.[66] Therefore, using short screening questionnaires for pregnant women in primary care is a worthwhile preventive measures, when combined with appropriate follow-up.

Routine screening questionnaires are less effective in women (see the note on sex differences above), necessitating the use of a lower cut-off or a screening test tailored for pregnant women. The T-ACE (see Box 25.5[67]) and the TWEAK (see Box 25.6[68]) are more sensitive screening for risky drinking during pregnancy than the MAST or the CAGE.

Box 25.5   The T-ACE questionnaire (Sokol 1989)[67]

T: **T**olerance – how many drinks does it take to make you feel high?

A: have people **A**nnoyed you by criticizing your drinking?

C: have you ever felt you ought to **C**ut down on your drinking?

E: **E**ye opener – have you ever had a drink first thing in the morning to steady your nerves or get rid of a hangover?

Scores are calculated as follows: a reply of "more than two drinks" to question T is considered a positive response and scores 2 points, and an affirmative answer to question A, C or E scores 1 point, respectively. A total score of 2 or more points on the T-ACE indicates a positive outcome for pregnancy risk drinking.

Box 25.6   The TWEAK questionnaire[68]

T: **T**olerance – how many drinks can you hold?

W: have close friends or relatives **W**orried or complained about your drinking in the past year?

E: **E**ye opener – do you sometimes take a drink in the morning when you get up?

A: **A**mnesia – has a friend or family member ever told you about things you said or did while you were drinking that you could not remember?

K (C): do you sometimes feel the need to **C**ut down on your drinking?

Scores are calculated as follows: a positive response to question T on Tolerance (i.e. consumption of more than five drinks) or question W on Worry yields 2 points each; an affirmative reply to question E, A or K scores 1 point each. A total score of 2 or more points on the TWEAK indicates a positive outcome for pregnancy risk drinking.

There are many factors that have to be kept in mind while screening for potential alcohol use problems during pregnancy. Some of these are outlined next.

- As many women alter their alcohol consumption after getting pregnant, more accurate measures of first-trimester drinking are obtained by enquiring about pre-pregnancy drinking patterns.[69]
- Women are also likely to deny or minimize their drinking during pregnancy, out of embarrassment.[70]
- Even moderate drinkers may underreport alcohol consumption during pregnancy.[71] In a study, 53% of the women who reported having more than 1.3 drinks per week during pregnancy reported higher levels of consumption when interviewed retrospectively.[72]
- Standard questions about quantity and frequency of alcohol consumption are unlikely to be helpful when screening pregnant women for alcohol use.

General management

There is no standard treatment for all patients who drink. Due to the high costs to health and society associated with hazardous alcohol consumption, it is essential to implement a strategy of early detection in the first level to *all* patients. It is essential to discern whether a patient has an alcohol use disorder or at-risk alcohol use, or if they drink within safe parameters.

Suitable treatment for any alcohol use disorder is determined by the patient's level of alcohol consumption and the associated health problems. The core of treatment rests on motivational interviewing (MI), brief interventions and cognitive-behavioural approaches.[73]

Stepped care approach

Because of the range of effective treatment methods that are available, and the complex socioeconomic nature of alcohol use disorders, services and interventions for alcohol use disorders have been classified in several different ways in various countries. However, recent models place an emphasis on developing stepped care models for service delivery, e.g. MoCAM (Models of Care for Alcohol Misusers),[74] with individual interventions belonging to different steps or tiers of varying intensities. The stepped care approach in alcohol use disorders is based on two key principles,[75,76] which are:

- the provision of the least restrictive and least costly intervention that will be effective for a person's presenting problems
- the use of a self-correcting mechanism that is designed to ensure that if an individual does not benefit from an initial intervention, a system of monitoring is in place to identify and provide a more appropriate and intensive intervention.

MoCAM in the UK recommends a four-tier framework with interventions belonging to tiers. Interventions are defined as individual elements of care (e.g. a brief intervention, assisted alcohol withdrawal or cognitive-behavioural therapy (CBT)) and, when taken together for each tier, are intended to comprise a programme of care for the individual. This model has been included by the National Institute for Health and Clinical Excellence (NICE) in England and Wales in its guidance on alcohol use disorders.[78] The division of tiers in this model are summarized in Table 25.1, to illustrate a sample evidence-based stepped care approach.[77]

Table 25.1 Models of Care for Alcohol Misusers (MoCAM)[74]	
Interventions	**Responsible agencies**
Tier 1 • Identification of alcohol misuse • Provision of information on sensible drinking • Simple brief interventions to reduce alcohol related harm • Referral of those with alcohol dependence or harm for more intensive interventions	These can be delivered by a wide range of staff in various settings, including: • emergency departments • primary care • acute hospitals • mental health services • criminal justice services • social services
Tier 2 This includes open-access facilities and outreach that provide: • alcohol-specific advice • information and support • extended brief interventions • triage assessment • referral of those with more serious alcohol-related problems for "care-planned" treatment *Note*: care-planned treatment refers to the process of planning and reviewing care within the context of structured alcohol treatment and this is located within Tier 3	• If staff have the appropriate competencies to deliver Tier 2 interventions, these can be delivered by the same range of agencies as Tier 1 interventions

continued overleaf

Table 25.1 Models of Care for Alcohol Misusers (MoCAM) – *continued*	
Interventions	**Responsible agencies**
Tier 3	
• Comprehensive assessment • Structured psychological interventions • Pharmacological interventions that aim to prevent relapse • Community-based assisted alcohol withdrawal • Day programmes • Specialist alcohol liaison with acute hospitals by specialist staff	• It relies on provision of community-based specialist alcohol misuse assessment, and alcohol treatment that is coordinated and planned • Tier 3 interventions are usually provided by staff working in specialist alcohol-treatment agencies • Interventions provided by primary care physicians often involve assisted alcohol withdrawal in the community or prescribing medication for relapse prevention • As with interventions in other tiers, staff need to have the relevant competence to be able to provide them safely and effectively
Tier 4	
• Comprehensive assessment • Inpatient assisted alcohol withdrawal • Structured psychosocial interventions provided in a residential setting, including residential rehabilitation. • "Wet" hostels, operating on a "harm-reduction" than an abstinence-oriented model of care, also fit within this tier	• These include the provision of residential, specialized alcohol treatments that are planned and coordinated, to ensure continuity of care and aftercare • Tier 4 interventions are usually provided by specialist alcohol inpatient or residential rehabilitation units • However, assisted alcohol withdrawal is often provided in other residential settings, including acute hospitals, mental health inpatient services, police custody and prisons, delivered by medical and other staff whose primary role is not specialist alcohol treatment

The American Society of Addiction Medicine (ASAM) has also developed criteria to define different types of services by defining four levels of care, which are: level I – outpatient treatment; level II – intensive outpatient treatment/partial hospitalization; level III – residential (medically monitored) treatment; level IV – medically managed intensive inpatient treatment.[78] ASAM levels III and IV both correlate with MoCAM tier 4 interventions.

Stepped care approaches in the treatment of alcohol use disorder have originated from increasing recognition that a wide spectrum of these disorders could respond to less-intensive brief interventions. The development of public health approaches and emerging evidence from randomized trials against the value of inpatient treatments have led to a recent shift towards community-based care with provision of early brief interventions by the primary care physician.

Brief motivational interventions

Brief intervention for alcohol problems is more effective than no intervention at all,[79–82] and can be as effective as more extensive interventions.[83,84] Brief intervention is designed to be conducted by health professionals who do not specialize in addictions treatment. The target population is mainly patients without alcohol dependence, although research has shown it to be effective in alcohol-dependent patients as well. The goal of brief intervention can range from safe moderate drinking to complete abstinence.[36,84,85] Complete abstinence is usually a preferred goal in alcohol-dependent individuals. The severity of the alcohol problem usually determines the approach and delivery of the brief intervention.

The key ingredients of brief interventions can be summarized by the acronym FRAMES: *Feedback*, *Responsibility*, *Advice*, *Menu* of strategies, *Empathy*, and *Self-efficacy*.[86]

In addition to these six elements, goal setting, follow-up, and timing are also found to be effective components in a successful brief intervention.[87]

Feedback of personal risk or impairment

The aim of this brief intervention is to provide patients with personalized feedback on their risks for harmful drinking, based on:

- current drinking patterns
- problem indicators (e.g. laboratory test results)
- sharing results of cognitive testing
- the medical consequences of their drinking.[79,80,87]

Evidence suggests that simply providing this feedback is enough to encourage a change in alcohol consumption.[88] Feedback delivered by impersonal means, for example using mail or the Internet, has also been shown to be effective, at least for short-term periods.[89]

Responsibility of the patient

Emphasizing the patient's responsibility and choice for reducing drinking improves self-perception of personal control.[90] In turn, this increases the motivation for behavioural change.[91]

Advice to change

Evidence suggests that behavioural change in drinking habits is more likely to happen when the advice to reduce or stop drinking is given in an explicit form.[90,92] During such consultations, the physician should express concern about the patient's current drinking and the related health risks, and may discuss guidelines for "low-risk" drinking.[93]

Menu of ways to reduce drinking

Offering a variety of strategies for changing drinking behaviour increases the likelihood that the patient will eventually choose one or more of them. Examples of such strategies are included in Box 25.7. Strategies can be presented to patients through self-help materials provided by health-care professionals and help may be given for carrying these strategies out.[37,81,94,95] Drinking diaries can be used to document the following:

- number of abstinent days
- number of drinking days
- number of drinks consumed on drinking days
- urges and temptations to drink
- situations wherein social pressure to drink was experienced
- alternatives to drinking.

Drinking diaries are most effective when such records are brief, factual and linked with specific situations.

Empathetic counselling

Delivery of brief interventions in a warm, reflective, and understanding style is much more effective than aggressive, confrontational or coercive approaches.[84,96]

Self-efficacy

Encouraging patients to rely on their own resources to bring about change in their drinking behaviour improves self-efficacy. Motivations-enhancing techniques can be used as part of brief interventions to encourage patients

Box 25.7 Examples for key elements of brief intervention

Feedback

- Inform the individual that his or her drinking may be contributing to a current medical problem, such as hypertension, or may increase the risk for certain health problems.[95]

Responsibility

- "No one can make you change or make you decide to change. What you do about your drinking is up to you."

Advice

- Express concern about the patient's current drinking and the related health risks.
- Discuss guidelines for "low-risk" drinking.[93]

Menu of strategies

- Setting a specific limit on alcohol consumption.
- Learning to recognize the antecedents of drinking.
- Developing skills to avoid drinking in high-risk situations.
- Planning ahead to limit drinking.
- Pacing one's drinking (e.g. sipping, measuring, diluting, and spacing drinks).
- Learning to cope with the everyday problems that may lead to drinking.[82,108,109]
- Drinking diaries to help patients monitor their abstinent days and the number of drinks consumed on drinking days.
- Recording instances when they are tempted to drink or experience social pressure to drink.
- Noting the alternatives to drinking that they use.

Empathy

- A warm, understanding and reflective style improves the efficacy of the brief intervention.
- Confrontational style reduces the efficacy of the brief intervention.

Self-efficacy

- Eliciting and reinforcing self-motivating statements, such as "I am worried about my drinking and want to cut back".
- Emphasizing the patient's strengths.

Goal setting

- Negotiate a formal drinking goal, which is specific, measurable, achievable, recordable and time limited.
- It may be presented in writing as a prescription from the doctor, or as a contract signed by the patient.

Follow-up

- Telephone calls from office staff.
- Repeat office visits.
- Repeat physical examinations.
- Regular laboratory tests.

Timing

- 12-point readiness-to-change questionnaire to match the intervention technique with the individual.

to develop, implement and commit to the plans to stop drinking and to be optimistic about their own ability to change.[83,97,98]

Establishing a drinking goal

Evidence suggests that patients are more likely to change their drinking behaviour when they actively participate in setting the drinking goals for themselves.[99,100] Collaboration between the patient and physician is important for setting effective drinking goals. Goals may be presented in writing as a prescription from the doctor, or as a contract signed by the patient.[79]

Follow-up

Following a successful delivery of brief interventions, it is important to provide follow-up to monitor the patient's progress and to provide ongoing support. Follow-up can be brief and specific and may take the form of telephone calls, repeat clinic visits, repeat physical examinations or laboratory tests.[79,80,101]

Timing

Behavioural change is most likely to happen when an individual recognizes the fact that they have a problem,[102,103] and believes in their own capacity to change.[104] Readiness to change is a significant predictor of changes in drinking behaviour.[105] Therefore, it is important to assess a patient's readiness to change at the start of a brief intervention. A 12-question "readiness to change" questionnaire[106] is a useful tool for matching brief intervention techniques with the individual's stage of readiness to change. This matching may be important; highly motivated individuals are more likely to derive benefit from a self-help manual with specific instructions,[107] whereas MI appears to be more effective than specific instructions in individuals with a lower motivation to change their drinking behaviour.[105]

The effectiveness of brief intervention

On an average, brief interventions reduce harmful drinking behaviour in about a quarter of non-dependent patients.[84] Assessment of drinking behaviour in itself can alter drinking behaviour in motivated individuals.[84] Brief interventions also appear to be useful for motivating alcohol-dependent patients to enter long-term alcohol treatment,[110] and can be as effective as specialized treatment approaches used in alcohol treatment units.[21,79,111,112] However, patients with more severe problems appear to benefit more from intensive treatment.[113]

Overall, variations of brief intervention techniques are effective for changing drinking behaviour in non-alcohol-dependent patients and are of benefit in motivating alcohol-dependent patients to enter long-term alcohol treatment. Brief interventions, therefore, are an important tool in the clinician's repertoire of treatment options in primary care settings.[114] However, brief intervention is not a single therapy but represents a collection of several different types of treatment interventions, with significant differences in the types of patients who can benefit from it, the time required to administer the intervention, and the cost.[114] Therefore, the clinician responsible for initiating brief interventions should carefully consider the choice of the intervention and the method of delivery, to decide which strategies best fit their situations.

Individual therapies

Success in a long-term recovery depends on changing individual expectations and behaviours towards alcohol. Principles from behavioural research, e.g. reinforcement and behaviour modelling, have been utilized by many treatment approaches for alcohol use disorder. In recent years, specific therapy approaches have been developed for alcohol use disorder, by combining behavioural principles of reinforcement and operant conditioning with existing treatment techniques.[115] Although they are primarily delivered in specialized treatment centres with trained staff, they can be adapted for use in primary care settings. A key use of behavioural therapy is in supplementing the ability of some individuals to quit drinking on their own (self-change). Simple behavioural approaches like goal setting, self-monitoring, analysis of drinking situations, and learning alternate coping skills can be easily learned by the individual, to drive the process of self-change. Other therapies, like couples and family therapies also aim to improve relationship factors by focusing on improving communication, avoiding conflicts and learning to solve problems that might otherwise lead to drinking. Provision of such treatment does not usually require a specialized setting and such therapies can be delivered in the primary care physician's office in an hour or less. Similar to brief interventions, matching an individual to the most appropriate therapy is important for improving the likelihood of a positive outcome from the treatment.

Mutual help groups

Mutual help groups (MHGs, such as Alcoholics Anonymous (AA)) remain the most commonly sought source of help for alcohol use disorders in many countries.[116] MHGs are typically groups of two or more individuals with a similar problem, who have a clear focus on supporting one another.[117] AA is an example of the largest group for alcohol use disorder, with a presence in most countries around the world, but similar groups catering to different populations with different needs and preferences also exist. The inherent flexibility and responsiveness of such groups make them easy to use.[118] Attendance requirements for MHGs are usually flexible, and timings are convenient or cleverly arranged, for example, at times of higher risk of a relapse to drinking (evening/weekends). Attending an AA meeting incurs no cost to the individual and is hugely cost effective when compared with similar provisions in the health-care service.[119] Outcomes achieved in some MHGs are comparable with more formal treatments.[120] Therefore, MHGs should be considered as an option for treatment whenever feasible. Twelve-step facilitation (TSF) therapy is a method that can be used by the health-care worker to encourage patients to attend MHGs. Evidence supports the value of active involvement of the physician in making arrangements for their patients to attend meetings or setting up introductions to group members.[121,122]

Assessment of comorbid health problems

Problems with alcohol use may have different presentations. Hence, screening questions may be helpful in a wide range of presentations. Heavy drinking is more common in men and those from low educational and socioeconomic backgrounds and in some professional groups. A history of new drinking should prompt questioning of changes in circumstances, as social stresses (workers, skilled professions), easy availability of alcohol (industry), significant life stresses, etc. may all trigger increased alcohol use. On the other hand, having a first-degree family relative with a history of alcohol problems may increase the risk for individuals.

Symptoms like low mood and anxiety (usually generalized anxiety or panic attacks) are often common presentation in those who misuse alcohol. The primary diagnosis of a depressive illness or an anxiety disorder might sometimes be unclear, as alcohol is used as self-medication to control mood, induce sleep or control anxiety. Paradoxically, long-term alcohol use may itself not only lead to adverse life events such as loss of employment, relationship problems, poverty, etc., but also cause a direct depressive effect on the nervous system. In discussion, people who drink excessively may minimize the contribution of their drinking and seek treatment for such symptoms as primary illnesses; however, when a concurrent alcohol problem is present, such a diagnosis must not be made at the first instance. On the other hand, when a pre-existing illness such as a depressive or an anxiety disorder is present and a person is using alcohol to control symptoms, treating the underlying cause will be important while simultaneously addressing the drinking.

A history of use of other substances should also be sought, not only at the initial assessment but at reviews; so it is important to check if the patients have substituted alcohol with other drugs – this sometimes includes benzodiazepines. Other drugs can also be used in conjunction with alcohol to enhance its effects or to cope with the side-effects of other drugs such as while coming off a "high" after taking a stimulant. While the patient may not give a history of excessive alcohol use, a physical examination for a presentation of physical illness might give a clue about the physical health sequelae of chronic alcohol use, such as injuries, spider naevi, ascites, signs of portal hypertension, hepatomegaly (early) or cirrhosis (late) of the liver.

Investigations in alcohol use disorder

Alcohol-related health effects may be monitored with laboratory investigations. The common blood tests undertaken in alcohol use disorders are full blood count, haemoglobin concentration and liver and renal function tests. A macrocytic anaemia may result from alcohol-related folate deficiency or a microcytic picture may present marrow suppression or blood loss in chronic drinkers. The liver may remain normal in many cases; however, there may be abnormalities in liver enzymes, particularly a rise in GGT. In alcoholic hepatitis, the level of alanine aminotransferase (ALT) is often more than twice that of aspartate transaminase (AST). Associated pancreatitis may result in a raised serum amylase.

In the case of established chronic alcohol misuse and presenting health problems, specialist investigation can be used to diagnose and monitor health. Fatty liver is common and detected by an ultrasound scan. The gastrointestinal effects of portal hypertension, which occurs late in chronic alcohol use, include hepatosplenomegaly that may be detected, although the liver appearance may continue to be normal for a very long time even in presence of deranged liver enzymes. Cirrhosis is detected by a nodular appearance on ultrasonography. Endoscopy may be used to investigate and treat oesophageal varices.

Elevated blood pressure and arrhythmia may indicate cardiovascular effects, and an electrocardiogram (ECG) can be done. Basic screening tests for cognition can be used to screen and monitor for memory deficits.

Medications

Commonly used medicines to treat alcohol dependence include:[123]

- disulfiram
- naltrexone (oral, extended release)
- acamprosate
- topiramate.

There are many promising new compounds targeting certain brain systems, which are being researched for use in alcohol withdrawal and relapse prevention.[124,125] Medications can be combined with behavioural treatments, with good results.[126] Recent research has focused on assessing the appropriate level of brief interventions to use in combination with pharmacotherapy, and establishing the best methods to improve medication adherence. Such approaches include adherence planning, problem-solving, and teaching strategies. Maintenance of contact with patients and teaching adherence techniques appear to correlate well with successful treatment of alcohol use disorder with pharmacotherapy. These factors are especially well suited to settings where doctors maintain ongoing relationships with their patients – i.e. primary care settings.[126]

Detecting and managing alcohol use disorder across the lifespan

The nature and characteristics of alcohol use disorder change over the life span. Young adults, including college students, are more prone to binge-drinking behaviour and therefore more likely to present with alcohol toxicity, drink-driving crashes, and disruptive or violent behaviour secondary to alcohol use.[127] On the other hand, moderate drinkers in older age groups are more at risk of harmful drug interactions due to alcohol. In addition, there are notable differences in the pattern of alcohol use across the human life span.[128] Early onset of drinking behaviour predicts a serious problem with alcohol in later life. Therefore, it is important to understand the influence of alcohol on individuals across different life stages, in order to design effective approaches for diagnosing, treating and preventing alcohol use disorders. Exploring the biological, psychological and social effects of alcohol use on individuals at different stages of development helps us to tailor and refine the brief interventions. It also enables the health-care professional to conceptualize the seemingly complex relationship of alcohol with biology and the environment.

The embryo and fetus

Alcohol-related birth defects are collectively known as fetal alcohol spectrum disorder (FASD). FASD represents a large proportion of preventable birth defects. Fetal alcohol syndrome (FAS) is the most severe form of FASD and is characterized by a range of learning and behavioural problems in addition to its characteristic physical abnormalities. In addition, prenatal exposure to alcohol increases the risk of developing an alcohol and other drug use disorder later in life.[129]

Adolescence

Consuming alcohol during adolescence (12–17 years of age) may affect development of the brain, especially the hippocampus which is involved in learning and memory.[130,131] Heavy episodic (binge) drinking behaviour is more common in adolescents than adults.[132] This is due to certain social factors (greater independence, peer pressure) and biological factors (less sensitive to negative effects of alcohol, such as increased sleepiness and lack of coordination).[132] However, adolescents are more sensitive for impairment in performance for complex tasks, e.g. driving, making adolescent alcohol use especially dangerous.[133,134]

Young adults

The risk of alcohol use disorder increases in this period (18–29 years of age). It is usually a time of transition in most cultures across the world. When compared with all other age groups, young adults aged 18–24 years are most at risk for alcohol use disorders and have the highest proportion of alcohol-related deaths.[135,136] This group is also likely to drink heavily, regardless of their sex, ethnicity or employment status. It also makes them more vulnerable to psychiatric conditions related to life transitions, such as depression and anxiety. Drinking is associated with risk-taking behaviours that might put people at increased risk for legal and social harm.[137]

Midlife

Most young adults will drink less as they transition into midlife (30–59 years of age) but some continue to drink heavily.[138] The biological consequences of heavy drinking e.g. alcoholic liver disease, pancreatitis, cardiovascular sequelae, alcohol-related brain disorders, and other adverse effects upon the endocrine and immune system, are most likely to emerge during this time.[138] Individuals in midlife are more likely to seek treatment for alcohol dependence.[138]

Older adults

Amongst all age groups, older adults tend to drink the least amount of alcohol.[139] However, with gradually increasing life spans worldwide, alcohol use disorders in older adults are an emerging health issue.[140] Moreover, newer generations are consuming more alcohol than previous generations, suggesting a future rise in alcohol use disorders in this age group as the current population ages.[140,141] As alcohol metabolism in the body slows down with age, older adults are more at risk of health conditions that can be exacerbated by alcohol – stroke, hypertension, neurodegeneration, memory loss, mood disorders and cognitive or emotional problems.[142] In addition, as older adults are more likely to take medications, the risk for dangerous drug interactions is substantially more in this age group.[143] Alcohol also increases the metabolism of most of psychiatric medications by inducing liver enzymes, thereby decreasing the effectiveness of such medications.[143] It is important to note that older adults tend to respond better to treatment that takes place in groups of people of similar ages.[144] Interventions that help in engaging social support systems for the individual, e.g. family therapy, are noted to be effective in this age group.[145–147] Pharmacotherapy for alcohol use disorder does not appear to have good evidence to support its use in older adults without additional social interventions.[148] Current literature suggests that the most beneficial treatment for alcohol use disorders in older adults may be education about the dangers of alcohol use.[149] The outcomes in this age group are also dependent on the age of onset of drinking behaviour, with an early drinking age linked with a poorer treatment outcome.[150–154]

Managing recovery

Management of recovery is an important part of any successful treatment programme for alcohol use disorder. Some factors that prevent an individual from entering treatment can also make them reluctant to continue with the treatment programmes. Dropping out of treatment can happen at any stage of the treatment. Traditionally, community treatment for alcohol use disorder is divided into two main phases. The first phase includes an intensive outpatient treatment of brief interventions (frequency: 2–3 sessions per week, duration: 1–2 months). It is followed by a continuing-care phase (self-help meetings). However, this does not fit well with the chronic nature of alcohol problems, which typically involve cycles of abstinence, relapse and treatment. Newer approaches have been designed to provide a continuum of care throughout the treatment period, with no clear distinction between the intensive and follow-up phases.[155,156] New evidence also suggests the value of interventions lasting up to a year and favours active engagement of the individual through various means – telephone calls, home visits and online communication tools.[157] Involvement of individuals' immediate support network, i.e. family, friends, and employers, has been demonstrated to be more successful in achieving the desired treatment outcomes.[129] Current trends in community treatment of alcohol use disorder are also focusing on finding innovative means to encourage engagement with treatment. Incentivizing engagement with treatment, i.e. a provision of monetary rewards, housing support, employment and alcohol-free social activities, are being explored to prevent individuals from dropping out of treatment. Individual preferences for the type and intensity of their treatment are increasingly being used to tailor such programmes to meet individuals' needs. The likelihood of relapse of alcohol use disorder can change throughout the treatment programme, and programmes should have the ability to detect and adapt to such changes. Use of emerging technologies, such as smartphones and Internet-based tools can also play a role in identifying such fluctuations in individual needs. Evidence is accruing to suggest that emerging technologies are improving access to services and promoting the effectiveness of treatment.[130]

Recognition and management of withdrawal and delirium tremens

Alcohol withdrawal syndrome

Alcohol withdrawal syndrome is the cluster of symptoms seen on significantly reducing or stopping alcohol consumption after prolonged periods of excessive use. Unlike most withdrawals from other chemical agents, alcohol withdrawal syndrome can be fatal. The symptoms of alcohol withdrawal can range from life-threatening seizures[158,159] and delirium tremens (DTs), to mild tremulousness, anxiety, hyperactivity, nausea, sweating, hypertension and mild pyrexia. They typically occur within 6–48 hours after the last drink and peak at 12–30 hours. Research evidence is unequivocal about the estimates of the incidence of serious consequences of alcohol withdrawal, with many studies indicating it to be as high as 50%. However, given the life-threatening nature of some of the symptoms, it is important to treat everyone who is suffering from alcohol withdrawal.

A thorough medical evaluation should be used to form the primary basis of the decision to choose a drug-administration technique for use in individual patients. Withdrawal severity scales should be used to complement, not replace, a thorough clinical evaluation. A thorough clinical examination should include an assessment for the following:

- hypoglycaemia
- subdural haematoma
- hepatic encephalopathy
- concurrent infections (lungs, skin, urinary)
- history of recurrent epilepsy.

The presence of any of the above would require a treatment in an acute hospital setting.

DTs, which occur in less than 5% cases of alcohol withdrawal, have the following features:

- agitation
- extreme anxiety and confusion
- delusions and sensory hallucinations
- coarse tremor
- sweating
- tachycardia
- pyrexia/high grade pyrexia
- metabolic acidosis.

The syndrome of DTs involves a severe overactivity of the autonomic nervous system (excito-neurotoxicity),[160–163] and it typically begins between 2 and 4 days after the last drink.[164] Overactivity of the sympathetic nervous system leads to increased production of the potentially neurotoxic hormones cortisol and noradrenaline (norepinephrine), with cortisol being specifically toxic to hippocampal neurons.[165] Therefore, repeated untreated alcohol withdrawals may lead to direct damage to the hippocampus, a part of the brain that is particularly important for memory and control of affective states. Repeated untreated alcohol withdrawals appear to have a cumulative effect and increase the risk of having withdrawals of increased severity in future.[166]

Presence of the symptoms of DTs indicates a medical emergency, as it is associated with an untreated mortality of 15%. Therefore it should be treated in acute medical settings.

Minor symptoms of alcohol withdrawal can be managed in community settings by the primary care physician and there seems to be good evidence to support the effectiveness of community-based detoxification. However, a brief admission to an inpatient unit should be considered if there is a risk of developing withdrawal complications.

The drugs of choice for treating withdrawal are the benzodiazepines, especially chlordiazepoxide, diazepam, oxazepam and lorazepam.[167] Lorazepam is particularly useful while treating alcohol withdrawal with a coexisting liver disease, as it is not metabolized by the liver. Usually a lower dose of the benzodiazepines is needed in women, elderly individuals, and those with a lower than average body weight. Administering decreasing doses of the chosen benzodiazepine over the period of alcohol withdrawal has traditionally been recommended.[168] An alternative approach can be a "loading dose strategy", which includes giving a dose of diazepam every 1 to 2 hours until withdrawal symptoms abate.[169] Because of the long half-life of diazepam and its metabolites, there is usually no need for further medication. This strategy simplifies treatment, protects against seizures, and eliminates a possible reinforcement of drug-seeking behaviour.

Seizures associated with alcohol withdrawal are usually self-limiting in nature. However, administration of diazepam by slow intravenous injection or rectally might be required in some cases. Intractable seizures or status epilepticus is a medical emergency, requiring acute intervention and further work-up by specialists.

Conclusion

The last three decades have witnessed the emergence of several new tools and techniques to address alcohol use disorder. Greater acknowledgement of alcohol use disorder as a complex problem with intractable social, economic and medical factors has led to development of various integrated approaches and newer models of treatment. Care providers are now increasingly prescribing medications and brief interventions to support individuals in changing their drinking behaviours. Options to seek help have multiplied, leading to a greater patient and provider choice, including self-help groups, brief interventions, behavioural therapies and pharmacotherapy. Internet and mobile web-based approaches are being tapped into to provide a 24-hour 7-day access to interventions and support.

However, undiagnosed and untreated alcohol use disorder is still a significant problem worldwide. Only a small minority of individuals are able to access appropriate treatment.[170] Although some individuals do recover on their own without formal treatment, many find themselves in a chronic cycle of remission and relapse with alcohol problems, which repeats throughout their lives. Therefore, introduction of innovative approaches to improve access to treatment still has an important role in helping people modify their drinking behaviour.[23] Improving diagnosis, better screening and provision of brief interventions in a variety of settings including primary care clinics has been effective in addressing some of the issues.

Individuals with alcohol use disorder differ in their degree of severity, the nature of their co-occurring conditions, and social systems. Making care more responsive to these factors still remains a challenge. Emerging technologies like Internet and mobile applications are likely to make some of these goals easier and more cost effective. The existing treatment framework – pharmacotherapy, brief interventions and MHGs – has been shown to have a significant impact on service delivery. Primary care settings offer a promising environment for incorporating both alcohol use disorder and mental health services, as they improve the reach and are perceived as less stigmatizing.[171] Future trends in treatment of alcohol use disorder are more likely to shift in the direction of integrated care in primary care settings.[172]

References

1   *ICD-10 classification of mental and behavioral disorders*. Geneva, World Health Organization, 1992.

2   *Mental health policy implementation guide: dual diagnosis good practice guide*. London, Department of Health, 2002.

3   Williams BT, Drummond DC. The Alcohol Problems Questionnaire: reliability and validity. *Drug and Alcohol Dependence*, 1994, 35:239–243.

4   *Diagnostic and statistical manual of mental disorders*, 4th ed (DSM-IV). Washington, American Psychiatric Association, 1994.

5   *Global status report on alcohol and health.* Geneva, World Health Organization, 2011 (WHO, http://www.who.int/entity/substance_abuse/publications/global_alcohol_report/msbgsruprofiles.pdf, accessed 3 January 2012).

6   Chisholm D et al. Reducing the global burden of hazardous alcohol use: a comparative cost-effectiveness analysis. *Journal of Studies on Alcohol,* 2004, 65:782–793.

7   Edwards G and Gross MM. Alcohol dependence: provisional description of a clinical syndrome. *BMJ,* 1976, 1:1058–1061.

8   Schuckit MA, Hesselbrock V. Alcohol dependence and anxiety disorders: what is the relationship? *American Journal of Psychiatry,* 1994, 151:1723–1734.

9   Babor TF et al. *The Alcohol Use Disorders Identification Test. Guidelines for use in primary health care.* Geneva, World Health Organization, 1992.

10   Rehm J et al. Global burden of disease and injury and economic cost attributable to alcohol use and alcohol-use disorders. *The Lancet,* 2009, 373:2223–2233.

11   World Health Organization. *Global Information System on Alcohol and Health (GISAH)* (http://www.who.int/substance_abuse/activities/gisah/en/index.html, accessed 2 December 2011).

12   *Strategies to reduce the harmful use of alcohol, Sixty First World Health Assembly, Report by the Secretariat.* Geneva, World Health Organization, 2008 (http://apps.who.int/gb/ebwha/pdf_files/A61/A61_13-en.pdf, accessed 3 January 2012).

13   Regier DA et al. Co-morbidity of mental disorders with alcohol and other drug abuse. Results from the Epidemiologic Catchment Area (ECA) Study. *JAMA,* 1990, 264:2511–2518.

14   Weaver T et al. Comorbidity of substance misuse and mental illness in community mental health and substance misuse service. *British Journal of Psychiatry,* 2003, 183:304–313.

15   Demirbas H et al. An examination of suicide probability in alcoholic in-patients. *Alcohol and Alcoholism,* 2003, 38:67–70.

16   Merrill J et al. Alcohol and attempted suicide. *British Journal of Addiction,* 1992, 87:83–89.

17   McCloud A et al. Relationship between alcohol use disorders and suicidality in a psychiatric population: in-patient prevalence study. *British Journal of Psychiatry,* 2004, 184:439–445.

18   Department of Health; University of London. St George's. Division of Mental Health. Section of Addictive Behaviour; Kable Limited; MORI Social Research Institute; Alcohol Needs Assessment Research Project (ANARP). *The 2004 national alcohol needs assessment for England.* London, Department of Health, 2005 (http://www.dh.gov.uk/en/Publicationsandstatistics/Publications/PublicationsPolicyAndGuidance/DH_4122341, accessed 3 January 2012).

19   Holder HD, Blose JO. Typical patterns and cost of alcoholism treatment across a variety of populations and providers. *Alcoholism: Clinical and Experimental Research,* 1991, 15:190–195.

20   Wurtze SE et al. Cost effectiveness of brief interventions for reducing alcohol consumption. *Social Science and Medicine,* 2001, 52:863–870.

21   Babor TF, Higgins-Biddle JC. *Brief intervention for hazardous and harmful drinking: a manual for use in primary care.* Geneva, World Health Organization, 2001.

22   Cohen E et al. Alcohol treatment utilization: findings from the National Epidemiologic Survey on Alcohol and Related Conditions. *Drug and Alcohol Dependence,* 2007, 86:214–221.

23   Huebner RB, Kantor LW. Advances in alcoholism treatment. *Alcohol Research and Health,* 2011, 33:295–299.

24   Tucker JA. Natural resolution of alcohol-related problems. *Recent Developments in Alcoholism,* 2003, 16:77–90.

25   Parhar KK et al. Offender coercion in treatment: a meta-analysis of effectiveness. *Criminal Justice and Behavior,* 2008, 35:1109–1135.

26   Klingemann H, Gmel G, eds. *Mapping the social consequences of alcohol consumption.* Dordrecht, Kluwer Academic Publishers, 2001.

27   Sobell LC, Cunningham JA, Sobell MB. Recovery from alcohol problems with and without treatment: prevalence in two population surveys. *American Journal of Public Health,* 1996, 86:966–972.

28   Simpson CA, Tucker JA. Temporal sequencing of alcohol-related problems, problem recognition, and help-seeking episodes. *Addictive Behaviors,* 2002, 27:659–674.

29 Narrow WE et al. Use of services by persons with mental and addictive disorders. Findings from the National Institute of Mental Health Epidemiologic Catchment Area Program. *Archives of General Psychiatry*, 1993, 50:95–107.

30 Wild TC, Roberts AB, Cooper EL. Compulsory substance abuse treatment: an overview of recent findings and issues. *European Addiction Research*, 2002, 8:84–93.

31 Codd RT Cohen BN. Predicting college student intentions to seek help for alcohol abuse. *Journal of Social and Clinical Psychology*, 2003, 22:168–191.

32 George AA, Tucker JA. Help-seeking for alcohol-related problems: social contexts surrounding entry into alcoholism treatment or Alcoholics Anonymous. *Journal of Studies on Alcohol*, 1996, 57:449–457.

33 Longabaugh R et al. Network support for drinking. In: Longabaugh R, Wirtz PW, eds. *Project MATCH hypotheses: results and causal chain analyses* Bethesda, MD: National Institute on Alcohol Abuse and Alcoholism, 2001:260–275 (Project MATCH Monograph Series, Vol. 8).

34 Institute of Medicine. *Broadening the base of treatment for alcohol problems. Report of a Study by a Committee of the Institute of Medicine, Division of Mental Health and Behavioral Medicine.* Washington, DC: National Academy Press, 1990.

35 Arnaout B, Petrakis I. Diagnosing co-morbid drug use in patients with alcohol use disorders. *Alcohol Research and Health*, 2008, 31:148–154.

36 O'Connor PG, Schottenfeld RS. Patients with alcohol problems. *New England Journal of Medicine*, 1998, 338:592–602.

37 Israel Y et al. Screening for problem drinking and counseling by the primary care physician-nurse team. *Alcoholism: Clinical and Experimental Research*, 1996, 20:1443–1450.

38 Fleming M. Screening and brief intervention in primary care settings. *Alcohol Research and Health*, 2004/2005, 28:57–62.

39 Taj N, Devera-Sales A, Vinson DC. Screening for problem drinking: does a single question work? *Journal of Family Practice*, 1998, 46:328–335.

40 Ewing JA. Detecting alcoholism: the CAGE questionnaire. *JAMA*, 1984, 252:1905–1907.

41 Fiellin DA, Reid MC, O'Connor PG. Screening for alcohol problems in primary care: a systematic review. *Archives of Internal Medicine*, 2000, 160:1977–1989.

42 Saunders JB et al. Development of the Alcohol Use Disorders Identification Test (AUDIT): WHO Collaborative Project on Early Detection of Persons with Harmful Alcohol Consumption–II. *Addiction*, 1993, 88:791–804.

43 Reinert DF, Allen JP. Alcohol Use Disorders Identification Test (AUDIT): a review of recent research. *Alcoholism: Clinical and Experimental Research*, 2002, 26:272–279.

44 Kokotailo PK et al. Validity of the Alcohol Use Disorders Identification Test in college students. *Alcoholism: Clinical and Experimental Research*, 2004, 28:914–920.

45 Chung T et al. Screening adolescents for problem drinking: performance of brief screens against DSM–IV alcohol diagnoses. *Journal of Studies on Alcohol*, 2000, 61:579–587.

46 Selzer ML. The Michigan Alcoholism Screening Test: the quest for a new diagnostic instrument. *American Journal of Psychiatry*, 1971, 127:1653–1658.

47 Pokorny AD, Miller BA, Kaplan HB. The brief MAST: a shortened version of the Michigan Alcoholism Screening Test. *American Journal of Psychiatry*, 1972, 129:118–121.

48 Reid MC, Fiellin DA, O'Connor PG. Hazardous and harmful alcohol consumption in primary care. Archives of Internal Medicine, 1999, 159:1681–1689.

49 Ebrahim SH et al. Alcohol consumption by pregnant women in the United States during 1988–1995. *Obstetrics and Gynecology*, 1998, 92:187–192.

50 Graham AW, Fleming MS. Brief interventions. In: Graham AW, Schultz TK, Wilford BB, eds. *Principles of addiction medicine*, 2nd ed. Chevy Chase, MD, American Society of Addiction Medicine, Inc., 1998:615–630.

51 Urbano-Marquez A et al. The greater risk of alcoholic cardiomyopathy and myopathy in women compared with men. *JAMA*, 1995, 274:149–154.

52 Hanna E et al. Dying to be equal: women, alcohol, and cardiovascular disease. *British Journal on Addiction*, 1992, 87:1593–1597.

53   Bradley KA et al. (1998) Alcohol screening questionnaires in women: a critical review. *JAMA*, 1998, 280:166–171.

54   Knott DH et al. Decision for alcohol detoxification: a method to standardize patient evaluation. *Postgraduate Medicine*, 1981, 69:65–78.

55   Wiehl WO, Hayner G, Galloway G. Haight Ashbury Free Clinics drug detoxification protocols, Part 4: Alcohol. *Journal of Psychoactive Drugs*, 1994, 26:57–59.

56   Sullivan JT et al. Assessment of alcohol withdrawal: the revised Clinical Institute Withdrawal Assessment for Alcohol scale (CIWA-Ar). *British Journal of Addiction*, 1989, 84:1353–1357.

57   Naranjo CA et al. Nonpharmacologic intervention in acute alcohol withdrawal. *Clinical Pharmacology and Therapeutics*, 1983, 34:214–219.

58   Young GP et al. Intravenous phenobarbital for alcohol withdrawal and convulsions. *Annals of Emergency Medicine*, 1987, 16:847–850.

59   Charness ME, Safran RM, Perides G. Ethanol inhibits neural cell-adhesion. *Journal of Biological Chemistry*, 1994, 269:9304–9309.

60   Wong EV et al. Mutations in cell adhesion molecule L1 cause mental retardation. *Trends in Neuroscience*, 1995, 18:168–172.

61   Ikonomidou C et al. Ethanol-induced apoptotic neurodegeneration and fetal alcohol syndrome. *Science*, 2000, 287:1056–1060.

62   Jacobson JL, Jacobson SE. Prenatal alcohol exposure and neurobehavioral development. *Alcohol Health and Research World*, 1994, 18:30–36.

63   Sampson PD et al. Prenatal alcohol exposure, birthweight, and measures of child size from birth to 14 years. *American Journal of Public Health*, 1994, 84:1421–1428.

64   Kelly SJ, Day N, Streissguth AP. Effects of prenatal alcohol exposure on social behavior in humans and other species. *Neurotoxicology and Teratology*, 2000, 22:143–149.

65   Stratton K, Howe C, Battaglia F, eds. *Institute of Medicine summary: fetal alcohol syndrome*. Washington, DC, National Academy Press, 1996.

66   Windham GC et al. Moderate maternal alcohol consumption and the risk of spontaneous abortion. *Epidemiology*, 1997, 8:509–514.

67   Sokol RJ, Martier SS, Ager JW. The T-ACE questions: practical prenatal detection of risk-drinking. *American Journal of Obstetrics and Gynecology*, 1989, 160:863–871.

68   Chan AK et al. The TWEAK test in screening for alcoholism/heavy drinking in three populations. *Alcoholism: Clinical and Experimental Research*, 1993, 6:1188–1192.

69   Day NL, Cottreau CM, Richardson GA. Epidemiology of alcohol, marijuana, and cocaine use among women of childbearing age and pregnant women. *Clinical Obstetrics and Gynecology*, 1993, 36:237–245.

70   Morrow-Tlucak M et al. Underreporting of alcohol use in pregnancy: relationship to alcohol. *Alcoholism: Clinical and Experimental Research*, 1989, 13:399–401.

71   Verkerk PH. The impact of alcohol misclassification on the relationship between alcohol and pregnancy outcome. *International Journal of Epidemiology*, 1992, 21(suppl.):S33–S37.

72   Jacobson SW et al. Maternal recall of alcohol, cocaine, and marijuana use during pregnancy. *Neurotoxicology and Teratology*, 1991, 13:535–540.

73   Schuckit MA. Alcohol-use disorders. *The Lancet*, 2009, 373:492–501.

74   Department of Health. *Models of care for alcohol misusers*. London, The Stationery Office, 2006.

75   Davison G. Stepped care: doing more with less? *Journal of Consulting and Clinical Psychology*, 2000, 68:580–585.

76   Sobell M, Sobell L. Stepped care as a heuristic approach to the treatment of alcohol problems. *Journal of Consulting and Clinical Psychology*, 2000, 68:573–579.

77   Alcohol-use disorders: diagnosis, assessment and management of harmful drinking and alcohol dependence. London, National Institute for Health and Clinical Excellence, 2009 (CG115) (www.nice.org.uk/guidance/CG115, accessed 4 January 2012).

78   Mee-Lee D et al., eds. *ASAM patient placement criteria for the treatment of substance-related disorders, second edition-revised* (ASAM PPC-2R). Chevy Chase, MD, American Society of Addiction Medicine, Inc., 2001.

79 Fleming MF et al. Brief physician advice for problem alcohol drinkers. A randomized controlled trial in community-based primary care practices. *JAMA*, 1997, 277:1039–1045.

80 Kristenson H et al. Identification and intervention of heavy drinking in middle-aged men: Results and follow-up of 24–60 months of long-term study with randomized controls. *Alcoholism: Clinical and Experimental Research*, 1983, 7:203–209.

81 Wallace P, Cutler S, Haines A. Randomised controlled trial of general practitioner intervention in patients with excessive alcohol consumption. *BMJ*, 1988, 297:663–668.

82 World Health Organization Brief Intervention Study Group. A cross-national trial of brief interventions with heavy drinkers. *American Journal of Public Health*, 1996, 86:948–955.

83 Edwards G et al. Alcoholism: a controlled trial of "treatment" and "advice". *Journal of Studies on Alcohol*, 1977, 38:1004–1031.

84 Bien TH, Miller WR, Tonigan JS. Brief interventions for alcohol problems: a review. *Addiction*, 1993, 88:315–336.

85 Graham K et al. Should alcohol consumption measures be adjusted for gender differences? *Addiction*, 1998, 93:1137–1147.

86 Miller WR, Sanchez VC. Motivating young adults for treatment and lifestyle change. In: Howard G, ed. *Issues in alcohol use and misuse in young adults*. Notre Dame, IN, University of Notre Dame Press, 1993:55–82.

87 Heather N et al. Evaluation of a controlled drinking minimal intervention for problem drinkers in general practice (the DRAMS scheme). *Journal of the Royal College of General Practitioners*, 1987, 37:358–363.

88 Moyer A et al. Brief interventions for alcohol problems: a meta-analytic review of controlled investigations in treatment-seeking and non-treatment-seeking populations. *Addiction*, 2002, 97:279–292.

89 Larimer ME, Cronce JM. Identification, prevention, and treatment: A review of individual-focused strategies to reduce problematic alcohol consumption by college students. *Journal of Studies on Alcohol*, 2002, 14(Suppl.):148–163.

90 Edwards G. Alcohol policy and the public good. *Addiction*, 1997, 92(Suppl.):S73–S79.

91 Miller PM, Mastria MA. *Alternatives to alcohol abuse: a social learning model*. Champaign, IL, Research Press Co., 1977.

92 Orford J, Edwards G. *Alcoholism*. Oxford: Oxford University Press, 1977.

93 National Institute on Alcohol Abuse and Alcoholism. *The physicians' guide to helping patients with alcohol problems*. Bethesda, MD, US Department of Health and Human Services, Public Health Service, National Institutes of Health, 1995 (NIH Publication No. 95-3769).

94 Anderson P, Scott E. The effect of general practitioners' advice to heavy drinking men. *British Journal of Addiction*, 1992, 87:891–900.

95 Chick J, Lloyd G, Crombie E. Counselling problem drinkers in medical wards: a controlled study. *BMJ*, 1985, 290:965–967.

96 Miller WR, Rollnick S. *Motivational interviewing: preparing people to change addictive behavior*. New York, Guilford Press, 1991.

97 Project MATCH Research Group. Matching alcoholism treatments to client heterogeneity: Project MATCH posttreatment drinking outcomes. *Journal of Studies on Alcohol*, 1997, 58:7–29.

98 Burge SK et al. An evaluation of two primary care interventions for alcohol abuse among Mexican-American patients. *Addiction*, 1997, 92:1705–1716.

99 Miller WR. Motivation for treatment: a review with special emphasis on alcoholism. *Psychological Bulletin*, 1985, 98:84–107.

100 Ockene JK et al. A residents' training program for the development of smoking intervention skills. *Archives of Internal Medicine*, 1988, 148:1039–1045.

101 Persson J, Magnusson PH. Early intervention in patients with excessive consumption of alcohol: a controlled study. *Alcohol*, 1989, 6:403–408.

102 DiClemente CC et al. The process of smoking cessation: an analysis of precontemplation, contemplation, and preparation stages of change. *Journal of Consulting and Clinical Psychology*, 1991, 59(2):295–304.

103 Prochaska JO, DiClemente CC. Stages and processes of self-change of smoking: Toward an integrative model of change. *Journal of Consulting and Clinical Psychology*, 1983, 51:390–395.

104 Bandura A. *Social learning theory*. Englewood Cliffs, NJ: Prentice-Hall, 1977.

105 Heather N, Rollnick S, Bell A. Predictive validity of the Readiness to Change Questionnaire. *Addiction*, 1993, 88:1667–1677.

106 Rollnick S et al. Development of a short "readiness to change" questionnaire for use in brief, opportunistic interventions among excessive drinkers. *British Journal of Addiction*, 1992, 87:743–754.

107 Spivak K, Sanchez-Craig M, Davila R. Assisting problem drinkers to change on their own: Effect of specific and non-specific advice. *Addiction*, 1994, 89:1135–1142.

108 Sanchez-Craig M. Random assignment to abstinence or controlled drinking in a cognitive-behavioral program: short-term effects on drinking behavior. *Addictive Behaviors*, 1980, 5:35–39.

109 Sanchez-Craig M, Spivak K, Davila R. Superior outcome of females over males after brief treatment for the reduction of heavy drinking: replication and report of therapist effects. *British Journal of Addiction*, 1991, 86:867–876.

110 Wutzke SE, Conigrave KM, Saunders, JB et al. The long-term effectiveness of brief interventions for unsafe alcohol consumption: a 10-year follow-up. *Addiction*, 2002, 97:665–675.

111 Kaner EFS et al. Effectiveness of brief alcohol interventions in primary care populations. *Cochrane Database of Systematic Reviews*, 2007, (2):CD004148.

112 Beich A, Thorsen T, Rollnick S. Screening in brief intervention trials targeting excessive drinkers in general practice: systematic review and meta-analysis. *BMJ*, 2003, 327:536–540.

113 Beich A, Gannik D, Malterud K. Screening and brief intervention for excessive alcohol use: qualitative interview study of the experiences of general practitioners. *BMJ*, 2002, 325:870–873.

114 *Brief intervention for alcohol problems. Alcohol Alert No. 43*. Rockville, MD, National Institute on Alcohol Abuse and Alcoholism, 1999.

115 Witkiewitz K, Marlatt A. Behavioral therapy across the spectrum. *Alcohol Research and Health*, 2011, 33:313–319.

116 United States Department of Health and Human Services, Substance Abuse and Mental Health Services Administration, Office of Applied Studies. *National Survey on Drug Use and Health (NSDUH)*. Ann Arbor, MI, Inter-university Consortium for Political and Social Research, 2007 (ICPSR23782-v2).

117 Humphreys K. *Circles of recovery: self-help organizations for addictions*. Cambridge: Cambridge University Press, 2004.

118 Kelly JF, Yeterian JD. The role of mutual-help groups in extending the framework of treatment. *Alcohol Research and Health*, 2011, 33:350–355.

119 Humphreys K, Moos RH. Reduced substance-abuse-related health care costs among voluntary participants in Alcoholics Anonymous. *Psychiatric Services*, 1996, 47:709–713.

120 Ouimette PC, Moos RH, Finney JW. Influence of outpatient treatment and 12-step group involvement in one-year substance abuse treatment outcomes. *Journal of Studies on Alcohol*, 1998, 59:513–522.

121 Sisson RW, Mallams JH. The use of systematic encouragement and community access procedures to increase attendance at Alcoholics Anonymous and Al-Anon meetings. *American Journal of Drug and Alcohol Abuse*, 1981, 8:371–376.

122 Tonigan JS, Connors GJ, Miller WR. Participation and involvement in Alcoholics Anonymous. In: Babor TF, Del Boca FK, eds. *Treatment matching in alcoholism*. New York: Cambridge University Press, 2003:184–204.

123 Krishnan-Sarin S, O'Malley S, Krystal JH. Treatment implications: using neuroscience to guide the development of new pharmacotherapies for alcoholism. *Alcohol Research and Health*, 2008, 31:400–407.

124 Addolorato G et al. Effectiveness and safety of baclofen for maintenance of alcohol abstinence in alcohol-dependent patients with liver cirrhosis: randomised, double-blind controlled study. *The Lancet*, 370:915–1922.

125 Anton RF et al. Efficacy of a combination of flumazenil and gabapentin in the treatment of alcohol dependence: relationship to alcohol withdrawal symptoms. *Journal of Clinical Psychopharmacology*, 2009, 29:334–342.

126 O'Malley SS, O'Connor PG. Medications for unhealthy alcohol use: across the spectrum. *Alcohol Research and Health*, 2011, 33:300–312.

127 Hungerford D et al. Feasibility of screening and intervention for alcohol problems among young adults in the ED. *American Journal of Emergency Medicine*, 2003, 21:14–22.

128 Jackson JS, Williams DR, Gomberg ESL. A life-course perspective on aging and alcohol use and abuse among African Americans. In: Gomberg ESL, Hegedus AM, Zucker RA, eds. *Alcohol problems and aging*. Bethesda, MD, National Institute on Alcohol Abuse and Alcoholism, 1998:63–87 (NIDA Research Monograph No. 33. NIH Pub. No. 98-4163).

129 Hannigan JH et al. A 14-year retrospective maternal report of alcohol consumption in pregnancy predicts pregnancy and teen outcomes. *Alcohol*, 2010, 44:583–594.

130 De Bellis MD et al. Hippocampal volume in adolescent–onset alcohol use disorders. *American Journal of Psychiatry*, 2000, 157:737–744.

131 Spear L. Adolescent brain and the college drinker: Biological basis of propensity to use and misuse alcohol. *Journal of Studies on Alcohol*, 2002(Suppl. 14):71–81.

132 Weitzman ER, Nelson TF, Wechsler H. Taking up binge drinking in college: The influences of person, social group, and environment. *Journal of Adolescent Health*, 2003, 32:26–35.

133 Zador PL, Krawchuk SA, Voas RB. Driver–related relative risk of driver fatalities and driver involvement in fatal crashes in relation to driver age and gender: an update using 1996 data. *Journal of Studies on Alcohol*, 2000, 61:387–395.

134 *Alcohol and transportation safety. Alcohol Alert No. 52*. Rockville, MD, National Institute on Alcohol Abuse and Alcoholism, 2001.

135 National Highway Traffic Safety Administration. Traffic safety facts 2003 annual report: early edition. Washington, DC, US Department of Transportation, 2004.

136 Schulenberg J et al. Development matters: taking the long view on substance abuse etiology and intervention during adolescence. In: Monti PM, Colby SM, O'Leary TA, eds. *Adolescents, alcohol, and substance abuse: reaching teens through brief interventions*. New York, Guilford Press, 2001:19–57.

137 Kimberly L et al. Alcohol use in early adolescence: the effect of changes in risk taking, perceived harm and friends' alcohol use. *Journal of Studies on Alcohol*, 2005, 66:275–283.

138 *Alcohol research: a lifespan perspective. Alcohol Alert No. 74*. Rockville, MD, National Institute on Alcohol Abuse and Alcoholism, 2008.

139 Johnson I. Alcohol problems in old age: a review of recent epidemiological research. *International Journal of Geriatric Psychiatry*, 2000, 15:575–581.

140 O'Connell H et al. Alcohol use disorders in elderly people–redefining an age old problem in old age. *BMJ*, 2003, 327:664.

141 American Medical Association. *Alcoholism in the elderly. Council on Scientific Affairs, American Medical Association. JAMA*, 1996, 275:797–801.

142 Reid MC, Anderson PA. Geriatric substance use disorders. *Medical Clinics of North America*, 1997, 81:999–1016.

143 Scott RB, Mitchell MC. Aging, alcohol and the liver. *Journal of the American Geriatrics Society*, 1988, 36:255–265.

144 Kofoed LL et al. Treatment compliance of older alcoholics: an elder-specific approach is superior to "mainstreaming". *Journal of Studies on Alcohol*, 1987, 48:47.

145 Dunlop J. Peer groups support seniors fighting alcohol and drugs. *Aging*, 1990, 361:28–32.

146 Atkinson RM, Tolson RL, Turner JA. Factors affecting treatment compliance of older male problem drinkers. *Journal of Studies on Alcohol*, 1993, 54:102–106.

147 Lemke S, Moos RH. Prognosis of older patients in mixed-age alcoholism treatment programs. *Journal of Substance Abuse Treatment*, 2002, 22:33–43.

148 Dar K. Alcohol use disorders in elderly people: fact or fiction? *Advances in Psychiatric Treatment*, 2006, 12:173–181.

149 Norton ED. Counseling substance abusing older adults. *Educational Gerontology*, 1998, 24:373–390.

150 Gulino C, Kadin M. Aging and reactive alcoholism. *Geriatric Nursing*, 1986, 7:148–151.

151 Menninger JA. Assessment and treatment of alcoholism and substance related disorders in the elderly. *Bulletin of the Menninger Clinic*, 2002, 66:166–184.

152 Adams SL, Waskel SA. Late onset of alcoholism among older Midwestern men in treatment. *Psychological Reports*, 1991, 68:432.

153 Brennan PL, Moos RH. Late life drinking behaviour. *Alcohol Health and Research World*, 1996, 20:197–205.

154 Schutte KK, Brennan L, Moos RH. Remission of late-life drinking problems: a 4-year follow up. *Alcoholism: Clinical and Experimental Research*, 1994, 18:835–844.

155 McKay JR. Continuing care research: what we have learned and where we are going. *Journal of Substance Abuse Treatment*, 2009, 36:131–145.

156 McKay JR, Hiller-Sturmhofel SH. Treating alcoholism as a chronic disease: Approaches to long-term continuing care. *Alcohol Research and Health*, 2011, 33:356–370.

157 Cunningham JA, Kypros K, McCambridge J. The use of emerging technologies in alcohol treatment. *Alcohol Research and Health*, 2011, 33:320–326.

158 Isbell H et al. An experimental study of the etiology of rum fits and delirium tremens. *Quarterly Journal of Studies on Alcohol*, 1955, 16:1–33.

159 Ng SK et al. Alcohol consumption and withdrawal in new-onset seizures. New England Journal of Medicine, 1988, 319:666–673.

160 Hoffman PL et al. N-methyl-D-asparate receptors and ethanol: inhibition of calcium flux and cyclic GMP production. *Journal of Neurochemistry*, 1989, 52:1937–1940.

161 Lovinger DM, White G, Wright FF. Ethanol inhibits NMDA-activated ion current in hippocampal neurones. *Science*, 1989, 243:1721–1724.

162 Suzdak PD et al. A selective imidazobenzodiazepine antagonist of ethanol in the rat. Science, 1986, 234:12243–1247.

163 Morrow AL et al. Chronic ethanol administration alters gamma-aminobutyric acid, pentobarbitol and ethanol-induced 36CL-uptake in cerebral cortical synaptoneurosomes. *Journal of Pharmacology and Experimental Therapeutics*, 1988, 246:158–164.

164 Victor M. Diagnosis and treatment of alcohol withdrawal states. *Practical Gastroenterology*, 1983, 7:6–15.

165 Sapolsky RM, Krey LC, McEwen BS. The neuroendocrinology of stress and aging: The glucocorticoid cascade hypothesis. *Endocrine Reviews*, 1986, 7:284–301.

166 Ballenger JC, Post RM. Kindling as a model for alcohol withdrawal syndromes. *British Journal of Psychiatry*, 1978, 133:1–14.

167 Liskow BI, Goodwin DW. Pharmacological treatment of alcohol intoxication, withdrawal and dependence: a critical review. *Journal of Studies on Alcohol*, 1987, 48:356–370.

168 Rosenbloom A. Emerging treatment options in the alcohol withdrawal syndrome. *Journal of Clinical Psychiatry*, 1988, 49(12 Suppl.):28–31.

169 Sellers EM et al. Diazepam loading: simplified treatment of alcohol withdrawal. *Clinical Pharmacology Therapeutics*, 1983, 34:822–826.

170 Dawson DA et al. Recovery from DSM-IV alcohol dependence: United States, 2001–2002. *Addiction*, 2005, 100:281–292.

171 Sterling S, Chi F, Hinman A. Integrating care for people with co-occurring alcohol and other drug, medical, and mental health conditions. *Alcohol Research and Health*, 2011, 33:338–359.

172 Institute of Medicine Committee on Crossing the Quality Chasm: Adaptation to Mental Health and Addictive Disorders. *Improving the quality of health care for mental and substance use conditions: Quality Chasm Series*. Washington DC: National Academies Press, 2006.

26 Drug use disorder in primary care mental health

Mohammed Abou-Saleh, Pedro Camacho and Nuzhat Anjum

Key messages

- The burden of substance misuse is great. It is a global public mental health problem with a substantial personal burden for affected individuals and their families; it produces significant economic and social hardships and contributes to crimes that affect society as a whole.

- Substance misuse commonly occurs with comorbid mental and physical health problems. Integrated primary care services help ensure that people are treated in a holistic manner, meeting their complex health and social care needs.

- The treatment gap for substance misuse is the greatest among mental disorders in all countries, particularly middle- and low-income countries. There is a significant gap between the prevalence of these mental disorders, on one hand, and the number of people receiving treatment and care, on the other. Primary care for mental health helps close this gap.

- Primary care for substance misuse improves access, and when care is integrated into primary care, people can access services closer to their homes, thus keeping their families together and maintaining their daily activities. Primary care for substance misuse also facilitates community outreach, health promotion, and long-term monitoring and management of affected individuals.

- Primary care for substance misuse and mental health promotes respect of human rights, including the right to treatment, and services delivered in primary care minimize stigma and discrimination.

- Primary care for substance misuse is effective, affordable and cost effective, especially when integrated with secondary care and social care in the community.

Introduction

Psychoactive substances, frequently known as psychoactive drugs, are substances that, when consumed, have the ability to change an individual's mental processes (e.g. consciousness, mood, thinking, motivation, etc.). Psychoactive substances exert their actions on brain systems that normally exist to regulate an individual's functions of mood, thoughts, and motivations.[1,2] Not all psychoactive substances have addictive potential. Of these, some are legal and others are not – psychiatric medications are psychotropic drugs and have a legal status, but not all of them have addictive potential.

Psychoactive substances have been used in religious ways, for medicinal purposes, or for recreational use. Our ancestors developed empiric knowledge about the pharmacological effects of certain chemical substances, obtained through their own experiences during their lives. Cannabis has been largely consumed by Islamic cultures; coca leaf was chewed in Southern America (i.e. to diminish fatigue); and opium was used to relieve pain. Human capacity to concentrate and synthesize more potent compounds facilitated a smooth transition from medicinal or recreational use to a morbid addictive pattern. In the 19th and 20th centuries, use of illicit psychoactive substances was moderately widespread, particularly among young adults. The capacity of these substances to induce joy or pleasure (positive reinforcement) or to relieve psychological distress (negative reinforcement) encourages individuals to use them repeatedly. Repetitive use, genetic vulnerability and other environmental issues can contribute to some individuals developing addiction, mental illness (i.e. depression or psychosis) or a medical disease outside the central nervous system (e.g. acute myocardial infarction induced by cocaine). Their illegal status may also add an appeal in particular risk-taking subcultures.[3]

Epidemiology of substance misuse

The World Mental Health (WMH) surveys in 28 countries[4] have shown an interquartile range (IQR) of lifetime *Diagnostic and Statistical Manual of Mental Disorders* (DSM-IV)[5] disorder prevalence estimates (combining anxiety, mood, externalizing, and substance use disorders) of 18.1% to 36.1%. The IQR of 12-month prevalence estimates was 9.8% to 19.1%.[4] Survival analysis showed the median and IQR of age of onset is very early for some anxiety disorders (range = 7–14 years, IQR = 8–11 years) and impulse control disorders (median = 7–15 years, IQR = 11–12 years). The distribution of age of onset is later for mood disorders (median = 29–43 years, IQR = 35–40 years), other anxiety disorders (median = 24–50 years, IQR = 31–41 years), and substance use disorders (median = 18–29 years, IQR = 21–26 years). Median and IQR lifetime prevalence estimates are (ranges): anxiety disorders 4.8% to 31.0% (IQR = 9.9–16.7%), mood disorders 3.3% to 21.4% (IQR = 9.8–15.8%), impulse control disorders 0.3% to 25.0% (IQR = 3.1–5.7%), substance use disorders 1.3% to 15.0% (IQR = 4.8–9.6%).[6]

Between 155 and 250 million people around the world (3.5% to 5.7% of the population aged 15–64 years) used illicit substances at least once in 2008. Cannabis involves the largest number (129–190 million people), followed by amphetamine-type substances, cocaine and opiates. Problem drug users were recently defined as "those who inject drugs and/or are considered dependent, facing serious social and health consequences as a result".[7] Applying this definition, in 2008 between 16 and 38 million people were problem drug users (10–15% of all people who used drugs that year). However, only between 12% and 30% of them had received treatment over the last year, which means that between 11 and 33.5 million problem drug users did not receive treatment. Treatment services for distinct drugs vary markedly across different regions of the world and frequently change over time. In recent years, the greatest demand for treatment in Europe and Asia was for opiates. For the Americas it was cocaine, and for Africa-Oceania it was cannabis. Over the last decade, the demand for cannabis treatment has increased in Europe, South America and Oceania; demand for cocaine treatment has declined in the Americas (mainly North America), while it has increased in Europe.[8]

Data from the first 17 countries participating in the World Health Organization's (WHO's) World Mental Health (WMH) Survey Initiative involved 85052 in the Americas (Colombia, Mexico, United States of America (USA)), Europe (Belgium, France, Germany, Italy, Netherlands, Spain, Ukraine), Middle East and Africa (Israel, Lebanon, Nigeria, South Africa), Asia (Japan, People's Republic of China), and Oceania (New Zealand).[6] The WHO Composite International Diagnostic Interview (CIDI) was used to assess the prevalence and correlates of a wide variety of mental and substance disorders. Cannabis use in the USA and New Zealand (both 42%) was far higher than in any other country. The USA was also an outlier in cocaine use (16%). Men were more likely than women to have used drugs; and not only were younger cohorts more likely to use all drugs, but the male–female gap was found to be closing in more recent cohorts. The period of risk for drug initiation also appears to be lengthening further into adulthood among more recent cohorts. Associations with sociodemographic variables were consistent across countries, as were the curves of incidence of lifetime use.[7]

Use of mental health services for anxiety, mood and substance disorders in 17 countries in the WHO world mental health surveys was also investigated.[7] The number of respondents using any 12-month mental health services (57 (2%; Nigeria) to 1477 (18%; USA)) was generally lower in low-income than in middle- and high-income countries, and the proportion receiving services tended to correspond to a country's percentages of gross domestic product spent on health care.[9,10] The study concluded that unmet needs for mental health treatment are pervasive and especially concerning in lower-income countries and that alleviation of these unmet needs will require expansion and optimum allocation of treatment resources.

The common co-occurrence of substance misuse and other psychiatric disorders and their intricate relationships have led to major community-based epidemiological studies in the USA, which have shown high rates of current and lifetime comorbidity. Moreover, studies of clinical populations conducted in North America, Europe and Australia, have shown even higher rates of comorbidity.[11]

The relatively recent recognition of this comorbidity can be attributed to a number of factors. Firstly, drug abuse services have developed separately from general psychiatric services, with little interface between them. Second, the move from hospital to community care for treatment of people with severe mental disorders has exposed them to the risk of developing alcohol and drug problems, and thus compounding their psychopathology and disabilities. Third, there is a high risk for self-harm and harm to people in the community in two distinct populations: the seriously mentally ill within general psychiatric services and those with severe personality disorders within addiction services. This has resulted in a tendency to disown these problems within the service concerned, together with an expectation that patients belong to the counterpart service. The aetiology of this high prevalence is unclear and opinions have varied on the reasons for this comorbidity, but the association is most commonly explained by either a causal relationship or shared aetiological factor(s) underlying both disorders. Moreover, the large variation in prevalence rates has focused attention on the challenge of defining this phenomenon, leading to improved diagnostic instruments and further research on their complex and intricate relationships.

The aetiology of drug misuse

The aetiology of drug misuse has been well elucidated, with identification of both risk and protective factors. As summarized in the National Institute for Health and Clinical Excellence (NICE) guideline,[12] there is robust evidence for aetiological factors of peer drug use, availability of drugs and also elements of family interaction, including parental discipline and family cohesion, as significant risk factors for drug misuse.[13] In particular, traumatic family experiences such as childhood neglect, homelessness or abuse increase the likelihood that the individual will develop problems with drugs later on in life.[14] Studies of twins, families and individuals who have been adopted suggest that vulnerability to drug misuse may also have a genetic component,[15] although it is unclear whether repeated use is primarily determined by genetic predisposition, or whether socioeconomic and psychological factors lead an individual to try drugs and then later to use them compulsively. Risk factors for heavy, dependent drug use are much more significant when they occur together rather than individually.

The effects of many illicit drugs are mediated via various brain circuits, in particular the mesolimbic systems, which have evolved to respond to basic rewards (such as food and sexual intercourse) to ensure survival. A diverse range of substances, including opioids, stimulants and cannabis, as well as alcohol and nicotine, all appear to produce euphoric effects via increasing levels of dopamine (a neurotransmitter) in the nucleus accumbens.[16] This has been well demonstrated in imaging studies of the human brain.[17] Euphoria resulting from use then potentiates further use, particularly for those with a genetic vulnerability (see later). Chronic drug use may produce long-lasting changes in the reward circuits, including reductions in dopamine receptor levels,[20] and these contribute to the clinical course of drug dependence, including craving, tolerance and withdrawal.[18] In addition, other types of neurotransmitter systems (for example, opioids, glutamates and cannabinoids) are implicated in the misuse of specific drugs.

Relevance in primary care

Psychotropic substances are important in primary care, not only because some have the potential to trigger dependence, but also because they generate high costs economically and in terms of health, family and work. This chapter focuses on illicit psychoactive substances, while issues related to alcohol use are discussed in Chapter 25.

Substance misuse is a common mental health problem in people attending primary care, reflecting its common occurrence in the general population. However, the need for treatment is often not met, as these individuals go undetected, which contributes to poor clinical and social outcomes.

Echoing the importance of primary care, the WHO *World Health Report* 2008[19] noted that the vision of primary care for mental health has not yet been realized in most countries, and advocated for the renewal and integration of mental health into primary care. Lack of political support, inadequate management, overburdened health services and, at times, resistance from policy-makers and health workers have hampered the development of services.

The neglect of substance misuse issues continues, despite documentation of their high prevalence and the substantial burden these disorders impose on individuals, families, communities and health systems when left untreated. The neglect also continues despite good evidence for the availability of effective treatments that can be successfully delivered in primary care settings.

The WHO-Wonca (World Organization of Family Doctors) publication, *Integrating mental health into primary care: a global perspective*[20] explained the rationale that applies to substance misuse:

- the burden of mental disorders is great
- mental and physical health problems are interwoven
- the treatment gap for mental disorders is enormous
- primary care for mental health enhances access
- primary care for mental health promotes respect of human rights
- primary care for mental health is affordable and cost effective
- primary care for mental health generates good health outcomes.

Most of the evidence for successful provision of treatment for drug misuse in primary care derives from research in high-income countries.[21–23] However, in a collaborative study on substitution therapy for opioid dependence and HIV/AIDS (human immunodeficiency virus/acquired immunodeficiency syndrome) in less-resourced countries in Asia (China, Indonesia and Thailand), Eastern Europe (Lithuania, Poland, and Ukraine) and the Middle East (Iran),[24] all countries demonstrated significant and marked reductions in reported heroin and other illicit opioid use; HIV (and other blood-borne virus) exposure risk behaviours associated with use of injected drugs; and criminal activity; and demonstrated substantial improvement in drug users' physical and mental health.

Treatment of drug misuse in primary care

There is good scope for the extension of services for drug misusers in primary care.[21,23] Firstly, there are benefits such as easy access, less stigma and early intervention. Second, the development of community-based specialized services has provided opportunities for effective liaison and shared care, and effective models have emerged (e.g. the Edinburgh and Glasgow schemes).[25,26] Third, more general practitioners (GPs), particularly those who are more recently qualified, are willing to provide care for drug misusers with the support of specialist services.

A successful liaison between primary care and specialist services depends on real communication, jointly agreed protocols (including care planning), patient contracts with appropriate sanctions, and regular formal reviews against treatment goals. With appropriate training and remuneration, methadone maintenance does have a role in general practice settings, particularly for limited periods of time, in the achievement of non-drug-related goals (such as dealing with relationship problems, or unemployment). Finally, since GPs accept medical and legal responsibility for anything they prescribe, they must have the final say, and this must be accepted by specialist services.

The development of services for substance misusers in developing countries has been slow or non-existent. National mental health programmes promoted by WHO have often referred to the growth of substance misuse in developing countries and the need for developing addiction services. Few countries that have developed addiction services have targeted the complex needs of those with severe addictions. In Saudi Arabia, the Al-Amal group of addiction treatment hospitals has been established to provide detoxification treatment and social rehabilitation.

Alcohol services are often provided by mainstream mental health services. Drug treatment has been confined to detoxification for people with opiate addiction, but not maintenance treatment. There has been widespread resistance to introducing methadone maintenance treatment for people with opiate addiction, including those with injecting drug use. This has been related to the rather puritanical attitude that maintenance treatment with addictive therapeutic drugs replaces one addiction with another, and that abstinence should be the sole aim of treatment. WHO has promoted flexible and comprehensive approaches to the treatment of addictions in developing countries, including the provision of care and services in primary care.

The *gold standard approach* to management of drug misuse in primary care is guided by the principles of good practice adapted to the treatment needs of drug misusers in a locality and all relevant attributes including cultural aspects. Good practice in the treatment of drug problems is evidence based, and any intervention has to fit into the whole system of health and social care, including the availability of specialist services. What has evolved in practice in high-income countries is a separate provision of drug addiction treatment services from mainstream mental health services. This has been related to the predominance of drug misusers in criminal justice settings, the stigma associated with illicit drug use being such they are shunned by society, their families and health professionals, and the constraints and restriction of prescribing controlled drugs such as methadone for opiate users. There has also been limited capacity and capability within non-specialist medical services, particularly primary care. This approach has developed in high-income countries, while middle- and low-income countries have rudimentary or no provision of drug treatment services, including specialist services.

The scene had changed in recent decades in high-income countries with a change in the philosophy of care and increasing emphasis placed on a harm-reduction approach to dealing with drug misuse – i.e. to reduce the harm drugs cause to physical and mental health and social functions, and to reduce crime. There have also been dramatic advances in both pharmacological and psychosocial treatment, with strong evidence for their effectiveness and cost-effectiveness. Models of care have been well established in high-income countries, with increasing integration with primary care. These models have resulted in shared collaborative care between specialist and primary care services,[21] with evidence for their effectiveness. However, there have been no similar service developments in low-income countries, and the proposed gold standard approach is based on the global drive for providing integrated mental health services in primary care.[20]

A good approach has recently been advocated and promoted by the Global Movement of Mental Health.[27] For middle- and low-income countries, it is proposed to adopt the packages of care for alcohol use disorders,[28] which should broadly apply to the care of drug use disorders. These can be summarized as follows:

- *alcohol use disorders* – conditions that range from hazardous and harmful alcohol use to alcohol dependence – are a low priority in low- and middle-income countries, despite causing a large health burden
- most alcohol-related harm is attributable to hazardous/harmful drinkers who make disproportionate use of primary health-care systems, but often go undetected and untreated for long periods, even though brief, easily delivered interventions are effective in this group of people
- health-care systems in low- and middle-income countries currently focus on providing tertiary care services for the treatment of dependence (where there is often a poor outcome). This focus needs to shift towards the cost-effective strategy of providing brief interventions for early alcohol use disorders
- effective evidence-based combinations of psychosocial and pharmacological treatments for alcohol use disorders are available in low- and middle-income countries, but are costly to implement. Policy-makers need to ensure that people with alcohol use disorders are offered the most appropriate services, using stepped care solutions that start with simple, structured advice for risky drinkers and progress to specialist treatment services for more serious alcohol use disorders
- low-and middle-income countries also need to improve their implementation of proven population-level preventive measures, to reduce the health burden due to alcohol use disorders. An international Framework Convention on Alcohol Control may help them do this.

Assessment of drug misuse in primary care

The core value or guiding principle for the management of substance misuse and dependence is that people with substance use disorders have the same entitlement to health and social care as other patients. It is the responsibility of all health professionals involved in their care to provide for their general health and social needs, as well as for their drug-related problems, through evidence-based interventions, including harm-reduction approaches.[23,29]

A good assessment should be thorough and comprehensive, with the purpose of identifying the nature and severity of any drug-related problem, understanding its causes, and assessing its consequences, to establish the strengths and weaknesses of patients and their conditions.

A good assessment will enable formulation of the diagnosis, which comprises medical and psychiatric diagnosis, as well as appropriate investigations, including psychological and social assessments.

A good formulation will result in a comprehensive treatment and care plan, addressing the patient's immediate needs, risk factors, and short-term and long-term management, including social rehabilitation for optimal integration into normal community living.

The aims of assessment are to:

- treat any emergency or acute problem
- confirm that the patient is taking drugs (history, examination, and urine analysis)
- assess the degree of dependence
- identify complications of drug misuse and assess risk behaviour
- identify other medical, social and mental health problems
- give advice on harm minimization, including, if appropriate, access to sterile needles and syringes, testing for hepatitis and HIV, and immunization against hepatitis B
- determine a patient's expectations regarding treatment and the degree of motivation to change
- assess the most appropriate level of expertise required to manage the patient (this may alter over time)
- refer/liaise appropriately (i.e. shared care, specialist or specialized generalist care, or other forms of psychological care, where appropriate)
- determine the need for substitute medication – in the case of the GP, this should be with advice from a specialist, ideally through shared care arrangements
- in private practice, establish that the patient is able to pay for treatment through legitimate means.

Identification and assessment of drug misuse (NICE guidelines)[30,31]

Asking questions about drug misuse

- In mental health and criminal justice settings (in which drug misuse is known to be prevalent), routinely ask service users about recent legal and illicit drug use, including the type, method of administration, quantity and frequency.
- In settings such as primary care, general hospitals and emergency departments, consider asking people about recent drug use if they have symptoms that suggest the possibility of drug misuse, such as:
  - acute chest pain in a young person
  - acute psychosis
  - mood and sleep disorders.

Initial assessment

- When making an assessment and developing and agreeing a care plan, consider the service user's:
  - medical, psychological, social and occupational needs
  - history of drug use
  - experience of previous treatment, if any
  - goals in relation to his or her drug use
  - treatment preferences.
- When delivering and monitoring the care plan:
  - agree the plan with the service user
  - maintain a respectful and supportive relationship with the service user
  - help the service user to identify when he or she is vulnerable to drug misuse, and explore alternative coping strategies
  - ensure that all service users have full access to a wide range of services
  - remember the importance of maintaining the service user's engagement with services

- review regularly the care plan of a service user receiving maintenance treatment, to ascertain whether detoxification should be considered
- collaborate with other care providers.

■ Use biological testing (for example, of urine or oral fluid) as part of a comprehensive assessment of drug use, but do not rely on it as the sole method of treatment.

Assessment of drug misuse and coexisting mental health problems

Assessment of drug misuse and coexisting mental health problems including serious mental illness is guided by the NICE guidelines for both disorders,[30,31] and has been reviewed.[32,33]

It is important for primary care practitioners to suspect and exclude physical causes for presenting symptoms, including acute intoxication, withdrawal, and side-effects from medications. Primary care also plays a role in screening for physical comorbidities that have a high rate of incidence in individuals with substance misuse and psychosis, including liver damage, blood-borne viruses, cognitive changes, and nutritional deficiencies, particularly where dependent drinking and injecting drug use is suspected.

It will usually be helpful to make an assessment of the individual's social support networks of family, friends and occupation and the degree to which the individual's networks are predicated around drinking or drug-use activities. Carers may also need an assessment of their needs. Where significant substance use is detected in primary care, the practitioner will usually need to assess the extent to which this substance use is problematic to the individual and those they come into contact with, including children, and whether there is physical or psychological dependence on the substance.[34]

The Global Mental Health Assessment Tool – Primary Care Version

The Global Mental Health Assessment Tool – Primary Care Version (GMHAT/PC) is a computerized clinical assessment tool developed to assess and identify a wide range of mental health problems in primary care. It generates a computer diagnosis, a symptom rating, a self-harm risk assessment, and a referral letter. The inter-rater reliability (kappa coefficient) based on symptom scores between a psychiatrist and a GP using the GMHAT/PC was alcohol misuse 1.00, anxiety 0.79, depression 0.82, drug misuse 1.00, eating disorder 0.66, phobia 0.83 and psychosis 0.78.[35]

The GMHAT/PC has already been translated into a number of languages of low- and middle-income countries. This method aims to improve the recognition of mental illness in primary care and initiation of appropriate treatments by increasing the skills of primary care workers. The use of computers could be a restriction, but the programme is being developed to allow installation on a touch-screen PDA, making it easy to use anywhere. Patients on the whole have received the GMHAT/PC assessment well and said they found it helpful as it covered more aspects of their mental health than the usual consultation.[35] As it covers a wide range of mental disorders including alcohol and drug misuse, it should prove useful in their early and accurate detection.

Sharma et al.,[36] using a Hindi version showed that other health professionals such as psychologists, and possibly others with some training, can use the computer-assisted GMHAT/PC program in different cultures for making a valid assessment and diagnosis of mental disorders. Studies carried out in the United Kingdom of Great Britain and Northern Ireland (UK) showed that nurses can use the GMHAT/PC in detecting mental disorders accurately in primary care and general health settings.[37] It was reassuring to find that the GMHAT/PC questions in Hindi were easy to understand by all the subjects interviewed, from rural as well as urban areas, to detect psychopathology in that population. The mean duration of the interview of around 16 minutes, similar to earlier UK studies, makes it feasible in routine assessments in primary care and general health settings in India. The GMHAT/PC interviews were very well received by the subjects as well the interviewers. It was a novelty in the clinic and some other patients requested that their mental health should also be checked by the computer assessment.

High mental health morbidity has a particularly adverse effect on general health and social well-being in the population of low- and middle-income countries. Given that the identification of mental health problems is vital to improve the outcome in many chronic illnesses, it is essential to improve their recognition rates. In an extensive review, Patel et al. highlighted that common mental health conditions such as depression, schizophrenia, alcohol misuse, etc., can be treated effectively in low- and middle-income countries.[38] A tool such as the GMHAT/PC can assist health and voluntary sector workers in detecting and managing mental health conditions, using its pathways of care, derived from evidence-based guidelines. It also adds to the skills of primary care health workers in detecting mental disorders more accurately. In addition to assisting in diagnosing mental disorders, the GMHAT/PC would also help with planning evidence-based treatments, as the pathways of care and guidelines are part of the program. This will give more chance to follow the treatment guidelines compared to current practice.

The use of computers in routine clinical practice is still a challenge in low- to middle-income countries. However, diminishing costs have led to increased availability and use of computers even in remote areas of India. The experience of using the GMHAT/PC in India suggests that its use in routine practice can be cost-effective for the following reasons: it takes on average about 15 minutes to cover all common mental disorders including substance misuse, and it records the information necessary to lead to useful clinical output. Any mental health-care professional (not necessarily psychiatrists) with adequate training can use it. Therefore, the GMHAT/PC could be a useful tool in implementing mental health programmes in all countries and would be particularly useful in low-income countries.

Treatment of drug misuse

A comprehensive assessment will produce a comprehensive treatment and care plan.[23,29] Ultimately, the aim is to enable patients to change their lifestyle so that they can lead life without the use of substances and can be free from all constraints and disabilities.

Assessment of a patient's readiness for change is a core intervention. The assessment of this readiness to change is based on the cycle of change of Prochaska and DiClemente,[39] wherein the substance user goes through the following:

- *precontemplation stage*: no change is being considered
- *contemplation stage*: the user becomes ambivalent towards drug use
- *determination*: the user decides to take steps
- *action*: change is started
- *maintenance*: the user consolidates the change achieved.

Drug users, however, often experience relapses into substance use and the cycle starts again. Based on the assessment of readiness to change, the counsellor attending to the drug user, and using motivational interviewing, will provide interventions to enhance the user's motivation by providing information during the precontemplation phase, increasing ambivalence during contemplation, exploring options during determination, working out practical strategies during action, working out relapse prevention during maintenance, and, finally, avoiding demoralization during relapse into substance misuse.

The aims of the treatment are as follows:

- to assist patients to remain healthy until they receive appropriate care/support so that they can achieve a drug-free life
- to reduce the use of illicit or unprescribed drugs; deal with problems relating to drug misuse; and reduce the dangers associated with drug misuse, particularly the risk of HIV, hepatitis B/C, and other blood-borne infections
- to reduce the duration of episodes of drug misuse; reduce the chance of future relapse into drug misuse; and reduce the need for criminal activity to finance drug misuse
- to reduce the risk of prescribed drugs being diverted to the illegal drug market; and stabilize the patient, where appropriate, on a substitute medication to alleviate withdrawal symptoms
- to improve overall personal, social, and family functions.

Treatment is subdivided into psychological and pharmacological therapies, and the optimal treatment plan will provide tailor-made combined psychosocial and pharmacological treatments matching the substance user's physical, psychiatric, psychological and social needs.

A wide range of psychological treatments have been developed in recent decades and are based on psychological theories of addictive behaviour, including conditioning and cognitive theories.

The goals of treatment are best conceived as a hierarchy of goals, including the following: reduction of psychological, social, and other problems directly related to drug use; reduction of psychological, social, and other problems not directly attributable to drug use; reduction of harmful or risky behaviours associated with drug use (e.g. sharing injecting equipment); attainment of less chaotic, non-dependent, or no problematic drug use; abstinence from main problem drugs; and abstinence from all drugs.

Psychosocial treatments

The primacy of psychosocial treatments of addictions is related to their established effectiveness and, importantly, to the provision of a context for comprehensive treatment, including pharmacotherapy.[13]

Moreover, psychosocial treatment is the treatment of choice for stimulant and cannabis misuse, and non-dependent alcohol and drug use, since there are no effective pharmacological treatments for these disorders. It is also useful for the treatment of comorbid psychiatric disorders such as anxiety and depressive disorders, and related social problems.

Elements of psychosocial treatment include the following: provision of information, structure for care, family involvement, facilitation of engagement and retention in treatment, self-help groups, and a counselling style that is non-judgemental, empowering, and enhancing of self-esteem and self-efficacy (see Box 26.1).

"The Matrix": summary of the psychological therapies evidence base in drug misuse

As discussed, psychological interventions are the mainstay of treatment of substance misuse in health-care settings including primary care. "The Matrix" is a guide to planning and delivering evidence-based psychological therapies within NHS Boards in Scotland.[40] It has been produced to help NHS service providers. The Matrix is intended to provide a summary of the information on the evidence base for the effectiveness of particular psychological therapies for particular service user groups based on Scottish Intercollegiate Guidelines Network (SIGN) and NICE guidelines. Table 26.1 summarizes the evidence base for the effectiveness of psychological treatments for substance misuse, using the following definitions:

- *level of severity*: a description of the level of severity of illness and an indicator of the potential level of functioning
- *level of service*: where service users are most likely to be treated most effectively
- *intensity of intervention*: low-intensity interventions are standardized interventions aimed at transient or mild mental health problems, with limited effect on functioning. High-intensity/specialist interventions denote a formal psychological therapy delivered by a relatively specialist psychological therapist, and are aimed at common mental health problems with more significant effect on functioning
- *what intervention?* The interventions are those that are recommended by guideline development groups such as NICE and SIGN
- *level of evidence*: this is the level of evidence of efficacy that is reported in published national guidelines.[41]

Pharmacological treatment of substance misuse

Pharmacotherapy of addictions has been the mainstay of treatment since the introduction of methadone for opiate addiction. This established the British model comprising methadone detoxification and maintenance, with the latter indication becoming more established when a harm-reduction approach was widely adopted to combat the spread of HIV, which was later extended to reduce other harms, including social harm and drug-related crimes. The other well-established – albeit more recently introduced – drug is buprenorphine, which is used for both opiate detoxification and maintenance, and is a safe and effective treatment for opiate addiction, when delivered in specialist and general practice settings;[31] it is recommended in NICE guidelines

- *Behavioural therapy*: a structured therapy focusing on changing behaviours and on environmental factors that trigger maladaptive behaviour.

- *Cue-exposure treatment*: a structured treatment involving exposure to drug-related cues that have been associated with past drug use.

- *A period without consumption of the drug*: this is intended to lead to a reduction (or habituation) of reactivity to drug cues and, thus, to a reduced likelihood of relapse.

- *Community-reinforcement approach*: a behavioural approach that focuses on what clients find rewarding in their social, occupational, and recreational life; it aims to help them change their lifestyle and social environment to support long-term changes in behaviour whereby substances use is less rewarding that non-use.

- *Contingency management*: also known as voucher-based therapy, this aims to encourage adaptive behaviour by rewarding the client for attaining goals (e.g. no use of illicit drugs as checked by urine screens) and by not rewarding them when these goals are unmet (e.g. illicit drug use); vouchers can usually be exchanged for consumer goods.

- *Cognitive therapy*: a structured therapy using cognitive techniques (e.g. challenging a person's negative thoughts) and behavioural techniques (e.g. behavioural experiments and activity planning) to change maladaptive thoughts and beliefs.

- *Cognitive-behavioural therapy* (CBT): a combination of both cognitive and behavioural therapies.

- *Relapse prevention*: uses several CBT strategies to enhance clients' self-control and to prevent relapse; it highlights problems that clients may face and develops strategies that they can use to deal with high-risk situations.

- *Motivational interviewing*: a focused approach aiming to enhance motivation for stopping substance use by exploring and resolving individuals' ambivalence about change.

- *Motivational enhancement therapy*: a brief intervention based on motivational interviewing, which also incorporates 'check-up' assessment and feedback.

- *Twelve-step approaches*: interventions used by self-help organizations such as Alcoholics Anonymous and Narcotics Anonymous; these are based on a philosophy that adopts an illness model and sees substance use as stemming from an innate vulnerability; individuals must acknowledge their addiction and the harm it has caused to themselves and others; they must also accept their lack of control over use and that, thus, the only acceptable goal is abstinence.

- *Other approaches*: the involvement of partners and family through marital and family therapies builds on the known social context of substance use; there are also various forms of counselling, group therapy, and milieu therapy.

Adapted from Abou-Saleh MT. Substance use disorders: recent advances in treatment and models of care. *Journal of Psychosomatic Research*, 2006, 61(3):305–310, under the terms of the Click-Use Licence.[23]

for opioid detoxification.[31] Other new treatments include lofexidine (for opiate detoxification), naltrexone,[42] and methadone and buprenorphine for the management of opioid dependence.[43]

NICE guidelines: opioid detoxification[31]

- Detoxification should be a readily available treatment option for people who are opioid dependent and have expressed an informed choice to become abstinent.

- In order to obtain informed consent, staff should give detailed information to service users about detoxification and the associated risks, including:
  - the physical and psychological aspects of opioid withdrawal, including the duration and intensity of symptoms, and how these may be managed
  - the use of non-pharmacological approaches to manage or cope with opioid withdrawal symptoms
  - the loss of opioid tolerance following detoxification, and the ensuing increased risk of overdose and death from illicit drug use that may be potentiated by the use of alcohol or benzodiazepines

Table 26.1 Matrix of psychological treatments in substance misuse

Level of severity	Level of service	Intensity of intervention	What intervention?	Level of evidence
Mild	Opportunistic contact	Low	Opportunistic brief intervention (motivationally based)	
Mild to moderate: cannabis use with comorbid anxiety and/or depression; stimulant use with comorbid anxiety and/or benzodiazepine use with panic disorder	Primary care/ secondary care	High	CBT; group CBT + gradual tapering (10 weeks)[41]	
Moderate to severe: stimulant use	Community/inpatient/ residential/criminal justice	High	Contingency management; behavioural couples therapy	A[41]
Moderate to severe: stimulants with comorbid anxiety and/or depression	Primary care/ community	High	CBT	A[41]

- the importance of continued support, as well as psychosocial and appropriate pharmacological interventions, to maintain abstinence, treat comorbid mental health problems and reduce the risk of adverse outcomes (including death).

■ Methadone or buprenorphine should be offered as the first-line treatment in opioid detoxification. When deciding between these medications, health-care professionals should take into account whether the service user is receiving maintenance treatment with methadone or buprenorphine; if so, opioid detoxification should normally be started with the same medication, according to the preference of the service user.

Methadone and buprenorphine for the management of opioid dependence[43]

■ Methadone and buprenorphine (oral formulations), using flexible dosing regimens, are recommended as options for maintenance therapy in the management of opioid dependence.

■ The decision about which drug to use should be made on a case by case basis, taking into account a number of factors, including the person's history of opioid dependence, their commitment to a particular long-term management strategy, and an estimate of the risks and benefits of each treatment made by the responsible clinician in consultation with the person. If both drugs are equally suitable, methadone should be prescribed as the first choice.

■ Methadone and buprenorphine should be administered daily, under supervision, for at least the first 3 months. Supervision should be relaxed only when the patient's compliance is assured. Both drugs should be given as part of a programme of supportive care.

Naltrexone for the management of opioid dependence[42]

■ Naltrexone is recommended as a treatment option in detoxified formerly opioid-dependent people who are highly motivated to remain in an abstinence programme.

■ Naltrexone should only be administered under adequate supervision to people who have been fully informed of the potential adverse effects of treatment. It should be given as part of a programme of supportive care.

- The effectiveness of naltrexone in preventing opioid misuse in people being treated should be reviewed regularly. Discontinuation of naltrexone treatment should be considered if there is evidence of such misuse.

Drug misuse primary care liaison service for opiate addiction

Primary care teams in high-income countries have been increasingly enabled to provide competent assessments and treatments for people with heroin and cocaine misuse, using evidence-based pharmacological treatments such as detoxification/assisted withdrawal and replacement treatments (methadone or buprenorphine), with key working and low-intensity psychosocial interventions such as motivational interviewing. See the resources on the (UK) Substance Misuse Management in General Practice web site for treatment approaches for all drug problems that can be managed in primary care.[44]

These treatments are optimally provided within shared care schemes with specialist addiction services. Such primary care liaison services are hardly ever provided in low-income countries, for a number of reasons: prohibition of use and licensing, poor capacity (skills) and capability (personnel) in primary care settings, and poor access to specialist treatment services, which are also poorly provided.

The Department of Health in the UK defines shared care as:

> The joint participation of specialists and GPs (and other agencies as appropriate) in the planned delivery of care for patients with a drug misuse problem, informed by an enhanced information exchange beyond routine discharge and referral letters. It may involve the day-to-day management by the GP of the patient's medical needs in relation to his or her drug misuse. Such arrangements would make explicit which clinician was responsible for different aspects of the patient's treatment and care. These may include prescribing substitute drugs in appropriate circumstances.[45]

Our local experience in south west London, the Substance Misuse Primary Care Liaison Service (SMPCL) in Wandsworth provides a direct clinical and liaison support service to GPs who are engaged in the treatment of adult users of opiates and/or cocaine or alcohol, to a problematic or dependent level. While the service will treat problematic drug users as a priority, it also has a remit to work with general practice in treating other drugs of abuse, including dependence on benzodiazepines, cannabis and other substances. The SMPCL provides services for:

- patients with short histories of drug misuse
- patients currently being prescribed substitute opiates by specialist services, who have achieved stability, and who are compliant with their treatment programme
- patients being discharged from prison who are stable on a substitute opiate prescription
- patients undergoing planned community detoxification
- patients withdrawing from crack cocaine and needing symptomatic treatment/psychosocial interventions.

Care planning, coordination and care management processes (including risk assessment and outcome measurement)

The SMPCL service forms part of the local integrated drug treatment response and will provide support to general practice for those treated under the substance misuse or alcohol enhanced service, with a range of services and support functions including:

- conducting initial triage assessments to ascertain the suitability of clients for treatment in a primary care setting, and advice on appropriate treatment regimes
- comprehensive and holistic assessment, including risk and mental health assessment and care planning – as well as preparation for treatment interventions
- dose reductions and adjustments to those under the care of key workers. This includes the role of the alcohol nurse in nurse prescribing, with close contact of the GP clinical lead

- providing expertise for GPs on assessment, management and care planning for patients who have mental health problems and problematic alcohol/drug consumption
- liaising with specialist prescribing services for further assessment if required, and, where appropriate, for stabilization before referral back to the GP for ongoing prescribing
- supporting community detoxification plans under supervision
- supporting access to other required interventions, including:
  - comprehensive assessment and care management
  - structured counselling
  - housing, welfare benefits and education training and employment
  - structured day care
  - residential rehabilitation
- preparing clients for discharge from treatment as appropriate, including the development of an after-care programme
- promoting health through brief interventions, motivational interviewing, empowering patients, and offering appropriate health education, information and advice to patients, relatives and carers
- providing a harm-reduction focus for harmful drinkers, particularly those with long-term alcohol-related disease and long-term injecting drug use.

Assessment and treatment of cannabis misuse in primary care

Cannabis use is the most common drug problem worldwide and presents in all health settings including primary care. Despite high levels of use, only 6% of those seeking treatment for substance misuse in England cite cannabis as their major drug of concern, and for most of those with cannabis use disorders, their presenting complaint is not their cannabis use;[46] common presentations include:

- respiratory problems, such as exacerbation of asthma, chronic obstructive airways disease, wheeze or prolonged cough, or other chest symptoms
- mental health symptoms, such as anxiety, depression, paranoia, panic, depersonalization, exacerbation of an underlying mental health condition
- problems with concentration while studying, or with employment and relationships
- difficulties stopping cannabis use
- legal or employment problems (arising from use of cannabis).

Cannabis use is associated with significant harms: acute intoxication risks, chronic effects, and risks in special populations; a recent review[46] provided an evidence-based approach for identifying and responding to cannabis use disorders, and pathway for a decision-making process for assessing the common affective symptoms in primary care. While there are no pharmacological interventions for cannabis misuse, brief psychosocial interventions are effective, and guidance is provided for the treatment of withdrawal symptoms and advising for patients on reducing their risk of harm from cannabis.

Management of benzodiazepine dependence in primary care

Benzodiazepine misuse and dependence remains a common problem in primary care. The prevalence of benzodiazepines use remains important worldwide. While the trend for their prescribing has been for more careful use in high-income countries, their use in low-income countries remains a growing and overlooked problem.

Benzodiazepines are highly effective as short-term treatment for anxiety and insomnia, but long-term prescribing may result in adverse effects on cognitive abilities, memory problems, mood swings and overdoses if mixed with other drugs, all of which could outweigh their benefits.[47] Benzodiazepines are potentially addictive drugs and dependence can develop within a few weeks or months of regular use.

The current management of benzodiazepines withdrawal syndrome consists of:

- adequate treatment of continuing symptoms of depression or anxiety
- utilization of a gradual taper schedule
- switching the patient to an equivalent dose of a long half-life benzodiazepine if difficulty is encountered in tapering off therapy with short half-life benzodiazepines.[48]

A recent Cochrane review of pharmacological interventions for management of benzodiazepine monodependence in outpatient settings concluded that gradual tapering was preferable to abrupt discontinuation and suggested the potential value of carbamazepine as an effective intervention for benzodiazepine gradual taper discontinuation.[49] It is imperative that this persistent problem is dealt with in primary care, where it is often started through injudicious prescribing by GPs. Alternative pharmacological treatments for anxiety and sleep problems should be considered, such as selective serotonin reuptake inhibitors (SSRIs). Lader et al. found that there is no clear evidence for the optimum rate of tapering, and schedules vary from 4 weeks to several years.[47] They recommended withdrawal in less than 6 months, as otherwise the withdrawal process can become the morbid focus of the patient's experience. Substitution of diazepam for another benzodiazepine can be helpful, at least logistically, as diazepam is available in a liquid formulation. Psychological interventions range from simple support through counselling to expert CBT. Patients with complex psychiatric presentations of comorbid psychiatric disorders, and those with co-dependence on alcohol, require referral and treatment in specialist settings.

The importance of primary care workforce attitudes for optimal outcomes

Substance misusers presenting for treatment generally show ambivalent attitudes towards their treatment: some show a clear conviction of their need to suspend or diminish consumption, but others are reluctant. It is therefore crucial for health professionals to show an understanding and empathic attitude, and to be respectful and sympathetic to the person's difficulty in tackling their drug problem.

Moreover, health professionals should anticipate that a majority of patients may suffer recurrences in their addictive behaviour, undergoing lapses and relapsing into drug use. Health professionals dealing with these patients employ motivational client-centred interventions to enable them to be more insightful and more willing to change One can use expressions such as: "I understand the difficulty you have in stopping or reducing substance use. I am here to help and work with you to deal with the problem, and step by step you will be able to overcome the problem and recover".

Clinicians should also be sensitized to the epidemiological data, risk factors and consequences of substance misuse. As stated in previous sections, substance misuse is among the 20 risk factors for death and disability worldwide.[50] The harmful effects of substance misuse are not limited to dependent misuse. Hazardous or harmful substance use are also associated with a wide variety of social, financial, legal and relationship problems for individuals and their families, and their burden may be greater than that associated with dependent use.[51] Occasional or non-problematic use can be defined as "lower risk"; "moderate risk" is associated with more regular use; and "high risk" with dependence. It is relatively easy for clinicians to identify "high-risk" or dependent users, but primary care workers should be familiar with screening and brief interventions techniques for dealing with low- and moderate-risk users. These techniques are also useful for helping these substance misusers, who are often not motivated to ask for help on their own.[51]

In order to increase the likelihood of obtaining patient consent to screening and give accurate answers about substance use, health professionals should:[51]

- show that they are listening carefully
- be friendly and non-judgemental
- show sensitivity and empathy
- provide information about screening
- carefully explain the reasons for asking about substance use

- maintain confidentiality
- link the screening proposed to the presenting complaint (where it is relevant)
- be flexible and sensitive to patient needs.

There is evidence for an association between duration of treatment and improved outcomes. Primary care staff are reminded that imposing arbitrary time limits on treatment duration does not enhance treatment outcomes.[52,53]

The key stakeholders necessary to deliver the "gold standard approach"

Substance misuse is a complex condition that affects different strata of society. These problems are not confined to addiction, but are also relevant to sporadic use. The treatment gap for substance use disorders remains considerable, despite the availability of cost-effective prevention and treatment programmes.[10] Therefore, programmes and strategies to mitigate the effects of substance misuse require the participation of broad sectors of society.

According to WHO,[54] 51.5% of countries have specialized treatment services as the main setting for the treatment of drug use disorders; and only 10% of countries report primary care to be the most commonly used setting for treatment of alcohol and drug use disorders. In low-income countries, mental health services are the main setting for treatment of alcohol and drug use disorder, and specialized treatment services gain importance as a country's income level rises.

Nongovernmental organizations and self-help movements are crucial in closing the intervention gap by preventing harmful use of alcohol and drugs, aggravation of dependency syndromes and subsequent health and social consequences; they are also important for rehabilitation strategies.[55] Self-help groups provide free support and are easily accessible, and patients can learn to self-regulate their emotional responses and behaviour, based on their own needs. The primary care team, including medical practitioners, nurses, psychologists and social workers, should have a major role in screening for substance use, detecting early disease stages, and hazardous and harmful use of alcohol, while psychiatrists and addiction specialists, should be involved in the treatment of more severe cases.[55]

Likewise, primary care staff can conduct activities in conjunction with self-help groups and civil associations. The joint actions can ensure that a larger sector of the population has adequate awareness to generate a social climate conducive to healthy lifestyles, and thus a smaller number of subjects would use addictive substances, thus closing the treatment gap.

Health promotion and prevention of drug misuse in primary care

Primary care offers optimal opportunities for promoting a healthy lifestyle and well-being and for prevention of substance misuse. While the evidence for what works in this setting is minimal, good approaches have been introduced and evaluated. Importantly these issues have been addressed in the WHO global *mental health Gap Action Programme* (mhGAP).[56]

Substance misuse is the most preventable mental health problem, and primary care is the optimal setting for delivering preventative interventions. In a brief overview, Medina-Mora (2005) referred to the Declaration of Demand Reduction that recognized the need to:[57]

- assess the problem, in order to base prevention on a regular evaluation of the nature and magnitude of substance abuse and related consequences
- tackle the problem, from discouraging initial use to reducing the negative health and social consequences, education, public awareness, early intervention, after-care and social reintegration, early assistance and access to services for those in need
- forge partnerships, through the promotion of a community-wide participatory and partnership approach as the basis for accurate assessment of the problem and formulation and implementation of appropriate programmes, integrated into broader social welfare and health-promotion policies and preventive education programmes

- focus on special needs of the population in general and of specific subgroups, with an emphasis on youth
- send the right message (the information utilized in educational and prevention programmes should be clear, scientifically accurate and reliable, culturally valid, timely and, where possible, tested on a target population).

The scope of prevention includes selective preventive interventions aimed at subgroups of the population whose risk of developing the disorder is significantly higher than average. The preventive interventions indicated target high-risk individuals who are identified as having minimal but detectable early signs or symptoms of the disorder. Early intervention with individuals who have experimented with substances but are not severely dependent and may therefore be "re-educated" through learning interventions is recommneded, as well as treatment of dependence, relapse prevention and social reintegration.

The evidence base for what works advocates the use of multiple-component programmes (school, family, community),[58] particularly if they are incorporated into a wider perspective of healthy lifestyles rather than emphasizing what is forbidden or dangerous. As summarized by Medina-Mora,[57] information alone has proved to be insufficient and better results have been observed when programmes include skills training components and when they can intervene in more than one of the steps in the chain from substance availability to having the opportunity to use substances, experimenting, continuous use, and different levels of dependence and abstinence.

The US National Institute of Drug Abuse has developed a list of principles for prevention, drawn from long-term research studies on the origins of substance abuse behaviours and the common elements of effective prevention programmes.[59] These include the following:

- prevention programmes should enhance protective factors and reverse or reduce risk factors, and while risk and protective factors can affect people of all groups, they may have a different effect depending on a person's age, sex, ethnicity, culture, and environment
- programmes should be tailored to address risks specific to population characteristics
- prevention programmes should be long term, with repeated interventions (i.e. booster programmes) to reinforce the original prevention goals.

Implementing these interventions in primary care involves improving capacity for screening, early detection and diagnosis and providing appropriate interventions within an integrated health and social care pathway for people with substance misuse, including those with comorbid mental health problems, who are particularly vulnerable. The latency between the onset of the primary mental disorder and that of the subsequent substance dependence gives a window of opportunity for preventive interventions: for most mental disorders, this latency period is 5–8 years.[57]

Commissioning services for mental disorders and coexisting substance misuse

A "dual diagnosis" of mental disorders and coexisting substance misuse is recognized as being common in both mental health and drug/alcohol misuse services. Service users with such problems have increased rates of service use, and worse clinical and social outcomes. Drug or alcohol misuse may exacerbate mental health problems; equally, psychiatric disorders can lead to problematic drug or alcohol use. Assessing which condition is the "primary" or "secondary" diagnosis can be difficult and can act as a barrier to accessing services, potentially leaving service users to "fall between the gaps".

The challenge for commissioners to overcome barriers relies on commissioning and developing services that can provide accurate assessment of individual need, shared/integrated care pathways, evidence-based skills mix and operational knowledge of local services.

For this reason, commissioners need to ensure dual diagnosis has a high profile when services are commissioned and that the needs of the individual are paramount within flexible treatment systems that can address complex and changing needs.

The commissioning cycle

The usual commissioning cycle should be followed. It is important that local definitions of dual diagnosis are initially agreed by all relevant agencies. A comprehensive needs assessment of the population to ascertain the scale and nature of the need for dual diagnosis should be undertaken; gaps in provision should be identified; and a suitable model that takes account of the local need, context and treatment systems should be designed and agreed.

Where services are commissioned for drug and alcohol use or mental health problems, commissioners should ensure the specification is clear about the requirement to meet the needs of dual diagnosis of service users, with appropriate evidence-based interventions relevant to the treatment tier (including primary care, tier 1 of the models of care of the service)[60] and that the skill set of the workforce is adequate to meet the need identified.

Skills

Guidance about appropriate staff capabilities to meet dual diagnosis need can be found in the publication *Closing the gap*.[61] Opportunities are explored for developing flexible partnerships with a variety of organizations to meet the training and support needs of the workforce in providing safe and effective care to service users with a dual diagnosis.[62]

The abilities of provider staff to screen, accurately assess (including risk assessment) and build care plans, provide appropriate interventions, follow-up assertively, and provide after-care/reintegration opportunities should be the main priority and clearly outlined in the service specifications.

The training needs of primary care staff should be included in dual diagnosis training strategies. They need to be clear about the level of comorbidity their service can safely address, when to ask for help, and how to access drug and alcohol or mental health services when appropriate.

Training costs can be reduced by joint funding between organizations and areas or by "skill sharing", where staff from drugs projects train mental health teams and vice versa. This has the added benefit of eroding some of the barriers and misunderstandings between services. Higher-level education courses on dual diagnosis are now available at some colleges, and provider agencies should be encouraged to take up this specialist training.

Where appropriate, some areas may wish to consider dual diagnosis "champions" within services, who raise awareness and take steps to ensure the workforce is adequately skilled.

Multi-agency working

It is often the case that multiple agencies are involved in the care of an individual with dual diagnosis. It is therefore important that communications are regular and clear, multi-agency reviews are undertaken, and appropriate referrals are made to services, with clearly understood criteria. Criteria need to be inclusive not exclusive of people with complex needs such as dual diagnosis. Joint working arrangements should be clear and protocols in place.

Integrated care pathways should be developed and made clear to all stakeholders, including service users themselves.

The primary outcomes for these initiatives are based on the premise that improving the commissioning and contractual agreements will improve services for patients with a dual diagnosis. Improvements made in the commissioning processes and systems will lead to better outcomes and create efficiencies in the system.

Conclusions and future opportunities

Substance misuse is a common mental health problem in individuals presenting in primary care. However, it is often hidden and goes undetected by primary care health professionals. This is attributed to the stigma attached to substance misuse, particularly illicit drug use, and to insufficient clinical and therapeutic skills and competencies in the primary care team. Once recognized, these patients can be treated, in view of the availability of effective psychosocial and pharmacological interventions. Again, the lack of capacity in therapeutic interventions in primary care staff is a major barrier for minimal provision.

Treatment of substance misuse in primary care settings is a major global priority for scaling-up treatment and preventative interventions, and for addressing the treatment gap and implementing the recommendation of the WHO mhGAP programme.[56] This is imperative action for implementation in all countries, particularly low-income ones; there is a serious shortage of specialist services and skilled health-care professionals in low-income countries, who are often restricted to working in custodial institutional care settings.

There is a dire need for a global initiative to address the unmet treatment needs of people with substance misuse disorder, on par with other mental disorders as recommended by the WHO-Wonca global programme for integrating mental health care into primary care.[19]

Integrating mental health and substance misuse services into primary care generates good health and social outcomes at reasonable costs. It is imperative that general primary care systems are strengthened by their integration with secondary mental health and specialist substance misuse services, as well as social care for recovery and improvement to patients' quality of life.

References

1   *Lexicon of alcohol and drug terms*. Geneva, World Health Organization, 2004 (http://whqlibdoc.who.int/publications/9241544686.pdf, accessed 6 December 2011).

2   *Neuroscience of psychoactive substance use and dependence*. Geneva, World Health Organization, 2004. (http://www.who.int/substance_abuse/publications/en/Neuroscience.pdf, accessed 6 December 2011).

3   Crocq MA. Historical and cultural aspects of man's relationship with addictive drugs. *Dialogues in Clinical Neuroscience*, 2007, 9:355–361.

4   Kessler RC et al. The global burden of mental disorders: an update from the WHO World Mental Health (WMH) surveys. *Epidemiologia e Psichiatria Sociale*, 2009, 18:23–33.

5   *Diagnostic and statistical manual of mental disorders*, 4th ed, text revision (DSM-IV-TR). Washington, American Psychiatric Association, 2000.

6   Kessler RC et al. Lifetime prevalence and age-of-onset distributions of mental disorders in the World Health Organization's World Mental Health Survey Initiative. *World Psychiatry*, 2007, 6(3):168–176.

7   Degenhardt L et al. Toward a global view of alcohol, tobacco, cannabis, and cocaine use: findings from the WHO World Mental Health Surveys. *PLoS Medicine*, 2008, 5:e141.

8   United Nations Office on Drugs and Crime. *World Drug Report 2010*. New York, United Nations Publication Sales, 2010 (http://www.unodc.org/documents/wdr/WDR_2010/World_Drug_Report_2010_lo-res.pdf, accessed 6 December 2011).

9   Wang PS et al. Use of mental health services for anxiety, mood, and substance disorders in 17 countries in the WHO world mental health surveys. *The Lancet*, 2007, 370(9590):841–550.

10 Wang PS, Angermeyer M, Borges G. 2007. Delay and failure in treatment seeking after first onset of mental disorders in the World Health Organization's World Mental Health Survey Initiative. *World Psychiatry*, 2007, 6:177–185.

11 Abou-Saleh MT, Janca A. The epidemiology of substance misuse and comorbid psychiatric disorders. *Acta Neuropsychatrica*, 2004, 16:3–8.

12 *Drug misuse: psychosocial intervention*. London, National Institute for Health and Clinical Excellence, 2007 (CG51) (http://www.nice.org.uk/nicemedia/live/11812/35975/35975.pdf, accessed 6 December 2011).

13 Frisher M et al. Substance misuse and psychiatric illness: prospective observational study using the general practice research database. Journal of *Epidemiology and Community Health*, 2005, 59(10):847–850.

14 Kumpfer KL, Bluth B. Parent/child transactional processes predictive of resilience or vulnerability to "substance abuse disorders". *Substance Use and Misuse*, 2004, 39:671–698.

15 Prescott CA, Madden PA, Stallings MC. Challenges in genetic studies of the etiology of substance use and substance use disorders: introduction to the special issue. *Behavior Genetics*, 2006, 36:473–482.

16 Dackis C, O'Brien C. Neurobiology of addiction: treatment and public policy ramifications. *Nature Neuroscience*, 2005, 8:1431–1436.

17 Volkow ND et al. Reinforcing effects of psychostimulants in humans are associated with increases in brain dopamine and occupancy of D(2) receptors. Journal of Pharmacology and Experimental Therapeutics, 1999, 291:409–415.

18 Lingford-Hughes A, Nutt D. Neurobiology of addiction and implications for treatment. *British Journal of Psychiatry*, 2003, 182:97–100.

19 *The World Health report 2008. Now more than ever.* Geneva, World Health Organization, 2008 (http://www.who.int/whr/2008/en/, accessed 12 December 2011).

20 World Health Organization and Wonca. *Integrating mental health into primary care. A global perspective.* Geneva, World Health Organization, 2008.

21 Abou-Saleh MT, Miller J. The management of drug misuse in primary care. *Primary Care Psychiatry*, 1999, 5:49–56.

22 Strang J et al. The prescribing of methadone and other opioids to addicts: national survey of GPs in England and Wales. *British Journal of General Practice*, 2005, 55:444–451.

23 Abou-Saleh MT. Substance use disorders: recent advances in treatment and models of care. *Journal of Psychosomatic Research*, 2006, 61:305–310.

24 Lawrinson P et al. Key findings from the WHO collaborative study on substitution therapy for opioid dependence and HIV/AIDS. *Addiction*, 2008, 103(9):1484–1492.

25 Greenwood J. Creating a new drug service in Edinburgh. *BMJ*, 1990, 300:587–589.

26 Hutchinson SJ et al. One-year follow-up of opiate injectors treated with oral methadone in a GP-centred programme. *Addiction*, 2000, 95:1055–1068.

27 Chisholm D et al.; Lancet Global Mental Health Group. Scale up services for mental disorders: a call for action. *The Lancet*, 2007, 370:1241–1252.

28 Benegal V, Chand PK, Obot IS. Packages of care for alcohol use disorders in low- and middle-income countries. *PLoS Medicine*, 2009, 6:e1000170.

29 Department of Health and the Devolved Administrations. *Drug misuse and dependence: UK guidelines on clinical management.* London: The Department of Health (England), The Scottish Government, Welsh Assembly Government and Northern Ireland Executive, 2007 (http://www.nta.nhs.uk/uploads/clinical_guidelines_2007.pdf, accessed 6 December 2011).

30 *Drug misuse: psychosocial interventions.* London, National Institute for Health and Clinical Excellence, 2007 (CG51) (http://guidance.nice.org.uk/CG51, accessed 12 December 2011).

31 *Drug misuse: opioid detoxification.* London, National Institute for Health and Clinical Excellence, 2007 (CG52) (http://guidance.nice.org.uk/CG52, accessed 12 December 2011).

32 Psychosis with coexisting substance misuse. London, National Institute for Health and Clinical Excellence, 2011 (CG120) (http://www.nice.org.uk/guidance/CG120/NICEGuidance, accessed 12 December 2011).

33 Abou-Saleh MT. Dual diagnosis: management within a psychosocial context. *Advances in Psychiatric Treatment*, 2004, 10:352–360.

34 *Psychosis with coexisting substance misuse.* London: National Institute for Health and Clinical Excellence, 2011 (CG120) (http://www.nice.org.uk/nicemedia/live/13414/53691/53691.pdf, accessed 6 December 2011).

35 Sharma VK et al. The Global Mental Health Assessment Tool–Primary Care Version (GMHAT/PC). Development, reliability and validity. *World Psychiatry*, 2004, 3:115–119.

36 Sharma VK et al. The Global Mental Health Assessment Tool-validation in Hindi: a validity and feasibility study. *Indian Journal of Psychiatry*, 2010, 52:316–319.

37 Sharma VK et al. Mental health diagnosis by nurses using the Global Mental Health Assessment Tool: a validity and feasibility study. *British Journal of General Practice*, 2008, 58:411–416.

38 Patel V et al. Treatment and prevention of mental disorders in low-income and middle-income countries. *The Lancet*, 2007, 370:991–1005.

39 Prochaska JO, Norcross JC, DiClemente CC. *Changing for good: the revolutionary program that explains the six stages of change and teaches you how to free yourself from bad habits.* New York, W Morrow, 1994.

40 *Mental Health in Scotland. "The Matrix". A Guide to delivering evidence-based psychological therapies in Scotland.* Edinburgh, The Scottish Government, 2008 (http://www.evidenceintopractice.scot.nhs.uk/media/131943/nes-matrix.pdf, accessed 6 December 2011).

41 *Psychological therapies matrix – February 2009.* Edinburgh, The Scottish Government, 2009 (http://www.scotland.gov.uk/Topics/Health/health/mental-health/servicespolicy/matrixfeb2009, accessed 12 December 2011).

42 *Naltrexone for the management of opioid dependence.* London: National Institute for Health and Clinical Excellence, 2007 (CG115) (http://www.nice.org.uk/nicemedia/live/11604/33812/33812.pdf, accessed 6 December 2011).

43 *Methadone and buprenorphine for the management of opioid dependence.* London: National Institute for Health and Clinical Excellence, 2007 (CG114) (http://www.nice.org.uk/nicemedia/live/11606/33833/33833.pdf).

44 Substance Misuse Management in General Practice (http://www.smmgp.org.uk/index.php, accessed 6 December 2011).

45 *Reviewed shared care arrangements for drug misusers.* London; Department of Health, 1995 (Executive letter; EL (95)114.

46 Winstock AR, Ford C, Witton J. Assessment and management of cannabis use disorders in primary care. *BMJ*, 2010, 340:c1571.

47 Lader M, Tylee A, Donoghue J. Withdrawing benzodiazepines in primary care. *CNS Drugs*, 2009, 23:19–34.

48 Schweizer E et al. Carbamazepine treatment in patients discontinuing long-term benzodiazepine therapy. Effects on withdrawal severity and outcome. *Archives of General Psychiatry*, 1991, 48:448–452.

49 Denis C et al. Pharmacological interventions for benzodiazepine mono-dependence management in outpatient settings. *Cochrane Database of Systematic Reviews*, 2006, (3):CD005194.

50 *Global health risks: mortality and burden of disease attributable to selected major risks.* Geneva, World Health Organization, 2009.

51 Humeniuk RE et al. World Health Organization 2010 *Brief intervention. The ASSIST-linked brief intervention for hazardous and harmful substance use. Manual for use in primary care.* Geneva, World Health Organization, 2010 (whqlibdoc.who.int/publications/2010/9789241599399_eng.pdf, accessed 12 December 2011).

52 Brewer DD et al. A meta-analysis of predictors of continued drug use during and after treatment for opiate addiction. *Addiction*, 1998, 93:73–92.

53 Magura S et al. Program quality effects on patient outcomes during methadone maintenance: a study of 17 clinics. *Substance Use and Misuse*, 1999, 34:1299–1324.

54 Babor TF, Stenius K. Treatment of substance use disorders within health services. In: *WHO ATLAS on substance use. Resources for the prevention and treatment of substance use disorders.* Geneva, World Health Organization, 2010:23–55 (www.who.int/substance_abuse/activities/msbatlaschtwo.pdf, accessed 13 December 2011).

55 Medina-Mora ME. Can science help close the treatment gap? *Addiction*, 2010, 105:15–16.

56 *mhGAP: Mental Health Gap Action Programme: scaling up care for mental, neurological and substance use disorders.* Geneva, World Health Organization, 2008.

57 Medina-Mora ME. Prevention of substance abuse: a brief overview. *World Psychiatry*, 2005, 4:25–30.

58 National Institute on Drug Abuse. *Preventing drug use among children and adolescents. A research-based guide.* Rockville, National Institute on Drug Abuse, 1997 (NIH Publication No. 97-4212).

59 National Institute on Drug Abuse, National Institutes of Health US Department of Health and Human Services. *Principles of drug addiction treatment: a research-based guide.* Rockville, National Institute on Drug Abuse, 2009 (NIH Publication No. 09-4180) (http://www.nida.nih.gov/podat/podatindex.html, accessed 13 December 2011).

60 *Models of care for treatment of adult drug misusers: Update 2006.* London, National Treatment Agency for Substance Misuse, 2006 (http://www.nta.nhs.uk/uploads/nta_modelsofcare_update_2006_moc3.pdf, accessed 13 December 2011).

61 Hughes L. *Closing the gap: a capability framework for working effectively with combined mental health and substance misuse problems (dual diagnosis)*. Lincoln, Centre for Clinical and Academic Workforce Innovation, 2006 (http://eprints.lincoln.ac.uk/729/1/uoa12eh05.pdf, accessed 6 December 2011).

62 Care Services Improvement Partnership. *Dual diagnosis; developing capable practitioners to improve services and increase positive service user experience*. London, Department of Health and Care Services Improvement Partnership, 2008 (http://www.nmhdu.org.uk/silo/files/developing-capable-practitioners-to-improve-services.pdf, accessed 6 December 2011).

Part VII

Childhood disorders in primary care mental health

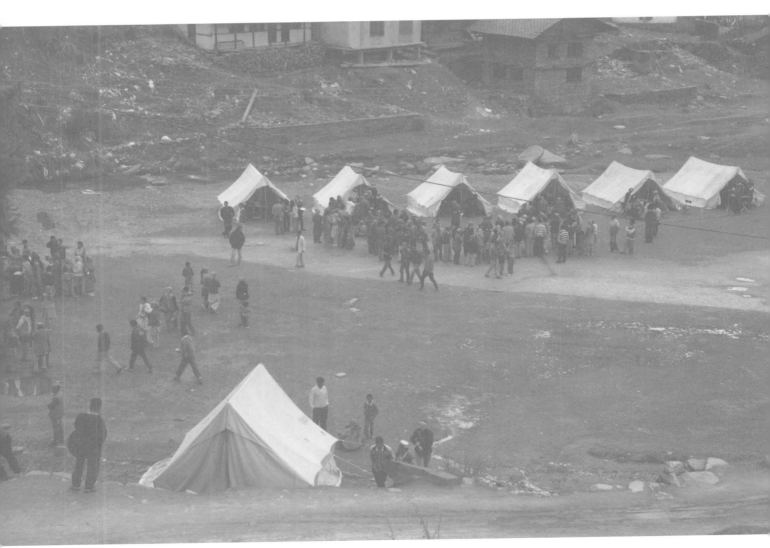

27 Development and psychopathology in infancy and early childhood

Jen-Yu Chou and Jung-Chia Su

Key messages

- The infant–parent relationship has a decisive influence on infants' mental health and development. Assessment and intervention are therefore important for a young child before maladaptive behaviour patterns emerge and the development is derailed.

- From the start of pregnancy, maternal mental status can have profound impact on the fetal brain. After birth, the brain development of infants is continuously affected by the experience of relating to their parents.

- Parents' early experience with their own caregiver and how they make sense of it influence their ability to take on parenting roles.

- Each child has unique temperament traits. The match or mismatch between the child's temperament and that of the parents has crucial impact on parenting and parent–child interaction.

- Assessment of infants and young children should include information regarding pregnancy, birth, social support, parental mental health, the infant's social-emotional development, parent–child relationship, the child's individual characteristics and other developmental risk factors.

Introduction

Human development takes place not in a vacuum but within multiple contexts, which include the constitutional contexts of an infant's temperament, sensory processing and neurobiology; the environmental contexts of family, community and culture; and the mediating context of the infant–caregiver relationship.[1] Directly or indirectly, these contexts dynamically interact with one another and are therefore continuously changing.[1]

With a particular set of inborn tendencies, the infant transforms continuously through interaction with the environment, which, in turn, is challenged and changed by the infant.[2] When a child encounters environmental or constitutional difficulties and tries to adapt, deviation from the normal developmental framework may occur and psychopathologies may develop.[3]

Since all humans start life as babies whose survival is dependent on a caring adult,[4] the infant–caregiver relationship works as a mediator between the contexts of development.[5] Simultaneously moulding and being moulded by other contexts, the infant–caregiver relationship shapes an infant's normal development and the formation of psychopathology, and is therefore the major focus of assessment and intervention in the contexts that can be changed and thus be subject to clinical intervention.[6]

This chapter focuses on the developmental contexts, psychopathologies in infancy and early childhood, and assessment and early intervention in primary health care. Because of the inconsistency in literature regarding definition of an age range, infancy and early childhood in this chapter broadly refer to those who are aged under 4 or 5 years.

The infant–caregiver relationship

The adaptive relationship

During the first year of life, an infant's emotional self-regulation is largely dependent on the caregiver's affect-related vocal and facial mirroring to the infant's behaviour.[7] When experiencing unbearable body sensations, urges or feelings, the infant needs, and usually elicits, the caregiver's assistance to resume to a calm state.[8] This mutual regulation has been understood by various authors as attunement,[9] mirroring,[10] containing,[11] or holding.[12]

It is important for parents to respond to their infant's affect expression by accurately producing the same expression and therefore mirroring the infant's internal experience; to differentiate fantasy from reality, the infant needs the parents to mirror in a playful, or marked manner.[13] This capability of marked mirroring supports the infant's feeling of security and capacity for self-regulation,[14] gradually allowing the infant to reflect on himself as an intentional being,[15] to develop an internal sense of hopefulness and curiosity,[16] and to think his own thoughts and feel his own feelings.[17] This "mentalizing" capacity, emerging from a relationship that is adaptive to the infant's need, provides strong support for development and protection against trauma.[18]

Attachment

Attachment theory explains a systematic method to assess and classify the parent–child relationship.[19] Since the work of Bowlby,[19] four categories of attachment have been identified: secure, avoidant, ambivalent/resistant and disorganized.[20,21]

A securely attached child is able to explore while using the caregiver as a secure base and becomes distressed when separated from the caregiver, but can be consoled and explore again after reunion.[20] Children in this category demonstrate higher self-esteem and positive affect and more harmonious connections with siblings and other adults.[22,23]

Children with insecure attachment patterns show limited (avoidant) or extreme (ambivalent) emotions when the mother is absent. At reunion, they run away from the mother or are difficult to comfort. Insecure attachments are associated with depression, anxiety, hostility and psychosomatic illness in later development.[24] Among the three types of insecure attachment, disorganized attachment is probably the most concerning. Children with disorganized attachment do not establish coherent attachment strategies and show disoriented behaviours. Disorganized attachment in infancy is found to be highly associated with hostility and aggression in later development.[25]

Intergenerational transmission of relationship

Infants internalize the experiences with their primary caregivers and carry them into later relationships.[26] Caregivers who were traumatized in infancy may be unable to respond appropriately to their infant's anxiety or engage in intrusive behaviours. It is well accepted that the way in which parents make sense of their own childhood experience has a profound effect on how they parent their children.[27] Affected by their internalized malevolent attachment figures or a past traumatic experiences, the caregiver is unable to see the actual infant and to establish a secure attachment.[28,29] As a result, their early attachment patterns transmit to the attachment type of their infants.[30]

Environmental contexts

Pregnancy

Pregnancy is an extraordinary situation for a woman and can be a stressful time for all parents.[31] During pregnancy, the mother experiences a vast number of rapid changes in her biological, psychological and social conditions.[32] This period of time has a great and lasting impact on the well-being of both mother and infant.

For example, the mother's representations of attachment during pregnancy predicts her infant's attachment pattern one year postpartum.[33]

While pregnancy is a risk factor for mental disorders in women, mothers with previous or current mental disorders are at particular risk in the adaptation to pregnancy.[34] The combined point prevalence ranges from 6.5% to 12.9% for depression at different trimesters of pregnancy,[35] and from 3% to 7% for post-traumatic stress disorder (PTSD).[36]

In addition, anxieties caused by unintended pregnancy, previous abortion and concerns about infertility[37] may also make the pregnancy overwhelming for the mother[38] and interfere with the infant's later attachment.[39] For women with severe or multiple risk factors, immediate intervention may be required.

Family and parental functioning

Maladaptive parenting

When the caregiver is withdrawn, intrusive or unpredictable, the infant may develop early defence mechanisms that have detrimental effects.[40] To gain attention from the unresponsive (lack of mirroring) caregiver, the infant may intensify his efforts and appear aggressive.[41] The infant may also subsequently respond to new situations anticipating that disruptive behaviour is necessary to gain attention. The infant may, alternatively, become precociously self-sufficient, overly controlling and unable to get in touch with feelings of dependency.[42]

Infants may become withdrawn and passive in order to maintain a feeling of continuity and security with intrusive parents,[43] and have poor affect regulation with parents who over-identify with the child's perspective (lack of marking).[44] All of these may be predictive of aggression, depression and other psychopathology.[45]

Adolescent mothers

Although some research has shown that adolescent mothers are less sensitive and responsive to their infants,[46] adolescents vary widely in parenting behaviours.[47] For example, although the requirements of parenting are usually in conflict with teenagers' developmental needs, some adolescent mothers find motherhood an achievement that they are unable to find elsewhere.[48] Furthermore, in some countries adolescent motherhood is the norm. It is therefore important for clinicians to consider the unique internal and external resources of each individual adolescent mother, including their possible underprivileged background, which may compound the perinatal and postpartum stress.[49] It is also important to pay attention to their relationships with the father of the infant, which determines the father's involvement and mediates between father–child contact and child functioning,[49] and relationships with their own mother, which can be a major resource of support, advice and modelling.[50]

Mental disorders in parents

Maternal depression

While as many as 80% of new mothers experience "postpartum blues",[51] 19.2% of women have a major depressive episode during the first 3 months postpartum.[35] Mothers with depression may be unresponsive, intrusive or unpredictable. This impaired maternal functioning contributes to adverse infant development and later psychopathology.[52] It is therefore very important for primary health practitioners to identify maternal depression as early as possible.

Maternal substance abuse

Maternal substance abuse has been a widespread concern through the world.[53] For example, approximately 10% of neonates in the United States of America are exposed to alcohol and 5% to illicit drugs.[54] Maternal substance abuse has a detrimental impact on infant development, through effects on the fetus[55] and impairment of parental functioning.[56] For example, children who are frequently left with multiple temporary caretakers while their parents pursue drug use may have insecure attachment and develop indiscriminate sociability.[54]

Exposure to violence

It is estimated that 300 million children worldwide are victims of sexual exploitation, domestic violence, armed conflicts or other forms of abuse.[57] Furthermore, the media and Internet have become increasingly important sources of exposure to violence.[58] Young children in particular are unable to distinguish media presentations from real experiences. These exposures to violent trauma, maltreatment and violence are associated with various developmental, emotional and behavioural problems.[59–61]

Children in the first years of life are the most vulnerable, not only because the majority of abuse happens during these years but also because exposure to violence during this time has severe impacts on the developing brain and mind.[62] Furthermore, since very young children experience the world from the maternal holding environment,[63] violence or war that affect the mother's ability to provide safety or that separate the infant from the mother will put the child at serious risk.[64]

Because parental functioning has the potential to inhibit or promote infant regulation and resilience,[65] profound damage to almost all areas of subsequent development takes place when the caregiver is the source of threat.[66] Therefore, it is important for primary health practitioners to evaluate parents' behaviour, their mental state and their awareness of their child's condition in situations involved with violence.[67]

The school, community, culture and policy

The broader environmental contexts of housing quality, neighbourhood, preschool, community, culture, and policy are also important.[68] Poverty, low socioeconomic status (SES) and residence in an economically disadvantaged neighbourhood each independently predict children's poor cognitive functioning and higher levels of social-emotional problems.[69]

Poverty and environmental risks

Children growing up in poverty are exposed to a higher likelihood of parental divorce,[70] poor parenting,[71] family disruption,[72] crime in their neighbourhood,[73] aggressive peers,[74] poor social support,[75] less parental involvement in school,[76] poor quality of child care[77] and impoverished library, computer, Internet,[78] and other home learning resources.[79]

Physically, they are also exposed to more noise, toxins and pollution;[68] more likely to live in accommodation of poor quality,[80] or located in areas under threat of natural disasters;[81] and more likely to have greater exposure to television,[82] insufficient nutrition,[83] and hazardous street traffic.[84]

Furthermore, mothers with a low income may have limited childcare options. While there is no consistent finding regarding the relationship between preschool types and child development,[85] the quality of preschool provision does have a strong impact on cognitive and social development.[86] Exposure to one or more of the above-mentioned risk factors has been found by a large number of research studies to have detrimental effects on children's cognitive, social-emotional and physical well-being.[87]

Foster care

Prior to entering a foster family, foster children often experience disruptions from primary caregivers, who they are simultaneously connected to and fearful of.[88] The confused child is likely to have patterns of behaviour that are confusing to the foster parents.

Non-attachment and indiscriminate sociability are common presentations.[89] Because of the disruption and the earlier maltreatment experience, infants and toddlers in foster care may have difficulty in forming new relationships.[90] For every foster parent, therefore, forming a way to communicate and to become the child's "go-to person" is a goal of prime priority.[91] Indiscriminate sociability, overly familiar behaviours with strangers for example, is also common among children in foster care, especially when there are or have been multiple placements or multiple caregivers.

Constitutional contexts

Neurobiology

It has been widely accepted that the basic structure of the brain develops in the early months of fetal life and that changes in connectivity and function occur in the first postnatal years.[92] While a diverse repertoire of synapses with complex and idiosyncratic patterns develops during the very early stages of life, the strength of synaptic connections is selectively modified later by experiences, including the quality and quantity of internal and external stimuli.[93] Therefore, starting from a very early stage in pregnancy, maternal mental status may have profound impact on the fetal brain.[92] Although a detailed account of fetal and infant neurobiology is beyond the scope of this chapter, it is important to note that not only the child's genetic make-up but also his/ her experiences play significant roles in brain development,[2,94] and thus early intervention could significantly alter the trajectory of a psychopathology.

Sensory processing

The way in which the nervous system receives, interprets and responds to internal and external sensory stimuli differs from person to person.[95] From birth onwards, an infant's responses to touch, taste, movement, sight, sound and body position continuously affect their caregiver's understanding and response.[96] It is difficult for parents to understand children with abnormalities of sensory processing. For example, a hypersensitive infant may seem fearful/cautious or negative/defiant; a hyposensitive infant may look uninterested; a sensory-seeking infant may appear impulsive.[97] Therefore, the sensory-processing abnormalities cause symptoms (e.g. difficulties in sleep, eating, emotion) both directly and through interfering with the infant–caregiver relationship.

Temperament

Temperament, the constitutional differences in emotion, attention, negative reactivity, self-regulation, sociability, rhythmicity and activity level that make each child unique,[89] are noticeable early in life.[99] Research has shown that specific temperament traits have direct or indirect effects on a child's behaviour problems and social functioning.[100]

It has been increasingly accepted that a child's temperament influences parenting and parent–child interactions,[101] and that the match or mismatch of the child's temperament with the caregiver plays an important role. Several factors might moderate the effects of temperament on social development. For example, changes in parenting may lead to changes in child temperament;[102] one component of the temperament (e.g. capacity for self-regulation) may enable the child to moderate another component (e.g. negative reactivity).

Prematurity

Premature birth can be a traumatic event for parents, leading to long-term anxiety, depression,[103] and PTSD reactions.[104] They often experience the infant's birth as a sudden interruption that is too shocking and painful to think of.

Firstly, the child's health is constantly threatened by uncertainties, which may delay their parents' psychological[105] or material investment[106] in the infant. Second, the parents may feel less intimacy with the preterm infant, who has limited ability to engage, or they may misunderstand the infant's behaviour as rejecting. Third, the mother may feel guilty for failing to carry the infant to term,[107] and thus become withdrawn in order to avoid guilty feelings, or she may intrusively search for reassuring responses from the infant. All of these are harmful to the formation[108] and maintenance[109] of parent–infant attachment.

Therefore, preterm infants are subject not only to the profound changes occurring in their brain,[110] and the intrusive medical procedures that inflict pain, stress and separation from parents,[111] but also to parents who are overwhelmed by uncertainties brought about by their birth.

Overall, children born preterm demonstrate difficulties in cognitive, attention, sensory and motor functions,[112] as well as withdrawal behaviour and difficulties with self-regulation in infancy.[113] These problems also persist into childhood[114] and adolescence.[115]

Autism and mental retardation in infancy

In the first[116] and second[117] years of life, infants with autistic disorders show atypical social interaction (e.g. eye contact and joint attention), sensory processing and motor development, patterns of temperament (e.g. marked passivity and decreased positive affect and activity level), repetitive movements, posturing or mannerisms, and delayed language expression and comprehension.

In spite of the fact that many parents have concerns about these manifestations,[118] and that children with autism can be reliably diagnosed by 2 years of age,[119] there is still a significant delay in identification and intervention, partly because of the diagnostic difficulties of autism during the early years of life.[120]

Similar delay in identification and intervention is also present with less severe mental retardation, due to parents' uncertainty about "what is normal" and the poor validity and reliability of IQ tests for infancy.[119] This delay, however, is less significant with severe mental retardation, where a higher percentage of instances are associated with genetic syndromes.[121]

Infants and young children with mental retardation or autism may pose significant challenges to parenting and become a source of stress in the family.[122] It is therefore important to evaluate the impact of the disorders on other family members.

The use of screening measures could also help parents as well as primary health clinicians to identify and understand subtle developmental problems and find help. Useful tools for primary practitioners (see Table 27.1) include the Brief Infant Toddler Social and Emotional Assessment (BITSEA)[123] and the Ages and Stages Questionnaires – Social Emotional (ASQ-SE).[124]

Table 27.1 Screening measures for primary health care

Measure	Age range, months	Time to complete, minutes	Areas screened
Ages and Stages Questionnaire – Social Emotional (ASQ-SE)[124]	3–66	10–15	Self-regulation, compliance, communication, adaptive behaviours, autonomy, affect and interaction with people
Brief Infant-Toddler's Social and Emotional Assessment (BITSEA)[123]	12–36	7–10	Emerging social-emotional problems in behaviour, emotions, and relationships, as well as language development across settings

Psychopathologies in infancy and early childhood

Classification

Researchers and clinicians have debated on whether to classify mental disorders in infancy and early childhood.[125] There are three concerns: (1) it is difficult to identify and measure symptoms because of the rapid change during this period;[126] (2) diagnoses locate problems in the infant and neglect the infant–caregiver relationship;[127] and (3) the label of a disorder may have an adverse impact on the child's image.[128]

Nevertheless, a common language is urgently needed because of the growing knowledge of early psychopathologies, the rapidly increasing use of psychopharmacological treatments among young children,[129] and the methodological needs in epidemiology.[130]

The revised version of Zero to Three's *Diagnostic Classification of Mental Health and Developmental Disorders of Infancy and Early Childhood* (*DC: 0–3R*) was designed to address this need.[97] It describes meaningful symptom patterns and related events or developmental features in the first 4 years of life. To make sure that clinicians have the constitutional, environmental and relational contexts in mind, it follows a multi-axial scheme. The five axes focus on clinical disorders (Axis I), relationship classification (Axis II), medical and developmental disorders and conditions (Axis III), psychosocial stressors (Axis IV) and emotional and social functioning (Axis V).

Epidemiology

Accumulating clinical evidence has shown that the social-emotional and behavioural problems identified in children aged 0–3 years persistently impair their development and mental health.[131] However, with the exception of autism,[132] very few studies have investigated the prevalence and course of psychopathology for this age group.[133]

In research based on the Copenhagen Child Cohort 2000,[134] Skovgaard and colleagues identified infants in the community aged under 10 months, with problems in eating (30.0%), sleeping (20.0%), defecation (16.0), gross motor function (14.1%), general development (13.0%), language (11.7%), and mother–child relationship,[135] and children aged 18 months with DC: 0–3 Axis I (18%) diagnosis, including regulatory disorder (7.1%), MSDD (3.3%), disorders of affect (2.7%), eating disorder (2.4%), sleeping disorder (1.4%), and adjustment disorder (0.9%), and with Axis II (8.5%) diagnosis of relationship disorders.[136]

Infant mental health practice in primary health care

Infants and young children are seen regularly in primary health care rather than mental health settings.[137] Primary health-care professionals therefore play a crucial role in infant mental health.

Assessment in a regular health visit

With infants and young children, assessment involves evaluation of both strengths and vulnerabilities[138] in individuals as well as contexts, and does not necessarily require a diagnosis.[139] Starting with the regular prenatal visits, information about pregnancy, social support, and parental mental health can be gathered;[138] during the postpartum period, the evaluation should focus on the infant's social-emotional development, infant–caregiver relationship and other developmental risk factors.

To obtain first-hand information in the "here and now" situation, information gathering involves techniques of routine clinical history taking, empathetic listening, open-ended and specific questions, and participant observation.[137]

Social-emotional development

Young children's behaviours are highly variable. Parents, teachers and other adults tend to have very different experiences of and responses to behaviours in infancy and early childhood.[140] Therefore, assessment should include information from multiple sources.[141] Since parents tend to be unaware of, and thus do not seek help for, their very young children's behavioural problems,[142] the standardized screening tests should be used with caution.[143]

Nevertheless, standardized parent-report screening tests could help identify social-emotional developmental problems,[144] and help primary care providers to become familiar with developmental issues (see Table 27.1). The DC: 0–3R also provides a guideline for assessing emotional and social functioning.

Parental functioning and mental health

Although the child's behaviour rather than parental difficulties is usually the presenting issue in primary health care, it is still important to evaluate parental mental illnesses and parents' ability to actively attend to the infant's anxiety without intrusively imposing their own anxiety on the infant. There are several screening tools that could be used in primary care settings, including The US Preventive Health Task Force Two-Question Depression Screener[145] and The Edinburgh Postnatal Depression Scale.[146]

Routines in a health visit naturally provide good opportunities to observe children's response and parents' function as a "secure base" in stressful situations.[147] When abnormalities in shared attention, mutual regulation, and communication between the parents and the child are noted, it is important to assess the developmental contexts. Although reluctance to talk about sensitive social-emotional issues is common, a good doctor–patient relationship usually help parents express their concerns.[148] It is also common for primary care practitioners to over-identify with the infant and/or the parent and to have strong emotions towards them. While the transference/countertransference situation is informative in understanding the internal conflicts and external struggles of the parents and the child, consultations with or referrals to mental health professionals may be necessary when the emotions are intense.

Intervention and referral

Intervention

It has been well accepted in relation to child development, that adequate and appropriate intervention should be in place as early as possible.[149] In routine practice, primary care practitioners can provide help through various ports of entry.[150] Comments to parents about their interaction with the child could help them to reflect upon their own internal representations and to recognize their child as a dependent but intentional being. Moreover, providing information regarding normal development and problematic behaviours is also an important support for parents with doubts.[137]

Referral

When there are multiple or persistent risks or disturbances, referral to infant mental health professionals is indicated. Since referrals to infant mental health services are frequently associated with difficulties, including financial concerns, limited service availability, physicians' reluctance to present concerns to parents, and stigma regarding mental health services, it is important for primary care practitioners to have a long-term relationship with infant mental health service providers and to accumulate experiences in the referral collaboration.[137]

The role of primary care professional is summarized in Box 27.1.

Box 27.1   What can be done in general practice?

What the GP as a clinician can do

1   Assess parental functioning in routine practice
2   Assess the child's emotional development with the above-mentioned screening tools
3   Assess other environmental, constitutional and relational risk factors
4   Establish a supportive alliance with parents and listen to their concerns
5   Provide information regarding normal child development and problematic behaviour
6   Make referral when necessary

What others in the primary care team (e.g. health visitor etc.) can do

1   Identify environmental, constitutional and relational risk factors early
2   Apply screening tools when necessary
3   Establish a supportive alliance with parents and listen to their concerns
4   Provide information regarding normal child development and problematic behaviours

What the wider community (e.g. social services, schools, playgroups) can do

1   Provide parents in need with financial support
2   Provide better access to medical, psychiatric and child-care services
3   Form supportive groups for parents in the community

What the caregivers can be supported to do

1   To understand and protect the baby's normal developmental need
2   To recognize the baby as a separate but intentional being
3   To separate their own needs from the baby's

Refer to a child psychiatrist or an infant mental health professional when:

1   a severe risk factor or multiple risk factors are noted
2   the child's emotional development is delayed
3   the caregiver's anxiety is intense and cannot be relieved

---

References

1 Zeanah CH. *Handbook of infant mental health*, 3rd ed. New York, Guilford Press, 2009.

2 Jurist EL, Slade A, Bergner S. *Mind to mind: infant research, neuroscience and psychoanalysis*. New York, Other Press, 2008.

3 Fischer KW et al. Psychopathology as adaptive development along distinctive pathways. *Development and Psychopathology*, 1997, 9:749–779.

4 Spitz RA. *The first year of life; a psychoanalytic study of normal and deviant development of object relations*. New York, International Universities Press, 1965.

5 Singer LT et al. Effects of infant risk status and maternal psychological distress on maternal-infant interactions during the first year of life. *Journal of Developmental and Behavioral Pediatrics*, 2003, 24:233–241.

6 Gerhardt S. *Why love matters: how affection shapes a baby's brain*. Hove, East Sussex; New York, Brunner-Routledge, 2004.

7 Beebe B, Lachmann FM. The contribution of mother-infant mutual influence to the origins of self- and object-representations. *Psychoanalytic Psychology*, 1988, 5:32.

8 Bettes BA. Maternal depression and motherese: temporal and intonational features. *Child Development*, 1988, 59:1089–1096.

9 Stern DN. *The interpersonal world of the infant: a view from psychoanalysis and developmental psychology*. New York, Basic Books, 1985.

10 Kohut H. *The analysis of the self*. New York, International Universities Press, 1971.

11 Bion WR. *Elements of psycho-analysis*. New York, Basic Books Pub. Co, 1963.

12 Winnicott DW. The theory of the parent–infant relationship. *International Journal of Psycho-analysis*, 1962, 43:238–239.

13 Fonagy P et al. *Affect regulation, mentalization, and the development of the self*. New York, Other Press, 2002.

14 Bretherton I, Munholland KA. Internal working models in attachment relationship: elaborating a central construct in attachment therory. In: Cassidy J, Shaver PR, eds. *Handbook of attachment: theory, research, and clinical applications*, 2nd ed. New York, Guilford Press, 2008:102–130.

15 Fonagy P, Target M. Mentalization and the changing aims of child psychoanalysis. Psychoanalytic Dialogues, 1998, 8:27.

16 Greenspan SI, Wieder S. *Infant and early childhood mental health: a comprehensive, developmental approach to assessment and intervention*. Washington, DC, American Psychiatric Publications, 2006.

17 Bion WR. *Learning from experience*. London, Heinemann, 1962.

18 Fonagy P, Target M. Attachment, trauma, and pscyhoanalysis: where psychoanalysis meets neuroscience. In: Jurist EL, Slade A, Bergner S, eds. *Mind to mind: infant research, neuroscience and psychoanalysis*. New York, Other Press, 2008:15–49.

19 Bowlby J. *Attachment and loss: Vol. 1: Attachment*. London, Hogarth Press and the Institue of Psycho-Analysis, 1969.

20 Ainsworth M et al. *Patterns of attachment: a psychological study of the strange situation*. Hillsdale, NJ, Lawrence Erlbaum, 1978.

21 Main M, Solomon, J. Procedures for identifying infants as disorganized/disoriented during the Ainsworth Strange Situation. In: Greenberg DC, Cummings EM, eds. *Attachment during the preschool years: theory, research and intervention*. Chicago, University of Chicago Press, 1990:121–160.

22 Volling BL, Belsky J. The contribution of mother–child and father–child relationships to the quality of sibling interaction: a longitudinal study. *Child Development*, 1992, 63:1209–1222.

23 Weinfield N et al. The nature of individual differences in infant–caregiver attachment. In: Shaver JCPR, ed. *Handbook of attachment: theory, research and clinical application*. New York, Guilford, 1999:68–88.

24 Kobak R, Sceery, A. Attachment in late adolescence: working model, affect regulation and perceptions of self and others. *Child Development*, 1988, 59:135–146.

25 Shaw D et al. Early risk factors and pathways in the development of early disruptive behavior problems. *Development and Psychopathology*, 1996, 8:21.

26 Sroufe L, Fleeson, J. The coherence of family relationships. In: Hinde RA, Stevenson-Hinde J, eds. *Relationships within families: mutual influences.* New York, Oxford Press, 1988:27–47.

27 Siegel DJ, Hartzell M. *Parenting from the inside out: how a deeper self-understanding can help you raise children who thrive.* New York, JP Tarcher/Putnam, 2003.

28 Lyons-Ruth K, Jacobvitz D. Attachment disorganization: genetic factors, parenting contexts, and developmental transformation from infancy to adulthood. In: Cassidy J, Shaver PR, editors. *Handbook of attachment: theory, research, and clinical applications,* 2nd ed. New York, Guilford Press, 2008:666–697.

29 Fraiberg S, Adelson E, Shapiro V. Ghosts in the nursery. A psychoanalytic approach to the problems of impaired infant–mother relationships. *Journal of the American Academy of Child Psychiatry,* 1975, 14:387–421.

30 Belsky J. The developmental and evolutionary psychology of intergenerational transmission of attachment. In: Carter CS et al., eds. *Attachment and bonding: a new synthesis.* Cambridge, MA, The MIT Press, 2005:169–198.

31 Stern DN, Bruschweiler-Stern N. *The birth of a mother: how the motherhood experience changes you forever.* New York, BasicBooks, 1998.

32 Slade A et al. The Psychology and psychopathology of pregnancy: reorganization and transformation. In: Zeanah CH, eds. *Handbook of infant mental health,* 3rd ed. New York, Guilford Press, 2009:22–39.

33 Fonagy P, Steele H, Steele M. Maternal representations of attachment during pregnancy predict the organization of infant–mother attachment at one year of age. *Child Development,* 1991, 62:891–905.

34 Condon JT, Corkindale C. The correlates of antenatal attachment in pregnant women. *British Journal of Medical Psychology,* 1997, 70:359–372.

35 Gavin NI et al. Perinatal depression: a systematic review of prevalence and incidence. *Obstetrics and Gynecology,* 2005, 106:1071–1983.

36 Morland L et al. Posttraumatic stress disorder and pregnancy health: preliminary update and implications. *Psychosomatics,* 2007, 48:304–308.

37 Bennetta SM et al. The scope and impact of perinatal loss: current status and future directions. *Professional Psychology: Research and Practice,* 2005, 36:180–187.

38 Boswell S. *Understanding your baby.* London and Philadelphia, Jessica Kingsley Publishers, 2004.

39 Ispa JM et al. Pregnancy acceptance, parenting stress, and toddler attachment in low-income black families. *Journal of Marriage and Family,* 2007, 69:1–13.

40 Emanuel L. Disruptive and distressed toddlers: the impact of undetected maternal depression on infants and young children. In: Emanuel LB, ed. *"What can the matter be?": therapeutic interventions with parents, infants, and young children.* London, Karnac Books, 2008:136–150.

41 Tronick EZ, Gianino AF, Jr. The transmission of maternal disturbance to the infant. *New Directions for Child Development,* 1986, 34:5–11.

42 Bick E. The experience of the skin in early object-relations. *International Journal of Psycho-analysis,* 1968, 49:484–486.

43 Cohn JF et al. Face-to-face interactions of depressed mothers and their infants. *New Directions in Child Development,* 1986, 34:31–45.

44 Gergely G. The obscure object of desire: 'nearly, but clearly not, like me': contingency preference in normal children versus children with autism. *Bulletin of the Menninger Clinic,* 2001, 65:411–426.

45 Cummings EM, Keller PS, Davies PT. Towards a family process model of maternal and paternal depressive symptoms: exploring multiple relations with child and family functioning. *Journal of Child Psychology and Psychiatry,* 2005, 46:479–489.

46 Osofsky JD, Hann DM, Peebles CD. Adolescent parenthood: risks and opportunities for parents and infants. In: Zeanah CH, ed. *Handbook of infant mental health.* New York, Guilford Press, 1993:106–119.

47 Wakschlag LS, Hans SL. Ealy parenthood in context: Implications for development and intervention. In: Zeanah CH, ed. *Handbook of infant mental health,* 2nd ed. New York, Guilford Press, 2000:129–144.

48 McMahon M. *Engendering motherhood: identity and self-transformation in women's lives.* New York, Guilford Press, 1995.

49   Coley RL, Chase-Lansdale PL. Adolescent pregnancy and parenthood. Recent evidence and future directions. *The American Psychologist*, 1998, 53:152–166.

50   Brubaker SJ, Wright C. Identity transformation and family caregiving: narratives of African American teen mothers. *Journal of Marriage and Family*, 2006, 68:1214–1228.

51   O'Hara MW et al. Prospective study of postpartum blues. Biologic and psychosocial factors. *Archives of General Psychiatry*, 1991, 48:801–806.

52   Goodman SH, Brand SR. Infants of depressed mothers: vulnerabilities, risk factors, and protective factors for the later development of psychopathology. In: Zeanah CH, ed. *Handbook of infant mental health*, 3rd ed. New York, Guilford Press, 2009:153–170.

53   Jain L. Maternal substance abuse. *Indian Journal of Pediatrics*, 1998, 65:283–289.

54   Boris NW. Parental substance abuse. In: Zeanah CH, ed. *Handbook of infant mental health*, 3rd ed. New York, Guilford Press, 2009.

55   Chen WJ et al. Alcohol and the developing brain: neuroanatomical studies. *Alcohol Research and Health*, 2003, 27:174–180.

56   Wolock I, Magura S. Parental substance abuse as a predictor of child maltreatment re-reports. *Child Abuse and Neglect*, 1996, 20:1183–1193.

57   UNICEF. *The state of the World's children 2005 – childhood under threat*. New York, UNICEF, 2004.

58   Stein AH, Friedrich IK. Television content and young children's behavior. In: Murray JP, Rubinstein EA, Comstock GA, eds. *Television and social behavior. Volume 2: Television and social learning*. Rockville, MD, National Institute of Mental Health, 1972:202–317.

59   Dube SR et al. Childhood abuse, household dysfunction, and the risk of attempted suicide throughout the life span: findings from the Adverse Childhood Experiences Study. *JAMA*, 2001, 286:3089–3096.

60   Manly JT et al. Dimensions of child maltreatment and children's adjustment: contributions of developmental timing and subtype. *Development and Psychopathology*, 2001, 13:759–782.

61   Lieberman AF, Van Horn P, Ozer EJ. Preschooler witnesses of marital violence: predictors and mediators of child behavior problems. *Developmental Psychopathology*, 2005, 17:385–396.

62   McEwen BS. Early life influences on life-long patterns of behavior and health. *Mental Retardation and Developmental Disabilities Research Review*, 2003, 9:149–154.

63   Winnicott DW. *The maturational processes and the facilitating environment; studies in the theory of emotional development*. New York, International Universities Press, 1965.

64   Freud A, Burlingham D. *War and children*. New York, Medical War Books, 1943.

65   Scheeringa MS, Zeanah CH. A relational perspective on PTSD in early childhood. *Journal of Traumatic Stress*, 2001, 14:799–815.

66   Cicchetti D et al. Stage-salient issues: a transactional model of intervention. *New Directions in Child Development*, 1988, 39:123–145.

67   Coates SW, Rosenthal JL, Schechter DS. *September 11: trauma and human bonds*. Hillsdale, NJ, Analytic Press, 2003.

68   Evans GW. The environment of childhood poverty. *The American Psychologist*, 2004, 59:77–92.

69   McLoyd VC. Socioeconomic disadvantage and child development. *The American Psychologist*, 1998, 53:185–204.

70   Reid I. *Social class differences in Britain: life-chances and life-styles*, 3rd ed. London, Fontana Press, 1989.

71   Newson J, Newson E. *Patterns of infant care in an urban community*. Baltimore, Penguin Books, 1965.

72   Emery RE, Laumann-Billings L. An overview of the nature, causes, and consequences of abusive family relationships. Toward differentiating maltreatment and violence. *The American Psychologist*, 1998, 53:121–135.

73   Sampson RJ, Raudenbush SW, Earls F. Neighborhoods and violent crime: a multilevel study of collective efficacy. *Science*, 1997, 277:918–924.

74   Sinclair J et al. Encounters with aggressive peers in early childhood: frequency, age differences, and correlates of risk for behavior problems. *International Journal of Behavioral Development*, 1994, 17:675–696.

75   Conger R, Elder GH. *Families in troubled times: adapting to change in rural America*. New York, A de Gruyter, 1994.

76   Benveniste L, Carnoy M, Rothstein R. *All else equal: are public and private schools different?* New York, Routledge Falmer, 2003.

77   Loeb S et al. Child care in poor communities: early learning effects of type, quality, and stability. *Child Development*, 2004, 75:47–65.

78   Becker HJ. Who's wired and who's not: children's access to and use of computer technology. *The Future of Children*, 2000, 10:44–75.

79   Smith JR, Brooks-Gunn J, Klehanov P. Consequences of living in poverty for young children's cognitive and verbal ability and early school achievement. In: Duncan GJ, Brooks-Gunn J, eds. *Consequences of growing up poor*. New York, Russell Sage Foundation, 1997:132–189.

80   Timmer DA, Eitzen DS, Talley KD. *Paths to homelessness: extreme poverty and the urban housing crisis*. Boulder, Westview Press, 1994.

81   Bartlett S. Children's experience of the physical environment in poor urban settlements and the implications for policy, planning and practice. *Environment and Urbanization*, 1999, 11:63–73.

82   Larson RW, Verma S. How children and adolescents spend time across the world: work, play, and developmental opportunities. *Psychological Bulletin*, 1999, 125:701–736.

83   Alaimo K et al. Food insufficiency, family income, and health in US preschool and school-aged children. *American Journal of Public Health*, 2001, 91:781–786.

84   Macpherson A, Roberts I, Pless IB. Children's exposure to traffic and pedestrian injuries. *American Journal of Public Health*, 1998, 88:1840–1843.

85   Clarke-Stewart A, Gruber CP, Fitzgerald LM. *Children at home and in day care*. Hillsdale, NJ, L Erlbaum Associates, 1994.

86   Peisner-Feinberg ES et al. The relation of preschool child-care quality to children's cognitive and social developmental trajectories through second grade. *Child Development*, 2001, 72:1534–1553.

87   Evans GW, English K. The environment of poverty: multiple stressor exposure, psychophysiological stress, and socioemotional adjustment. *Child Development*, 2002, 73:1238–1248.

88   Rubin DM et al. Placement stability and mental health costs for children in foster care. *Pediatrics*, 2004, 113:1336–1341.

89   Zeanah CH, Jr., Smyke AT. Attachment disorders in relation to deprivation. In: Rutter M et al., eds. *Rutter's child and adolescent psychiatry*, 5th ed. Malden, MA, Blackwell Publishers, 2008:906–915.

90   Dozier M, Bick J. Changing caregivers: coping with early adversity. *Pediatric Annals*, 2007, 36:205–208.

91   Smyke AT, Breidenstine AS. Foster care in early childhood. In: Zeanah CH, ed. *Handbook of infant mental health*, 3rd ed. New York, Guilford Press, 2009:500–515.

92   Sheridan M, Nelson CA. Neurobiology of fetal and infant development: implication for infant mental health. In: Zeanah CH, ed. *Handbook of infant mental health*, 3rd ed. New York, Guilford Press, 2009:40–58.

93   Edelman GM, Tononi G. *A universe of consciousness: how matter becomes imagination*. New York, NY, Basic Books, 2000.

94   Edelman GM. *Second nature: brain science and human knowledge*. New Haven, Yale University Press, 2006.

95   Dunn W. A Sensory processing approach to supporting infant–caregiver relationship. In: Sameroff AJ, McDonough SC, Rosenblum K, eds. *Treating parent–infant relationship problems: strategies for intervention*. New York, Guilford Press, 2004:152–187.

96   DeGangi GA, Porges SW, Sickel RZ, Greenspan SI. Four-year follow-up of a sample of regulatory disordered infants. *Infant Mental Health Journal*, 1993, 14:330–343.

97   Zero to Three. *DC:0–3R: Diagnostic classification of mental health and developmental disorders of infancy and early childhood, revised edition*. Washington, DC, Zero To Three Press, 2005.

98   Sanson A, Hemphill S, Smart D. Temperament and social development. In: Smith PK, Hart CH, eds. *Blackwell handbook of childhood social development*. Oxford; Malden, MA, Blackwell Publishers, 2002:97–116.

99 De Pauw SS, Mervielde I. Temperament, personality and developmental psychopathology: a review based on the conceptual dimensions underlying childhood traits. *Child Psychiatry and Human Development*, 2010, 41:313–329.

100 Sanson A, Hemphill S, Smart D. Connections between temperament and social development: a review. *Social Development*, 2004, 13:142–170.

101 Lytton H. Child and parent effects in boys' conduct disorder: a reinterpretation. *Developmental Psychology*, 1990, 26:683–697.

102 van den Boom DC. The influence of temperament and mothering on attachment and exploration: an experimental manipulation of sensitive responsiveness among lower-class mothers with irritable infants. *Child Development*, 1994, 65:1457–1477.

103 Miles MS et al. Depressive symptoms in mothers of prematurely born infants. *Journal of Developmental and Behavioral Pediatrics*, 2007, 28:36–44.

104 Jotzo M, Poets CF. Helping parents cope with the trauma of premature birth: an evaluation of a trauma-preventive psychological intervention. *Pediatrics*, 2005, 115:915–919.

105 Taylor J. A fetish is born: sonographers and the making of the public fetus. In: Taylor JS, Layne LL, Wozniak DF, eds. *Consuming motherhood*. New Brunswick, NJ, Rutgers University Press, 2004:187–210.

106 Scheper-Hughes N. *Death without weeping: the violence of everyday life in Brazil*. Berkeley, University of California Press, 1992.

107 Holditch-Davis D, Miles MS, Belyea M. Feeding and non-feeding interactions of mothers and prematures. *Western Journal of Nursing Research*, 2000 , 22:320–334.

108 Levy-Shiff R, Sharir H, Mogilner MB. Mother- and father-preterm infant relationship in the hospital preterm nursery. *Child Development*, 1989, 60:93–102.

109 Minde K et al. Effect of neonatal complications in premature infants on early parent-infant interactions. *Developmental Medicine and Child Neurology*, 1983, 25:763–777.

110 Nix CM, Ansermet F. Prematurity, risk factors, and protective factors. In: Zeanah CH, ed. *Handbook of infant mental health*, 3rd ed. New York, Guilford Press, 2009:180–196.

111 Cohen M. *Sent before my time: a child psychotherapist's view of life on a neonatal intensive care unit*. London, Tavistock Clinic, 2003.

112 Bhutta AT et al. Cognitive and behavioral outcomes of school-aged children who were born preterm: a meta-analysis. *JAMA*, 2002, 288:728–737.

113 Wolf MJ et al. Neurobehavioral and developmental profile of very low birthweight preterm infants in early infancy. *Acta Paediatrica*, 2002, 91:930–938.

114 Anderson P, Doyle LW. Neurobehavioral outcomes of school-age children born extremely low birth weight or very preterm in the 1990s. *JAMA*, 2003, 289:3264–3272.

115 Dahl LB et al. Emotional, behavioral, social, and academic outcomes in adolescents born with very low birth weight. *Pediatrics*, 2006, 118:e449–459.

116 Zwaigenbaum L et al. Behavioral manifestations of autism in the first year of life. *International Journal of Developmental Neuroscience*, 2005, 23:143–152.

117 Chawarska K et al. Autism spectrum disorder in the second year: stability and change in syndrome expression. *Journal of Child Psychology and Psychiatry*, 2007, 48:128–138.

118 Samms-Vaughan M, Franklyn-Banton L. The role of early childhood professionals in the early identification of autistic disorder. *International Journal of Early Years Education*, 2008, 16:75–84.

119 Carr T, Lord C. Autism spectrum disorders. In: Zeanah CH, ed. *Handbook of infant mental health*, 3rd ed. New York, Guilford Press, 2009:549–563.

120 Autism and Developmental Disabilities Monitoring Network Surveillance Year 2002 Principal Investigators. Prevalence of autism spectrum disorders – autism and developmental disabilities monitoring network, 14 sites, United States, 2002. *Suveillance Summaries, Morbidity and Mortality Weekly*, 2007, 56:12–28.

121 Heikura U et al. Etiological survey on intellectual disability in the northern Finland birth cohort 1986. *American Journal of Mental Retardation*, 2005, 110:171–180.

122 Crnic KA, Friedrich WN, Greenberg MT. Adaptation of families with mentally retarded children: a model of stress, coping, and family ecology. *American Journal of Mental Deficiency*, 1983, 88:125–138.

123 Briggs-Gowan MJ et al. The Brief Infant-Toddler Social and Emotional Assessment: screening for social-emotional problems and delays in competence. *Journal of Pediatric Psychology*, 2004, 29:143–155.

124 Squires J, Bricker DD, Twombly E. *Ages & stages questionnaires, social-emotional (ASQ:SE): a parent-completed, child-monitoring system for social-emotional behaviors.* Baltimore, MD, PH Brookes Publishing Co, 2002.

125 Angold A, Egger HL. Psychiatric diagnosis in preschool children. In: DelCarmen-Wiggins R, Carter A, eds. *Handbook of infant, toddler, and preschool mental health assessment.* Oxford; New York, Oxford University Press, 2004:123–140.

126 Egger HL, Angold A. Classification of psychopathology in early childhood. In: Zeanah CH, ed. *Handbook of infant mental health*, 3rd ed. New York, Guilford Press, 2009:285–300.

127 Burke MG. Depression in preschool children. *Journal of the American Academy of Child and Adolescent Psychiatry*, 2003, 42:263–264; author reply 4–5.

128 McClellan JM, Speltz ML. Psychiatric diagnosis in preschool children. *Journal of the American Academy of Child and Adolescent Psychiatry*, 2003, 42:127–128; author reply 8–30.

129 Zito JM et al. Trends in the prescribing of psychotropic medications to preschoolers. *JAMA*, 2000, 283:1025–1030.

130 DelCarmen-Wiggins R, Carter AS. Introduction – assessment of infant and toddler mental health: advances and challenges. *Journal of the American Academy of Child and Adolescent Psychiatry*, 2001, 40:8–10.

131 Carter AS, Briggs-Gowan MJ, Davis NO. Assessment of young children's social-emotional development and psychopathology: recent advances and recommendations for practice. *Journal of Child Psychology and Psychiatry*, 2004, 45:109–134.

132 Chawarska K, Klin A, Volkmar FR. *Autism spectrum disorders in infants and toddlers: diagnosis, assessment, and treatment.* New York, Guilford Press, 2008.

133 Egger HL, Angold A. Common emotional and behavioral disorders in preschool children: presentation, nosology, and epidemiology. *Journal of Child Psychology and Psychiatry*, 2006, 47:313–337.

134 Skovgaard AM et al. Predictors (0–10 months) of psychopathology at age 1½ years – a general population study in The Copenhagen Child Cohort CCC 2000. *Journal of Child Psychology and Psychiatry*, 2008, 49:553–562.

135 Skovgaard AM. [Markers of mental health problems based on public health nurses' assessments of 0- to 1-year-old children: the Copenhagen County Child Cohort 2000]. *Ugeskrift for Laeger*, 2007, 169:1006–1010.

136 Skovgaard AM et al. The prevalence of mental health problems in children 1(1/2) years of age – the Copenhagen Child Cohort 2000. *Journal of Child Psychology and Psychiatry*, 2007, 48:62–70.

137 Zeanah PD, Gleason MM. Infant Mental Health in Primary Health Care. In: Zeanah CH, ed. *Handbook of infant mental health*, 3rd ed. New York, Guilford Press, 2009:549–563.

138 Hagan JF, Shaw JS, Duncan PM. *Bright futures: guidelines for health supervision of infants, children, and adolescents*, 3rd ed. Elk Grove Village, IL, American Academy of Pediatrics, 2008.

139 Emde RN, Bingham RD, Harmon RJ. Classification and the diagnostic process in infancy. In: Zeanah CH, ed. *Handbook of infant mental health.* New York, Guilford Press, 1993:225–235.

140 Zeanah CH, Boris NW, Scheeringa MS. Psychopathology in infancy. *Journal of Child Psychology and Psychiatry*, 1997, 38:81–99.

141 Clark R, Tluczek A, Gallagher KC. Assessment of parent-child early relational disturbances. In: DelCarmen-Wiggins R, Carter A, eds. *Handbook of infant, toddler, and preschool mental health assessment.* Oxford; New York, Oxford University Press; 2004:25–60.

142 Glascoe FP. Parents' evaluation of developmental status: how well do parents' concerns identify children with behavioral and emotional problems? *Clinical Pediatrics*, 2003, 42:133–138.

143 Carter AS et al. Parent reports and infant-toddler mental health assessment. In: Zeanah CH, ed. *Handbook of infant mental health*, 3rd ed. New York, Guilford Press, 2009:233–251.

144 Earls MF, Hay SS. Setting the stage for success: implementation of developmental and behavioral screening and surveillance in primary care practice – the North Carolina Assuring Better Child Health and Development (ABCD) Project. *Pediatrics*, 2006, 118:e183–188.

145 Olson AL et al. Brief maternal depression screening at well-child visits. *Pediatrics*, 2006, 118:207–216.

146 Cox JL, Holden JM, Sagovsky R. Detection of postnatal depression. Development of the 10-item Edinburgh Postnatal Depression Scale. *British Journal of Psychiatry*, 1987, 150:782–786.

147 Bowlby J. *A secure base: parent–child attachment and healthy human development*. New York, Basic Books, 1988.

148 Heneghan AM, Mercer M, DeLeone NL. Will mothers discuss parenting stress and depressive symptoms with their child's pediatrician? *Pediatrics*, 2004, 113:460–467.

149 Stallard P. Review: school based prevention and early intervention programmes reduce anxiety. *Evidence Based Mental Health*, 2009, 12:116.

150 Stern DN. *The motherhood constellation: a unified view of parent–infant psychotherapy*. New York, Basic Books, 1995.

28 Child mental health in primary care

Yen-Hsun Huang, Pei-Chin Lee and Vincent Chin-Hung Chen

Key messages

- The general practitioner (GP) plays an important role in early recognition of children with mental health problems and in guiding families to diagnostic and intervention services.

- Child mental disorders, frequently seen by a GP in primary care settings, include autism spectrum disorder, intellectual disabilities/mental retardation, attention deficit hyperactivity disorder, disruptive behavioural disorder (i.e. oppositional defiant disorder and conduct disorder) and tic disorder.

- Child and adolescent mental disorders have similar prevalence rates across different ethnocultural groups. Most patients have a high rate of other comorbid psychiatric disorders and deserve close evaluation.

- Cultural relevance and contextual understanding are important for evaluation of child and adolescent mental disorders. Mental disorders should be defined as dynamic responses to social/environmental impairments rather than as rigid diagnostic labels.

- Global diversity in national policy and services for child and adolescent mental health are observed, as well as barriers to care. Strategies to promote child and adolescent mental health include a holistic mental health framework and cooperation between the family, community, nongovernmental organizations, school systems and medical resources.

Introduction

According to the World Health Organization (WHO), mental health disorders are one of the leading causes of disability worldwide. Most adult or adolescent psychiatric disorders occur in childhood or are increased by childhood adversities.[1] The prevalence of child and adolescent psychiatric disorders is estimated to be around 12%, and these disorders are among those ranked highest in the WHO's report of global burden of disease.[2]

A review of community studies found that worldwide, the prevalence rates for child and adolescent mental disorders range from 1.7% to 17.8%.[3] In addition to high prevalence rates of child mental disorders, rates of functional impairment are also very high.[4] A case-control study based on a global assessment of functioning found that all preschool children with behavioural disorders (100%) were impaired, as compared with 15.5% of those children without a disorder.[4,5]

Approximately 1 in 10 children and adolescents receive mental health services, but most of them receive primary care every year.[6] Therefore, the general practitioner (GP) plays an important role in early recognition of children with mental health problems and in guiding families to diagnostic and assessment resources, as well as intervention services.[7,8] Unlike specialists in child mental health care, GPs usually meet with parents and children when problems or symptoms are in an undifferentiated state and there are no clues as to the appropriate solutions.[9] Early identification needs knowledge of signs and symptoms, as well as appropriate developmental surveillance and problem- or disorder-specific screening.[10,11]

In spite of strong advocates from parent groups and professional organizations about the role of the GP in the early screening of child mental disorders,[7,12] a survey of 255 GPs in the United States of America

(USA) found that most (82%) routinely screened for general developmental delays, but only 8% screened for specific disorders such as autism spectrum disorder (ASD).[13] Lack of familiarity with tools (62%), referrals to a specialist (47%), or insufficient time and resources (32%) were the main reasons for not screening for mental disorders. Awareness of and familiarity with screening tools, continuing education of mental health services or providing additional resources to the GP are warranted to ensure that efficient referrals take place and that coordinated services for children with mental disorders are made readily available.

Mental disorders such as ASD, intellectual disabilities/mental retardation (ID/MR), attention-deficit hyperactivity disorder (ADHD), disruptive behavioural disorder (i.e. oppositional defiant disorder, ODD, and conduct disorder, CD), and tic disorder have high prevalence rates in childhood and are frequently seen by GPs in primary care settings.[14] This chapter will focus on addressing these childhood mental disorders in the primary care setting (i.e. ASD, ID/MR, ADHD, ODD, CD, and tic disorder). This will provide a more general picture of such disorders, their prevalence rates, the screening process, the appropriate tools to be used by the GP and evidence-based mental health services.

Autism spectrum disorder

Prevalence

The prevalence of autistic disorder is estimated to be around 7.1 per 10 000; that of pervasive developmental disorder 27.5 per 10 000; and that ASD 20.0 per 10 000.[15,16] ASD is more common in boys than in girls. A meta-analysis of 40 studies around the world found the prevalence of autistic disorder ranged from 0.7 to 60 per 10 000 and the prevalence of ASD ranged from 3.3 to 121 per 10 000.[15] Regional difference was analysed, with studies from Japan having significantly higher prevalence rates than North American studies (odds ratio (OR) = 3.60, 95% confidence interval (CI) = 1.73 to 7.46). However, even after controlling for study region, living area (urban versus rural/mixed; OR = 2.85, 95% CI = 1.47 to 5.53) and diagnostic criteria (*International Classification of Diseases* (ICD)-10 or *Diagnostic and Statistical Manual of Mental Disorders* (DSM)-IV versus others; OR= 3.48, 95% CI = 1.92 to 6.33) were also significantly associated with the estimated prevalence of autism.

Clinical picture and pattern

ASD is a lifelong developmental disorder characterized by severe deficits in reciprocal social interaction and communication and repetitive or stereotyped behaviour.[17] These criteria reflect the central role of deficits in social and stereotyped behaviour in children with ASD.[18] Problems with regard to social responsiveness, play behaviour and communication can be present in those as young as 6–12 months. Typical signs include a child's inability to make eye contact with others, share interests or pleasurable experiences, notice the absence of caregivers, or to respond to requests by using gestures or verbal communication.

Screening and detection

The National Initiative for Autism Screening and Assessment (NIASA)[12] and the American Academy of Pediatrics (AAP)[7] emphasize the importance of educating clinicians and families to help to identify children with ASD at an early stage. It is recommended to screen and diagnose ASD in three stages.[18,19] Autism-specific screening should be performed when children fail routine developmental assessment. Those who are positive in specific autism screening should be referred to a formal evaluation by an experienced multidisciplinary team. Screening measures that are easily administered, widely disseminated and have good psychometric properties[20–22] are summarized in Table 28.1.

Table 28.1 Screening measures for primary health care

Measure	Age range, months	Time to complete, minutes	Areas screened
General developmental screen			
Parents' Evaluation of Developmental Status (PEDS)[23]	0–95	2–10	Fine motor, gross motor, self-help, expressive language, receptive language and social-emotional
Ages and Stages Questionnaires, third edition (ASQ-3)[24]	1–66	10–15	Communication, gross motor, fine motor, problem-solving, and personal-social
Ages and Stages Questionnaire – Social and Emotional (ASQ-SE)[25]	3–60	10–15	Self-regulation, compliance, communication, adaptive behaviours, autonomy, affect and interaction with people
Autism-specific screening tool			
Checklist for Autism in Toddlers (CHAT)[26,27]	18	10–20	Symptoms of autism
The Modified Checklist for Autism in Toddlers (M-CHAT)[28]	18–42	10	Symptoms of autism
The Pervasive Developmental Disorders Screening Test, Second Edition (PDDST-II)[29]	12–48	10–20	Symptoms of autistic disorder, pervasive developmental delay, and Asperger's disorder

Intervention

The goals of intervention for children with ASD are to improve the child's functional independence, and quality of life through the acquisition of skills in the core deficit areas.[20,30] Intensive behavioural therapy and communication training are well studied and have strong evidence to support their effectiveness for children with ASD.[31,32] Argumentative and assistive communication might include a picture exchange communication system, sign language, and assistive technology, helping children with severe communication problems.[33] Parent-mediated behavioural interventions are valuable, where parents and children are trained with a highly structured behavioural model that is generalized to their everyday life,[34] and their efficacy has been found to be quite promising.[31,32] Provision of special education might include placement in an appropriate class with adequate support for learning, transition planning and vocational training. Curricula such as treatment and education of autistic and related communication handicapped children (TEACCH) are found to be effective in improving developmental and functional skills for ASD.[12,35,36]

Intellectual disabilities/mental retardation

Prevalence

The estimates of prevalence of ID/MR across countries and regions range from 2 to 85 per 1000 children.[37] Racial differences of prevalence of ID/MR are observed, with higher rates among African American children and Australian indigenous children compared with other ethnic groups.[38] However, both methodological issues (e.g. measures of intelligent quotient (IQ), demographic composition of the study participant) and family and social-cultural factors (e.g. poverty) may confound this finding. Higher prevalence rates are also observed in males and in rural areas.

Clinical picture and pattern

In the past decade, the diagnosis of MR has gone beyond the single measure of IQ and has been replaced by intellectual disabilities or ID/MR, to reflect the dynamic and holistic interactions between an individual with limited intellectual and adaptive skills within a personal specific contextual environment.[39] ID/MR is characterized by significantly subaverage intellectual functioning (an IQ of approximately 70 or below), onset before the age of 18 years and concurrent deficits in adaptive functioning.[17] Deficits in adaptive function are defined as problems in conceptual, social and practical adaptive skills.[40] The deficits of ID/MR might be related to impairment (i.e. performance incapacity), activity limitations, and participation restrictions (i.e. the opportunity to function) according to the International Classification of Functioning and Disability (ICIDH-2).[41] Subcategories differentiated by IQ scores are summarized in Table 28.2.

Table 28.2	Levels of intellectual disabilities/mental retardation[a]				
Level	**IQ range**	**Appropriate mental age (years)**	**Proportion of MR group, %**	**Prevalence[b]**	**Adult attainment**
Mild	50–70[c]	9–12	85	1.70	Literacy ++ Self-help skills ++ Good speech ++ Semi-skilled work +
Moderate	35–49	6–9	10	0.94–8	Literacy + Self-help skills ++ Domestic speech + Unskilled work with or without supervision +
Severe	20–34	3–6	3–4	0.38–7	Assisted self-help skills + Minimum speech + Assisted household chores +
Profound	<20	<2	1–2	0.30	Speech +/– Self-help skills +/–

Created from the works of Volkmar and Dykens[42] and Girimaji.[43]

++ definitely attainable; + attainable; +/– sometimes attainable.

[a] Based on ICD-10 and DSM-IV.

[b] Based on the studies of Gisslera and his colleagues[44] and Leonard and Wen.[38]

[c] DSM-IV allows for some clinical judgement in the diagnosis and levels of ID/MR, e.g. the upper IQ limit of ID/MR diagnosis could range from 70 to 75 and lower limit of mild ID/MR could range from 50 to 55.

Screening and detection

For children with moderate to profound ID/MR, early detection in infancy might take place when the child has physical or psychological signs that are accompanied with severe disability.[45] The GP might first notice signs of ID/MR by noting delayed milestones of development in many domains, poor ability to learn new things, poor self-care skills, and poor school performance.[43] Families might also complain of behaviour problems such as hyperactivity, inattention, impulsivity, self-injurious behaviour, or sleep/appetite disturbances.

Developmental screening, with checklists of adaptive function using a brief standardized tool can aid in the identification of children at risk of MR.[7,46] The PEDS, ASQ-3 and ASQ-SE are developmental screening tools recommended for children aged under 12 years. The Adaptive Behavioral Scale – school version second edition,[47] Adaptive Behavioral Scale – residential and community version second edition,[48] and Vineland Adaptive Behavior Scales[49] are appropriate and recommended for use in clinics.[50]

Intervention

Treatment of accompanying psychopathology or physical disorder (such as epilepsy) is similar to treatment of people without ID/MR, but needs to take into account the child's level of function and communication.[51] Education is crucial for children with ID/MR. For young preschool children with ID/MR, an early-intervention programme that delivers in a family-centered way is critical to address the developmental needs and simple self-care skills of children with ID/MR, in addition to parental support and education.[52] Direct, systematic instruction in academic learning, and functional training such as daily living skills is the most effective approach for children with ID/MR.[53] Inclusive education with appropriate special education support can provide social experience and curriculum for children with ID/MR, but a meta-analysis of different education studies for children with ID/MR found inconsistent results.[54]

Attention-deficit hyperactivity disorder

Prevalence

According to current data and related research, one of the most common childhood psychiatric disorders worldwide is clearly ADHD.[55] There are two main approaches used to define ADHD that are worth noting, one follows the DSM-IV,[17] and the other follows the ICD-10, using the name hyperkinetic disorder (HKD).[56] HKD details similar operational criteria for the disorder but it is more stringent. A number of studies have found that the prevalence rates of ADHD are higher if the DSM-IV criteria are used as opposed to ICD-10 criteria.[57] According to the literature reviews reported, the prevalence rates for ADHD vary from 0.5% to 26%; of course these rates are influenced by the type of diagnostic criteria used, patient sample size, geographic factors and information sources utilized.[58] A more recent review concluded that the worldwide pooled prevalence is estimated to be 5.29%.[59] Numerous reports have highlighted the increasing prevalence of ADHD and the increasing use of ADHD medication over the past 10 years.[60,61] A male preponderance and male to female ratio of approximately 3:1 has been estimated for rates of ADHD.[62]

Clinical picture and pattern

ADHD is characterized by inattention, hyperactivity and impulsiveness. The presentation of ADHD varies under different environments at different ages.[63] Short play sequences (less than 3 minutes), leaving activities before completion and not listening are typical presentations of inattention in preschool age. Children with ADHD at this age might move all the time like a whirlwind and cannot notice danger. School-age children with attention problem might be easily distracted, forgetful and disorganized compared with their peers. Children with hyperactivity and impulsiveness are restless and thoughtless. Therefore, they might break rules, interrupt group activities, act out of turn, and irritate their peers, classmates and adults. In adolescence and adulthood, people with ADHD show lack of foresight and planning, with difficulty in focusing on details of a task, as well as more accidents. Instead of motor hyperactivity, they are more in a subjective status of restlessness and poor self-control.

Some children with ADHD persist to have symptoms in adolescence and adulthood.[64] It is estimated that around 60% of ADHD symptoms, as well as various clinical and psychosocial impairments, are found in adult life. Based on a meta-analysis, 15% of children with ADHD retain the full diagnosis when they are 25 years old and half of them are in partial remission.[65] The prevalence rate of adults with ADHD is around 2.5%.[66] The predictors of persistent ADHD in adolescence and adulthood are the combined subtype of ADHD, more severe symptoms, comorbid disorders in childhood, psychosocial adversity, parental psychopathology and a family history of ADHD.[67,68] ADHD has a quite high rate of comorbid psychiatric disorders. According to one study, 40% of clinical cases have ODD, 34% have anxiety disorder, 14% have CD and 11% have tic disorder.[69] Furthermore, it is common that those with ADHD also suffer from adolescent substance abuse.[70]

Screening and detection

The AAP, the American Academy of Child and Adolescent Psychiatry (AACAP) and National Institute for Health and Clinical Excellence (NICE) have each outlined a number of recommendations with regard to the evaluation and diagnosis of children with suspected ADHD.[71-73] Based on a review of these institutions' guidelines, it is important to review a summary of the five key recommendations for evaluation of children with suspected ADHD. Firstly, a clear understanding of each patient's history and documented physical examination is vital. This should include, but not be limited to, the child's developmental history, history of learning difficulties, family history, hearing and vision examination, school assessment and so on. Second, discussions should take place with parents or caregivers and involved teachers, to obtain direct evidence of the suspected ADHD child's core symptoms, age of onset, duration and overall degree of impairment. Third, to adequately make a diagnosis of ADHD, the child is required to meet DSM-IV diagnostic criteria and the child's symptoms must be causing psychological and social/educational impairment in various settings. Fourth, any coexisting conditions also need to be assessed, such as anxiety disorder, depression, CD or ODD and so on. Lastly, although valuable, it is imperative that clinicians do not base their diagnosis of ADHD only on rating scales and/or observational data.

There are a number of rating scales that can be used for ADHD symptoms that are both efficient and cost-effective methods of collecting information in standard clinical practice. These include broad-band checklists and ADHD-specific measures. These broad-band rating scales gather information on a variety of types of child behavioural problems and comorbid symptoms, while ADHD-specific rating scales assess the main symptoms of ADHD. The rating scales examined are detailed in Table 28.3. Regardless of the obvious benefits of scales, such rating scales alone cannot establish a diagnosis.[72] Therefore, they should be interpreted with caution, within a clinical context, and be supplemented with detailed interview information.

Table 28.3 Screening measures for ADHD in the primary care setting

Measure	Age range, years	Time to complete, minutes	Areas screened
Group 1: ADHD-specific rating scales			
ADHD Rating Scale IV (ADHD-RS-IV)[74]	5–18	15–20	DSM-IV diagnostic criteria for ADHD
Swanson, Nolan, and Pelham IV questionnaire (SNAP-IV)[75]	6–18	10	DSM-IV diagnostic criteria for ADHD and other comorbid DSM diagnoses
Vanderbilt ADHD Rating Scale (VARS)[76,77]	Elementary school	10	DSM-IV diagnostic criteria for ADHD and other comorbid DSM diagnoses
Conners 3[78]	6–18	20	ADHD symptoms and common comorbid conditions
Conners EC (Early Childhood)[79]	2–6	25	Attention, hyperactivity, aggressive behaviour, anxiety, social functioning, atypical behaviour, mood and affect, physical symptoms, adaptive skills, communication, motor skills, play, cognition
Group 2: Broad-band assessments			
Behavior Assessment System for Children – 2nd edition (BASC-2)[80]	2–21	10–20	Activities of daily living, functional communication, adaptability, hyperactivity, aggression, leadership, anxiety, learning problems, attention problems, social skills, atypicality, somatization, CD, study skills, depression, withdrawal
Child Behavior Checklist (CBCL/6–18)[81]	6–18	15	Anxiety, depression, somatic complaints, withdrawn, social problem, attention problems, rule-breaking behaviour, aggressive behaviour, thought problems
Child Behavior Checklist (CBCL/1.5–5)[82]	1.5–5	15	Emotional reaction, anxiety, depression, somatic complaints, withdrawn, attention problems, aggressive behaviour, sleep problems

Intervention

Before any intervention begins, it is important to follow some key steps. Firstly, a clear explanation of this sometimes misunderstood disorder and its precise nature should be given to three groups: the affected child, related family members and the child's teachers. Offering simple advice is helpful in reducing the symptoms of these affected children.[63] If available, it is prudent to refer parents to group cognitive-behavioural therapy (CBT) sessions, encompassing both education and parenting skills; furthermore, children themselves also benefit from group CBT sessions and social skills training.[72] A number of proactive strategies have been implemented to help children with ADHD, and several have shown promising results; these include biofeedback, relaxation techniques, physical exercise, contingency management training by itself, or in conjunction with problem-solving, or working memory training, or with teacher psycho-education, and so on.[31,32]

In addition to psychological, behavioural and educational interventions, an important part of any comprehensive treatment plan should generally include some form of drug treatment. A number of ADHD-related reviews, in particular two recent ones[31,32] with regard to evidence-based intervention for ADHD children, clearly support the effectiveness of a combination of medication, behavioural therapy and self-verbalization. Certain stimulants, such as methylphenidate and dexamphetamine, are effective in controlling hyperactivity, aggression, comorbid CD and so on.[31] Second-line medications such as tricyclic antidepressants, non-cyclic antidepressants (e.g. atomoxetine), clonidine and carbamazepine are also widely used. When children with ADHD suffer from the comorbid conditions of depression and anxiety, the related literature supports the use of tricyclic antidepressants,[83] and for children with ADHD and tic disorder, the use of clonidine has been advocated in some reviews.[84]

Disruptive behavioural disorder

Prevalence

Disruptive behavioural disorders include CD and ODD. The prevalence of ODD and CD varies depending on the population, diagnostic criteria, instruments used, period considered (point or lifetime), and informant; thus, it is difficult to establish an accurate estimate. The prevalence of ODD was recently reported as ranging from 2.6% to 15.6%.[85] It has also been noted that before puberty, boys have a higher prevalence than girls of such disorders; however, during adolescence they have been shown to have equal prevalence.[85] The prevalence of CD ranges from 4% to 16% for boys and 1% to 9% for girls.[86] The male predominance with regard to CD remains consistent over development, while sex ratios narrow gradually in the mid-teens.[87] This suggests that most CD in females appears at older ages. Another study review taking place in the United Kingdom of Great Britain and Northern Ireland (UK) shows the prevalence of conduct problems has been significantly increasing over the past 25 years.[88]

Comorbid disorders are common in children with ODD and CD. In the UK, another community-based study of children with ODD showed that 14% had ADHD, 14% had anxiety disorder and 9% had depressive disorders.[89] A follow-up study in Ontario, Canada, taking place over a 4-year period, reported that 46% of children with CD had one other or more psychiatric disorders: hyperkinetic disorder was found in 35% and emotional disorder in 29%.[90] Somatoform disorder, substance disorder and learning disabilities are also highly prevalent among children with CD.[91,92] CD has a strong connection with psychiatric disorders that occur later in life, such as antisocial personality disorder, mood and anxiety disorders, and alcohol and substance use disorders.[93,94]

Clinical picture and pattern

Disruptive behaviours (conduct problems), which constitute a broad spectrum of behaviours, are one of the most common mental disorders associated with significant caregiver strain.[95] The cluster can be divided to two distinct areas of ODD and CD.[17] ODD has ongoing patterns of negative, disobedient and hostile behaviour towards authority figures; furthermore, such individuals have an inability to take responsibility for their own mistakes and continue to have issues with anger control. CD is defined by repeated severe antisocial and aggressive behaviour, including aggression towards both people and animals, property destruction, deceptiveness with regard to theft, and ongoing rule violation.[17]

The core symptoms of ODD/CD may be observed as early as preschool and they rarely present for the first time after the age of 16 years;[17] both ODD and CD behaviours maintain a relatively stable pattern over time.[90,96,97] It is important to note that early onset (below the age of 10 years) associated with a course of conduct problems strongly correlates with a poor prognosis and an increased risk for comorbid disorders in adult life.[17,98,99] ODD is risk factor for CD and CD is predictor of antisocial personality disorder.[100,101] Although ODD, CD and adult antisocial personality disorder are regarded as a diagnostic progression series in severity of antisocial behaviour, the majority of cases of ODD and CD do not progress further.[91,101,102]

Screening and detection

Several methods and a number of informants are required, due to the heterogeneity of ODD/CD; thus, adequate assessments with multiple informants (e.g. parents, the patient, teachers, the police and social workers) concerning the different levels of the patient's impairment in multiple settings must be detailed to help clinicians to decide on the most effective treatment strategy. Such assessments include the use of clinical interviews, behavioural rating scales and direct behavioural observation.[103] Adequate evaluation of complementary risk factors and protective factors is also important when attempting to establish additional key intervention targets. Fortunately, with recent advances in developmental approaches to diagnosis, and assessment tools that help to examine conduct problems, clinicians are now able to make decision in a much shorter period of time. Some examples of such easy-to-use approaches are the Structured Assessment of Violence Risk in Youth (SAVRY),[104] Early Assessment Risk List for Boys (EARL-20B),[105] Early Assessment Risk List for Girls (EARL-21G),[106] and more. As previously mentioned, broad-band behavioural rating scales are also quite helpful when attempting to assess conduct behaviour, comorbid disorders and adjustment problems. The BASC-2,[80] the Achenbach System of Empirically Based Assessment (ASEBA),[81,82] the Conners Rating Scales (Conners 3),[78] and the Revised Behavior Problem Checklist (RBPC)[107] are all frequently used in clinical practice and for related research.

Intervention

The first line of treatment for ODD and CD should be structured psychosocial intervention. Recent evidence-based reviews suggest that cognitive-behavioural treatments for parents, children, teachers, peers and other members of the school are effective.[108,109] The first-line approach to help affected young children is parent training. Direct child-training approaches are generally reserved for older children with a greater capacity for learning.[109] Some studies have suggested that multisystem treatment approaches, including CBT approaches, behavioural therapies, parent training, pragmatic family therapies and pharmacological interventions, are superior to typical community services.[110] One of the key challenges is that the moderators and predictors of psychosocial treatment outcome are highly inconsistent in a number of studies. In addition, several other influences can moderate response, such as caregivers' management skills, parents' marital status, maternal depression, paternal substance use, youth deviant peer association, and comorbidity.[111,112]

Psychopharmacological treatment is a useful adjuvant treatment for comorbid disorders and target symptoms, but is insufficient alone when attempting to manage and treat CD.[113] Stimulant medications, such as alpha-agonists, and atomoxetine have been found to be quite effective to reduce aggression in CD that is comorbid with ADHD.[114-116] Low doses of risperidone have been reported as being effective for patients with CD who have a good tolerance.[117] Furthermore, some short-term studies showed lithium, divalproex sodium and antidepressants were also effective in reducing aggression.[118-120]

Tic disorder

Prevalence

It has been estimated that 4.8–24% of school-age children have tics,[121,122] and that 0.4–3.8% have Tourette's disorder.[123,124] The international prevalence of Tourette's disorder has been estimated to be approximately 1%, according to a review study.[125] Males are more likely to have tics than females (male to female ratio: 4.3:1).[126] Another study showed that 88% of Tourette's disorder patients had comorbidities, and that the most common comorbidities were ADHD (60%) and obsessive–compulsive disorder (OCD; 59%).[126] An increasing number of hereditary relationships among these three disorders have been reported.[127,128] Thus, the combination of tics, ADHD and OCD is often called "the Tourette's syndrome triad".[129] Tics are also comorbid with developmental disorders such as ID/MR, ASD and Asperger's disease.[130] Also, boys with tics are generally more likely to have ADHD, while girls with tics are more likely to have OCD.[131]

Although this disorder has been researched extensively and well examined in western society, the characteristics and features of tics are less well known in other cultures. One cross-cultural study showed that demography, family history, clinical features, comorbidity and treatments are quite similar across various cultures.[132]

Clinical picture and pattern

A "tic" is a stereotyped repetitive movement (i.e. motor tic) or an utterance (i.e. vocal or phonic tic) that mimics some aspect of normal behaviour. Generally, tics will vary in intensity and forcefulness. Twitching, eye blinking, facial grimacing, head jerking, or shoulder shrugs are considered to be simple motor tics, and more complex tics mimic purposive behaviours such as facial expressions or gestures of the arm and head. Vocal tics range from sniffing, coughing sounds to complex vocalizations and speech. According to the DSM-IV diagnostic system, tic disorders can be categorized into three major categories: transient tic disorder, chronic motor or vocal tic disorder, and Tourette's disorder.[17] Transient tic disorder is characterized by one or more simple motor or vocal tics that wax and wane in severity for at least one month. If a tic lasts for more than one year, it is defined as chronic motor or vocal tic disorder. Diagnostic criteria of Tourette's disorder include the presence of both motor and vocal tics, with a duration of at least one year and onset before the age 18 years.

The age of onset is typically between 3 and 8 years.[133] For Tourette's disorder, motor tics typically appear first, usually followed by vocal tics 1–2 years later. Research has shown that vocal tics will seldom appear without previous onset of motor tics.[134] The most common tics involve the face and then the arms, and the common vocal tics include inarticulate utterances, coprolalia and echolalia.[135] Typically, patients with Tourette's disorder have several different types of tics and these different types will wax and wane over time. Tics usually increase in situations involving stress and decrease when children concentrate on certain tasks, especially tasks that interest them.

Tics tend to improve in early adulthood after reaching their most severe levels around the preadolescence age.[133,136] They usually resolve in approximately one-third of cases, with another one-third becoming less severe, but for the remaining one-third the tics are sadly lifelong. There are no known reliable predictors of outcome at this time.[133,137] By the age of 10 years, most children with tics are aware of premonitory urges such as a feeling of tightness, tension, itching of the focal area or having sense of discomfort and anxiety that can be relieved by performing the tics.[138] These premonitory urges and the consummatory phenomenon contribute to individual patients' sense that tics can initially be partially suppressed voluntarily, but the urge and impulse accumulate until the tics are released.

Screening and detection

The guiding principle of initial assessment is to screen for tics and coexisting disorders by examining a patient's history, conducting a thorough neurological examination, and investigating the developmental process. Many patients require treatment for both tics and comorbid disorders such as OCD and ADHD. Therefore, paying close attention to each individual's adaptive function, identifying impairment and distress, is crucial when deciding on further treatment.[139] The Yale Global Tic Severity Scale (YGTSS)[140] is a clinician-rated, semi-structured scale that helps to evaluate motor and phonic symptoms. Utilizing this scale, a clinician can rate motor and vocal tics according to their number, frequency, intensity, complexity and interference, on a 6-point ordinal scale.

Intervention

As the majority of tics experienced by patients are mild and not disabling, both waxing and waning, providing effective education and supportive suggestions to patients, caregivers or related family members and school teachers is usually sufficient. A key focus should be placed on strengthening the child's self-confidence and self-esteem.[129] When tics do become disabling, behaviour therapy or pharmacotherapy is clearly indicated. Habit-reversal treatment (one type of CBT) was reported to be effective in a randomized trial.[141] It focused on relaxation, self-monitoring, contingency management, inconvenience review, awareness training and competing response. Alpha-2-agonists such as clonidine and guanfacine have a good effect on tics with cormorbid ADHD.[142–144] Antipsychotics are more potent and have a more predictable effectiveness. Classical antipsychotics including haloperidol, pimozide and tiapride, and atypical antipsychotics including risperidone, olanzapine, ziprasidone and aripiprazole also have documented efficacy.[145–150] Treatments will generally begin with a low dose given before sleep. Botulinum toxin injection and deep brain stimulation surgery are also therapeutic options for patients who are refractory to medication treatment.[151,152]

Global diversity in care delivery for children with mental disorders

Diagnosis and assessment

Conventional child psychiatry is broadly based on biomedical and western cultural perspectives, whereas literature addressing non-western and non-medical knowledge in child psychiatry remains relatively sparse.[153,154] While it is recognized that the prevalence rates and patterns of general child and adolescent mental disorders are similar across different ethnocultural groups, it is also clear that some cross-cultural presentations may vary in detail.[153–159] Some standardized child dimensional assessment instruments, including the ASEBA[81,82] and the Strengths and Difficulties Questionnaire(SDQ)[160] have been translated into more than 70 languages and have been found to be acceptable by respondents from many different cultures.[161] Multicultural research with regard to these assessment instruments has revealed that the distributions of problems of children and adolescents from differential cultural societies overlap considerably, except for some differences in particular items and scales.[161]

In caring for children and adolescents with mental disorders, it is important to have a clear cultural contextual understanding. Disorders of mental functioning should be defined as dynamic responses to social/environmental impairments rather than as a rigid diagnostic labels.[153] The degree of impairment and the inability of the individual to participate in society are more important than diagnosis of the specific disorder.[153] GPs are also advised to take the cultural context into account in order for the assessment process and treatment plan to be acceptable.[162] DSM-IV cultural formulation is useful when organizing and conceptualizing the cultural factors in the assessment and treatment of children and adolescents.[163] This is structured into five main categories: (1) identity of the individual; (2) explanations of the illness; (3) factors associated with the psychosocial environment and levels of functioning; (4) relationship between the individual and the service providers; and (5) overall cultural assessment for diagnosis and care.[17]

Cultural sensitivity and appropriateness are crucial for all service contexts.[155] There are no easy guidelines but the main requirement is to be aware of the various needs of the patients. In high-income countries, it has been suggested that mental health teams be comprised of members from several different ethnocultural backgrounds, as well as from several different professional disciplines, in order to support the diverse cultural child psychiatric population.[164] When assessing potential patients in areas with limited resources, service providers should consider broader categories of disorders rather than the narrower disease definitions. It is vital to make use of available existing personnel and services in order to recognize the patients who potentially need treatment or to refer them for further assessment by personnel with more experience and time.[153]

Barriers to care

Several barriers around the world inhibit care for children with mental disorders.[153,165] Critical barriers include transportation, limited resources (including financial, trained personnel and facilities), lack of public knowledge about child mental disorders, lack of ability to communicate effectively in the patient's native language and stigma among children, families and treatment providers.[153] With questionnaires received from 66 countries globally, the WHO Atlas Project studying child and adolescent mental health resources found stigma was identified as a barrier in 68.1% of countries,[165] with a greater prevalence (80.0%) in high-income countries than in low-income countries (37.5%). Transportation and lack of care resources were identified as the most significant barriers in low-income countries.

Policy and programmes

National policy on child and adolescent mental health is a commitment of the government to the well-being of its nation's youth and provides a comprehensive framework to develop services.[166] As the Atlas Project has pointed out, having a child and adolescent mental health policy does not mean that a country has an identifiable service programme.[165] The countries with the highest proportion of children and adolescents in their population are the countries most likely to be lacking in a child and adolescent mental health policy and service programmes. The smallest percentage of countries reported to have child and adolescent mental health national policy and service programmes was among the lowest-income countries compared with the percentages reported in higher-income countries. However, there is worldwide variability in the presence of national policy and service programmes for child and adolescent mental health.[166] The African Region, for example, has the most limited national policy and fewest service programmes but countries like South Africa and Mozambique have very comprehensive models of child mental health care, comparable to the best in any region of the world.[165]

Service system

About 10–20% of children and adolescents are identified as needing mental health services, in both high-income and low-income countries.[167] However, the range of coverage and quality of services for youth are generally worse than those for adults, even in well-resourced regions such as Europe.[168] Also, while the service gap in high-income countries is very large, the situation is even worse in low-income countries worldwide.[165] Global variability in the service gap is also observed. Countries with highly developed child and adolescent mental health services, such as those in Scandinavian regions and Israel, meet about 80% of service needs, but others among high-income countries have only 20% provision.

A trend toward the development of specialized services for specific disorders, such as ADHD and autism, is reported in the Eastern Mediterranean and the Region of the Americas.[165] Specifically, parental advocacy, the dissemination of new knowledge, and the influence of the pharmaceutical industry contribute to development of disorder-specific services.

Although ADHD is a well-recognized childhood mental disorder worldwide, psychostimulants are prohibited or unavailable in about half of all countries.[165] There is no essential drug list for child psychotropic medications in more than 70% of the countries that the WHO Atlas project surveyed.

School-based consultation or services are critical for school-aged children with mental disorders. However, although some countries have excellent model programmes,[168] most high-income and low-income countries do not have sound school services for children with mental disorders.[165]

Strategies to promote child and adolescent mental health

Several strategies have been proposed to promote child and adolescent mental health care.[169,170] A holistic mental health framework is crucial to include a broader range of stakeholder groups at all levels. The WHO's guidelines for child and adolescent mental health care[153] are a useful reference. Prevention of problems or disorders, and promotion of well-being or health should be targeted, with achievable goals.

Family, community, nongovernmental organizations and school systems should be strengthened, while specialist capacity in child and adolescent mental health should be developed.[169] Professionals at all levels, including teachers, school counsellors, social workers, GPs, paediatricians, child psychologists and psychiatrists, should be included for comprehensive and efficacious intervention. However, for low- and middle-income countries, low-cost community resources (i.e. parents, children, adolescents, GPs, teachers, grass-root workers and volunteers) may be more affordable and sustainable.[170] Telepsychiatry and the Internet are seen as promising ways to deliver intervention, with training of care providers and clients.

Advocacy and awareness work in the community is warranted to remove social barriers. A preliminary school-based project to increase awareness of child and adolescent mental health has had promising results in nine countries of various economic levels across five continents.[171]

References

1   Insel TR, Fenton WS. Psychiatric epidemiology: it's not just about counting anymore. *Archives of General Psychiatry*, 2005, 62:590–592.

2   Costello EA, Egger H, Angold A. 10-year research update review: the epidemiology of child and adolescent psychiatric disorders: I. methods and public health burden. *Journal of the American Academy of Child and Adolescent Psychiatry*, 2005, 44:972–986.

3   Merikangas KR et al. Epidemiology of mental disorders in children and adolescents. *Dialogues in Clinical Neuroscience*, 2009, 11:7–20.

4   Egger HL, Angold A. Common emotional and behavioral disorders in preschool children: Presentation, nosology, and epidemiology. *Journal of Child Psychology and Psychiatry*, 2006, 47:313–337.

5   Keenan K et al. DSM-III-R disorders in preschool children from low-income families. *Journal of the American Academy of Child and Adolescent Psychiatry*, 1997, 36:620–627.

6   Kramer T, Garralda EA. Child and adolescent mental health problems in primary care. *Advances in Psychiatric Treatment*, 2000, 6:287–294.

7   American Academy of Pediatrics. Policy statement: Identifying infants and young children with developmental disorders in the medical home: an algorithm for developmental surveillance and screening. *Pediatrics*, 2006, 118:405–420.

8   Committee on Pediatric Workforce. Reaffirmed policy statement – Pediatric primary health care. *American Academy of Pediatrics*, 2010, 127:397.

9   Rakel RE. The family physician. In: Rakel RE, ed. *Textbook of family medicine*. Philadelphia, PA, Elsevier, 2007:3–14.

10   Committee on Children With Disabilities. The pediatrician's role in the diagnosis and management of autistic spectrum disorder in children. *Pediatrics*, 2001, 107:1221–1226.

11   Council on Children With Disabilities. Identifying infants and young children with developmental disorders in the medical home: an algorithm for developmental surveillance and screening. *Pediatrics*, 2006, 118:405–420.

12   National Initiative for Autism. *National Autism Plan for Children (NAPC): Plan for the identification, assessment, diagnosis and access to early interventions for pre-school and primary school aged children with autism spectrum disorders (ASD)*. London, The National Autistic Society, 2003.

13   Dosreis S et al. Autism spectrum disorder screening and management practices among general pediatric providers. *Developmental and Behavioral Pediatrics*, 2006, 27:S88–S94.

14   Garralda ME, Bowman FM, Mandalia S. Children with psychiatric disorders who are frequent attenders to primary care. *European Child and Adolescent Psychiatry*, 1999, 8:34–44.

15   Williams JG, Higgins JPT, Brayne CEG. Systematic review of prevalence studies of autism spectrum disorders. *Archives of Disease in Childhood*, 2006, 91:8–15.

16   Fombonne E. Epidemiological surveys of autism and other pervasive developmental disorders: an update. *Journal of Autism and Developmental Disorders*, 2003, 33:365–382.

17   *Diagnostic and statistical manual of mental disorders*, 4th ed, text revision (DSM-IV-TR). Washington, American Psychiatric Association, 2000.

18   Barbaresi WJ, Katusic SK, Voigt RG. Autism: a review of the state of the science for pediatric primary health care clinicians. *Archives of Pediatric and Adolescent Medicine*, 2006, 160:1167–1175.

19   Filipek PA et al. Practice parameter: screening and diagnosis of autism. *Neurology*, 2000, 55:468–479.

20   Levy SE, Mandell DS, Schultz RT. Autism. *The Lancet*, 2009, 374:1627–1638.

21   Mawlea E, Griffiths P. Screening for autism in pre-school children in primary care: systematic review of English language tools. *International Journal of Nursing Studies*, 2006, 43:623–636.

22   Robins DL, Dumont-Matieu TM. Early screening for autism spectrum disorders: update on the Modified Checklist for Autism in Toddlers and other measures. *Developmental and Behavioral Pediatrics*, 2006, 27:S111–S119.

23   Glascoe FP. Collaborating with parents: using parents' evaluations of developmental status to detect and address developmental and behavioral problems. *Journal of Developmental and Behavioral Pediatrics*, 1999, 20:187–188.

24 Squires J, Bricker D. *Ages & Stages Questionnaires®, Third Edition (ASQ-3™) A parent-completed child-monitoring system*. Baltimore, MD, Brookes, 2009.

25 Squires J, Bricker DD, Twombly E. *Ages & Stages Questionnaires, social-emotional (ASQ:SE): a parent-completed, child-monitoring system for social-emotional behaviors*. Baltimore, MD, Brookes, 2002.

26 Baron-Cohen S et al. Psychological markers in the detection of autism in infancy in a large population. *British Journal of Psychiatry*, 1996, 168:158–163.

27 Baron-Cohen S, Allen J, Gillberg C. Can autism be detected at 18 months – the needle, the haystack, and the CHAT. *British Journal of Psychiatry*, 1992, 161:839–843.

28 Robins DL et al. The Modified Checklist for Autism in Toddlers: an initial study investigating the early detection of autism and pervasive developmental disorders. *Journal of Autism and Developmental Disorders*, 2001, 31:131–144.

29 Siegel B. *Pervasive Developmental Disorders Screening Test-II (PDDST-II)*. San Antonio, TX, Harcourt Assessment Inc., 2004.

30 Myers SM, Johnson CP. Management of children with Autism Spectrum Disorders. *Pediatrics*, 2007, 120:1162–182.

31 The Werry Centre. *Evidence-based age-appropriate interventions – a guide for child and adolescent mental health services (CAMHS)*, 2nd ed. Auckland, The Werry Centre for Child and Adolescent Mental Health Workforce Development, 2010.

32 *Evidence-based child and adolescent psychosocial interventions*. Elk Grove Village, IL, American Academy of Pediatrics, 2011 (http://www.aap.org/commpeds/dochs/mentalhealth/docs/CR%20Psychosocial%20Interventions.F.0503.pdf, accessed 10 December 2011).

33 Paul R. Interventions to improve communication in autism. *Child and Adolescent Psychiatric Clinics of North America*, 2008, 17:835–856.

34 Ingersoll B. The effect of a parent-mediated imitation intervention on spontaneous imitation skills in young children with autism. *Research in Developmental Disabilities*, 2007, 28:163–175.

35 Eikeseth S. Outcome of comprehensive psycho-educational interventions for young children with autism. *Research in Developmental Disabilities*, 2008, 30:158–178.

36 Mesibov GB, Shea V, Schopler E. *The TEACCH approach to autism spectrum disorders*. New York, Springer Publishers, 2005.

37 Roeleveld N, Zielhuis GA, Gabreels F. The prevalence of mental retardation: A critical review of recent literature. *Developmental Medicine and Child Neurology*, 1997, 39:125–132.

38 Leonard H, Wen X. The epidemiology of mental retardation: challenges and opportunities in the new Millennium. *Mental Retardation and Developmental Disabilities Research Reviews*, 2002, 8:117–134.

39 Shevell MI. Present conceptualization of early childhood neurodevelopmental disabilities. *Journal of Child Neurology*, 2010, 25:120–126.

40 American Association on Mental Retardation. *Mental retardation: definition, classification and systems of support*. Washington DC, American Association on Mental Retardation, 2002.

41 *International classification of functioning, disability and health*. Geneva, World Health Organization, 2001.

42 Volkmar FR, Dykens E. Mental retardation. In: Rutter M, Taylor E, eds. *Child and adolescent psychiatry*, 4th ed. Oxford, Blackwell Publishing, 2002:697–722.

43 Girimaji SC. Clinical practice guidelines for the diagnosis and management of children with mental retardation. *Indian Journal of Psychiatry*, 2005 (http://www.indianjpsychiatry.org/cpg/cpg2008/CPG-CAP_05.pdf, accessed 30 January 2012).

44 Gisslera M et al. Health registers as a feasible means of measuring health status in childhood – a 7-year follow-up of the 1987 Finnish birth cohort. *Paediatric and Perinatal Epidemiology*, 1998, 12:437–455.

45 Winner M. *Children with exceptionalities in Canadian classrooms. Children with intellectual disabilities*, 8th ed. Ontario, Pearson, 2008.

46 Myrbakk E, von Tetzchner S. Screening individuals with intellectual disability for psychiatric disorders: comparison of four measures. *American Journal of Mental Retardation*, 2008, 113:54–70.

47 Lambert N, Nihira K, Leyland H. *Adaptive Behaviour Scale – school version*, 2nd ed. Washington, DC, American Association of Mental Retardation, 1993.

48   Nihiri K, Leyland H, Lambert N. *Adaptive Behavioral Scale – residential and community version*, 2nd ed. Austin, TX, Pro-ed, 1993.

49   Sparrow S, Balla D, Cicchetti D. *Vineland Adaptive Behavior Scales*. Pine Circle, MN, American Guidance Service, 1984.

50   Carr A, O'Reilly G. Diagnosis, classification and epidemiology. In: Carr A et al., eds. *The handbook of intellectual disability and clinical psychology practice*. London, Routledge, 2007:1–49.

51   Timimi S, Dwivedi K. Child and adolescent psychiatry. In: Puri B, Treasaden I, ed. *Psychiatry: an evidence-based text*. London, Edward Arnold, 2010.

52   Malone DM, Boat M. Early childhood intervention. In: Wehman P, McLaughlin PJ, Wehman T, eds. *Intellectual and developmental disabilities: toward full community inclusion*. Austin, TX, Pro-ed; 2005:51–92.

53   Kauffman JM, Hung LY. Special education for intellectual disability: current trends and perspectives. *Current Opinion in Psychiatry*, 2009, 22:452–456.

54   Graves P, Tracy J. Education for children with disabilities: The rationale for inclusion. *Journal of Paediatrics and Child Health*, 1998, 34:220–225.

55   Remschmidt H. Global consensus on ADHD/HKD. *European Child and Adolescent Psychiatry*, 2005; 14: 127–37.

56   *The ICD-10 classification of mental and behavioural disorders: clinical descriptions and diagnostic guidelines*. Geneva, World Health Organization, 1992.

57   Goodman R et al. The Development and Well-Being Assessment: description and initial validation of an integrated assessment of child and adolescent psychopathology. *Journal of Child Psychology and Psychiatry*, 2000, 41:645–655.

58   Singh I. Beyond polemics: science and ethics of ADHD. *Nature Reviews. Neuroscience*, 2008, 9:957–964.

59   Polanczyk G et al. The worldwide prevalence of ADHD: a systematic review and metaregression analysis. *American Journal of Psychiatry*, 2007, 164:942–948.

60   Centers for Disease Control and Prevention. Increasing prevalence of parent-reported attention-deficit/hyperactivity disorder among children – United States, 2003 and 2007. *MMWR: Morbidity and Mortality Weekly Report*, 2010, 59:1439–1443.

61   Castle L et al. Trends in medication treatment for ADHD. *Journal of Attention Disorders*, 2007, 10:335–342.

62   Heptinstall E, Taylor, E. Sex difference and their significance. In: Sandberg S, ed. *Hyperactivity and attention disorders of childhood*, 2nd ed. Cambridge, Cambridge University Press, 2002.

63   Tayor E, Sonu-Barke E. Disorder of attention and activity. In: Rutter M et al., eds. *Rutter's child & adolescent psychiatry*, 5th ed. Oxford, Wiley-Blackwell, 2008:521–542.

64   Biederman J, Mick E, Faraone SV. Age-dependent decline of symptoms of attention deficit hyperactivity disorder: impact of remission definition and symptom type. *American Journal of Psychiatry*, 2000, 157:816–818.

65   Faraone SV, Biederman J, Mick E. The age-dependent decline of attention deficit hyperactivity disorder: a meta-analysis of follow-up studies. *Psychological Medicine*, 2006, 36:159–165.

66   Simon V et al. Prevalence and correlates of adult attention-deficit hyperactivity disorder: meta-analysis. *British Journal of Psychiatry*, 2009, 194:204–211.

67   Lara C et al. Childhood predictors of adult attention-deficit/hyperactivity disorder: results from the World Health Organization World Mental Health Survey Initiative. *Biological Psychiatry*, 2009, 65:46–54.

68   Biederman J et al. Predictors of persistence and remission of ADHD into adolescence: results from a four-year prospective follow-up study. *Journal of the American Academy of Child and Adolescent Psychiatry*, 1996, 35:343–351.

69   Jensen PS et al. Findings from the NIMH Multimodal Treatment Study of ADHD (MTA): implications and applications for primary care providers. *Journal of Developmental and Behavioral Pediatrics*, 2001, 22:60–73.

70   Wilens TE et al. Does stimulant therapy of attention-deficit/hyperactivity disorder beget later substance abuse? A meta-analytic review of the literature. *Pediatrics*, 2003, 111:179–185.

71	Committee on Quality Improvement Subcommittee on Attention-Deficit/Hyperactivity Disorder. Clinical practice guideline: Diagnosis and evaluation of the child with attention-deficit/hyperactivity disorder. *Pediatrics*, 2000, 105:1158–1170.

72	Atkinson M, Hollis C. NICE guideline: attention deficit hyperactivity disorder. *Archives of Disease in Childhood. Education and Practice Edition*, 2010, 95:24–27.

73	Dulcan M. Practice parameters for the assessment and treatment of children, adolescents, and adults with attention-deficit/hyperactivity disorder. American Academy of Child and Adolescent Psychiatry. *Journal of the American Academy of Child and Adolescent Psychiatry*, 1997, 36(10 Suppl.):85S–121S.

74	DuPaul GJ et al. ADHD Rating Scale–IV: checklists, norms, and clinical interpretation. New York, Guilford Press, 1998.

75	Swanson JM. *School-based assessments and intervention for ADD students*. Irvine, KC Publishing, 1992.

76	Wolraich ML et al. Teachers' screening for attention deficit/hyperactivity disorder: comparing multinational samples on teacher ratings of ADHD. *Journal of Abnormal Child Psychology*, 2003, 31:445–455.

77	Wolraich ML et al. Psychometric properties of the Vanderbilt ADHD diagnostic parent rating scale in a referred population. *Journal of Pediatric Psychology*, 2003, 28:559–567.

78	Conners CK. *Conners 3 manual*. New York, Multi-Health Systems, 2008.

79	Conners CK. *Conners early childhood manual*. New York, Multi-Health Systems, 2009.

80	Reynolds CR, Kamphaus RW. *BASC-2: Behavior Assessment System for Children*, 2nd ed. Circle Pines, MN, American Guidance Service, 2004.

81	Achenbach TM, Rescoria LA. *Manual for the school-age forms and profiles*. Burlington, University of Vermont, Department of Psychiatry, 2001.

82	Achenbach TM, Rescoria LA. *Manual for the ASEBA preschool forms & profiles*. Burlington, VT, University of Vermont, Research Center for Children, Youth, & Families, 2000.

83	Biederman J et al. A double-blind placebo controlled study of desipramine in the treatment of ADD: III. Lack of impact of comorbidity and family history factors on clinical response. *Journal of the American Academy of Child and Adolescent Psychiatry*, 1993, 32:199–204.

84	Hunt RD, Capper L, O'Connell P. Clonidine in child and adolescent psychiatry. *Journal of Child and Adolescent Psychopharmacology*, 1990, 1:87–102.

85	Boylan K et al. Comorbidity of internalizing disorders in children with oppositional defiant disorder. *European Child and Adolescent Psychiatry*, 2007, 16:484–494.

86	Olsson M. DSM diagnosis of conduct disorder (CD) – a review. *Nordic Journal of Psychiatry*, 2009, 63:102–112.

87	Moffitt TE. *Sex differences in antisocial behaviour: conduct disorder, delinquency, and violence in the Dunedin longitudinal study*. Cambridge, Cambridge University Press, 2001.

88	Collishaw S, Maughan B, Goodman R, Pickles A. Time trends in adolescent mental health. *Journal of Child Psychology and Psychiatry*, 2004, 45:1350–1362.

89	Angold A, Costello EJ. Toward establishing an empirical basis for the diagnosis of oppositional defiant disorder. *Journal of the American Academy of Child and Adolescent Psychiatry*, 1996, 35:1205–1212.

90	Offord DR et al. Outcome, prognosis, and risk in a longitudinal follow-up study. *Journal of the American Academy of Child and Adolescent Psychiatry*, 1992, 31:916–923.

91	Loeber R et al. Oppositional defiant and conduct disorder: a review of the past 10 years, part I. *Journal of the American Academy of Child and Adolescent Psychiatry*, 2000, 39:1468–1484.

92	Carroll JM et al. Literacy difficulties and psychiatric disorders: evidence for comorbidity. *Journal of Child Psychology and Psychiatry*, 2005, 46:524–532.

93	Moss HB, Lynch KG. Comorbid disruptive behavior disorder symptoms and their relationship to adolescent alcohol use disorders. *Drug and Alcohol Dependence*, 2001, 64:75–83.

94	Myers MG, Brown SA, Mott MA. Preadolescent conduct disorder behaviors predict relapse and progression of addiction for adolescent alcohol and drug abusers. *Alcoholism, Clinical and Experimental Research*, 1995, 19:1528–1536.

95	Bussing R et al. Child temperament, ADHD, and caregiver strain: exploring relationships in an epidemiological sample. *Journal of the American Academy of Child and Adolescent Psychiatry*, 2003, 42:184–192.

96   Cohen P, Cohen J, Brook J. An epidemiological study of disorders in late childhood and adolescence – II. Persistence of disorders. *Journal of Child Psychology and Psychiatry*, 1993; 34:869–77.

97   Lahey BB et al. Four-year longitudinal study of conduct disorder in boys: patterns and predictors of persistence. *Journal of Abnormal Psychology*, 1995, 104:83–93.

98   Robins LN, McEvoy LT. Conduct problems as predictors of substance abuse. In: Robins LN, Rutter M, eds. *Straight and deviant pathways from childhood to adulthood*. New York, Cambridge University Press, 1990:182–204.

99   Lavigne JV et al. Oppositional defiant disorder with onset in preschool years: longitudinal stability and pathways to other disorders. *Journal of the American Academy of Child and Adolescent Psychiatry*, 2001, 40:1393–400.

100 Turgay A. Aggression and disruptive behavior disorders in children and adolescents. *Expert Review of Neurotherapeutics*, 2004, 4:623–632.

101 Lahey BB et al. Instability of the DSM-IV Subtypes of ADHD from preschool through elementary school. *Archives of General Psychiatry*, 2005, 62:896–902.

102 Rowe R et al. The relationship between DSM-IV oppositional defiant disorder and conduct disorder: findings from the Great Smoky Mountains Study. *Journal of Child Psychology and Psychiatry*, 2002, 43:365–373.

103 McMahon RJ, Frick PJ. Evidence-based assessment of conduct problems in children and adolescents. *Journal of Clinical Child and Adolescent Psychology*, 2005, 34:477–505.

104 Borum R, Bartel P, Forth A. *Manual for the Structured Assessment of Violence Risk in Youth (SAVRY)*. Tampa, Florida, University of South Florida, 2002.

105 Augimeri L et al. *The Early Assessment of Risk List for Boys (EARL-20B)*. Toronto, Earlscourt Child and Family Centre, 2001

106 Levene KS et al. *Assessment Risk List for Girls (EARL-21G)*. Toronto, Earlscourt Child and Family Centre, 2001.

107 Quay HC, Peterson DR. *Revised Behavior Problem Checklist-PAR Edition: professional manual*. Odessa, FL, Psychological Assessment Resources, 1996.

108 Brestan EV, Eyberg SM. Effective psychosocial treatments of conduct-disordered children and adolescents: 29 years, 82 studies, and 5272 kids. *Journal of Clinical and Child Psychology*, 1998, 27:180–189.

109 Eyberg SM, Nelson MM, Boggs SR. Evidence-based psychosocial treatments for children and adolescents with disruptive behavior. *Journal of Clinical Child and Adolescent Psychology*, 2008, 37:215–237.

110 Webster-Stratton C, Reid MJ, Hammond M. Treating children with early-onset conduct problems: intervention outcomes for parent, child, and teacher training. *Journal of Clinical Child and Adolescent Psychology*, 2004, 33:105–124.

111 Eddy JM, Chamberlain P. Family management and deviant peer association as mediators of the impact of treatment condition on youth antisocial behavior. *Journal of Consulting and Clinical Psychology*, 2000; 68: 857–63.

112 Beauchaine TP, Webster-Stratton C, Reid MJ. Mediators, moderators, and predictors of 1-year outcomes among children treated for early-onset conduct problems: a latent growth curve analysis. *Journal of Consulting and Clinical Psychology*, 2005, 73:371–388.

113 Steiner H. Practice parameters for the assessment and treatment of children and adolescents with conduct disorder. American Academy of Child and Adolescent Psychiatry. *Journal of the American Academy of Child and Adolescent Psychiatry*, 1997, 36(10 Suppl.):122S–139S.

114 Klein RG et al. Clinical efficacy of methylphenidate in conduct disorder with and without attention deficit hyperactivity disorder. *Archives of General Psychiatry*, 1997, 54:1073–1080.

115 Spencer T et al. An open-label, dose-ranging study of atomoxetine in children with attention deficit hyperactivity disorder. *Journal of Child and Adolescent Psychopharmacology*, 2001, 11:251–265.

116 Kemph JP et al. Treatment of aggressive children with clonidine: results of an open pilot study. *Journal of the American Academy of Child and Adolescent Psychiatry*, 1993, 32:577–581.

117 Findling RL et al. A double-blind pilot study of risperidone in the treatment of conduct disorder. *Journal of the American Academy of Child and Adolescent Psychiatry*, 2000, 39:509–516.

118 Donovan SJ et al. Divalproex treatment for youth with explosive temper and mood lability: a double-blind, placebo-controlled crossover design. *American Journal of Psychiatry*, 2000, 157:818–820.

119 Malone RP et al. A double-blind placebo-controlled study of lithium in hospitalized aggressive children and adolescents with conduct disorder. *Archives of General Psychiatry*, 2000, 57:649–654.

120 Soller MV, Karnik NS, Steiner H. Psychopharmacologic treatment in juvenile offenders. *Child and Adolescent Psychiatric Clinics of North America*, 2006, 15:477–499.

121 Snider LA et al. Tics and problem behaviors in schoolchildren: prevalence, characterization, and associations. *Pediatrics*, 2002, 110:331–336.

122 Khalifa N, von Knorring AL. Prevalence of tic disorders and Tourette syndrome in a Swedish school population. *Developmental Medicine and Child Neurology*, 2003, 45:315–319.

123 Wong CK, Lau JT. Psychiatric morbidity in a Chinese primary school in Hong Kong. *Australian and New Zealand Journal of Psychiatry*, 1992; 26: 459–466.

124 Kurlan R et al. Prevalence of tics in schoolchildren and association with placement in special education. *Neurology*, 2001, 57:1383–1388.

125 Robertson MM. The prevalence and epidemiology of Gilles de la Tourette syndrome. Part 1: the epidemiological and prevalence studies. *Journal of Psychosomatic Research*, 2008, 65:461–472.

126 Freeman RD et al. An international perspective on Tourette syndrome: selected findings from 3,500 individuals in 22 countries. *Developmental Medicine and Child Neurology*, 2000, 42:436–447.

127 Pauls DL et al. Gilles de la Tourette's syndrome and attention deficit disorder with hyperactivity. Evidence against a genetic relationship. *Archives of General Psychiatry*, 1986, 43:1177–1179.

128 Comings DE, Comings BG. Tourette's syndrome and attention deficit disorder with hyperactivity: are they genetically related? *Journal of the American Academy of Child and Adolescent Psychiatry*, 1984, 23:138–146.

129 Kurlan R. Clinical practice. Tourette's syndrome. *New England Journal of Medicine*, 2010, 363:2332–2338.

130 Ringman JM, Jankovic J. Occurrence of tics in Asperger's syndrome and autistic disorder. *Journal of Child Neurology*, 2000, 15:394–400.

131 Pauls DL, Leckman JF. The inheritance of Gilles de la Tourette's syndrome and associated behaviors. Evidence for autosomal dominant transmission. *New England Journal of Medicine*, 1986, 315:993–997.

132 Staley D, Wand R, Shady G. Tourette disorder: a cross-cultural review. *Comprehensive Psychiatry*, 1997, 38:6–16.

133 Leckman JF et al. Course of tic severity in Tourette syndrome: the first two decades. *Pediatrics*, 1998, 102:14–19.

134 Robertson MM. The Gilles de la Tourette syndrome: the current status. *British Journal of Psychiatry*, 1989, 154:147–169.

135 Abuzzahab FS, Anderson FO. Gilles de la Tourette's syndrome: crosscultural analysis and treatment outcome. In: Abuzzahab FS, Anderson FO, eds. *Gilles de la Tourette's syndrome: international registry*. St Paul, MN, Mason, 1976 :71–79.

136 Leckman JF. Tourette's syndrome. *The Lancet*, 2002, 360(9345):1577–1586.

137 Singer HS, Walkup JT. Tourette syndrome and other tic disorders. Diagnosis, pathophysiology, and treatment. *Medicine (Baltimore)*, 1991, 70:15–32.

138 Leckman JF, Walker DE, Cohen DJ. Premonitory urges in Tourette's syndrome. *American Journal of Psychiatry*, 1993, 150:98–102.

139 Leckman JF et al. Yale approach to assessment and treatment. In: Leckman JF, Cohen DJ, eds. *Tourette's syndrome tics, obsession, compulsions: developmental psychopathology and clinical care*. New York, John Wiley and Sons, 1998:285–309.

140 Leckman JF et al. The Yale Global Tic Severity Scale: initial testing of a clinician-rated scale of tic severity. *Journal of the American Academy of Child and Adolescent Psychiatry*, 1989, 28:566–573.

141 Deckersbach T et al. Habit reversal versus supportive psychotherapy in Tourette's disorder: a randomized controlled trial and predictors of treatment response. *Behaviour Research and Therapy*, 2006, 44:1079–1090.

142 Tourette's Syndrome Study Group. Treatment of ADHD in children with tics: a randomized controlled trial. *Neurology*, 2002, 58:527–536.

143 Leckman JF et al. Clonidine treatment of Gilles de la Tourette's syndrome. *Archives of General Psychiatry*, 1991, 48:324–328.

144 Scahill L et al. A placebo-controlled study of guanfacine in the treatment of children with tic disorders and attention deficit hyperactivity disorder. *American Journal of Psychiatry*, 2001, 158:1067–1074.

145 Shapiro E et al. Controlled study of haloperidol, pimozide and placebo for the treatment of Gilles de la Tourette's syndrome. *Archives of General Psychiatry*, 1989, 46:722–730.

146 Eggers C, Rothenberger A, Berghaus U. Clinical and neurobiological findings in children suffering from tic disease following treatment with tiapride. *European Archives of Psychiatry and Neurol Sciences*, 1988, 237:223–229.

147 Bruggeman R et al. Risperidone versus pimozide in Tourette's disorder: a comparative double-blind parallel-group study. *Journal of Clinical Psychiatry*, 2001, 62:50–56.

148 Stephens RJ, Bassel C, Sandor P. Olanzapine in the treatment of aggression and tics in children with Tourette's syndrome – a pilot study. *Journal of Child and Adolescent Psychopharmacology*, 2004, 14:255–266.

149 Sallee FR et al. Ziprasidone treatment of children and adolescents with Tourette's syndrome: a pilot study. *Journal of the American Academy of Child and Adolescent Psychiatry*, 2000, 39:292–299.

150 Liu YY et al. [A control study of aripiprazole and tiapride treatment for tic disorders in children]. *Zhongguo Dang Dai Er Ke Za Zhi*, 2010, 12:421–424.

151 Simpson DM et al. Assessment: botulinum neurotoxin for the treatment of movement disorders (an evidence-based review): report of the Therapeutics and Technology Assessment Subcommittee of the American Academy of Neurology. *Neurology*, 2008, 70:1699–1706.

152 Maciunas RJ et al. Prospective randomized double-blind trial of bilateral thalamic deep brain stimulation in adults with Tourette syndrome. *Journal of Neurosurgery*, 2007, 107:1004–1014.

153 *Caring for children and adolescents with mental disorders: setting WHO directions*. Geneva, World Health Organization, 2003.

154 Leckman JF, Leventhal BL. Editorial: a global perspective on child and adolescent mental health. *Journal of Child Psychology and Psychiatry*, 2008, 49:221–225.

155 Nikapota A, Rutter M. Sociocultural/ethnic groups and psychopathology. In: Rutter M et al., eds. *Rutter's child & adolescent psychiatry*, 5th ed. Oxford, Wiley-Blackwell, 2009:199–211.

156 Costello EJ et al. The Great Smoky Mountains Study of Youth. Goals, design, methods, and the prevalence of DSM-III-R disorders. *Archives of General Psychiatry*, 1996, 53:1129–1136.

157 Roberts RE, Roberts CR, Xing Y. Prevalence of youth-reported DSM-IV psychiatric disorders among African, European, and Mexican American adolescents. *Journal of the American Academy of Child and Adolescent Psychiatry*, 2006, 45:1329–1337.

158 Goodman A, Patel V, Leon DA. Child mental health differences amongst ethnic groups in Britain: a systematic review. *BMC Public Health*, 2008, 8:258.

159 Angold A et al. Psychiatric disorder, impairment, and service use in rural African American and white youth. *Archives of General Psychiatry*, 2002, 59:893–901.

160 Goodman R. The Strengths and Difficulties Questionnaire: a research note. *Journal of Child Psychology and Psychiatry*, 1997, 38:581–586.

161 Achenbach TM et al. Multicultural assessment of child and adolescent psychopathology with ASEBA and SDQ instruments: research findings, applications, and future directions. *Journal of Child Psychology and Psychiatry*, 2008, 49:251–275.

162 Rousseau C, Measham T, Bathiche-Suidan M. DSM IV, culture and child psychiatry. *Journal of the Canadian Academy of Child and Adolescent Psychiatry*, 2008, 17:69–75.

163 Ecklund K, Johnson WB. Toward cultural competence in child intake assessments. *Professional Psychology: Research and Practice*, 2007, 38:356–362.

164 Measham T, Rousseau C, Nadeau L. The development and therapeutic modalities of a transcultural child psychiatry service. *Canadian Child and Adolescent Psychiatry Review*, 2005, 14:68–72.

165 *Altas of child and adolescent mental health resources: Global concerns: Implications for the future.* Geneva, World Health Organization, 2005.

166 Shatkin JP, Belfer ML. The global absence of child and adolescent mental health policy. *Child and Adolescent Mental Health*, 2004, 9:104–108.

167 *The World Health Report 2001 – mental health: new understanding, new hope.* Geneva, World Health Organization, 2001.

168 Levav I et al. Psychiatric services and training for children and adolescents in Europe: Results of a country survey. *European Child and Adolescent Psychiatry*, 2004; 13: 395–401.

169 Patel V et al. Promoting child and adolescent mental health in low and middle income countries. *Journal of Child Psychology and Psychiatry*, 2008, 49:313–334.

170 Graeff-Martins AS et al. Diffusion of efficacious interventions for children and adolescents with mental health problems. *Journal of Child Psychology and Psychiatry*, 2008, 49:335–352.

171 Hoven CW et al. Worldwide child and adolescent mental health begins with awareness: A preliminary assessment in nine countries. *International Review of Psychiatry*, 2008, 20:261–270.

29 Adolescent mental health in primary care

Vincent Chin-Hung Chen, Shou-Hung Huang and Meng-Chih Lee

Key messages

- About one-third to one-quarter of children and adolescents develop a mental disorder. However, only 20–25% of the affected children and adolescents receive treatment.
- The emergence of adolescent mental disorders encompasses interaction of biological vulnerability, psychological characteristics and sociocultural influence.
- The role of primary care for mental health problems includes early identification, offering treatment for less severe problems, and pursuing health promotion and problem prevention.
- In low- and middle-income countries, strategies to improve services for child and adolescent mental disorder include the provision of adequate advocacy tools to reveal the burden; poverty alleviation; health-awareness programmes; enforcing legislation; training centres within the region; partnerships with professionals in developed countries; integration for the training, continuing supervision and support of general practitioners and paediatricians in the detection and treatment of mental disorders; developing widescale community and primary health-care-based capacities; and building non-specialist capacities.
- Collaboration with mental professionals and community services is helpful and new technology makes collaboration more feasible.

Introduction

Up to 50% of all adult mental disorders have their onset in adolescence,[1] but treatment typically occurs years later.[2] Globally, about one-third to one-quarter of children and adolescents develop a *Diagnostic and Statistical Manual of Mental Disorders* (DSM) mental disorder,[3] with suicide being the third leading cause of death in adolescents.[4] However, only 20–25% of affected children and adolescents receive treatment.[5] Furthermore, affected adolescents tend to have severe physical symptoms and higher exposure to illicit drugs.[6]

The epidemiological data for mental disorders are similar among children and adolescents in industrialized countries and less developed areas.[7] The prevalence of mental disorders range from 9.4% in south India, 12.5% in Sao Paulo, Brazil, 13% in China, 14% in Khartoum, Sudan, 15% in north-central Nigeria, to 16% in Ibadan, Nigeria.[8] However, there is a wide range of differences globally in terms of policy and care resources.[4] There is still a significant lag in the development of mental health resources for children and adolescents in low-income countries,[9] many of which have no "specific focal point" for organized services and data collection in child and adolescent mental health.[8] For example, there is fewer than one psychiatrist per 100 000 people in most countries in South-East Asia and fewer than one per million in countries in sub-Saharan Africa.[8]. Omigbodun suggests that support for development of child mental health services in these areas requires "the provision of adequate advocacy tools to reveal the burden, poverty alleviation, health awareness programmes, enforcing legislation, training centers within the region, and partnerships with professionals in developed countries".[8] Patel et al. stated that developing a service structure like those used in resource-rich areas is not feasible for children and adolescents in low- and middle-income countries.[9] They suggested several strategies to improve services for child and adolescent mental disorder in low- and middle-income countries, including: (1) integration for the training, continuing supervision and support of general practitioners (GPs) and paediatricians in the detection and treatment of child and adolescent mental disorders; (2) developing widescale community and primary health-care-based capacities; and (3) building non-specialist capacities.[9]

It is estimated that rates of psychiatric disorders in attenders in primary care are also high: 1 in 4 of 7–12 year olds; 4 in 10 of 13–16 year olds.[10] GPs are at the forefront of being able to identify mental health problems at the first encounter and being able to either offer or serve as gateways to appropriate services.[11] It has been suggested that the role of primary care as it relates to mental health problems encompasses:[12]

1   early identification of mental health problems
2   offering treatment for less severe problems
3   pursuing health promotion and problem prevention.

This chapter gives an overview of mental disorders commonly emerging among adolescents, including depression, anxiety, schizophrenia substance use and suicidal behaviours. Information for primary physicians including prevalence, pattern, detection, intervention and referral principles are described. Some other mental disorders, such as attention-deficit hyperactivity disorder (ADHD) and conduct disorder, which often emerge in childhood and continue to manifest in adolescence, are discussed in Chapter 28.

The prevalence of mental disorders

Depressive disorders

Major depressive disorder (MDD) is a debilitating condition that has been increasingly recognized among youth, particularly adolescents. According to one recent review,[3] the current prevalence of MDD among children and adolescents worldwide ranges from 0.6% to 3.0%. Another review revealed that the prevalence of current or recent depression among adolescents is 6% worldwide and the lifetime prevalence of MDD among adolescents may be as high as 20% in North America.[13] MDD is also associated with early pregnancy, decreased school performance, and impaired work, social, and family functioning during young adulthood.[13]

Anxiety disorders

The median prevalence rate of all anxiety disorders reported in a recent review was 8% worldwide, with an extremely wide range of estimates.[14] Another recent review found community prevalence estimates ranged from 3.1% to 17.5% for the point prevalence of diagnosis of any anxiety disorder in children and adolescents, across multiple international epidemiological studies.[15] Generalized anxiety disorder (GAD) and social anxiety disorder (SAD) are the two most prevalent mental disorders in adolescents.[16] The published data support either a chronic and persistent course or a relapsing and remitting course when anxiety disorders are diagnosed in childhood and adolescence.[17]

Schizophrenia

Schizophrenia is a chronic and severely disabling disorder and usually emerges in late adolescence or early adulthood.[18] Schizophrenia occurring before the age of 17 years is considered "early-onset schizophrenia", while onset before 13 years is termed "very early-onset schizophrenia".[18] Very early-onset schizophrenia is estimated to occur less than one in 30 000.[19] The prevalences have been estimated to be 0.9 per 10 000 at 13 years of age and 17.6 per 10 000 at 18 years of age.[20]

Substance use disorder

Substance use disorder is one of the most prevalent psychiatric disorders. The median estimate of alcohol or drug abuse or dependence in community surveys of adolescents in high-income countries is 5%, with a range from 1 to 24%.[21] The National Comorbidity Survey – Adolescent Supplement (2010) in the United States of America (USA) showed the lifetime prevalence based on DSM-IV diagnostic criteria was 6.4% for alcohol abuse/

dependence, 8.9% for drug abuse/dependence and 11.4% for any substance abuse/dependence.[22] Substance use disorder among adolescents is a worldwide problem and is just as important in low-income countries as in western countries.[1] However, studies from low-income countries are relatively limited.[9] Behrendt et al. postulated that concurrent use of substances is important for the association between the age of first use and the speed of transition to substance use disorders.[23] It is also suggested that an earlier age of onset of substance use is related to greater severity of dependence.[24] Therefore, it is important to intervene early in substance use disorders in adolescents.

Suicide

Every year, over one million children and adolescents attempt suicide, and increasing numbers of youth in the USA have suicidal thoughts.[25] A systematic review of 128 studies showed the mean proportion of adolescents reporting lifetime prevalence of attempted suicide was 9.7% (95% confidence interval (CI) = 8.5% to 10.9%), and 29.9% (95% CI = 26.1% to 33.8%) of adolescents reported suicidal ideation.[26] A lower prevalence of some suicidal phenomena was found for Asian populations.[26] Because such distressed youth are most likely to visit them, family physicians occupy a crucial role in the assessment and treatment of suicidal youth.[27] However, it has been noted by a research study that primary care physicians fail to identify 83% of the suicidal adolescent cases.[28] Furthermore, adolescents with physical problems like asthma have higher suicide mortality than those without such problems.[29] Therefore, it is essential to train primary care physicians in the recognition and management of suicidal youth.

Integrated models (biopsychosocial model) for understanding mental disorders: suicidal behaviour as an example

The emergence of mental disorder encompasses interaction of biological vulnerability, psychological characteristics and sociocultural influence. A model of integration of biopsychosocial factors gives the clinician a basis for understanding and treating mental disorders. For example, several different psychological models have been proposed for understanding suicidal behaviour. These include psychodynamic models, impulsivity of personality, dichotomous thinking and cognitive rigidity, impaired problem-solving, hopelessness, over-general autobiographical memory, and biases in future judgement.[30] Poor problem-solving is a well-recognized feature of deliberate self-harm and also a target of recent intervention studies. Problem-solving can be more difficult in the face of impulsivity, concrete thinking and hopelessness.[31]

From the psychodynamic aspect, Freud asserted that most people cope with the loss of a loved person through the process of mourning. However, for some people the experience is unbearable and generates enormous anger. The individual feels ambivalence but preserves the mental image of the loved person by internalization and it becomes part of the ego. Feelings of anger are transformed into self-censure and the wish to self-harm, because it is impossible to express these feelings towards the lost object.[30] Williams et al. draw together the threads of contemporary researchers in their proposed "cry of pain" model, which sees suicidal behaviour as an attempt to escape from a feeling of entrapment, a feeling of being both "defeated" and "closed in".[30] Early in the sequence, where escape potential is threatened but not yet eliminated, escape attempts will be characterized by high levels of activity, anger and protest, such as deliberate self-harm. When people believe they cannot escape from an external situation or internal turmoil, and that there is no hope of rescue, lethal deliberate self-harm and completed suicide will happen.[30] Williams et al. have suggested that some cognitive styles are likely to make people vulnerable to these responses.[32] The first is attention bias, which makes people focus on negative environmental cues and tend to sense the defeat/rejection feeling. Second, the strategy of over-general memory prevents people from recalling past experiences in sufficient detail to develop problem-solving strategies (problem-solving is thought to be an important deficit among suicide victims).[31] Third, suicidal individuals are less likely to be able to generate examples of future positive events than controls, and this is a possible mechanism of hopeless feeling, an important risk factor for suicide.[32]

Mann et al. have proposed a more comprehensive model, the stress-diathesis model, to explain the complex interaction between a variety of risk factors in connection to suicide.[33] This model argues that the risk for suicidal acts is determined not merely by an acute stressor but also by an underlying diathesis (predisposition). This diathesis may be reflected in tendencies to experience more suicidal ideation or to be more impulsive and, therefore, more likely to act on suicidal feelings.[33] Genetic factors and acquired susceptibility, early traumatic life experiences, chronic illness (especially of the central nervous system), chronic alcohol and substance abuse, and other factors like raised cholesterol can contribute to development of the diathesis.[34] Acute mental disorder or somatic illness, severe abuse of alcohol or drugs, or social or family problems can all act as stresses to provoke the diathesis.[34]

To expand the stress-diathesis model, Wasserman adds the dimensions of protective factors (such as good family relationship) and suicidal communication (the dynamics between the suicidal individual and his/her family and other key persons). Thus, suicide outcomes depend on the interaction of risk factors, protective factors and the response of significant others when individuals communicate their suicidal tendency.[34]

Clinical presentation

Contact with GPs is an important opportunity for the early identification of affected children and adolescents, which could promote early treatment or referral to specialist services.[10] Evaluation of psychosocial and health risk factors may also help the GP to identify child psychiatric disorders.[10] These factors may include adolescents with persistent functional symptoms, those who are markedly disabled or impeded by physical complaints, those with peer-relationship difficulties and those with mothers in poor mental health.[35] The principles for diagnosis of mental disorders based on underlying rules encompass (1) *psychopathology*: symptoms with significant severity and duration; (2) *functional impairment*: problems related to academic/job performance, interpersonal and family relationships; and (3) *exclusion criteria*: symptoms not caused by drug or substance use or organic problems. In this section, some clues related to symptoms for adolescent mental disorder are described.[36]

Depressive disorders

Major depression

This is characterized by a combination of symptoms such as depressed mood, low energy and poor concentration that interfere with the ability to work, study, sleep, eat, and enjoy once-pleasurable activities.[37] The atypical representation of depression as irritable mood easily confuses the diagnosis among adolescents.[36] An episode of depression might occur only once, but more commonly occurs several times in a lifetime.

Dysthymia

This is a less severe type of depression involving long-term, chronic symptoms that are not disabling but keep an individual from functioning well or from feeling good.[37] Symptoms include problems with sleeping or eating, fatigue, poor concentration, low self-esteem and feelings of hopelessness.[36]

Anxiety disorders

There are associations between anxiety disorders and other mental disorders. The high frequency of comorbidity between anxiety disorders and mood disorders has even led to consideration of a developmental continuity between the two disorders, with early anxiety predicting later development of depression in adulthood.[3] The most likely periods of onset for anxiety disorders are: (1) middle childhood for separation anxiety and specific phobias; (2) late childhood for overanxious disorder; (3) middle adolescence for social phobia; (4) late adolescence for panic disorder: and (5) early adulthood for GAD and obsessive–compulsive disorder (OCD).[38] Few distribution differences are found among ethnic groups and social classes.[39] Guidelines proposed from Columbia University describing the essential symptoms of anxiety disorders are presented in Table 29.1.[37] However, for a proper diagnosis, the criteria of the ICD-10 or DSM-IV-TR (Text Revision)[36] need to be applied.

Table 29.1 Pattern of anxiety disorders

Disorder	Symptoms
Generalized anxiety	Constant, exaggerated, worrisome thoughts, physical symptoms, and tension about routine life events and activities. Sufferers almost always anticipate the worst, even though there is little reason to expect it.
Specific phobia	Extreme, disabling, and irrational fear of something that poses little or no actual danger. Avoidance of feared objects or situations can result in unnecessary, limiting accommodations.
Separation anxiety	Unreasonable fears about leaving home and parents. Serious educational or social problems can develop if away from school and friends for an extended period of time.
Social phobia	Overwhelming and disabling fear of scrutiny, embarrassment, or humiliation in social situations, which leads to avoidance of many potentially pleasurable and meaningful activities.
Panic	Repeated episodes of intense fear appearing without warning. Physical symptoms include chest pain, heart palpitations, shortness of breath, dizziness, abdominal distress, feelings of unreality, and fear of dying.
Agoraphobia	Anxiety about being in open spaces or situations from which escape might be difficult (or embarrassing), or in which help might not be available in the event.
Obsessive–compulsive	Patterns of repetitive thoughts and behaviours that are distressing but extremely difficult to overcome.
Post-traumatic stress	Persistent symptoms that occur after a traumatic event. Nightmares, flashbacks, emotional numbness, depression, anger, irritability, distractedness, and being easily startled are common symptoms.

Adapted, with permission, from *Guidelines for child and adolescent mental health referral*, 2nd ed. New York, Columbia University, Department of Child and Adolescent Psychiatry, 2003.[37]

Schizophrenia

The diagnostic criteria of early-onset schizophrenia are similar to those for adults. In adolescents, social or intellectual deterioration may present itself as a failure to achieve expected levels of interpersonal, academic or occupational achievement.[36,40] The clinical presentation encompasses positive symptoms (an excess or distortion of normal functioning, including hallucination, delusion, disorganized speech, disorganized or catatonic behaviour) and negative symptoms (including affective flattening – restrictions in the range and intensity of emotional expression; alogia – defect of the fluency and productivity of thought and speech; avolition – restricted initiation of goal-directed behaviour).[36] The presentation of schizophrenia differs little between disorders in adulthood and adolescence. In younger adolescents, the content may even relate to childhood themes of ghosts, monsters or film and TV characters.[40] In addition, early-onset schizophrenia is associated with worsening cognitive performance and functional outcomes.[41] Schizophrenia causes lifelong impairment, and more than half of affected individuals require continuous support; 10–15% ultimately commit suicide, and many become homeless.[19]

Substance use disorders

According to the DSM diagnostic system, abuse is defined as adverse consequences (such as law, physical, relationship, and job problems) related to the repeated use of substances. Dependence is a loss of control, or preoccupation with the substance along with tolerance, withdrawal, and compulsive drug-taking behaviour.[36] The most commonly abused substances among adolescents include alcohol, nicotine, cannabis, amphetamines and the derivatives (MDMA (3,4-methylenedioxymethamphetamine) or ecstasy), cocaine, hallucinogens (phencyclidine, LSD (lysergic acid diethylamide), mescaline), inhalants (glue-sniffing, toluene-sniffing), opiates (heroin), sedatives and tranquillizers (barbiturates, sleeping pills, benzodiazepine), ketamine and anabolic steroids.[42] Abuse problems in adolescents have been shown to be more complicated than in adults.[42] Firstly, less withdrawal is noted due to the relatively shorter time of use. Second, more complex psychosocial issues are noted in adolescents. Some adolescents develop substance use problems due to subgroup culture and others due to school failure and social exclusion caused by specific learning disorder. Third, other adolescent mental disorders should be always considered. Self-medication has been reported to be related to affective disturbances and ADHD.[42] There is an extremely high prevalence of suicide attempts in substance users.[43]

Suicide

Suicidal behaviours include those that have fatal and non-fatal outcomes. The term suicidal behaviour includes the most "clear-cut" act of completed suicide, together with a heterogeneous spectrum of self-harm that ranges from highly lethal attempts (in which survival is the result of good fortune) to low-lethality attempts that occur in the context of a social crisis and contain a strong element of an appeal for help.[44] The terminology used to describe a fatal outcome of suicidal behaviour is always suicide, but there are several terminologies for non-fatal behaviour, including suicide attempt, parasuicide and deliberate self-harm. The problem of whether suicide intent exists always arises in the various definitions of non-fatal suicidal behaviour. Hawton et al. have discussed in detail the problems of definition and proposed three important issues when defining deliberate self-harm.[45] The first is when to include the deliberate ingestion of excess amounts of alcohol or drugs of abuse alone. A second is whether repetitive self-mutilation should be included. The third issue is the intent involved in the act.[45] The authors suggest that the inclusion of self-harm arising from alcohol or substance use alone needs to be assessed and decided on by a clinician; they argue that repetitive self-mutilation should be included because it is also related to future suicide risk,[46] and is difficult to distinguish from acts that are repeated less frequently;[45] finally, they choose to define deliberate self-harm irrespective of intent because it often involves mixed intent, and in many cases suicide intent may be low or absent.[47] Self-mutilation is used to describe serious bodily mutilation without suicidal intent.[31] Repetitive superficial bodily harm without suicidal intent is also known as self-injurious behaviour or self-wounding.[31] Young people tend to choose less fatal methods,[48] but more easily harm themselves repetitively.[49]

Screening and detection

The current practice of reliance on adolescents themselves or on parental complaints and standard physician interview has been found to underidentify adolescent depression.[25] It has also been revealed that as many as 83% of those attempting suicide are not identified by health-care providers as a danger to themselves, even when examined by primary care clinicians in the months before their attempt.[25]

Written screening tools may be completed prior to meeting with the practitioner, which can save time and target areas to focus on during the appointment.[17,50] The goal of screening is to identify those who have the condition of interest (true positives) from those who do not have the condition (true negatives).[25] However, the high false-positive rate (adolescents who screen positive but do not have the condition) still hinders precise case-finding, especially for the low-prevalence problems, such as suicide.[13,25,51] There is debate over the potential harms of false positives, such as stigma and increased strain on health-care resources.[52] Interviews can provide the clinician with more detailed information to make a diagnosis.[50] A thorough assessment should include recording a history of the problem, family history, other psychiatric disorders, family life, neighbourhood environment, school life, peer relationships, current medication and substance use. In addition, the clinician should have an understanding of the patient's past medical history for both physical and mental health problems, family history, medication use, prescription and non-prescription drugs, development (including school performance and diagnosis of ADHD), and suicidal ideation.[50] Organic conditions that might cause symptoms include infections and endocrine or neurological disorder.[50] Feelings of guilt, worthlessness, hopelessness and suicidal ideation are unlikely to be a direct result of a medical condition, and individuals expressing these feelings should be evaluated for depression.[53]

Some reviews summarize useful screening instruments for primary physicians to detect mental problems among adolescents; these are discussed next.

Depressive disorders

Harmin et al. have described some commonly used tools for screening depression,[50] including the Beck Depression Inventory II (BDI, for 13–18 years), the Patient Health Questionnaire – Adolescent version (PHQ-A, for 13–18 years), the Children's Depression Inventory (for 7–17 year olds), the Pediatric Symptom Checklist (for 3–16 years) and the Guidelines for Adolescent Preventative Services Questionnaire (for 11–21 years). Other instruments like the CES-D (Center for Epidemiological Studies – Depression Scale), the CIS-R (Revised Clinical Interview Schedule) and the SDQ (Strengths and Difficulties Questionnaire) have also been proposed by another review.[13]

Anxiety disorders

Rockhill et al. have comprehensively introduced related screening scales for the adolescent anxiety disorders.[17]

- The Pediatric Symptom Checklist (PSC) and PSC-17: for 3–16 years; this rates cognitive, emotional and behavioural problems.
- The Youth-Reported Pediatric Symptom Checklist (Y-PSC): for 11 years and older; this is a youth self-report version of the PSC.
- The Behavior Assessment System for Children-2 (BASC- 2), parent, and teacher: for 2–21 years; this is a broad-band behaviour questionnaire.
- BASC-2 Self-Report of Personality (SRP): for 8–25 years; this is a youth self-report of thoughts and feelings.
- The Child Behavior Checklist (CBCL) and Teacher Report Form (TRF) anxiety (panic/somatic, separation anxiety, social phobia, general anxiety, and school phobia): for 1.5–5 years and 6–18 years; this is a broad-band behaviour questionnaire.
- Youth self-report: for 11–18 years; this is a youth self-report broad-band behaviour questionnaire.
- The Screen for Child Anxiety Related Emotional Disorders – Revised (SCARED-R): for 7 years and older; this is for anxiety (panic/somatic, separation anxiety, social phobia, general anxiety, and school phobia).
- The Multidimensional Anxiety Scale for Children (MASC): for 8–19 years; this is for anxiety (physical symptoms, social anxiety, harm avoidance, separation/panic).
- The Fear Survey Schedule for Children – Revised: for 7–18 years; this is for childhood fears (fear of failure/criticism, fear of the unknown, fear of injury and small animals, fear of danger/death, and fear of medical situations).
- Children's Yale-Brown Obsessive–Compulsive Scale – Child Report and Parent Report: for 5–17 years; this is for symptoms of OCD and severity of obsessions and compulsions.
- Trauma symptom checklist for children: for 8–16 years; this is for post-traumatic stress disorder (PTSD; anxiety, depression, anger, post-traumatic stress, dissociation and sexual concerns).

Schizophrenia

Efforts have been increasingly focused on improving early detection and prevention of schizophrenia in high-risk individuals, due to the heavy burden of schizophrenia on patients and their caregivers.[19] Research has concentrated on young people with ultra high risk for schizophrenia, characterized by attenuated positive symptoms, brief limited intermittent psychotic symptoms, and/or genetic risk factors with functional decompensation.[19] Self-reported psychotic symptoms (delusion or hallucination) in childhood are often a marker of an impaired developmental process and should be actively assessed.[54] A formal physical examination, including a comprehensive neurological assessment, needs to be considered in every case, to exclude an underlying physical illness, such as epilepsy, cerebral tumour or other space-occupying lesion or neurodegenerative disorder.[40] One recent review provided useful criteria to differentiate adolescent schizophrenia from other medical disorders.[55] Psychotic symptoms due to substance misuse are frequently suspected in adolescents, and urine or hair analysis for illicit drugs should be undertaken.[40]

Substance use disorders

Leccese et al. have provided a comprehensive review for scales of adolescent substance use,[56] including the Adolescent Drinking Index (ADI), the Adolescent Drug Involvement Scale (ADIS), the Drug and Alcohol Problem Quick Screen (DAP), Drug Use Screening Inventory – Revised (DUSI-R), the Personal Experience Screening Questionnaire (PESQ), the Problem Oriented Screening Instrument for Teenagers (POSIT), the Rutgers Alcohol Problem Index (RAPI) and the Teen Addiction Severity Index (T-ASI). Other new instruments like the Substances and Choices Scale (SACS) and the CAGE-AID (CAGE questionnaire Adapted to Include Drugs) are brief and valid tools for detecting substance use disorder among adolescents.[57,58]

Suicide

In addition to interviewing the suicidal child or adolescent, collateral information should be obtained from others who know the youth, such as a parent. The individual's level of risk of suicide needs to be assessed.

Information regarding suicide risk to be assessed includes:[59] characteristics of the adolescent – sex, age, lives alone, psychotic thinking, suicidal ideation, suicidal plan, and history of previous suicide attempts (lethality and motivating feelings). Family history, current mental health of the parent and the context of the support system are also important.

High-risk situations include adolescents with a plan or recent suicide attempt with a high probability of lethality; suicide intent; current agitation or severe hopelessness; and impulsivity and severe dysphoric mood associated with bipolar disorder, major depression, psychosis, or a substance use disorder.[60]

For the screening, Horowitz et al. have provided an overview for screening tools for suicide.[25] Some useful instruments such as the Columbia Suicide Screen, Suicide Risk Screen, DISC-IV (Diagnostic Interview Schedule for Children), and Risk of Suicide Questionnaire are introduced.[25] Another useful summary of knowledge about adolescent suicide is reported by Shain et al.[60]

Interventions

Two recent reviews have summarized suggestions for intervention in adolescent mental disorders. Among them, American Academy of Pediatrics summarizes the intervention strategies according to level of evidence.[61] Another comprehensive review from New Zealand categorizes the treatment according to best-supported ("well-established") interventions and promising ("probably efficacious") interventions (see Tables 29.2–29.4).[57]

Depressive disorders

Evidence level of treatment: depressive disorders [61]

- Best support: CBT, CBT and medication, CBT with parents, family therapy
- Good support: client-centred therapy, expressive writing/journalling/diary, interpersonal therapy, relaxation

A treatment matrix is presented in Table 29.2.[57]

Another review focusing on the treatment for adolescent depression in primary care settings finds that SSRIs, psychotherapy and combined treatment are effective in increasing response rates and reducing depressive symptoms.[13] SSRIs may be associated with a small increased risk of suicidality (ideation or attempts) and should only be considered if judicious clinical monitoring is possible.[13] The United States (US) Food and Drug Administration (FDA) recommends that adolescents taking fluoxetine have a psychiatric follow-up weekly for 4 weeks, every other week for the next 4 weeks, and once a month thereafter.[62] One randomized controlled trial aimed to test the effectiveness of a quality-improvement intervention for adolescent depression in primary care clinics.[63] The programme included (1) care managers helping primary practitioners in evaluation and treatment of depression; (2) CBT training provided to care managers; (3) patients and clinicians together

Table 29.2 Treatment matrix: depressive disorders

Treatment	Treatments in childhood and adolescence[a,b]
Interpersonal therapy	Best-supported (well-established) intervention, although evidence is inconclusive in achieving remission
Cognitive-behavioural therapy (CBT)	Best-supported (well-established) intervention although recent studies suggest that further evaluation may be required
Systemic family therapy, other family therapies	Promising: needs further evaluation
Medication (psychological therapies should be considered as first line of treatment)	Selective serotonin reuptake inhibitors (SSRIs): fluoxetine – promising (probably efficacious, needs close monitoring). Recent results show improvements when combined with CBT
Social skills training	Not well evaluated. Appears effective in the recovery phase

[a] Best-supported ("well-established") interventions: at least two scientifically defensible group-design studies conducted by different investigative teams, or more than nine single-case designs, treatment manuals and strong experimental designs.

[b] Promising ('probably efficacious') interventions: at least two studies demonstrating the intervention to be more effective than a no-treatment control group, or several single-case studies, as well as manuals that prescribe the intervention.

Reproduced, with permission, from *Evidence-based age-appropriate interventions – a guide for child and adolescent mental health services (CAMHS)*. Auckland, The Werry Centre for Child and Adolescent Mental Health Workforce Development, 2010.[57]

making treatment modality choices; and (4) education for practitioners regarding the evaluation, management and pharmacological and psychosocial treatment of depression. The results showed that after interventions, patients under treatment present lower depression and higher mental health-related quality of life.[63]

Anxiety disorders

Evidence level of treatment: anxiety disorders[61]

- Best support: CBT, CBT and medication, CBT with parents, education, exposure, modelling
- Good support: assertiveness training, CBT for child and parent, family psycho-education, hypnosis, relaxation
- Moderate support: contingency management, group therapy

A treatment matrix is presented in Table 29.3.[57]

There is substantial evidence supporting the application of CBT and SSRIs for anxiety disorders among children.[17] Although SSRIs are associated with a small increase of suicide ideation risk in adolescents, their risk/benefit ratio in paediatric anxiety disorders is favourable with appropriate monitoring.[17] In contrast to the amount of evidence regarding treatment efficacy in mental health settings, one recent review revealed that there has been no research regarding the outcomes for anxiety disorders in paediatric primary care settings.[64] In these settings, evaluation of the effectiveness of manual-based CBT carried out by mental health practitioners, prescription of SSRIs by paediatricians, and collaborative models of providing treatments for anxiety disorders in adolescents are all badly needed.[64]

Schizophrenia

The first episode represents specific challenges, including clarifying the diagnosis, psycho-education and establishing rapport with the patient and their family.[19] Treatment with antipsychotics is the main strategy to treat adolescent schizophrenia. There are two recent useful reviews addressing the effects and side-effects of antipsychotics for early-onset schizophrenia.[19,65] The atypical antipsychotics include risperidone, clozapine,

Table 29.3	Treatment matrix: anxiety disorders
Disorder	**Treatments across all ages – childhood and adolescence**[a,b]
Generalized anxiety disorder	No best-supported ("well-established") treatments
	Promising ("probably efficacious") are: CBT, family anxiety management, modelling, in vivo exposure, relaxation training and reinforced practice
OCD	No best-supported treatments
	Promising: SSRIs, clomipramine – enhanced with psychosocial therapies; CBT – accepted for clinical use but limited studies. More effective when coupled with family therapy; family therapy and response prevention appear to be effective, but have not been adequately evaluated
Agoraphobia	No best-supported treatments or promising treatments at this time
Panic disorder	No best-supported or promising treatments at this time
Specific phobia	Best-supported are: participant modelling and reinforced practice
	Promising treatments are: systematic desensitization and CBT
Social phobia	No best-supported or promising treatment at this time
	Group therapy incorporating education and cognitive strategies is accepted for clinical use, although not adequately evaluated
Separation anxiety	No best-supported treatments
	Promising treatments are: CBT, family anxiety management, in vivo exposure, relaxation training and reinforced practice

[a] Best-supported ("well-established") interventions: at least two scientifically defensible group-design studies conducted by different investigative teams, or more than nine single-case designs, treatment manuals and strong experimental designs.

[b] Promising ('probably efficacious') interventions: at least two studies demonstrating the intervention to be more effective than a no-treatment control group, or several single-case studies, as well as manuals that prescribe the intervention.

Reproduced, with permission, from *Evidence-based age-appropriate interventions – a guide for child and adolescent mental health services (CAMHS)*. Auckland, The Werry Centre for Child and Adolescent Mental Health Workforce Development, 2010.[57]

quetiapine, aripiprazole, olanzapine and ziprasidone. Among these, risperidone, quetiapine, aripiprazole and olanzapine were approved by the US FDA for treating schizophrenia in adolescents aged 13–17 years.[66] One recent article showed antipsychotics can improve psychotic symptoms, while atypical antipsychotics did not demonstrate superior efficacy over typical antipsychotics for early-onset schizophrenia.[19] Typical antipsychotics were accompanied by high rates of side-effects, such as extrapyramidal symptoms, sedation and elevated prolactin levels. Atypical antipsychotics readily caused weight gain, abnormal prolactin elevation, sedation and metabolic effects.[19] In general, children and adolescents have a higher risk of side-effects than adults.[67] Polypharmacy also contributes to risks.[19]

Following the resolution of acute episodes, emphasis shifts to prevention of relapse. Psychosocial interventions are needed to improve adherence to treatment, coping with stressors and return to school.[19] Rehabilitation programmes encompass relapse prevention, assistance in meeting educational or vocational goals, and long-term health-maintenance issues.[19]

Substance use disorders

A treatment matrix is presented in Table 29.4.[57]

Table 29.4 Treatment matrix: substance use disorders

Treatment: medication	Use in adolescence[a,b]
Methadone	Moderately recommended: best supported
Naltrexone	Moderately recommended: best supported
Medication for comorbid conditions	Needs further evaluation; insufficient evidence about the effect on substance abuse/dependence – important regarding use for dependence
Disulfiram	Not recommended unless there is serious dependence where other treatments have been tried
Psychological: structural strategic family therapy	Best supported
Motivational interviewing	Promising: probably efficacious
CBT and behavioural approaches	Promising: probably efficacious
Multisystemic therapy	Promising: probably efficacious
Prevention programmes	Promising: support for skills-oriented resilience-building programmes
Interpersonal and psychodynamic therapy	Needs further evaluation – anecdotal evidence of their use

[a] Best-supported ("well-established") interventions: at least two scientifically defensible group-design studies conducted by different investigative teams, or more than nine single-case designs, treatment manuals and strong experimental designs.

[b] Promising ('probably efficacious') interventions: at least two studies demonstrating the intervention to be more effective than a no-treatment control group, or several single-case studies, as well as manuals that prescribe the intervention.

Reproduced, with permission, from *Evidence-based age-appropriate interventions – a guide for child and adolescent mental health services (CAMHS)*. Auckland, The Werry Centre for Child and Adolescent Mental Health Workforce Development, 2010.[57]

Suicide

Steele et al. have provided a useful review of intervention strategies for suicide; the following findings are put forward:[59]

- the first step is to assess whether hospitalization is needed. If no alliance can be formed or if the youth is psychotic or impulsive, hospitalization should be strongly considered
- no-suicide contracts are unreliable
- the support of the family in ongoing treatment should be obtained whenever possible and may help with adherence to treatment
- dialectical behaviour therapy is helpful when available, and fluoxetine combined with CBT has been helpful for suicidal ideation as well as depressed mood
- interpersonal therapy is useful for depressed adolescents but has not yet been shown to benefit suicidal ideation or behaviour
- there is a small amount of evidence that family therapy is beneficial in reducing suicidal ideation in teenagers without major depressive illness
- treatment modalities (including psychotherapy) and preventive strategies (including school-based interventions, gatekeeper and primary practitioner training, and treatment of psychiatric disorders) are considered in the light of existing evidence.[59]

Shain provides additional strategies to deal with suicide behaviours, including removal of lethal methods (such as firearms and lethal medication), maintaining contact, and treating underlying psychiatric disorders.[60]

Psychiatry/primary care collaboration

Although GPs may serve as the first frontier for identifying and intervening in adolescent mental disorders, referrals for further mental health services are sometimes expected. The American Academy of Child and Adolescent Psychiatry has proposed the following criteria for a practitioner to consider when making a decision about whether to refer adolescent patients:

- an emotional or behavioural problem constitutes a threat to the safety of the child/adolescent or the safety of those around him/her
- there is a significant change in an adolescent's emotional or behavioural functioning for which there is no obvious or recognized precipitant
- in addition to an adolescent's emotional or behavioural problems, the primary caretaker has serious emotional impairment or substance abuse problems
- an emotional or behavioural problem causes significant disruption in day-to-day functioning or reality contact
- when a child or adolescent is hospitalized for treatment of a psychiatric illness
- there is no meaningful improvement after 6–8 weeks' treatment
- diagnostic issues may be related to an organic aetiology or complex mental health/legal issues
- there is a history of abuse, neglect and/or removal from home, with current significant symptoms as a result of these actions
- the symptom picture and family psychiatric history suggests that treatment with psychotropic medication may result in an adverse response
- there is only a partial response to a course of psychotropic medication or treatment with more than two psychotropic medications
- a chronic medical condition is associated with behaviour that seriously interferes with the treatment of that condition.[68]

A report from the Massachusetts Child Psychiatry Access Project (MCPAP) programme, a system for child psychiatry/primary care collaboration, provides Massachusetts paediatric primary care clinicians with rapid access to child psychiatry expertise, education and referral assistance.[69] The strategies include immediate telephonic child psychiatry consultation, direct face-to-face child psychiatry consultation, care coordination, and educational services. Data on participation and utilization over 3.5 years from 1 July 2005, to 31 December 2008 were collected. Primary care clinician surveys assessed satisfaction and impact on access to care, encompassing perception of access to care, ability to meet the needs of patients with mental health problems, timeliness of access to a child psychiatrist, and satisfaction with MCPAP consultative services. The results showed paediatric primary care clinicians contacted the MCPAP mainly for diagnostic questions (34%), identifying community resources (27%) and consultation regarding medication (27%).[69] The rate of primary care clinicians who reported that they are usually able to meet the needs of psychiatric patients increased from 8% to 63%. Consultations were reported to be helpful by 91% of primary care clinicians.[69] New technology, such as the application of telemedicine technology allows provision of outpatient mental health consultation and clinical services to communities with little access to mental health care.[70] This "virtual mental health clinic" could deliver specialist consultations, clinical services, and educational experiences to physicians primary-care clinics in poor resource-poor areas.[70]

Conclusion

Adolescent mental disorders are prominent worldwide and in primary care settings. GPs are at the front line to screen and help these adolescents. A variety of scales are available to help identify individuals who are at risk, but further confirmation for diagnosis is warranted. Collaboration with mental professionals and community services is helpful, and new technology makes collaboration more feasible. Although several evidence-based intervention models have been developed among mental health services, further studies to confirm their feasibility and effectiveness in the primary care setting is needed.

References

1   Belfer ML. Child and adolescent mental disorders: the magnitude of the problem across the globe. *Journal of Child Psychology and Psychiatry*, 2008, 49:226–236.

2   Kessler RC et al. Age of onset of mental disorders: a review of recent literature. *Current Opinion in Psychiatry*, 2007, 20:359–364.

3   Merikangas KR, Nakamura EF, Kessler RC. Epidemiology of mental disorders in children and adolescents. *Dialogues in Clinical Neurosciences*, 2009, 11:7–20.

4   Belfer ML. A global perspective on child and adolescent mental health. Editorial. *International Review of Psychiatry*, 2008, 20:215–216.

5   American Academy of Child and Adolescent Psychiatry Committee on Health Care Access and Economics Task Force on Mental Health. Improving mental health services in primary care: reducing administrative and financial barriers to access and collaboration. *Pediatrics*, 2009, 123:1248–1251.

6   Kramer T, Garralda ME. Psychiatric disorders in adolescents in primary care. *British Journal of Psychiatry*, 1998, 173:508–513.

7   Giel R et al. Childhood mental disorders in primary health care: results of observations in four developing countries. A report from the WHO Collaborative Study on Strategies for Extending Mental Health Care. *Pediatrics*, 1981, 68:677–883.

8   Omigbodun O. Developing child mental health services in resource-poor countries. *International Review of Psychiatry*, 2008, 20:225–235.

9   Patel V et al. Promoting child and adolescent mental health in low and middle income countries. *Journal of Child Psychology and Psychiatry*, 2008, 49:313–334.

10 Kramer T, Garralda ME. Child and adolescent mental health problems in primary care. *Advances in Psychiatric Treatment*, 2000, 6:287–294.

11 Eapen V, Jairam R. Integration of child mental health services to primary care: challenges and opportunities. *Mental Health in Family Medicine*, 2009, 6:43–48.

12 Bower P et al. The treatment of child and adolescent mental health problems in primary care: a systematic review. *Family Practice*, 2001, 18:373–382.

13 Williams SB et al. Screening for child and adolescent depression in primary care settings: a systematic evidence review for the US Preventive Services Task Force. *Pediatrics*, 2009, 123:e716–735.

14 Costello EJ, Egger H, Angold A. 10-year research update review: the epidemiology of child and adolescent psychiatric disorders: I. Methods and public health burden. *Journal of the American Academy of Child and Adolescent Psychiatry*, 2005, 44:972–986.

15 Pine DS et al. Challenges in developing novel treatments for childhood disorders: lessons from research on anxiety. *Neuropsychopharmacology*, 2009, 34:213–228.

16 Costello EJ et al. Prevalence and development of psychiatric disorders in childhood and adolescence. *Archives of General Psychiatry*, 2003, 60:837–844.

17 Rockhill C et al. Anxiety disorders in children and adolescents. *Current Problems in Pediatric and Adolescent Health Care*, 2010, 40:66–99.

18 Mattai AK, Hill JL, Lenroot RK. Treatment of early-onset schizophrenia. *Current Opinion in Psychiatry*, 2010, 23:304–310.

19 Beitchman JH. Childhood schizophrenia. A review and comparison with adult-onset schizophrenia. *Psychiatric Clinics of North America*, 1985, 8:793–814.

20 Gillberg C et al. Teenage psychoses – epidemiology, classification and reduced optimality in the pre-, peri- and neonatal periods. *Journal of Child Psychology and Psychiatry*, 1986, 27:87–98.

21 Costello EJ et al. Prevalence of psychiatric disorders in childhood and adolescence. In: Levin BL, Petrila J, Hennessy KD, eds. *Mental health services: a public health perspective*, 2nd ed. Oxford, Oxford University Press, 2004:111–128.

22 Merikangas KR et al. Lifetime prevalence of mental disorders in US adolescents: results from the National Comorbidity Survey Replication – Adolescent Supplement (NCS-A). *Journal of the American Academy of Child and Adolescent Psychiatry*, 2010, 49:980–989.

23 Behrendt S et al. Transitions from first substance use to substance use disorders in adolescence: is early onset associated with a rapid escalation? *Drug and Alcohol Dependence*, 2009, 99:68–78.

24 Chen VC et al. Severity of heroin dependence in Taiwan: reliability and validity of the Chinese version of the Severity of Dependence Scale (SDS[Ch]). *Addictive Behaviors*, 2008, 33:1590–1593.

25 Horowitz LM, Ballard ED, Pao M. Suicide screening in schools, primary care and emergency departments. *Current Opinion in Pediatrics*, 2009, 21:620–627.

26 Evans E et al. The prevalence of suicidal phenomena in adolescents: a systematic review of population-based studies. *Suicide and Life-Threatening Behavior*, 2005, 35:239–250.

27 Davidson S, Manion IG, eds. *Canadian youth mental health and illness survey: survey overview, interview schedule and demographic cross tabulations*. Ottawa, Canadian Psychiatric Association, 1993.

28 Clark D. Suicidal behaviour in childhood and adolescence: recent studies and clinical implications. *Psychiatric Annals*, 1993, 23:271–283.

29 Kuo CJ et al. Asthma and suicide mortality in young people: a 12-year follow-up study. *American Journal of Psychiatry*, 2010, 167:1092–1099.

30 Williams JMG, Pollock LR. The psychology of suicidal behaviour. In: Hawton K, Heeringen K, eds. *The international handbook of suicide and attempted suicide*. Chichester, John Wiley & Sons, Ltd, 2000: 79–94.

31 Skegg K. Self-harm. *The Lancet*, 2005, 366:1471–1483.

32 Williams JMG, Pollock LR. Psychological aspects of the suicidal process. In: Heeringen KV, ed. *Understanding suicidal behaviour: the suicidal process approach to research, treatment and prevention*. Chichester, John Wiley & Sons Ltd, 2001:76–93.

33 Mann JJ et al. Toward a clinical model of suicidal behavior in psychiatric patients. *American Journal of Psychiatry*, 1999, 156:181–189.

34 Wasserman D. *Suicide – an unnecessary death*. London, Duntiz, 2001:13–27.

35 Garralda ME, Bowman FM, Mandalia S. Children with psychiatric disorders who are frequent attenders to primary care. *European Child and Adolescent Psychiatry* 1999, 8:34–44.

36 *Diagnostic and statistical manual of mental disorders*, 4th ed, text revision (DSM-IV-TR). Washington, American Psychiatric Association, 2000.

37 *Guidelines for child and adolescent mental health referral*, 2nd ed. New York, Columbia University, Department of Child and Adolescent Psychiatry, 2003.

38 Pine DS et al. The risk for early-adulthood anxiety and depressive disorders in adolescents with anxiety and depressive disorders. *Archives of General Psychiatry*, 1998, 55:56–64.

39 Merikangas KR et al. Vulnerability factors among children at risk for anxiety disorders. *Biological Psychiatry*, 1999, 46:1523–1535.

40 Clark AF. Proposed treatment for adolescent psychosis. 1: Schizophrenia and schizophrenia-like psychoses. *Advances in Psychiatric Treatment*, 2001, 7:16–23.

41 Kao YC, Liu YP. Effects of age of onset on clinical characteristics in schizophrenia spectrum disorders. *BMC Psychiatry*, 2010, 10:63.

42 Michael Rutter, Taylor E, eds. *Child and adolescent psychiatry*, 4th ed. Chichester, Wiley-Blackwell, 2005.

43 Chen VC et al. Suicide attempts prior to starting methadone maintenance treatment in Taiwan. *Drug and Alcohol Dependence*, 2010, 109:139–143.

44 Stengel E. *Suicide and attempted suicide*. New York, Aronson, 1974.

45 Hawton K et al. Monitoring deliberate self-harm presentations to general hospitals. *Crisis*, 2006, 27:157–163.

46 Cooper J et al. Suicide after deliberate self-harm: a 4-year cohort study. *American Journal of Psychiatry*, 2005, 162:297–303.

47 Hjelmeland H et al. Why people engage in parasuicide: a cross-cultural study of intentions. *Suicide and Life-Threatening Behavior*, 2002, 32:380–393.

48 Chen VC et al. A community-based study of case fatality proportion among those who carry out suicide acts. *Social Psychiatry and Psychiatric Epidemiology*, 2009, 44:1005–1011.

49 Chen VC et al. Non-fatal repetition of self-harm: population-based prospective cohort study in Taiwan. *British Journal of Psychiatry*, 2010, 196:31–35.

50 Hamrin V, Magorno M. Assessment of adolescents for depression in the pediatric primary care setting. *Pediatric Nursing*, 2010, 36:103–111.

51 Shaffer D et al. The Columbia Suicide Screen: validity and reliability of a screen for youth suicide and depression. *Journal of the American Academy of Child and Adolescent Psychiatry*, 2004, 43:71–79.

52 Sanci L, Lewis D, Patton G. Detecting emotional disorder in young people in primary care. *Current Opinion in Psychiatry*, 2010, 23:318–323.

53 Richardson LP, Katzenellenbogen R. Childhood and adolescent depression: the role of primary care providers in diagnosis and treatment. *Current Problems in Pediatric and Adolescent Health Care*, 2005, 35:6–24.

54 Polanczyk G et al. Etiological and clinical features of childhood psychotic symptoms: results from a birth cohort. *Archives of General Psychiatry*, 2010, 67:328–338.

55 Lauterbach MD, Stanislawski-Zygaj AL, Benjamin S. The differential diagnosis of childhood- and young adult-onset disorders that include psychosis. *Journal of Neuropsychiatry and Clinical Neurosciences*, 2008, 20:409–418.

56 Leccese M, Waldron HB. Assessing adolescent substance use: a critique of current measurement instruments. *Journal of Substance Abuse Treatment*, 1994, 11:553–563.

57 *Evidence-based age-appropriate interventions – a guide for child and adolescent mental health services (CAMHS)*. Auckland, The Werry Centre for Child and Adolescent Mental Health Workforce Development, 2010.

58 Couwenbergh C et al. Screening for substance abuse among adolescents validity of the CAGE-AID in youth mental health care. *Substance Use and Misuse*, 2009, 44:823–834.

59 Steele MM, Doey T. Suicidal behaviour in children and adolescents. Part 2: treatment and prevention. *Canadian Journal of Psychiatry*, 2007, 52(6 Suppl. 1):35S–45S.

60 Shain BN. Suicide and suicide attempts in adolescents. *Pediatrics*, 2007, 120:669–676.

61 *Evidence-based child and adolescent psychosocial interventions*. Vintage, IL, American Academy of Pediatrics, 2011 (http://www.askferc.org/uploads/docs/resources/evidence_based_child_interventions_aap.pdf , accessed 11 December 2011).

62 *FDA labeling change request letter for antidepressant medications*. Silver Spring, FDA, 2009 (http://www.fda.gov/Drugs/DrugSafety/InformationbyDrugClass/ucm096352.htm, accessed 11 December 2011).

63 Asarnow JR et al. Effectiveness of a quality improvement intervention for adolescent depression in primary care clinics: a randomized controlled trial. *JAMA*, 2005, 293:311–319.

64 Sakolsky D, Birmaher B. Pediatric anxiety disorders: management in primary care. *Current Opinion in Pediatrics*, 2008, 20:538–543.

65 Kumra S et al. Efficacy and tolerability of second-generation antipsychotics in children and adolescents with schizophrenia. *Schizophrenia Bulletin*, 2008, 34:60–71.

66 Mathis MV. *Atypical antipsychotics and pediatrics. Background and update on June 9–10 2009 Psychopharmacological Drugs Advisory Committee Meeting*. Silver Springs, FDA, 2009 (http://www.fda.gov/downloads/AdvisoryCommittees/CommitteesMeetingMaterials/PediatricAdvisoryCommittee/UCM193200.pdf, accessed 22 January 2012).

67 Correll CU et al. Recognizing and monitoring adverse events of second-generation antipsychotics in children and adolescents. *Child and Adolescent Psychiatric Clinics of North America*, 2006, 15:177–206.

68 *When to seek referral or consultation with a child and adolescent psychiatrist*. Washington DC, American Academy of Child and Adolescent Psychiatry, 2008 (http://www.aacap.org/cs/root/physicians_and_allied_professionals/when_to_seek_referral_or_consultation_with_a_child_and_adolescent_psychiatrist, accessed 22 January 2012).

69 Sarvet B et al. Improving access to mental health care for children: the Massachusetts Child Psychiatry Access Project. *Pediatrics*, 2010, 126:1191–1200.

70 Neufeld JD et al. The e-Mental Health Consultation Service: providing enhanced primary-care mental health services through telemedicine. *Psychosomatics*, 2007, 48:135–141.

Part VIII

Acquired neurocognitive disorders of old age in primary care mental health

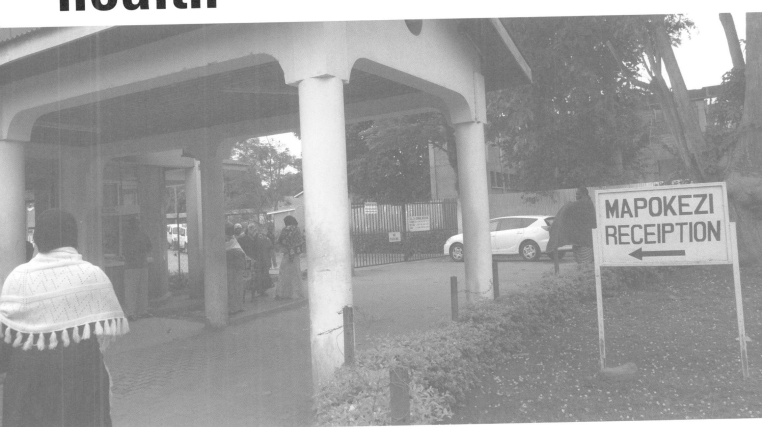

30 Dementia in primary care mental health

Carlos Augusto de Mendonça Lima, José Miguel Caldas de Almeida, Steve Iliffe and Jill Rasmussen

Key messages

- Dementia accounts for 11.2% of years lived with disability of people aged 60 years or older, and patients with dementia have a substantially shortened life expectancy. The total estimated cost of dementia worldwide was US$604 billion in 2010.

- In many countries, the current configuration of services for people with dementia will not cope with the consequences of the demographic shift that is now under way: primary care will need to adopt a more active role.

- Primary care professionals need to acquire new skills, particularly around psychosocial interventions and the development of systematic care packages and pathways.

- Primary care practitioners can effectively master the diagnostic task in the early stages of dementia syndrome, once they know what it is they are facing, and what resources they can call upon.

- This chapter contributes to increasing the knowledge of primary care professionals on the diagnosis and management of dementia in primary care.

Introduction

Dementia is a major public health problem worldwide. It is one of the most common diseases in the elderly, affecting an increasing number of people in both high-income and low-income countries. It causes enormous suffering, disability and mortality to individuals, represents a huge burden to their families, and accounts for high costs to society.

According to the *World Health Report 2003*, dementia accounts for 11.2% of years lived with disability of people aged 60 years or older – more than stroke (9.5%), cardiovascular disease (5%) or all types of cancer (2.4%).[1] Dementia is also associated with mortality: patients with dementia have a substantially shortened life expectancy; the average survival after diagnosis is 8 years.[1]

Dementia represents enormous costs for society. The total estimated costs of dementia worldwide were US$604 billion in 2010.[3] These costs include those of informal care (unpaid care provided by families and other caregivers), direct medical care costs (primary care, hospital care) and direct social care costs (community care, residential care, nursing home care, food supply, etc.).

In high-income countries, where 35–50% of the people with dementia live in care homes,[4] direct social care costs account for more than half of the total costs. In low- and middle-income countries, where the large majority of people with dementia live at home and depend on the care provided by their families, informal care costs represent two-thirds of the total costs. Overall, the costs of direct medical care represent a small part of all costs worldwide (around 16%), while the costs of informal care and the direct costs of social care amount to 42% of all costs worldwide. A large majority of the total global costs of dementia (89%) are incurred in high-income countries, 10% in middle-income countries and less than 1% in low-income countries. However, less than half of the people with dementia live in high-income countries, 40% live in middle-income countries and 14% live in low-income countries.[3]

From a clinical perspective, dementia can be described as a "group of usually progressive neurodegenerative brain disorders characterized by intellectual deterioration and more or less gradual erosion of mental and later physical function, leading to disability and death".[5] Dementia syndrome occurs in Alzheimer disease, in cerebrovascular diseases and in other conditions primarily or secondarily affecting the brain.

Dementia can affect people of any age. However, it is most common in the elderly. One of the major characteristics of dementia is the progressive decline experienced by the patient. The rate of this decline depends on various factors: type of dementia, general health condition, quality of care and social support.

An adequate response to the needs of people with dementia and their families requires a combination of health and social care interventions, including day care and residential care. Primary care is an essential component of the care provided to people with dementia, from early primary prevention, early detection and treatment to treatment in the most advanced stages of the illness.

Epidemiology

In the last 20 years, several important epidemiological studies in dementia have been carried out across the world. Most of these studies were conducted in Europe and the United States of America (USA). However, the available data do allow the prevalence of dementia in the different regions of the world to be estimated. The authors of the World Alzheimer Report 2009 conducted a systematic review of the global prevalence of dementia, identifying 147 studies in different regions of the world.[6] According to this review, 35.6 million people were estimated to suffer from dementia worldwide. Due to demographic changes, it is estimated that the number of people with dementia will almost double every 20 years, to 65.7 million in 2030 and 115.4 million in 2050. The average estimated prevalence of dementia for those aged 60 years or over, in all regions, is 4.7%. High-income countries have a higher prevalence of dementia than low-income countries. According to authors of the World Alzheimer Report 2009,[6] the crude prevalence rates in Western Europe and North America for those aged 60 years and over are 7.2% and 6.9 %, while in low-income countries, due to demographic differences, the prevalence is significantly lower: for instance, 2.6% in Africa and 3.9% in Asia.[6] However, a much more significant increase is expected in these countries in the near future, compared to high-income countries. While Europe and North America are expected to experience an increase of 40% and 63% respectively, in the next 20 years, a 117% growth is expected in East Asia and a 134–146% growth in Latin America. In 2010, of all people with dementia, more than half (58%) lived in low-income countries, a number that is expected to rise to 71% in 2050.[3]

Of all types of dementia, Alzheimer disease is the most common, particularly among older people and women, accounting for around 60% of all cases. Vascular dementia and dementia with Lewy bodies account for around one-third of all cases, while frontotemporal dementia is a common form in cases of early onset.[4] Other causes of dementia include neurodegenerative diseases, such as Huntington disease, and toxic and metabolic disorders, such as alcohol-related dementia.

The prevalence rate increases with age. According to an analysis conducted by the EURODEM (European Community Concerted Action on the Epidemiology and Prevention of Dementia) Group,[7] in the age group 65–70 years, rates varied between 1.2% and 4.7%, while between 75 and 84 years, rates were between 4.5% and 18.3%, and after 85 years rates varied between 11.5% and 39%. Regarding sex differences, the same study showed higher prevalence in women in all age groups, except in the age group 65–69 years, which showed a higher rate in men.

Coping with the dementia challenge

A historical perspective

Older persons' well-being and health have been two major goals of medicine since its beginning. However, collection and reporting of complete clinical and psychopathological descriptive observations in this group only started at the end of the 18th century.[8]

In 1830, it was observed that older persons could present some specific types of mental deterioration and that these could be associated with changes in some structures of the brain. At this time, the concept of dementia had more a forensic meaning than a medical one. The term was used to refer to all states of acquired intellectual disabilities resulting in psychosocial incapacity.[9,10]

The concept of senile dementia was only created by the end of the 19th century, with the development of neurobiology. Alzheimer disease became the model for all senile dementia.[11] This resulted in inclusion of incorrect age boundaries and exclusion of non-cognitive symptoms in the diagnostic criteria of senile dementia; these have only recently been revised.

In some high-income countries, the development of specific programmes and services to care for older persons with mental disorders depended on the local context. The majority of these countries used already existing departments of psychiatry, neurology or even gerontology. This process mainly occurred after the second World War, according to specific opportunities and local political will. This tendency was still present in the beginning of the 1970s.[12]

Since then, there has been a growing interest in dementia because of several different factors that together created the possibility to change the way we care for people with the disorder and support their natural caregivers. The extraordinary growth in the number of older people in the global population – and not only in high-income countries – is just one of these factors, with consequences for society values, transactions and economics and in terms of the epidemiological distribution of health (and mental health) problems.

Meanwhile, different disciplines in the field of neurosciences have been making significant contributions to our understanding of the underlying pathological processes of the different types of dementias. Researchers have developed biological models that form the basis of the progress in therapeutic strategies.

In consequence, some drugs have become available to help people with dementia and thereby reduce the burden for their families. Although these treatments cannot cure dementia, they can significantly improve patients' quality of life and change the course of dementia, and have contributed to create new strategies of care.

The introduction of diagnostic criteria in the nosology of mental health disorders at the end of 1980s helped health professionals to diagnose dementia in the same way in every country of the world. Comparative studies (at clinical, epidemiological level, etc.) among different countries and cultures became much more reliable and robust.

In conjunction with these changes, a better understanding of the natural course of dementia contributed to the development of neuropsychological tools that are used for different purposes, from the simple screening tool to the more sophisticated assessments of specific impairments. The contribution of neuropsychology is important to help in the early diagnosis of dementia, to define the different stages of the disorder, to quantify the follow-up and to identify specific care needs.

Complementing this knowledge, the development of neuroimaging has provided an extraordinary tool to identify possible neurological causes for dementias, helping the diagnostic process and understanding of the evolution of dementia. The search for dementia biomarkers and methods of genetic testing are other contributions that shape the way we will manage people with dementia in the future; there are associated ethical questions that are not yet completely resolved.

Finally, the best way to approach the complexity of dementia is through multidisciplinary collaboration, which requires recognition and respect of the boundaries of each discipline and establishment of new forms of collaboration. This also includes partnership with credible groups of service consumers that have assumed a significant role of advocacy and have influence with policy-makers and authorities.

All this progress has resulted in two complementary strategies to manage people with dementia in different health settings:

- the proposal of practice guidelines as a result of consensus among experts representing different groups of interest

- the development of policies, programmes and services in an effort to efficiently meet the need of care of persons with dementia and support them in a public health framework.

Guidelines

Only three examples of guidelines will be mentioned here. They are not exhaustive but they have significantly contributed to inspire several others. The American Psychiatric Association (APA) published a *Practice guideline for the treatment with Alzheimer's disease and other dementias* in 2007.[13] It was not intended to be construed or to serve as a standard of medical care but rapidly became a reference among specialists. The guideline was developed according to a well-established APA methodology and process, which includes:

- a comprehensive literature review
- development of evidence tables
- initial drafting of the guideline by a work group that includes psychiatrists with clinical and research expertise in dementia
- production of multiple revised drafts with widespread review; 22 organizations and 64 individuals submitted significant comments
- approval by the APA Assembly and Board of Trustees
- planned revisions at regular intervals.

The International Psychogeriatric Association gave a contribution with its *Consensus statement on defining and measuring treatment benefits in dementia*.[14] This statement was generated by an international group representing caregivers, organizations and professionals with expertise in dementia. The purpose was to make recommendations in order to help future research into drugs to treat dementia. The complexity of assessing individuals with dementia in order to demonstrate the efficacy of treatments justifies a multidimensional assessment, which is also useful in a clinical context. It should use clear, predefined diagnostic and severity criteria and outcome measures, which include functional and executive capacity. Outcomes should include effects on people with dementia with regard to cognition, behavioural and psychological symptoms, quality of life, global assessments, and activities of daily living, and it must be tailored to the education and culture of the participants. Outcomes can also appropriately encompass effects on caregivers. Despite considerable recent progress and several 'candidate' biomarkers, none is yet satisfactory for determining diagnosis, severity, progression or prediction of response.

Finally, the World Health Organization (WHO) published the *mhGAP intervention guide for mental, neurological and substance use disorders in non-specialized health settings* (MIG).[15] This has been developed for use in non-specialized health-care settings. It is aimed at health-care providers working at first- and second-level facilities. These health-care providers may be working in a health centre or as part of the clinical team at a district-level hospital or clinic. They include general physicians, family physicians, nurses and clinical officers. The MIG is brief, in order to facilitate interventions by busy non-specialists in low- and middle-income countries. It describes in detail *what to do* but does not go into descriptions of *how to do it*. It is not the intention of the MIG to cover service development. Although the MIG is to be implemented primarily by non-specialists, specialists may also find it useful in their work. In addition, specialists have an essential and substantial role in training, support and supervision. The MIG indicates where access to specialists is required for consultation or referral. Creative solutions need to be found when specialists are not available in the district. Specialists would also benefit from training on public health aspects of the programme and service organization. One of the chapters of the MIG specifically concerns dementia, with recommendations for assessment and management, including how to identify dementia, and it describes the possible psychosocial and pharmacological interventions.

Organizing programmes and services

Clinical specialists in dementia are a scarce resource and they should not play a role in the first-line care of people with this disorder. In several countries, the model of care is more orientated towards acute rather than chronic conditions. A consequence of this is a lack of respect for basic principles of distributive justice; there is a high risk of non-respect of the equity of care principle, with access to care depending upon means to pay. The same is often true for the distribution of resources between rural and urban areas.[16]

Figure 30.1 shows the distribution of WHO regions in the world according to the percentage of countries with mental health programmes and the proportion of older persons living in each of these regions. The high disparity among these regions is evident but the reasons are complex and they depend in part on how countries allocate resources to the care of older persons.[17]

These health inequities in a social group, the social gradient in health within countries, and the marked health inequities between countries are caused by *the unequal distribution of power, income, goods, and services, globally and nationally, the consequent unfairness in the immediate, visible circumstances of people's lives – their access to health care, schools, and education, their conditions of work and leisure, their homes, communities, towns, or cities – and their chances of leading a flourishing life.* This unequal distribution of health-damaging experiences is not caused by "natural" reasons and is the result of a *toxic combination of poor social policies and programmes, unfair economic arrangements, and bad politics.* So, social determinants of health are constituted by the structural determinants and conditions of daily life and are responsible for the majority of health inequities between and within countries. Older people are at risk of being one of the groups that are most vulnerable to these social determinants and need particular protection against their negative consequences. With three overall recommendations for action on the social determinants of health (improve daily living conditions; tackle the inequitable distribution of power, money and resources; and measure and understand the problem and assess the impact of action), the WHO Commission on Social Determinants of Health (CSDH) aspires to reduce the world health inequities in a generation.[18,19]

The development of services for people with dementia needs to be tailored to suit the health-systems context. The ethics of health care require that governments take initial planning steps, now. The one certainty is that in the absence of clear strategies and policies, the elderly will absorb increasing proportions of the resources devoted to health care.[20]

Three documents can be cited that exemplify the effort to recommend a comprehensive strategy to develop programmes and services for people with dementia; this list also is not exhaustive. The first is a consensus

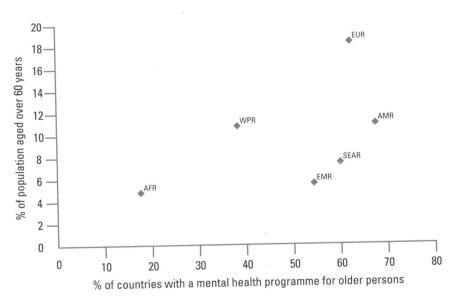

Figure 30.1 Distribution of the different WHO regions according to the proportion of persons with more than 60 years and the proportion of countries with a mental health programme for the older persons

AFR = African Region; AMR = Region of the Americas; EMR = Eastern Mediterranean Region; EUR = European Region; SEAR = South-East Asia Region; WPR: Western Pacific Region.

Reproduced, with permission, from de Mendonça Lima CA, Kühne N, Buschfort R. ATLAS: mapping mental health resources for old persons in the world. *Psychogeriatria Polska*, 2004, 1(3):167–174[17]

statement jointly organized by WHO and the World Psychiatry Association (WPA) on organization of care for the elderly with mental disorders.[21] Although the statement is not specifically aimed at the needs of people with dementia, it does also concern older patients with this disorder. According to this document, the following components should ideally be the responsibility of specialized teams of trained health-care professionals.

Community mental health teams

The community mental health team (CMHT) may consist of doctors, psychiatric nurses, psychologists, social workers, therapists and secretaries. Referral to the CMHT is usually from primary care. The main responsibilities of the CMHT are specialist assessment, investigation and treatment of people in their home setting.

Inpatient services

Acute inpatients units need to provide specialist assessment and treatment. This may in some cases include rehabilitation before return to the community.

Day hospitals

This is an acute service that offers assessment and treatment to older people who can be maintained at home, supported by the multidisciplinary team.

Outpatient services

These provide assessment, diagnosis and treatment for people who are fit enough to live in the community and get to and from the hospital base. Outpatient services should be close to the inpatient and day-patient units. They may involve memory clinics and mobile clinics.

Hospital respite care

Hospital beds may be used to provide a respite service for people with behavioural problems, in order to give their carers a break and enable care at home to continue as long as possible.

Continuing hospital care

Care for life in a hospital setting may be required for people with dementia and difficult associated behavioural problems. Such care should be provided in as relaxed and homely an environment as possible, with carers encouraged to participate.

Liaison services

Consultations and/or liaison services should be provided between facilities for people with dementia and those serving general and geriatric medicine, general psychiatry, residential facilities and social agencies. This relationship should be of a reciprocal nature.

Primary care

The primary care team has the initial responsibility for identifying, assessing and managing mental health problems in older people. The decision to refer to the CMHT is usually made in primary care.

Community and social support services

These are services (both formal and informal) to enable the elderly person to remain at home. This includes a range of activities provided by voluntary or government/social services:

- respite facilities: a range of short-term, time-limited services both inside and outside the home (residential services, other carers, day programmes) to support the carers
- residential care: for those patients whose physical, psychological, and/or social dependencies make living at home no longer possible, a spectrum of residential facilities should be provided. These range from supported accommodation with low-level supervision, to medium-level care facilities and to full nursing facilities.

Prevention

The team caring for people with dementia should engage in prevention of relapse of behavioural disorders by careful follow-up. They should also identify the risk factors in the elderly and ensure these are effectively managed by appropriate medical and social strategies.

Another contribution to the organization of care was presented by Alzheimer's Disease International during its 20th annual conference held in 2004 in Kyoto, Japan.[16] It presents the minimum actions required for dementia care in three scenarios, depending on the level of each country's resources. This was developed in 10 key areas using a public health framework developed by WHO. This strategy suggests a feasible, pragmatic series of actions and objectives for health systems at all levels of development (see Table 30.1).

Finally, some countries have developed national strategies to face the dementia challenge. In 2008, France allocated 1.6 billion euros for the French Alzheimer Plan. In 2009, the Department of Health in the United Kingdom of Great Britain and Northern Ireland (UK) published its *Living well with dementia: a National Dementia Strategy*.[22] This is a comprehensive strategy that aims to transcend existing boundaries between health and social care and the third sector, between service providers and people with dementia and their carers. The vision is for a system where all people with dementia have access to care and support that they would benefit from. It is intended that the fear and stigma associated with dementia will decrease. Families affected by dementia will know where to go for help and what services to expect; the quality of care will be high and of equal quality wherever they might live; and people will seek help early for problems with memory and be encouraged to do so. Knowledge is power with respect to diagnosis, and it gives those affected and their families an understanding of what is happening and the ability to make choices themselves. Making the diagnosis early on in the illness means that there is the chance to prevent future problems and crises and to benefit more from positive interventions.

Care for people with dementia: the role of primary care

Across the world, the family remains the cornerstone of care for older people who have lost the capacity for independent living.[16] However, stereotypes abound and have the potential to mislead. In high-income countries with their comprehensive health and social care systems, the vital caring role of families, and their need for support, is often overlooked. In low- and middle income countries, the reliability and universality of the family care system is often overestimated. People with dementia in these countries typically live in large households, with extended families. But these are widely perceived as under threat from the social and economic changes that accompany economic development and globalization.[23] Some of the contributing factors include the following:

- changing attitudes towards older people
- the education of women and their increasing participation in the workforce
- migration
- declining fertility in the course of the demographic transition.

Primary care professionals are in a unique position to change this situation by improving the detection and management of dementia. In high-income countries, the evidence suggests that primary care doctors and nurses can make a dementia diagnosis with reasonable accuracy during a typical consultation.[24] These findings cannot be generalized to low- and middle-income countries, for various reasons: lower number of health professionals, less training in elderly medicine and fewer care options, among others. There is therefore an urgent need to develop specific policies and programmes aimed at training primary care professionals in low- and middle-income countries in the formal diagnosis and management of dementia. According to WHO recommendations:[24]

> Non specialist health care providers should seek to identify possible cases of dementia in the primary health care setting and in the community after appropriate training and awareness raising. Brief informant assessment and cognitive tests should be used to assist in confirming these cases. For a formal dementia diagnosis, a more detailed history, medical review and mental state examination should be carried out to exclude other common causes of cognitive impairment and decline. Training should be provided to non-specialist health care providers to diagnose dementia at first or second level health care.

Table 30.1 Minimum actions required for dementia care

Overall recommendations	Scenario A: low level of resources	Scenario B: medium level of resources	Scenario C: high level of resources
1 Provide treatment in primary care	Recognize dementia care as a component of primary health care	Develop locally relevant training materials	Improve the effectiveness of management of dementia in primary health care
	Include the recognition and treatment of dementia in training curricula of all health personnel	Provide refresher training to primary care physicians (100% coverage in 5 years)	Improve referral patterns
	Provide refresher training to primary care physicians (at least 50% coverage in 5 years)		
2 Make appropriate treatments available	Increase the availability of essential drugs for the treatment of dementia and associated psychological and behavioural symptoms	Ensure availability of essential drugs in all health-care settings	Provide easier access to newer drugs (e.g. anticholinesterase agents) under public or private treatment plans
	Develop and evaluate basic educational and training interventions for caregivers	Make effective caregiver interventions generally available	
3 Give care in the community	Establish the principle that people with dementia are best assessed and treated in their own homes	Initiate pilot projects on integration of dementia care with general health care	Develop alternative residential facilities
	Develop and promote standard needs assessments for use in primary and secondary care	Provide community care facilities (at least 50% coverage with multidisciplinary community teams, day care, respite and inpatient units for acute assessment and treatment)	Provide community care facilities (100% coverage)
	Initiate pilot projects on development of multidisciplinary community care teams, day care and short-term respite care	According to need, encourage the development of residential and nursing-home facilities, including a regulatory framework and system for staff training and accreditation	Give individualized care in the community to people with dementia
	Move people with dementia out of inappropriate institutional settings		

4 Educate the public	Promote public campaigns against stigma and discrimination Support nongovernmental organizations in public education	Use the mass media to promote awareness of dementia, foster positive attitudes, and help prevent cognitive impairment and dementia	Launch public campaigns for early help seeking, recognition and appropriate management of dementia
5 Involve communities, families and consumers	Support the formation of self-help groups Fund schemes for nongovernmental organizations	Ensure representation of communities, families, and consumers in policy-making, service development and implementation	Foster advocacy initiatives
6 Establish national policies, programmes and legislation	Revise legislation based on current knowledge and human rights considerations Formulate dementia care programmes and policies: • legal framework to support and protect those with impaired mental capacity • inclusion of people with dementia in disability benefit schemes • inclusion of caregivers in compensatory benefit schemes Establish health and social care budgets for older persons	Implement dementia care policies at national and subnational levels Establish health and social care budgets for dementia care Increase the budget for mental health care	Ensure fairness in access to primary and secondary health-care services, and to social welfare programmes and benefits
7 Develop human resources	Train primary health-care workers Initiate higher professional training programmes for doctors and nurses in geriatric psychiatry and medicine Develop training and resource centres	Create a network of national training centres for physicians, psychiatrists, nurses, psychologists and social workers	Train specialists in advanced treatment skills

continued overleaf

Dementia in primary care mental health

Table 30.1 Minimum actions required for dementia care – *continued*

Overall recommendations	Scenario A: low level of resources	Scenario B: medium level of resources	Scenario C: high level of resources
8 Link with other sectors	Initiate community, school and workplace dementia-awareness programmes Encourage the activities of nongovernmental organizations	Strengthen community programmes	Extend occupational health services to people with early dementia Provide special facilities in the workplace for carers of people with dementia Initiate evidence-based mental health promotion programmes in collaboration with other sectors
9 Monitor community health	Include dementia in basic health information systems Survey high-risk population groups	Institute surveillance for early dementia in the community	Develop advanced monitoring systems Monitor the effectiveness of preventive programmes
10 Support more research	Conduct studies in primary health-care settings on the prevalence, course, outcome and impact of dementia in the community	Institute effectiveness and cost–effectiveness studies for community management of dementia	Extend research on the causes of dementia Carry out research on service delivery Investigate evidence on the prevention of dementia

Reproduced, with permission, from 3.1: Dementia. In: *Neurological disorders: public health challenges.* Geneva, World Health Organization, 2006:42–54.

Primary care professionals can also have a major role in the physical assessment and prescription of psychotropic medicines and other medication. Finally, they can support families and other informal carers to cope with psychological stress, using counselling and psycho-educational interventions.

Diagnosis of dementia in primary care

There is increasing interest in earlier diagnosis of dementia syndrome for three reasons. The first is the ageing of the population, and the consequent rising prevalence of dementia. The second reason is the increasing cost of care for people with dementia, and finally there are the perceived benefits of early recognition and intervention, for the person with dementia and their carer. Given the disease burden, it is not surprising that national governments and third-party payers for health care are focusing on better management of dementia syndrome. Early intervention to reduce downstream costs of treatment is therefore an attractive proposition. Primary care is seen as the place in which early identification could occur, in the course of routine care. There are, however, substantial problems in making this a reality.

Delayed recognition

Dementia syndrome is underdiagnosed and undertreated in primary care in many (possibly all) countries.[25,26] For example, in the USA an estimated 50% of primary care patients with dementia are not recognized by their primary care physicians as having the disease.[27]

The insidious and very variable development of dementia syndrome makes its recognition problematic for primary care practitioners of all disciplines. Communication difficulties, problems with spatial awareness and the impaired ability to perform activities of daily living independently may arise before short-term memory losses become apparent. Missed appointments and issues around drug compliance are also common.[28] Changes in personality and/or mood may lead primary care physicians to make an initial diagnosis of depression rather than dementia, and initiate treatments that may be ineffective or even harmful in that they exacerbate cognitive impairment. This is not an elementary diagnostic error on the practitioner's part, because the two conditions share characteristics, and depression may coexist with dementia, creating a complicated clinical scenario in which the practitioner is uncertain about how to interpret the symptom pattern.

Early recognition

Is earlier recognition of dementia syndrome worthwhile? The evidence suggests that there are tangible benefits to earlier recognition of dementia, at least for some people, but caution is needed in this context, because most evidence of patients' and carers' perceptions has been collected from clinic populations – that is, those diagnosed – rather than from community populations, which include those not yet diagnosed. We shall return to this topic later, because there are grounds to believe that not all symptomatic patients (or their families) seek early diagnosis.

Many primary care practitioners have an understandable fear that they may damage their patients by incautious or erroneous diagnosis and precipitate a catastrophic response. This fear may be exaggerated, but it is not without foundation. Nevertheless, earlier disclosure of the diagnosis seems to be what people with dementia want,[29] and what younger professionals want to give.[30] The benefits of making a diagnosis include ending uncertainty about the cause of symptoms and changes in behaviour in the person with early dementia, with a consequent better understanding of problems on the part of family members and other carers; opening access to appropriate psychological and social support; promoting positive coping strategies in the affected person and those around them; and facilitating planning and the fulfilment of short-term goals.[31–34] There is also the potential for using cholinesterase inhibitor medication in those individuals with dementia who have Alzheimer disease, to modify symptoms to some extent, at least for a period of time, and perhaps delay the need for a patient to relocate to a care home.

Enhancing skills in primary care

The insidious nature of dementia means that it is most likely to present as a problem in primary care but, as we have seen, there are obstacles to its earlier recognition. Considerable efforts have been made to enhance the diagnostic skills of primary care practitioners through educational interventions, with some limited successes.[35] Because of the time constraints in primary care consultations, the focus has been on development of brief screening tests for assessing cognitive function. These include the General Practitioner Assessment of Cognition (GPCOG),[36] the Mini-Cog Assessment Instrument,[37] the Memory Impairment Screen (MIS),[38] and the Six-Item Cognitive Impairment Test (6CIT).[39] The Memory Alteration Test (MAT) tests verbal, episodic and semantic memory, and appears to distinguish early Alzheimer disease from mild cognitive impairment.[40] These instruments have been found to be as clinically and psychometrically robust as the longer and more time-consuming Mini Mental State Examination (MMSE), and therefore more appropriate for use in primary care.[41]

However, despite the availability of primary-care-friendly tests of cognitive function, there has been little evidence of improvement in the recognition of and response to dementia syndromes in primary care. The UK evidence is particularly compelling, with evidence of little shift in general practitioner (GP) confidence and attitudes about dementia diagnosis and management, from the early educational interventions[42] and the UK Audit Commission at the end of the 1990s,[43] to later independent researchers[44] and the UK National Audit Office in 2007.[45] A recent retrospective study of a large cohort of patients diagnosed with dementia also showed little variation in incident diagnoses over the same period.[46]

The reasons for this failure to change clinical practice are unclear, but may include practitioners' attitudes, time factors, case-load and reimbursement mechanisms. There appears to be great variation between practitioners, with some taking the view that primary care is the only consistent source of help for people with dementia, while others adopt a nihilistic stance, arguing that "nothing can be done" for the patient with dementia. Time factors and the size of case-load do seem to have an impact on clinical performance, disadvantaging people with early, and difficult-to-recognize, changes in cognition. Studies from different settings have advanced the plausible argument that the problem of underdiagnosis is probably due to the interaction of case-complexity, shortage of time and the negative effects of reimbursement systems.[47,48] However, there is also considerable evidence that the main problem does not lie in a lack of diagnostic skills, but rather a lack of the resources for clinical management that their patients with dementia need. The difficulty for primary care is that it is encouraged to meet the needs of patients with dementia and their carers, in situations where psychosocial resources are inadequate and the effectiveness of medication very limited in power and duration.

There is considerable evidence for this conclusion. Studies of family doctors' diagnostic abilities show high levels of competence in those studied. In particular, vignette studies suggest that GPs tend to overdiagnose rather than underdiagnose dementia.[49] Clinical management skills are lacking, and do not appear to improve with education.[50] Confidence in working with people with dementia is low;[45] referral to specialists is rapid (once the syndrome is recognized), with a strong tendency (in the UK) to transfer responsibility for continuing care away from general practice and toward specialist services.[51] Support services for people with dementia are viewed by primary care practitioners as insufficient in quantity, variable in quality, and often difficult to access or coordinate.[44] Finally, "therapeutic nihilism" persists as a minority opinion.[52,53]

The limits of education

There is evidence to support the argument that suboptimal recognition of dementia in primary care reflects the paucity of responses available; nevertheless, the primary focus in many countries is on professional development (rather than service provision). This leads to a concentration on educational interventions. The view that the performance of primary care physicians in diagnosis and management of dementia syndromes can be improved by education and the provision of brief assessment tools is based on three false premises. The first is that generalists have more difficulty in diagnosing dementia than specialists, although there are good grounds to believe the contrary (see above). The second is that a quick test of cognitive function will help the diagnostic process more than any other approach. The third is that the behaviour of primary care clinicians is determined by clinical encounters, and not by whole systems of care. The counter argument is that therapeutic responses are shaped by available therapies, in the broadest definition of this term. Absent or inadequate specialist or social care support can have a negative effect on motivation to identify and respond to patients' problems. What matters is the whole system available to support patients with dementia. When primary care practitioners know that they have access to the expertise they need to support patients with dementia, and their families, through a progressive neurodegenerative disease, they will prioritize the acquisition of diagnostic and management skills. While both general education about dementia and specific training in the use of brief cognitive assessment tools undoubtedly have merits, they are not the solution to the problem of underrecognition of dementia in the community.

The specialist perspective on dementia syndrome has an inhibitory effect on our understanding of it. There is a tendency to underestimate how slowly the cognitive changes suggestive of dementia syndrome diverge from those of normal ageing, and how dementia emerges through the personality of the individual over the course of time. The description that follows of the trajectory of Alzheimer disease, the commonest dementia subtype, illustrates this. In addition, specialists often fail to understand the diagnostic process as it occurs in primary care, thinking of it as something similar to the linear processes that (they believe) they follow when making a diagnosis in a clinic.

The emergence of dementia

A review of cognitive markers in preclinical Alzheimer disease suggests that impairment in multiple cognitive domains is observable several years before a clinical diagnosis is made. The observed cognitive deficits in the early stages are not qualitatively different from those seen in normal ageing, suggesting continuity rather than discontinuity from normal ageing to preclinical dementia.[54] Using the findings of longitudinal studies, we can create a model of the transition from normal ageing to Alzheimer disease, as shown in Figure 30.2. The red line shows the very slow reduction in global cognitive function during ageing. The blue line represents the cohort that deviates away from the ageing norm, slowly over many years, until it becomes truly distinguishable from the larger population as having dementia syndrome. This model has five ill-defined and variable time phases.

Phase A is a long period (a decade or more) in which some cognitive functions (especially linguistic ability and general intelligence) deteriorate more than might be expected. Phase B is a decompensation phase in which global cognitive deterioration occurs, especially in episodic memory, executive functioning, verbal ability, visuospatial skills, attention and perceptual speed. Phase C is a period of relative stability in cognitive function, in which information transfer from temporary to permanent memory decreases, a change that is exacerbated with increasing cognitive demands.[55] These changes in cognitive function are matched by changes in multiple brain structures and functions, and in brain size. This phase can be called "mild cognitive impairment" (MCI), but there is a considerable overlap in cognitive performance between normal ageing and this impaired state,

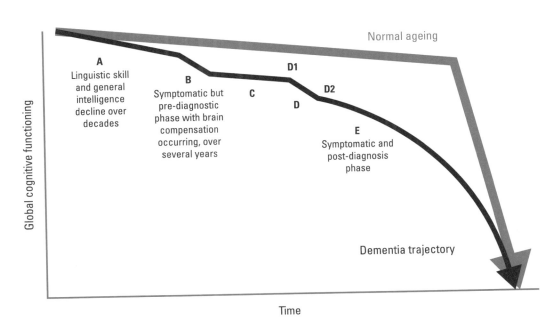

Figure 30.2   A model of the transition from normal ageing to Alzheimer disease

making routine screening for MCI in primary care impractical. Recognition of phase B is particularly hampered by the lack of impact of cognitive losses on everyday life, since brain plasticity and behavioural and social compensatory mechanisms operate to protect the affected individual.

The second downturn (phase D) is the beginning of rapid decline in cognitive function, lasting between 2 and 5 years (phase E).[46] This is clinically obvious dementia. Compensatory mechanisms presumably fail, perhaps because semantic memory (the store of facts and general knowledge) and implicit memory (the non-conscious influence of past experience on subsequent performance) become degraded.[56] Average survival from this point is 5 years, during which symptoms increase and capabilities are lost.[57] At present, diagnosis tends to occur at point D2 on the trajectory, some months after the precipitous decline begins; educational and awareness-raising efforts are designed to bring this recognition point forward in time, towards D1.

Understanding diagnostic thinking in primary care

Diagnosis is often presented in algorithm form as a linear process of testing patients with specific signs or symptoms, to identify a cause so that treatment can begin. Such linear thinking leads to the overemphasis on brief tools for assessing cognitive function already noted. This does not work in primary care, where pattern recognition and the use of "illness scripts" (more or less complex representations of diseases) are used in non-linear pathways to find the most probable explanations for presenting symptoms.[58] The diagnosis of any slowly evolving, long-term illness in primary care is made on the basis of more than one consultation, using an iterative and dynamic hypothetico-deductive diagnostic process that allows the family physician to generate and test hypotheses repeatedly over time.[59] Cognitive function tests can help with this process, and it is sensible to use one that fits into a busy work schedule, but such tests do not and cannot substitute for pattern recognition.

The first stage of diagnosing dementia is, therefore, the suspicion that it may be emerging (*the trigger phase*). This suspicion is often "triggered" by a symptom within the patient's story, or in a report from someone who knows the patient well. Early potential triggers may be related to loss of function rather than to memory loss, but these will be missed if the illness script does not contain functional loss as part of the dementia pattern.[60,61]

A specific problem with dementia syndrome is that all those involved – patients, families and primary care physicians – may be reluctant to diagnose a serious and largely unmodifiable disease loaded with a huge burden of stigma. Physicians may hesitate to label a patient as such,[62] and family members may gradually take over social roles from the patient, protecting him or her from decompensation in daily life, without necessarily being aware of the significance of their actions.[60]

The cognitive impairments that slowly accumulate in dementia syndrome do so within complex personalities, themselves embedded in social relationships. Dementia becomes a concern, and help is sought when cognitive losses can no longer be accommodated and create a problem in everyday life. A telling study of "late" diagnoses in older people from a rural community in Italy demonstrates how dementia syndrome functioned like a physical disability. Traditional respect shown towards older people was only overcome when the family economy was disrupted by the cognitive losses of the individual with dementia. Once family members had to take time off from work to attend to the older person, dementia emerged as a problem needing a solution.[63]

Diagnosis of dementia in the primary care setting

Cognitive assessment tests of the kind described next are not sufficient in themselves to reach a diagnosis of dementia. A detailed history by the primary care physician is required, including a comprehensive assessment of the patient's symptoms and concerns, and an account of their psychological state, behaviour and functioning obtained from their family, carers or other informants. Current guidance from the UK recommends that the primary care physician performs some routine investigations (blood screening for vitamin B_{12} deficiency, hypothyroidism, diabetes, renal failure and abnormal calcium levels, and possibly a chest X-ray and electrocardiogram (ECG)), before referring the patient for a specialist secondary care assessment.[5]

Memory clinics are increasingly being established to provide specialist centres for such an assessment. Evaluation of one such specialist memory clinic service in England has revealed high patient satisfaction and a two-fold increase in successful engagement with ethnic minority patients, who appear to be underserved by traditional services.[64]

The second step in the diagnostic process – usually taken in specialist settings – excludes potentially treatable pathologies like brain tumours or normal-pressure hydrocephalus, and includes detailed neurocognitive assessment and a computerized tomography (CT) scan. This will allow the subtyping of dementia that is important for both prognosis and treatment, particularly because of tendencies in primary care to underdiagnose Alzheimer disease,[65] the only one of the dementias where symptom modification with medication is possible.

Disclosure

Primary care practitioners need to understand that the experience of memory assessment (as described above) can induce shame and distress, even before the formal disclosure of a diagnosis. This distress can lead to people trying to maintain their sense of identity, which in turn can be perceived by professionals as "covering up" or "loss of insight".[66–68] Careful preparation of the person with suspected dementia, by their family physician or primary care nurse, may help minimize this type of reaction to assessment. During the assessment and diagnostic process, people should routinely be asked if they wish to know the diagnosis and with whom this should be shared.[32,69] Immediately after the disclosure of the diagnosis, support groups can promote well-being, allowing people to explore the experience of dementia in a safe setting.[70]

The majority of people with mild dementia wish to know their diagnosis,[71] and all primary care practitioners should assume that the diagnosis will be discussed with the person with dementia, unless there are clear reasons not to do so. Adjustment to the diagnosis is easier in a supportive social context, which primary care can offer because of the longstanding relationships between professionals and patients. The skills needed are the ability to anticipate and respond to shock, fear and grief, and these skills are widespread in primary care. Nonetheless, clinicians may find this task emotionally difficult, and may require their own support with such therapeutic work.[72]

People who have been informed of their diagnosis of dementia sometimes report that this disclosure process is badly handled, that little information is provided, or that little or no follow-up occurs.[73] A systematic review of the literature about sharing the diagnosis of dementia[31] suggests that failure to share, or provision of vague information about the diagnosis, is experienced as confusing and upsetting for some people with dementia and their families. The tasks of primary care, then, are to revisit the diagnosis with patients, to check their understanding and the information that they need, and to provide regular follow-up. People with learning disabilities are at higher risk of developing dementia syndrome (see later), and are a special case. They too should be told their diagnosis of dementia, and those supporting them (including primary care practitioners) should have access to specialist clinical advice and support about information sharing with people with learning difficulties.[74]

Psychosocial support: reframing dementia

The fear of triggering individual distress, denial and withdrawal from contact with services is one factor that inhibits practitioners from discussing dementia as a diagnosis,[52] and the clinical skills needed to manage this diagnostic transition may be lacking in primary care. This skill gap needs to be closed, because one of the major advantages of engaging people psychologically at an early stage of cognitive decline or dementia, in primary care, is to develop a trusting relationship while cognition and insight remain relatively intact. Listening to patients' experiences and providing simple cognitive or behavioural coping strategies have been found to be beneficial.[75]

Cognitive behavioural therapy (CBT) with people with mild to moderate dementia can be useful for overcoming catastrophic thinking and depressive withdrawal. Focusing on a patient's beliefs and attitudes about dementia, exploring the source and affect associated with unhelpful or inaccurate beliefs, and providing accurate verbal and written information can be helpful with the acceptance of a diagnosis. The use of CBT techniques allows a person-centred approach, which can help reduce fears that others will "find out" the diagnosis, and that a rapid deterioration in abilities plus the emergence of socially embarrassing behaviour, are imminent.[33]

The techniques used include combinations of reality orientation, memory strategies and reframing – all therapeutic techniques that address the anxiety and distress of individuals "terrified" by the diagnosis. In cognitive reframing, "stupidities" are relabelled as "difficulties" and catastrophic thoughts can be reformulated into more normalized terms. Reframing offers primary care practitioners an easily understood and applied method of working with people with dementia and their families. It appears to be more effective in promoting coping strategies in carers than individual problem-solving approaches or group interventions.[76]

Knowledge transfer: providing information in primary care

Primary care practitioners should ensure that people with newly diagnosed dementia and members of their family receive accurate details of local support.[43] Clinicians, people with dementia and their family members have different concerns, and primary care practitioners need to be sensitive to these different agendas. People with financial problems may find caregiving particularly difficult and may benefit from early referral to financial or debt advice agencies.[77] When working with people from minority ethnic communities, where terms like dementia may not be widely known, practitioners should draw on specialist support and publications.[78,79]

Support for carers

Carers of people with dementia experience depressed mood, report higher caregiving burden and have worse general health than carers of patients with other chronic diseases.[36] There is some evidence that carers can be reluctant to seek professional help,[80,81] but carer depression is one of the determinants of relocation of the person with dementia to a nursing home.[82] Primary care practitioners should, therefore, adopt a case-finding approach to carers of people with dementia and a problem-solving stance towards their situation.[83]

The experience of care-giving burden depends largely upon the carer's coping strategies, their sense of loneliness and their perceived lack of accessible support, rather than "objective" measure of tasks and responsibilities.[84,85] Supporting positive coping strategies and promoting problem-solving behaviour appear effective in reducing depression in carers,[86] and primary care practitioners can have an important role here because of their close contact with the person with dementia and their family. Nevertheless, it is important to keep a sense of proportion, for while interventions for people with dementia living at home are appreciated by carers, they do not reduce perceived caregiving burden.[87,88] People with dementia are more likely to be referred for specialist assessment when carer stress (often linked to behavioural and psychological symptoms of dementia) is identified.[89]

Comorbidities and dementia

Compared to cognitively intact older people, those with dementia have significantly reduced survival.[46,90,91] This increased mortality in patients with dementia is thought to be due to the presence of comorbid vascular diseases (including congestive heart failure, ischaemic heart disease and cerebrovascular disease) and diabetes.[92,93] For example, the incidence of recurrent stroke in patients with dementia is double that in cognitively intact patients.[94] The extent to which comorbid conditions are more frequent, and underdiagnosed, in people with dementia is debated.[95–97] The few studies that have investigated the management of comorbid diseases such as acute myocardial infarction,[98] recurrent stroke[99] and atrial fibrillation[100] suggest suboptimal care for those with dementia. Primary care practitioners should therefore aim for optimal treatment of cardiovascular risk factors and existing comorbidities in people with dementia, to optimize their quality of life, at least during the early to middle phases of the disease. In the later phase, when blood pressure falls and weight decreases, treatment approaches need to be reviewed.

Management of people with dementia in primary care

Currently the only available pharmacological strategies are:

- secondary prevention to try to delay the onset in people at risk of dementia: e.g. patients with diabetes or cardiovascular disease

- symptomatic treatments for people diagnosed with dementia.

In the future, it is hoped that both preventative and disease-modifying treatments will become available.

Goals of treatment

The main goals of treatment for dementia are:

- symptomatic improvement
- slowing or arrest of symptom progression
- maintaining patient and family/carer quality of life.

The response to an intervention can be considered as stabilization or improvement of symptoms. This can occur in three areas – cognition, activities of daily living (basic and instrumental) and global assessment by the patient and/or carer(s). In the more advanced stages of the disease, changes in cognitive performance are less relevant and also more difficult to quantify.

Principles of treatment

It is important that patients with dementia:

- are under regular review; this is usually coordinated by primary care, but frequently involves shared care pathways with secondary care, who are involved in supervising and assessing the response to pharmacological treatments
- have an ongoing "treatment plan", with defined goals, that considers both pharmacological and non-pharmacological treatment options
- have medical care integrated with education and support; such integration also applies to families and carers
- have optimal management of comorbid physical conditions
- have appropriate end-of-life care.

Preventing dementia in primary care

Although there are no current treatments to prevent dementia, there is a growing body of evidence that suggests minimizing risk factors (diabetes, cardiovascular risk factors), eating a healthy diet and maintaining physical and cognitive abilities and emotional well-being, can help delay the appearance of symptoms of dementia.[101]

Physical activity

Studies have found that older adults who are physically active may experience slower rates of cognitive decline. Perhaps some of the most compelling evidence comes from new analyses of the Framingham study that show one hour per day of moderate or heavy physical activity is associated with a 45% lower risk of developing dementia.[102] There are also additional benefits on stroke and cardiovascular disease, higher high-density lipoprotein and cholesterol levels, a reduced risk for colon cancer, and lower overall rates of mortality. Inclusion of physical activity, a low-cost, low-risk, and readily available intervention, as part of a public health strategy could have important implications for delaying memory loss.

Diet

A variety of studies have suggested a benefit of diet on cognitive impairment. Evidence from the Dietary Approaches to Stop Hypertension (DASH) diet suggests higher scores for cognitive functioning are associated with four food categories – whole grains, vegetables, low-fat dairy foods and nuts and beans.[103] Evidence about the potential benefit of omega-3-fatty acids is conflicting. Studies conducted in healthy elderly individuals with age-related cognitive decline suggest a benefit, while evidence from a study in mild/moderate Alzheimer disease suggested no benefit.[103]

More research is needed before one can confidently say which and how much of these foods may be beneficial and how long one needs to adhere to such a diet for benefit.

Mild cognitive impairment

MCI is a stage where people have mild symptoms that do not meet diagnostic criteria for dementia. Such people are at increased risk for development of dementia, particularly if their symptoms are associated with agitation, depression and apathy.[104] Results of studies with cholinesterase inhibitors and vitamin E in MCI patients have shown no benefit in reducing the risk of developing AD.[105]

Pharmacological interventions

Of the dementia syndromes, Alzheimer disease has been most studied with respect to assessment of potential symptomatic and disease-modifying therapies. As well as the hallmark pathology of amyloid plaques and tangles, Alzheimer disease is characterized by selective degeneration of cholinergic neurons. Other neurotransmitters (glutamate) and other processes (inflammatory and oxidative stress mechanisms) are also known to be associated with disturbances in neurotransmitter function that can contribute to the cognitive deficits seen in Alzheimer disease.[106] Cholinergic deficiencies have also been identified in Parkinson dementia.

To date, the main focus of pharmacological treatment for dementia, particularly mild and moderate Alzheimer disease (including Down syndrome), has been drugs that target augmentation of the cholinergic system by inhibiting the action of the enzyme cholinesterase. Three cholinesterase inhibitors are approved for use in mild to moderate Alzheimer disease – donepezil, galantamine and rivastigmine. The only other class of drug approved for use in Alzheimer disease is the N-methyl-D-aspartic acid (NMDA) receptor antagonist, memantine, which prevents excessive stimulation of the glutamate system. Memantine is approved for use in moderate to severe Alzheimer disease.

The cholinesterase inhibitors have also been studied in MCI, vascular dementia, frontotemporal dementia and dementia with Lewy bodies. An overview of evidence for drug treatments (approved and non-approved) in dementia is shown in Table 30.2 and Table 30.3 presents dosing regimes for drugs approved for use in Alzheimer disease.

Table 30.2 Overview of evidence for drug treatments for dementia[a]

	Level of evidence	Recommendation
Alzheimer disease		
Cholinesterase inhibitors: donepezil; galantamine; rivastigmine	Type 1a evidence for the efficacy of cholinesterase inhibitors for mild to moderate Alzheimer disease	A
	Type 2b evidence to support the switching from one cholinesterase inhibitor to another if the first is not tolerated or is ineffective	
NMDA receptor antagonist: memantine	There is type 1a evidence for the efficacy of memantine for moderate to severe Alzheimer disease	A
	There is type 1b evidence for adding memantine to a cholinesterase inhibitor	
Dementia with Lewy bodies and Parkinson disease dementia	Type 1b evidence supports treatment with cholinesterase inhibitors in Lewy body dementia and Parkinson disease dementia, including neuropsychiatric symptoms	A
	Type 1b evidence for memantine	

Table 30.2 Overview of evidence for drug treatments for dementia – *continued*

	Level of evidence	Recommendation
Vascular dementia	Type 1b evidence supports the use of cholinesterase drugs and memantine in the treatment of cognitive impairment in dementia, although effect sizes are small and may not be clinically significant	A
Other drugs		
Ginkgo biloba	Type 1b evidence for a modest effect in the treatment of cognitive impairment in dementia; effect sizes are small and may not be clinically significant	A
Vitamin B_{12}/folate	No evidence to suggest that vitamin B_{12} and folate are effective in the routine treatment of Alzheimer disease. Trials are ongoing, which may provide type 1a evidence	B
Oestrogens	Conflicting evidence over the use of oestrogens in dementia; type 2a evidence of a protective effect and 1b of a harmful effect. Until further evidence is available, oestrogens should not be prescribed for preventing or treating dementia	B
Anti-inflammatory drugs	Type 1a evidence that a variety of anti-inflammatory drugs do not produce benefit in Alzheimer disease	A
Antioxidants	Type 1b evidence of a delay in progression of Alzheimer disease with high-dose vitamin E alone, but not when combined with selegiline	B
Statins	Type 1a evidence of no effect of statins in the prevention of dementia	A

[a] Adapted, with permission, from Burns A, O'Brien J. Clinical practice with anti-dementia drugs: a consensus statement from British Association for Psychopharmacology. *Journal of Psychopharmacology*, 2006, 20(6):732–755.[107]

Level of evidence

1a: Evidence from meta-analysis of randomized controlled trials.

1b: Evidence from at least one randomized controlled trial.

2a: Evidence from at least one well-designed controlled study without randomization.

2b: Evidence from at least one other type of well-designed quasi-experimental study.

3: Evidence from well-designed non-experimental descriptive studies such as comparative studies, correlation studies, case-studies.

4: Evidence from expert committee reports or opinions and of clinical experiences of respected authorities.

Grade of recommendation

A: Required: at least one randomized controlled trial as part of the body of literature of overall quality and consistency addressing specific recommendation (evidence levels 1a and 1b).

B: Availability of well-conducted clinical studies but no randomized clinical trials on the topic of recommendation (includes evidence levels 2a, 2b and 3).

C: Evidence obtained from expert committee reports and/or clinical experiences of respected authorities (evidence level 4).

D: Indicates absence of directly applicable clinical studies of good quality.

Table 30.3 Dosing of drugs approved for Alzheimer disease

Drug/indication	Dose	Comment
Mild/moderate Alzheimer disease		
Donepezil[a]	5–10 mg once daily	Tablets and orodispersible tablets
		Reports of syncope and seizures associated with heart block
Galantamine	16–24 mg/day as twice daily (bd) dosage	Titrate from 4 mg bd, maintaining this dose for 4 weeks
		Tablets and oral solution
Rivastigmine	6–12 mg/day as bd dosage	Titrate from 3 mg daily, maintaining this dose for 2 weeks
		Transdermal
Moderate/severe Alzheimer disease		
Memantine	20 mg as bd dosage	Oral drops, solution and tablets
		Titrate from 5 mg at weekly intervals

[a] Donepezil high dose 23 mg.[110]

The most commonly occurring adverse events with cholinesterase inhibitors are nausea, vomiting, diarrhoea and weight loss; and with memantine, dizziness, headache, constipation, somnolence and hypertension. Patients showing no benefit with one cholinesterase inhibitor may show better tolerance or efficacy with a different drug in this class, or, in moderate or severe dementia, to a combination of cholinesterase inhibitor and memantine.[108,109] The cholinesterase inhibitors and memantine are available in a variety of formulations suitable for patients with swallowing difficulties.

Vascular and mixed dementias

Vascular dementia, previously known as multi-infarct dementia, has many aetiologies including multiple infarcts, episodes of hypotension, leukoaraiosis and haemorrhage. There is increasing recognition that vascular dementia coexists with other causes of dementia, particularly Alzheimer disease, which has resulted in the term "mixed dementia". The majority of elderly individuals with dementia have evidence of a mixed picture of cerebrovascular disease, vascular dementia and Alzheimer disease.[111–115] The co-occurrence of these features has resulted in a change of thinking from vascular dementia to the concept of vascular cognitive impairment.[116]

The main focus for the treatment of vascular dementia should be optimal treatment of the underlying cause(s); e.g. essential hypertension, diabetes, atrial fibrillation.

Both the cholinesterase inhibitors and memantine have been studied in vascular and mixed dementias. Data from two double-blind, placebo-controlled trials with donepezil and one with galantamine, in patients with probable and possible vascular dementia and mixed dementia have shown modest benefits on cognition and activities of daily living.[117–120] In similar patient populations, memantine showed some benefit on cognition and reduction of caregiver burden, with no associated major side-effects.[121–124] However, questions remain about the clinical relevance of the effects and how much of the benefits are due to the drugs' effect on coexistent Alzheimer disease.

Dementia with Lewy bodies and Parkinson disease dementia

Patients with dementia with Lewy bodies and Parkinson disease dementia pose particular challenges in clinical management, due to the presence of cognitive, motor and psychiatric symptoms. Psychiatric and cognitive symptomatology is frequently underrecognized and undertreated.[125,126] The combination of psychiatric pathology and side-effects of drugs prescribed for the cognitive, motor and psychiatric symptoms has been referred to as the "motion–emotion conundrum".

Cognitive symptoms

Clinical trials have been carried out with rivastigmine,[127,128] donepezil[129] and memantine in dementia with Lewy bodies and Parkinson disease dementia,[130,131] and rivastigmine is approved for Parkinson disease dementia. Currently there are no approved treatments for dementia with Lewy bodies.

Rivastigmine is associated with significant improvements in cognitive, neuropsychiatric and functional symptoms in both dementia with Lewy bodies and Parkinson disease dementia.[130,132] The effects on cognition and functional symptoms were of a similar magnitude to those seen in Alzheimer disease. Evidence from studies with memantine suggests some global clinical benefit in both dementia with Lewy bodies and Parkinson disease dementia, with a suggestion of a larger effect in Parkinson disease dementia.[131]

Motor symptoms

Levodopa monotherapy is the preferred option, due to concerns about inducing confusion and psychosis with other anti-Parkinsonian medications (selegiline, amantadine, catechol-O-methyltransferase (COMT) inhibitors, anticholinergics and dopamine agonists). The clinical response to levodopa is often less dramatic in patients with dementia with Lewy bodies than in patients with idiopathic Parkinson disease.[133]

Sleep problems

See below.

Frontotemporal dementia

Treatment strategies focus mainly on managing the psychiatric and behavioural symptoms. Antidepressants, such as the selective serotonin reuptake inhibitors (SSRIs) and trazodone may reduce the associated behavioural problems. Antipsychotic drugs are sometimes used, but issues of side-effects that increase mortality are similar to those seen in other dementias (see section of neuropsychiatric symptoms below). Patients experiencing language difficulties may benefit from speech therapy.

Other pharmacological aspects of the treatment of dementia

Dementia should not be regarded as a cognitive disorder alone. Varying levels of psychiatric symptoms frequently occur, with depression and anxiety being more frequent in the mild and moderate phases of illness, and hallucinations and delusions in the moderate and severe phases. Association with neurological issues also needs to be recognized; e.g. Parkinsonism (most frequently seen in dementia with Lewy bodies) and the increased risk of seizures.

Neuropsychiatric or behavioural and psychological symptoms of dementia

Behavioural and psychological symptoms of dementia present as three main syndromes – agitation, psychosis and mood disorders.[134] An overview of the risk/benefit of the available treatments for these symptoms is given in Table 30.4.

Agitation and aggression

Before specific pharmacological treatments are considered for agitation and aggression, potential physical causes, such as infections, pain, dehydration, sensory impairments (vision, hearing – see later), and environmental causes (lack of sensory stimulation, see non-pharmacological interventions below) should be excluded. Non-pharmacological interventions (psychological therapy, aromatherapy and light therapy see later) should be considered first line for symptoms that occur infrequently, only arise under specific circumstances or are unlikely to put patients at risk to themselves or others. Carers should be asked to monitor symptoms (including keeping a diary) and the patient's response to interventions.

Patients with symptoms that fail to respond to non-pharmacological treatment and/or present a safety concern should be referred to secondary care. In circumstances where there is acute distress and the risk of harm, short-term treatment with an atypical antipsychotic may still be considered the best option.[135,136] In less acute situations, management with cholinesterase inhibitors and/or memantine, antidepressants or anticonvulsants should be considered.[135]

Table 30.4 Risk/benefit of pharmacological treatment of behavioural and psychological symptoms of dementia[a]

Trials conducted	Evidence	Major adverse effects	Interpretation
Typical antipsychotics	Significant but modest advantage over placebo for behavioural symptoms Meta-analysis for haloperidol indicated improvement for aggression, but not in other symptoms	Parkinsonism, dystonia, tardive dyskinesia, QTc interval prolongation, significant increase in mortality compared with atypicals (≤180 days risk ratio = 1.37)	Adverse events make the use of typical antipsychotics inadvisable in people with Alzheimer disease
Atypical antipsychotics	Significant benefit in the treatment of aggression over 12 weeks	Parkinsonism, sedation, increased mortality(1.5–1.7-fold), increased cerebrovascular adverse events	Probably still the best option for short-term treatment (6–12 weeks) of aggression that is severe, persistent and treatment resistant. Serious adverse events are a major contraindication to long-term therapy
Cholinesterase inhibitors	No benefit in agitation over 12 to 24 weeks	Generally well tolerated, gastrointestinal symptoms (nausea and vomiting) are the most frequent adverse events	Evidence from the total pool of trials suggests an overall effect on behavioural and psychological symptoms of dementia over 6 months; the main benefits are probably for anxiety and apathy rather than aggression and agitation
Memantine	Benefit in irritability, lability, agitation and aggression and psychosis over 3 to 6 months in individual studies, meta-analysis and pooled analyses	Very well tolerated; low risk of hypertension	Promising treatment, but a prospective study in patients with clinically significant agitation is required
Antidepressants	Trazodone meta-analysis – insufficient evidence of efficacy Citalopram: equivalence to other active treatments in active comparator trials, with efficacy over placebo in one small placebo-controlled trial Sertraline: significant benefit for agitation in post hoc analysis in placebo-controlled randomized controlled trial	Generally well tolerated; hyponatraemia can occur with SSRIs	Evidence base for SSRIs is encouraging, but preliminary; large placebo-controlled trials of long duration are urgently needed

Trials conducted	Evidence	Major adverse effects	Interpretation
Anticonvulsants	Carbamazepine: significant improvement in behavioural symptoms in one of two randomized controlled trials with overall benefit confirmed in meta-analysis. Sodium valproate: Cochrane review – cannot be tolerated in clinically effective doses Gabapentin: evidence very preliminary	Carbamazepine: good tolerability in the short-term; drug–drug interactions a potential concern; potential to impair balance and increase risk of falls; mortality does not seem to be increased	Promising treatment option; larger and longer trials needed; long-term safety needs to be established; further work needed to determine if a preferential response is shown in agitated patients with concurrent affective symptoms

[a] Adapted, by permission from Macmillan Publishers Ltd: Ballard CG et al. Management of agitation and aggression associated with Alzheimer disease. *Nature Reviews Neurology* 5:245–255, copyright 2009.[135]

Extreme caution is recommended for use of typical and atypical antipsychotics in patients with Lewy body and Parkinson dementias, where neuroleptic sensitivity reactions are seen in up to 50% of patients exposed to such agents.[131,132]

Psychotic symptoms

Delusional symptoms are common, while full-blown psychosis is rare. Common presentations include thinking someone is stealing things, and misidentification, such as when a patient feels that their living place is not their home.[137] Antipsychotics are the mainstay of treatment for psychosis. However, in long-term treatment, typical and atypical antipsychotics are associated with a significant increase in cardiovascular events and mortality (see Table 30.4). Patients with significant psychotic symptoms should be referred to secondary care.

Mood disorders (depression and emotional liability) in dementia

Depression is commonly found in association with dementia and the two may be linked in a number of ways. De novo depression in an elderly person can be the first manifestation of a dementing illness. Patients can become depressed and/or emotional and frustrated at the lack of ability to perform tasks that they previously found relatively easy. On the other hand, depression can be associated with:

- poor concentration or executive function
- impairment associated with concomitant medications, e.g. analgesics
- pseudodementia
- concurrent medical illnesses, e.g. stroke, Parkinson disease, excessive alcohol.

There is no clear correlation between the severity of dementia and the severity of depression.[138] Patients with dementia can also exhibit sudden changes in mood that are usually precipitated by frustration or minor events.

The characteristics of depression in people with dementia are generally similar to those in individuals without dementia. As it is often very difficult to obtain an accurate history from the patient themselves, primary care physicians need to enquire of carers and family members about core symptoms: e.g. sleep disturbance, poor appetite, anxiety, decreased activity and inability to experience pleasure, especially in activities that were previously pleasurable.

There is little evidence from prospective randomized clinical trials evaluating antidepressants in depression associated with dementia.[139] The general impression from the evidence is that some patients respond well to antidepressants, with the best evidence for the SSRIs sertraline and citalopram. Tricyclic antidepressants should be avoided because anticholinergic effects can worsen confusion.

Psychological treatments, particularly CBT should be considered for people with mild dementia. Patients who fail to respond to therapy, or where there is uncertainty about the diagnosis, should be referred to secondary care.

Epilepsy in dementia

A number of studies have demonstrated that dementia is a risk factor for developing seizures and epilepsy. People with dementia have a 5 to 10 times greater risk of developing seizures compared with age-matched controls.[140-142] Between 8% and 22% of patients with Alzheimer disease will have a seizure, which will usually be complex partial or generalized tonic clonic.[143] Patients with dementia who develop seizures should be referred to a neurologist for careful assessment that includes blood tests, a CT scan or magnetic resonance imaging (MRI), and an electroencephalogram (EEG) to assess the seizure type and any other underlying cause for the seizure. From these tests, an anti-epileptic medication will be selected to help control the seizures.

The choice of anti-epileptic drug depends on a number of factors:[144]

- kinetics in the elderly
- potential side-effects
- risk for drug–drug interactions.

Non-pharmacological treatments that decrease behavioural problems (see non-pharmacological interventions below) may also help to decrease the risk of seizures.

Sleep problems

Sleep problems are common in people with dementia and may be caused by a number of factors:

- diet: too much caffeine, alcohol
- environmental: room too hot, lack of daytime activity
- medical causes: side-effects of medication (analgesics); painful conditions, e.g. arthritis, angina; congestive heart failure; disruption of the sleep–wake cycle
- psychological issues: depression, disturbing dreams.

It is important to identify the contributory factors to the sleep disorder and manage those appropriately. Hypnotics are not recommended due to the risks for confusion, sedation and falls. A form of melatonin (Circadin®) has been approved recently for the short-term treatment of primary insomnia in patients aged 55 years or over. Trials are ongoing to evaluate the efficacy of Circadin® in patients with mild to moderate Alzheimer disease.

Dementia with Lewy bodies is associated with a number of sleep disorders: REM sleep behaviour disorder, restless legs syndrome, periodic limb movements of sleep and excessive daytime sleepiness. REM sleep behaviour disorder can be treated with clonazepam 0.25 mg at bedtime, titrated slowly, monitoring for both efficacy and side-effects.[128]

Drug–drug interactions

In older people, adverse drug reactions, including interactions, are a common cause of admission to hospital and are an important cause of morbidity and death. As most adverse drug reactions in the elderly are predictable and therefore potentially avoidable, good communication is pivotal in developing an effective therapeutic partnership with the patient and with fellow health professionals.

Elderly patients are at increased risk of drug–drug interactions, not only because they are likely to be taking multiple medications but also because of factors such as age-related changes in pharmacokinetics and pharmacodynamics, frailty, greater inter-individual variability and reduced homoeostatic mechanisms.

Other types of interactions to consider include:

- drug–disease, drug–nutrition and drug–herbal products.
- over-the-counter products that may cause major side-effects, e.g. non-steroidal anti-inflammatory medicines, sedating antihistamines, sedatives and H2 blockers.

Points to consider

- Where possible, avoid long-acting drugs and drugs with active metabolites, especially those with metabolites with a long-half-life.
- When introducing a drug, start low and go slow but do achieve a therapeutic dose.
- For patients with renal and/or hepatic impairment, always check the product labelling for recommendations about dose adjustments.
- Reversible cognitive impairment is common with opioid analgesics and other drugs with sedative side-effects.
- Patients with dementia are prone to delirium when given medications with cholinergic effects – tricyclic antidepressants.
- There is an increased risk of falls with benzodiazepines and sedating hypnotics, and drugs that are associated with postural hypotension.
- Constipation is worsened by calcium, calcium channel blockers and anticholinergics.

Non-pharmacological interventions

There is an increasing body of evidence demonstrating the benefit of non-pharmacological interventions in dementia, particularly for the management of agitation and aggression and other behavioural and psychological symptoms of dementia. These interventions include psychological interventions, light and aromatherapy.

Psychological interventions

Psychological interventions that have been researched include reality orientation, validation therapy, reminiscence therapy, "Snoezelen" therapy or multisensory stimulation, simulated-presence therapy structured activity, music therapy and environmental manipulation. A systematic review by Livingston et al. concluded that validation therapy is both practical and has some efficacy.[145] A "tool-box" of psychological interventions that can be individualized has shown benefit in agitation.[146]

Aromatherapy

There is accumulating evidence for the benefit of lavender and Melissa (lemon balm) oils in the management of agitation.[147–149] Melissa oil is formulated into a base cream and applied twice daily, and lavender oil is used as an aroma-stream. Aromatherapy has a role where there is no immediate high-level risk to the patient or others from agitation.

Light therapy

Mood and behavioural disturbances, as well as circadian rhythm disturbance, are known to be associated with dementia. Light therapy given in the morning is beneficial in the management of agitation,[150] and light combined with melatonin increases daytime wake time and activity levels and strengthens the sleep–wake cycle.[151]

End-of-life care

Dementia is often *not* viewed by health professionals and family and carers as a terminal illness in the same way as cancer; indeed even if people can appreciate that dementias are progressive, incurable diseases, families and clinicians may continue to have difficulty viewing them as causing death. As a result, in many cases, patients have not received appropriate support in the final stages of their illness.

End-of-life care for patients with dementia is complex and best viewed in a similar way to palliative care.

The assessment and management of patients with severe dementia (non-ambulatory, loss of meaningful conversation, dependent in most or all activities of daily living), requires a broad and thoughtful approach, gathering information from all available sources (carer, family). There are often readily treatable causes of increased confusion or delirium and challenging behaviour, e.g. inadequate hydration, painful conditions. As with any elderly person, individuals with dementia are susceptible to painful conditions (arthritis, osteoporosis, urinary tract infections). Indeed, a recent study of people with dementia who exhibited challenging behaviour found that in 75% of cases the behaviour responded to analgesics.[152]

When a patient reaches the severe stage of dementia, there are additional factors that predict a 50% risk of mortality:[153,154]

- hip fracture
- multiple pressure sores
- need for insertion of a feeding tube
- pneumonia
- recurrent infections
- weight loss of 10% or more.

Primary care also has an important role in oversight of the health of family and carers and support in bereavement.

Mental capacity

People who lack mental capacity need someone else to manage their legal, financial and health affairs. A recent WPA Section of Old Age Psychiatry consensus statement made provision for people to choose someone not only to manage their finances and property should they become incapable, but also to make health and welfare decisions on their behalf.[155]

It is important that those involved in the care of people with dementia appreciate the medicolegal aspects around mental capacity and the importance of "advance decisions". An "advance decision" allows a person to state what forms of treatment and support they would or would not like should they become unable to decide for themselves in future. This is an opportunity for individuals and their families to discuss and document treatment preferences towards the end of life while the person still has reasonable capacity. People with dementia need to be confident that their end-of-life wishes will be respected and that they will be supported and cared for in a coordinated and planned way so that they die in the place and in the manner that they have chosen.

Primary care physicians have an important role to play in discussing with families of patients with dementia consideration of a more palliative approach to care and away from diagnostic procedures and treatments that may cause more burdens than benefits and therefore not be in the patient's best interests. They play a key role when decisions are needed about interventions such as hospitalization, antibiotics, intravenous fluid or enteral nutrition. Discussions about care should consider a patient's prior wishes, the agreed-upon goals of therapy, and the risk/benefit of the treatment options.

Considerations about provision of dementia care

Primary care faces a significant challenge in delivering safe, quality, cost-effective care for the elderly in general and people with dementia in particular. The needs of this patient population are complex; they suffer from a range of chronic medical conditions, receive multiple medications including psychotropic drugs, display a wide range of behavioural and psychological symptoms, and have high utilization of health- and social care systems. Limitations of primary health-care provision include insufficient time for review, difficulty accessing community resources with expertise in dementia care, poor communication between health, social and community care, and absence of support from an interdisciplinary dementia care team.[156]

An example of what a collaborative dementia care programme should include is:[156]

- a feasible dementia identification and diagnosis process, including a reliable tool for periodic needs assessment and evaluation of ongoing therapy
- pharmacological and psychosocial interventions that prevent or reduce the family caregiver's psychological and physical burden
- self-management tools to enhance the patient and the caregiver skills in managing dementia disability and navigating the health-care system
- pharmacological interventions for care recipients that target the cognitive, functional, behavioural and psychological symptoms of dementia, such as:

- enhancement of the patient's cholinergic system via prescribing cholinesterase inhibitors and decreasing exposure to medication with anticholinergic effects
- improvement in medication adherence
- reduction in cerebrovascular risk factors such hypertension, diabetes and hyperlipidaemia
- prevention and management of delirium, depression and psychosis superimposed on dementia
- case management and coordination with community resources including adult day care, respite care and support groups
- modification of the patient's physical home environment to accommodate dementia disability
- an increasing focus on palliative care needs as the illness progresses, including advance care planning, attentive management of pain and other symptoms, avoidance of burdensome and undesired medical treatments, and eventual discussion of referral to a hospice.

Primary care has a vital role to play in:

- minimizing risks factors for dementia by optimizing care of diabetes and cardiovascular disease during adult life
- early recognition and diagnosis of dementia
- signposting patients and their families to help and support throughout the course of illness but particularly at the time of diagnosis. Charitable organizations such as the Alzheimer's Association provide a range of services that GPs need to be aware of
- coordinating the management of people with dementia, including optimizing management of physical comorbidities
- recognizing the specific needs of people with dementia who also have sensory impairments and learning disabilities (see below).

Populations with specific needs

There are certain groups of people with dementia who need additional consideration:

- early-onset dementia, which is often familial
- learning disability
- people from minority ethnic groups, rural, island or traveller communities
- people with sight and hearing impairments.

Learning disability

There is no evidence that dementia affects people with learning disabilities differently from how it affects other people. However, the early stages are more likely to be missed or misinterpreted – particularly if several professionals are involved in the person's care. The person with dementia may find it hard to express how they feel their abilities have deteriorated, and problems with communication may make it more difficult for others to assess change.

It is essential that people who understand the person's usual methods of communication are involved when a diagnosis is being explored – particularly where the person involved does not use words to communicate.

All individuals with a learning disability have some increased risk for dementia:[157]

- 50 years and over: 13%
- 65 years and over: 22%.

Down syndrome and Alzheimer disease

About 20% of people with learning disability have Down syndrome and this patient group is at particular increased risk of Alzheimer disease. Data suggest that the following percentages of people with Down syndrome have dementia:[158]

- 30–39 years: 2%

- 40–49 years: 9.4%
- 50–59 years: 36.1%
- 60–69 years: 54.5%.

Visual impairment

One in 10 people over the age of 75 years has a significant visual impairment. There are 2 million people in the UK who self-define as having a sight problem or seeing difficulty and, of these, the majority are aged over 65 years.[159] The Royal National Institute for the Blind and Alzheimer's Society have formed a special interest group on dementia and sight loss[160] in order to:

- develop a better understanding of issues for older people with sight loss and dementia
- influence policy and practice within both organizations
- develop and disseminate materials that contribute to good practice.

Deafness

Approximately one in seven people in the UK have a hearing problem and the number is rising as more people live well into old age.[160] Most people gradually lose their hearing, as they get older, with significant increases from the age of 50 years; 71% of the over-70 population are deaf or have a significant hearing loss. Consequently, many people with dementia also have hearing loss, and some will have been deaf from an early age. The challenges of coping with dementia are made much worse when the person cannot hear properly.

Important principles to remember when working with people with dementia who are also deaf are:

- try to keep communication channels open; it is not acceptable to write the person off and assume that they are unable to understand you and have nothing important to tell you
- deaf people rely more on visual clues in day-to-day life, so making sure that the person is wearing clean, up-to-date spectacles is essential
- everyone is different, so adopt an individual approach to communication
- sometimes you will not be sure if you have been successful or not – but you still must not give up; keeping an open mind is essential.

Helpful ways of speaking include:

- get the person's attention before you start speaking
- make sure the person can see your face clearly and that it is well lit
- get onto the same level, so they are not having to look up or down
- do not shout or raise your voice! This will distort your speech making it more difficult to understand. It may also make you sound angry or impatient, and can be painful to the deaf person
- choose a quiet place or minimize background noise
- say clearly what the conversation is about
- keep the message simple
- speak a little more slowly than usual, but keep the natural rhythms of your speech; this will help the person with lip reading
- do not over-exaggerate your words as you speak
- if the person is having difficulty understanding, try using different words to express your meaning
- if the person is comfortable with reading, you can also try writing down your message.

Remember that some patients have both visual AND hearing impairment.

Non-verbal communication

The following are some ideas for making the most of non-verbal communication for people with hearing loss or learning disability:[161]

- try to be relaxed and friendly – smile!

- avoid any signals that might make you seem impatient
- make sure that the person can see your face clearly – don't sit or stand with your back to the window or other source of light
- do not cover your mouth with your hand or anything else while you speak
- use eye contact to hold the person's attention
- use gestures to back up what you mean, but avoid moving your hands around too much, as this can be distracting
- use your fingers to give important details like numbers
- get close enough to the person to have a conversation, but not so close they feel crowded
- if it seems appropriate, touch can also be useful
- use objects or pictures to help the person to understand what you are telling or asking them.

Collaboration and integration of services and implications for commissioning

Primary care needs far greater support, together with collaboration and integration of services to provide the appropriate type of care at the right time to both patients and their families and carers throughout the course of dementia. This is exemplified in the 17 key objectives of the National Dementia Strategy for England (see Figure 30.2).[22]

- *Objective 1*: improving public and professional awareness and understanding of dementia. Public and professional awareness and understanding of dementia to be improved and the stigma associated with it addressed. This should inform individuals of the benefits of timely diagnosis and care, promote the prevention of dementia, and reduce social exclusion and discrimination. It should encourage behaviour change in terms of appropriate help seeking and help provision.
- *Objective 2*: good-quality early diagnosis and intervention for all. All people with dementia to have access to a pathway of care that delivers: a rapid and competent specialist assessment; an accurate diagnosis, sensitively communicated to the person with dementia and their carers; and treatment, care and support provided as needed following diagnosis. The system needs to have the capacity to see all new cases of dementia in the area.
- *Objective 3*: good-quality information for those with diagnosed dementia and their carers. Providing people with dementia and their carers with good-quality information on the illness and on the services available, both at diagnosis and throughout the course of their care.
- *Objective 4*: enabling easy access to care, support and advice following diagnosis. A dementia adviser to facilitate easy access to appropriate care, support and advice for those diagnosed with dementia and their carers.
- *Objective 5*: development of structured peer support and learning networks. The establishment and maintenance of such networks will provide direct local peer support for people with dementia and their carers. It will also enable people with dementia and their carers to take an active role in the development and prioritization of local services.
- *Objective 6*: improved community personal support services. Provision of an appropriate range of services to support people with dementia living at home and their carers. Access to flexible and reliable services, ranging from early intervention to specialist home-care services, which are responsive to the personal needs and preferences of each individual and take account of their broader family circumstances. Accessible to people living alone or with carers, and people who pay for their care privately, through personal budgets or through local authority-arranged services.
- *Objective 7*: implementing the Carers' Strategy. Family carers are the most important resource available for people with dementia. Active work is needed to ensure that the provisions of the Carers' Strategy are available for carers of people with dementia. Carers have a right to an assessment of their needs and can be supported through an agreed plan to support the important role they play in the care of the person with dementia. This will include good-quality, personalized breaks. Action should also be taken to strengthen support for children who are in caring roles, ensuring that their particular needs as children are protected.

- *Objective 8*: improved quality of care for people with dementia in general hospitals. Identifying leadership for dementia in general hospitals, defining the care pathway for dementia there and the commissioning of specialist liaison older people's mental health teams to work in general hospitals.
- *Objective 9*: improved intermediate care for people with dementia. Intermediate care that is accessible to people with dementia and that meets their needs.
- *Objective 10*: considering the potential for housing support, housing-related services and telecare to support people with dementia and their carers. The needs of people with dementia and their carers should be included in the development of housing options, assistive technology and telecare. As evidence emerges, commissioners should consider the provision of options to prolong independent living and delay reliance on more intensive services.
- *Objective 11*: living well with dementia in care homes. Improved quality of care for people with dementia in care homes by the development of explicit leadership for dementia within care homes, defining the care pathway there, the commissioning of specialist in-reach services from community mental health teams, and through inspection regimes.
- *Objective 12*: improved end-of-life care for people with dementia. People with dementia and their carers to be involved in planning end-of-life care that recognizes the principles outlined in the Department of Health End of Life Care Strategy. Local work on the End of Life Care Strategy to consider dementia.
- *Objective 13*: an informed and effective workforce for people with dementia. Health and social care staff involved in the care of people who may have dementia to have the necessary skills to provide the best quality of care in the roles and settings where they work. To be achieved by effective basic training and continuous professional and vocational development in dementia.
- *Objective 14*: a joint commissioning strategy for dementia. Local commissioning and planning mechanisms to be established to determine the services needed for people with dementia and their carers, and how best to meet these needs. These commissioning plans should be informed by the World Class Commissioning guidance for dementia developed to support this strategy.
- *Objective 15*: improved assessment and regulation of health and care services and of how systems are working for people with dementia and their carers. Inspection regimes for care homes and other services that better assure the quality of dementia care provided.
- *Objective 16*: a clear picture of research evidence and needs. Evidence to be available on the existing research base on dementia in the UK and gaps that need to be filled.
- *Objective 17*: effective national and regional support for implementation of the strategy. Appropriate national and regional support to be available to advise and assist local implementation of the strategy. Good-quality information to be available on the development of dementia services, including information from evaluations and demonstrator sites.

Achievement of these goals has important implications for commissioning of services (primary, secondary, community and social care) for people with dementia. As described in the National Dementia Strategy,[22] to achieve this there is a need to:

- encourage help seeking and help offering (referral for diagnosis) by changing public and professional attitudes, understanding and behaviour
- make early diagnosis and treatment the rule rather than the exception. This will be achieved by locating the responsibility for the diagnosis of mild and moderate dementia in a specifically commissioned part of the system that can (1) make the diagnoses well; (2) break those diagnoses sensitively and well to those affected; and (3) provide individuals with immediate treatment, care and peer and professional support as needed
- enable people with dementia and their carers to live well with dementia by the provision of good quality of care for all with dementia, from diagnosis to the end of life, in the community, in hospitals and in care homes.

Conclusion

In many countries, the current configuration of services for people with dementia will not cope with the consequences of the demographic shift that is now under way. Primary care, which has traditionally deferred to specialist provision for diagnosis and management of people with dementia, will need to adopt a more active role. This will entail the acquisition of new skills, particularly around psychosocial interventions, and the development of systematic care packages and pathways.

Improving the ability of primary care practitioners to identify dementia syndrome depends, therefore, on recognition of the necessary preconditions for acquiring new skills. First, there need to be solutions to the problems that dementia syndrome generates. Memory assessment services are needed, as are psychosocial supports and therapies. The latter are particularly important, given the limited pharmacological therapies available. Whole-system changes would need to include policy changes at the macro level of funding bodies, efforts at systematization of care at the meso level of specialist service providers, and educational interventions aimed at individual professionals and work groups at the micro level. These changes would be different in different jurisdictions, depending on funding streams, the presence or absence of a gatekeeper function in primary care, and the availability in the community of other disciplines, like clinical psychology.

Second, practitioners' pattern-recognition abilities need to be enhanced and their illness scripts made richer and deeper. The perception that dementia syndrome is primarily a disorder of memory needs to be modified, to take into account subtler changes like loss of executive functions (anticipation, planning), as well as more obvious functional losses like difficulties with once-easy tasks – making a phone call, using a cash machine, working the remote control on the television. Educational interventions need to be built around these principles. Finally, the natural history of dementia syndrome needs to be understood as a disorder that breaks away from normal ageing, and breaks through compensatory psychological and social mechanisms. The diagnostic task is rarely an easy one in the early stages of dementia syndrome, but it is one that primary care practitioners can master once they know what it is they are facing, and what resources they can call upon.

References

1   *World Health Report 2003 – shaping the future*. Geneva, World Health Organization, 2003.

2   Ritchie K, Lovestone S. The dementias. *The Lancet*, 2002, 360:1759–1766.

3   *World Alzheimer Report 2010. The Global economic impact of dementia*. London, Alzheimer's Disease International, 2010.

4   *Dementia UK*. London, Alzheimer's Society, 2007.

5   National Institute for Health and Clinical Excellence (NICE). *Dementia. a NICE-SCIE guideline on supporting people with dementia and their carers in health and social care*. London, British Psychological Society and the Royal College of Psychiatrists, 2007.

6   *World Alzheimer Report 2009*. London, Alzheimer's Disease International, 2009.

7   Lobo A et al. Prevalence of dementia and major subtypes in Europe: a collaborative study of population-based cohorts. *Neurology*, 2000, 54:S4–S9.

8   Busse EW. Scope and development in the twentieth century. In: Copeland JRM et al., eds. *Principles and practice of geriatric psychiatry*. Chichester: John Wiley & Sons Ltd, 2002:7–8.

9   Berrios GE. Alzheimer's disease: a conceptual history. *International Journal of Geriatric Psychiatry*, 1990; 5: 355–365.

10 Berrios GE. A conceptual history in the nineteenth century. In: Copeland JRM et al., eds. *Principles and practice of geriatric psychiatry*. Chichester: John Wiley & Sons Ltd, 2002:3–6.

11 Dillman R. *Alzheimer's disease. The concept of disease and the construction of medical knowledge*. Amsterdam, Thesis Publishers, 1990.

12 de Mendonça Lima CA et al. Psiquiatria Geriátrica: origens históricas de uma subespecialidade da psiquiatria. *Arquivos Brasileiros de Psiquiatria, Neurologia e Medicinal Legal*, 2006, 100:26–33.

13 American Psychiatric Association. *Practice guideline for the treatment with Alzheimer's disease and other dementias*, 2nd ed. Washington DC, American Psychiatric Press, 2007.

14 Katona C et al., on behalf of the Consensus Group. International Psychogeriatric Association consensus statement on defining and measuring treatment benefits in dementia. *International Psychogeriatrics*, 2007, 19:345–354.

15 *mhGAP intervention guide for mental, neurological and substance use disorders in non-specialized health settings*. Geneva, World Health Organization, 2010 (http://www.who.int/mental_health/mhgap/evidence/en/, accessed 11 December 2011).

16   3.1: Dementia. In: *Neurological disorders: public health challenges*. Geneva, World Health Organization, 2006:42–54.

17   de Mendonça Lima CA, Kühne N, Buschfort R. ATLAS: mapping mental health resources for old persons in the world. *Psychogeriatria Polska*, 2004, 1:167–174.

18   *Closing the gap in a generation. Health equity through action on the social determinants of health. Final Report of the Commission on Social Determinants of Health*. Geneva, World Health Organization, 2008.

19   de Mendonça Lima CA. Social determinants of health and promotion of mental health in old age. In: Bährer-Kohler, ed. *Social determinants and mental health*. New York, Nova Science Publishers, Inc., 2011.

20   Kalache A. Ageing is a Third World problem too. *International Journal of Geriatric Psychiatry*, 1991, 6:617– 618.

21   World Health Organization and World Psychiatric Association. *Organizing services for the elderly with mental disorders. A technical consensus statement*. Geneva, World Health Organization, 1997 (WHO/MSA/MNH/MND/97.3).

22   Department of Health (DH/SCLG&CP/SCPI/SR). *Living well with dementia: a National Dementia Strategy*. Leeds, Department of Health, 2009.

23   Tout K. *Ageing in developing countries*. Oxford, Oxford University Press, 1989.

24   World Health Organization. Dementia. *Evidence-based recommendations for management of dementia in non-specialized health settings. mhGAP Evidence Resource Center*. Geneva, WHO Mental Health GAP Action Programme (mhGAP), 2010 (http://www.who.int/mental_health/evidence/mhGAP_intervention_guide/en/index.html, accessed 11 December 2011).

25   Pucci E et al. General practitioners facing dementia: are they fully prepared? *Neurological Sciences*, 2004, 24:384–389.

26   Vernooij-Dassen M et al. and the INTERDEM group. Factors affecting the timely recognition and diagnosis of dementia in primary care across eight European states: a modified focus group study. *International Journal of Geriatric Psychiatry*, 2005, 20:1–10.

27   Boustani M et al. Screening for dementia in primary care: a summary of the evidence for the US preventive services task force. *Annals of Internal Medicine*, 2003, 138:927–937.

28   Bamford C et al. Can primary care record review facilitate earlier diagnosis of dementia? *Family Practice*, 2007, 24:108–116.

29   Jha A, Tabet N, Orrell M. To tell or not to tell – comparison of older patients' reaction to their diagnosis of dementia and depression. *International Journal of Geriatric Psychiatry*, 2001; 16: 879–885.

30   Sullivan K, O'Conor F. Should a diagnosis of dementia be disclosed? *Aging & Mental Health*, 2001, 5:340–348.

31   Bamford C et al. Disclosing a diagnosis of dementia: a systematic review. *International Journal of Geriatric Psychiatry*, 2004, 19:151–169.

32   Pratt R, Wilkinson H. A psychosocial model of understanding the experience of receiving a diagnosis of dementia. *Dementia*, 2003, 2:181–199.

33   Husband HJ. The psychological consequences of learning a diagnosis of dementia: three case examples. *Aging and Mental Health*, 1999, 3:179–183.

34   Smith AP, Beattie BL. Disclosing a diagnosis of Alzheimer's disease: patients and families' experiences. *Canadian Journal of Neurological Sciences*, 2001, 28(Suppl. 1):S67–S71.

35   Koch T, Iliffe S. Changing practice in the diagnosis and management of dementia in primary care. *British Journal of General Practice*, 2011, 61:514–515.

36   Brodaty H, Green A. Who cares for the carer? The often forgotten patient. *Australian Family Physician*, 2002, 31:833–836.

37   Borson, S et al. The mini-cog: a cognitive 'vital signs' measure for dementia screening in multi-lingual elderly. *International Journal of Geriatric Psychiatry*, 2000, 15:1021–1027.

38   Buschke H et al. Screening for dementia with the Memory Impairment Screen. *Neurology*, 1999, 52:231–238.

39   Brooke P, Bullock R. Validation of the 6 item Cognitive Impairment Test. *International Journal of Geriatric Psychiatry*, 1999, 14:936–940.

40 Rami L et al. Screening for amnestic mild cognitive impairment and early Alzheimer's disease with M@T (Memory Alteration Test) in the primary care population. *International Journal of Geriatric Psychiatry*, 2007, 22:294–304.

41 Milne A et al. Screening for dementia in primary care: a review of the use, efficacy and quality of measures. *International Psychogeriatrics*, 2008, 3:431–458.

42 Iliffe S, Manthorpe J, Eden A. Sooner or later? Issues in the early diagnosis of dementia in general practice: a qualitative study. *Family Practice*, 2003, 20:376–381.

43 *Forget me not*. London, Audit Commission, 2002.

44 Turner S et al. General practitioners' knowledge, confidence & attitudes in the diagnosis and management of dementia. *Age and Ageing*, 2004, 33:461–467.

45 National Audit Office. *Improving services and support for people with dementia*. London, The Stationery Office, 2007.

46 Rait G et al. Survival of people with a clinical diagnosis of dementia in primary care. *BMJ*, 2010, 341:c3584.

47 Stoppe G et al. Physicians competence regarding the early diagnosis of dementia: differences between family physicians and primary care neuropsychiatrists in Germany. *Psychiatrische Praxis*, 2007, 34:134–138.

48 Hinton L et al. Practice constraints, behavioural problems and dementia care: primary care physicians perspectives. *Journal of General Internal Medicine*, 2007, 22:1625–1627.

49 O'Connor D et al. Do general practitioners miss dementia in elderly patients? *BMJ*, 1988, 297:1107–1110.

50 Downs M et al. Effectiveness of educational interventions in improving detection and management of dementia in primary care: a cluster randomized controlled study. *BMJ*, 2006, 332:692–695.

51 Wilcock J et al. Concordance with clinical practice guidelines for dementia in general practice. *Aging & Mental Health*, 2009, 13:155–161.

52 Iliffe S, Wilcock J. The identification of barriers to the recognition of and response to dementia in primary care using a modified focus group method. *Dementia*, 2005, 4:12–23.

53 Iliffe S, Wilcock J, Haworth D. Obstacles to shared care for patients with dementia: a qualitative study. *Family Practice*, 2006, 23:353–362.

54 Bäckman L et al. Multiple cognitive deficits during the transition to Alzheimer's disease. *Journal of Internal Medicine*, 2004, 256:195–204.

55 Small BJ et al. Cognitive deficits in preclinical Alzheimer's disease. *Acta Neurologica Scandinavica*, 2003, 107(S179):29–33.

56 Spaan PEJ, Raaijmakers JGW, Jonker C. Alzheimers's disease versus normal ageing: a review of the efficiency of clinical and experimental memory measures. *Journal of Clinical and Experimental Neuropsychology*, 2003, 25:216–233.

57 Xie J, Brayne C, Matthews FE. Survival times in people with dementia: analysis from population based cohort study with 14 year follow-up. *BMJ*, 2008, 336:258–262.

58 Feltovitch PJ, Barrow HS. Issues of generality in medical problem solving. In: Schmidt HG, de Volder ML, eds. *Tutorials in problem-based learning*. Van Gorcum, Assen, 1884:128–142.

59 de Lepeleire J, Heyrman J. Diagnosis and management of dementia in primary care at an early stage: the need for a new concept and an adapted structure. *Theoretical Medicine and Bioethics*, 1999, 20:215–228.

60 de Lepeleire J, Heyrman J, Buntinx F. The early diagnosis of dementia: triggers, early signs and luxating events. *Family Practice*, 1998, 15:431–436.

61 de Lepeleire J et al. How do general practitioners diagnose dementia. *Family Practice*, 1994, 11:148–152.

62 Downs M, Bowers B. Caring for people with dementia. *BMJ*, 2008, 336:225–226.

63 Antonelli Incalzi R et al. Unrecognised dementia; sociodemographic correlates. *Aging (Milano)*, 1992, 4:327–332.

64 Banerjee S et al. Improving the quality of care for mild to moderate dementia; an evaluation of the Croydon Memory Service Model. *International Journal of Geriatric Psychiatry*, 2007, 22:782–788.

65 Maeck L, Haak S, Knoblauch A, Stoppe G. Early diagnosis of dementia in primary care: a representative eight year follow-up study in Lower Saxony, Germany. *International Journal of Geriatric Psychiatry*, 2007, 22:23–31.

66 Keady J, Nolan M, Gilliard J. Listen to the voices of experience. *Journal of Dementia Care*, 1995, 3:15–17.

67 Cheston R, Jones K, Gilliard J. Group psychotherapy and people with dementia. *Aging and Mental Health*, 2003, 7:452–461.

68 Cheston R, Jones K, Gilliard J. Remembering and forgetting: group with people who have dementia. In: Adams T, Manthorpe J, eds. *Dementia care*. London, Arnold, 2003:124–149.

69 Pinner G, Bouman WP. What should we tell people about dementia? *Advances in Psychiatric Treatment*, 2003, 9:335–341.

70 Cheston R, Jones K. A place to work it all out together. *Journal of Dementia Care*, 2000, 8:22–24.

71 de Lepeleire J, Buntinx F, Aertgeerts B. Disclosing the diagnosis of dementia: the performance of Flemish general practitioners. *International Psychogeriatrics*, 2004, 16:421–428.

72 Arber A, Gallagher A. Breaking bad news revisited: the push for negotiated disclosure and changing practice implications. *International Journal of Palliative Nursing*, 2003, 9:166–172.

73 Clare, L. Managing threats to self: awareness in early stage Alzheimer's disease. *Social Science and Medicine*, 2003, 57:1017–1029.

74 Kerr D, Wilkinson H. *The know: implementation good practice – information and tools for anyone supporting people with a learning disability and dementia*. York, Joseph Rowntree Foundation, 2005.

75 Adams WL et al. Physicians' perspectives on caring for cognitively impaired elders. *The Gerontologist*, 2005, 45:231–239.

76 Lavoie JP et al. Understanding the outcomes of a psycho-educationaal group intervention for caregivers of persons with dementia living at home: a process evaluation. *Aging and Mental Health*, 2005, 9:25–34.

77 Schneider J et al. Eurocare: a cross-national study of co-resident spouse caters for people with Alzheimer's disease: I – factors associated with carer burden. *International Journal of Geriatric Psychiatry*, 1999, 14:651–661.

78 Adamson J. Awareness and understanding of dementia in African/Caribbean and South Asian families. *Health and Social Care in the Community*, 2001, 6:391–396.

79 Bowes A, Wilkinson H. We didn't know it would get that bad: South Asian experiences of dementia and the service response. *Health and Social Care in the Community*, 2003, 11:387–396.

80 Toseland R et al. Predictors of health and human services use by persons with dementia and their family caregivers. *Social Science and Medicine*, 2002, 55:1255–1266.

81 Brodaty H, Thompson C, Fine M. Why caregivers of people with dementia and memory loss don't use services. *International Journal of Geriatric Psychiatry*, 2005, 20:537–546.

82 Grasel E. When home care ends – changes in the physical health of informal caregivers caring for dementia patients: a longitudinal study. *Journal of the American Geriatric Society*, 2002, 50:843–849.

83 Bridges-Webb C. Dementia care in general practice. What can the BEACH survey tell us? *Australian Family Physician*, 2002, 31:381–383.

84 Schultz R et al. Dementia caregiver intervention research: in search of clinical significance. *Gerontologist*, 2002, 42:589–602.

85 Bertrand R, Fredman L, Saczinski J. Are all caregivers created equal? Stress in caregivers to adults with and without dementia. *Journal of Ageing and Health*, 2006, 18:534–551.

86 Zanetti O et al. Depressive symptoms of Alzheimers caregivers are mainly due to personal rather than patient factors. *International Journal of Geriatric Psychology*, 1998, 13:358–367.

87 Sorensen S, Pinquart M, Duberstein P. How effective are interventions with caregivers? An updated meta-analysis. *Gerontologist*, 2002, 42:356–372.

88 Gitlin L et al. Effects of multicomponent interventions on caregiver burden and depression: the REACH multisite initiative at 6 month follow-up. *Psychology and Ageing*, 2003, 18:361–374.

89 Bruce D et al. Communication problems between dementia carers and general practitioners: effect on access to community services. *Medical Journal of Australia*, 2002, 177:186–188.

90 Molsa PK, Marttila RJ, Rinne UK. Long-term survival and predictors of mortality in Alzheimer's disease and multi-infarct dementia. *Acta Neurologica Scandinavica*, 1995, 91:159–164.

91 Fitzpatrick AL et al. Survival following dementia onset: Alzheimer's disease and vascular dementia. *Journal of Neurological Science*, 2005, 229–230:43–49.

92   Gambassi G et al. Predictors of mortality in patients with Alzheimer's disease living in nursing homes. *Journal of Neurology, Neurosurgery and Psychiatry*, 1999, 67:59–65.

93   Larson EB et al. Survival after initial diagnosis of Alzheimer's disease. *Annals of Internal Medicine*, 2004, 140:501–509.

94   Moroney JT et al. Dementia after stroke increases the risk of long-term stroke recurrence. *Neurology*, 1997, 48:1317–1325.

95   Schubert CC et al. Comorbidity profile of dementia patients in primary care: are they sicker? *Journal of the American Geriatric Society*, 2006, 54:104–109.

96   Zekry D et al. Demented versus non-demented very old inpatients: the same comorbidities but poorer functional and nutritional status. *Age and Ageing*, 2008, 37:83–89.

97   Fu C et al. Comorbidity in dementia. *Archives of Pathology and Laboratory Medicine*, 2004, 128:32–38.

98   Sloan FA et al. The effect of dementia on outcomes and process of care for Medicare beneficiaries admitted with acute myocardial infarction. *Journal of the American Geriatric Society*, 2004, 52:173–181.

99   Moroney JT et al. Treatment for the secondary prevention of stroke in older patients: the influence of dementia status. *Journal of the American Geriatric Society*, 1999, 47:824–829.

100   Gurwitz JH et al. Atrial fibrillation and stroke prevention with warfarin in the long-term care setting. *Archives of Internal Medicine*, 1997, 157:978–984.

101   Ritchie K et al. Designing prevention programmes to reduce incidence of dementia: prospective cohort study of modifiable risk factors. *BMJ*, 2010; 341:c3885.

102   Tan ZS et al. Physical activity and the risk of dementia: the Framingham Study. Abstract 01-01-03. In: *Alzheimer's Association International Conference on Alzheimer's Disease*, New Orleans, 15 July 2010.

103   Wengreen H. DASH diet adherence scores and cognitive decline and dementia among aging men and women: Cache County study of Memory Health and Aging. In: *Alzheimer's Association International Conference on Alzheimer's Disease*, Vienna, 14 July 2009.

104   Geda. Agitation, depression, apathy predictors of progression from MCI to dementia. Abstract 01-05-05. In: *Alzheimer's Association International Conference on Alzheimer's Disease*, Honolulu, 11 July 2010.

105   Petersen RC et al. Vitamin E and donepezil for the treatment of mild cognitive impairment. *New England Journal of Medicine*, 2005, 352:2379–2388.

106   Schachter AS, Davis KL. Alzheimer's disease. *Dialogues in Clinical Neuroscience*, 2000, 2:91–100.

107   Burns A, O'Brien J. Clinical practice with anti-dementia drugs: a consensus statement from British Association for Psychopharmacology. *Journal of Psychopharmacology*, 2006, 20(6):732–755.

108   Cummings JL. Managing psychosis in patients with Parkinson's disease. *New England Journal of Medicine*, 1999, 340:801–803.

109   Tariot PN et al. Memantine treatment in patients with moderate to severe Alzheimer disease already receiving donepezil: a randomized controlled trial. *JAMA*, 2004, 291:317–324.

110   Schwartz LM, Woloshin S. How the FDA forgot the evidence: the case of donepezil 23 mg. *BMJ*, 2012, 344:e1086.

111   Snowdon DA et al. Brain infarction and the clinical expression of Alzheimer disease. The Nun Study. *JAMA*, 1997, 277:813–817.

112   Bowler JV et al. Fallacies in the pathological confirmation of the diagnosis of Alzheimer's disease. *Journal of Neurology, Neurosurgery and Psychiatry*, 1998, 64:18–24.

113   Holmes C et al. Validity of current clinical criteria for Alzheimer's disease, vascular dementia and dementia with Lewy bodies. *British Journal of Psychiatry*, 1999, 174:45–50.

114   Lim A, Tsuang D, Kukull W. Clinico-neuropathological correlation of Alzheimer's disease in a community-based case series. *Journal of the American Geriatric Society*, 1999, 47:564–569.

115   Neuropathology Group of the Medical Research Council Cognitive Function and Ageing Study (MRC CFAS). Pathological correlates of late-onset dementia in a multicentre, community-based population in England and Wales. *The Lancet*, 2001, 357:169–175.

116   Hachinski VC, Bowler JV. Vascular dementia. *Neurology*, 1993, 43:2159–2160.

117   Erkinjuntti T et al. Efficacy of galantamine in probable vascular dementia and Alzheimer's disease combined with cerebrovascular disease: a randomised trial. *The Lancet*, 2002; 359: 1283–1290.

118 Black S et al. and the Donepezil 307 Vascular Dementia Study Group. Efficacy and tolerability of donepezil in vascular dementia: positive results of a 24-week, multicenter, international, randomized, placebo-controlled clinical trial. *Stroke*, 2003, 34:2323–2330.

119 Bowler JV. Acetylcholinesterase inhibitors for vascular dementia and Alzheimer's disease combined with cerebrovascular disease. *Stroke*, 2003, 34:584–586.

120 Wilkinson D et al. and the Donepezil 308 Study Group. Donepezil in vascular dementia. *Neurology*, 2003, 61:479–486.

121 Winblad B, Poritis N. Memantine in severe dementia: results of the 9M-Best Study (benefit and efficacy in severely demented patients during treatment with memantine). *International Journal of Geriatric Psychiatry*, 1999, 14:135–146.

122 Orgogozo JM et al. Efficacy and safety of memantine in patients with mild to moderate vascular dementia: a randomized, placebo-controlled trial (MMM 300). *Stroke*, 2002, 33:1834–1839.

123 Wilcock G, Mobius HJ, Stoffler A. A double-blind, placebo-controlled multicentre study of memantine in mild to moderate vascular dementia (MMM500). *International Clinical Psychopharmacology*, 2002, 17:297–305.

124 Areosa SA, Sherriff F. Memantine for dementia. *Cochrane Database of Systematic Reviews*, 2003, (3):CD003154.

125 Cummings JL et al. Behavioral effects of memantine in Alzheimer disease patients receiving donepezil treatment. *Neurology*, 2006, 67:57–63.

126 Kao AW et al. Cognitive and neuropsychiatric profile of the synucleinopathies: Parkinson disease, dementia with Lewy bodies, and multiple system atrophy. *Alzheimer Disease and Associated Disorders*, 2009, 23:365–370.

127 Emre M et al. Rivastigmine for dementia associated with Parkinson's disease. *New England Journal of Medicine*, 2004, 351:2509–2519.

128 McKeith IG et al., for the Consortium on DLB. Dementia with Lewy bodies: diagnosis and management: third report of the DLB Consortium. *Neurology*, 2005, 65:1863–1872.

129 Thomas AJ et al. A comparison of the efficacy of donepezil in Parkinson's disease with dementia and dementia with Lewy bodies. *International Journal of Geriatric Psychiatry*, 2005, 20:938–944.

130 Emre M et al. Memantine for patients with Parkinson's disease dementia or dementia with Lewy bodies: a randomised, double-blind, placebo-controlled trial. *The Lancet Neurology*, 2010, 9:969–977.

131 Aarsland D et al. Memantine in patients with Parkinson's disease dementia or dementia with Lewy bodies: a double-blind, placebo-controlled, multicentre trial. *The Lancet Neurology*, 2009, 8:613–618.

132 McKeith I et al. Efficacy of rivastigmine in dementia with Lewy bodies: a randomised, double-blind, placebo-controlled international study. *The Lancet*, 2000, 356:2031–2036.

133 Molloy S et al. The role of levodopa in the management of dementia with Lewy bodies. *Journal of Neurology, Neurosurgery and Psychiatry*, 2005, 76(9):1200–1203.

134 Lyketsos CG. Neuropsychiatric symptoms (behavioural and psychological symptoms of dementia) and the development of dementia treatments. *International Psychogeriatrics*, 2007, 19:409–420.

135 Ballard CG et al. Management of agitation and aggression associated with Alzheimer disease. *Nature Reviews Neurology* 2009, 5:245–255.

136 *Donepezil, galantamine, rivastigmine and memantine for the treatment of Alzheimer's disease.* London, National Institute for Health and Clinical Excellence, 2011 (TA217).

137 Devanand DP et al. The course of psychopathologic features in mild to moderate Alzheimer's disease. *Archives of General Psychiatry*, 1997, 54:257–263.

138 Harwood D et al. Depressive symptoms in Alzheimer's disease: an examination among community-dwelling Cuban American patients. *American Journal of Geriatric Pychiatry*, 2000, 8:84–91.

139 Bains J, Birks JS, Dening TR. The efficacy of antidepressants in the treatment of depression in dementia. *Cochrane Database of Systematic Reviews*, 2002, (4):CD003944.

140 Hauser WA et al. Seizures and myoclonus in patient's with Alzheimer's disease. *Neurology*, 1986, 36:1226–1230.

141 Hesdorffer DC et al. Dementia and adult onset unprovoked seizures. *Neurology*, 1996, 46:727–730.

142 Mendez M, Lim G. Seizures in elderly patients with dementia: epidemiology and management. *Drugs and Aging*, 2003, 20:791–803.

143 Amatniek JC et al. Incidence and predictors of seizures in patients with Alzheimer's disease. *Epilepsia*, 2006, 47:867–872.

144 Jenssen S, Schere D. Treatment and management of epilepsy in the elderly demented patient. *American Journal of Alzheimer's Disease and Other Dementias*, 2010, 25:18–26.

145 Livingston G et al., and the Old Age Task Force of the World Federation of Biological Psychiatry. Systematic review of psychological approaches to the management of neuropsychiatric symptoms of dementia. *American Journal of Psychiatry*, 2005, 162:1996–2021.

146 Cohen-Mansfield J, Libin A, Marx MS. Non-pharmacological teatment of agitation: a controlled trial of systematic individualised intervention. *The Journals of Gerontology Series A Biological Sciences Medical Sciences*, 2007, 62:908–916.

147 Ballard CG et al. Aromatherapy as a safe and effective treatment for the management of agitation in severe dementia: the results of a double-blind placebo-controlled trial with Melissa. *Journal of Clinical Psychiatry*, 2002, 63:553–558.

148 Akhondzadeh S et al. *Melissa officinalis* extract in the treatment of patients with mild to moderate Alzheimer's disease: a double-blind, placebo-controlled randomized trial. *Journal of Neurology, Neurosurgery and Psychiatry*, 2003, 74:863–866.

149 Lin PW et al. Efficacy of aromatherapy (*Lavandula angustifolia*) as an intervention for agitation in dementia: a cross-over randomised trial. *International Journal of Geriatric Psychiatry*, 2007, 22:405–410.

150 Thorpe L et al. Bright light therapy for demented nursing home patients with behavioral disturbance. *American Journal of Alzheimer's Disease and Other Dementias*, 2000, 15:18–26.

151 Dowling GA et al. Melatonin and bright-light treatment for rest-activity disruption in institutionalized patients with Alzheimer's disease. *Journal of the American Geriatrics Society*, 2008, 56:239–246.

152 Hesebo et al. Efficacy of treating pain to reduce behavioural disturbances in residents of nursing homes with dementia: cluster randomised clinical trial, *BMJ*, 2011, 343:d4065.

153 Lynn J. Serving patients who may die soon and their families: the role of hospice and other services. *JAMA*, 2001, 285:925–932.

154 Morrison RS, Siu AL. Survival in end-stage dementia following acute illness. *JAMA*, 2000, 284:47–52.

155 Katona C et al. World Psychiatric Association section of old age psychiatry consensus statement on ethics and capacity in older people with mental disorders. *International Journal of Geriatric Psychiatry*, 2009, 24:1319–1324.

156 Boustani M et al. Can primary care meet the biopsychosocial needs of older adults with dementia? *Journal of General Internal Medicine*, 2007, 22:1625–1627.

157 Cooper S. A high prevalence of dementia amongst people with learning disabilities not attributed to Down's syndrome. *Psychological Medicine*, 1997, 27:609–616.

158 Prasher VP. Age specific prevalence, thyroid dysfunction and depressive symptomatology in adults with Down's syndrome and dementia. *International Journal of Geriatric Psychiatry*, 1995, 10:25–31.

159 RNIB. *Sight problems. Changing the way we think about blindness.* London, RNIB, 2009 (http://www.rnib.org.uk/livingwithsightloss/Documents/sight_problems_guide.pdf, accessed 21 January 2012).

160 Alzheimer's Society. *Dementia and sight loss interest group* (http://forum.alzheimers.org.uk/showthread.php?17232-Dementia-and-sight-loss-new-interest-group, accessed 22 December 2011).

161 Alzheimer Scotland. *Dementia and deafness: what you need to know* (www.alzscot.org/pages/info/deafness.htm, accessed 22 December 2011).

Part IX

Physical health and mental illness

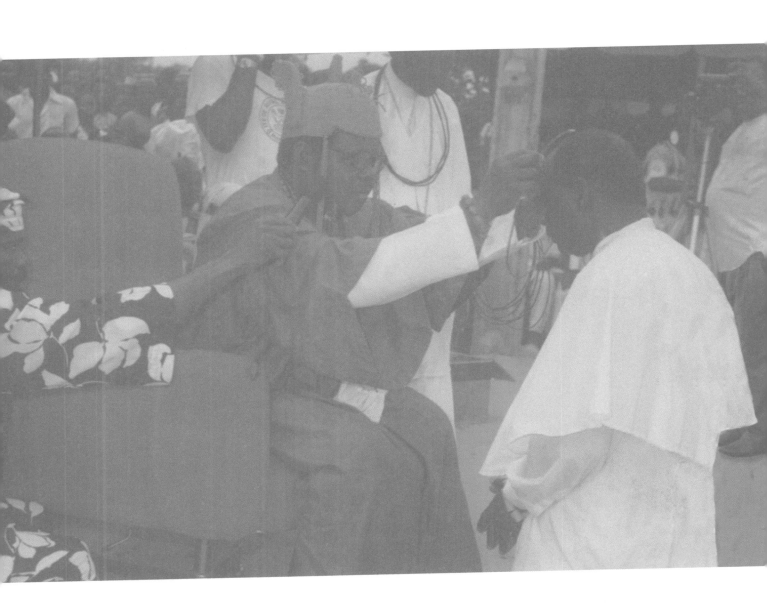

31 Mental disorders due to physical illness at the interface: practical considerations

Sherry Katz-Bearnot, Olatunji F Aina, Karinn Glover, Francis Ibe Ojini, Janna Gordon-Eliot

Key messages

- Physical illnesses may present as mental illnesses. Patients with new onset of psychiatric symptoms should be evaluated for medical problems.
- Endocrinological derangements are particularly likely to present with psychiatric symptoms.
- Psychiatric morbidity complicates the treatment of medical illness.
- Delirium is underrecognized as a physiological derangement presenting as a psychiatric symptom. The treatment of delirium requires correction of the underlying medical problem.
- Alcohol withdrawal is also underrecognized in the medical setting. The treatment of this dangerous disorder is complicated by comorbid medical conditions, organ failure and medication interactions.

Introduction

Primary health care (PHC) is essential to health-care services worldwide. It is defined as a system of health care based on practical, scientifically sound, and socially acceptable methods, made universally accessible to individuals and families at affordable costs. PHC includes preventive, curative and rehabilitative services.[1]

The 2008 WHO monograph *Primary health care, now more than ever* reviews the need for primary health care worldwide.[2] The report emphasizes the need for integration of mental health services into primary care services in order for patients to receive comprehensive and individualized care.

Patients with affective, cognitive, and behavioural symptoms present themselves, or are brought by their families, to the attention of the medical system. They are seen in a variety of settings with a wide range of available resources, staffed by clinicians with many different types of training. In all cases, the presenting complaint, whether manifestly physical or behavioural, is the "entry ticket" to the medical system. The majority of this monograph is focused on psychiatric illness and psychosocial problems presenting to the primary care clinician, which may present as physical illness, psychiatric illness or a combination of the two.[2] In high-resource settings, where primary and secondary care services are available at district general hospitals, psychiatric consultation-liaison services may also exist. In low-resource settings, and where district general hospital services do not exist, primary care clinicians must be prepared to evaluate these symptoms and plan appropriate treatments. Wherever the patient initially presents, it is essential to make a full physical and psychological assessment.

This chapter aims to educate all first contact physicians about affective, cognitive and behavioural symptoms that may be mistaken for psychiatric illness, but are, in fact, psychiatric manifestations of physical illness. Prompt recognition of such syndromes can be life saving.

We hope to increase awareness of mental illness in the context of medical illness and provide practical guidelines for the diagnosis and treatment of a selection of commonly encountered clinical syndromes, symptoms and illnesses commonly encountered in primary care. The chapter covers a range of disorders with neuropsychiatric presentations, including infectious diseases (including acquired immunodeficiency syndrome (AIDS)-related neuropsychiatric conditions), neurological disorders (including delirium and pain syndromes), endocrinological disorders (including thyroid diseases, diabetes and other endocrinopathies) and alcohol use and withdrawal disorders in the medically ill, as well as including a short discussion of the differential diagnosis of fatigue. It is not an encyclopaedic contribution; there are several excellent textbooks devoted to this topic providing more complete coverage of the field of consultation-liaison psychiatry and psychosomatic medicine. These are listed in the "Further reading" section at the end of the chapter. We have chosen a small number of common syndromes that may be diagnosed and treated in high- and low-resource settings, including district general hospitals, medical care homes, rural health stations or nurse-led clinics.

Mental disorders at the interface: epidemiology

Epidemiological studies have shown varying prevalence figures for psychiatric morbidities presenting in primary care. The WHO collaborative studies in the early 1980s showed that 17.7% of patients attending rural primary care clinics in several low-income countries had treatable psychological problems.[3] In the absence of adequate specialist services, the de facto mental health system is the primary care system.

De Girolamo and Bassi,[4] reviewing epidemiological surveys of psychiatric disorders in the community and in primary care, noted that few low-income countries have been involved in such surveys. In such countries, particularly in Africa, "functional" somatic symptoms appear to be overrepresented in primary care patients. Furthermore, certain somatic symptoms seem to have a cultural specificity. For example, complaints of crawling sensations or feelings of internal heat are more common in Africa than elsewhere.

In a study of primary care clinic attendees by Berardi et al.,[5] the estimated prevalence of *International Classification of Diseases* (ICD)-9 psychiatric disorders and subthreshold disorders was 12.4% and 18.0% respectively. The three most common psychiatric disorders were generalized anxiety, major depression and neurasthenia.

In more recent studies, 30% of primary care patients were shown to meet DSM-IV-TR diagnostic criteria for psychiatric disorders,[6] and two-thirds of patients with psychiatric illness were seen in primary care facilities. In epidemiological studies of medium- and high-income countries, the most common psychiatric syndromes seen in primary care facilities continue to be depression, anxiety, alcohol abuse and impaired cognitive functioning.

According to a report by the Lancet Global Mental Health Group,[7] many physical illnesses increase the risk of mental disorders. Such comorbidities complicate help-seeking behaviour on the part of the patient, making it difficult to assign an accurate diagnosis and select the best available treatment.

In addition, psychiatric comorbidity with medical illness may aggravate the course of medical illness (e.g. by interfering with compliance), causing increased distress and increasing costs. "Circular comorbidity", the phenomenon of medical morbidity increasing psychiatric morbidity and psychiatric morbidity further increasing medical comorbidity, is discussed in greater detail below.

It is more difficult to find epidemiological data about the prevalence of medical illnesses presenting as psychiatric disorders, and the attendant increase in morbidity, which is the particular focus of this chapter. For example, anxiety has been reported in 12–79% of patients who are ultimately diagnosed with Cushing's disease. Such a wide range in the reported incidence data is unhelpful. When available, such data will be addressed in the section for each disorder.

Diagnosis of mental disorders due to physical illness at the interface

The best tool for diagnosis of mental disorders due to physical illness is an informed and attuned clinician with enough time to talk to the patient.

The ideal is a detailed clinical history, as well as thorough physical and mental status examinations. In recognition that actual work conditions vary from the ideal, much interest has developed in finding screening instruments for psychiatric disorders in primary care. Studies have shown that the use of screening tools increases detection of mental disorders by 47%.[8]

Screening tests may be administered by clinicians or completed by patients themselves. Self-reports are more efficient, saving clinicians' time, but are only practical if the patient is able to read and fill out the form, and paper and writing implements are available. Examples of screening instruments relevant to the conditions discussed here are mentioned in the text. A detailed discussion of screening tools appears elsewhere in this book.

In settings where consultation-liaison psychiatric services are available, a summary of the diagnosis, treatment and recommendations for follow-up care should routinely be sent to the primary care clinician to ensure continuity of care.

Selected physical illnesses and comorbid mental disorders at the interface

This section describes a range of physical health problems that may present with psychological symptoms, and mental health problems that may present as a physical health problem to a physician, and brings together a range of conditions covered in other chapters of this book.

Endocrine and metabolic disorders

Endocrine and metabolic disorders have numerous psychiatric sequelae, while psychiatric illness and some psychiatric treatments can, in turn, negatively affect endocrine and metabolic homeostasis. We will discuss the interrelationship between such medical conditions and a range of psychiatric symptoms and disorders. Guidelines for the general practitioner (GP) managing psychiatric issues in the primary care setting and at the interface will be reviewed. Table 31.1 presents the information in summary form.

Diabetes

An increased prevalence of several psychiatric disorders has consistently been found in individuals with diabetes. Depression is up to three times more common in these patients (both type 1 and type 2) than in the general population, and individuals with depression may be at increased risk of developing diabetes. Depressed patients with diabetes have higher rates of poor glucose control (higher haemoglobin A_{1c} (HbA_{1c})) and diabetic complications, including nephropathy, retinopathy and cardiovascular disease. They also have higher mortality rates. Ludman et al. found that depressive symptoms better predicted the severity of diabetic morbidity than did the patient's hemoglobin A_{1c} values or the actual number of diabetes complications.[9]

The relationship between diabetes and depression is bidirectional and may result from an interaction of biological and behavioural changes. It is possible that diabetes causes biological alterations (via inflammatory changes and neurobiological mechanisms) that contribute to the development of depression. The poorer the disease control, the higher the risk for depression and the more severe the depressive symptoms. Some have hypothesized that microvascular changes from diabetes (notably in cerebral white matter) may contribute to depressive disorders.

The psychological burden of diabetes symptoms and the psychosocial effects of living with chronic illness can both cause and perpetuate depression. Depression itself may predispose – through poor self-care, unhealthy lifestyle choices and inadequate utilization of medical care and social support – to the development, or worsening, of diabetes. One could hypothesize a relationship in which depression predisposes to poorer diabetes outcome, which, in turn, exacerbates the depression.

It has been consistently found that individuals with diabetes who report more stress in their lives have poorer glycaemic control. Stress appears to affect health outcome through alterations in adrenergic and other neurohormonal processes that impact glucose regulation, as well as through an increase in negative behaviours (dietary, exercise, etc.) and impaired self-maintenance.

There is evidence that reduction in depressive symptoms, through treatment with antidepressant medication or cognitive-behavioural therapy (CBT) may be associated with improvements in metabolic parameters, such as HbA_{1c} values.

Physicians should suspect depression in patients with impaired adherence to treatment or poor glycaemic control. The evidence would indicate that identification and treatment of depression might enhance health outcomes, while efforts to improve glycaemic control and limit the complications of diabetes may have a positive impact on mood and overall well-being.

Individuals with schizophrenia and bipolar disorder may have up to a three-fold increased risk of diabetes (largely type 2 diabetes) compared to the general population. It is thought that this effect is modulated predominantly by the higher rates of obesity in these patient groups. The use of antipsychotic agents is associated with significant metabolic consequences, including dyslipidaemia, obesity and insulin resistance. The elevated rates of diabetes in individuals taking antipsychotic medications appear to be modulated by both weight gain and the agents' direct effects on insulin regulation. Other negative behaviours common in patients with chronic mental illness, such as tobacco use and inactivity, may also contribute to the development of diabetes.

Eating disorders may predispose to, or develop as a consequence of, diabetes; disordered eating has a negative impact on overall outcome for individuals with diabetes. Binge-eating disorders may result in, or exacerbate, type 2 diabetes, through obesity and high carbohydrate intake. In cultures with an emphasis on thinness and a preoccupation with media images, the heightened focus on eating, food choices and body image may predispose individuals with diabetes to eating disorders. Adolescent girls and young women with type 1 diabetes are more likely to have disturbed eating behaviours compared to others in their age group. This population is also more susceptible to eating disorder-related behaviours, such as insulin restriction for weight loss. Polonsky et al. found that 40% of women with diabetes aged between 15 and 30 years reported such behaviours.[10] In patients with diabetes, evidence of poor glycaemic control (e.g. end-organ damage, elevated HbA_{1c}) may be an early indication of disordered eating behaviour. In working with patients for whom there is such concern (including concern about insulin restriction), useful questions for the patients might include: "Do you ever change your insulin dose or skip insulin doses to influence your weight?" and "How often do you take less insulin than prescribed?"[11]

Thyroid disorders

The vast majority of patients with hypothyroidism have depressive symptoms; in fact depression may be one of the earliest manifestations of hypothyroidism. Hypothyroidism can be associated with low energy, anxiety and cognitive dysfunction, symptoms that can also be found in depression. Psychotic symptoms may develop in severe hypothyroidism (myxoedema madness). Patients with bipolar disorder are also more likely to have thyroid abnormalities, with the rapid-cycling subtype being highly correlated with hypothyroidism. Lithium administration for bipolar disorder can itself cause hypothyroidism, and thyroid function tests should be part of routine health screening in patients taking lithium.

Hyperthyroidism, most commonly due to Graves' disease, is associated with a variety of psychiatric symptoms, including anxiety, irritability, depression, mania, psychosis and cognitive impairment. The presentation may vary according to age, with younger patients exhibiting agitation, and older individuals appearing withdrawn (known as "apathetic hyperthyroidism").

Hashimoto's encephalopathy is a rare syndrome associated with high antithyroid antibody concentrations, and may present with a variety of neuropsychiatric manifestations including seizures, psychosis and delirium.

Resolution of psychiatric symptoms due to thyroid dysfunction requires, first and foremost, reversal of the underlying thyroid dysfunction and restoration of the euthyroid state. Pharmacologic treatment targeting specific symptoms (e.g. antidepressants for depression, mood stabilizers for mania, antipsychotic agents for psychosis or delirium) may also be needed in the acute management, though these treatments will not be adequate for remission of the symptoms if the thyroid disorder is not adequately addressed.

Treatment with exogenous steroids, disorders of the adrenal glands and the hypothalamic-pituitary-adrenal axis

Elevated levels of cortisol and other glucocorticoids, as found in Cushing's syndrome, can cause a myriad of psychiatric symptoms and syndromes. The leading cause of Cushing's syndrome is exogenous corticosteroid administration, a mainstay of treatment for inflammatory and autoimmune illnesses. Exogenous steroids may produce insomnia, mood changes (irritability, depressed mood or mania), psychosis and cognitive changes (deficits in learning and memory). They are the leading cause of secondary mania in medical patients. Anxiety symptoms are present in most cases of Cushing's syndrome. Cognitive impairment in Cushing's syndrome probably develops as a consequence of modulation of glucocorticoid receptors in the neocortex and hippocampus. The effects appear to be dose and duration related, with acute pulse-dosing of steroids being associated with manic symptoms and low-dose chronic use more commonly causing a depressive syndrome.

Reversal of the underlying hypercortisolism is necessary for the treatment of psychiatric syndromes secondary to Cushing's syndrome. There is some evidence that cognitive symptoms emerging during the course of Cushing's disease may persist indefinitely, even after the hypercortisolaemia is fully treated.

Adrenal insufficiency, due to Addison's disease or corticotropin deficiency, can also cause a number of psychiatric disturbances, such as apathy, withdrawal and general mental impoverishment. Frank psychosis may be a presenting symptom during Addisonian crisis.

Dysfunction of the hypothalamopituitary-adrenal (HPA) axis has been frequently cited in the pathophysiology of psychiatric disorders. Hypercortisolism can be considered a biological marker in depression, and it is suspected that HPA axis dysregulation and the development of depression are causally related. Depressed patients have been found to have elevated plasma levels of cortisol and adrenocorticotropic hormone (ACTH), with disruption of the characteristic diurnal pattern of secretion. Subjects with depression demonstrate an abnormal (non-suppressed) cortisol response to the dexamethasone-suppression test. It is suspected that dysfunctional signalling by mineralocorticoid and glucocorticoid receptors leads to an impaired negative feedback loop. Tests that evaluate diurnal secretion or suppressability, however, have not achieved clinical utility as screening tests for depression. Their use remains limited by concerns about false positives, false negatives and cost.

Gonadal and reproductive disorders

Psychiatric symptoms may develop in the context of gonadal dysfunction. Testosterone deficiency in men may present as a result of hypothalamic, pituitary or gonadal dysfunction. Medications such as methadone, treatments such as chemotherapy, and medical conditions, including hepatitis C and human immunodeficiency virus (HIV), may predispose to low-testosterone states. Hypogonadism in men has been associated with changes in mood and cognition, as well as an increased risk of depression. The role of testosterone supplementation in hypogonadal men for mood augmentation remains controversial. The expected benefits of treatment must be weighed against the potential risks of supplementation, including prostate disorders, blood hyperviscosity, liver toxicity and cardiovascular dysfunction.

In women, fluctuations in mood symptoms across the menstrual cycle, with significant worsening of depressive and anxiety symptoms during the luteal phase and associated impaired functioning, characterize premenstrual syndrome (PMS) and its more severe form, premenstrual dysphoric disorder (PMDD). Women who report premenstrual mood symptoms also appear to be more susceptible to psychiatric symptoms at other times of hormonal shifts, such as during or after pregnancy and in the perimenopausal period. For a diagnosis of PMDD to be made, the woman must report a persistent pattern (most cycles for at least one year) of five or more specified mood symptoms during the last week of the luteal phase, with improvement at the onset of the follicular phase, and absence of these symptoms during the week postmenses. These symptoms must also cause marked impairment in functioning or relationships.[7] To aid in diagnosis, the patient should be asked to perform prospective daily rating of mood across the menstrual cycle. A full psychiatric evaluation, to rule out other contributing psychiatric conditions, is another important element of the assessment.

Treatment of PMS includes behavioural measures, such as exercise, limiting caffeine and nicotine, and the practice of stress-reduction techniques. Supplementation with B vitamins, as well as calcium carbonate and vitamin D (see later), may also be useful. PMDD can be treated with antidepressants, such as selective serotonin reuptake inhibitors (SSRIs). SSRIs can be useful even when given for a few days from the late luteal phase into the early follicular phase, as well as in continuous dosing across the cycle. The combination of ethinylestradiol and drospirenone (marketed in different formulations as Yasmin®, Yaz® and Beyaz®) has been approved for treatment of PMDD in women wishing to use an oral contraceptive pill for prevention of pregnancy.

Anxiety and depressive disorders are common in women with polycystic ovary syndrome (PCOS). Psychiatric symptoms in this disorder may be related to patients' psychological responses to the physical effects of the disorder (including truncal obesity, hirsutism and infertility), in addition to the direct effects of neuroendocrine abnormalities (e.g. hyperinsulinaemia, increased levels of androgens). Women with PCOS may also have higher rates of bipolar disorder than the general population. Valproate appears to predispose to PCOS, but the association between PCOS and bipolar disorder may be independent of the effect of valproate.

Infertility is influenced by, and has a variety of effects on, psychiatric and psychological functioning. Psychiatric illness – through its modulation of the stress response and hormonal changes, as well as through alteration of behaviour (smoking, alcohol, nutritional and exercise factors) – influences fertility. Infertility, in turn, affects mental health, with up to 50% of women and 15% of men undergoing infertility evaluation or treatment assessing the process as being the most stressful event of their lives. In women with infertility, up to 50% may develop major depressive disorder, and 40% may be diagnosed with an anxiety disorder.[12] A sizable minority, 20% in one study,[13] may experience suicidal thinking. Medications used in infertility treatment may carry a range of psychiatric side-effects. Progesterones (particularly the non-synthetic, plant-derived preparations) may cause depressed mood, insomnia and fatigue. Clomiphene is associated with development of anxiety, insomnia and, rarely, psychosis.

Hormonal treatments used in the management of some cancers have been associated with psychiatric symptoms. Androgen deprivation with gonadotropin-releasing hormone (GnRH) antagonists may cause significant fatigue, as well as decreased libido, in men undergoing treatment for prostate cancer. Anti-oestrogen treatments, including agents such as tamoxifen, can lead to insomnia, irritability and depressive symptoms in some women. Antidepressants may have a role in the treatment of psychiatric side-effects, as well as hot flushes, in women taking tamoxifen.

Importantly, antidepressants that inhibit CYP 2D6 should be avoided in combination with tamoxifen, as they can reduce the effectiveness of tamoxifen (by preventing the conversion of the prodrug to the active form of the pharmaceutical) and have been connected to cases of cancer recurrence. The strongest 2D6 inhibitors, paroxetine, fluoxetine, duloxetine and bupropion, should be avoided in women taking tamoxifen, while the weak 2D6 inhibitor, venlafaxine, is the preferred choice for treating anxiety and depression in women on tamoxifen.

Other endocrinopathies

Phaeochromocytomas (catecholamine-secreting tumours) can produce intermittent anxiety and autonomic symptoms. Patients with these tumours have been misdiagnosed as having panic disorder, various neurological conditions, and substance intoxication or withdrawal.

Hyperprolactinaemia, either a consequence of treatment with antipsychotic medications and serotonin-modulating antidepressants, or the manifestation of a pituitary adenoma, may present with anxiety and depression.

Disorders of the parathyroid gland are associated with psychiatric symptoms through changes in calcium homeostasis. The most common cause of hypoparathyroidism is removal of the parathyroid glands during head and neck surgery (e.g. thyroid surgery). The development of hyperparathyroidism depends upon factors such as surgical technique, anatomical features, and presurgery vitamin D status. Ten per cent of total thyroidectomy patients have initial hypocalcaemia, but this condition becomes persistent in less than half of such patients.[14]

Hypercalcaemia due to hyperparathyroidism (a possible consequence of lithium treatment) can present with personality changes, apathy, anxiety, depressed mood and cognitive changes. Symptoms frequently resolve completely with treatment of the hypercalcaemia.

Several investigators have found a relationship between vitamin D deficiency and depression. Vitamin D metabolism may be involved in the pathophysiology of seasonal affective disorder (SAD). There has also been speculation about a causative role of vitamin D deficiency and calcium dysregulation in PMDD. The literature on vitamin D and mood disorders remains indeterminate, with limitations in the available studies.

Nonetheless, many investigators recommend that individuals with depressive symptoms be encouraged to take 1000–2000 IU of vitamin D daily and to obtain modest sunlight exposure. This recommendation is an example of a low-cost, low-risk intervention in primary care that may carry benefit for both mental and physical health.

Other metabolic disorders

Metabolic derangements of all types can present with a range of psychiatric symptoms and syndromes. Practitioners in the general medical setting should be attentive to signs and symptoms that might indicate negative behaviours or poor self-care, which may be early signs of mental illness. The general principle for treatment of psychiatric symptoms is that the underlying medical disorder should be addressed. This may completely resolve the associated psychiatric syndrome.

Patients with longstanding psychiatric illness who develop new signs of confusion or other cognitive deficits should be suspected of having an underlying medical process. Acute changes in cognition or sensorium are rarely due to a primary psychiatric condition.

Hyponatraemia may cause acute changes in mental status, and may present with confusion, psychosis and irritability. Psychogenic polydipsia should be suspected in hyponatraemic patients with chronic psychotic illnesses or mental retardation. The use of several different psychotropic medications (including mood stabilizers, antidepressants and antipsychotic agents) has been associated with the syndrome of inappropriate antidiuretic hormone secretion (SIADH).

Patients with eating disorders are susceptible to metabolic derangements such as hypokalaemia, which may manifest with fatigue and depressive symptoms. Hypomagnesaemia should also be considered in patients with anorexia nervosa, particularly during the refeeding process.

Patients who drink excessive amounts of alcohol may present with evidence of metabolic derangements and nutritional deficiencies that require immediate attention to preserve brain function. Thiamine deficiency, commonly found in patients who abuse alcohol, may lead to neurological and cognitive dysfunction. Thiamine supplementation is essential in patients suspected of drinking too much and having poor nutrition. Thiamine deficiency may lead to Wernicke's encephalopathy (ataxia, ophthalmoplegia, confusion and memory deficits), which may progress and become irreversible without prompt medical attention. Korsakoff's syndrome (a chronic amnestic and confabulatory disorder, developing as a late consequence of thiamine deficiency in chronic alcohol abusers) is rarely treatable once it has manifested, even with correction of the thiamine deficiency.

Hypomagnesaemia may also be found in patients with alcohol use disorder, and can manifest with anxiety, agitation, and cognitive changes, in addition to physical complications such as neuromuscular irritability, seizures and cardiac arrhythmias.

In older patients, or patients who are suspected of having poor nutrition or self-care, the clinician should have a low threshold for monitoring levels of cobalamin (vitamin B_{12}) and folate (vitamin B_9), especially in the presence of mood or cognitive symptoms. Vitamin B_{12} deficiency can have a range of neuropsychiatric consequences, including mood symptoms, psychosis, obsessive–compulsive symptoms, and cognitive impairment, as well as neurological findings such as posterior column signs. Folate deficiency can be associated with depressed mood. Folate and vitamin B_{12} deficiencies are linked with elevations in homocysteine, a risk factor for dementia. Folate deficiency is more common in individuals with psychiatric illness than in the general population, independent of the higher rate of alcohol disorders in this population. Depression secondary to folate deficiency may not respond well to antidepressant therapy, and appropriate treatment requires normalization of folate levels. Based on the high prevalence of vitamin B_{12} and folate deficiency in the elderly (due to a combination of nutritional and absorption factors), clinicians should consider supplementation in appropriate patients, as the cost is low and the risk of complications is virtually absent.

Table 31.1 Summary of medical illness, psychiatric morbidity, recognition and management for the primary care professional

Condition	Psychiatric presentation and comorbidity	Recognition and evaluation	Aspects of management
Diabetes mellitus	Depression; relationship with diabetes may be bidirectional/circular	May manifest as "poor adherence", changes in sleep or appetite, depressed or anxious mood	• Treating comorbid depression (e.g. antidepressant, CBT) may improve management of diabetes, and vice versa
	Schizophrenia and bipolar disorder (have higher rates of diabetes due to lifestyle factors and psychiatric medications)	Worsening glucose control when psychiatrically destabilized or with changes in psychiatric medications	• Screen for self-care behaviours, medication and dietary adherence • Monitor metabolic profiles • Communication with psychiatrist to optimize psychiatric regimen and minimize metabolic burden
	Eating disorders (restricting, insulin abuse, binge eating); relationship may be bidirectional/circular	Evidence of poor glycaemic control despite reports of good adherence; rapid changes in weight; preoccupation with food, calories, exercise, body shape/weight	• "Do you change your insulin dose to manage your weight?" • Consider food diaries, nutrition consult, referral to mental health provider
Thyroid disorders		Thyroid function studies and antithyroid antibodies	• Correction of thyroid dysfunction necessary to reverse the psychiatric symptoms • Concurrent treatment of psychiatric symptoms may be warranted if severe
Hypothyroidism	Depression, mania (rapid cycling); hypothyroidism may be related to lithium		
Hyperthyroidism	Anxiety, irritability, cognitive impairment, depression, psychosis		
Hashimoto's encephalopathy	Seizures, psychosis, delirium		

Disorder	Clinical features	Comments
Adrenal disorders		• Correction of the underlying adrenal abnormality, or minimize/ pulse exogenous steroids • Psychiatric medications (e.g. antidepressants, antipsychotics) may be warranted if symptoms are severe
Cushing's syndrome	Depression, anxiety, mania, psychosis, cognitive impairment	Evaluate source of the hypercortisolism (exogenous, endogenous)
Adrenal insufficiency	Apathy, withdrawal, psychosis	
Gonadal disorders		
Testosterone deficiency (men)	Depression, apathy, cognitive slowing	May be related to medications (methadone, chemotherapy) or medical conditions (hepatitis C and HIV) • The role of testosterone supplementation is controversial
Premenstrual dysphoric disorder (PMDD)	Persistent pattern (most cycles for ≥1 year) of ≥5 mood symptoms in the last week of the luteal phase • More severe form of PMS, with functional impairment • Women with PMDD may be more susceptible to psychiatric symptoms after pregnancy or perimenopausally	• Prospective daily mood charting may be useful • Exercise, limit caffeine, B vitamin and calcium supplementation; antidepressants, ethinylestradiol/ drospirenone (Yasmin®, Yaz® and Beyaz®)
Polycystic ovary syndrome (PCOS)	Anxiety and depressive disorders are common	Psychiatric symptoms + truncal obesity, hirsutism, infertility, insulin insensitivity • Avoid use of valproate, which may predispose to PCOS • Weight loss, exercise recommended
Other endocrine and metabolic disorders		• Correct the underlying medical cause or metabolic derangement
Phaeochromocytoma	Intermittent anxiety and autonomic symptoms	May be misdiagnosed as panic disorder, substance abuse

continued overleaf

Table 31.1 Summary of medical illness, psychiatric morbidity, recognition and management for the primary care professional – *continued*

Condition	Psychiatric presentation and comorbidity	Recognition and evaluation	Aspects of management
Hyperprolactinaemia	Anxiety and depression	May be a consequence of antipsychotic medications	
Hyperparathyroidism, hypercalcaemia	Apathy, anxiety, depressed mood, personality and cognitive changes	Hyperparathyroidism may result from lithium treatment	
SIADH/hyponatraemia	Confusion, irritability, psychosis	• May be a result of antidepressants, antipsychotics, antiepileptics • Monitor for psychogenic polydipsia	
Thiamine deficiency	Wernicke's encephalopathy (ataxia, ophthalmoplegia, cognitive impairment) Korsakoff's syndrome (amnesia, confabulation)	Suspect thiamine deficiency in alcohol abuse	
Vitamin B_{12} deficiency	Mood symptoms, psychosis, obsessive–compulsive symptoms, cognitive impairment	Suspect in alcohol abuse, elderly, poor nutrition	

Companion to Primary Care Mental Health

Endocrine/metabolic and psychiatric effects of medications

Table 31.2 illustrates the medications used to treat psychiatric disorders that may have negative endocrine and metabolic effects, and Table 31.3 shows the medications used for medical conditions that can lead to psychiatric symptoms and syndromes; these are reviewed next.

Mood stabilizers

Lithium salts, used most commonly in the treatment of bipolar disorder, can cause hypothyroidism and hyperparathyroidism, SIADH, nephrogenic diabetes insipidus and renal dysfunction via the mechanism of interstitial nephropathy or glomerular sclerosis. Long-term use of lithium can lead to irreversible end-stage renal disease in a small proportion of patients (0.2–0.7%).[15] The development of renal dysfunction is related to factors including age, the presence of other medical conditions, and episodes of lithium toxicity. Given the potential for renal disease as a result of lithium treatment, patients should have routine (at least yearly) renal function evaluation and adjustment of lithium to the lowest therapeutically effective dose. For those who develop evidence of renal impairment, use of adjunctive mood-stabilizing agents to allow for lowering or discontinuation of lithium, may be indicated.

Carbamazepine and oxcarbazepine, anticonvulsants used for mood stabilization, have been associated with SIADH in 5–40% of cases.[16] Valproate appears to carry an increased risk of polycystic ovary syndrome as well as decreased sodium.

Antidepressants

Serotonin-modulating antidepressants, such as SSRIs, can cause SIADH, at rates ranging from 0.5% to 32% of cases.[17] SSRIs can also have the effect of unmasking a silent phaeochromocytoma, probably via impaired reuptake of circulating catecholamines.

Recent concerns about long-term treatment with SSRIs have included an increased risk of low bone mineral density (BMD) and fractures, modulated by serotonin receptors on osteoblasts, osteoclasts and osteocytes. The increased rate of fractures may also be mediated by an increased risk of falls in individuals taking SSRIs. In one 5-year prospective study of over 5000 adults over the age of 50 years, the risk of fracture doubled with daily use of SSRIs.[18] Depression itself is associated with an increased risk of low BMD, in part due to depression-related behaviours, such as reduced exercise, dietary deficiencies and unhealthy habits, including smoking. Given these findings, a risk–benefit analysis should be considered in patients remaining on SSRIs long term, who are at risk of osteoporosis or fractures.

Antipsychotic agents

Antipsychotic medications, though life saving in many individuals with chronic psychiatric disorders, carry a range of significant metabolic side-effects, including obesity, glucose dysregulation and dyslipidaemia (affecting lipoproteins and triglycerides). Several of the second-generation (atypical) antipsychotics, including quetiapine, olanzapine and clozapine, are among the worst offenders in terms of weight gain and metabolic side-effects. The atypical agent risperidone has moderate impact on weight and metabolic dysfunction, while some of the first-generation (typical) agents, such as haloperidol, carry less risk. Two newer agents, ziprasidone and aripiprazole, appear to carry a reduced incidence of weight gain and metabolic disorders, and may be preferred in individuals with obesity, diabetes and dyslipidaemia. Close monitoring of metabolic parameters is essential in the management of patients taking antipsychotic medications. Emphasis on health-promoting dietary behaviours and physical activity, as well as efforts to minimize risk by keeping antipsychotic agents at their lowest effective dose and switching to agents with fewer metabolic side-effects, can be useful in decreasing the long-term health risks of chronic antipsychotic treatment. Antipsychotic agents are also associated with hyperprolactinaemia, as well as a small risk of hyponatraemia and SIADH.

The approach to the patient in clinical practice

A host of interrelationships exist between endocrine/metabolic and psychiatric disorders through biological mechanisms, behavioural changes, and treatment effects. The practitioner in the clinical setting should have a low threshold for screening for routine endocrine or metabolic dysfunction in patients presenting with psychiatric symptoms, especially if the symptoms are acute in onset, or do not fit easily into a well-known psychiatric syndrome. A thorough physical examination will reveal signs that help guide the practitioner in formulating a differential diagnosis. A patient presenting with depressed mood and fatigue, dry skin and constipation, for example, should alert the clinician to the possibility of hypothyroidism.

The physician-administered Primary Care Evaluation of Mental Disorders (PRIME-MD),[19] or the patient self-report version, the Patient Health Questionnaire (PHQ),[20] can be utilized in the primary care setting to identify mental disorders and symptoms. Positive results should trigger a response for psychiatric treatment or referral to a mental health-care provider. Tools such as the Problem Areas in Diabetes (PAID) scale, and the Diabetes Quality of Life (DQOL) measure can be particularly useful in screening patients with diabetes for whom psychiatric symptoms are suspected.[11]

Table 31.2 Medical morbidity of common psychotropic medications

Medication	Endocrine/metabolic side-effects
Lithium salts	• Hypothyroidism • Polydipsia • Interstitial nephritis
SSRI antidepressants	• SIADH • ↑ risk of low BMD and fractures • Unmasking of a silent phaeochromocytoma
Carbamazepine/oxcarbazepine	• SIADH
Valproic acid derivatives	• ↑ risk of polycystic ovarian syndrome
Antipsychotic medications	• Weight gain • Impaired glucose tolerance, diabetes • Dyslipidaemia • SIADH

Table 31.3 Psychiatric morbidity of common non-psychotropic medications

Medication	Psychiatric side-effects
Exogenous corticosteroids	• Mood changes (irritability, mania, dysphoria, lability) • Insomnia • Psychosis • Delirium
GNRH agonists	• Fatigue
Anti-oestrogen therapy	• Insomnia • Irritability • Depressive symptoms
Fertility treatments	• Sleep disturbances • Mood changes • Anxiety • Psychosis

Delirium: a medical symptom not a psychiatric illness

Delirium is a clinical syndrome characterized by an acute change in cognition and a disturbance of consciousness. It is a direct physiological consequence of a general medical condition, substance intoxication or withdrawal, use of medication, or a combination of these factors.

Delirium may be the harbinger of impending physiological decompensation. Prompt diagnosis and treatment of the underlying medical problem can therefore be life saving.

Delirium is very common, especially in the elderly. About 10–25% of patients in acute medical and surgical wards develop delirium. Such patients typically have markedly prolonged hospital stays, frequent associated complications, much higher in-hospital mortality rates and higher medical care costs.[21]

Pathogenesis of delirium

Delirium is commonly associated with medical and surgical illness, intoxication and withdrawal states, and central nervous system disease. Almost any severe acute medical or surgical condition, under the right circumstances, may cause delirium. Common causes may be divided into the categories of primary brain disorders (direct causes) and indirect causes, including systemic illness, medications, etc.

Primary brain disorders include head injury, stroke, increased intracranial pressure, central nervous system (CNS) infection, autoimmune disorders (either primary or post-infectious) and epilepsy. Systemic illnesses include metabolic disturbances such as hypo- and hyperglycaemia; infections such as urinary tract infection and pneumonia; endocrine disturbances such as hypo- and hyperthyroidism, hypo- and hyperparathyroidism; rheumatoid or other autoimmune disorders; cardiopulmonary, renal or hepatic failure; and metabolic or electrolyte derangements of any aetiology. Substance intoxication including alcohol and drug abuse, as well as withdrawal from such substances may lead to delirium. Delirium may also be seen with prescription or over-the-counter (OTC) medications, as well as from drug–drug interactions alone or in the presence of decreased organ function from underlying medical illnesses.

The pathophysiology of delirium is poorly understood, but it is likely that multiple mechanisms are involved. Possible mechanisms include cholinergic deficiency or failure of cholinergic transmission (a possible mechanism for delirium in some metabolic abnormalities and delirium caused by drugs); failure of cerebral oxidative metabolism (a possible mechanism for delirium in patients with pulmonary and cardiovascular diseases); and effects of cytokines on cerebral function (a possible mechanism for delirium in CNS and systemic infections).

Delirium can be regarded as a clinical syndrome resulting from the interconnection of several pathological mechanisms. The development of delirium is usually multifactorial and involves the interrelationship between a predisposed patient and exposure to triggering factors. Box 31.1 lists the factors that have been identified as predisposing to delirium and Box 31.2 lists those that independently precipitate delirium. The most important problems are infections, medication toxicity and cardiorespiratory and neurologic disorders.

Clinical features of delirium

The key features of delirium include:

- disturbance of consciousness: defined in the DSM-IV as reduced clarity of awareness of the environment
- inattention: reduced ability to focus, sustain, or shift attention; distractibility; and diminished concentration. Registration of new information is impaired, leading to disorientation and memory deficits
- perceptual disturbances: may include disturbances of the perception of shape (micropsia or macropsia), depersonalization, derealization, illusions and auditory or visual hallucinations
- disorders of sleep and wakefulness: the sleep/wake cycle is almost always disturbed, with marked periods of drowsiness or sleep in the day and insomnia at night.

The symptoms of delirium usually develop over hours to days and patients with delirium show unpredictable fluctuations in symptoms. Symptoms may be intermittent and are often worse at night (referred to clinically as "sundowning").

Three clinical subtypes of delirium have been described: hyperactive, hypoactive and mixed types.

Hyperactive delirium

This manifests with psychomotor hyperactivity and heightened arousal. The patient is disoriented, restless or agitated, may be aggressive, may have visual hallucinations, may repeatedly pull at clothing, and may attempt to get out of bed or to pull out catheters, monitors, or intravenous lines. It is usually easy to recognize hyperactive delirium, although it can occasionally be confused with a psychotic disorder.

Delirium tremens (DTs), an extreme form of alcohol withdrawal, comprises a combination of psychic and autonomic hyperactivity and is a form of hyperactive delirium. It usually manifests within 24–72 h after the last drink, but may be seen as late as 14 days from the last ingestion. Autonomic hyperactivity (tachycardia, hypertension, diaphoresis and even fever) is the earliest physiological manifestation, and may be subtle. Later manifestations are easier to diagnose and more obvious: such patients may be agitated, confused or frankly hallucinating. The hallucinations are frequently visual but may also include tactile (haptic) hallucinations, which are unusual in delirium from other causes but typical of DTs. Treatment of DTs constitute a medical emergency. (For other features of alcohol withdrawal and treatment of withdrawal, see Chapter 25 and the information on alcohol withdrawal later in this chapter.)

Hypoactive delirium

This is the most common presentation but it is (paradoxically) the type most likely to be overlooked or misdiagnosed. The clinical features of delirium are much less obvious than in a patient with hyperactive delirium. The patient is subdued, quietly confused, disoriented and apathetic, and the condition may be mistaken for depression, dementia or medication-induced somnolence. Such patients may appear to be sleeping and tend to be passed over during clinical rounds.

Mixed type

The patient fluctuates between hypoactive and hyperactive delirium.

Differentiating delirium from dementia

This is a common clinical dilemma. There is a strong interrelationship between delirium and dementia. Dementia is a strong risk factor for developing delirium, and delirium is associated with increased risk of developing dementia.

In dementia, the patient is usually alert (no clouding of consciousness) and engages well in conversation (no attention impairment) but is confused and disoriented in time and place. The onset of dementia is insidious and at presentation the illness may have been progressive for months or years. The sleep/wake cycle is usually normal in dementia.

Differentiating delirium from primary psychiatric disorder

An acute onset and fluctuating nature of delirium are key features in distinguishing it from primary psychiatric disorders. Psychotic disorders such as schizophrenia usually have a slow onset and chronic course. The sensorium is usually clear. Hallucinations are usually auditory rather than visual and delusions tend to be systematized, bizarre, and uninfluenced by the environment. Delusions in the delirious patient are usually fleeting and related to environmental stimuli, and may not be remembered. Acute onset of psychiatric symptoms without prior history of psychiatric illness (especially in persons aged 50 years or older), or the presence of medical illness, suggests delirium rather than a primary psychiatric disorder and should prompt a thorough medical work-up.

Making the diagnosis of delirium

The diagnosis of delirium is clinical and requires a high index of suspicion, especially in patients with hypoactive delirium who may manifest subtle signs. Since a detailed history is often difficult or impossible to obtain from a patient with delirium, it is necessary to rely on family members or caregivers for information. It is important to review the patient's past medical history and medications, including their use of alcohol or illicit drugs. Since delirium is a manifestation of a medical illness, physical examination of a patient with delirium should be thorough, paying attention to vital signs as well as a careful search for cardiorespiratory, neurological and infectious disorders.

Once a clinical diagnosis of delirium is established, laboratory studies are helpful in establishing the aetiologic factors. A complete blood count, electrolytes, blood glucose, renal and liver function tests, urinalysis, electrocardiogram, chest X-ray and oxygen saturation are recommended routine in patients with delirium. Additional investigations such as electroencephalography (EEG), lumbar puncture, HIV and syphilis serology, toxicology screen and brain imaging (computerized tomography (CT) or magnetic resonance imaging (MRI)) and other tests may be required, depending on the clinical circumstances.

The clinical diagnosis of delirium can be aided by screening instruments such as the Confusion Assessment Method (CAM). The CAM is recommended for routine use by the American Psychiatric Association[22] and the UK National guidelines.[23] It was designed to allow non-psychiatric clinicians to diagnose delirium quickly and accurately. The CAM diagnostic algorithm is based on four cardinal features of delirium: (1) acute onset and fluctuating course; (2) inattention; (3) disorganized thinking; and (4) altered level of consciousness. A diagnosis of delirium is made when features 1, 2 and either 3 or 4 are present. CAM has been shown to have high sensitivity and specificity in diagnosing delirium, which improves with further clinician training.[24] It should be noted that the CAM is not recommended for use as the sole means for identification of delirium in the clinical setting. Informed clinical assessment, combined with screening measures, is required to avoid missing the diagnosis, especially in hypoactive, subtle and atypical cases.

Management of delirium

Recognizing delirium is important because it is an indication of an underlying medical condition or drug toxicity that should be identified and addressed.

Four key steps in management are: identifying and addressing the underlying causes, maintaining behavioural control, preventing complications, and supporting functional needs.

Identifying and addressing underlying medical conditions

Pharmaceuticals are a common cause of delirium in the elderly. Cardiopulmonary conditions or incipient sepsis should be considered as possible causes. A review of current medications (including OTC medications), particularly psychotropic, narcotic, and anticholinergic medications, is necessary. The possibility of alcohol or sedative intoxication or withdrawal should be considered. Alcohol withdrawal syndrome should be suspected in every unexplained delirium. It may manifest itself when the patient has been hospitalized for some unrelated problem.

A careful history and thorough physical examination followed by some basic laboratory investigations will usually identify other common and readily treatable causes of delirium, such as mild infections (especially urinary tract infections) or dehydration, both of which may cause delirium in the elderly.

Maintaining behavioural control

Agitated psychotic behaviour in patients with delirium that is either hazardous for the patient or interferes with ongoing medical treatment is best managed with high-potency traditional antipsychotic medications such as haloperidol, or second-generation antipsychotics. Haloperidol is preferred because it has no anticholinergic properties, is rarely associated with hypotension or respiratory depression, and can be given orally, intramuscularly or intravenously. The dose of haloperidol depends on the patient's age and the severity of agitation. In most young adults with a mild to moderate degree of agitation, haloperidol can be initiated in a dose of 2–5 mg twice daily, but can be repeated every four hours as needed. Up to 10 mg of haloperidol can be used as starting dose in patients with severe agitation. The corresponding dose in elderly patients with mild to moderate agitation is 0.5–1 mg, and for severe agitation, up to 2 mg. If parenteral administration is used initially, the oral form should be substituted as soon as is practical. In emergency situations, 0.5 mg of haloperidol can be given every 30 minutes to 1 hour until the agitation is controlled.

Limited data suggest that second-generation antipsychotics have similar efficacy to haloperidol, with fewer side-effects than high-dose haloperidol. Reasonable starting dosages for these drugs in patients with delirium are risperidone 0.5 mg twice daily, olanzapine 5 mg daily and quatrain 25 mg twice daily.

Benzodiazepines such as diazepam and lorazepam are the agents of choice in treating alcohol withdrawal delirium. Guidelines for the treatment of alcohol withdrawal are presented in the section on alcohol use disorders later in this chapter and also discussed in Chapter 25.

When agitated patients stabilize, antipsychotics should be continued for a period of days to weeks, depending on the severity of the agitation and the dose required to achieve behavioural control. They should then be tapered slowly and cautiously discontinued. It used to be thought that delirium resolved promptly with the resolution of the underlying medical problem. This is not, however, always the case. Patients may continue to experience symptoms for many months after the acute illness and may require medication for persistent symptoms.

There is a tendency to use restraints on patients with hyperactive delirium. Physical restraints should be avoided as much as possible because they tend to increase agitation and have the potential to cause harm. However, if other measures to control a patient's behaviour are ineffective and it seems likely the patient, if unrestrained, may cause injury to themself or others, restraints can be used with caution. Patients who are restrained should be monitored closely and the restraint discontinued as soon as possible. A useful alternative to restraints may be constant observation by sitters or family members.

Environmental interventions can be helpful, particularly in relatively mild cases of delirium. Correcting sensory deficits with eyeglasses and hearing aids helps patients understand their surroundings and decreases agitation and paranoia. Providing an environment with adequate lighting, reduced noise, and with a visible clock and calendar may help to reduce disorientation and agitation. In addition, a room with a window will help to orient patients to diurnal clues and may limit disruption of the sleep/wake cycle. A nightlight may decrease nocturnal agitation and frightening illusions, or may make a patient less likely to sleep through the night. Family members can help in reassuring agitated patients, through frequent touching and verbal orientation, and should be encouraged to stay with the patient for as long as necessary. Although there are no randomized controlled trials of these interventions, they are relatively easy to carry out. Moreover, they can involve family members, who are often anxious to be involved in the patient's care.

Supportive care and prevention of complications

Supportive care includes attention to oral intake and prevention of aspiration, falls, and decubitus ulcers.

Drug–drug interactions

Primary care physicians should be aware of the drug–drug interactions that can occur and contribute to the manifestations of delirium, as well as the patient's response to treatment. The two major types of drug–drug interactions are pharmacodynamic interactions and pharmacokinetic interactions.

Pharmacodynamic drug–drug interactions are predictable as they occur as the sum of the synergy or antagonism of medications at the target receptors. Two examples of pharmacodynamic interactions that may cause delirium are: (1) amitriptyline and benztropine when given together have synergistic anticholinergic activity; urinary retention, constipation and dry mucosa are adjunctive clues (in addition to the delirium itself) to the increased anticholinergic state; (2) the combination of phenelzine, a monoamine oxidase inhibitor (MAOI), and paroxetine, an SSRI, can produce serotonin syndrome (serotonin toxicity) due to synergistic drug-induced increase in intrasynaptic serotonin. The patient presents with the triad of neuromuscular hyperactivity, autonomic hyperactivity and altered sensorium. An awareness of serotonin syndrome is crucial not only in avoiding this potentially lethal combination of medications but also in recognizing the clinical picture so that treatment can be promptly initiated.

Pharmacokinetic drug–drug interactions are more complex and occur through multiple mechanisms such as alteration in drug absorption, distribution, metabolism or excretion. By nature they are less predictable. Pharmacokinetic drug–drug interactions involve key enzymatic systems associated with drug metabolism. The two major systems are the cytochrome P450 system, consisting of enzymes that perform oxidative (phase I) metabolism of drugs and the uridine 5'-diphosphate glucuronosyltransferases (UGTs) involved in phase II conjugative drug metabolism. Some drugs act as inhibitors of these enzymes and impair their ability to metabolize their target substrates, thus producing increased blood levels of substrate medications. Some other drugs act as inducers and cause an increase in the production of these enzymes, leading to increased metabolism of the substrates of the particular enzymes (resulting in reduced blood levels of medications). There is a large range of drug–drug interactions involving the P450 and UGT systems and the clinician can consult tables of interactions available from multiple published and online sources. An exhaustive and accessible set of P450 tables and explanations can be found in the *Concise guide to drug interaction principles for medical practice:*

cytochrome P450s, UGTs, P-Glycoproteins.[25] The best defence against detrimental drug–drug interactions is the clinician's awareness and focused attention.

Prevention of delirium

Studies on delirium prevention are limited. The most successful approach to prevention appears to be the attenuation of modifiable risk factors in individual patients. Correction of dehydration, modification of unnecessary noise and stimuli, promotion of good sleep hygiene, removal of urinary catheters and physical restraints, use of eyeglasses and hearing aids, provision of orienting information, and early mobilization are recommended to reduce the incidence of delirium.

Delirium: summary

- Delirium is commonly associated with medical and surgical illness, intoxication and withdrawal states and CNS disease. It may be the earliest manifestation of systemic illness.

- Delirium is very common. Groups at high risk of developing delirium are the elderly, post-surgical patients, drug abusers and those with pre-existing brain damage.

- Recognizing delirium is important because it is an indication of an underlying medical condition or drug toxicity that must be identified and addressed.

- Delirium may be misdiagnosed as dementia, psychosis or somnolence, leading to further morbidity when the underlying causes of the delirium remain untreated. Inappropriate administration of medications compounds the problem.

- Management includes correctly diagnosing the cause, using supportive measures including psychotropic medications when indicated.

Box 31.1 Predisposing factors in delirium

Patient characteristics
- Age older than 65 years
- Male

Medical/pharmacological factors
- Severe illness
- Intensive care unit admission
- Multiple medications
- Dementia
- Depression
- Dehydration
- Alcoholism

Environmental/social factors
- Social isolation
- Vision or hearing impairment
- Functional dependence or immobility
- Sleep deprivation

Box 31.2 Precipitating factors in delirium

Infections

■ Intracranial: encephalitis, meningitis (toxic, viral, bacterial, spirochete, tick-borne, etc.)

■ Systemic: pneumonia, urinary tract infection, septicaemia, malaria, AIDS

Medications

■ Psychotropic drugs (anxiolytics, antidepressants, sedative-hypnotics, antipsychotics)

■ Anticholinergic drugs (antispasmodics, antihistamines, antiparkinsonian agents)

■ Anticonvulsants

■ Analgesics (narcotics, non-steroidal anti-inflammatory drugs (NSAIDs))

■ Antiarrhythmic drugs

■ Any medication or metabolite that crosses the blood–brain barrier

Metabolic

■ Hepatic failure, renal failure, hypoxia

Vascular

■ Shock, vasculitis

Neurologic

■ Stroke, hypertensive encephalopathy, seizures, CNS AIDS

Cardiorespiratory

■ Arrhythmia, heart failure, respiratory failure, myocardial infarction

Autoimmune

■ Primary CNS (e.g. paraneoplastic syndrome, other limbic encephalitides)

■ Systemic autoimmune disorder with CNS involvement (e.g. lupus cerebritis)

Endocrine

■ Hypoglycaemia, hyperglycaemia, hypothyroidism, hyperthyroidism

Surgery

■ Orthopaedic, cardiac

Trauma

■ Head injury, burns

Withdrawal/intoxication syndromes

■ Alcohol, illicit drugs, benzodiazepines

Others

■ Urinary catheter, physical restraints, pain

Alcohol use disorders in patients with medical illness

(Additional information about alcohol use disorder can be found in Chapter 25.)

Alcohol use disorders, which are prevalent in the practice of primary care medicine, are often comorbid with other medical conditions, complicating their identification and appropriate management.

Consider the case-study below.

Case-study

Ms A is a 63-year-old married woman, with a history of atrial fibrillation (maintained in sinus rhythm), peptic ulcer disease, hypercholesterolaemia and hypertension, who has been seeing her primary care provider, Dr Z, for the past 10 years. She presents one day complaining of "fluttering in my chest" and "the sweats". She tells Dr Z she is sure it is "just anxiety", or maybe related to symptoms of menopause. She reports that she has retired this year, adding "I know it was early, but my boss was always on at me about being late or making mistakes!" On review of her systems, she notes frequent heartburn, worse after eating. She has lost 10 lb since her last appointment 6 months ago. Incidentally, Dr Z notes a bruise on her knee, and Ms A explains that she fell the other day, "but it was just a silly fall, and I only slightly bumped my head!" Her pulse is irregular and fast at 125 beats per minute; blood pressure is 170/100 mmHg. She is noted to be mildly diaphoretic and with a fine hand tremor. Another bruise (of a different age) is found on her shoulder. She has mild epigastric tenderness on palpation.

Ms A is a woman with known medical problems now presenting with several medical complaints and physical findings. If not attuned to the possibility of alcohol use in all his patients, Dr Z might miss this diagnosis, attributing her recurrence of atrial fibrillation to her known risk for arrhythmia, her "heartburn" to her peptic ulcer disease, and the fall to just a "silly" mechanical incident. If Dr Z keeps alcohol use in his differential diagnosis, he might consider that the atrial fibrillation may have been induced by an alcohol binge, the heartburn may be alcoholic gastritis, and her elevated blood pressure may not just be worsening primary hypertension but a sign of alcohol withdrawal. Putting these things together, the tremor would fit in with a picture of withdrawal, the fall could be related to intoxication or imbalance problems due to cerebellar damage from alcohol or nutritional deficiencies (poor diet because of excessive drinking, which may also explain the weight loss), and even her "early retirement" might be a clue that her drinking had begun affecting her functioning at work. The health-care provider should not automatically assume an alcohol use disorder, but – importantly – without a high index of suspicion for the possibility of alcohol misuse, the clinician is at risk of missing it. If the above patient had been a young man with known substance abuse and no medical issues, Dr Z may have immediately considered an alcohol use disorder. Ms A, a typical patient in primary care, might not trigger the consideration of alcohol use disorder, because of her age, sex, marital status and multiple medical problems (which can obscure the findings of an alcohol use disorder). Missing the diagnosis of alcohol use disorder and active withdrawal, however, could be potentially life threatening, both acutely and chronically.

The diagnosis and management of patients with alcohol use disorder is discussed in detail in Chapter 25. A few points about the evaluation and management of patients with alcohol use disorder and multiple medical conditions are worth special mention. Concurrent medical conditions can confuse the picture of an alcohol use disorder and alcohol withdrawal. Baseline hypertension may mask the autonomic arousal of alcohol withdrawal. In such cases, other signs such as tachycardia, tremor (outstretched hands, tongue fasciculations), diaphoresis and hyperactive reflexes should be evaluated to expand the clinical data. Older individuals, or patients treated with antihypertensive medications such as beta-blockers, may not be able to mount a normal sympathetic response to alcohol withdrawal. In such cases, changes in mental status – mild confusion and inattentiveness, anxiety/agitation, or visual and tactile hallucinations – may be the only signs of withdrawal.

Patients with alcohol use disorder who also have comorbid medical conditions, or are elderly, are more prone to, and more sensitive to, the consequences of alcohol use. Parenteral repletion of thiamine and other B vitamins as well as magnesium should be prioritized in these patients. There should be a low threshold to request brain imaging, such as CT, to rule out new and old subdural bleeds, especially in patients with known bleeding risk or those on anticoagulant or antiplatelet therapies. For patients with cognitive impairment (which may be related to another process, such as Alzheimer disease, or may be more closely connected to alcohol use, including vascular dementia or Korsakoff's amnestic syndrome), the family and others should be interviewed about the patient's alcohol use.

The treatment for withdrawal, described in Chapter 25, can be applied to patients with comorbid medical conditions. Special attention to the patient's hepatic functioning is warranted; in patients with transaminitis or signs of more chronic liver impairment (such as low albumin or elevated coagulation factors), the clinician should consider the use of benzodiazepines with fewer active metabolites (such as temazepam, oxazepam or lorazepam). Medically ill patients may also be at increased risk for delirium as a result of withdrawal and/or the treatment of withdrawal (benzodiazepines). The clinician should be reluctant to consider outpatient management of alcohol withdrawal in patients at higher risk of complications, such as older patients and patients with medical comorbidities. Safety measures, such as raised bedrails and frequent monitoring, should be considered in these patients. Antipsychotic medications may be necessary to control agitated behaviours, although they should be used carefully. Antipsychotics have the potential to lower the seizure threshold and recent epidemiological studies have raised a concern for increased rates of death in elderly patients with dementia who were treated with antipsychotics.

Chronic pain syndromes and their role in increasing psychiatric morbidity

(Additional information about pain syndromes can be found in Chapter 21.)

Pain is one of the most frequent reasons patients consult a physician. Chronic pain is defined as pain that persists and is not alleviated by treatments that are often effective. Chronic pain may also be the major presentation in a patient with medically unexplained symptoms.

There is an increased occurrence of psychological disorders among persons with chronic pain, and this has an impact on their well-being and productivity.

Primary care physicians need to be aware of these psychological factors, since they significantly influence the prognosis and course of chronic pain, and account for a significant proportion of the disability in patients with chronic pain (see Box 31.3).

Box 31.3 Common pain disorders that are usually accompanied by psychiatric morbidity

- Chronic headache
- Trigeminal neuralgia
- Back pain
- Abdominal pain (irritable bowel syndrome)
- Pelvic pain
- Neuropathic pain
- Complex regional pain syndrome (reflex sympathetic dystrophy)
- Post-stroke pain
- Fibromyalgia
- Osteoarthritis
- Sickle cell disease "pain crises"

Psychiatric comorbidities in patients with pain syndromes

Chronic pain is associated with high rates of psychopathology, including sleep disorders, depression, anxiety, substance abuse and personality disorders.

Sleep disorder

Sleep disorder in patients with pain syndromes tends to be more of a disturbance in the quality of sleep rather than in the total duration of sleep. In general, the percentage of time spent in each sleep stage is not markedly different between patients with chronic pain and normal individuals. However, in patients with chronic pain, sleep is often more fragmented, with the overall sleep period broken down into several brief periods of sleep. This results in poor, non-refreshing sleep.

Depression

Depression has been shown to be an antecedent of chronic pain, a consequence of chronic pain, and a concomitant biological relative of chronic pain. In patients who have depression and chronic pain, if the pain is alleviated, the depression also improves and the reverse is also true.

Anxiety disorders

Patients with painful syndromes have an increased risk of anxiety disorders such as panic disorder, phobias, obsessive–compulsive disorder, post-traumatic stress disorder (PTSD) or generalized anxiety disorder.

PTSD has been strongly associated with chronic pain. PTSD is a prevalent disorder that has a significant impact on the quality of life for survivors of traumatic events such as combat injuries (military and civilian victims), motor vehicle crashes and childhood abuse. The residual effects of such traumatic events may be profound, and physical symptoms of pain may play a central role.

Substance abuse

Substance use disorders have been found to be more common among patients with chronic pain compared with those without chronic pain. The most commonly abused substances in chronic pain patients are alcohol and narcotics. Opioids are the most frequently prescribed drugs for the relief of moderate to severe chronic pain. The most important concern is the addictive potential of narcotic analgesics, although it is a more unusual phenomenon than previously believed. Screening tests such as the CAGE-AID screen (the CAGE questionnaire Adapted to Include Drugs, see Box 25.1) can be employed to aid in the identification of patients with chronic pain – patients who are at risk for substance abuse. In addition, patients on opioids should be clinically monitored for signs of abuse. Abuse-related behaviours include: reports of obtaining medications from multiple sources, forging or stealing prescriptions, or selling prescription medications.

Personality disorders

High rates of personality disorders have been documented among patients with chronic pain. Histrionic, dependent, paranoid and borderline personality disorders have been identified as the most common.

Management of pain/psychiatric disorder comorbidity

The treatment of chronic pain involves a comprehensive approach that includes providing an appropriate level of analgesia and rehabilitation measures. Total pain relief is less likely with chronic pain syndromes. The main treatment objectives, therefore, should be pain control and physical rehabilitation. The selection of pain-management modalities should be guided by the severity of the pain and the presence or absence of comorbidities. The WHO analgesic ladder is an appropriate guide to initiating pharmacotherapy.[26] The first step is the use of non-opioid medications such as paracetamol, NSAIDs, tricyclic antidepressants, anticonvulsants and topical preparations, in addition to other strategies, such as physiotherapy and massage. The second and third steps involve the use of opioids, which are necessary when other treatment measures have failed to provide sufficient pain control, and the quality of life is poor because of the pain.

The most common side-effect following chronic use of opioids is reduction of gastrointestinal motility, with consequent constipation. A prophylactic bowel regimen, including the use of stool softeners and laxatives, should be initiated at the start of opioid therapy.

Compound analgesic preparations that contain a simple analgesic (such as paracetamol or aspirin) with an opioid are available and can provide greater relief of pain than a non-opioid analgesic given alone. Patients should be cautioned against excessive use of these compounds, to avoid hepatotoxicity from high doses of paracetamol.

Primary care physicians also need to be able to address the psychosocial problems that may complicate pain. Patients with depression or anxiety who also have pain can be helped by antidepressants. Tricyclic antidepressants (TCAs) are effective treatments for depression and pain. They appear to have an analgesic effect apart from their antidepressant effects. The use of TCAs may be limited by their antimuscarinic side-effects. SSRIs are better tolerated but provide less benefit. The newer dual-action antidepressants, duloxetine and venlafaxine, which are serotonin and norepinephrine (noradrenaline) reuptake inhibitors, have been shown in clinical trials to alleviate pain and depressive symptoms. SSRIs are first-line medications in the treatment of PTSD.

Anti-epileptic drugs such as carbamazepine and gabapentin are effective in neuropathic pain conditions and are considered the most effective drugs in the treatment of trigeminal neuralgia and diabetic neuropathy. Pregabalin is a new anti-epileptic medication licensed for the treatment of peripheral and central neuropathic pain as well as generalized anxiety disorder.

Psychotherapy and physical rehabilitation

Psychotherapeutic approaches such as CBT can be employed in treating chronic pain and can reduce some of the distress associated with pain, and also foster adaptation.

Physical therapy may be useful in chronic pain and is a cornerstone treatment for patients with complex regional pain syndrome. An improvement in function despite pain and a return of the patient to a feeling of usefulness in the social context of family, work and community, are the key goals of rehabilitation in all forms of chronic pain disorders.

Pain syndromes: summary

- Pain, especially of the chronic variety, is commonly associated with psychiatric disorders.
- Depressive disorders, anxiety disorders, substance use disorders, sleep disorders and personality disorders have been identified as the most common psychiatric comorbidities.
- Comorbid psychiatric conditions account for a significant proportion of the disability in persons with chronic pain.
- Interventions targeting comorbid psychiatric conditions as well as medical conditions are better able to alleviate the suffering of patients with chronic pain syndromes than approaches targeting either alone.
- Narcotic analgesics have a defined place in the management of chronic pain, but it is incumbent on the physician to be aware of the potential for misuse and abuse.

Fatigue

(Additional information about chronic fatigue syndrome can be found in Chapter 21.)

Between one-quarter and one-third of patients seen by a primary care physician (PCP) in any given day complain of fatigue.[27–29] It is a non-specific symptom, but usually contains one or more of the following elements: a decrease in stamina to maintain an activity, a sense of weakness (in the absence of objective findings), and ultimately, a disinterest in initiating activities because of such difficulties. The ability to function at work, in the family, and in the community is impaired and the capacity to enjoy life is diminished.

Ultimately, one-third of these patients will be found to have a primary medical diagnosis; one-third of these patients will receive a primary psychiatric diagnosis; and less than 10% will be diagnosed as having chronic fatigue syndrome according to the official criteria of the Centers for Disease Control and Prevention (CDC).[30,31]

The most important diagnostic tools for the assessment of fatigue are old-fashioned and extremely low-tech. They consist of a good relationship with the patient and knowledge of the community context, a thorough history and a careful physical examination. Simple blood tests will rule in or rule out major disease entities. If these first assessments fail to point to an aetiology, it is not usual that one will be found.

Chronic fatigue syndrome

Chronic fatigue syndrome is discussed at length in Chapter 21. It is a CDC-standardized diagnosis,[31] and is intentionally restrictive. The purpose of creating this narrow, standardized, diagnosis is to have a homogeneous population for research purposes. Chronic fatigue syndrome is diagnosed in less than 10% of all patients presenting with fatigue.

Making the diagnosis

History and physical examination

The clinician should take particular note of the patient's general appearance and level of self-care, which are strong indicators of their level of functioning. Asking the patient to describe the fatigue using open-ended questions will help cultivate rapport. Particular attention should be paid to sleep patterns and sleep disruptions, as well as the possibility of non-restorative sleep. Taking a parallel history of the patient's life circumstances will also yield useful information about psychosocial stressors particular to the patient and family, as well as in the community. Most of the medical and psychological causes of fatigue noted in Box 31.4 yield positive findings in a thorough history and complete physical examination. Neurological and mental status examinations (with a simple cognitive examination) complete the assessment of patients with fatigue.

Box 31.4   Common causes for fatigue

Causes of insomnia or non-restorative sleep

- Sleep apneoa, restless legs syndrome, congestive heart failure, arrhythmia with palpitations, pulmonary disease (air hunger), conditions that cause pain, nausea, itching, or night sweats
- *Psychiatric conditions*: depression; PTSD with nightmares, anxiety/worry; substance intoxication or withdrawal.

Causes of weakness

- Anaemia, nutritional deficits, endocrinopathies (especially thyroid disease or Addison's disease), wasting syndromes (including HIV, chronic diarrhoea from any cause), neuromuscular syndromes, primary neurological disorders (stroke, multiple sclerosis) paraneoplastic syndromes, occult neoplasm, rheumatological diseases including lupus and rheumatoid arthritis, chronic infectious disease (tuberculosis)
- *Psychiatric conditions*: depression (weight loss from appetite loss, anergy), dementia syndromes

---

Laboratory assessments

Simple and relatively inexpensive laboratory tests will rule in or out most major illnesses causing fatigue. These include a complete blood count (haemoglobin, cell size and shape, white blood cell count and differential), serum glucose, basic electrolytes, renal function markers, liver function markers, thyroid function tests and erythrocyte sedimentation rate (or, when available, C-reactive protein). A chest X-ray is also a useful screening test.

If the history, physical examination and basic lab assessments do not yield results that focus on a particular disease entity or organ system, the likelihood is low that a cause for the fatigue will be determined at the time of the evaluation. While it is good news for the patient that no major disease has been discovered, it may be frustrating as well that no cause has been determined that might be easily corrected and the fatigue eliminated. Both aspects should be discussed with the patient, when the results of the assessment are being presented.

The main differential diagnosis, between physical and psychological causes of fatigue is not dichotomous and the relationship between physical symptoms and psychiatric illness may be indirect. For example: a reciprocal relationship exists between depression/anxiety and any physical illness causing pain. Pain causes insomnia and, eventually, depression; depression lowers the pain threshold and makes sleep even more difficult and less restorative, thus indirectly causing fatigue.

For the most part, patients are not averse to a psychological explanation for fatigue, as long as they feel neither disparaged nor that their symptoms have been minimized. Antidepressant medications may be a useful adjunctive treatment, whether or not a physical cause for the fatigue is determined. Recent studies have recommended psychotherapy with CBT and graded exercise therapy, a form of supervised physical reconditioning. These treatments have been demonstrated to improve function and decrease symptoms in patients presenting with fatigue.[32,33]

Infectious diseases

In low-income countries, infections arising from lack of clean water, poor hygiene, and insect vectors continue to represent a significant public health concern. Delayed presentation to treatment facilities leads to severe forms of infection at initial presentation, with delirium as a possible psychiatric complication. Examples of such infections include diarrhoeal diseases, pneumonia and meningitis.

Malaria is one the major killer diseases in low-income tropical countries and represents a particular threat to children and pregnant women. Notable psychiatric complications of malaria include cerebral malaria-induced delirium, as well as traumatic reactions to premature delivery and infant death. Virtually all antimalarial drugs carry some psychiatric morbidity, from disrupted sleep and vivid nightmares (Malarone® (atovaquone + proguanil hydrochloride), chloroquine) to frank psychosis (Lariam® (mefloquine)).

HIV/AIDS: an illness with significant and intertwined medical and psychiatric morbidity

PCPs caring for patients with HIV often treat a variety of comorbid mental disorders: mood disorders, anxiety disorders, psychotic disorders, substance use and abuse, and cognitive disorders. All have considerable bearing on antiretroviral therapy (ART) adherence as well as quality of life. It is imperative that the clinician is adept at assessing patients for the presence of mental illness and makes the treatment of mental illness part of the overall plan. The presence of a psychiatric disorder does not disqualify a patient from receiving ART.

Symptoms of mental illness may predate the acquisition of the virus and/or may be the result of HIV disease and associated conditions. The presence of mental illness may increase the risk of infection with, and transmission of, HIV and may also adversely affect medication adherence.

Recognizing and treating mental illness in the clinic setting

This section aims to provide the PCP with a framework for recognizing and treating mental illness in HIV patients in the clinic setting.

Recognizing mood disorders

Mood disorders include dysthymia, the more severe major depressive disorder (MDD) and bipolar disorder. Around the time of their HIV diagnosis, many patients report depressive symptoms, which may or may not reach the severity of MDD. After the immune system has declined in function, patients are at great risk for depression as well. Symptoms of MDD include: low mood, poor appetite with concomitant weight loss, insomnia, fatigue (symptoms that shadow the symptoms of advanced AIDS itself) as well as a sense of hopelessness, and on occasion, suicidality. It is important to make the distinction between MDD and dysthymia because untreated MDD can affect adherence. The PHQ-9 is an extremely useful, brief self-report instrument for depression screening in the primary care setting.[34]

The clinician should be alert for subtle symptoms of mania, which include irritability, restlessness and agitation. The more blatant symptoms of mania may be well known and described by family or community members, who can be educated to recognize them as the beginning of an episode that requires treatment: a period of seven or more days during which an individual has a decreased need for sleep (only 2–4 hours nightly), increased energy/restlessness, racing thoughts and rapid speech, irritability, increased risky behaviour and poor impulse control (e.g. having unprotected sexual intercourse with many partners, or gambling).

When evaluating a patient for depression, it is important to remember that bipolar disorder often presents with depressive symptoms. Patients who present with depressive symptoms should be asked if they have ever had symptoms of mania, as this determines the diagnosis and the appropriate treatment.

Recognizing anxiety disorders (including PTSD)

Anxiety often occurs in patients who are newly diagnosed and those who are coming to terms with their illness. Anxiety reaches pathologic severity (and should be actively treated) when it interferes with relationships, coping, and ability to function. Patients may present with somatic symptoms such as palpitations, muscle tension, shortness of breath, or lightheadedness, rather than explicitly state that they are anxious. These patients often induce anxiety in the clinician, which may be diagnostic. It is important to rule out medical causes for somatic symptoms and help the patient understand that anxiety has both emotional and physiological manifestations.

Special attention should be paid to patients presenting with PTSD. One study of 357 patients with HIV found that approximately 68% of women and 35% of men had been victims of sexual assault before the age of 15 years. Those with a history of assault reported greater anxiety and depression.[35] Given the extent of trauma among HIV patients, it is important that the PCP is sensitive to the level of mistrust that may affect the relationship with the provider and adherence to the medication regimen. It is also important to address the PTSD itself, because it might fuel further anxiety and depression.

Recognizing psychosis and psychotic illness

Psychosis is defined as delusions, hallucinations and disorganized speech and/or behaviour. It can include affective flattening or psychomotor agitation. Psychotic symptoms may present in a number of contexts and may have multiple aetiologies, including mental illness proper, as well as psychosis resulting from substance intoxication, substance withdrawal, and delirium.

Psychotic illnesses include schizophrenia, schizoaffective disorder and bipolar disorder. Distinguishing among them may be impossible when the patient is acutely psychotic. The diagnosis of schizophrenia may be made in the presence of the psychotic symptoms listed above. The onset of the disease is usually early adulthood and the diagnosis requires that symptoms be present for at least 6 months and cause significant impairment in social functioning. The psychosis of bipolar disorder and schizoaffective disorder is often of shorter duration, and features grandiosity and expansiveness not usually seen with schizophrenia. Bipolar patients tend to show mood lability, whereas patients with schizophrenia tend to have a flat affect. Schizoaffective disorder presents with some features of mood disorder combined with those of a psychotic disorder.

It is important to note that psychotic symptoms may occur in the context of ART use (particularly efavirenz) and in late-stage HIV/AIDS. New-onset delusions, disorientation, and fluctuating wakefulness are indicative of delirium (see earlier).

Recognizing substance-induced mental disorders

(A more comprehensive discussion of substance abuse evaluation and treatment can be found earlier in the chapter, as well as a short guide to alcohol use disorders in medically ill patients. See also Chapters 26 and 25 respectively.)

Patients often use substances to treat psychiatric symptoms. The physician must be vigilant for signs of substance intoxication and withdrawal (see Table 31.4). The best diagnostic tool is a high index of suspicion when patients present with anomalous symptom constellations. Urine and serum drug toxicology (when available) can be of great help in explaining the patient's symptoms. Medications associated with arrhythmias and QT prolongation should be avoided for patients suspected of using stimulants, while sedating medications should be avoided for patients suspected of using opiates.

Table 31.4 Basic signs and symptoms of intoxication and withdrawal of common drugs of abuse		
Drug	**Intoxication**	**Withdrawal**
Stimulants (cocaine, amphetamine, methamphetamine)	Diaphoresis, agitation, paranoia, psychosis, pupillary dilation	Intense dysphoria, depression
Opiates (heroin, morphine, prescription opiates)	Lethargy, sedation, pupillary constriction	Diaphoresis, intense anxiety, diarrhoea, vomiting, arthralgias, yawning, rhinorrhoea
Alcohol	Sedation, disinhibition, ataxia	Intense anxiety, tremors, diaphoresis, autonomic instability, delirium

Treatment guidelines: clinical "pearls"

Pharmacologic treatment of mental illness should take into account the following: pharmacokinetics, pharmacodynamics, side-effect tolerability, and drug–drug interactions.

Pharmacokinetics is defined as the characteristic absorption, distribution, metabolism and excretion of a pharmaceutical. Attention to pharmacokinetics is important for patients with end-organ damage such as liver or renal failure. For example, lithium should not be given to a patient with renal disease. A hepatically metabolized medication should be given in lower doses than recommended to a patient with impaired liver function. Cytochrome P450 inducers such as carbamazepine and phenytoin, or inhibitors such as fluoroquinolone antibiotics are the basis for many adverse drug–drug interactions, and are examples of pharmacokinetic interactions. Other inhibitors relevant to HIV patients include protease inhibitors, antifungals and macrolide antibiotics like erythromycin and clarithromycin. The benzodiazepines, midazolam and triazolam, as well as the antidepressant trazodone may reach toxic levels in the presence of protease inhibitors. Other important inducers are cigarette smoking, St John's wort and rifampin. See Table 31.5 for a guide to common drug–drug interactions between HIV treatments and psychiatric medications.

Pharmacodynamics describes the relationship between drugs and the molecular receptors with which it interacts. Receptors may be upregulated or downregulated by disease or medication. These factors should be taken into consideration when choosing treatment. For example, TCAs and MAOIs must never be administered at the same time or within 2 weeks of each other, as serotonin syndrome may occur.

When initiating any psychotropic medication, the patient should be started on a low dose, which is increased slowly to minimize side-effects and drug–drug interactions of both types. For example, multiple anticholinergic medications should be avoided. Consideration must also be made for body habitus and nutritional status (i.e. wasting). Patients with hypoalbuminaemia, liver disease and renal disease may have decreased drug binding of acidic and neutral drugs. Plasma concentrations of the free drug are increased and thus drug efficacy and toxicity are enhanced.

Treatment for depression

Medications such as citalopram and escitalopram have few reported drug–drug interactions and few side-effects. To minimize any potential side-effects, one may direct the patient to begin dosing with half of the lowest-strength tablet for 5 days and increase the dose slowly. Paroxetine is a more sedating antidepressant that often boosts appetite and may therefore be appropriate for patients with poor appetite and insomnia related to depression. Mirtazapine is another antidepressant that is useful for insomnia and poor appetite. Bupropion and venlafaxine have an activating quality and are therefore better taken during the day. Fluoxetine should be avoided, as it has a long half-life and is metabolized by both cytochromes 2D6 and 3A4, isoenzymes used by protease inhibitors.

Treatment for anxiety

Psychotherapy (individual, group, couples) is a mainstay of anxiety treatment and should be administered whether or not medication is prescribed. SSRIs are the main psychopharmacologic treatment for many anxiety disorders. Patients must be informed that the medication may take up to 2–4 weeks to fully treat the anxiety symptoms and that the medication must be taken every day in order to achieve the full effect. The following medications are commonly used for anxiety disorders: sertraline (panic disorder, PTSD); fluoxetine (panic disorder); and paroxetine (panic disorder, generalized anxiety disorder, PTSD). It is especially important to "start low and go slow" with activating medications such as sertraline and venlafaxine, as anxious patients are highly sensitive to the initial and temporary increase in agitation associated with these medicines.

Benzodiazepines such as clonazepam and lorazepam may be used to treat anxiety as the SSRI is being initiated. The benzodiazepine is then tapered over a 1–2-week period after the patient has reached a therapeutic dose of the SSRI. Use of benzodiazepines carries the risk of addiction in some patients, but all patients are subject to drug dependence including withdrawal phenomena and desensitization to medication effect (tachyphylaxis). While useful in the short term, benzodiazepines are generally to be avoided for long-term use. Alprazolam (Xanax®), in particular, with its rapid onset, short half-life, and exacerbation of symptoms as the medication wears off (rebound phenomenon) is a particularly poor choice for patients with any risk for addiction.

Buspirone, which is neither an SSRI nor a benzodiazepine, may be helpful for some patients with generalized anxiety disorder. Like the SSRI antidepressants, it requires 4–7 weeks to begin to work, and has no abuse potential. As it is a CYP450 3A4 substrate, grapefruit juice, macrolide antibiotics and antifungals such as ketoconazole will increase serum levels significantly. The initial dosage is 5 mg three times daily and it has been found effective at doses of 20 to 60 mg per day in two or three divided doses.

Treatment for bipolar disorder

Treatment for acute bipolar mania include the anti-epilepsy drug valproic acid, and second-generation antipsychotics like aripiprazole, olanzapine and ziprasidone. All may be used for long-term mood stabilization. It is best to avoid carbamazepine because its cytochrome P450 interactions complicate and sometimes prohibit the use of ART. Quetiapine has a particular indication for bipolar depression.

Lithium is an inexpensive treatment for bipolar disorder and is effective for suicidal patients. Dosing is based on the patient's weight and tolerance of side-effects, and blood levels must be monitored as the dose is being adjusted upward, and annually thereafter. Thyroid and renal function must be monitored every 6–12 months during treatment. Given the narrow therapeutic index, the PCP should be vigilant for signs of toxicity, which may be brought on by anything that compromises renal function or causes dehydration in a patient with HIV, such as a fever.

Treatment for psychosis

First-generation antipsychotics including haloperidol, fluphenazine and thorazine are all proven treatments for schizophrenia. The practitioner should be attuned to potential side-effects of antipsychotics, as patients with HIV/AIDS are at higher risk for extrapyramidal symptoms such as Parkinsonism, as well as akathisia.

Second-generation antipsychotics generally carry less risk of extrapyramidal side-effects but are often associated with weight gain, dyslipidaemia and glucose intolerance/diabetes. They are also considerably more expensive than first-generation antipsychotics. For patients with poor appetite and significant weight loss, a second-generation antipsychotic like olanzapine can be useful. On the other hand, patients with dyslipidaemia or diabetes can benefit from ziprasidone, as there is less risk of metabolic syndrome (though this agent is associated with a greater risk of QT prolongation relative to other second-generation antipsychotics and should therefore be used cautiously, if at all, with patients at risk for long QT and arrhythmia).

Wasting

Wasting is defined as unintentional loss of more than 10% of the body weight. It has multiple aetiologies in patients with HIV/AIDS: malabsorption; loss of appetite secondary to nausea; depression; and/or dementia. For patients with depression and comorbid wasting, mirtazapine and paroxetine are among the first choices for antidepressant medications as they tend to stimulate the appetite and are associated with weight gain. For patients with bipolar disorder or schizophrenia, olanzapine may be used for its associated weight gain. The clinician should use the side-effect profile to the advantage of the patient.

HIV-associated dementia

Little is known about the worldwide incidence and prevalence of HIV-associated dementia (HAD). The HIV virus is highly neurotropic and symptoms have been greatly reduced by the advent of triple therapy with antiretroviral medications, which lower viral load. Unfortunately, the neurocognitive sequelae of HIV are quite prevalent in populations that lack access to ART. HAD occurs chiefly among those who have had HIV for a number of years and have progressed to AIDS. In the primary care setting, HAD in its early stages presents with cognitive impairment, apathy, regression, psychosis, slow speech and tremor or psychomotor slowing. Studies in several countries including three African nations (Kenya, Uganda and Ethiopia) show depression to be a major psychiatric complication of HIV/AIDS.[36,37] Alternatively, patients with HIV may show signs of mania late in the course of their illness. This presentation is usually in the context of HAD and portends a grim outcome. In its later stages, HAD presents with mutism, incontinence, perseveration and severe regression. The Oral Trail Making test Part B[38] is a good screen for early HIV dementia and the Modified HIV Dementia Scale is a useful way to assess and monitor cognitive impairment.[39,40]

Management of HIV-associated dementia

When psychosis arises in the context of HAD, the first goal of treatment is to optimize ART to reduce the viral load. This may slow or even partially reverse HAD and its associated symptoms. Second-generation antipsychotics such as olanzapine, ziprasidone and risperidone are all generally effective at treating both the manic and psychotic aspects of HAD. Most SSRIs are safe for the depressive symptoms seen in HAD. The antidepressant bupropion should be avoided, as it tends to lower the seizure threshold.[41]

Table 31.5 HIV-related treatments: substrates, inhibitors, and inducers at cytochrome P450 isoenzymes 2D6 and 3A4

P450 enzyme	Common substrates	Common inhibitors	Common inducers
2D6	First-generation antipsychotics, TCAs, tramadol	Bupropion, fluoxetine, paroxetine, ritonavir	Carbamazepine
3A4	Protease inhibitors, zolpidem, statins	Atazanavir, cimetidine, clarithromycin, ciprofloxacin	Carbamazepine, efavirenz, nevirapine, ritonavir, rifampin, St John's wort

Adapted from Cozza K, Williams SG, Wynn GH. 2008. Psychopharmacologic treatment issues in AIDS psychiatry. In: Cohen M, Gorman JM, eds. 2008. *Comprehensive textbook of AIDS psychiatry*. New York, Oxford University Press, 2008, Table 32.1 page 464, by permission of Oxford University Press, Inc.[42]

References

1   Thornicroft G et al. WPA guidance on steps, obstacles and mistakes to avoid in the implementation of community mental health care. *World Psychiatry*, 201, 9:67–77.

2   World Health Organization, 2008. The world health report 2008: primary health care now more than ever. Geneva, World Health Organization, 2008 (http://www.who.int/whr/2008/en/index.html, accessed 11 December 2011).

3   Ohaeri JU et al. The prevalence of psychiatric morbidity among adults attending at the five primary healthcare facilities of a rural community in Nigeria. *The Nigerian Postgraduate Medical Journal*, 1994, 1:12–16.

4   de Girolamo G, Bassi M. Community surveys of mental disorders: recent achievements and works in progress. *Current Opinion in Psychiatry*, 2003, 16:403–411.

5   Berardi D et al. Mental, physical and functional status in primary care attenders. *International Journal of Psychiatry in Medicine*, 1999, 29:133–148.

6   *Diagnostic and statistical manual of mental disorders*, 4th ed, text revision (DSM-IV-TR). Washington, American Psychiatric Association, 2000.

7   Prince M et al. No health without mental health. *The Lancet*, 2007, 370:13–31.

8   Pingitore D, Sansone RA. Using DSM-IV primary care version: a guide to psychiatric diagnosis in primary care. *American Family Physician*, 1998, 58:1347–1352.

9   Ludman EJ et al. Depression and diabetes symptom burden. *General Hospital Psychiatry*, 2004, 26:430–436.

10 Polonsky WH et al. Insulin omission in women with IDDM. *Diabetes Care*, 1994, 17:1178–1185.

11 Goebel-Fabbri A, Musen G, Levenson J. Endocrine and metabolic disorders. In: Levenson JL, ed. *The American Psychiatric Publishing textbook of psychosomatic medicine: psychiatric care of the medically ill*, 2nd ed. Washington, DC, American Psychiatric Publishing, Inc., 2011: 495–516.

12 Stewart D, Vigod S, Stotland N. Obstetrics and gynecology. In: Levenson JL, ed. *The American Psychiatric Publishing textbook of psychosomatic medicine: psychiatric care of the medically ill*, 2nd ed. Washington, DC, American Psychiatric Publishing, Inc., 2011: 733–760.

13 Kerr J, Brown C, Balen AH. The experiences of couples who have had infertility treatment in the United Kingdom: results of a survey performed in 1997. *Human Reproduction*, 1999, 14:934–938.

14   Khan MI, Waguespack SG, Hu MI. Medical management of postsurgical hypoparathyroidism. *Endocrine Practice*, 2010, 6:1–19.

15   Presne C et al. Lithium-induced nephropathy: Rate of progression and prognostic factors. *Kidney International*, 2003, 64:585–592.

16   Van Amelsvoort T et al. Hyponatremia associated with carbamazepine and oxcarbazepine therapy: a review. *Epilepsia*, 1994, 35:181–188.

17   Jacob S, Spinler SA. Hyponatremia associated with selective serotonin-reuptake inhibitors in older adults. *Annals of Pharmacotherapy*, 2006, 40:1618–1622.

18   Richards JB et al. Effect of selective serotonin reuptake inhibitors on the risk of fracture. *Archives of Internal Medicine*, 2007, 167:188–194.

19   Spitzer RL et al. Health-related quality of life in primary care patients with mental disorders. Results from the PRIME-MD 1000 Study. *JAMA*, 1995, 274:1511–1517.

20   Spitzer RL, Kroenke K, Williams JB. Validation and utility of a self-report version of PRIME-MD: the PHQ primary care study. Primary Care Evaluation of Mental Disorders. Patient Health Questionnaire. *JAMA*, 1999, 282:1737–1744.

21   Lanska DJ. Acute confusional states. In: Corey–Bloom J, David RB, eds. *Clinical adult neurology*, 3rd. ed. New York, Demos Medical Publishing, 2009: 185–200.

22   American Psychiatric Association. Practice guideline for the treatment of patients with delirium. *Amercian Journal of Psychiatry*, 1999, 156(5 Suppl.):1–20.

23   *The prevention, diagnosis and management of delirium in older people. National Guidelines*. London, Royal College of Physicians, 2006 (http://bookshop.rcplondon.ac.uk/contents/6be09b43-4f53-46ad-aa11-9bac401f3164.pdf, accessed 27 January 2012).

24   Wei LA et al. The Confusion Assessment Method (CAM): a systematic review of current usage. *Journal of the American Geriatric Society*, 2008, 56:823–830.

25   Cozza KL, Armstrong SC, Oesterheld JR. *Concise guide to drug interaction principles for medical practice: cytochrome P450s, UGTs, P-glycoproteins*, 2nd ed. Washington DC, American Psychiatric Publishing, Inc., 2003.

26   WHO pain ladder. In: Cancer pain relief, 2nd ed. Geneva, World Health Organization, 1996 (http://whqlibdoc.who.int/publications/9241544821.pdf, accessed 27 January 2012).

27   Bates DW et al. Prevalence of fatigue and chronic fatigue syndrome in a primary care practice. *Archives of Internal Medicine*, 1993, 153:2759–65.

28   Fuhrer R, Wessely S. The epidemiology of fatigue and depression: a French primary-care study. *Psychological Medicine*, 1995, 25:895–905.

29   Kroenke K, Arrington MR, Mangelsdorff AD. The prevalence of symptoms in medical outpatients and the adequacy of therapy. *Archives of Internal Medicine*, 1990, 150:1685–1689.

30   Kroenke K et al. Chronic fatigue in primary care. Prevalence, patient characteristics, and outcome. *JAMA*, 1988, 260:929–934.

31   Fukuda K et al. The chronic fatigue syndrome: a comprehensive approach to its definition and study. International Chronic Fatigue Syndrome Study Group. *Annals of Internal Medicine*, 1994, 121:953–959.

32   Rimes KA, Chalder T. Treatments for chronic fatigue syndrome. *Occupational Medicine (London)*, 2005, 55:32–39.

33   Whiting P et al. Interventions for the treatment and management of chronic fatigue syndrome: a systematic review. *JAMA*, 2001, 289:1360–1368.

34   Kroenke K, Spitzer RL, Williams JB. The PHQ-9: validity of a brief depression severity measure. *Journal of General Internal Medicine*, 2001, 16:606–613.

35   Kalichman SC et al. Emotional adjustment in survivors of sexual assault living with HIV-AIDS. *Journal of Traumatic Stress*, 2002, 15:289–296.

36   Petrushkin H, Boardman J, Ovuga E. Psychiatric disorders in HIV-positive individuals in urban Uganda. *Psychiatric Bulletin*, 2005, 29:455–558.

37   Byakika-Tusiime J et al. Longitudinal antiretroviral adherence in HIV+ Ugandan parents and their children initiating HAART in the MTCT-Plus family treatment model: role of depression in declining adherence over time. *AIDS and Behavior*, 2009, 13(Suppl. 1):S82–S91.

38 Ricker JH, Asselrod BN. Analysis of an oral paradigm for the Trail Making Test. *Assessment*, 1994, 1:51–55.

39 Ryan E, Byrd D. Neuropsychological evaluation. In: Cohen M, Gorman JM, eds. *Comprehensive textbook of AIDS psychiatry*. New York, Oxford University Press, 2008: 73–87.

40 Davis HF et al. Assessing HIV-associated dementia: modified HIV dementia scale versus the Grooved Pegboard. *The AIDS Reader*, 2002, 12:29–38.

41 Schatzberg A et al. *Manual of clinical pharmacology*, 7th ed. Washington DC, American Psychiatric Publishing Inc., 2010: 645.

42 Cozza K, Williams SG, Wynn GH. 2008. Psychopharmacologic treatment issues in AIDS psychiatry. In: Cohen M, Gorman JM, eds. 2008. *Comprehensive textbook of AIDS psychiatry*. New York, Oxford University Press, 2008: 464.

32 Physical health consequences of mental illness

André Tylee, Elizabeth Barley, Latha Hapugoda and Richard Holt

Key messages

- Patients with severe mental illness and depression die prematurely from physical disorders.
- Patients with severe mental illness need regular physical health checks to identify disorders.
- People with long-term physical conditions are many times more likely to have concurrent depression and anxiety disorders.
- There is good evidence that comorbid depression and anxiety can be treated and this can improve overall function.
- There is emerging evidence to show that treating comorbid depression can improve physical condition-specific outcomes.

Introduction

This chapter describes the many physical health consequences of severe mental illness (usually defined as schizophrenia and bipolar disorders) and the common comorbidity of long-term physical health conditions and depressive disorder. In the UK, over 15 million people have long-term physical health conditions, and the prevalence of depression in people with long-term conditions is often twice that of the normal population. In addition, with ageing populations, many people have several long-term physical health conditions and this increases the prevalence of depression further. Although there are some similarities between severe mental illness (SMI) and common mental health disorders such as depression, this chapter is organized into two sections because each area is a distinct public health issue. The first discusses SMI and physical health; the second discusses depression and physical health.

What this means for GPs

- Patients with SMI die 15 years prematurely.
- Patients with SMI have many physical conditions.
- Patients with SMI need organized case management.
- Patients with depressive disorder often have physical comorbidity.
- Patients with depressive disorder and long-term conditions need organized case management.

Severe mental illness and physical health

Introduction

Schizophrenia and bipolar disorder are chronic and debilitating psychiatric illnesses that affect ~1% of the population globally. Although the term has attracted criticism because it implies that other psychiatric illnesses are not severe, collectively, schizophrenia and bipolar illness are frequently referred to as "severe mental illness" (SMI).[1] SMIs, also known as psychotic disorders, are conditions that produce disturbances in thinking and perception that are severe enough to distort perception of reality.[2] A lifetime prevalence of schizophrenia and bipolar disorder has been reported to be around 1–2%.[1,3,4] Psychotic conditions affect around 2.5% of the European population in any one year.[5] In England, the national prevalence reported for the year 2009/2010 for patients registered in primary care was 0.7%, with a higher prevalence (0.9%) in London. Some local authority areas and primary care practices in London report higher rates (1.0% or more).[6]

SMIs are within the top 30 leading causes of years of life lost due to disability globally.[7] These conditions reduce employability and independent living.[8] Further, patients experience worse physical health and reduced life expectancy compared to the general population.[9] Conversely, poor physical health can have a negative effect on mental health. These challenges have a huge impact on the length and quality of people's lives and lead to substantial costs to society.[5]

Mortality related to severe mental illness and physical illness

People living with SMI are between one and a half and three times more likely to die in any one year compared to the general population, due to a combination of unnatural deaths (including suicides) and natural causes that are mainly treatable. Unnatural causes contribute to 40% of the excess mortality experienced by people with schizophrenia, and individuals with SMI are 8.4 times more likely than the general population to commit suicide. Sixty per cent of the excess deaths in people with SMI are caused by physical illness, with the commonest cause of death being cardiovascular disease (CVD).[5] People with schizophrenia and bipolar disorder die at least 10 years younger than members of the general population and experience an average 25-year shorter life expectancy.[5,10–12]

The standardized mortality rates (SMRs) in schizophrenia have been increasing during recent decades.[11,13] The median SMRs for the 1970s, 1980s and 1990s were 1.8, 3.0 and 3.2 respectively; the widening mortality gap is concerning, particularly as much of this excess mortality is preventable through assertive management of comorbid physical illness.[12,14] A similar trend in SMR ranging from 1.2 to 2.5 has been documented in studies among people with bipolar disorder.[15] A more recent study from the United States of America (USA) reported a significantly ($P < 0.001$) increased mortality among people with schizophrenia or schizoaffective disorder compared to an age- and sex-matched general population; patients were followed until 2005, for a median of 23.5 years.[16] People affected with bipolar disease[17] and schizophrenia have twice the risk of death due to heart disease compared to the general population.[14]

Evidence indicating an increasing trend in SMR from CVD is of concern. A community cohort study in the United Kingdom of Great Britain and Northern Ireland (UK) indicated that CVD-related mortality in schizophrenia increased from 1981 to 2006. The SMR in 1981–1986 was 129 (95% confidence interval (CI) = 27 to 377) and 350 (95% CI = 186 to 598) in 2001–2006. The relative risks for the two periods were 0.76 (95% CI = 0.19 to 3.12) and 1.52 (95% CI = 0.57 to 4.07) respectively.[18] Smokers had a higher SMR ($P < 0.002$) for CVD (379; 95% CI = 311 to 459) compared to non-smokers (194; 95% CI = 125 to 286), and 70% of the excess deaths due to natural causes were attributed to smoking. This highlights the importance of prevention and appropriate management of CVD risk factors, including measures to reduce the exposure to active and passive smoking.

The effects of physical comorbidity in SMI are significant, not only due to severely reduced life expectancy and the huge impact on the quality of life of affected individuals and their family members, but also due to rising costs of health and social care.[19,20] In the European Region, the cost of poor mental health due to lost opportunities to obtain paid work and unpaid activities, including caring responsibilities and household tasks, account for more than two-thirds of the total cost.[5] Considering the predicted demographic growth and socioeconomic changes over the next few decades in the European Union (EU), the potential cost of health and social care due to SMI is likely to increase significantly.[5] Clinical programmes aimed at reducing cardiovascular risk factors, and evidence-based interventions in reducing inequalities in health care could help reduce the burden of avoidable deaths as well as limiting excessive cost for the health-care economy.

Comorbidity associated with severe mental illness

Comorbidity associated with SMI has been investigated extensively, dating back to mid-19th century.[12] There is consistent evidence that people with SMI are at an increased risk of a wide range of medical comorbidity. Using a large population-based sample of commercially insured adults with schizophrenia in the USA,[19] Carney et al. reported in 2006 that one-third of the study population (average age 40 years) had three or more long-term medical conditions, nearly three times more than controls (33.2% versus 12.1%). Only 29% of people had no claims for somatic comorbidities, compared with 54% of controls.

A cross-sectional comparative study in the USA reported 74% of people with SMI had a chronic physical health problem, while 50% had two or more conditions. Chronic pulmonary disease was most common, with a prevalence of 31%.[21] More than 50% of hospitalized patients with schizophrenia in the USA had one or more comorbid psychiatric or general medical conditions.[22] The most common conditions in this group were cardiovascular, pulmonary, neurological and endocrine diseases,[19] and individuals in this group were three times more likely to have diabetes and twice as likely to have CVD as the general population. A review of people with schizophrenia undertaken by Leucht et al. in 2007 found that these individuals are at a higher risk of developing CVD, diabetes, sexual dysfunction, tuberculosis, osteoporosis and dental health problems.[23]

There may be differences between SMIs in the prevalence, time of onset and type of physical illness co-occurring among this group of patients. For example, a retrospective cohort study in the USA, among patients receiving primary care, showed that earlier onset of risk factors and heart disease was noted among individuals with schizophrenia compared to those with affective psychosis and healthy controls. Patients with schizophrenia had increased relative risk for obesity and congestive heart failure, while patients with affective psychoses had increased risk for diabetes.[23] A higher prevalence of hypertension was reported in a nationally representative sample of people with schizophrenia in the USA,[24] and in a review by De Hert et al.[9] However, a meta-analysis of 12 papers by Osborn et al. in 2008 did not find any significant increase in hypertension among people with SMI.[25] This finding is consistent with the findings of Carney et al.[19] The above findings indicate that up-to-date knowledge of comorbid physical illness and SMI is critical for primary care clinicians to enable prevention, early diagnosis and treatment, in order to decrease associated morbidity and mortality and improve the prognosis of people with SMI.[24,26]

Factors contributing to increased comorbidity of physical illness in severe mental illness

Numerous studies have documented that many factors contribute to increased physical illness among people with SMI, including environmental, mental illness-related, medication-related, system-related (such as stigma about mental illnesses), and physician-related factors such as overshadowing and lack of expertise in identifying physical illness in patients with SMI.[19,23,27–29]

A familial link between mental illness was first suggested by Henry Maudsley in 1879, when he stated "Diabetes is a condition that occurs in families in which insanity prevails". This astute clinical observation has been replicated by more modern studies that show there is a high prevalence of metabolic abnormalities in the first-degree relatives of people with SMI. Between 17% and 50% of people with schizophrenia have a family history of type 2 diabetes.[30] Although this association may result from a shared familial environment, genome-wide association studies have suggested a shared genetic linkage between diabetes and both schizophrenia and bipolar disorder.[31]

Both the early and adult environment may contribute to the comorbidity. It is now well recognized that term infants who have a lower birth weight are at increased risk of developing a number of physical illnesses such as CVD, diabetes and osteoporosis in adulthood. Recent studies have also indicated that low birth weight is also a risk factor for adult mental illness.[32]

In adulthood, individuals with schizophrenia tend to consume diets that have higher fat and refined sugar content than the general population, while their fruit, fibre and vegetable intake is low.[33,34] This, coupled with decreased physical activity, may explain the increased prevalence of obesity in people with schizophrenia and predispose the individual to diabetes and CVD. Other important adult environmental factors linking the two conditions include smoking and urbanization.

It is unclear to what extent SMI per se directly increases the risk of diabetes and CVD, but metabolic abnormalities in association with altered body composition have been found in some but not all studies of antipsychotic-naive individuals with first-episode psychosis. Individuals with untreated psychosis have chronic elevations in stress hormones, which may increase the long-term risk of diabetes, obesity and CVD.[35]

The effect of second-generation antipsychotics on the morbidity and mortality of patients with SMI has been widely debated. There is clear evidence that people with SMI are at a higher risk of cardiometabolic dysfunction and antipsychotic-medication-related side-effects, such as increase in weight and metabolic disorders. It is argued that the advantages of antipsychotic medication resulting in reduction of symptoms need to be balanced against the associated side-effects. However, there is variation in the way patients respond to their medication and the degree of side-effects they experience. Therefore, clinical decision-making, initial assessment and regular review of side-effects and appropriate management using guidance are key to reducing the risk and improving clinical outcomes.[1,36] A large-scale 11-year cohort study in Finland, using 66 881 patients with schizophrenia reported that cumulative exposure to any antipsychotic drug for 7–11 years did not widen the gap in life expectancy between the patient group and the general population. The gap in life expectancy in 1996 was 25 years, compared to 22.5 years in 2006. Patients exposed to antipsychotics had a lower death rate (0.81, 95% CI = 0.77–0.84) compared to those with no drug use. The observed decline in the gap in life expectancy was in spite of a substantial increase in use of second-generation antipsychotics, from 12.6% in 1996 to 64% in 2006. There was an inverse relationship between duration of treatment and mortality. Clozapine use resulted in substantial reduction in mortality compared to other antipsychotics.[37]

Higher prevalence of mortality risk factors among people with SMI

People affected with schizophrenia experience high levels of all the top six World Health Organization (WHO) mortality risk factors – raised blood pressure, smoking, high blood glucose, sedentary lifestyle, obesity and dyslipidaemia, in that order, all of which are modifiable.[38] Compared to 33% in the general population in the UK, 61% and 46% of people with schizophrenia and bipolar disorder (respectively) smoke;[39] as a consequence, smoking-related premature death, heart disease and respiratory disorders are more common among people with SMI. A meta-analysis of studies across 20 countries demonstrated a consistent association between schizophrenia and current smoking (weighted average odds ratio (OR) = 5.9; 95% CI = CI 4.9 to 5.7).[40] The findings of Halbreich et al. in 1996 relating to smoking behaviour are consistent with the above.[41] This study further indicated that people with schizophrenia consumed higher-fat lower-fibre diets and engaged in less physical activity than the general population.[41] Halbreich and colleagues also found similar results relating to dietary habits among people with schizophrenia.[41] Consistent with the above findings, Fagiolini and Goracci in 2009[42] and Paton et al. in 2004[43] reported that less physical activity, unhealthy eating habits and smoking were more common among patients with SMI. A more recent community cohort study on individuals with schizophrenia reported a 73% rate of smoking (among those whose smoking status was recorded), which was twice that of the general population,[18] and further increases their risk of morbidity and mortality from physical illness.

Cardiovascular disease and severe mental illness

People with SMI have nearly twice the normal risk of dying from CVD.[18] More than two-thirds of patients with schizophrenia, compared with approximately one-half in the general population, die of coronary heart disease (CHD). The excess cardiovascular mortality associated with schizophrenia and bipolar disorder is attributed in part to an increased risk of the modifiable CHD risk factors: unhealthy lifestyles, obesity, smoking, diabetes, hypertension and dyslipidaemia.[1,9,24,44–46]

Despite the higher prevalence of the above risk factors and metabolic risks associated with antipsychotic drugs,[47] many patients with SMI have limited access to general health care, with less opportunity for CVD risk screening and prevention than would be expected in a non-psychiatric population.[1,26] Although many of these chronic conditions may be unavoidable given the current wealth of knowledge, many deaths in SMI are considered avoidable.[14,48] Increasing evidence shows that out of a range of contributing factors, disparities in health-care access and delivery are important contributors to excess mortality among people with SMI.[49] Reducing these risk factors requires a multidisciplinary holistic approach to enhance mental and physical well-being, in order to reduce the risk of physical comorbidity.[5]

Management of cardiovascular disease in primary care

An understanding of the risks of medical comorbidity is crucial for both primary care clinicians and patients with schizophrenia, in order to provide benefit from effective prevention, early diagnosis and timely care. This will improve the prognosis and outcomes of patients with SMI.[50]

The National Institute for Health and Clinical Excellence (NICE) Clinical Guidelines 82[33] and 67[51] provide guidance for assessment and management of cardiovascular risk among patients with SMI and place the responsibility for the management of physical health within primary care.

The Quality and Outcomes Framework related to severe mental illness

The Quality and Outcomes Framework (QOF),[52] a financial reward system to encourage primary care clinicians to provide high-quality care, was introduced in the UK in 2004, as part of the primary care contractual arrangements. The QOF covers four domains including clinical and patient experience. There are over 100 indicators, of which five are related to SMI as shown in Box 32.1. Currently, NICE has the responsibility for managing an independent process for developing and reviewing clinical and health improvement indicators on the QOF.[52] Primary care trusts (PCTs) in England have the responsibility for supervision and auditing of the QOF system. Elsewhere in the UK, health boards in Scotland, regional boards in Northern Ireland, and local health boards in Wales are responsible for this role.

Box 32.1   QOF indicators related to mental health[53]

- *MH 6:* The percentage of patients with schizophrenia, bipolar affective disorder and other psychoses on the register who have a comprehensive care plan documented in the records agreed between individuals, their family and/or carers as appropriate (Target – 50%)

- *MH 7:* The percentage of patients with schizophrenia, bipolar affective disorder and other psychoses who do not attend the practice for their annual review who are identified and followed up by the practice team within 14 days of non-attendance (Target – 90%)

- *MH 9:* The percentage of patients with schizophrenia, bipolar affective disorder and other psychoses with a review recorded in the preceding 15 months (in the review there should be evidence that the patient has been offered routine health-promotion and prevention advice appropriate to their age, sex and health status) (Target – 90%)

- *Smoking 3:* The percentage of patients with any or any combination of the following conditions: coronary heart disease, stroke or transient ischaemic attack (TIA), hypertension, diabetes, chronic obstructive pulmonary disease (COPD), chronic kidney disease (CKD), asthma, schizophrenia, bipolar affective disorder or other psychoses, whose notes record smoking status in the previous 15 months. (Target – 90%)

- *Smoking 4:* The percentage of patients with any or any combination of the following conditions: coronary heart disease, stroke or TIA, hypertension, diabetes, COPD, CKD, asthma, schizophrenia, bipolar affective disorder or other psychoses, who smoke, whose notes contain a record that smoking-cessation advice or referral to a specialist service, where available, has been offered within the previous 15 months (Target – 90%)

The QOF financial reward system has been reported as a cost-effective use of resources for a substantive proportion of general practitioner (GP) practices for most indicators that can be assessed.[54] However, primary care clinicians can "exception report" patients from an indicator for a number of reasons, which include:

- the patient not attending for a review or declining treatment
- the treatment is clinically inappropriate for a patient or the patient has been diagnosed recently or registered with the practice recently.

These criteria leave room for some clinicians to inappropriately "exception report" patients despite the fact that these patients may have a greater need for primary care compared to those who attend for regular review. This often includes patients needing high support and living in supported accommodation.

Just over a half a per cent of registered patients in England are being followed up or treated for a severe mental health problem in primary care. London[55] has a significantly higher proportion of registered patients receiving follow-up for SMI (0.6%) and follow-up and related quality of care varies across GP practices within the same

PCT areas within England. Therefore, assessment and management of cardiovascular risk factors and diabetes as part of the care of patients with SMI need to be improved by adopting proactive approaches to reduce variation across GP practices.

However, GPs cannot achieve this alone, as they are fully occupied with their current roles and have limited capacity to take on extra roles. There is a need to expand and train the workforce within general practice to include other staff such as practice nurses. Already, current UK evidence suggests that these nurses can play a key role in developing preventive activity within general practice.

A recent paper reported that some socioeconomically disadvantaged groups were more likely to be "exception reported" when these patients have failed to reply to primary care invitations or when they have refused to attend for review.[56] The authors recommend that primary care clinicians identify these patients proactively and review them appropriately to help achieve best outcomes through appropriate clinical care.[56] This is likely to be even more relevant to people with SMI, considering the socioeconomic and communication barriers they confront in responding in a timely manner, or complying with invitations to attend regular review, despite the fact that their need of care could be higher than that of others without SMI. However, this area needs to be researched further to obtain a clear picture and address variation if found. Working relationships between primary care, cardiologists, diabetologists and other specialists need to be strengthened to provide coordinated and seamless care.[1]

Clinical implications

- Primary care physicians should use proactive approaches to ensure that patients with SMI are not disadvantaged, by specifically targeting them in general practice with innovative and outreach approaches. This should include those in supported accommodation.

- Priorities are training of primary care clinicians, and administrative staff in practices, to address the barriers such as stigma and sociocultural aspects, and also close collaboration with sectors who are well equipped to work with these disadvantaged groups.

- Primary care clinicians should be provided with specific training to update their knowledge on psychiatry, in order to manage SMI patients more effectively within primary care.

- Health promotion needs be targeted at carers and family members as well, to enable them to reduce lifestyle risk factors in individuals with psychiatric illness at periods of relapse.

Diabetes and SMI

Diabetes mellitus was one of the first chronic diseases to be recognized in people with schizophrenia and in patients who use antipsychotic drugs.[28] There is evidence from studies in the USA and Europe that the prevalence of diabetes in people with schizophrenia and bipolar illness is about 10–15%, equivalent to a 2–3-fold increase compared with the general population.[57] Carney et al.,[19] in a US-based study population of commercially insured young people, showed that schizophrenia was not only associated with an increased OR for diabetes, but also with an increase in diabetes-related complications compared with controls (OR 2.11, 95% CI = 1.36 to 3.28). It is acknowledged that there is a high prevalence of undiagnosed diabetes within the general population; however, the burden appears to be higher among people with SMI, among whom up to 70% of all cases of diabetes are undiagnosed.[58] The particularly large number of undiagnosed cases of diabetes among this group of people may be due to the challenges they may encounter in accessing physical health services and their reluctance to volunteer symptoms.[1]

Much attention has been paid to the effect of antipsychotics on the risk of developing diabetes, but overall there is a dearth of high-quality studies examining whether the association is causative. Though a small number of individuals have developed diabetes soon after commencing treatment with antipsychotics, the risk overall seems low and most people on antipsychotic treatment will not develop diabetes as a result of their treatment.[59]

Table 32.1 summarizes the results from a number of studies that show the prevalence and OR of diabetes mellitus among patients with SMI. It can be seen that diabetes is more prevalent among patients with schizophrenia and patients on treatment with antipsychotic medication.

Table 32.1 The prevalence and odds ratio (OR) of diabetes mellitus among patients with severe mental illness

Study	Result
Retrospective analysis of data and interviews of large populations of persons with schizophrenia and the general population from 1991 to 1996 in the USA[60]	Diabetes was more prevalent among patients with schizophrenia even before the advent of atypical antipsychotic drugs.
Retrospective cohort study of 59 089 conventional antipsychotic users; 9053 atypical antipsychotic users; and 1 491 548 controls from a UK general practice database from 1994 to 2002[61]	Treatment with antipsychotics is associated with an increased risk of developing diabetes. The hazard ratio of diabetes mellitus in conventional antipsychotic users and atypical antipsychotic users was 1.9 and 2.9 respectively.
Retrospective cohort study in a general practice database of 2071 patients on haloperidol, 266 patients on olanzapine, 567 patients on risperidone, 109 patients on quetiapine and 6012 controls, from 1996 to 2002 in Italy[62]	Treatment with antipsychotics is associated with an increased risk of developing diabetes. The hazard ratio of diabetes mellitus in patients on haloperidol was 12.4; olanzapine was 20.4; risperidone was 18.7; and quetiapine was 33.7.
Case-control study of 424 newly diagnosed diabetes mellitus patients versus 1522 controls in the UK General Practice Research Database from 1994 to 1999[63]	Treatment with antipsychotics increased the risk of developing diabetes. OR = 1.7 of incident diabetes mellitus in patients with current antipsychotic use.

There is an increased rate of obesity among those with SMI,[64,65] and they are at higher risk of obesity-related morbidity. As a consequence of obesity, the patient's self-esteem is likely to be reduced and there may be poor concordance with psychiatric treatment.[66] On the other hand, obesity could be a risk factor for developing SMI. A population survey of data in the USA found that people who are obese are at 50% higher risk of developing bipolar disorder, while the increased risk of having panic disorders or agoraphobia is 25%.[67]

A combination of sedentary lifestyle, poor dietary behaviour and psychiatric medication contribute to this condition.[8] Significant weight gain is a side-effect of all antipsychotic medication but especially clozapine and olanzapine.[68] With second-generation antipsychotics, however, the weight gain varies with the individual, thus making predictions about weight change difficult. The risk of weight gain seems higher in those with tendency to overeat in time of stress, those with past history of obesity, first-episode patients and younger individuals. The most reliable predictor of weight gain appears to be weight gain in the early weeks of treatment.[69]

Challenges

A higher rate of lifestyle risk factors, poor access and lack of coordination of psychiatric services and medical management are all issues that leave these patients with undetected medical conditions. It has been reported repeatedly that half of all long-term conditions go unrecognized in patients with schizophrenia.[1,19,70,71] People with SMI are also less likely than healthy individuals to report physical symptoms spontaneously.[50] When they do present, stigma and their lack of social skills make it less likely they will receive good care.[72] Studies suggest that mental health professionals often miss medical illnesses in their patients with SMI and rarely undertake physical examinations of these patients.[73]

Clinical implications

Though prevention and management of obesity in people with SMI is difficult, it can be tackled. There is sufficient evidence from studies that behaviour change through advice about physical activity and diet is as effective in weight reduction or prevention of weight gain among patients with SMI as it is in the general population.[66] In most studies, the effectiveness of these behaviour-change programmes was brought about by group interventions that created peer support. Expert groups recommend the need for all patients with SMI who are overweight or obese to be provided with or referred to diet and exercise counselling or specialist weight-management programmes, particularly at the commencement of treatment with a second-generation antipsychotic.[74]

Chronic obstructive pulmonary disease and severe mental illness

COPD accounts for nearly 60% of all smoking-attributable disease.[75] It is hugely underdetected nationally, regionally and at GP practice level in the UK. People with SMI are likely to be at high risk for developing this disease because of their higher rate of smoking, which is a modifiable risk factor. Underdetection among people with SMI may be even greater because of lack of awareness of symptoms of COPD, added to communication barriers that exist even when this group comes into contact with primary care.

Himelhoch et al. reported a 22.6% prevalence of COPD among those with SMI compared to 5% for COPD in the general US population for a similar age group.[76] In the SMI group, 60.5% were current smokers – significantly above the national average.[76] Another UK review also reported higher rates of COPD among patients with schizophrenia compared to control groups.[77]

Table 32.2 summarises the results of studies of the prevalence of COPD in patients with SMI.

Table 32.2 Summary of studies showing the prevalence and odds ratio of COPD among patients with severe mental illness	
Study	**Result**
Cross-sectional comparative study involving 147 patients with SMI in a cross-sectional comparative study of Medicaid claims from 1996 to 2000 in USA[21]	74% of the patients were treated for a chronic physical illness, and chronic pulmonary disease was most prevalent (31%).
Literature review of 1074 patients with schizophrenia or schizoaffective disorder versus 726 262 controls from 1996 to 2002[23]	COPD, complicated diabetes mellitus, hypothyroidism, hepatitis C and arthritis were more prevalent in the schizophrenia or schizoaffective group. OR = 1.88 (95% CI = 1.51 to 2.32), 2.11 (95% CI = 1.36 to 3.28), 2.62 (95% CI = 2.09 to 3.28), 7.54 (95% CI = 3.55 to 15.99) and 1.40 (95% CI = 1.04 to 1.89), respectively.

Clinical implications

The NICE clinical guideline on COPD provides evidence-based interventions for delivering care for patients with COPD in primary care.[78] Screening of high-risk groups for COPD through spirometry is a key clinical requirement of this guideline. A higher prevalence of smoking is mainly responsible for COPD, and other respiratory conditions are more prevalent among patients with SMI, highlighting the need for improved interventions on smoking among high-risk groups such as patients with SMI.

Severe mental illness and osteoporosis

Osteoporosis is a major public health concern among people with SMI. Some studies have found decreased bone mineral density (osteopenia or osteoporosis) in people with schizophrenia compared to normal controls.[79–82] One reason for this finding is that many antipsychotic drugs increase the serum prolactin concentration. A sedentary lifestyle and lack of exercise on account of decreased spontaneity and other negative symptoms that are frequent in schizophrenia; smoking, alcohol and drug abuse; dietary and vitamin deficiencies; decreased exposure to sunshine; and polydipsia inducing electrolyte imbalance have all been mentioned as factors that may lead to reduced bone mineral density.[41] The problems of osteoporosis in people with schizophrenia remain serious, although preventive measures that should be implemented include an adequate diet, weight-bearing exercise, oestrogen- or testosterone-replacement therapy as necessary, and the avoidance of prolactin-increasing antipsychotic drugs where possible. There is evidence that people with schizophrenia receive less care for their osteoporosis than age-matched controls.[83]

Clinical implications

Dual X-ray absorptiometry (DEXA) may not be readily available in all health systems and there are no guidelines on screening for osteoporosis by DEXA in people with SMI. It appears reasonable to consider

DEXA for people who have mental illness as well as other risk factors. It is, however, imperative for people with SMI to be given advice about the need for adequate intake of calcium and vitamin D. They should also be given advice about the importance of regular weight-bearing exercise. Pharmacological therapy with bisphosphonates can also be given to people with mental illness who have low bone mineral density, in the same way as it is prescribed for the general population. As peak bone mineral density is often not reached until the early 20s, it is advisable to avoid treating younger patients with prolactin-raising antipsychotics, in order to reduce their risk of developing osteoporosis later in life. It is reasonable to use the oral contraceptive pill in amenorrhoeic premenopausal women, in order to maintain skeletal integrity if it is not possible to change or reduce the dose of their antipsychotic medication.[79]

Hypothyroidism and severe mental illness

An increased occurrence of hypothyroidism among patients with schizophrenia was first indicated in a population-based study using commercially insured people in the USA (OR = 2.62%, 95% CI = 2.09 to 3.28).[19] However, this finding may not be applicable to non-insured populations and racial and ethnic minority groups.[19] Analysis of National Hospital Discharge Survey (NHDS) data in the USA showed that acquired hypothyroidism was nearly three times more prevalent among discharged patients with a primary diagnosis of schizophrenia,[24] although reasons for this association remain unclear.

Severe mental illness and the prevalence of human immunodeficiency virus, hepatitis B and hepatitis C

People with SMI are at significantly increased risk for infection with human immunodeficiency virus (HIV), hepatitis C virus or both. Increased rates of HIV infection in patients with SMI have been reported; one study conducted in the USA reported rates almost eight times (3.1% versus 0.4%) that of the general population.[78] Though there is insufficient evidence to prove that rates of infection with hepatitis B (HBV) and C (HCV) virus are also higher among people with SMI, the same study suggests HBV prevalence and HCV prevalence could be about 5 and 11 times (respectively) higher than in the general population.[84]

Although overall sexual activity is lower in people with SMI, those who are sexually active tend to engage in higher-risk behaviour than the general population. This probably reflects an inadequate knowledge and understanding of the risks of HIV and hepatitis. It is thought that the emotional instability associated with mental illness, as well as factors such as homelessness encountered by these people, increase high-risk behaviour for infection.[85,86] The risk of infection is also thought to be higher in women than men.[87,88]

Clinical implications

It is clearly important that a person with mental illness understands the danger of engaging in high-risk sexual activity. The delivery of relevant factual information is often insufficient to bring about behavioural changes that reduce the risk of exposure and transmission and so there is a responsibility to encourage the practice of safe sex. Prevention services should develop sexual health education and other prevention interventions tailored to suit people with SMI.[87-89] Also, provision of high-quality and effective clinical care for people with SMI needs to be ensured at all levels of care.

For those who develop either HIV or hepatitis, effective pharmacotherapy exists, and antipsychotics and highly active antiretroviral treatments for HIV can be used together successfully.

Severe mental illness and cancer

Patients with SMI are known to be at increased risk of mortality from cancer.[90] This increased risk may be attributable to the physical, psychological and social problems associated with their poor mental state. As mentioned, this group of people are less likely to report symptoms and follow up treatment adequately. Results from a study of 933 women with psychiatric illness and 44 195 women without psychiatric illness aged 50–64 years conducted in the UK from 1996 to 1998, showed that women who had multiple detentions (OR = 0.40; 95% CI = 0.29 to 0.55) and diagnosis of psychosis (OR = 0.33; 95% CI = 0.18 to 0.61) were less likely to attend screening for breast cancer.

Clinical implications

Health-care personnel involved in the care of people with mental illness should be more proactive at ensuring that people with mental illness attend cancer screening programmes and follow-up sessions when due.

Physical comorbidity and severe mental illness among racial and ethnic minority groups

Previous sections highlighted the inequalities experienced by the SMI population compared to non-SMI groups. However, there is increasing evidence that some groups within the SMI population such as ethnic minority groups, socioeconomically deprived and older populations experience more physical health problems. For example, a nationally representative sample in the USA indicated that SMI disproportionately affects a greater percentage of ethnic minority groups compared to those with other disorders and those with no psychiatric condition.[91] In addition. they are more likely to have a higher prevalence of SMI and experience poor access to care.[91-93] Consistent with the above, the Clinical Antipsychotic Trials in Intervention Effectiveness (CATIE) study also demonstrated that ethnic minority groups with SMI had a higher percentage of patients with abnormal metabolic conditions who did not receive treatment, compared to non-ethnic minorities with SMI.[94] The percentage of participants who had dyslipidaemia, hypertension and diabetes who were not treated was 88.2%, 62.4% and 30.2% respectively, although racial and ethnic groups reported higher rates for all three conditions – 96%, 79% and 50% respectively.[94] Sociocultural factors, economic deprivation and social exclusion associated with ethnic minority groups are likely to be partly responsible for these disparities. On the other hand, higher predisposition to develop diabetes and hypertension among some ethnic minority groups (people with South Asian and Black Caribbean origin respectively) may also be a contributing factor for this variation.[95-97]

The influence of culture on clinical care for people with severe mental illness and somatic comorbidity

Culture has a great influence on health behaviour. It affects perceptions, the way of coping with physical and mental illness, the way people access health care and the way of interacting with clinicians through influencing the expectations and preferences of both parties.[98-100] This is particularly relevant for people with SMI with cognitive and social impairment, who are confronted with more cultural issues, such as stigma.[101] For example, a study undertaken within six community mental health organizations in Manhattan serving a diverse group of ethnic minority groups with SMI provided insight into how cultural elements within patients, providers and systems influenced patient experience.[102] Participants included service users (66), clinicians (25), administrators (21) and families/carers. Multiple methods of data collection were used, including participant observation, and analytical rigour was obtained through triangulation of sources of data, audit trail and consultation with experts. The authors concluded that efforts to join up mental health and primary care need to be designed around the culture of the organization, considering the cultural factors and clarifying clear lines of responsibility for different professionals to provide seamless care for patients from a diverse range of demographic backgrounds. They also emphasized the need to recognize and overcome service users' mistrust, through provision of culturally competent communication skills training for providers to ensure effective patient–clinician interactions.[102] The findings were used to develop a conceptual framework (see Figure 32.1). This demonstrates how an existing health-care intervention or a new intervention could be made culturally competent to enhance the physical health of people with SMI.

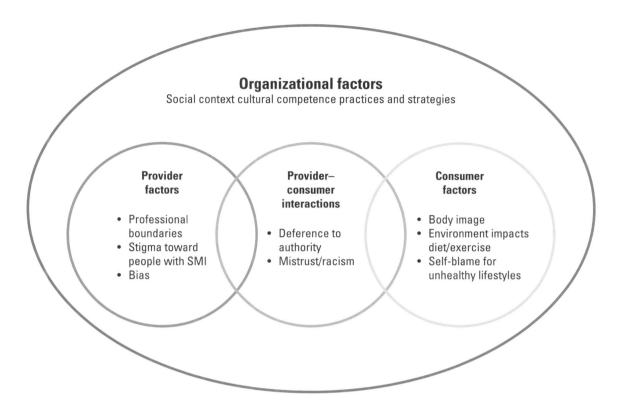

Figure 32.1 Cultural elements in the health care of people with severe mental illness. Adapted, with permission, from Cabassa LJ. NYS Center of Excellence for Cultural Competence New York State Psychiatric Institute Department of Psychiatry, Columbia University New York State Office of Mental Health: Bureau of Cultural Competence. *Improving the physical health of Latinos and African Americans with serious mental illnes*s. Webinar Series sponsored by New York State Office of Mental Health: Bureau of Cultural Competence (http://nyspi.org/culturalcompetence/what/documents/ImprovingthePhysicalHealthofLatinosandAfrican AmericanswithSeriousMentalIllness.pdf)[102]

Incompatibility between the social context of an organization (which includes professional boundaries, service user–clinician interaction and patient factors) and an innovative service development could have a negative impact on delivering and maintaining the sustainability of a service. Hence, any service redesign needs to identify cultural factors influencing the patient, provider and patient–provider interaction.[102]

Interventions aimed at patients with severe mental illness and physical comorbidity

Mental illness accounts for approximately 12% of the current global disease burden and it is predicted that this figure will rise to approximately 15% by 2020, with much of the burden being projected to occur in low-income countries.[7] Some argue that the consequences of mental ill-health could be even greater in these countries, considering the higher level of stigma and myths, combined with an absence of community safety networks.[103]

Considering the negative impact of the current and increasing burden of medical conditions among people with SMI, there is a strong need for policy-makers and professional bodies to place greater emphasis on primary and secondary prevention, detection of risk factors, and early diagnosis and intervention for physical illness in this patient group.[9]

Higher occurrence of physical illness comorbidity among patients with severe mental disorder

Previous sections provide convincing evidence on existing inequalities among patients with SMI and comorbid medical conditions. However, it is of concern that some subgroups within this wider mental health patient population experience even higher levels of disadvantage in terms of higher incidence, late detection of physical illness, reduced access to services, suboptimal quality of care, and worse clinical outcomes.[110–112] Some of these groups include black and minority ethnic (BME) groups, older people, women, the prison population and asylum seekers.[113–115]

A prospective case-control study, Aetiology and Ethnicity of Schizophrenia and Other Psychoses (AeSOP), undertaken over a 2-year period from 1997 among 16–64-year-old residents in Nottingham, south east London and Bristol, showed that BME groups had a significantly higher incidence rate of bipolar affective disorder compared to their white counterparts.[110] UK evidence also indicates that black ethnic groups are more likely to be inpatients and to have been admitted through crisis routes with more complex care pathways compared to their counterparts.[111] The variation partly explained the greater use of specialist care.[111]

Lifestyle interventions in improving the physical health of people with severe mental illness

Encouraging healthy lifestyle behaviours is a vital component in the process of recovery from SMI.[112] Implementing appropriately designed well-planned, culturally sensitive interventions that facilitate patients with SMI to engage in physical activity, healthy eating and weight-management behaviour is a vital component in promoting physical health in this group. However, some authors argue that ethnic minorities are not well represented in research on lifestyle interventions among this group and that adequate consideration has not been given to cultural and language-related issues.[113] This is particularly relevant as there is consistent evidence from the UK and the USA that certain ethnic minority groups are at a higher risk of developing SMI and also diabetes and CVD.[58,114]

The ability of people with SMI to achieve healthy lifestyle changes and experience substantive improvement in their health and well-being is well recognized.[112] A number of intervention studies aimed at addressing patient-, clinician- and system-related barriers have demonstrated promising results and these are discussed next.

Primary Care Access, Referral and Evaluation (PCARE) study

PCARE, a randomized controlled trial (RCT) to test a population-based care-management intervention designed to improve primary medical care in community mental health settings through a pioneering model, provided promising results.[115] This study included 407 patients with SMI receiving mental health care in a community mental health centre, who were randomly assigned to either the medical care-management intervention or routine care. The intervention consisted of two trained care managers providing support in overcoming patient-, clinician- and system-related barriers by facilitating improved access to primary care through a combination of advocacy, education and helping patients to overcome logistical barriers to access care. No direct medical services were provided. Self-management skills of patients were developed using motivational interviewing techniques rather than persuading them to change behaviours. This process also involved goal setting and action plans agreed with patients, relating to medical care or lifestyle behaviour change, as well as assisting patients to engage as active partners in managing their own health issues. Assessment of the quality of primary care was undertaken at baseline and one-year follow-up using evidence-based indicators across four domains of primary care, which included:

- physical examination
- screening tests
- vaccinations
- education, including lifestyles and self-examination.

There were significant improvements in the quality and outcomes of primary care in the PCARE intervention group at one-year follow-up.

Members of the intervention group:

- were more likely to have a primary care provider (71.2% versus 51.9%)
- were exposed to twice the rate of preventive interventions in primary care (58.7% versus 21.8%)
- experienced a higher proportion of quality cardiometabolic care (34.9% versus 27.7%)
- demonstrated significant improvements in quality of life related to mental health.

Furthermore, detection of previously undiagnosed physical illness was significantly greater in the intervention group (11.9%) than in the usual care group (1.8%) (χ^2 = 10.75, P = 0.005). Hypertension and hyperlipidaemia were the most commonly found newly detected conditions. These findings suggest that care management is a promising approach for improving medical care for patients treated in community mental health settings.

Community Care of North Carolina

Through structured partnership working between funding bodies, primary care clinicians, and local healthcare providers, community health networks could have a place in the holistic management of patients with SMI. Such an intervention was implemented by the Community Care of North Carolina (CCNC) for patients with chronic illnesses on Medicaid. With this approach, the CCNC was able to realize savings, especially in emergency department utilization, outpatient care and pharmacy.[116] The CCNC successfully combined:

- linking patients to a medical home
- ensuring quality improvement among participating practices
- appointing case managers to help follow up on treatment recommendations and lifestyle changes as advised by the primary care clinician for high-risk patients
- intervention planning and measurement of success
- providing a statewide programme while still maintaining local control.

The local control was a vital aspect of the programme because it encouraged regional creativity and ownership, which sustained the programme.

Bipolar disorder medical care model

In an RCT conducted between March and June 2006 in Pittsburgh USA, a combined programme of patient education on self-management, behavioural change to reduce cardiovascular risk factors and encouragement of provider engagement delivered as a bipolar disorder medical care model in 27 patients with bipolar disorder demonstrated a slowing down of the deterioration in physical health-related quality of life compared to 31 patients with bipolar disorder who received usual care (t = 2.01, df = 173, P = 0.04).[20] A vital intervention could be the involvement of case/care managers who actively followed up on cases in both programmes. To overcome the identified challenge of poor clinical integration in the care of people with SMI, a conceptual framework for integrated care that includes information-sharing among health-care providers with a shared understanding of goals and roles, all working together in order to meet all the health-care needs of the patient effectively, is likely to work.[117]

Health-promotion interventions

Though there is a dearth of quantitative evidence that lifestyle modifications including smoking cessation, physical activity and healthy diet programmes can reduce mortality in patients with SMI, it is most likely that members of this group also have the potential to benefit, as lifestyle modification has been proven to work in the general population.[38] Increasing evidence shows that individualized, dedicated and innovative interventions to address barriers confronted by patients with SMI, to promote patient engagement and boost self-confidence could foster those achieving beneficial effects from such interventions.[8]

A systematic literature review undertaken by the New York State Psychiatric Institute to examine the impact of lifestyle interventions on health outcomes of people with SMI found promising results that lifestyle interventions could be effective for people with SMI.[113] Twenty-two eligible studies carried out in the USA between 1980 and 2009 were reviewed; nine were RCTs. For 12 studies (54.6%), participants comprised only those with schizophrenia or schizoaffective disorders, while the rest included other conditions including major depression and anxiety disorders in addition to the previous two conditions. Nine studies (40.9%) were small-scale single-site, efficacy trials, with only one study recruiting 309 participants. All interventions were aimed at improving knowledge, developing skills and supporting sustainable behaviours relating to healthy eating, physical activity and weight management, using a range of health-care staff delivering the interventions – both individual and group based. All lifestyle interventions were derived from previously existing initiatives aimed at the general population (e.g. Diabetes Prevention Programme and Weight Watchers). Most interventions included a range of behaviour-change techniques, including goal-setting, problem-solving, motivational counselling, assertiveness training, rewards/token reinforcements and risk/benefit comparisons, and involved interactive and fun-based methods to meet the cognitive and motivational impairment of people with SMI, using a media mix. Statistically significant improvements relating to CVD risk factors including systolic and diastolic blood pressure, blood glucose, triglycerides and/or central obesity were evident in six out of 12 studies investigating the impact of lifestyle interventions on cardiovascular risk factors. Similarly, statistically significant weight reductions were observed among those who received a structured lifestyle intervention, and treatment in 10 out of 18 studies involving interventions aimed at weight management. Only studies with interventions lasting between 24 and 48 weeks demonstrated significant weight loss.[113]

"In SHAPE" personalized health-promotion intervention

A one-year pilot called "In SHAPE", a personalized multifaceted health-promotion intervention aimed at improving diet and physical activity behaviour, involving 76 adults with SMI, delivered in community mental health settings in New Hampshire USA, showed significant improvements in lifestyle-related behaviour and reported improvements in mental health functioning and negative symptoms.[118] The programme was based on the assumption that compliance and the effectiveness and efficiency of interventions are improved when they are personalized to meet the needs, abilities and preferences of the service users. Social inclusion and community integration were integral to the intervention, which was delivered by "health mentors" – fitness trainers who were provided with adequate knowledge of SMI and additionally trained on goal setting, motivational interviewing and healthy eating behaviours. Intervention was provided in mainstream community settings over a period of 9 months.[118]

Interventions involved the following:

- personalized fitness and diet plans jointly agreed between the health mentor and the participant, based on each individual's initial assessment of fitness status, personal fitness goals, dietetic behaviour and preferred type of physical activity and the setting
- weekly one-to-one sessions with participants to review the progress of behaviour change and goals, in order to skill them up to address the motivational challenges they faced and to reinforce and acknowledge positive changes in behaviour
- instructing participants how to accommodate the challenges of cognitive social handicaps commonly seen among patients with SMI
- funding to use local physical activity facilities
- incentives for achieving fitness and healthy eating goals and motivational celebrations
- proactive outreach to encourage re-engagement of dropouts whenever necessary.

Compared to the baseline assessment, post-intervention comparison at 9 months showed a significant increase in the level of exercise, vigorous activity and leisure walking ($P < 0.01$) and a trend towards improved readiness to reduce calorie intake ($P < 0.053$). Reflecting these changes, the waist circumference of participants decreased significantly from the baseline value (103.8 ± 15.9 cm versus 100.6 ± 20.1 cm at 9 months $P = 0.046$). Further, satisfaction with physical fitness also improved by an average of 0.8 points on a Likert scale rating, with statistically significant improvement from the baseline (2.7 ± 1.4 and 3.5 ± 1.6 at 9 months, $P = 0.001$). Moreover, mental health functioning (measured by the SF-12 MCS (Short Form 12-item Mental Component Summary)) also improved ($P = 0.024$), together with a reduction in the severity of negative symptoms ($P = 0.003$). However, there was no significant reduction in blood pressure among 13 participants included in this part of the analysis (6.3 ± 18.5 mmHg reduction in systolic blood pressure (effect size = -0.49).[118]

Success factors for behaviour change in "In SHAPE"

A subsequent qualitative investigation nested within the above quantitative study was undertaken by Shiner et al. in 2008, to examine which components of the intervention participants perceived as most influential in achieving improvements in physical activity behaviour.[8] Eight participants out of 24 who had achieved improvement were used for this analysis, which involved one-hour individual interviews. Three main themes emerged regarding participants' views of what led to their success in the intervention:

- personalized interventions to encourage engagement in the programme

- relationships established with health mentors
- strengthened self-confidence facilitated through different approaches.

Basic primary care plus wellness training: health-promotion intervention

An RCT using a health-promotion intervention – basic primary care plus wellness training delivered over a period of 12 months for people with SMI – showed significant changes compared to a group who received only basic primary care. Intervention was aimed at addressing the cognitive deficits of patients by skilling them in self-management. A total of 309 participants were recruited to the study during a short-term residential treatment programme, and assessment of perceived health status (SF -36), global assessment of function and self-efficacy was undertaken at baseline and at 6, 12 and 18 months through interviews. Analysis, undertaken by using multilevel regression to investigate differences by group across time while controlling for health-related confounding factors, showed that people with SMI had significantly better improvements in perceived health status (SF-36) and general health scales.[119]

Key points from previous research

The above examples provide details of some of the interventions undertaken to address the patient-, provider- and system-related barriers experienced by patients with SMI in order to improve access to services for this group with a greater need compared to those without these conditions. These interventions have recognized that people with SMI could make changes to their behaviours to benefit their health and well-being, as suggested by Richardson et al.[112] Interventions have included personalization, better integration of services, and enhancement of communication, training and education for health-care professionals, provision of incentives for achieving goals, financial support to attend services, care planning and coordination. Although these studies were mainly based in the USA, which limits generalizability, the concepts used and barriers addressed are similar to those in other countries, particularly in relation to integrated working,[120] personalization, coordination, care planning, self-management, proactive outreach and rewarding achievements in behaviour change. The financial assistance provided for participants of the In SHAPE intervention is noteworthy, as people with SMI generally experience financial difficulties due to poor employability. In addition, these approaches required multidisciplinary partnership work across organizational boundaries and innovative and culturally sensitive initiatives to target hard-to-reach groups, who experience poor access and suboptimal quality of care, to ensure existing inequalities are narrowed.

Conclusions

People with SMI have increased risk of physical comorbidity and premature death compared to the general population. The most commonly observed long-term conditions are diabetes, obesity, CVD and COPD. These patients also experience significantly higher rates of the WHO-recognized mortality risk factors, including smoking, hypertension, high cholesterol and physical inactivity, all of which are modifiable. Further, they experience disparities in access to and receipt of optimal clinical care compared to those without SMI. Suboptimal care is caused by a number of clinician-, system- and patient-related factors, which could be addressed through effective strategies. These include integration of mental health and primary care with a clear line of responsibility; care coordination, emphasizing the need for clinicians to look proactively for early signs of SMI-related physical illness, minimizing medication-related side-effects through initial assessment; regular monitoring of cardiometabolic disorders in primary care; and appropriate referral to lifestyle services.

Improving knowledge on continuing inequalities related to SMI and physical illness, and training of administrators and clinicians on culturally appropriate communication skills would facilitate effective use of existing services to improve clinical and patient outcomes. While emphasis on adherence to evidence-based guidance and protocols in provision of care plays a significant role, clinicians need to make sure the services are equitable for diverse and disadvantaged communities, if necessary by provision of outreach care. Addressing patient-related factors through education; skilling patients to overcome barriers; personalization of services; goal setting; care planning; self-management; rewarding achievements; and continuous support through peer educators, care managers and health mentors would ensure continuity of care and enhance the quality of care and outcomes. This group of patients deserves the best care to compensate for a range of adverse factors affecting their quality of life and ability to live to their full potential. Increasing evidence on effective interventions provides promising results, and medical professionals have a duty to make sure this evidence is put into practice to make a difference to these patients' lives and to ensure mental health care is affordable.

Depression and physical health

Introduction

It is well recognized that depression and physical illness are strongly associated: good physical health contributes to mental well-being, and vice versa. Higher rates of depression have been found in populations with a wide range of chronic physical diseases, including, respiratory, renal, coronary and vascular disease, epilepsy, Parkinson disease, HIV/AIDS and cancer.[121,122] Furthermore, people who have depression as well as a physical illness are at risk of worse outcomes, including increased mortality.[116]

An expert panel of European clinicians and policy-makers[5] has concluded that, despite the wealth of research evidence, the bidirectional impacts of mental health on physical health have not been recognized well enough and that this has led to both missed opportunities for intervention and the creation of gaps in the care of certain groups of people. Physically ill people may not receive treatment for their depression and the physical health of those with diagnosed depression may be neglected.[122]

In the UK, recognition of this problem has led to the development of guidelines for the management of depression in adults with chronic physical health problems,[122] and, for a brief time, to the provision of incentives for GPs to screen for depression in CHD and diabetes. In low- and middle-income countries, where commonly over 75% of people with mental disorders receive no treatment or care at all, and less than 2% of the health budget is spent on mental health,[123] consideration of the mental health of people with a physical illness is likely to be a low priority.

Physical consequences of depression

Rates of depression

Depression as a primary diagnosis is common, with a lifetime prevalence ranging from 2% to 15%.[124,125] In primary care, rates are higher because the population studied is mainly presenting with health problems. In a review of 118 studies assessing the accuracy of GPs' diagnoses of depression,[126] the prevalence of depression for adults aged 18 to 65 years was 18.4%; this increased to 27.6% when older adults (>65 years) were included. The prevalence varied between countries, being highest in the Netherlands (13.5% to 33.3%) and lowest in Australia (5.0% to 17.0%).[120]

Morbidity

Worldwide, depression is a major cause of disease burden, accounting for almost 12% of the total years lived with disability.[124] Depression ranks third among the leading causes of disability worldwide. In terms of overall burden of disease, worldwide and unipolar depression makes the third largest contribution to this burden; in low-income countries it is the eighth largest contributor.[127] For women, however, depression is the leading cause of disease burden in both high-income and low- and middle-income countries. There are effective pharmacological and psychological treatments for depression. Antidepressant drugs are tolerated by most, but they are not without adverse effects. Older drugs – tricyclic antidepressants (TCAs) are especially associated with dry mouth, constipation and dizziness. These effects are lower in people taking selective serotonin reuptake inhibitors (SSRIs), which are the current preferred option, but nausea, diarrhoea, anxiety, agitation, insomnia, nervousness and headache are more common with these drugs.[118] Sexual dysfunction has been reported as a side-effect of all antidepressants,[129] which may impact greatly on quality of life.

As well as negative emotions, depression is associated with a wide range of impacts on physical and psychosocial functioning, both at home and in the workplace.[130] Adverse effects on functioning and quality of life are seen in both major depression and milder forms of the disorder.[131] Other impacts of depression that contribute to disability and reduced quality of life are insomnia, daytime sleepiness and fatigue.[132] Cognitive dysfunction may also be a problem, especially in terms of reduced attention and executive function.[132] Many people with depression also report somatic symptoms, including pain.[133]

Mortality

People with depression are at a greater risk of early death. In a meta-analysis of 25 studies,[134] which included 106 628 people who were depressed, who had an overall relative risk of dying of 1.81 (95% CI = 1.58 to 2.07) was found in depressed compared to non-depressed people. A further important finding of this study was that the increased risk exists not only in major depression, but also in subclinical forms of depression.[134] The rate of excess mortality from depression in a study of more than 60 000 Norwegians[135] was found to be similar to that from smoking in the general population.[5] Depression should therefore be considered as a life-threatening disorder. Depression is a major risk factor for suicide. About 21% of people with depressive disorders will attempt suicide; many will be successful.[136] On average, about 800 000 people commit suicide every year, of whom 86% are in low- and middle-income countries.[137] Worldwide, suicide accounts for nearly 1% of all deaths, and nearly two-thirds of these occur in people who have a depressive disorder.[136]

Depression, in common with other mental disorders, may also be associated with adverse health behaviours, such as smoking, poor diet and lack of exercise, which may lead to reduced quality of life, increased risk of disease and, eventually, death. Approximately 60% of the excess mortality associated with depression is explained by physical ill health.[5] People with depression may be less likely to access health care for treatment or screening because of social isolation, fear of stigma and concerns about "wasting the doctor's time";[123] they may also be less motivated to adhere to treatment regimens.[138] Depression may also be associated with physiological changes that increase the risk of disease and death. Depressive disorders have been found to adversely affect endocrine, neurologic and immune responses by increasing sympathetic tone, decreasing vagal tone and causing immunosuppression.[134] Inflammatory markers and hypothalamic-pituitary-adrenal axis dysregulation[121] have also been associated with depressive symptoms. In a longitudinal study of 4681 older adults (aged 65 years or more) without diabetes,[139] a single report of high depressive symptoms, an increase in symptoms with time, and persistently high symptoms over time were each associated with an excess incidence of diabetes. These associations persisted even when controlling for known risk factors for diabetes, such as body mass index, physical activity, cigarette smoking, alcohol intake, and C-reactive protein level. Similarly, people with depression are also at increased risk of CHD. Two systematic reviews have shown that depression among healthy individuals increases the risk of subsequent CHD by approximately 60% (RR = 1.64), even after controlling for other cardiac risk factors.[140,141] The exact mechanisms that predispose individuals with depression to physical illness are not understood fully and more research is needed.

Comorbidity: physical illness and depression

People with physical illness are also at increased risk of becoming depressed

In people with comorbid physical illness, the prevalence of depression is increased compared with the general population.[142,143] In a study of more than 245 000 people in 60 countries, an average of between 9.3% and 23.0% of participants with one or more chronic physical diseases had comorbid depression.[143] An increased incidence of depression has been reported in people with a wide range of chronic physical conditions, and rates of depression vary between them. In diabetes and CHD, rates of depression are particularly increased, with depression twice as prevalent as in the general population.[144,145]

Increased morbidity in depression comorbid with physical illness

When depression is comorbid with physical illness, morbidity is increased; in the above study,[143] it was consistent across countries and people with different demographic characteristics that those with depression comorbid with one or more chronic diseases had worse health scores than those with angina, arthritis, asthma or diabetes alone. Those with diabetes and depression were most disabled.[143]

People with comorbid depression and physical illness have worse outcomes than those with either condition alone.[146] For instance, depression in individuals with established CHD predicts further coronary events (OR = 2.0) and greater impairment in health-related quality of life.[144,147] There is also evidence that individuals who develop depression following acute coronary syndrome, as opposed to those with depression that predates the acute coronary syndrome, may be at particularly high risk of worse cardiac outcomes.[148–150] Furthermore, concurrent physical illness is known to reduce the likelihood of major depression being recognized by GPs,[151,152] so individuals with both conditions may not receive appropriate care.

Increased mortality in depression comorbid with physical illness

For a range of physical illnesses, findings suggest an increased risk of death when comorbid depression is present.[153] For example, depressed individuals with CHD are more than twice as likely to die as those with CHD alone.[145,147] An association between comorbid depression and an increased risk of death has been found in heart failure, even after controlling for disease severity.[154,157] There is also consistent evidence of increased mortality in those with comorbid depression and diabetes,[158,159] chronic kidney disease[160] or cancer.[161] The severity of depression is important, with those with more severe depression at greatest risk of death. For instance, in a 3-year follow-up study of 4154 patients with diabetes,[159] minor depression was associated with a 1.67-fold increase in mortality, and major depression was associated with a 2.30-fold increase compared with non-depressed patients and after adjustment for age, sex, race/ethnicity and educational attainment. Similarly, in an 18-month follow-up study of 958 hospitalized patients with heart failure,[162] severe, but not moderate, depressive symptoms were found to be associated with heart failure readmission and survival. An increased risk of 1.3–1.5 was observed, and a linear association between depression (Center for Epidemiological Studies – Depression Scale (CES-D)) scores and heart failure readmission and mortality.

The above studies consider increased mortality from physical illness, but European studies have shown that people with depression and comorbid physical illness are also at greater risk of suicide.[5] This is particularly the case for people with cancer, who have at least a 50% greater risk of suicide than the general population, with the risk being considerably higher in the first year following diagnosis and for men.[163–165] Increased risk of suicide has also been found in Swedish patients who had undergone surgery for gastric or duodenal ulcers.[166]

The mechanisms behind the association between depression and either mortality or morbidity in physical illness are not fully understood.[160] Either diminished health-care behaviour or physiological impairment, or a combination of the two, may be important. Similar mechanisms to those seen for people with SMI may play a role; for example, people with depression tend to be less active and eat less healthy diets.[167,168]

Several studies have found depression to be associated with reduced adherence to medical treatments; however, others have not found this association or have found it only in relation to some aspects of adherence.[160] This is likely to be because adherence behaviour is complex, especially in relation to multifactorial treatment regimens.[160] There are some data suggesting that antidepressants may increase the risk of diabetes. A recent nested cohort study from Finland reported that people with continuing use of antidepressants had double the risk of diabetes, although this study was not able to disentangle the contribution of the antidepressant from that of the illness.[169] A UK case-control study of people with depression, however, found an 84% increased risk of diabetes in people with recent long-term use of antidepressants, with no difference between SSRIs and TCAs.[170] Certain combinations of antidepressants, such as SSRIs and TCAs may increase the risk of diabetes further but this finding may reflect diabetes occurring in a higher-risk group, because those with more severe depression are more likely to need combination therapy. Certain antidepressants, for example mirtazapine, are associated with weight gain, which may increase the long-term risk of diabetes. Physiological antecedents may also be important, but there is limited understanding of these. For example, acute psychological stress may increase cortisol and catecholamine secretion and the circulating concentration of a number of inflammatory cytokines, such as interleukin (IL)-6 and tumour necrosis factor (TNF)-α, which may in turn worsen insulin resistance and increase the risk of diabetes. Similarly in CVD, it has been suggested that immune functioning and inflammation may mediate the link with depression,[171] but more research is needed to explain this.

The impact of illness on daily living may also be a factor. A cross-sectional survey of 20 183 community-dwelling Australian adults aged 60 years and over[172] suggests that the level of impairment associated with the physical illness may be a more important determinant of the risk of depression.

Interventions for depression in physical illness

There are effective treatments for depression;[122] however, additional burden from comorbid physical illness may impact on their effectiveness. There are a number of well-conducted systematic reviews of studies of the effectiveness of a range of interventions for depression comorbid with physical illness. These include participants with both depressive symptoms and clinically diagnosed depression. The studies included in the reviews, and discussed next, tend to have been conducted largely in high-income countries, especially the UK and USA.

Antidepressants for physically ill people

A recent Cochrane review (search date 2009) of antidepressants for depression in physically ill people included 51 RCTs, with a total of 3603 participants with a wide range of physical health problems.[173] Forty-four RCTs including 3372 participants contributed data towards the efficacy analyses. Overall, pooled efficacy data for the primary outcome (efficacy 6–8 weeks after randomization) provided an OR of 2.33, 95% CI = 1.80 to 3.00, $P < 0.00001$ (25 studies, 1674 patients) favouring antidepressants. Antidepressants were also more efficacious than placebo at the other time points. At 6–8 weeks, fewer patients receiving placebo dropped out compared to patients treated with an antidepressant. Dry mouth and sexual dysfunction were more common in patients treated with an antidepressant. The authors concluded that antidepressants are superior to placebo in treating depression in physical illness, although it is likely that publication and reporting biases exaggerated the effect sizes obtained. Further research is required to determine the comparative efficacy and acceptability of particular antidepressants in this population.

Psychological treatments for depression in cancer patients

A Cochrane review (search date 2005) of psychotherapy for depression among incurable cancer patients found 10 RCTs with 780 participants.[174] Data from six studies were used for meta-analyses (292 patients in the psychotherapy arm, 225 in the control arm). Among these six studies, four used supportive psychotherapy, one cognitive-behavioural therapy (CBT), and one problem-solving therapy. Compared with treatment as usual, psychotherapy was associated with a significant decrease in depression score (standardized mean difference = −0.44, 95% CI = −0.08 to −0.80). None of the studies focused on patients with clinically diagnosed depression. The authors concluded that evidence from RCTs of moderate quality suggest that psychotherapy is useful for treating depressive states in advanced cancer patients. However, none of the evidence supports the effectiveness of psychotherapy for patients with clinically diagnosed depression. Two other reviews with the same search date considered pharmacological treatments in patients with a range of cancer prognoses.[175,176] The first[175] included 24 RCTs (3348 participants), the second[176] included 10 RCTs (1199 participants) and one cohort study (60 participants). Both found little evidence for the effectiveness of psychotherapeutic interventions.

Pharmacological treatments for depression in cancer patients

The two above reviews[175,176] also considered the use of pharmacological treatments for depression in cancer; the first concluded there was some evidence of effectiveness of pharmacological interventions for cancer patients with depression but that there was a paucity of data on tolerability.[175] The other review found little evidence for pharmacological interventions.[177] This is consistent with a recent Cochrane review (search date 2009) of pharmacological treatment of depression in patients with a primary brain tumour,[177] which did not identify any relevant studies.

Heart disease and depression

Coronary heart disease

A Cochrane review (search date 2004) identified 36 trials (12 841 participants) of psychological interventions for CHD.[178] Seventeen of these were of stress management. Overall, a small reduction in depression and anxiety was found, but there was no effect on total or cardiac mortality or on revascularization.

A very recent review (search date 2011) identified 16 trials of psychological and pharmacological interventions for depression comorbid with CHD.[179] It found a small, but clinically meaningful effect of psychological interventions and SSRIs on depression outcomes in CHD patients. No effects on mortality rates or cardiac events were found. However, the evidence was considered sparse due to few high-quality trials and the heterogeneity of populations and interventions tested.

Heart failure

A Cochrane review (search date 2003) of psychological interventions for depression in heart failure did not identify any relevant trials.[180] A subsequent review (search date 2007) of CBT for depression in heart failure, found 10 RCTs (3138 participants).[181] However, the included trials were of poor quality and the evidence presented was insufficient to recommend CBT as a treatment for depressive symptoms in these patients.

Renal disease and depression

A Cochrane review (search date 2004) of physical measures (e.g. antidepressants, electroconvulsive therapy (ECT)) for treating depression in dialysis patients found a small RCT (12 participants) of fluoxetine versus placebo in depressed patients on chronic dialysis.[182] There was no significant difference in depression scores between the treatment and control groups. Another Cochrane review (search date 2003) considered psychosocial interventions for depression in dialysis patients but found no relevant RCTs.[183]

Parkinson disease and depression

A Cochrane review (search date 2001) of therapies for depression in Parkinson disease found no trials of ECT or psychological therapy.[184] Three RCTs (106 participants) were found that tested antidepressant drugs; however, these provided insufficient data to determine their effectiveness and safety in Parkinson disease.

Chronic obstructive pulmonary disease and depression

One systematic review (search date 2006) examined CBT for anxiety and depression in COPD and found three RCTs ($n = 165$) and one non-randomized controlled trial ($n = 8$).[185] This limited evidence suggests that CBT, when used with exercise and education, could contribute to significant reductions in anxiety and depression in patients with clinically stable and severe COPD. However, further trials are needed to confirm this.

Stroke and depression

A Cochrane review (search date 2008) of interventions for treating depression after stroke identified 16 RCTs (1655 participants) of 17 varied interventions (13 pharmaceutical agents, four trials of psychotherapy).[186] This concluded that there is some evidence of benefit of pharmacotherapy in terms of a complete remission of depression and an improvement in depression rating scales, but there was also evidence of an associated increase in adverse events. There was no evidence of benefit of psychotherapy.

Epilepsy and depression

A Cochrane review (search date 2007) of psychological treatments for epilepsy included three trials with depression as an outcome.[187] Two of these found CBT to be effective in reducing depression, among people with epilepsy with a depressed affect, while the other did not. The authors conclude that there is insufficient evidence to support the use of psychological therapies in epilepsy.

HIV/AIDS and depression

A review (search date 2005) of seven RCTs (494 participants) of antidepressant medication concluded that this is efficacious in treating depression in men seen in outpatients who are positive for the HIV.[188] Women and ethnic minorities were underrepresented in the included studies, so the findings cannot be generalized to all individuals with depression who are HIV-positive. In a later review (search date 2006),[189] the same authors identified eight RCTs (665 participants) of group psychotherapy for depressive symptoms in HIV-infected individuals. They concluded that group psychotherapy may reduce depressive symptoms in patients infected with HIV, but, again, the results may not be applicable to women. Finally, a review (search date 2005) of CBT for HIV-positive persons' mental health and immune functioning identified 15 controlled trials.[190] These indicated that CBT plus stress management skills training delivered in at least 10 sessions is efficacious in improving depression (and other psychological states) in people living with HIV.

Impact and delivery of interventions for depression and physical health outcomes

Management of depression in physical illness may be expected to lead to improved physical health outcomes through improved health behaviours or because of the dual role of inflammation or immunopathology in depression and many physical illnesses.[121] Systematic reviews have been conducted of the evidence for the effectiveness of a range of pharmacological and psychological interventions for depression comorbid with a variety of long-term physical illnesses (cancer, heart disease, renal disease, Parkinson disease, COPD, stroke, epilepsy and HIV/AIDS). However, findings have been mixed and in many cases there is a lack of trials. In conditions where there is evidence that depression has been improved following intervention (e.g. cancer, heart disease, HIV/AIDS), there is as yet little evidence that this has resulted in better physical health outcomes. This may be because more complex treatments are needed. A recent trial of coordinated care management, an enhanced depression care intervention which provides depression-severity-related treatment guidance, found improvements in both depression and control of medical disease in patients with either or both heart disease and diabetes (n = 214).[191] These improvements were seen at 12 months; longer-term studies are needed to determine the effect on actual morbidity and mortality. Nevertheless, improvement of depression is an important goal. Effective drug and psychosocial treatments and interventions are needed to address the factors that may link depression and poor physical health, such as adverse health behaviours, social problems and impaired functioning. Effective drug and psychosocial treatments can be delivered by primary care staff. In most high-income countries, evidence-based guidelines have long been available for the management of depression in people with or without physical illness. An extensive set of treatment guidelines for mental disorders (including depression), which are also suitable for low- and middle-income countries, has recently been published by WHO (WHO 2008) as part of their programme.[123] Furthermore, many of the factors that may predispose physically ill people to depression, such as impaired functioning and social isolation, are amenable to management by primary care staff. The UK Government's latest mental health strategy promotes greater use of services, such as social clubs and advice agencies, that are not traditionally considered to fall within the mental health sphere but that help enhance well-being.[192] However, there is now some debate as to how the physical consequences of mental illness are best managed in primary care.

Models of mental health care delivery in primary care settings

A balanced care model which is essentially community-based, but in which hospitals play an important backup role has been recommended for optimal mental health-care provision.[193] In most countries, primary care acts as the "gatekeeper" to care in specialist settings.[194] Due to the high level of resources needed for specialist mental health services, it has been argued that low-resource countries should focus on establishing and improving mental health services within primary care settings, using specialist services only as a backup, and that medium-income countries should provide some additional components such as outpatient clinics, community mental health teams, acute inpatient care, long-term community-based residential care and occupational care.[193] In the UK, those with SMI are likely to be referred for specialist care, whereas most people with common mental disorders are treated solely in primary care. Four models of mental health-care delivery in this setting have been described:[195] training of primary care staff; "replacement/referral"; "consultation-liaison"; and "collaborative care". Evidence for the effectiveness of these models comes mostly from Europe, (especially the UK) and the USA, and usually involves participants whose mental health problem is their primary diagnosis, rather than people with physical ill health and comorbid mental health problems.

Training of primary care staff

Training of primary care staff may involve providing training in improving prescribing, implementing guideline-based care or providing skills in psychological therapy. Systematic reviews have found that most types of training (such as passive dissemination of guidelines and short-term courses) were ineffective in improving outcome in patients. By contrast, more intensive training for GPs in psychosocial interventions may be beneficial.[195]

Replacement/referral

In this model, specialists working within primary care, for instance psychological therapists, mental health nurses or social workers, are given the primary responsibility for management of the mental health problem. A Cochrane review identified 42 studies of the effects of such "on-site mental health workers".[196] Thirty-seven studies were in Europe (35 UK, 1 the Netherlands, 1 West Germany), the rest were in the USA, Australia, New

Zealand or Sri Lanka. Overall, on-site mental health workers were found to reduce the number of consultations with primary care professionals, psychotropic prescribing, prescribing costs and rates of referral to off-site mental health services in those seen by on-site mental health workers. However, these effects were small and not consistent across studies. The cost–benefit of on-site mental health workers could not be determined from the available evidence.

Consultation-liaison

This involves mental health specialists entering into an ongoing educational relationship with primary care clinicians, to support them in caring for individual patients.[195] Evidence from systematic review indicates that this model may change clinician behaviour, but there is no evidence of benefit to the wider practice population.[195]

Collaborative care

This is structured care that involves a greater role of non-medical specialists to augment primary care.[195] Systematic review evidence shows that in the USA, collaborative care, compared with usual care, is beneficial for patients with depression.[197] A subsequent well-conducted RCT suggests this may also be the case in the UK.[198] However, the provision of mental health services within primary care has often been found to be less than optimal.[199] In Europe, mental health training for primary care staff is often insufficient.[5] Improvement in primary care mental health provision may be facilitated by ensuring that there are sufficient numbers of primary care staff – regulating training, organizing adequate and ongoing supervision of primary care staff by mental health professionals and addressing staff attitudes; and by developing and managing coordinated support networks with specialized community mental health services and other relevant sectors.[5]

However, in low- and middle-income countries, where there is reduced access not only to mental health specialists, but also often to primary care professionals, alternative approaches may be needed. "Task-shifting", where lay workers are trained to deliver evidence-based interventions, has been shown to provide promising benefits in low- and middle-income countries in promoting immunization uptake and breastfeeding, improving tuberculosis (TB) treatment outcomes, and reducing child morbidity and mortality when compared to usual care.[200] In mental health, three cluster randomized trials have used lay workers to deliver evidence-based psychological therapy for depression in low- and middle-income countries.[201] In Goa, India, a collaborative-stepped care intervention found improved recovery rates at 6 months for patients with depression and anxiety ($n = 2796$). This effect was seen in public primary care settings, which are characterized by a collective clinic-centred model of care, but not in private primary care settings characterized by a personalized client-centred model of care.[202] In Uganda, adapted interpersonal therapy delivered in individual and group settings reduced the prevalence of depression at 6 months in adults reporting or diagnosed with major depressive disorder ($n = 248$).[203] Similarly, in Pakistan, a CBT-based intervention was found to reduce the prevalence of depression in women in the third trimester of pregnancy ($n = 903$).[204] These studies suggest that greater use of lay workers may help improve mental health care in countries where health-care professionals are scarce; a Cochrane review is planned to assess this.[205] Whether lay workers can deliver interventions that address mental health problems comorbid with physical illness also needs to be tested. Other barriers to provision of mental health care in low- and middle-income countries, such as inadequate investment in mental health care, mental health-related stigma and acceptability of mental health treatments,[201] may also need to be addressed. It is possible, however, that mental health interventions delivered in the context of physical illness may be perceived as carrying less stigma.

References

1   Holt RIG, Peveler RC. Review on diabetes and cardiovascular risk in severe mental illness: a missed opportunity and challenge for the future. *Practical Diabetes International*, 2010, 27:79–84.

2   McManus S et al. *Adult psychiatric morbidity in England, 2007: results of a household survey*. Leeds, NHS Information Centre for Health and Social Care Information Centre, 2009.

3   Kendler KS et al. Lifetime prevalence, demographic risk factors and diagnostic validity of nonaffective psychosis as assessed in a US community sample. The National Comorbidity Survey. *Archives of General Psychiatry*, 1996, 53:1022–1031.

4   Goodwin G et al. ECNP consensus meeting. Bipolar depression. Nice, March 2007. *European Neuropsychopharmacology*, 2008, 18:535–549.

5   *Mental and Physical Health Charter*. Brussels, The Mental and Physical Health Platform, 2009. (http://ec.europa.eu/health/mental_health/eu_compass/policy_recommendations_declarations/mh_charter_en.pdf, accessed 23 December 2011).

6   NHS Information Centre. *The Quality and Outcomes Framework database* (http://www.ic.nhs.uk/services/prescribing-support-unit-psu/using-the-service/reference/datasets/the-quality-and-outcomes-framework-database, accessed 23 December 2011).

7   Murray C, Lopez A, eds. *The global burden of disease*. Boston, Harvard School of Public Health, WHO and the World Bank, 1996.

8   Shiner B et al. Learning what matters for patients: qualitative evaluation of a health promotion program for those with serious mental illness. *Health Promotion International*, 2008, 23:275–282.

9   De Hert M et al. Cardiovascular disease and diabetes in people with severe mental illness position statement from the European Psychiatric Association (EPA), supported by the European Association for the Study of Diabetes (EASD) and the European Society of Cardiology (ESC). *European Psychiatry*, 2009, 24:412–424.

10   Parks J et al. *Morbidity and mortality in people with serious mental illness*. Alexandria VA, National Association of State Mental Health Programme Directors, 2006 (13th Technical Report) (http://www.nasmhpd.org/general_files/publications/med_directors_pubs/Technical%20Report%20on%20Morbidity%20and%20Mortality%20-%20Final%2011-06.pdf, accessed 23 December 2011).

11   Brown S. Excess mortality of schizophrenia: a meta-analysis. *British Journal of Psychiatry*, 1997, 171:502–508.

12   Santhouse A, Holloway F. Physical health of patients in continuing care. *Advances in Psychiatric Treatment*, 1999, 5:455–462.

13   Osby U et al. Mortality and causes of death in schizophrenia in Stockholm County, Sweden. *Schizophrenia Research*, 2000, 45:21–28.

14   Saha S, Chant D, McGrath J. A systematic review of mortality in schizophrenia – is the differential mortality gap worsening over time? *Archives of General Psychiatry*, 2007, 64:1123–1131.

15   Angst F et al. Mortality of patients with mood disorders: follow-up over 34–38 years. *Journal of Affective Disorders*, 2002, 68:167–181.

16   Capasso RM et al. Mortality in schizophrenia and schizoaffective disorder: an Olmsted County, Minnesota cohort: 1950–2005. *Schizophrenia Research*, 2008, 98:287–294.

17   Osby U et al. Excess mortality in bipolar and unipolar disorder in Sweden. *Archives of General Psychiatry*, 2001, 58:844–850.

18   Brown S et al. Twenty-five year mortality of a community cohort with schizophrenia, *British Journal of Psychiatry*, 2010, 196:116–121.

19   Carney CP, Jones L, Woolson RF. Medical comorbidity in women and men with schizophrenia: a population-based controlled study. *Journal of General Internal Medicine*, 2006, 21:1133–1137.

20   Kilbourne AM et al. Improving medical psychiatric outcomes among individuals with bipolar disorder: a randomized controlled trial. *Psychiatric Services*, 2008, 59:760–768.

21   Jones DR et al. Prevalence, severity, and co-occurrence of chronic physical health problems of persons with serious mental illness. *Psychiatric Services*, 2004, 55:1250–1257.

22   Green AI et al. Detection and management of comorbidity in patients with schizophrenia. *Psychiatric Clinics of North America*, 2003, 26:115–139.

23   Leucht S et al. Physical illness and schizophrenia. A review of the literature. *Acta Psychiatrica Scandinavica*, 2007, 116:317–333.

24   Weber NS et al. Psychiatric and general medical conditions comorbid with schizophrenia in the National Hospital Discharge Survey. *Psychiatric Services*, 2009, 60:1059–1067.

25   Osborn DP et al. Relative risk of diabetes, dyslipidaemia, hypertension and the metabolic syndrome in people with severe mental illnesses: systematic review and metaanalysis. *BMC Psychiatry*, 2008, 8:84.

26   Balf G et al. Metabolic adverse events in patients with mental illness treated with antipsychotics: a primary care perspective. *Primary Care Companion to the Journal of Clinical Psychiatry*, 2008, 10:15–24.

27 Phelan M, Stradins L, Morrison S. Physical health of people with severe mental illness: can be improved if primary care and mental health professionals pay attention to it. *BMJ*, 2001, 322:433–434.

28 Oud MJT, Meyboom-de Jong. Somatic diseases in patients with schizophrenia in general practice: their prevalence and health care. *BMC Family Practice*, 2009, 10:32.

29 McDaid D. Mental health reform: Europe at the crossroads. *Health Economics, Policy and Law*, 2008, 3:219–228.

30 Holt RJ, Bushe C, Citrome L. Diabetes and schizophrenia: are we any closer to understanding the link? *Journal of Psychopharmacology*, 2005, 19(6 Suppl.):56–65.

31 Gough SC, O'Donovan MC. Clustering of metabolic comorbidity in schizophrenia: a genetic contribution? *Journal of Psychopharamcology*, 2005, 19(6 Suppl.) 47–55.

32 Susser E et al. Schizophrenia after prenatal famine. Further evidence. *Archives of General Psychiatry*, 1996, 53:25–31.

33 Hack M et al. Behavioural outcomes and evidence of psychopathology among very low birth weight infants at age 20 years. *Pediatrics*, 2004, 114:932–940.

35 McCreadie RG, Scottish Schizophrenia Lifestyle Group. Diet, smoking and cardiovascular risk in people with schizophrenia: descriptive study. *British Journal of Psychiatry*, 2003, 183:534–539.

35 Ryan MC, Collins P, Thakore JH. Impaired fasting glucose tolerance in first-episode, drug-naïve patients with schizophrenia. *American Journal of Psychiatry*, 2003, 160:284–289.

36 Deakin B et al. The physical health challenges in patients with severe mental illness: cardiovascular and metabolic risks. *Journal of Psychopharmacology*, 2010, 24:1–8.

37 Tiihonen J et al. 11-year follow-up of mortality in patients with schizophrenia: a population-based cohort study (FIN11 study). *The Lancet*, 2009, 374:620–627.

38 Wildgust HJ, Beary M. Review: are there modifiable risk factors which will reduce the excess mortality in schizophrenia? *Psychopharmacology*, 2010, 24(4 Suppl.):37–50.

39 *Schizophrenia. Core interventions in the treatment and management of schizophrenia in adults in primary and secondary care (update)*. London, National Institute for Health and Clinical Excellence, 2009 (CHG82).

40 De Leon J, Diaz FJ. A meta-analysis of worldwide studies demonstrates an association between schizophrenia and tobacco smoking behaviors. *Schizophrenia Research*, 2005, 76:135–157.

41 Halbreich U, Palter S. Accelerated osteoporosis in psychiatric patients: possible pathophysiological processes. *Schizophrenia Bulletin*, 1996, 22:447–454.

42 Fagiolini A, Goracci A. The effects of undertreated chronic medical illnesses in patients with severe mental disorders. *Journal of Clinical Psychiatry*, 2009, 70(Suppl. 3):22–29.

43 Paton C et al. Obesity, dyslipidaemias, and smoking in an inpatient population treated with antipsychotic drugs. *Acta Psychiatrica Scandinavica*, 2004, 110:299–305.

44 Correll CU. Balancing efficacy and safety in treatment with antipsychotics. *CNS Spectrums*, 2007, 12(10 Suppl. 17):12–20, 35.

45 Hennekens CH et al. Schizophrenia and increased risks of cardiovascular disease. *American Heart Journal*, 2005, 150:1115–1121.

46 Amaddeo F et al. Avoidable mortality of psychiatric patients in an area with a community-based system of mental health care. *Acta Psychiatrica Scandinavica*, 2007, 115:320–325.

47 Fleischhacker WW et al. Comorbid somatic illnesses in patients with severe mental disorders: clinical, policy, and research challenges. *Journal of Clinical Psychiatry*, 2008, 69:514–519.

48 McDermott S et al. Heart disease, schizophrenia, and affective psychoses: epidemiology of risk in primary care. *Community Mental Health Journal*, 2005, 41:747–755.

49 Lawrence D, Kisely S. Inequalities in healthcare provision for people with severe mental illness. *Journal of Psychopharmacology*, 2010, 24(11 Suppl.):61–68.

50 Jeste DV et al. Medical comorbidity in schizophrenia. *Schizophrenia Bulletin*, 1996, 22:413–427.

51 *Lipid modification. Cardiovascular risk assessment and the modification of blood lipids for the primary and secondary prevention of cardiovascular disease*. London, National Institute for Health and Clinical Excellence, 2008 (CG67). www.nice.co.uk

52 *Quality and Outcomes Framework*. London, Department of Health, 2010 (http://www.dh.gov.uk/en/Healthcare/Primarycare/PMC/Quality/OutcomesFramework/index.htm, accessed 23 December 2011).

53 *nGMS Quality & Outcomes Framework 2009–2010*. London, Department of Health, 2010 (http://www. primarycaretraining.co.uk/news/ngms-qof-guidance/, accessed 23 December 2011).

54 Walker S et al. Value for money and the Quality and Outcomes Framework in primary care in the UK NHS. *British Journal of General Practice*, 2010, 60:e213–220.

55 The London Health Observatory (www.lho.org.uk, accessed 23 December 2011).

56 Simpson CR et al. Are different groups of patients with stroke more likely to be excluded from the new UK general medical services contract? A cross-sectional retrospective analysis of a large primary care population. *BMC Family Practice*, 2007, 8:56.

57 Holt RIG, Peveler RC, Byrne CD. Schizophrenia, the metabolic syndrome and diabetes. *Diabetic Medicine*, 2004, 21:515–523.

58 Subramaniam M, Chong SA, Pek E. Diabetes mellitus and impaired glucose tolerance in patients with schizophrenia. *Canadian Journal of Psychiatry*, 2003, 48:345–347.

59 Holt RIG, Peveler RC. (2006b) Antipsychotic medication. *Diabetes, Obesity and Metabolism*, 2006, 8:125–135.

60 Dixon L et al. Prevalence and correlates of diabetes in national schizophrenia samples. *Schizophrenia Bulletin*, 2000, 26:903–912.

61 Carlson C et al. Diabetes mellitus and antipsychotic treatment in the United Kingdom. *European Neuropsychopharmacology*, 2006, 16:366–375.

62 Sacchetti E et al. Incidence of diabetes in a general practice population: a database cohort study on the relationship with haloperidol, olanzapine, risperidone or quetiapine exposure. *International Clinical Psychopharmacology*, 2005, 20:33–37.

63 Kornegay CJ, Vasilakis-Scaramozza C, Jick H. Incident diabetes associated with antipsychotic use in the United Kingdom general practice research database. *Journal of Clinical Psychiatry*, 2002,63:758–762.

64 Dickerson FB et al. Obesity among individuals with serious mental illness. *Acta Psychiatrica Scandinavica*, 2006, 113:306–313.

65 De Hert M et al. Metabolic syndrome in people with schizophrenia: a review. *World Psychiatry*, 2009, 8:15–22.

66 Pendlebury J et al. Long-term maintenance of weight loss in patients with severe mental illness through a behavioural treatment programme in the UK. *Acta Psychiatrica Scandinavica*, 2007, 115:286–294.

67 Simon GE et al. Association between obesity and psychiatric disorders in the US adult population. *Archives of General Psychiatry*, 2006, 63:824–830.

68 Allison DB et al. Antipsychotic-induced weight gain: a comprehensive research synthesis. *American Journal of Psychiatry*, 1999, 156:1686–1696.

69 Holt RI, Peveler RC. Obesity, serious mental illness and antipsychotic drugs. *Diabetes Obesity and Metabolism*, 2009, 11:665–679.

70 Bernardo M et al. Low level of medical recognition and treatment of cardiovascular risk factors in patients with schizophrenia in Spain. *Schizophrenia Research*, 2006, 81:176–177.

71 Kilbourne AM et al. Recognition of co-occurring medical conditions among patients with serious mental illness. *Journal of Nervous and Mental Disease*, 2006, 194:598–602.

72 Glodman LS. Medical illness in patients with schizophrenia. *Journal of Clinical Psychiatry*, 1999, 60(Suppl. 21):10–15.

73 Felker B, Yazell JJ, Short D. Mortality and medical comorbidity among psychiatric patients: a review. *Psychiatric Services*, 1996, 47:1356–1363.

74 Consensus development conference on antipsychotic drugs and obesity and diabetes. *Diabetes Care*, 2004, 27:596–601.

75 Hyland A et al. *Cigarette smoking-attributable morbidity by state*. Buffalo, Roswell Park Cancer Institute, 2003.

76 Himelhoch S et al. Prevalence of chronic obstructive pulmonary disease among those with serious mental illness. *American Journal of Psychiatry*, 2004, 161:2317–2319.

77 Filik R et al. The cardiovascular and respiratory health of people with schizophrenia. *Acta Psychiatrica Scandinavica*, 2006, 113:298–305.

78   *Chronic obstructive pulmonary disease (update).* London, National Institute for Health and Clinical Excellence, 2010 (CG101).

79   Holt RI, Peveler RC. Antipsychotics and hyperprolactinaemia: mechanisms, consequences and management. *Clinical Endocrinology*, 2011, 74:141–147.

80   Zhang-Wong JH, Seeman MV. Antipsychotic drugs, menstrual regularity and osteoporosis risk. *Archives of Women's Mental Health*, 2002, 5:93–98.

81   Bilici M et al. Classical and atypical neuroleptics, and bone mineral density, in patients with schizophrenia. *International Journal of Neuroscience*, 2002, 112:817–828.

82   Meaney AM et al. Effects of long-term prolactin-raising antipsychotic medication on bone mineral density in patients with schizophrenia. *British Journal of Psychiatry*, 2004, 184:503–508.

83   Bishop JR et al. Osteoporosis screening and treatment in women with schizophrenia: a controlled study. *Pharmacotherapy*, 2004, 24:515–521.

84   Rosenberg SD et al. Prevalence of HIV, hepatitis B, and hepatitis C in people with severe mental illness. *American Journal of Public Health*, 2001, 91:31–37.

85   McKinnon K. Sexual and drug risk behavior. In: Cournos F, Balakar N, eds. *AIDS and people with severe mental illness: a handbook for mental health professionals.* New Haven, CN, Yale University Press, 1996:17–56.

86   Coverdale JH, Turbott SH. Risk behaviors for sexually transmitted infections among men with mental disorders. *Psychiatric Services*, 2000, 51:234–238.

87   Carey MP, Carey KB, Kalichman SC. Risk for human immunodeficiency virus (HIV) infection among persons with severe mental illnesses. *Clinical Psychology Review*, 1997, 17:271–291.

88   Carey MP, Carey KB, Weinhardt LS. Behavioural risk for HIV infection among adults with a severe and persistent mental illness: patterns and psychological antecedents. *Community Mental Health Journal*, 1997, 33:133–142.

89   Weinhardt LS et al. HIV risk reduction in the seriously mentally ill. Pilot investigation and call for research. *Journal of Behavior Therapy and Experimental Psychiatry*, 1997, 28:87–95.

90   Brown S, Inskip H, Barraclough B. Causes of the excess mortality of schizophrenia. *British Journal of Psychiatry*, 2000, 177:212–217.

91   McAlpine DD, Mechanic D. Utilisation of specialty mental health care among persons with severe mental illness: the roles of demographics, need, insurance and risk. *Health Services Research*, 2000, 35:277–292.

92   Harris KM, Edlind MJ, Larson S. Racial and ethnic differences in the mental health problems and use of mental health care. Medical Care, 2005, 43:775–784.

93   Bardsley M, Lowdell C. *Health and minority ethnic groups. A discussion paper.* Produced for the London Health Strategy by the Health of Londoners Project, Directorate of Public Health East London and The City Health Authority. London, The Health of Londoners Project, 1999.

94   Nasrallah HA et al. Low rates of treatment for hypertension, dyslipidemia and diabetes in schizophrenia: data from the CATIE schizophrenia trial sample at baseline. *Schizophrenia Research*, 2006, 86:15–22.

95   Bhopal R, Hayes L, White M. Ethnic and socio-economic inequalities in coronary heart disease, diabetes and risk factors in Europeans and South Asians. *Journal of Public Health*, 2002, 24:95–105.

96   Raleigh VS. Diabetes and hypertension in Britain's ethnic minorities: implications for the future of renal services. *BMJ*, 1997, 314:209.

97   Cappuccio FP. Ethnicity and cardiovascular risk:variations in people of African ancestry and South Asian origin. *Journal of Human Hypertension*, 1997, 11:571–576.

98   Caprio S et al. Influence of race, ethnicity, and culture on childhood obesity: implications for prevention and treatment. *Obesity*, 2008, 16:2566–2577.

99   Kleinman A, Benson P. Anthropology in the clinic: the problem of cultural competency and how to fix it. *PLoS Medicine*, 2006, 3:e294.

100 Whitley R. Cultural competence, evidence-based medicine and evidence-based practices. *Psychiatric Services*, 2007, 58:1588–1590.

101 Cabassa LJ, Ezell JM, Lewis-Fernandez R. Lifestyle interventions for adults with serious mental illness: a systematic literature review. *Psychiatric Services*, 2010, 61:774–782.

102 Cabassa LJ. NYS Center of Excellence for Cultural Competence New York State Psychiatric

Institute Department of Psychiatry, Columbia University New York State Office of Mental Health: Bureau of Cultural Competence. *Improving the physical health of Latinos and African Americans with serious mental illness.* Webinar Series sponsored by New York State Office of Mental Health: Bureau of Cultural Competence (http://nyspi.org/culturalcompetence/what/documents/ImprovingthePhysicalHealthofLatinosandAfricanAmericanswithSeriousMentalIllness.pdf, accessed 1 February 2012).

103 Gureje O, Olley BO, Ephraim-Oluwanuga O. Do beliefs about causation influence attitudes to mental illness? *World Psychiatry,* 2006, 5:104–107.

104 Bresnahan M et al. Geographical variation in incidence, course and outcome of schizophrenia: a comparison of developing and developed countries. In: Murray RM et al., eds. *The epidemiology of schizophrenia.* Cambridge, Cambridge University Press, 2003:5–17.

105 Harrison G et al. Severe mental disorder in Afro-Caribbean patients: some social, demographic and service factors. *Psychological Medicine,* 1989, 19:683–696.

106 Pinto R, Ashworth M, Jones R. Schizophrenia in Black Caribbeans living in the UK: an exploration of underlying causes of the high incidence rate. *British Journal of General Practice,* 2008, 58:429–434.

107 Dowrick C et al. Researching the mental health needs of hard-to-reach groups: managing multiple sources of evidence. *BMC Health Services Research,* 2009, 9:226.

108 Fazel M, Wheeler J, Danesh J. Prevalence of serious mental disorder in 7000 refugees resettled in western countries: a systematic review. *The Lancet,* 2005, 365:1309–1314.

109 Bhui K, Shanahan L, Harding G. Homelessness and mental illness: a literature review and a qualitative study of perceptions of the adequacy of care. *International Journal of Social Psychiatry,* 2006, 52:152–165.

110 Kennedy LT et al. Incidence of bipolar affective disorder in three UK cities: results from the AeSOP study. *British Journal of Psychiatry,* 2005, 186:126–131.

111 Bhui K et al. Ethnic variations in pathways to and use of specialist mental health services in the UK: systematic review. *British Journal of Psychiatry,* 2003, 182:105–116.

112 Richardson CR et al. Integrating physical activity into mental health services for persons with serious mental illness. *Psychiatric Services,* 2005, 56:324–331.

113 *Improving the physical health of people with serious mental illness: a systematic review of lifestyle interventions: a report from the NYS Center of Excellence for Cultural Competence at the New York State Psychiatric Institute.* New York, NY, NYS Center of Excellence for Cultural Competence, 2010.

114 Hellerstein DJ et al. Assessing obesity and other related health problems of mentally ill Hispanic patients in an urban outpatient setting. *The Psychiatric Quarterly,* 2007, 78:171–181.

115 Druss BG et al. A randomized trial of medical care management for community mental health settings: The Primary Care Access, Referral, and Evaluation (PCARE) study. *American Journal of Psychiatry,* 2010, 167:151–159.

116 Steiner BD et al. Community Care of North Carolina: improving care through community health networks. *Annals of Family Medicine,* 2008, 6:361–367.

117 Horvitz-Lennon M, Kilbourne AM, Pincus HA. From silos to bridges: meeting the general health care needs of adults with severe mental illnesses. *Health Affairs,* 2006, 25:659–669.

118 Van Citters AD et al. A pilot evaluation of the In SHAPE individualized health promotion intervention for adults with mental illness. *Community Mental Health Journal,* 2010, 46:540–552.

119 Chafetz L et al. Clinical trial of wellness training: health promotion for severely mentally ill adults. *Journal of Nervous and Mental Disease,* 2008, 196:475–483.

120 Caffel J, Bartley S. *A rapid review of the mental illness directed enhanced service in Wales.* Cardiff, National Public Health Service for Wales, 2009.

121 Steptoe A, ed. *Depression and physical illness.* Cambridge, Cambridge University Press, 2007.

122 *Depression: the treatment and management of depression in adults.* London, National Institute for Health and Clinical Excellence, 2009 (CG90).

123 *mhGAP: Mental Health Gap Action Programme: scaling up care for mental, neurological and substance use disorders.* Geneva, World Health Organization, 2008.

124 Ustun TB, Chatterji S. Global burden of depressive disorders and future projections. In: Dawson A, Tylee A, eds. *Depression: social and economic timebomb.* London, BMJ Books, 2001:31–32.

125 Ustun TB et al. Global burden of depressive disorders in the year 2000. *British Journal of Psychiatry*, 2004, 184:386–392.

126 Mitchell AJ, Vaze A, Rao S. Clinical diagnosis of depression in primary care: a meta-analysis. *The Lancet*, 2009, 374:609–619.

127 *The global burden of disease: 2004 update*. Geneva, World Health Organization, 2008.

128 Trindade E, Menon D. *Selective serotonin reuptake inhibitors (SSRIs) for major depression. Part I. Evaluation of the clinical literature*. Ottawa, Canadian Coordinating Office for Health Technology Assessment, 1997 August Report 3E. *Evidence-based Mental Health*, 1998, 1:50.

129 Taylor D, Paton C, Kapur S, eds. *The Maudsley prescribing guidelines in psychiatry*, 11th ed. Chichester, Wiley Blackwell, 2012.

130 Greer TL, Kurian BT, Trivedi MH. Defining and measuring functional recovery from depression. *CNS Drugs*, 2010, 24:267–284.

131 Judd LL et al. Psychosocial disability during the long-term course of unipolar major depressive disorder. *Archives of General Psychiatry*, 2000, 57:375–380.

132 Veiel HO. A preliminary profile of neuropsychological deficits associated with major depression. *Journal of Clinical and Experimental Neuropsychology*, 1997, 19:587–603.

133 Simon GE et al. An international study of the relation between somatic symptoms and depression. *New England Journal of Medicine*, 1999, 341:1329–1335.

134 Cuijpers P, Smit F. Excess mortality in depression: a meta-analysis of community studies. *Journal of Affective Disorders*, 2002, 72:227–236.

135 Mykletun A et al. Levels of anxiety and depression as predictors of mortality: the HUNT study. *British Journal of Psychiatry*, 2009, 195:118–125.

136 Sartorius N. The economic and social burden of depression. *Journal of Clinical Psychiatry*, 2001, 62(Suppl.15):8–11.

137 World Health Organization. *10 facts on mental health* (http://www.who.int/features/factfiles/mental_health/mental_health_facts/en/index2.html, accessed 23 December 2011).

138 Carney RM et al. Major depression and medication adherence in elderly patients with coronary artery disease. *Health Psychology*, 1995, 14:88–90.

139 Carnethon MR et al. Longitudinal association between depressive symptoms and incident type 2 diabetes mellitus in older adults. The Cardiovascular Health Study. *Archives of Internal Medicine*, 2007, 167:802–807.

140 Bultmann U et al. Depressive symptoms and the risk of long-term sickness absence: a prospective study among 4747 employees in Denmark. *Social Psychiatry and Psychiatric Epidemiology*, 2006, 41:875–880.

141 Wulsin LR, Singal BM. Do depressive symptoms increase the risk for the onset of coronary disease? A systematic quantitative review. *Psychosomatic Medicine*, 2003, 65:201–210.

142 Noel PH et al. Depression and comorbid illness in elderly primary care patients: impact on multiple domains of health status and well-being. *Annals of Family Mediicne*, 2004, 2:555–562.

143 Moussavi S et al. Depression, chronic diseases, and decrements in health: results from the World Health Surveys. *The Lancet*, 2007, 370:851–858.

144 Anderson RJ et al. The prevalence of comorbid depression in adults with diabetes: a meta-analysis. *Diabetes Care*, 2001, 24:1069–1078.

145 Davidson W et al. Assessment and treatment of depression in patients with cardiovascular disease: National Heart, Lung, and Blood Institute Working Group report. *Psychosomatic Medicine*, 2004, 68:645–650.

146 Benton T, Staab J, Evans DL. Medical co-morbidity in depressive disorders. *Annals of Clinical Psychiatry*, 2007, 19:289–303.

147 Barth J, Schumacher M, Herrmann-Lingen C. Depression as a risk factor for mortality in patients with coronary heart disease: a meta-analysis. *Psychosomatic Medicine*, 2004, 66:802–813.

148 Dickens C et al. New onset depression following myocardial infarction predicts cardiac mortality. *Psychosomatic Medicine*, 2008, 70:450–455.

149 Grace SL et al. Effect of depression on five-year mortality after an acute coronary syndrome. *American Journal of Cardiology*, 2005, 96:1179–1185.

150 Van Melle JP et al. Prognostic association of depression following myocardial infarction with mortality and cardiovascular events: a meta-analysis. *Psychosomatic Medicine*, 2004, 66:814–822.

151 Tylee AT, Freeling P, Kerry S. Why do general practitioners recognise major depression in one woman patient yet miss it in another? British Journal of General Practice, 1993, 43:327–330.

152 Freeling P et al. Unrecognised depression in general practice. *British Medical Journal (Clinical Research)*, 1985, 290:1880–1883.

153 Cassano P, Fava M. Depression and public health. An overview. *Journal of Psychosomatic Research*, 2002, 53:849–857.

154 Faris R et al. Clinical depression is common and significantly associated with reduced survival in patients with non-ischaemic heart failure. *European Journal of Heart Failure*, 2002, 4:541–551.

155 Jiang W et al. Relationship between depressive symptoms and long-term mortality in patients with heart failure. *American Heart Journal*, 2007, 154:102–108.

156 Murberg TA et al. Depressed mood and subjective symptoms as predictors of mortality in patients with congestive heart failure: a two-year follow-up study. *International Journal of Psychiatry in Medicine*, 1999, 29:311–326.

157 Vaccarino V et al. Depressive symptoms and risk of functional decline and death in patients with heart failure. *Journal of the American College of Cardiology*, 2001, 38:199–205.

158 Zhang X et al. Depressive symptoms and mortality among persons with and without diabetes. *American Journal of Epidemiology*, 2005, 161:652–660.

159 Katon WJ et al. The association of comorbid depression with mortality in patients with type 2 diabetes. *Diabetes Care*, 2005, 28:2668–2672.

160 Chilcot et al. Depression in end-stage renal disease: current advances and research. *Seminars in Dialysis*, 2010, 23:74–82.

161 Pinquart M, Duberstein PR. Depression and cancer mortality: a meta-analysis. *Psychological Medicine*, 2010, 40:1797–1810.

162 Lesman-Leegte et al. Depressive symptoms and outcomes in patients with heart failure: data from the COACH study+. *European Journal of Heart Failure*, 2009, 11:1202–1207.

163 Innos K et al. Suicides among cancer patients in Estonia: a population-based study. *European Journal of Cancer*, 2003, 39:2223–2228.

164 Robinson D et al. Suicide in cancer patients in South East England from 1996 to 2005: a population-based study. *British Journal of Cancer*, 2009, 101:198–201.

165 Misono S et al. Incidence of suicide in persons with cancer. *Journal of Clinical Oncology*, 2008, 26:4731–4738.

166 Bahmanyar S et al. Risk of suicide among operated and non-operated patients hospitalized for peptic ulcers. *Journal of Epidemiology and Community Health*, 2009, 63(12):1016–1021.

167 Goodwin RC. Association between physical activity and mental disorders among adults in the United States. *Preventative Medicine*, 2003, 36:698–703.

168 Ciechanowski PS, Katon WJ, Russo JE. Depression and diabetes: impact of depressive symptoms on adherence, function, and costs. *Archives of Internal Medicine*, 2000, 160: 3278–3285.

169 Andersohn F et al. Long-term use of antidepressants for depressive disorders and the risk of diabetes mellitus. *American Journal of Psychiatry*, 2009, 166:591–598.

170 Brown LC et al. Type of antidepressant therapy and risk of type 2 diabetes in people with depression. *Diabetes Research and Clinical Practice*, 2008, 79:61–67.

171 Lesperance F et al. The association between major depression and levels of soluble intercellular adhesionmolecule 1, interleukin-6, and C-reactive protein in patients with recent acute coronary syndromes. *American Journal of Psychiatry*, 2004, 161:271–277.

172 Pfaff JJ et al. Medical morbidity and severity of depression in a large primary care sample of older Australians: the DEPS-GP project. *Medical Journal of Australia*, 2009, 190(7 Suppl.):S75–S80.

173 Rayner L et al. Antidepressants for depression in physically ill people. *Cochrane Database of Systematic Reviews*, 2010, (3):CD007503.

174 Akechi T et al. Psychotherapy for depression among incurable cancer patients. *Cochrane Database of Systematic Reviews*, 2008, (2):CD005537.

175 Williams S, Dale J. The effectiveness of treatment for depression/depressive symptoms in adults with cancer: a systematic review. *British Journal of Cancer*, 2006, 94:372–390.

176 Rodin G et al. Supportive Care Guidelines Group of Cancer Care Ontario Program in Evidence-based Care. The treatment of depression in cancer patients: a systematic review. *Supportive Care in Cancer*, 2007, 15:123–136.

177 Rooney A, Grant R. Pharmacological treatment of depression in patients with a primary brain tumour. *Cochrane Database of Systematic Reviews*, 2010, (3):CD006932.

178 Rees K et al. Psychological interventions for coronary heart disease. *Cochrane Database of Systematic Reviews*, 2004, (2):CD002902.

179 Baumeister H, Hutter N, Bengel J. Psychological and pharmacological interventions for depression in patients with coronary artery disease. *Cochrane Database of Systematic Reviews*, 2011, (9):CD008012.

180 Lane DA, Chong AY, Lip GYH. Psychological interventions for depression in heart failure. *Cochrane Database of Systematic Reviews*, 2005, (1):CD003329.

181 Dekker RL. Cognitive behavioral therapy for depression in patients with heart failure: a critical review. *Nursing Clinics of North America*, 2008, 43:155–170.

182 Rabindranath KS et al. Physical measures for treating depression in dialysis patients. *Cochrane Database of Systematic Reviews*, 2005, (2):CD004541.

183 Rabindranath KS et al. Psychosocial interventions for depression in dialysis patients. *Cochrane Database of Systematic Reviews*, 2005, (3):CD004542.

184 Ghazi-Noori S et al. Therapies for depression in Parkinson's disease. *Cochrane Database of Systematic Reviews*, 2003, (2):CD003465.

185 Coventry PA, Gellatly JL. Improving outcomes for COPD patients with mild-to-moderate anxiety and depression. A systematic review of cognitive behavioural therapy. *British Journal of Health Psychology*, 2008, 13:381–400.

186 Hackett ML et al. Interventions for treating depression after stroke. *Cochrane Database of Systematic Reviews*, 2008, (4):CD003437.

187 Ramaratnam S, Baker GA, Goldstein LH. Psychological treatments for epilepsy. *Cochrane Database of Systematic Reviews*, 2008, (3):CD002029.

188 Himelhoch S, Medoff DR. Efficacy of antidepressant medication among HIV-positive individuals with depression: a systematic review and meta-analysis. *AIDS Patient Care and STDs*, 2005, 19:813–822.

189 Himelhoch S, Medoff D R, Oyeniyi G. Efficacy of group psychotherapy to reduce depressive symptoms among HIV-infected individuals: a systematic review and meta-analysis. *AIDS Patient Care and STDs*, 2007, 21:732–739.

190 Crepaz N et al. Meta-analysis of cognitive-behavioral interventions on HIV-positive persons' mental health and immune functioning. *Health Psychology*, 2008, 27:4–14.

191 Katon WJ et al. Collaborative care for patients with depression and chronic illnesses. *New England Journal of Medicine*, 2010, 363:2611–2620.

192 *New horizons: a shared vision for mental health*. London, Department of Health, 2009.

193 Thornicroft G, Tansella M. *What are the arguments for community-based mental health care?* Copenhagen, WHO Regional Office for Europe (Health Evidence Network report, 2003 (http://www.euro.who.int/document/E82976.pdf, accessed 23 December 2011).

194 *The World Health Report 2001. Mental Health: new understanding, new hope*. Geneva, World Health Organization, 2001.

195 Bower PJ, Gilbody S. Managing common mental health disorders in primary care: conceptual models and evidence base. *BMJ*, 2005, 330:839–842.

196 Harkness EF, Bower PJ. On-site mental health workers delivering psychological therapy and psychosocial interventions to patients in primary care: effects on the professional practice of primary care providers [update of *Cochrane Database of Systematic Reviews*, 2000, (3):CD000532]. *Cochrane Database of Systematic Reviews*, 2009, (1):CD000532.

197 Gilbody S et al. Collaborative care for depression: a systematic review and cumulative meta-analysis. *Archives of Internal Medicine*, 2006, 166:2314–2321.

198   Richards DA et al. Collaborative care for depression in UK primary care: a randomized controlled trial. *Psychological Medicine*, 2008, 38:279–287.

199   Gilbody S et al. Educational and organisational interventions to improve the management of depression in primary care: a systematic review. *JAMA*, 2003, 289:3145–3151.

200   Lewin S et al. Lay health workers in primary and community health care for maternal and child health and the management of infectious diseases. *Cochrane Database of Systematic Reviews*, 2010, (3):CD004015.

201   Patel V et al. Improving access to psychological treatments: Lessons from developing countries. *Behaviour Research and Therapy*, 2011, 49:523–528.

202   Patel V et al. Effectiveness of an intervention led by lay health counsellors for depressive and anxiety disorders in primary care in Goa, India (MANAS): A cluster randomised controlled trial. *The Lancet*, 2010, 376:2086–2095.

203   Verdeli H et al. Adapting group interpersonal psychotherapy for a developing country: experience in rural Uganda. *World Psychiatry*, 2003, 2:114–120.

204   Rahman A et al. Cognitive behaviour therapy-based intervention by community health workers for mothers with depression and their infants in rural Pakistan: a cluster randomised controlled trial. *The Lancet*, 2008, 372:902e909.

205   van Ginneken N et al. Non-specialist health worker interventions for mental health care in low- and middle-income countries (protocol). *Cochrane Database of Systematic Reviews*, 2011, (5):CD009149.

33 Multimorbidity in primary care mental health

Todd M Edwards, Igor Švab, Gabriel Ivbijaro, Joseph Scherger, David D Clarke and Gene A Kallenberg

Key messages

- Multimorbidity is defined as patient complexity resulting from interactions in the presentation, course, treatment and outcomes associated with multiple biological *and* mental health problems, including substance misuse and social problems.
- Multimorbidity is linked to many adverse health consequences.
- It is important to assess patients with multimorbidity for their adverse childhood experiences.
- Complexity theory recognizes that simply counting the number of chronic conditions is insufficient because it obscures the interactions among co-occurring biological, psychological and social challenges, and interactions between the patient, family and health-care system.
- The patient-centred medical home (PCMH) concept has much potential for patients with multimorbidity, but it will not reach its full potential without also addressing the important component of multimorbidity that derives from patients' mental health needs. More than just patient-centredness, the integration of mental health services will enable the PCMH to meet its goals of enhanced access, coordinated care and high-quality care.
- For primary care to be effective in managing complex patients with multimorbidity, it has to adopt an approach that enables the clinician to quantify complexity and allocate resources according to the individual's cumulative need, taking into account diversity and ethnicity. This can be enhanced with a stepped care approach.
- The management of multimorbidity is more successful if a self-management programme is in place.
- There is a growing need for development of training programmes to teach primary care physicians and mental health professionals to work together in teams to treat complex patients.

Introduction

A gentleman, who is a long-distance lorry driver, presented to his general practitioner (GP) with a 4-week history of feeling anxious and not sleeping and has lost interest in his personal hygiene. He is also worried about his family and future, especially as he has recently been diagnosed with and is receiving treatment for tuberculosis. He informed his GP that his daughter is aged 14 years and attending secondary school, where his wife works as a dinner lady.

This type of presentation highlights the experience of multimorbidity and the complexities of primary care mental health.

Management of multiple chronic health conditions is an increasingly common challenge. Due to longer life expectancy and demographic change, the number of people with two or more chronic illnesses has increased and is expected to increase further in the future; multimorbidity is becoming a rule, rather than an exception. In the United States of America (USA), for example, more than 25% of patients have two or more chronic conditions,[1] which frequently include mental health problems such as substance use disorders, mental illnesses, disorders of cognitive impairment, and developmental disabilities. Studies from several countries confirm that patients with multimorbidity comprise a significant portion of family doctors' patients.[2]

A standard definition of multimorbidity has been elusive; no clear definition has been able to capture the clinical burden of the endless number of possible disease combinations.[2,3] The related and more common term, comorbidity, has been defined by Feinstein as "any distinct additional entity that has existed or may occur during the clinical course of a patient who has the index disease under study".[4] In this definition, it is not clear which condition would be considered the index disease and which the comorbid condition.[5] Starfield defined comorbidity as the concurrent existence of one or more unrelated conditions in an individual with any given condition, and multimorbidity as the co-occurrence of biologically unrelated illnesses.[6] Multimorbidity has been defined by others as multiple chronic health problems in an individual,[7–9] without any reference to a primary or index condition.[10] Although counting the number of illnesses is a simple of way of documenting the occurrence of multimorbidity, we agree with Starfield, who stated "total morbidity is not the same as the sum of different diseases".[11]

More recently, the term "patient complexity" has emerged to underscore the biopsychosocial demands associated with multiple health conditions, including family, socioeconomic, cultural, spiritual, environmental and doctor–patient relationship issues.[5,12] The term "complexity" recognizes that simply counting the number of chronic conditions is insufficient because it obscures the interactions among co-occurring biological, psychological and social challenges. For example, a 43-year old African-American man visits his primary care physician with a presentation of uncontrolled type 2 diabetes, obesity, unemployment, depression, crystal methamphetamine addiction and social isolation. He feels helpless to change his life due to physical and emotional stress and a lack of needed support and resources. This patient represents how we define *multimorbidity*: "patient complexity resulting from interactions in the presentation, course, treatment and outcomes associated with multiple biological and mental health problems, including substance misuse and social problems (e.g. family distress)". We will use the term "multimorbidity" in this chapter rather than the more traditional and conventional term "comorbidity", in order the capture the patient complexity described above. However, some of the concepts that apply to multimorbidity are common to comorbidity.

Primary care is commonly the medical home for complex patients. Patients seek guidance from their family doctors to manage medically explained and unexplained symptoms in multiple biological systems, psychological and relational distress, and the stress associated with many social conditions, including homelessness and poor social support. The variation of problem interactions arising from multimorbidity presents challenges for the individual primary care clinician. Most multimorbid patients require coordinated and holistic treatment, often involving other caregivers or health professionals. To treat patients with multimorbidity, it is not enough to know specific approaches to single diseases. One must also be able to use knowledge and clinical wisdom to weigh the importance and interaction of different health issues, the relative benefits of treatment options, as well as patient preferences, in order to develop a shared treatment plan. Primary care physicians are best suited to deal with this complex challenge, because of their unique breadth of knowledge and negotiating skills and their typical long-term relationship with their patients.

In this chapter, we will describe (1) the challenges and burden associated with multimorbidity, particularly the combination of mental health issues that can best be addressed in primary care; (2) the optimal systems for management of multimorbidity; and (3) specific treatment strategies for multiproblem patients and their family members. First, we will address the prevalence and then the adverse health consequences associated with multimorbidity.

The prevalence of multimorbidity

The lack of a standard definition and the challenges of studying complex clusters of chronic conditions have resulted in a dearth of good data on the prevalence of multimorbidity. The research has come from high-income countries and primarily focuses on comorbidities with a specific index disease rather than an examination of all co-occurring chronic conditions.[13] The research specifically examining the occurrence of multiple-occurring chronic conditions is inconsistent. In most studies, multimorbidity is defined as two or more chronic medical conditions and does not include mental health problems. None of the studies collected data from medical records, and almost half the studies were limited to an elderly population.

Despite the inconsistencies, some trends are apparent. Firstly, the prevalence rate of multimorbidity is large, estimated to be 21% in 2005, and growing,[14] which may be partly due to lower thresholds for diagnosis and inclusion of new diagnoses.[11] Second, multimorbidity is the norm, not the exception, in older patients; age has the strongest association with multimorbidity.[15] Fortin and colleagues reviewed studies from around the world and predictably found that the prevalence of multimorbidity increases with age and is substantial among older adults.[16] A study of older adults in Sweden found the prevalence of multimorbidity was as high as 55%, with significantly higher rates found among the oldest-old, lower-educated persons, and women.[17] As the primary care patient population continues to age, GPs and their colleagues will need to be prepared for increasing numbers of patients with multimorbidity, many of whom will be coping with the additional side-effects of pharmacological interventions used in treatment of mental illness.

Third, multimorbidity is a growing concern among younger populations. A 2005 Canadian study of primary care patients estimated the prevalence of multimorbidity by counting the number of medical conditions and using the Cumulative Illness Rating Scale (CIRS) to consider the severity of illness.[2,18] Results showed that nearly 50% of patients aged between 45 and 64 years of age had five or more chronic conditions. Younger patients in lower socioeconomic groups are especially vulnerable to multimorbidity. Finally, multimorbidity is more common in socially deprived populations. According to Barnett et al.,[15] middle-aged patients in the most deprived group have similar multimorbidity to older patients in the most affluent group.

Increases in multimorbidity have significant consequences for primary care and secondary care, in relation to both consultation rates and expenditure. Multimorbidity is associated with increases in the costs of care, hospitalizations and adverse events.[19] When patients present to primary care with coexisting medically complex health problems, the chances of referral significantly increase, even when the patient has a common condition.[20] According to Starfield et al.,[21] receiving care from multiple specialists is associated with higher costs, more procedures and more medications. The current interventions used to treat multimorbidity place a significant financial burden on health-care systems, which raises important questions about the appropriate role of specialists in the management of patients with multimorbidity.[11]

Adverse health consequences associated with multimorbidity

Multimorbidity is linked to many adverse health consequences,[1,14,19,22–24] including physical disability, use of multiple medications, increased risk for adverse drug events, mortality,[13,25–28] functional impairment,[29–34] hospitalizations[35] and the onset of additional health problems.[36] As discussed earlier, multimorbidity is also associated with increased referral to secondary care, increased health-care costs[37,38] and health-care utilization, such as the number of physician encounters, rate of hospitalization, length of hospital stay and drug intake.[3,13] Multimorbidity poses a threat to quality of life, which decreases with increasing severity of physical and psychiatric diagnoses.[39,40] Social support is a valuable resource for increasing quality of life in patients with multimorbidity. A growing body of literature demonstrates that *providing* emotional support to others is more beneficial that *receiving* emotional support.[41,42]

Links to childhood trauma

Several dimensions of poorer health and social functioning in adulthood have been linked to childhood stress. Felitti and colleagues' Adverse Childhood Experiences (ACE) Study in 1998 surveyed 18 000 people undergoing routine check-ups to learn if their childhood experience had included trauma, such as (1) physical, emotional or child abuse; (2) domestic violence; or (3) drug and alcohol misuse.[43] The study also asked about a variety of health and social outcomes, which were then correlated with the trauma scores. With higher childhood trauma scores, patients were many times more likely to:

- have multiple physical symptoms
- smoke or have emphysema or heart disease
- have a sexually transmitted disease or hepatitis

- use intravenous drugs or misuse alcohol
- suffer from depression or have attempted suicide
- have diabetes or be obese
- be divorced or a victim of violence from an intimate partner
- have multiple sexual partners or an unintended pregnancy.

Nicolaidis et al. studied 380 women in an American medical clinic.[44] Their survey asked about physical or sexual childhood abuse and assessed the impact of physical or sexual abuse in childhood on physical symptoms. A remarkable 36% of their subjects reported having been abused as children. On a measure of physical symptoms, the group who had been abused as children had a 37% higher score than those who had not been abused. The former group also had a mean 50% higher score on a measure of depression; 55% of this group had at least mild symptoms of depression, compared to 28% of the group who had not been abused.

Zielinski surveyed 5000 American adults for their childhood history of physical abuse, sexual abuse, severe neglect and any maltreatment.[45] Those who had this history were compared with those who did not, with respect to their employment status, income level and health-care utilization. The results showed that adults who experienced any form of maltreatment as children were twice as likely to be unemployed as those who experienced no maltreatment. The group that experienced physical abuse was 2.4 times more likely to be unemployed than those with no maltreatment. For those who experienced more than one form of maltreatment, the ratio was 2.9. In parallel with this, the proportion living in poverty was 1.6 times higher in those physically abused, two times higher if severely neglected and 2.8 times higher if subjected to multiple forms of maltreatment. A history of childhood trauma is an important area for assessment in patients coping with multimorbidity.

Links to psychological distress

Multimorbidity commonly includes a range of mental health problems, such as anxiety and depressive symptoms.[29,46] In a study of family practice patients, Fortin and colleagues found that a simple count of chronic diseases was not associated with psychological distress, but psychological distress did increase with the severity of multimorbidity,[39] which is consistent with the research on quality of life already discussed. Primary care plays a central role in identifying and managing psychological distress in patients coping with multiple chronic conditions.

Complexity and primary care

Primary care has been described as the "somatic symptom superhighway".[47,48] Primary care physicians manage patients with medical illness in multiple biological systems (e.g. cardiovascular, pulmonary, and renal systems) with a clear organic explanation, as well as medically unexplained symptoms (e.g. fatigue, headache, back pain), in a system designed primarily to manage acute, episodic problems in visits to solo doctors or the emergency room.[47] In a 2010 article in *The New Yorker*, Dr Atul Gawande summed up the poor fit between complex patients and our current health-care systems:[49]

> For a thirty-year-old with a fever, a twenty-minute visit to the doctor's office may be just the thing. For a pedestrian hit by a minivan, there's nowhere better than an emergency room. But these institutions are vastly inadequate for people with complex problems: the forty-year-old with drug and alcohol addiction; the eighty-four-year-old with advanced Alzheimer's disease and a pneumonia; the sixty-year-old with heart failure, obesity, gout, a bad memory for his eleven medications, and half a dozen specialists recommending different tests and procedures. It's like arriving at a major construction project with nothing but a screwdriver and a crane.

The patients described by Dr Gawande, who are very familiar to primary care doctors, are also frequently coping with a myriad of psychological, relationship and social issues, such as depression, anxiety, marital discord, unemployment, caregiver burden and neighbourhood crime.[47,50] Relationship and social stress may be much more threatening to recovery than the illness itself,[47] by either exacerbating current health problems or contributing to the development of new conditions. For example, an adult daughter caring for her mother with Alzheimer disease or a father's uncertainty about his ability to remain in the family home due to financial problems depletes the emotional resources necessary to follow sound medical advice. Assistance from human service organizations (e.g. educational, vocational, spiritual) is frequently needed or already involved.[47]

Medical training is not structured to address this patient complexity. For the last 300 years, scientific thinking has been dominated by the influence of Newtonian science, where the dominant metaphor has been the machine. Using Newton's theories, problems can be broken into their parts to be understood, and cause and effect are directly linked. Such a theoretical approach can be helpful in many areas of clinical practice.[51] Figure 33.1 shows how consultations can be simple, complicated, complex or chaotic, depending on the certainty of the doctor (x axis) and the agreement between the doctor and the patient (y axis).[52] In primary care, where complexity is the daily landscape, many recommendations from evidence-based medicine are unlikely to apply in a straightforward manner.

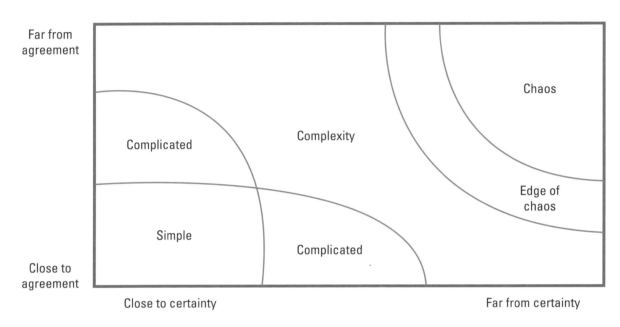

Figure 33.1 The Stacey matrix. Adapted, with permission, from Zimmerman B. *Ralph Stacey's agreement and certainty matrix.* Edgeware – Aides, Plexus Institute, Toronto, Schulich School of Business, York University, 2001 (http://www.plexusinstitute.com/edgeware/archive/think/main_aides3.html)

In addition to cause-and-effect thinking, another unhelpful paradigm is the Cartesian view that mind and body are separate entities, which are diagnosed and treated separately.[53] This separation has many manifestations in modern medicine and in our current health-care systems (e.g. "carved out" mental health services in the USA, the frequency of missed diagnoses of depression, patients being told unexplained symptoms are "all in your head"). As discussed earlier, primary care patients present with a mix of chronic medical and mental health conditions that are impacted by a variety of characteristics, such as culturally informed health beliefs.[54] How health-care professionals interact with culturally diverse patients also impacts health behaviours and outcomes. Patient preferences for relational style vary across diverse cultural groups and are associated with patient engagement in treatment, increased adherence, and improved patient outcomes and reference.[55] These complex presentations require medical and mental health-care professionals to adjust communication patterns with diverse patients and embrace the idea that mind and body are an integrated, related whole.[53]

The science of complex adaptive systems provides a paradigm for responding to the challenges of health care in the 21st century, where clinical practice, organization, information management, research, education and professional development are interdependent and built around multiple self-adjusting and interacting systems.[56] In complex systems, unpredictability and paradox are ever present; some things will remain unknowable. Complexity requires a more comprehensive, coordinated, team-based, and patient-centred approach to usual care and decision-making for important health conditions – including mental health conditions – and coordinating that care in a way that patients understand and accept.[47,57]

The following examples illustrate common complexity in primary care:

- patient 1: a 55-year-old obese man with recently discovered arterial hypertension, who is a smoker and has an enlarged prostate, who claims that he is under stress at work
- patient 2: a 55-year-old man with type 2 diabetes and chronic liver failure due to his alcoholism. The patient is unemployed and is physically abusing his wife and children. He claims that he is violent because he is under stress.

In both cases, medical and mental health problems are intertwined; each problem exacerbates another problem. A patient-centred, collaborative care approach for both of the patients described above has the potential to adequately address complexity. The only strategies that will prevent either of the complex patients from becoming "difficult patients" is primary care doctors appropriately recognizing and managing their interacting problems as early as possible,[47] and collaborating with other professionals, particularly in terms of handling the anxiety, alcoholism, and, most challengingly, the abuse issues. Such an approach requires a specific kind of health-care system, which we describe next.

Optimal health-care systems for multimorbidity

Successful programmes to manage complex patients must overcome a variety of health-care systems challenges, including fragmentation of the delivery system, misaligned incentives, a focus on acute problems, and a lack of team-based care. Much of the care of persons with chronic diseases has been centred on concepts of individual disease management. That standard, however, may not be sufficiently comprehensive for persons with multiple chronic conditions, diseases or disabilities.[58]

The degree of difficulty in both coping and caring increases substantially for patients with multimorbidity. Conflicting recommendations have been documented in approximately 17% of those with multimorbidity, who can be seeing up to seven different physicians. Patient differences in treatment preferences, financial/social supports, health literacy, and the presence of psychological symptoms like depression (up to 50%) also contribute. Providers are less well trained to handle many of the complex needs of their patients, including the management tasks of patient education, working with and assessing the needs of caregivers, coordinating services, and participating in interdisciplinary team-based care. In addition, multimorbid patients confirm that these challenges are greater than those experienced by patients with single diseases.[58]

Policy-makers agree that a multidisciplinary approach with a community orientation, based on a continuous, personalized doctor–patient relationship is the method of choice. The model of community-oriented primary care (COPC), where multidisciplinary teams serve a defined population is not new. The first COPC in former Yugoslavia dates from 1926.[59] The principles of COPC were modified in order to suit different health-care systems in Europe, often adopting different names. Unfortunately, in many countries (e.g. Soviet Union), the original idea of COPC was changed into a system of poli-clinics, with fragmentation of services, which did not happen in other countries, such as the United Kingdom of Great Britain and Northern Ireland (UK). The difference lies in the importance of family medicine. The countries with good family medicine have managed to keep the qualities of COPC; the countries without it have problems with coordination of care. The lesson is clear: for community-oriented health care to be successful, you need family doctors to coordinate all the services. Many of these ideas are beginning to take hold in the USA.

The patient-centred medical home

In the USA, attention has focused on the patient-centred medical home (PCMH) as one of the key delivery-system components that can coordinate patient-focused, highly integrated health care. PCMHs will focus on primary care delivery and coordination of more sophisticated services provided by other more specialized and technical components of vertically integrated systems, which some are calling "accountable care organizations". The PCMH movement has captured the hopes of primary care physicians in the USA, who, after witnessing more than a decade of decline in America, feel that primary care is poised for a comeback if better reimbursement, greater recognition and increased medical student interest can be accomplished. A rational and affordable health-care system depends on a healthy foundation of primary care. The medical home model, with its patient-centred coordination of care, seems to be just the right concept on which to pin the hopes of both primary care and patients with multimorbidity.

Primary care in the USA enjoyed a period of rapid growth in the 1990s, riding the wave of managed care. It was a period of cost reduction based on primary care physicians serving as "gatekeepers". The gatekeeper model was doomed to fail, however, among an American public that demands choice over where it gets health care and resists external limits to the amount of that health care, even as they are not yet willing, as a society, to pay for it. Tied together as they were, through the characterization of the "gatekeeper" enforcing those limits, the popularity of primary care declined along with that of managed care. In cynical terms, one might say that today's medical home model is the gatekeeper over again with nicer words, but now it is in a new era where supply and cost limitations are newly understood and palpable in the setting of nearly 10% unemployment and the deepest recession since the Great Depression.

Managed care's gatekeepers and today's PCMHs share the strategy of asking patients to have their comprehensive care coordinated in a single primary care environment and become subject to real financial limits to the amount of care that can be delivered. Recent innovations in primary care, such as coordinated chronic illness care, multidisciplinary team approaches, and health information technology, combine to offer new processes of care that were not understood or available 15 years ago, and they have the potential of increasing the cost-effectiveness of care as well. These innovations, coupled with the unsustainable costs associated with unchecked growth in the volume and inefficiency of care delivery, plus the increasing multimorbidity needs of an ageing population offer hope that the PCMH will not suffer the fate of its predecessor "gatekeepers".

In 2007, the major US primary care organizations agreed on a set of guiding principles for the PCMH, which are presented next.[60]

- Personal physician: each patient has an ongoing relationship with a personal physician trained to provide first contact, continuous and comprehensive care.
- Physician-directed medical practice: the personal physician leads a team of individuals at the practice level who collectively take responsibility for the ongoing care of patients.
- Whole-person orientation: the personal physician provides all the patient's health care or arranges care with other qualified professionals for all stages of life, acute care, chronic care, preventive services and end-of-life care.
- Care is coordinated and/or integrated across all elements of the complex health-care system (e.g. subspecialty care, hospitals, home health agencies, nursing homes) and the patient's community (e.g. family, public and private community-based services). Care is facilitated by registries, information technology, health information exchange and other means, to ensure that patients get the indicated care when and where they need and want it, in a culturally and linguistically appropriate manner.
- Quality and safety are hallmarks of the medical home:
  - practices advocate for their patients to attain optimal, patient-centred outcomes that are defined by a care-planning process driven by a compassionate, robust partnership between physicians, patients and the patient's family
  - evidence-based medicine and clinical decision-support tools guide decision-making
  - physicians in the practice accept accountability for continuous quality improvement through voluntary engagement in performance measurement and improvement
  - patients actively participate in decision-making, and feedback is sought to ensure patients' expectations are being met
  - information technology is utilized appropriately to support optimal patient care, performance measurement, patient education and enhanced communication
  - practices go through a voluntary recognition process by an appropriate nongovernmental entity, to demonstrate that they have the capabilities to provide patient-centred services consistent with the medical home model
  - patients and families participate in quality-improvement activities at the practice level.
- Enhanced access to care is available through systems such as open scheduling, expanded hours and new options for communication between patients, their personal physician and practice staff.
- Payment appropriately recognizes the added value provided to patients who have a PCMH.

These principles describe the innovations necessary in primary care to achieve improved coordination of care and better outcomes. All the principles are progressive, except one that sticks out as a commitment to the past

– physician-directed care. The crafters of these principles continue to believe in the primacy of the doctor–patient relationship and the positive therapeutic effect of ongoing continuity between patient and physician.

Is the PCMH, with its commitment to physician-directed care, really patient centred? It depends on what one means by patient-centred care. To some, being patient centred means that the focus is on the patient, not just the disease. Another view is to put the patient on the care team, even at the centre of the team.[61] In the Institute of Medicine report, *Crossing the quality chasm*, patient centred is one of the six aims for quality health care, and the report defines it as care that encompasses qualities of compassion, empathy and responsiveness to the needs, values and expressed preferences of the individual patient.[62] Shared decision-making has emerged as a desired care model, especially when the evidence is not completely clear what tests and treatments are preferred, such as with screening and treatment for breast or prostate cancer. In such situations, patient preference becomes paramount and often drives the medical decision-making. These concepts allow for patient centredness through their more active and engaged participation, while converting the traditional physician control over medical practice into the role of expert collaborator and coach.

The PCMH concept has much to offer patients with multimorbidity, but it will not reach its full potential without addressing mental health needs.[63,64] More than just patient centredness, the integration of mental health services will enable the PCMH to meet its goals of enhanced access and coordinated and high-quality care.[65] Mental health professionals in the PCMH, what some are labelling "collaborative care", will have the ability to assist any primary care patient, either through a traditional referral system or by immediately assisting with care in coordination with other health-care professionals as they are in the process of seeing their patients. When the primary care physician detects emotional stress, a formal mental health diagnosis, or a health behaviour change need, they can perform a "warm handoff" during the visit to the embedded mental health professional, which is more likely to result in patients receiving timely mental health services compared with usual referral to similar, but distant carved-out services. While more studies are needed to deepen the support for collaborative services across the full range of mental health needs, there is strong evidence that such care improves outcomes for patients with depression – one of the most common mental health diagnoses in primary care. Additional potential benefits of collaborative care include (1) improved sensitivity and accuracy of mental health problem identification among partnering primary care physicians; (2) contributions to increased screening, detection and intervention; and (3) possibly earlier prevention of mental health and substance use issues.

The success of these interdisciplinary and community-oriented approaches is due to the fact that an increasing percentage of the population requires specialized, multidimensional support to achieve patient-centred goals. New technologies (e.g. web-based electronic communication and telemedicine) and models of care delivery (e.g. coordination with community resources and promotion of patients' self-management skills described in the next section) may provide opportunities to improve this support.[66] The challenges for the future will be to help practices achieve improvements in patient-specific goals in ways that are both cost effective and efficient.

Treatment of multimorbidity in primary care

"Staffing up"

The complexity arising from multimorbidity presents challenges for the primary care clinician. It is impossible for one clinician to possess all the skills to manage this complexity simply by using a stepped care approach. Enhancing the primary care team skill mix and collaboration with other mental health and social agencies are essential to achieve the best outcomes. In Chapter 7 of this volume, Riba and colleagues describe how to manage the interface between mental health and medicine in primary care and highlight several models of collaborative care. Research is emerging that shows the benefits of collaborative care. For example, Katon et al. found that a collaborative care intervention involving nurse care managers and physicians integrating the management of medical and psychological illnesses improved both medical outcomes and depression in depressed patients with diabetes, coronary heart disease or both.[67]

Skill mix in primary care can be attained through either delegation or diversification. Delegation is when a task formerly performed by a professional is delegated to someone outside the profession but within the team who traditionally would not have provided that service, such as depression care managers. This provides the professional more time for complex and specialized tasks. Diversification occurs when (1) primary care services are enhanced through the recruitment of a new type of workforce; or (2) primary care team members increase the breadth of their original training by developing expertise in a new field or technique.

The outcome of this approach is to diversify the skills within the team so that a wider range of interventions can be delivered to those with multimorbidity and complexity. It also provides cost containment through the efficiencies realized by empowering other members of the workforce across professional boundaries to "staff up" or work at the top of their skill level – to provide the intervention at a cheaper unit cost. The skill mix can be held within the immediate primary care team or in collaboration with other primary care teams in the same locality. This results in improved quality of care, as staff with the appropriate skills can be deployed to deliver their intervention most effectively, so enabling complexity to be better managed within the team.[68-71]

Skill mix is applicable to high-, medium- and low-income countries. However, there may be a need for legislation or regulation to enable workers to carry out tasks not previously performed by their professional group. In the UK, for example, nurses, optometrists, pharmacists, physiotherapists, podiatrists and radiographers are able to prescribe medication through a framework termed a patient group direction (PGD),[72] described in Chapter 12 of this book. The World Health Organization (WHO) *Mental health atlas 2005* describes a scarcity of secondary care mental health resources and low numbers of mental health professionals in low- and medium-income countries.[73] Increased use of delegation and diversification by family doctors working in low- and medium-income countries, supported by an appropriate governance framework is recommended so that they can better cater for the complex needs of mental health patients. The WHO *Mental health atlas 2005* also recognizes a need for high-income countries to increase the development of skill mix, including increasing access to non-medical doctor prescribing and the use of other health-care workers to reduce cost and better utilize available economic resources.[73]

Stepped care

The stepped care model provides a framework for the organization and provision of services from the least intrusive, most effective intervention to the most restrictive or intrusive intervention in a graded way, depending on needs and complexity,[74] within the pyramid of health.[75] Many patients with mental disorders suffer multiple simultaneous conditions, which may be physical health problems, comorbid mental health disorders or issues arising from social disadvantage. Some of the complexity may be associated with behavioural manifestations of mental disorder such as overactivity, agitation, accidental and non-accidental injuries; or with cognitive impairment, movement disorders, pseudo-Parkinsonism, substance misuse, housing problems, employment issues, and relationship issues. All these problems need to be identified, assessed and addressed by the family doctor, their extended primary care teams, the wider support networks in the community and secondary care mental health teams, and in low- and medium-income countries through other workers.

The Department of Health in the UK has developed a model to address the complexity of mental health presentations.[76] This combines a number of features of illness and disability to describe the complexity of any given individual mental health presentation by using a description of the symptoms of illness and diagnosis, impairment, associated risks and course of the illness. When these features are combined, the individual is assigned to a cluster of mental disorders. This methodology is particularly useful in primary care as it addresses mental health difficulties in a holistic way, taking account of the core illness while acknowledging physical and psychiatric comorbidity and including the wider social determinants of health such as living conditions and individual vulnerability to self and others.

For primary care to be effective in managing complex patients with multimorbidity, it has to adopt an approach that enables the clinician to quantify complexity and allocate resources according to the individual's cumulative need, taking into account diversity and ethnicity. This can be enhanced with a stepped care approach to mental health issues, while recognizing that supporting self-care is paramount in each step within the model. Each of the conditions identified must be treated to its optimal potential, using local and national evidence-based guidelines, recognizing that medication may lead to interactions or side-effects that can worsen other comorbid conditions. It is essential to have good communication and good record keeping with patients and all the agencies involved in supporting care and this may require data-sharing protocols to be in place.

Table 33.1 presents a proposed stepped care model for complex multimorbid mental health presentations.

Table 33.1 Proposed stepped care model for complex multimorbid mental health presentations

Steps	Focus of intervention	Nature of intervention
Step 4: high risk	• All patients with two or more conditions • At least one identified mental health problem • Severe disability • Has a clearly identifiable risk characteristic, such as imminent thoughts or plans relating to self-harm (or harm to others) or suicide	• Treatment of identified conditions • Need to collaborate with local specialist services • Combined use of primary, secondary and tertiary care resources through case management • Psychological therapy, e.g. cognitive-behavioural therapy (CBT) • Expert patient programme to improve self-care techniques • Use of skill mix available in the primary care setting • Family interventions • Shared care/collaborative care with other community providers e.g. charitable organizations, nongovernmental organizations (NGOs), etc. • Appointment of health advocate from primary care skill mix
Step 3: moderate risk	• All patients with two or more conditions • At least one identified mental health problem • Moderate disability • Has non-specific thoughts or ideas regarding harm to self or others, e.g. regrets that self-harm failed to lead to death, but no intention to undertake further self-harm	• Treatment of identified conditions • Psychological therapy, e.g. CBT • Expert patient programme to improve self-care techniques • Use of skill mix available in the primary care setting • Family interventions • Shared care/collaborative care with other community providers, e.g. charitable organizations, NGOs, etc. • Appointment of health advocate from primary care skill mix
Step 2: low–moderate risk	• All patients with two or more conditions • At least one identified mental health problem • Mild disability • No thoughts or plans regarding harm to self or others.	• Treatment of identified conditions • Psychological therapy, e.g. CBT • Expert patient programme to improve self-care techniques • Use of skill mix available in the primary care setting
Step 1: low risk	• All uncomplicated patients with two or more conditions • Low or no disability • To be screened for comorbid mental and physical health conditions • No thoughts or plans regarding harm to self or others.	• Assessment and screening • Treatment of identified conditions • Support • Information about illness including coping and self-management strategies through readily available community resources using skill mix available within the community and primary care workforce • Problem-solving techniques • Monitoring • Promotion of self-care activities

Finally, in recognition of the fact that patients spend only a relatively small percentage of their time with any of the health-care team members, and the vast majority of their time in their own living environment, teaching them self-management skills is paramount for success in managing multimorbidity. Self-management, which teaches skills to carry out treatment plans, guides behaviour change, and promotes emotional support, increases the likelihood of success in the management of chronic diseases.[77–80] In the USA, health-related behaviours are associated with 40% of avoidable morbidity and mortality.[81] Self-management consists of the following components outlined by Bayless et al.:[82]

- engaging in activities that promote physical and psychological health
- interacting with health-care providers and adhering to treatment recommendations, monitoring health status and making associated care decisions
- managing the impact of the illness on physical, psychological and social functioning.[83,84]

Patients with multimorbidity require a different approach to self-management in comparison to patients with single diseases. A significantly higher percentage of patients with multimorbidity compared to those with single morbidity receive care from multiple health-care professionals, including nurses, physician's assistants, psychologists, social workers, nutritionists and pharmacists,[85] which often means understanding and implementing multiple, and sometimes conflicting, care plans. This complexity demands a self-management approach that is tailored to individual patients, incorporates support for both disease-specific and general self-management skill sets,[82] and encourages continuous communication between health-care professionals.

The literature has identified numerous barriers to the effective implementation of self-management strategies. Three studies explored potential barriers for patients with multiple morbidities. Participants in these studies reported the following: insufficient awareness of resource support, transportation problems, financial constraints (e.g. lack of insurance coverage), compound effects of diseases and medications, persistent depressive symptoms, and feeling overwhelmed by a single illness.[58,86,87] When barriers are minimized or eliminated, potentially useful approaches to supporting self-management include motivational interviewing to explore and resolve ambivalence in the patient,[88] and collaborative goal setting and treatment planning.[89] Collaborative goal setting and treatment planning that includes reflective listening, validation of the patient's point of view, curiosity, clear explanations, and summarizing statements by the doctor is associated with positive patient outcomes.[90]

Conclusions

A recurring theme in this chapter is the importance of patient-centred care and collaboration between health-care professionals to effectively manage a range of biological and psychosocial issues in primary care. To treat complex patients, members of the health-care team need to closely collaborate and likely relinquish some autonomy.[91] How will the workforce be prepared to provide this kind of multidisciplinary, collaborative care for complex patients?

There is a growing need for the development of programmes to teach physicians and mental health professionals to work together in teams.[92] Such programmes establish an educational environment for collaboration that includes the following attributes described by Miller and Cohen-Katz:[91]

- *mindfulness:* openness to new ideas
- *respectful interaction:* mutually valued interchange
- *heedful interrelating:* awareness of one's own role and that of others
- *channelled effectiveness:* appropriate use of diverse communication
- *mix of social and task relatedness:* conversations about work, family and friends
- *diversity:* respect for differences
- *trust:* belief that you can depend on others.

PCMHs, as well as other community-oriented health-care systems, can provide the educational environment to improve physician skills in leadership, teamwork, patient education and communication.[93,94] In addition, such training can help mental health professionals overcome their tendency to work in isolation, and increase their flexibility in the ways they deliver care.[95] Primary care environments that nurture a culture of collaboration will significantly benefit all health-care professionals and the patients they serve.

References

1   Anderson G. *Chronic care: making the case for ongoing care.* Princeton, NJ, Robert Woods Johnson Foundation, 2010.

2   Fortin M et al. Prevalence of multimorbidity among adults seen in family practice. *Annals of Family Medicine*, 2005, 3:223–228.

3   Schafer I et al. The German multicare-study: patterns of multimorbidity in primary health care – protocol of a prospective cohort study. *BMC Health Services Research*, 2009, 9:145.

4   Feinstein AR. Pre-therapeutic classification of co-morbidity in chronic disease. *Journal of Chronic Disease*, 1970, 23:455–468.

5   Valderas JM et al. Defining comorbidity: implications for understanding health and health services. *Annals of Family Medicine*, 2009, 7:357–363.

6   Starfield B. *Diseases, comorbidity, and multimorbidity in primary care. Primary care course.* Cape Town, The Johns Hopkins University, 2007.

7   Fortin M et al. Multimorbidity's many challenges. *BMJ*, 2007, 334: 1016–1017.

8   Mercer SW, Watt GMC. The inverse care law: clinical primary care encounters in deprived and affluent areas of Scotland. *Annals of Family Medicine*, 2007, 5:503–510.

9   van den Akker M, Buntinx F, Knottnerus JA. Comorbidity or multimorbidity: what's in a name. a review of the literature. *European Journal of General Practice*, 1996, 2:65–70.

10 Bayliss EA et al. Processes of care desired by elderly patients with multimorbidities, *Family Practice*, 2008, 25:287–293.

11 Starfield B. Challenges to primary care from co- and multi-morbidity. *Primary Health Care Research and Development*, 2011, 12:1–2.

12 Peek CJ, Baird MA, Coleman E. Primary care for patient complexity, not only disease. *Families, Systems and Health*, 2009, 27:287–302.

13 Gijsen R et al. Causes and consequences of comorbidity: a review. *Journal of Clinical Epidemiology*, 2001, 54:661–674.

14 Vogeli C et al. Multiple chronic conditions: prevalence, health consequences, and implications for quality, care management, and costs. *Journal of General Internal Medicine*, 2007, 22:391–395.

15 Barnett K. Understanding the relationship between multi-morbidity and socioeconomic deprivation. In: *The Scottish School of Primary Care Annual Conference, "Thinking global", Edinburgh, 19–20 April 2011* (http://www.sspc.ac.uk/events/sspc%20kbarnett.pdf, accessed 28 December 2011).

16 Fortin M et al. Relationship between multimorbidity and health-related quality of life of patients in primary care. *Quality of Life Research: An International Journal of Quality of Life Aspects of Treatment, Care and Rehabilitation*, 2006, 15:83–91.

17 Marengoni A et al. Prevalence of chronic diseases and multimorbidity among the elderly population in Sweden. *American Journal of Public Health*, 2008, 98:1198–1200.

18 Linn BS, Linn MW, Gurel L. Cumulative illness rating scale. *Journal of the American Geriatric Society*, 1968, 16:622–626.

19 Wolff JL, Starfield B, Anderson G. Prevalence, expenditures, and complications of multiple chronic conditions in the elderly. *Archives of Internal Medicine*, 2002, 162:2269–2276.

20 Forrest CB, Reid RJ. Prevalence of health problems and primary care physicians' specialty referral decisions. *Journal of Family Practice*, 2001, 50:427–432.

21 Starfield B et al. Ambulatory specialist use by nonhospitalized patients in US health plans: correlates and consequences. *Journal of Ambulatory Care Management*, 2009, 32:216–225.

22 Hwang W et al. Out-of-pocket medical spending for care of chronic conditions. *Health Affairs*, 2001, 20:267–278.

23 Warshaw G. Introduction: advances and challenges in care of older people with chronic illness. *Generation*, 2006, 30:5–10.

24 Lee TA et al. Mortality rate in veterans with multiple chronic conditions. *Journal of General Internal Medicine*, 2007, 22:403–407.

25 Hoffman C, Rice D, Sung H. Persons with chronic conditions: their prevalence and costs. *JAMA*, 1996, 276:1473–1479.

26 Field TS et al. Risk factors for adverse drug events among older adults in the ambulatory setting. *Journal of the American Geriatric Society*, 2004, 52:1349–1354.

27 Oldridge NB et al. Prevalence and outcomes of comorbid metabolic and cardiovasclar conditions in middle- and older age adults. *Journal of Clinical Epidemiology*, 2001, 54:928–934.

28 Charlson M et al. Validation of a combined comorbidity index. *Journal of Clinical Epidemiology*, 1994, 47:1245–1251.

29 Berkanovic E, Hurwicz ML. Rheumatoid arthritis and comorbidity. *The Journal of Rheumatology*, 1990, 17:888–892.

30 Dunlop DD et al. Arthritis prevalence and activity limitations in older adults. *Arthritis and Rheumatism*, 2001, 44:212–221.

31 Guralnik JM et al. Maintaining mobility in late life: demographic characteristics and chronic conditions. *American Journal of Epidemiology*, 1993, 137(8):845.

32 Rozzini R et al. Geriatric index of comorbidity: validations and comparison with other measures of comorbidity. *Age and Ageing*, 2002, 31:277–285.

33 Verbrugge LM, Lepkowski JM, Imanaka Y. Comorbidity and its impact on disability. *The Milbank Quarterly*, 1989, 67:450–484.

34 Verbrugge LM, Lepkowski JM, Konkol LL. Levels of disability among U.S. adults with arthritis. *Journal of Gerontology: Social Sciences*, 1991, 46:S71–S83.

35 Elixhauser A et al. *Hospitalization in the United States, 1997*. Rockville, MD, Agency for Healthcare Research and Quality, 2000 (AHRQ Publication No. 00-0031; HCUP Fact Book No. 1).

36 Gabriel SE, Crowson CS, O'Fallon WM. Comorbidity in arthritis. *Journal of Rheumatology*, 1999, 26:2475–2479.

37 Michelson H, Bolund C, Brandberg Y. Multiple chronic health problems are negatively associated with health related quality of life (HRQoL) irrespective of age. *Quality of Life Research: An International Journal of Quality of Life Aspects of Treatment, Care and Rehabilitation*, 2000, 9:1093–1104.

38 Starfield B et al. Comorbidity and the use of primary care and specialist care in the elderly. *Annals of Family Medicine*, 2005, 3:215–222.

39 Fortin M, Bravo G, Hudon C. Psychological distress and multimorbidity in primary care. *Annals of Family Medicine*, 2006, 4:417–422.

40 Gamma A, Angst J. Concurrent psychiatric comorbidity and multimorbidity in a community study: gender differences and quality of life. *European Archives of Psychiatry and Clinical Neuroscience*, 2001, 251:43–46.

41 Warner L et al. Giving and taking – differential effects of providing, receiving and anticipating emotional support on quality of life in adults with multiple illnesses. *Journal of Health Psychology*, 2010, 15:660–670.

42 Schwartz C, Sendor M. Helping others helps oneself: response shift effects in peer support. *Social Science and Medicine*, 1999, 48:1563–1575.

43 Felitti VJ et al. Relationship of childhood abuse and household dysfunction to many of the leading causes of death in adults. The Adverse Childhood Experiences (ACE) study. *American Journal of Preventive Medicine*, 1998, 14:245–258.

44 Nicolaidis C et al. Differences in physical and mental health symptoms and mental health utilization associated with intimate-partner violence versus childhood abuse. *Psychosomatics*, 2009, 50:340–346.

45 Zielinski DS. Child maltreatment and adult socioeconomic well-being. *Child Abuse and Neglect*, 2009, 33:661–665.

46 Crabtree H et al. The Comorbidity Symptom Scale: a combined disease inventory and assessment of symptom severity. *Journal of the American Geriatrics Society*, 2000, 48:1674–1678.

47 Peek CJ. Collaborative care: aids to navigation. In: *Collaborative Care Research Network (CCRN), Research development conference, 8–9 October 2009, Denver, CO, USA* (http://www.aafp.org/online/en/home/clinical/research/natnet/get-involved/ccrn-info/ccrnconference.html, accessed 28 December 2011).

48   Sobel DS. Improving health outcomes through collaborative care: "out of the Box" healthcare strategies. In: *Institute of Behavioral Healthcare, Third National Primary Care Behavioral Healthcare Summit. Chicago, 10–12 November 1997* (http://www.acponline.org/clinical_information/journals_publications/ecp/augsep98/detect.htm, accessed 28 December 2011).

49   Gawande A. The hot spotters: can we lower medical costs by giving the neediest patients better care? *The New Yorker*, January 24 2011.

50   Fries JF et al. Reducing health care costs by reducing the need and demand for medical services. *New England Journal of Medicine*, 1993, 329:321–325.

51   Innes AD, Campion P, Griffiths F. Complex consultations and the "edge of chaos". *British Journal of General Practice*, 2005, 55:47–52.

52   Stacey RD. *Strategic management and organisational dynamics: the challenge of complexity*, 3rd ed. London, Pitman Publishing, 1999.

53   McDaniel SH, Campbell TL, Seaburn DB. Principles for collaboration between health and mental health providers in primary care. *Family Systems Medicine*, 1995, 13:283–298.

54   Ivbijaro G, Kolkiewicz L, Palazidou E. Mental health in primary care: ways of working – the impact of culture. *Primary Care Mental Health*, 2005, 3:47–53.

55   Mulvaney-Day NE et al. Preferences for relational style with mental health clinicians: A qualitative comparison of African American, Latino, and Non-Latino White patients. *Journal of Clinical Psychology*, 2011, 67:31–44.

56   Plsek PE, Greenhalgh T. Complexity science: the challenge of complexity in health care. *BMJ*, 2001, 323:625–628.

57   Švab I. Take home message from the president of Wonca Europe. *Primary care*, 2010, 10:13.

58   Bayliss EA, Ellis JL, Steiner JF. Barriers to self-management and quality-of-life outcomes in seniors with multimorbidities. *Annals of Family Medicine*, 2007, 5:395–402.

59   Borovečki A, Belicza B, Orešković S. 75th anniversary of Andrija Stampar School of Public Health – what can we learn from our past for our future? *Croatian Medical Journal*, 2002, 43:371–373.

60   American Academy of Family Physicians, American Academy of Pediatrics, American College of Physicians, American Osteopathic Association. *Joint principles of the patient-centered medical home*, 2007 (http://www.aafp.org/online/etc/medialib/aafp_org/documents/policy/fed/jointprinciplespcmh0207.Par.0001.File.tmp/022107medicalhome.pdf, accessed 22 December 2011).

61   Berenson RA et al. A house is not a home: keeping patients at the center of practice redesign. *Health Affairs*, 2008, 27:1219–1230.

62   Institute of Medicine, Committee on the Quality of Health Care in America. *Crossing the quality chasm: a new health system for the 21st century*. Washington, DC, National Academy Press, 2001.

63   Croghan TW, Brown JD. *Integrating mental health treatment into the patient centered medical home*. Rockville, MD, Agency for Healthcare Research and Quality, US Department of Health and Human Services, 2010.

64   de Gruy FV, Etz RS. Attending to the whole person in the patient-centered medical home: the case for incorporating mental healthcare, substance abuse care, and health behavior change. *Families, Systems and Health*, 2010, 28:298–307.

65   Hunter CL, Goodie JL. Operational and clinical components for integrated-collaborative behavioural healthcare in the patient-centered medical home. *Families, Systems and Health*, 2010, 28:308–321.

66   Bayliss EA et al. Supporting self-management for patients with complex medical needs: recommendations of a working group. *Chronic Illness*, 2007, 3:167–175.

67   Katon WJ, Lin EHB, Von Korff M. Collaborative care for patients with depression and chronic illnesses. *New England Journal of Medicine*, 2010, 363:2611–2620.

68   *Discussion paper 3: Determining skill mix in the health workforce: guidelines for managers and health professionals*. Geneva, World Health Organization, 2000.

69   Buchan J, Dal Poz MR. Skill mix in health care workforce: reviewing the evidence. *Bulletin of the World Health Organization*, 2002, 80:575–580.

70   Kernick D, Scott A. Economic approaches to doctor/nurse skill mix: problems, pitfalls, and partial solutions. *British Journal of General Practice*, 2002, 52:42–46.

71 Buchan J, Calman L. *OECD Health Working Paper No. 17: skill-mix and policy change in the health workforce: nurses in advanced roles.* Paris, Organisation for Economic Co-operation and Development, 2005.

72 *Non-medical prescribing by nurses, optometrists, pharmacists, physiotherapists, podiatrists and radiographers: a quick guide for commissioner.* Liverpool, National Prescribing Centre, 2010.

73 *Mental health atlas 2005,* rev ed. Geneva, World Health Organization, 2005.

74 Chew-Graham C. NICE has modified its stepped-care model for treating depression. *Guidelines in Practice,* 2009, 12:1–7.

75 World Health Organization and Wonca. *Integrating mental health into primary care. A global perspective.* Geneva, World Health Organization, 2008.

76 *Clustering booklet. For use in Mental Health Payment by Results evaluation work (Jul–Dec 2010).* London, Department of Health, 2010.

77 Bodenheimer T et al. Patient self-management of chronic disease in primary care. *JAMA,* 2002, 288:2469–2475.

78 National Collaborating Centre for Mental Health. *Depression: the NICE guideline on the treatment and management of depression in adults.* London: The British Psychological Society and The Royal College of Psychiatrists, 2010.

79 Wagner EH. Managed care and chronic illness: health services research needs. *Health Services Research,* 1997, 32:702–714.

80 Katon W et al. Rethinking practitioner roles in chronic illness: the specialist, primary care physician and the practice nurse. *General Hospital Psychiatry,* 2001, 23:138–144.

81 Mokdad AH et al. Actual causes of death in the United States, 2000. *JAMA,* 2004, 291:1238–1245.

82 Bayliss EA et al. Supporting self-management for patients with complex medical needs: recommendations of a working group. *Chronic Illness,* 2007, 3:167–175.

83 Clark NM et al. Self-management of chronic disease by older adults: a review and questions for research. *Journal of Aging Health,* 1991, 3:3–27.

84 Wagner EH, Austin BT, Von Korff M. Improving outcomes in chronic illness. *Managed Care Quarterly,* 1996, 4:12–25.

85 Noel PH et al. The challenges of multimorbidity from the patient perspective. *Journal of General Internal Medicine,* 2007, 22:419–424.

86 Bayliss EA et al. Descriptions of barriers to self-care by persons with comorbid chronic diseases. *Annals of Family Medicine,* 2003, 1:4–7.

87 Jerant AF, von Friederichs-Fitzwater MM, Moore M. Patients' perceived barriers to active self-management of chronic conditions. *Patient Education and Counseling,* 2005, 57:300–307.

88 Resnicow K et al. Motivational interviewing in health promotion: it sounds like something is changing. *Health Psychology,* 2001, 21:444–451.

89 Wagner EH et al. Finding common ground: patient-centeredness and evidence-based chronic illness care. *Journal of Alternative Complementary Medicine,* 2005, 11:S7–S15.

90 Beck RS, Daughtridge R, Sloane PD. Physician–patient communication in the primary care office: a systematic review. *Journal of the American Board of Family Practice,* 2002, 15:25–38.

91 Miller WL, Cohen-Katz J. Creating collaborative learning environments for transforming primary care practices now. *Families, Systems and Health,* 2010, 28:334–347.

92 Blount FA, Miller BF. Addressing the workforce crisis in integrated primary care. *Journal of Clinical Psychology in Medical Settings,* 2009, 16:113–119.

93 Bohmer RMJ. 2010. Managing the new primary care: the new skills that will be needed. *Health Affairs,* 2010, 29:1010–1014.

94 Rieselbach RE, Crouse BJ, Frohna JG. Teaching primary care in community health centers: addressing the workforce crisis for the underserved. *Annals of Internal Medicine,* 2010, 152:118–122.

95 Edwards TM, Patterson J. Supervising family therapy trainees in primary care medical settings: context matters. *Journal of Marital and Family Therapy,* 2006, 32:33–43.

Index

dysthymia 87, 245, 288, 324, 566, 634

Early Assessment Risk List for Boys (EARL-20B) 541
Early Assessment Risk List for Girls (EARL-21G) 541
early childhood 9, 10–12, 272, 273
Early Head Start programme 35
Eating Attitudes Test (EAT) 439
eating disorders 421–44
    aetiology 425–7
    assessment 427–36
    diagnosis 422–4
    epidemiology 424–5
    key messages 421
    mental disorders at the interface 614, 617
    overview 421–2, 440
    sociocultural factors 427
    treatment 436–40
echolalia 542
ecstasy 557
Edinburgh Postnatal Depression Scale
    (EPDS-10) 365, 369, 373, 375–7, 525
education
    dementia 582–3
    determinants of health and mental health 13, 15
    prevention of episodes of mental disorder 35, 36,
      37
    suicidality 191, 192
    Tackling Stigma Framework 57–8
Edwards, G 471
efavirenz 635
effectiveness 58, 144, 146
efficiency 144, 146
Egypt 102, 103
Ekers, D 26, 327
elderly patients see older adults
electroconvulsive therapy (ECT) 25, 230, 349
Eliot, TS 83
emotion-based coping style 392
empathy 69, 82, 83, 85, 481–2
empirically supported treatment (EST) 396, 399
employment 13, 14, 37, 271, 303–4
empowerment 17, 38
encouragement 68, 69–71, 72
endocrine and metabolic disorders 613–28
Endocrine Society of America 448
end-of-life care 66, 595–6
End of Life Care Strategy 600
endogenous opioids 427
endorphins 267
engagement session 400–2, 400–2
Engel, George 117
England 56–9, 242, 251–3 see also UK
enhanced care 26
enhanced specialist referral (ESR) 25
"enhanced usual care" 25

environment
    the consultation 156
    determinants of health and mental health 6, 8, 10,
      11
    environmental interventions 270–1
    ethics 91
    infancy and early childhood 522
EPDS see Edinburgh Postnatal Depression Scale
epilepsy 87, 89, 105, 594, 660
Equality Act (2010) 450
equity 50, 82, 146
erythromycin 636
escitalopram 215, 289, 298, 299, 300, 330
EST see empirically supported treatment
Estonia 182
ethics 80–94
    abuse of psychiatry 86–7
    context 91–2
    diagnostic consultation 161–2
    how could things be better? 92
    illness, disease and health: the mental
      dimension 83–4
    impossibility of precise diagnosis 84
    journey to being a patient 84–5
    key messages 80
    listening and hearing 89–91
    mad or bad 85–6
    mind and body 88–9
    moral luck 86
    sensibility and insight 88
    somatization 89
    stigma 88
    traditional ethical perspectives 80–3
ethnicity
    advocacy and overcoming stigma 49, 56, 60
    determinants of health and mental health 15, 17
    environmental interventions 270
    severe mental illness and physical health 650, 652
    suicidality 179
EURODEM (European Community Concerted
    Action on the Epidemiology and Prevention of
    Dementia) Group 572
Europe 28, 255–6
European Association for the Study of Diabetes 350
European Psychiatric Association 350
European Society of Cardiology 350
evaluation of primary care mental health 138–52
    background 139–40
    collaborative care 32–3
    evaluation focus and objectives 146–7
    evaluation research design 147–9
    evaluation theories 144–5
    health services evaluation frameworks 145–6
    key concepts 140–4
    key messages 138

I–Thou relation 69

Jackson, JL 389, 409
James, William 65, 66
Jamtland study 191
Japan 17, 179, 191
job satisfaction 14
JOBS programme 37
Johnson, SK 390, 391, 392, 393
Josephson, AM 70
Judaism 179
Judeo–Christian ethics 81
Jung, Carl 66
Junger, G 161
justice 82

Kalabay, L. 126
Kaltenthaler, E 26
Kaner, EFS 37
Kaplan, AS 431, 437
Kates, N 32
Katon, W 33, 192, 679
Kehoe, Nancy 73
Kendrick, T 26, 324
Kenya 103–4, 108, 127
Kessler, D 26
Kessler, R 288
ketamine 558
King's Fund 259
Kirsch, I 169
Kleinman, A 169
Koenig, HG 68
Kohler, L 394
Konig, H-H 27
Korsakoff's syndrome 617, 630
Kraepelin, Emil 353
Kroenke, K 388, 409
Kubler-Ross, Elizabeth 71

labiaplasty 452
Lader, M 509
Lalonde Report (1976) 6
Lambert, MJ 398
lamotrigine 229, 231, 235
The Lancet 28, 50, 127, 421
Lancet Global Mental Health Group 612
language 57, 90, 91
Lariam® 634
Lasegue, Charles 421
Latino patients 390
laughter 267
Launer, J 402
lavender 595
learning disabilities 99, 540, 597, 598
Leccese, M 560

Lee, A 129
Lee, David 351
Leeds Dependence Questionnaire (LDQ) 476
Leiknes, KA 391
lemon balm oils 595
Leucht, S 643
levels of systemic collaboration 119–21
Levine, SB 448
levodopa 591
Lieberman, JA 397
life-course framework 8
LIFE Curriculum 54
life expectancy 62, 63, 644
life-review techniques 38
life-stages 10–18
    adolescence 12–13
    adulthood 13–17
    old age 17–18
    pregnancy and early childhood 10–12
lifestyle behaviours 15, 37, 652
light therapy 349, 595
Lin, EHB 321
Lipowski, ZJ 388
listening 68, 69, 72, 73, 89–91, 390
literacy 15, 37
lithium
    bipolar disorder 231, 233–4, 344–5, 347
    disruptive behavioural disorder 541
    mental disorders at the interface 621, 622, 637
    prescribing principles 209, 222, 231, 233–4, 237
Lithuania 13, 179
liver cirrhosis 472, 484
Liverpool University Neuroleptic Side-effect Rating
    Scale (LUNSERS) 209
Livingston, G 595
Living well with dementia 577
lofepramine 216, 222
London 251–3, 270
London School of Economics 242
looked-after children 12
lorazepam 231, 299, 488, 625, 630, 636
low birth weight 10, 11, 643
low-income countries
    determinants of health and mental health 18–21,
        27–9, 30
    intervention models 369–72
    managing the interface in primary care 122,
        126–7
    perinatal mental health 367
    prevalence of mental health disorders 98
    public health aspects 102, 107–8
    schizophrenia 357
    suicidality 196–7
low-intensity psychosocial interventions 244, 327–9
Luoma, JB 188

phaeochromocytomas 616, 619, 621
phalloplasty 452
pharmacodynamics 626, 636
pharmacokinetics 626–7, 636
phenelzine 222, 300, 301, 626
phobias
  adolescent mental health 556, 557
  anxiety 286, 293, 296, 301
  chronic pain syndromes 631
  cost-effective treatments 26
PHQ *see* Patient Health Questionnaire
physical abuse 15, 72, 674, 675
physical activity
  anxiety 295
  dementia 587
  depression 220, 326, 329
  determinants of health and mental health 15, 25
  heath promotion 653, 654
  interventions across the life course 35, 38
  social and environmental interventions 267, 274
physical health and mental illness 609–86
  mental disorders due to physical illness at the
    interface 611–40
  multimorbidity in PCMH 672–86
  physical health consequences of mental
    illness 641–71
physical health consequences of mental illness 641–
  71
  cancer and SMI 649–50
  cardiovascular disease and SMI 644–6
  comorbidity associated with severe mental
    illness 643–4
  COPD and SMI 648
  depression and physical health 656–61
  diabetes and SMI 646–7
  HIV and hepatitis and SMI 649
  hypothyroidism and SMI 649
  influence of culture on clinical care in SMI 650–1
  interventions 651–5
  key messages 641
  models of mental health care delivery 661–2
  mortality related to severe mental illness and
    physical illness 642
  osteoporosis and SMI 648–9
  overview 641
  prevalence of mortality risk factors in SMI 644
  racial and ethnic minority groups and SMI 650
  severe mental illness and physical health 641–2,
    655–6
physical restraints 626
physiotherapists 238
Pignone, MP 23
pimozide 543
pining 311
placebo effect 304

PMDD *see* premenstrual dysphoric disorder
pneumonia 634
poetry 90
poisoning 181, 183
policy 101–2
political influence 86
political violence 85
pollution 522
polycyclic aromatic hydrocarbons (PAHs) 236
polycystic ovary syndrome (PCOS) 616, 619, 621
polypharmacy 209
population health approach 141
Positive Parenting Programme (PPP) 272
positive regard 85
Posmontier, B 367
postnatal depression 11, 24, 367
postnatal support groups 274
"postpartum blues" 521
postpartum psychosis 368
post-traumatic stress disorder (PTSD)
  adolescent mental health 557, 559
  chronic pain syndromes 631, 632
  depression 325
  epidemiology 286
  evaluation and diagnosis 291
  HIV/AIDS 634–5
  infancy and early childhood 12, 521
  pharmacological treatment 300–1
  prevalence of mental health disorders 98
  psychological treatment 296–7
  social change 268
poverty
  childhood trauma 675
  determinants of health and mental health 8–11,
    13–15, 18
  interventions across the life course 37
  perinatal mental health 369
  pregnancy and early childhood 10, 11, 522
  prevalence of mental health disorders 98
  social and environmental interventions 269, 270
  "structural violence" 85
practice administrators 59
practice nurses 26, 59
prayer 68, 71
pregabalin 298, 299, 300, 632
pregnancy
  alcohol use disorder 476, 478
  bipolar disorder 227
  determinants of health and mental health 10–12,
    15
  environmental contexts 520–1
  interventions across the life course 34–5
  perinatal mental health 365, 367, 368
  tobacco use disorder 467
prematurity 10, 11, 523

self-care 53–4, 73
self-efficacy 481–2
self-esteem 15, 84
self-harm 180, 181, 182, 224, 473, 558
self-help 211, 221, 244, 275–6
self-help books 275, 296
self-help groups 243, 294–5, 510
self-instructional training (SIT) 288
self-management 273–4, 682
semantic memory 584
Semrad, Elvin 69
sensibility 88
sensory processing 523
separation anxiety 557, 562
The serenity prayer 71
serotonergic genes 426
serotonin 10, 38, 169, 459
serotonin and noradrenaline reuptake inhibitors
    (SNRIs) 220, 289, 298, 300, 632
serotonin syndrome 216, 626, 636
sertraline
    anxiety 298, 300, 301
    bipolar disorder 342
    dementia 593
    depression 215, 329, 330
    eating disorders 438
    HIV/AIDS 636
severe mental illness (SMI)
    cancer and SMI 649–50
    cardiovascular disease and SMI 644–6
    comorbidity associated with severe mental
        illness 643–4
    COPD and SMI 648
    diabetes and SMI 646–7
    HIV and hepatitis 649
    hypothyroidism and SMI 649
    influence of culture on clinical care in SMI 650–1
    interventions 651–5
    models of mental health care delivery 661–2
    mortality related to severe mental illness and
        physical illness 642
    osteoporosis and SMI 648–9
    physical health consequences 641–71
    prevalence of mortality risk factors in SMI 644
    racial and ethnic minority groups and SMI 650
    severe mental illness and physical health 641–2
    shared care 30
Severity of Alcohol Dependence Questionnaire
    (SADQ-C) 476
sex differences *see* gender differences
sexual abuse 15, 635, 675
sexual behaviour 84, 106, 649
sexual dysfunction 303, 656
Shain, BN 560
shared care 29, 30, 31–2, 123, 507

shared decision-making 293–4
Sharma, VK 31, 502
Shear, K 314
Shickle, D 161
shifted outpatient clinic 141
Shinkfield, AJ 147
Shortell, SM 407
SIADH *see* syndrome of inappropriate antidiuretic
    hormone secretion
side-effects 209, 213–14, 298
Side-Effects Scale/Checklist for Antipsychotic
    Medication (SESCAM) 209
Sifneos, PE 395
SIGN *see* Scottish Intercollegiate Guidelines
    Network
Silagy, C 460
Silber, TJ 388
Simkin, S 182
Simon, GE 32, 33
sincerity 82
sinusitis 321
Six-Item Cognitive Impairment Test (6CIT) 582
skill mix 250, 679, 680
skin problems 320, 321
Skovgaard, AM 525
sleep deprivation therapy 349
sleep disorder 594, 630–1
sleep hygiene 25, 220, 326
Slovenia 126, 191
slums 270
Sluyter, Dean 71
SMI *see* severe mental illness
Smit, F 25
Smith, M. 143
smoking
    adolescent mental health 557
    advocacy 52
    COPD and SMI 648
    mortality rate 99
    pregnancy 10
    prevalence 457, 458
    resilience 267
    smoking cessation 235–7, 458–67
"Snoezelen" therapy 595
SNRIs *see* serotonin and noradrenaline reuptake
    inhibitors
social and environmental interventions 265–80
    cultural and traditional factors 267–8
    environmental interventions 270–1
    epidemiology 266
    healthy behaviour 274–5
    implications for mental health promotion and
        prevention 277–8
    implications for workforce 276–7
    key messages 265